Handbook of Experimental Pharmacology

Continuation of Handbuch der experimentellen Pharmakologie

Vol. 74

Antiepileptic Drugs

Contributors

L. Beani · C. Bianchi · S. Caccia · B. E. Dwyer · M. J. Eadie
L. S. Freer · H.-H. Frey · B. B. Gallagher · S. Garattini
G. D. Gladding · R. C. Griggs · R. Hess · T. A. Holliday · E. F. Hvidberg
D. Janz · G. L. Jones · I. Jurna · W. P. Koella · R. Kretzschmar
H. J. Kupferberg · W. Löscher · B. S. Meldrum · E. Perucca
E. Przegaliński · A. Richens · J. E. Riggs · H. Schäfer · D. Schmidt
M. Schmutz · E. A. Swinyard · H. J. Teschendorf · C. G. Wasterlain
G. H. Wimbish · K. Wiśniewski · D. M. Woodbury

Editors

H.-H. Frey and D. Janz

Springer-Verlag
Berlin Heidelberg New York Tokyo 1985

Professor Dr. HANS-HASSO FREY
Laboratorium für Pharmakologie und Toxikologie
Fachbereich Veterinärmedizin
Freie Universität Berlin
Koserstraße 20, D-1000 Berlin 33

Professor Dr. DIETER JANZ
Abteilung für Neurologie
Klinikum Charlottenburg
Spandauer Damm 130
D-1000 Berlin 19

With 54 Figures

ISBN-13: 978-3-642-69520-9 e-ISBN-13: 978-3-642-69518-6
DOI: 10.1007/978-3-642-69518-6

Library of Congress Cataloging in Publication Data. Main entry under title: Antiepileptic drugs. (Handbook of experimental pharmacology; vol. 74) Includes bibliographical references and index. 1. Anticonvulsants. 2. Epilepsy–Chemotherapy. I. Beani, L. II. Frey, H.-H. (Hans-Hasso), 1927–. III. Janz, Dieter. IV. Series: Handbook of experimental pharmacology; v. 74. [DNLM: 1. Anticonvulsants. 2. Epilepsy. W1 HA51L v. 74/QV 85 A6281] QP905.H3 vol. 74[RM322] 615.'1 s [616.8'53061] 84-5608
ISBN-13: 978-3-642-69520-9

Softcover reprint of the hardcover 1st edition 1985

Typesetting, printing, and bookbinding: Brühlsche Universitätsdruckerei, Giessen
2122/3130-543210

List of Contributors

L. Beani, Istituto di Farmacologia, Università di Ferrara, Via Fossato di Mortara 23-64B, I-44100 Ferrara

C. Bianchi, Istituto di Farmacologia, Università di Ferrara, Via Fossato di Mortara 23-64B, I-44100 Ferrara

S. Caccia, Istituto di Ricerche Farmacologiche „Mario Negri", Via Eritrea 62, I-20157 Milano

B. E. Dwyer, Epilepsy Research Laboratory (111N-1), VA-Medical Center, 16111 Plummer Street, Sepulveda, CA 91343, USA

M. J. Eadie, Department of Medicine, University of Queensland, Clinical Sciences Building, Royal Brisbane Hospital, Brisbane, 4029, Australia

L. S. Freer, Department of Medicine, Rhode Island Hospital, Coventry, RI 02816, USA

H.-H. Frey, Laboratorium für Pharmakologie und Toxikologie, Fachbereich Veterinärmedizin, Freie Universität Berlin, Koserstr. 20, D-1000 Berlin 33

B. B. Gallagher, Medical College of Georgia, School of Medicine, Department of Neurology, Augusta, GA 30912, USA

S. Garattini, Istituto di Ricerche Farmacologiche „Mario Negri", Via Eritrea 62, I-20157 Milano

G. D. Gladding, Epilepsy Branch, National Institute of Neurological and Communicative Disorders and Stroke, National Institutes of Health, Federal Building, Room 114, Bethesda, MD 20205, USA

R. C. Griggs, Department of Neurology, University of Rochester School of Medicine, Rochester, NY 14642, USA

R. Hess, Rütistraße 38, CH-8032 Zürich

T. A. Holliday, School of Veterinary Medicine, Department of Surgery, University of California, Davis, CA 95616, USA

E. F. Hvidberg, Department of Clinical Pharmacology, University Hospital, Rigshospitalet, 9 Blegdamsvej, DK-2100 Copenhagen, Denmark

D. Janz, Abteilung für Neurologie, Klinikum Charlottenburg, Spandauer Damm 130, D-1000 Berlin 19

G. L. Jones, Division of Neuropharmacology and Epileptology, Department of Physiology, University of Utah, Salt Lake City, UT 84108, USA

I. JURNA, Abteilung Neuropharmacologie, Institut für Pharmakologie und Toxikologie der Universität des Saarlandes, D-6650 Homburg/Saar

W. P. KOELLA, Buchenstr. 1, CH-4104 Oberwil

R. KRETZSCHMAR, Unternehmensbereich Pharma, BASF, Biologische Forschung und Entwicklung, Knoll AG, D-6700 Ludwigshafen

H. J. KUPFERBERG, Epilepsy Branch, National Institute of Neurological and Communicative Disorders and Stroke, Neurological Disorders Program, National Institutes of Health, Federal Building 36/SD-19, Bethesda, MD 20205, USA

W. LÖSCHER, Laboratorium für Pharmakologie und Toxikologie, Fachbereich Veterinärmedizin, Freie Universität Berlin, Koserstr. 20, D-1000 Berlin 33

B. S. MELDRUM, Institute of Psychiatry, University of London, De Crespigny Park, London SE5 8AF, Great Britain

E. PERUCCA, Università di Pavia, Istituto di Farmacologia Medica, Piazza Botta 10, I-27100 Pavia

E. PRZEGALIŃSKI, Polish Academy of Sciences, Institute of Pharmacology, 12 Smetna Street, PL-31-343 Krakow

A. RICHENS, Department of Pharmacology and Therapeutics, Welsh National School of Medicine, Heath Park, Cardiff CF4 4XN, Great Britain

J. E. RIGGS, West Virginia University, School of Medicine, Department of Neurology, Morgantown, WV 26506, USA

H. SCHÄFER, Scientific Division, Desitin-Werk Carl Klinke GmbH, Weg beim Jäger 214, D-2000 Hamburg 63

D. SCHMIDT, Freie Universität Berlin, Klinikum Charlottenburg, Abteilung für Neurologie, Spandauer Damm 130, D-1000 Berlin 19

M. SCHMUTZ, Biology Research, Pharmaceuticals Division, Ciba-Geigy AG, K-125.14.04 CH-4002 Basel

E. A. SWINYARD, Departments of Biochemical Pharmacology and Toxicology and Pharmacology, College of Pharmacy and School of Medicine, University of Utah, Salt Lake City, UT 84112, USA

H. J. TESCHENDORF, Unternehmensbereich Pharma, BASF, Biologische Forschung und Entwicklung, Knoll AG, D-6700 Ludwigshafen

C. G. WASTERLAIN, Department of Neurology, UCLA School of Medicine, VA Medical Center, Neurology Service, 16111 Plummer Street, Sepulveda, CA 91343, USA

G. H. WIMBISH, Texas College of Osteopathic Medicine and Director, Institute of Forensic Medicine, Fort Worth, TX 76107, USA

K. WIŚNIEWSKI, Medical Academy, Institute of Pharmacology and Toxicology, Department of Pharmacology, Mickiewicza 2, PL-15-222 Bialystock 8

D. M. WOODBURY, Division of Neuropharmacology and Epileptology, University of Utah, College of Medicine, Salt Lake City, UT 84108, USA

Preface

Epileptic disorders need treatment for many years or even for life, and this makes a thorough understanding of the pharmacokinetics and possible hazards and side effects of the drugs used in treatment mandatory. During recent decades our knowledge in this field has considerably increased, not least as a result of the development of specific and sensitive methods for the determination of antiepileptic agents in biological material. The clinical pharmacology of this group of drugs has been studied extensively and can today be regarded as well established. This does not necessarily mean that drug treatment of epilepsy is without problems. For example, it has recently been shown that one of the newer antiepileptic drugs, greeted with great enthusiasm by clinicians, may in rare instances induce serious damage to the liver and the pancreas, and seems even to have a certain teratogenic potential.

Clinical problems should be understood as a challenge to the experimental pharmacologist, who should try to find explanations for the clinical hazards, and, if possible, show new ways in which better drugs might be developed. In recent years interest has focused on the importance of the inhibitory transmitter γ-aminobutyric acid (GABA) in the pathophysiology of epilepsy, and there have been a series of attempts to find useful antiepileptic drugs among substances interfering with GABA metabolism in the CNS. While the final success of these attempts cannot yet be judged, it seems worthwhile to assemble reports on the experimental pharmacology of the drugs presently in use in this volume in order to provide research workers interested in the field of antiepileptic drugs and in the treatment of the different forms of epilepsy with a comprehensive and critical review of our present knowledge. Beyond the general and individual pharmacology of antiepileptic drugs, this volume contains a fairly broad section dealing with the clinical pharmacology and practical use of these agents, an introductory section on epileptic diseases in man and animals, and a section concerned with the pathophysiological mechanisms active in these diseases. These mechanisms may provide important starting points for new approaches to the development of active and specific drugs. The editors hope that the structure of the volume will make it easy for the experimental pharmacologist and the clinician to find information which might not be obtained so simply and quickly from other sources.

A chapter on the electrophysiology of the epileptic nerve cell was planned but had to be omitted because it would have delayed publication considerably, and thus deprived the book of its topicality. The editors would like to use this opportunity to thank all contributing authors, especially for the patience with which they respected special wishes from the publisher and the editors and tolerated the delay that is all but unavoidable when a book is written by about 30 scientists from all over the world. We must also thank Professor HERKEN of the editorial board and the publisher for their sympathetic cooperation. Last but not least we thank the secretaries to the editors, Mrs. ANNE-EVA BARZ and Mrs. ILSEBILL BROOKES, without whose capable assistance the task would have been unsurmountable.

HANS-HASSO FREY
DIETER JANZ

Contents

Clinical Aspects of Epileptic Diseases

CHAPTER 1

Epilepsy: Seizures and Syndromes

D. JANZ

A. Definition 3
B. Epidemiology 3
C. Classification 5
D. Epileptic Seizures 5
E. Syndromes of Epilepsy 12
F. Age-Related Syndromes 12
I. Neonatal Convulsions (Neonatal Seizures) 12
II. Febrile Convulsions 13
III. Epilepsy with Infantile Spasms (West Syndrome, Infantile Spasms, Epilepsy with Propulsive Petit Mal) 13
IV. Epilepsy with Myoclonic-Astatic Seizures (Lennox-Gastaut Syndrome 15
V. Epilepsy with Frequent Absences (Friedmann Syndrome, Pyknolepsy) 17
VI. Epilepsy with Juvenile Myoclonic Jerks (Herpin-Janz Syndrome, Epilepsy with Impulsive Petit Mal, Juvenile Myoclonic Epilepsy) 18
VII. Awakening Epilepsy (Epilepsy with Nonfocal Grand Mal) . . 18
VIII. Benign Focal Epilepsy of Childhood [Benign Epilepsy of Children with Rolandic (Centrotemporal) Foci] 19
G. Age-Unrelated Epilepsy Syndromes 20
I. Epilepsies with Complex Focal (Psychomotor) Seizures (Temporal, Rhinencephalic, Limbic Epilepsy) 20
II. Epilepsies with Simple Focal Seizures (Neocortical Epilepsy, Epilepsy with Jacksonian Seizures, Adversive Seizures, Sensory Auras, Sensory Seizures) 21
III. Status Epilepticus 23
IV. Syndromes of Seizures Elicited by Sensory Stimuli (So-called Reflex Epilepsies) 24
References 26

CHAPTER 2

Electroencephalography. R. HESS. With 16 Figures

A. Introduction 35
B. Main Forms of Epileptiform Patterns 36
C. Focal Epileptiform Activity 39
D. Bilateral Epileptiform Patterns 42
E. Activation Procedures 46
F. Electrocorticography and Depth-recording 49
References 53

CHAPTER 3

Epilepsy in Animals. T. A. HOLLIDAY

A. Introduction 55
B. Acquired Epilepsies in Animals 55
C. Inherited Epilepsies in Animals 56
I. Photomyoclonic Seizures in the Baboon (*Papio papio*) 56
II. Inherited Epilepsy in Dogs 59
III. Inherited Epilepsy in Mongolian Gerbils (*Meriones unguiculatus*) . 66
IV. Inherited Epilepsy in Domestic Fowl 69
D. Concluding Remarks 71
References 72

Pathophysiology of Seizure Disorders

CHAPTER 4

Intermediary Metabolism. B. E. DWYER and C. G. WASTERLAIN
With 5 Figures

A. Introduction 79
B. Brain Energy Reserves and the Cell Redox Potential 79
I. Cerebral Energy Use During Seizures 79
II. Brain Redox Potential and Lactic Acidosis 84
C. Seizures and Glycolytic Flux 85
I. Regulation of Glycolysis: Phosphofructokinase 85
II. Hexokinase 86
III. Pyruvate Kinase 87
D. The Citric Acid Cycle and Epileptic Seizures 87
I. Energy Metabolism 87
II. Amino Acid Metabolism 87
III. Ammonia Metabolism 89
E. Free Fatty Acid Metabolism 90
F. Metabolic Mechanisms of Neuronal-Cell Damage During Status Epilepticus 90
I. Role of Extracerebral Factors 90
II. Role of Sustained Cell Firing 91
III. Role of Energy Failure 91

IV. Lactic Acidosis 92
V. Calcium "Cytotoxicity" 92
G. Epileptic Seizures in the Neonate 94
I. Mobilization of Glycogen Reserves 94
II. Limited Transport Capacity of the Blood-brain Barrier 94
References 96

CHAPTER 5

Monoamines and the Pathophysiology of Seizure Disorders. E. PRZEGALIŃSKI

A. Introduction 101
B. Catecholamines 103
I. Electrically Induced Seizures 103
II. Seizures Induced by Chemical Agents 110
III. Reflex Epilepsy Models 116
IV. Other Models of Epilepsy 119
C. Serotonin 120
I. Electrically Induced Seizures 120
II. Seizures Induced by Pentylenetetrazol 124
III. Reflex Epilepsy Models 125
D. Histamine 128
E. Conclusions 129
References 130

CHAPTER 6

Acetylcholine. C. BIANCHI and L. BEANI

A. Introduction 139
B. Effect of Cholinergic Drugs on Susceptibility to Seizures 139
C. Effect of Experimental and Spontaneous Seizures on the Cholinergic System 140
I. Electroshock and Convulsant Drugs 140
II. Spontaneous and Audiogenic Convulsions 141
III. Focal Epilepsy 142
D. Kindling and the Cholinergic System 144
E. Conclusions 146
References 147

CHAPTER 7

GABA and Other Amino Acids. B. S. MELDRUM. With 2 Figures

A. Introduction: Amino Acids as Neurotransmitters 153
B. Amino Acids Producing Inhibition 153
I. Introduction 153
II. GABA 156
III. Glycine 168
IV. Taurine 169

C. Amino Acids Producing Excitation 172
I. Dicarboxylic Amino Acids 172
II. Sulphinic and Sulphonic Acids 175
D. Concluding Remarks 176
I. Inherited Abnormalities of Amino Acid Metabolism and Epilepsy . 176
II. Amino Acids and Antiepileptic Drugs 176
References 177

CHAPTER 8

Prostaglandins. K. WIŚNIEWSKI and H.-H. FREY

A. Introduction 189
B. Effects of Prostaglandins on Experimentally Induced Convulsions . 190
C. Convulsant Effect of Prostaglandins 192
D. Release of Prostaglandins During Convulsions 192
E. Conclusions 193
References 193

General Pharmacology of Antiepileptic Drugs

CHAPTER 9

Chemical Constitution and Pharmacological Effect. H. SCHÄFER
With 1 Figure

A. Introduction 199
B. Five-Membered Heterocyclic Compounds 200
I. Hydantoins 200
II. Oxazolidinediones 208
III. Succinimides 209
C. Six-Membered Heterocyclic Compounds 217
I. Barbiturates and Other Compounds 217
II. Phenobarbital and Primidone 221
D. Acyl Ureas 222
E. Tricyclic Compounds: Carbamazepine 223
F. Benzodiazepines 227
G. Valproic Acid 231
H. Miscellaneous Compounds 234
References 236

CHAPTER 10

Biochemistry. G. L. JONES and D. M. WOODBURY

A. Introduction 245
B. Ionic Permeability 245
I. Effects on Sodium Conductance 245
II. Effects on Calcium Conductance 248
III. Effects on Potassium Conductance 251
IV. Effects on Chloride Conductance 252

C. Neurotransmitter Metabolism, Disposition, and Dynamics 252
I. Effects on Intracellular Processes Related to Transmitter Release . 252
II. Effects on Neurotransmitter Metabolism and Disposition 253
III. Effects on Receptor-Ionophore Dynamics 255
D. Perspective 258
References 259

CHAPTER 11

Tolerance and Dependence. H.-H. Frey

A. Introduction 265
B. Tolerance 265
I. Metabolic Tolerance 266
II. Functional Tolerance 268
III. Acute Tolerance 274
IV. Conclusions 275
C. Physical Dependence 275
I. Experimental Evidence 276
II. Clinical Evidence 277
III. Conclusions 278
References 278

CHAPTER 12

Animal Experimental Methods in the Study of Antiepileptic Drugs
W. P. Koella. With 4 Figures

A. Introduction 283
B. Models of Epileptiform Phenomena in Animals 285
I. Electrically Induced Seizures 286
II. Chemically Induced Ictal and Interictal States (Exclusive of Metals) 295
III. Focal Epileptogenesis Through Local Application of Metals or Metal Salts 303
IV. Local Freezing as Epileptogenic Factor 309
V. Models for Secondary and Progressive Epileptogenic Lesions . 311
VI. Animals with "Inborn" Epilepsy: Genetic Models 318
VII. Circadian Aspects 320
C. Some Nonsymptomatic Models 322
I. Biophysical Approach 322
II. Biochemical Approach 325
D. Discussion 325
I. Models for Screening 326
II. Testing for "Special Indications" 327
References 331

APPENDIX TO CHAPTER 12

Antiepileptic Drug Development Program
G. D. GLADDING, H. J. KUPFERBERG, and E. A. SWINYARD

A. Antiepileptic Drug Development Programm 341
B. Anticonvulsant Screening Project 341
I. Phase I 342
II. Phase II 342
III. Phase III 343
IV. Phase IV 343
V. Phase V 343
VI. Phase VI 346
VII. Phase VII 346
C. Toxicity/Selected Pharmacology Project 346
D. Primate Model of Epilepsy 346
E. Controlled Clinical Trials 347
References 347

Specific Pharmacology of Antiepileptic Drugs

CHAPTER 13

Hydantoins. G. L. JONES and G. H. WIMBISH. With 6 Figures

A. Introduction 351
B. Chemistry 352
I. Physicochemical Properties 352
II. Structure-Activity Relationships 353
III. Analytical Methods 358
C. Anticonvulsant Activity 361
I. Anticonvulsant Potency in Laboratory Animals 361
II. Anticonvulsant Potency in Man 369
III. Mechanism of Anticonvulsant Action 370
D. Other Central Nervous System Effects 375
E. Actions Outside the CNS 376
I. Cardiac Muscle 376
II. Smooth Muscle 376
III. Skeletal Muscle 378
IV. Other Actions 378
F. Pharmacokinetics 380
I. Absorption and Bioavailability 380
II. Distribution 383
III. Biotransformation 391
IV. Excretion 400
G. Drug Interactions 401
H. Toxicology 401
I. Acute Toxicity 401
II. Chronic Toxicity Studies 403

III. Teratogenic Effects 404
IV. Mutagenic Effects 405
V. Other Toxic Effects 405
References 406

CHAPTER 14

Barbituric Acid Derivatives. B. B. GALLAGHER and L. S. FREER
With 3 Figures

A. Introduction 421
B. Chemistry and Physicochemical Properties 421
I. Relationship of Molecular Structure to Anticonvulsant Activity . 422
II. Relationship of Acidic and Lipophilic Properties of Barbituric Acid Derivatives to CNS Activity 423
C. Analytical Methods for Determination of Barbituric Acid Derivatives in Biological Fluids and Tissues 425
D. Anticonvulsant Activity 426
E. Other CNS Effects 429
F. Pharmacodynamic Effects Outside the CNS 431
G. Pharmacokinetics 432
I. Absorption 432
II. Distribution 432
III. Metabolism 433
IV. Excretion 438
H. Drug Interactions 438
J. Toxicology 439
References 441

CHAPTER 15

Primidone. H.-H. FREY. With 1 Figure

A. Chemistry and Physicochemical Properties 449
I. Physicochemical Properties 449
II. Analytical Methods for Determination from Biological Material . 449
B. Anticonvulsant Activity 451
I. Anticonvulsant Efficacy in Laboratory Animals 451
II. Anticonvulsant Potency in Man 454
III. Mechanism of Anticonvulsant Action 455
C. Other Central Nervous System Effects 458
D. Pharmacodynamic Actions Outside the Central Nervous System . . . 459
E. Pharmacokinetics 459
I. Absorption 459
II. Distribution 460
III. Metabolism 462
IV. Elimination 465
F. Drug Interactions 466
G. Toxicology 468
I. Acute Toxicology 468

II. Chronic Toxicity Studies 469
III. Teratogenic Effect 469
IV. Mutagenic Effect 469
V. Other Toxic Effects 470
VI. Clinical Intoxications 470
References 470

CHAPTER 16

Carbamazepine. M. SCHMUTZ. With 2 Figures

A. Introduction 479
B. Chemistry and Physicochemical Properties 479
C. Anticonvulsant Activity 481
I. Anticonvulsant Activity in Rodent-Screening Tests 481
II. Anticonvulsant Activity in Further Animal Models 481
III. Pharmacological Effects Possibly Related to Anticonvulsant Activity 484
IV. Neurobiochemical Effects Possibly Related to Anticonvulsant Activity 485
V. Mechanisms of Action 488
D. Behavioral, Neurological, and Autonomic Effects 489
I. Antiaggressive and/or Anxiolytic Effects 489
II. Antineuralgic Effects 489
III. Antidiuretic Effects 490
IV. Effects on Alcohol-Withdrawal Symptoms 490
V. Antiarrhythmic Effects 490
VI. Antimaniacal Effects 491
VII. Other Effects 491
E. Pharmacokinetics 492
I. Absorption 492
II. Distribution 492
III. Metabolism 493
IV. Elimination 495
F. Drug Interactions 496
G. Toxicology 497
I. Acute Toxicity Studies 497
II. Subacute and Chronic Toxicity Studies 497
III. Reproduction Studies 497
IV. Mutagenicity Studies 498
V. Carcinogenicity Studies 498
References 498

CHAPTER 17

Valproic Acid. W. LÖSCHER. With 1 Figure

A. Chemistry and Physicochemical Properties 507
B. Antiepileptic Activity 508

I. Valproic Acid in Experimental Models of Epilepsy 508
II. Mechanism of Anticonvulsant Action of Valproic Acid 513
C. Central Nervous System Effects Besides the Anticonvulsant Effect . 517
D. Pharmacodynamic Properties Outside the Central Nervous System . 519
E. Pharmacokinetics 520
I. Absorption and Bioavailability 520
II. Distribution and Protein Binding 520
III. Elimination 522
F. Drug Interactions 525
I. Effect of Valproic Acid on Other Drugs 525
II. Effect of Other Drugs on Valproic Acid 526
G. Toxicity 526
References 528

CHAPTER 18

Oxazolidinediones. R. KRETZSCHMAR and H. J. TESCHENDORF

A. Introduction 537
B. Anticonvulsant Effects 537
I. Chemically Induced Convulsions 538
II. Electrically Induced Convulsions 540
III. Convulsions Produced by Other Methods 541
C. Central Nervous System Effects Besides the Anticonvulsant Effect . 541
I. Influence on the Electroencephalogram 542
II. Influence on Behavior 542
D. Biochemical Effects 543
I. Transmitter 543
II. Other Effects 543
E. Pharmacodynamic Properties Outside the Central Nervous System . 544
F. Pharmacokinetics 544
I. Absorption 544
II. Distribution 545
III. Metabolism 546
IV. Excretion 546
G. Interactions 547
H. Toxicity 547
References 548

CHAPTER 19

Succinimides. H. J. TESCHENDORF and R. KRETZSCHMAR

A. Introduction 557
B. Anticonvulsant Effects 558
I. Chemically Induced Convulsions 558
II. Electrically Induced Convulsions 560
III. Convulsions Induced by Other Methods 561
C. Central Nervous System Effects Besides the Anticonvulsant Effect . 562
I. Influence on the EEG 562

II. Influence on Behavior . . . 562
III. Effects on Neurochemical Processes . . . 563
D. Pharmacodynamic Properties Outside the Central Nervous System . 564
E. Pharmacokinetics . . . 565
I. Absorption . . . 565
II. Distribution . . . 565
III. Metabolism . . . 566
IV. Elimination . . . 567
F. Interactions . . . 568
G. Toxicity . . . 568
References . . . 569

CHAPTER 20

Benzodiazepines. S. CACCIA and S. GARATTINI. With 3 Figures

A. Introduction . . . 575
B. Chemical Structure of Benzodiazepines . . . 575
C. Methods of Determination . . . 576
D. Kinetics . . . 577
I. Absorption and Distribution . . . 577
II. Metabolism and Elimination Half-lives . . . 577
E. Anticonvulsant Properties . . . 581
F. Relationship Between Anti-Pentylenetetrazol Activity and Brain Concentrations of Benzodiazepines . . . 583
G. Relationship Between Benzodiazepine Concentrations in the Brain and High-Affinity Drug-Binding Sites . . . 585
References . . . 588

CHAPTER 21

Carbonic Anhydrase Inhibitors. J. E. RIGGS and R. C. GRIGGS

A. Introduction . . . 595
B. Anticonvulsant Effect . . . 595
C. Clinical Use and Limitations . . . 597
D. Toxicity . . . 598
References . . . 598

CHAPTER 22

Acetylurea Derivatives. E. A. SWINYARD

A. Introduction . . . 601
B. Chemistry . . . 601
I. Synthesis and Physicochemical Properties . . . 601
II. Structure-Activity Relations . . . 601
C. Experimental Pharmacology . . . 602
I. Anticonvulsant Activity . . . 602
II. Other Pharmacodynamic Properties . . . 604
III. Pharmacokinetics . . . 604

IV. Drug Interactions 605
V. Effects on Clinical Laboratory Tests 605
D. Toxicity 605
I. Acute Administration 605
II. Chronic Administration 606
E. Conclusions 608
References 608

CHAPTER 23

Electrophysiological Effects of Antiepileptic Drugs. I. JURNA

A. Introduction 611
B. Phenytoin 612
I. Neuronal Membranes 612
II. Synaptic Transmission 615
III. Brain 617
IV. Summary 619
C. Barbiturates 620
I. General Remarks 620
II. Membrane Excitability 620
III. Synaptic Transmission 621
IV. Spinal Cord 623
V. Brain 625
VI. Summary 627
D. Carbamazepine 627
I. Nerve Fibers 627
II. Synaptic Transmission 628
III. Brain 629
IV. Summary 630
E. Valproic Acid 630
I. Ganglia and Spinal Cord Neurons 630
II. Brain 630
III. Summary 632
F. Oxazolidinediones 632
I. Nerve Fibers and Ganglia 632
II. Spinal Cord 633
III. Synaptic Transmission in the Spinal Trigeminal Nucleus 633
IV. Brain 634
V. Summary 634
G. Succinimides 635
I. Synaptic Transmission 635
II. Brain: Focal Seizure Activity 636
III. Summary 636
H. Benzodiazepines 636
I. Facilitation of GABAergic Transmission 636
II. Excitable Membranes and Synaptic Transmission in the Periphery . 637
III. Spinal Cord 638

IV. Brain 640
V. Summary 644
J. Miscellaneous 644
I. Carboanhydrase Inhibition: Acetazolamide 644
II. Local Anesthetics 645
References 645

Clinical Pharmacology of Antiepileptic Drugs

CHAPTER 24

Clinical Pharmacokinetics of Antiepileptic Drugs
E. PERUCCA and A. RICHENS. With 6 Figures

A. Hydantoin Drugs 661
I. Phenytoin 661
II. Mephenytoin (Methoin) 671
III. Ethotoin 672
B. Barbiturates and Chemically Related Anticonvulsants 673
I. Phenobarbital (Phenobarbitone) 673
II. Methylphenobarbital (Mephobarbital) 676
III. Eterobarbital 678
IV. Primidone 678
C. Carbamazepine 681
D. Valproic Acid 689
E. Succinimides 693
I. Ethosuximide 693
II. Methsuximide 695
III. Phensuximide 696
F. Benzodiazepines 696
I. Diazepam 696
II. Clonazepam 701
G. Oxazolidinediones 702
I. Trimethadione (Troxidone) 702
II. Paramethadione 703
H. Acetazolamide 703
J. Sulthiame 704
K. Pheneturide 704
References 705

CHAPTER 25

Monitoring Antiepileptic Drug Levels. E. F. HVIDBERG

A. Introduction 725
B. Justification for Monitoring Plasma Concentration Levels of Antiepileptic Drugs 726
C. The Concept of the Therapeutic Level 727
D. Clinical Evaluation of Therapeutic Levels 728

E. Therapeutic Plasma Concentration Ranges for the Individual Antiepileptic Drugs . . . 729
I. Phenytoin . . . 729
II. Carbamazepine . . . 730
III. Phenobarbital . . . 733
IV. Primidone . . . 734
V. Ethosuximide . . . 735
VI. Benzodiazepines . . . 736
VII. Valproic Acid . . . 737
VIII. Other Antiepileptic Drugs . . . 739
F. Protein Binding and Monitoring Antiepileptic Drug Levels . . . 739
G. Monitoring Antiepileptic Drug Therapy by Measurements in Biological Fluids Other than Plasma . . . 741
I. General Considerations . . . 741
II. Monitoring Salivary Levels of Antiepileptic Drugs . . . 742
III. Monitoring Antiepileptic Drugs in Tears . . . 746
H. Active Metabolites and Monitoring Antiepileptic Drug Levels . . . 747
I. Phenytoin . . . 748
II. Carbamazepine . . . 748
III. Phenobarbital . . . 749
IV. Primidone . . . 749
V. Ethosuximide . . . 749
VI. Benzodiazepines . . . 749
VII. Valproic Acid . . . 750
J. Pharmacodynamic Aspects of Monitoring Antiepileptic Drug Levels . 750
K. Practical Problems of Monitoring Antiepileptic Drug Levels . . . 751
I. Timing of Sampling . . . 751
II. Handling of Blood Samples and Results . . . 752
L. Utilization of the Monitoring of Antiepileptic Drug Levels . . . 753
References . . . 755

CHAPTER 26

Clinical Use of Antiepileptic Drugs. M. J. Eadie. With 1 Figure

A. Introduction . . . 765
B. Use of Antiepileptic Drugs in Epilepsy . . . 765
I. Indications for the Use of Antiepileptic Drugs . . . 765
II. Aim of Antiepileptic Drug Therapy . . . 766
III. Selection of an Antiepileptic Drug . . . 767
IV. Use of Antiepileptic Drugs in Practice . . . 776
V. Combinations of Antiepileptic Drugs . . . 785
VI. Indications for Cessation of Antiepileptic Drug Therapy . . . 786
C. Use of Antiepileptic Drugs for Indications Other than Epilepsy . . . 787
I. Migraine . . . 787
II. Tic Douloureux . . . 787
III. Other Varieties of Pain . . . 787
IV. Hyperinsulinism . . . 787

V. Dyskinesia . . . 787
VI. Cardiac Arrhythmia . . . 788
VII. Myotonia . . . 788
VIII. Miscellaneous . . . 788
References . . . 788

CHAPTER 27

Adverse Effects. D. SCHMIDT

A. Introduction . . . 791
B. Mechanism of Adverse Effects . . . 791
I. Dose-Dependent Side Effects . . . 791
II. Drug-Induced Diseases . . . 792
C. Adverse Effects . . . 793
I. Adverse Effects of Individual Antiepileptic Drugs . . . 793
II. Antiepileptic Drug-Induced Diseases . . . 800
References . . . 818

CHAPTER 28

Antiepileptic Drug Interactions. E. PERUCCA and A. RICHENS
With 3 Figures

A. Interactions Affecting the Kinetics of Antiepileptic Drugs . . . 831
I. Drugs Which May Affect the Gastrointestinal Absorption of Antiepileptic Drugs . . . 831
II. Drugs Which May Affect the Plasma Protein Binding of Antiepileptic Drugs . . . 832
III. Drugs Which May Inhibit the Metabolism of Antiepileptic Drugs . 834
IV. Drugs Which Stimulate the Metabolism of Antiepileptic Drugs . 838
V. Drugs Which May Affect the Renal Excretion of Antiepileptic Drugs . . . 840
B. Interactions Affecting the Kinetics of Other Drugs . . . 841
I. Drugs Whose Gastrointestinal Absorption May Be Affected by Antiepileptic Drugs . . . 841
II. Drugs Whose Plasma Protein Binding May Be Affected by Antiepileptic Drugs . . . 841
III. Drugs Whose Metabolism May Be Inhibited by Antiepileptic Drugs . . . 842
IV. Drugs Whose Metabolism May Be Stimulated by Antiepileptic Drugs . . . 842
V. Interactions Resulting in Altered Drug Excretion in Urine . . . 845
References . . . 846

Subject Index . . . 857

Clinical Aspects of Epileptic Diseases

CHAPTER 1

Epilepsy: Seizures and Syndromes

D. JANZ

A. Definition

The term epilepsy refers to all pathological states or diseases which are characterized by recurrent epileptic seizures. Single epileptic seizures provoked only by occasional causes are termed occasional epileptic seizures. Epileptic seizures are characterized by paroxysmal changes in the sensory system, motor system, subjective well-being, and objective behavior caused by a sudden, excessive, rapid discharge of gray matter of some part of the brain (JACKSON 1931). The wide range of symptoms of epileptic seizures reflects the manifold functions of the brain in a pathologically distorted manner.

B. Epidemiology

The assumption that 5% of all people will have an epileptic seizure at least once in the course of their lives is scarcely an exaggeration since 3%–4% alone – according to a careful study 33/1,000 (HAUSER and KURLAND 1975) – have febrile seizures in the first 5 years of life. The incidence of neonatal convulsions varies from 0.5% to 1.4% (WOODBURY 1977). Although their incidence is unknown, other occasional epileptic seizures (*epileptische Gelegenheitsanfällle*) such as so-called stress convulsions (FRIIS and LUND 1974) are certainly not rare; the sampe applies to epileptic seizures after withdrawal of alcohol, barbiturates, and other drugs or in acute illnesses such as meningoencephalitis and in toxic conditions such as uremia or eclampsia.

A reliable study in Rochester, Minnesota, recorded epilepsy in the strict sense in 6.57 of 1,000 persons (HAUSER and KURLAND 1975). This included all people who had had at least two seizures not provoked by fever, alcoholism, or other occasional causes – at least one of them in the previous 5 years – or who were taking antiepileptic drugs.

The true prevalence, however, is probably higher as the figure does not include those patients who had previously only had minor seizures and who comprise about one-fifth of all patients with epilepsy in a clinical patient population (JANZ 1969). Nor does it include those with active epilepsy who for various reasons had not been to a doctor and who, according to a field study (ZIELINSKI 1974), comprise about one-third of all patients. Taking into account the assumption that even in a developed country about one-third of all patients with active epilepsy remain undiscovered, the US Plan for Nationwide Action on Epilepsy (US Department of Health, Education and Welfare 1977) assumes that epilepsy in the sense of recurrent seizures without occasional causes occurs in 1% of the population.

As regards the sociomedical significance, insofar as this can be expressed in figures, it can be assumed according to investigations and estimates that 0.25 (JANZ 1973) to 0.36/1,000 (US Department of Health, Education and Welfare 1977) of the population are hospitalized in institutions on account of epilepsy and that 3.33 (JANZ 1973) to 3.60/1,000 (US Department of Health, Education and Welfare 1977) of the population display particular medical and/or social problems on account of epilepsy. The remainder presumably live largely adjusted lives in their society and, insofar as they are in medical care, require no special diagnostic, therapeutic, or rehabilitative services.

The distribution of various types of epileptic seizures varies according to whether predominantly children or adults are affected. In children we find more cases of epilepsy with minor generalized seizures and in adults more cases of epilepsy with minor focal seizures.

In our patient population of a neurological hospital, epilepsy with only grand mal seizures was found in about 40%, epilepsy with major and minor seizures also in about 40%, and epilepsy with only minor seizures in about 20%. Epilepsies with minor focal seizures occurred in just under 40%, focal seizures with complex symptoms (psychomotor) being three times more frequent than those with simple symptoms (neocortical). In slightly less than 20% there were minor generalized seizures, whereby the propulsive seizures of West's syndrome (infantile spasms) and the myoclonic astatic seizures of the Lennox syndrome, together comprising just under 3%, are perhaps slightly underrepresented compared with a pediatric patient sample. Epilepsy with absences (of both pyknoleptic and nonpyknoleptic frequency) occurred in about 12% of the cases and epilepsy with myoclonic jerks of the impulsive petit mal type in slightly over 4% (Table 1).

Table 1. Distribution of different types of seizure in 6,500 patients seen in 20 years at the University Department of Neurology, Heidelberg. (JANZ 1969)

Type of seizure	With grand mal	Without grand mal	Total *n*	%
Propulsive seizures (infantile spasms)	59	55	114	1.8
Myoclonic astatic seizures	39	34	73	1.1
Pyknoleptic absences	336	169	505	7.8
Nonpyknoleptic juvenile absences	165	32	197	3.0
Impulsive petit mal (juvenile myoclonic jerks)	253	27	280	4.3
Complex focal seizures	1,265	725	1,990	30.6
Simple focal seizures	278	288	566	8.7
Pure grand mal	2,567		2,567	39.5
Unclassifiable	165	43	208	3.2
Total	5,127	1,373	6,500	100.0

C. Classification

Epilepsies are classified as idiopathic or symptomatic according to whether no cause is detected or whether a morphologically definable brain lesion can be found. Epileptic seizures can be subdivided into major seizures (grand mal) and minor seizures, both of which can be further classified as major seizures with focal or generalized onset and minor seizures with focal or generalized onset, depending on whether the clinical picture and the EEG begin with symptoms of focal or generalized discharges. According to the frequency of the seizures various types of course can be distinguished and are termed monoepilepsy (with a single seizure), oligoepilepsy (with occasional seizures), stationary epilepsy (when the frequency of seizures remains constant), and progressive epilepsy (seizures increasing in frequency). In the case of epilepsy with minor seizures the frequency of occurrence is usually further specified as spanioleptic (with sporadic seizures), pyknoleptic (with several seizures per day), or cycloleptic (with seizures occurring periodically in clusters). With regard to the manifestation age we speak of neonatal seizures; epilepsy in babies, infants, school-children, puberty, and adolescence; and so-called late-onset epilepsy; or simply of age-related and age-unrelated epilepsies.

Such distinctions provide certain pointers to the nature and cause of the seizures and to the prognosis of course and therapy. Thus seizures with focal onset, for example, are usually the expression of symptomatic epilepsy; oligoepilepsies are in general solitary epileptic seizures (*epileptische Gelegenheitsanfälle*); infantile epilepsy is often the result of pre- and perinatal brain lesions; and seizures occurring after the age of 20, if they do not result from a brain injury and are not alcohol withdrawal seizures, raise suspicion of a brain tumor. Particular types of seizure elicitation and a connection of seizures to certain situations can also serve as classification principles. Thus we speak of febrile convulsions, stress convulsions, reflex epilepsy, sleep epilepsy, and epilepsy on awakening. Etiological factors are the basis for the distinction between residual (after brain lesions) and processual (in progressive brain illnesses) epilepsy; topological factors are the basis for the distinction between focal epilepsy of the temporal lobe, focal epilepsy of the frontal lobe, and focal epilepsy of the parietal or occipital region.

Although proposals for an internationally uniform classification of epilepsy (MERLIS 1970) have not borne fruit, a classification of epileptic seizures accepted by the International League Against Epilepsy has been compiled (GASTAUT 1970) and was recently revised (DREIFUSS 1981) (Table 2).

D. Epileptic Seizures

The greatest step toward a rational treatment of epilepsy was the realization that the action of antiepileptic drugs depends not on the type of epilepsy but on the type of epileptic seizure. In 1945 LENNOX reported dramatic success in seizures of the so-called petit mal triade, which had until then been considered uncontrollable by a drug which had no effect on convulsive seizures. Since then the terms anticonvulsant drug and antiepileptic drug have ceased to be synonymous as since this experience we know that there are antiepileptic drugs without anticonvulsant

Table 2. Revised clinical and electroencephalographic classification of seizures. (DREIFUSS 1981)

I. Partial (focal, local) seizures

Partial seizures are those in which, in general, the first clinical and electroencephalographic changes indicate initial activation of a system of neurons limited to part of one cerebral hemisphere. A partial seizure is classified primarily on the basis of whether or not consciousness is impaired during the attack. When consciousness is not impaired, the seizure is classified as a simple partial seizure. When consciousness is impaired, the seizure is classified as a complex partial seizure. Impairment of consciousness may be the first clinical sign, or simple partial seizures may evolve into complex partial seizures. In patients with impaired consciousness, aberrations of behavior (automatisms) may occur. A partial seizure may not terminate, but instead progress to a generalized motor seizure. Impaired consciousness is defined as the inability to respond normally to exogenous stimuli by virtue of altered awareness and/or responsiveness.

There is considerable evidence that simple partial seizures usually have unilateral hemispheric involvement and only rarely have bilateral hemispheric involvement; complex partial seizures, however, frequently have bilateral hemispheric involvement.

Partial seizures can be classified into one of the following three fundamental groups:

A. Simple partial seizures
B. Complex partial seizures
   1. With impairment of consciousness at onset
   2. Simple partial onset followed by impairment of consciousness
C. Partial seizures evolving to generalized tonic-clonic convulsions (GTC)
   1. Simple evolving to GTC
   2. Complex evolving to GTC (including those with simple partial onset)

Clinical seizure type	EEG seizure type	EEG interictal expression
A. *Simple partial seizures* (consciousness not impaired)	Local contralateral discharge starting over the corresponding area of cortical representation (not always recorded on the scalp)	Local contralateral discharge
1. With motor signs		
(a) Focal motor with march		
(b) Focal motor with march (Jacksonian)		
(c) Versive		
(d) Postural		
(e) Phonatory (vocalization or arrest of speech)		
2. With somatosensory or special-sensory symptoms (simple hallucinations, e.g., tingling, light flashes, buzzing)		
(a) Somatosensory		
(b) Visual		
(c) Auditory		
(d) Olfactory		
(e) Gustatory		
(f) Vertiginous		
3. With autonomic symptoms or signs (including epigastric sensation, pallor, sweating, flushing, piloerection and pupillary dilatation)		

Table 2 (continued)

4. With psychic symptoms (disturbance of higher cerebral function). These symptoms rarely occur without impairment of consciousness and are much more commonly experienced as complex partial seizures		
(a) Dysphasic		
(b) Dysmnesic (e.g., déjàvu)		
(c) Cognitive (e.g., dreamy states, distortions of time sense)		
(d) Affective (fear, anger, etc.)		
(e) Illusions (e.g., macropsia)		
(f) Structured hallucinations (e.g., music, scenes)		
B. *Complex partial seizures* (with impairment of consciousness; may sometimes begin with simple symptomatology)	Unilateral or, frequently bilateral discharge, diffuse or focal in temporal or frontotemporal regions	Unilateral or bilateral generally asynchronous focus; usually in the temporal or frontal regions
1. Simple partial onset followed by impairment of consciousness		
(a) With simple partial features (A.1–A.4) followed by impaired consciousness		
(b) With automatisms		
2. With impairment of consciousness at onset		
(a) With impairment of consciousness only		
(b) With automatisms		
C. *Partial seizures evolving to secondarily generalized seizures* (This may be generalized tonic-clonic, tonic, or clonic)	Above discharges become secondarily and rapidly generalized	
1. Simple partial seizures (A) evolving to generalized seizures		
2. Complex partial seizures (B) evolving to generalized seizures		
3. Simple partial seizures evolving to complex partial seizures evolving to generalized seizures		

II. Generalized seizures (convulsive or nonconvulsive)

Generalized seizures are those in which the first clinical changes indicate initial involvement of both hemispheres. Consciousness may be impaired and this impairment may be the initial manifestation. Motor manifestations are bilateral. The ictal electroencephalographic patterns initially are bilateral, and presumably reflect neuronal discharge which is widespread in both hemispheres.

Table 2 (continued)

Clinical seizure type	EEG seizure type	EEG interictal expression
A. 1. *Absence seizures*	Usually regular and symmetrical 3 c/sec but may be 2–4 c/sec spike-and-slow-wave complexes and may have multiple spike-and-slow-wave complexes. Abnormalities are bilateral	Background activity usually normal although paroxysmal activity (such as spikes or spike-and-slow-wave complexes) may occur. This activity is usually regular and symmetrical
(a) Impairment of consciousness only (b) With mild clonic components (c) With atonic components (d) With tonic components (e) With automatisms (f) With autonomic components (b through f may be found alone or in combination)		
2. *Atypical absence*	EEG more heterogeneous; may include irregular spike-and-slow-wave complexes, fast activity or other paroxysmal activity. Abnormalities are bilateral but often irregular and asymmetrical	Background usually abnormal: paroxysmal activity (such as spikes or spike-and-slow-wave complexes) frequently irregular and asymmetrical
May have: (a) Changes in tone that are more pronounced than in A.1 (b) Onset and/or cessation that is not abrupt		
B. *Myoclonic seizures* Myoclonic jerks (single or multiple)	Polyspike and wave, or sometimes spike and wave or sharp-and-slow waves	Same as ictal
C. *Clonic seizures*	Fast activity (10 c/sec or more) and slow waves; occasional spike-and-wave patterns	Spike-and-wave or polyspike-and-wave discharge
D. *Tonic seizures*	Low voltage, fast activity or a fast rhythm of 9–10 c/sec or more decreasing in frequency and increasing in amplitude	More or less rhythmic discharges of sharp and slow waves, sometimes asymmetrical. Background is often abnormal for age
E. *Tonic-clonic seizures*	Rhythm at 10 or more c/sec decreasing in frequency and increasing in amplitude during tonic phase, interrupted by slow waves during clonic phase	Polyspike and waves or spike and wave, or, sometimes, sharp and slow wave discharges

Table 2 (continued)

Clinical seizure type	EEG seizure type	EEG interictal expression
F. *Atonic seizures* (Astatic) (combinations of the above may occur, e.g., B and F, B and D)	Polyspikes and wave or flattening or low-voltage fast activity	Polyspikes and slow wave

III. Unclassified epileptic seizures

Includes all seizures that cannot be classified because of inadequate or incomplete data and some that defy classification in hitherto described categories. This includes some neonatal seizures, e.g., rhythmic eye movements, chewing, and swimming movements.

IV. Addendum

Repeated epileptic seizures occur under a variety of circumstances:

1. as fortuitous attacks, coming unexpectedly and without any apparent provocation; 2. as cyclic attacks, at more or less regular intervals (e.g., in relation to the menstrual cycle, or the sleep-waking cycle); 3. as attacks provoked by: (a) nonsensory factors (fatigue, alcohol, emotion, etc.), or (b) sensory factors, sometimes referred to as "reflex seizures."

Prolonged or repetitive seizures (status epilepticus). The term "status epilepticus" is used whenever a seizure persists for a sufficient length of time or is repeated frequently enough that recovery between attacks does not occur. Status epilepticus may be divided into partial (e.g., Jacksonian), or generalized (e.g., absence status or tonic-clonic status). When very localized motor status occurs, it is referred to as epilepsia partial continua.

action. Therefore, in the development of new drugs we must not only investigate substances with anticonvulsant action but must also look for antiepileptic drugs which act specifically on various seizures types. From the pharmacodynamic point of view even the latest version of the seizure classification accepted by the International League Against Epilepsy is by no means ideal. As it was compiled with the help of relatively objective techniques of seizure monitoring it is, however, the best of the classifications presently available for the purposes of clinical pharmacology. Whe therefore quote here in part the definitions of the various seizure types given by the Commission for Classification and Terminology of the International League Against Epilepsy (DREIFUSS 1981, see Table 2):

Partial (Focal, local) Seizures

The fundamental distinction between simple partial seizures and complex partial seizures is the presence or the impairment of the fully conscious state.

A. Partial seizures

1. *With motor signs.* Any portion of the body may be involved in focal seizure activity depending on the site of origin of the attack in the motor strip. Focal motor seizures may remain strictly focal or they may spread to contiguous cortical areas producing a sequential involvement of body parts in an epileptic "march". The seizure is then known as a Jacksonian seizure. Consciousness is usually preserved, however, the discharge may spread to those structures whose participation is likely to result in loss of consciousness and generalized convulsive movements. Other focal motor attacks may be versive with head turning to one side, usually contraversive to the discharge. If speech is involved, this is either in the form of speech arrest or occasionally vocalization. Occasionally a partial dysphasia is seen in the form of epileptic palilalia with involuntary repetition of a syllable or phrase.

2. *Seizures with autonomic symptoms* such as vomiting, pallor, flushing, sweating, piloerection, pupil dilatation, boborygmi and incontinence may occur as simple partial seizures.

3. *With somatosensory or special sensory symptoms.* Somatosensory seizures arise from those areas of cortex subserving sensory function, and they are usually described as pins and needles or a feeling of numbness. Occasionally a disorder of proprioception or spatial perception occurs. Like motor seizures, somatosensory seizures also may march and also may spread at any time to become a complex partial or generalized tonic-clonic seizure as in A1. Special sensory seizures include visual seizures varying in elaborateness and depending on whether the primary or association areas are involved, from flashing lights to structured visual hallucinatory phenomena, including persons, scenes, etc. (see A4f). Like visual seizures, auditory seizures may also run the gamut from crude auditory sensation to such highly integrated functions as music (see A4f). Olfactory sensations, usually in the form of unpleasant odors, may occur.

Gustatory sensations may be pleasant or odious taste hallucinations.

Vertiginous symptoms include sensations of falling in space, floating, as well as rotatory vertigo in a horizontal or vertical plane.

4. *With psychic symptoms* (disturbance of higher cerebral function). These usually occur with impairment of consciousness (i.e. complex partial seizures).

a) Dysphasia – this was referred to earlier.
b) Dysmnesic symptoms – a distorted memory experience such as a distortion of the time sense, a dreamy state, a flashback or a sensation as if a naive experience had been experienced before, known as déjà vu, or as if a previously experienced sensation had not been experienced, known as jamais-vu, may occur.
c) Cognitive disturbance may be experienced. These include dreamy states, distortions of the time sense, sensations of unreality, detachment or depersonalization.
d) With affective symptomatology. Sensation of extreme pleasure or displeasure, as well as fear and intense depression with feelings of unworthiness and rejection, may be experienced during seizures...
e) Illusions. These take the form of distorted perceptions in which objects may appear deformed. Polyoptic illusions such as monocular diplopia, distortions of size, macropsia or micropsia, or of distance may occur. Similarly, distortions of sound, including microacusia and macroacusia may be seen. Depersonalization, as if the person were outside his body, may occur. Altered perception of size or weight of a limb may be noted.
f) Structured hallucinations. Hallucinations may occur as manifestations or perceptions without a corresponding external stimulus and may affect somatosensory, visual, auditory, olfactory, or gustatory senses.

B. Seizures with complex symptomatology, automatisms

Ictal epileptic automatisms usually represent the release of automatic behavior under the influence of clouding of consciousness that accompanies a generalized or partial epileptic seizure (confusional automatisms). They may occur in complex partial seizures as well as in absence seizures. Postictal epileptic automatisms may follow any severe epileptic seizure, especially a tonic-clonic one, and are usually associated with confusion.

Drowsiness or somnolence implies a sleep state from which the patient can be aroused to make appropriate motor and verbal responses. In stupor, the patient may make some spontaneous movement and can be aroused by painful or other vigorously applied stimuli to make avoidance movements. The patient in confusion makes inappropriate responses to his environment and is disoriented as regards place or time or person.

Aura. The aura is that portion of the seizure which occurs before consciousness is lost and for which memory is retained afterwards. It may be that, as in simple partial seizures, the aura is the whole seizure. Where consciousness is subsequently lost, the aura is, in fact, the signal symptom of a complex partial seizure.

Generalized Seizures

A. Absence seizures

The hallmark of the absence attack is a sudden onset, interruption of ongoing activities, a blank stare, possibly a brief upward rotation of the eyes. If the patient is speaking, speech is slowed or interrupted; if walking, he stands transfixed; if eating, the food will stop on its way to the mouth. Usually the patient will be unresponsive when spoken to. The attack lasts from a few seconds to half a minute and evaporates as rapidly as it commenced.

1. *Absence with impairment of consciousness only.*
2. *Absence with mild clonic components.* Here the onset of the attack is indistinguishable from the above but clonic movements may occur in the eyelids, at the corner of the mouth or in other muscle groups which may vary in severity from almost imperceptible movements to generalized myoclonic jerks.
3. *Absence with atonic components.* Here there may be a diminution in tone of muscles subserving posture as well as in the limbs leading to drooping of the head, occasionally slumping of the trunk, dropping of the arms and relaxation of the grip.
4. *Absence with tonic components.* Here during the attack tonic muscular contraction may occur, leading to increase in muscle tone which may affect the extensor muscles or the flexor muscles symmetrically or asymmetrically. If the patient is standing the head may be drawn backward and the trunk may arch. This may lead to retropulsion.
5. *Absence with automatisms...* Purposeful or quasi-purposeful movements occurring in the absence of awareness during an absence attack are frequent and may range from lip licking, swallowing, to clothes fumbling or aimless walking.

B. Tonic-clonic seizures

The most frequently encountered of the generalized seizures are the generalized tonic-clonic seizures, often known as grand mal. Some patients suffering with this experience a vague ill-described warning, but the majority lose consciousness without any premonitory symptoms. There is a sudden sharp tonic contraction of muscles and when this involves the respiratory muscles there is stridor, a cry or moan and the patient falls to the ground in the tonic state, occasionally injuring himself in falling. He lies rigid on the ground and during this stage tonic contraction inhibits respiration and cyanosis may occur. The tongue may be bitten and urine may be passed involuntarily. This tonic stage then gives way to clonic convulsive movements lasting for a variable period of time and during this stage small gusts of grunting respiration may occur between the convulsive movements but usually the patient remains cyanotic and saliva may froth from the mouth. At the end of this stage deep inspiration occurs and all the muscles relax, after which the patient remains unconscious for a variable period of time and often stiff and sore all over. He then frequently goes into a deep sleep and when he awakens feels quite well apart from soreness and frequently headache.

Myoclonic Seizures. [Myoclonic jerks (single or multiple)]. Myoclonic jerks are sudden, brief, shock-like contractions which may be generalized or confined to the face and trunk or to one or more extremities or even to individual muscles or groups of muscles. Myoclonic jerks may be rapidly repetitive or relatively isolated.

Many instances of myoclonic jerks and action myoclonus are not classified as epileptic seizures. The myoclonic jerks of myoclonus due to spinal cord disease, dyssynergia cerebellaris myoclonica, subcortical segmental myoclonus, paramyoclonus multiplex and opsoclonus-myoclonus syndrome must be distinguished from epileptic seizures.

Clonic Seizures. Generalized convulsive seizures occasionally lack a tonic component and are characterized by repetitive clonic jerks. As the frequency diminishes the amplitude of the jerks does not. The post-ictal phase is usually short.

Tonic Seizures. To quote Gowers, a tonic seizure is "a rigid, violent muscular contraction, fixing the limbs in some strained position. There is usually deviation of the eyes and of the head towards one side, and this may amount to rotation involving the whole body and may actually cause the patient to turn around, even two or three times. The features are distorted; the color of the face, unchanged at first, rapidly becomes pale and then flushed and ultimately livid as the fixation of the chest by the spasms stops the movements of respiration. The eyes are open or closed; the conjunctiva is insensitive; the pupils dilate widely as cyanosis comes on. As the spasm continues, it commonly changes in its relative intensity in different parts, causing slight alterations in the position of the limbs."

Atonic Seizures. A sudden diminution in muscle tone occurs which may be fragmentary, leading to a head drop with slackening of the jaw, the dropping of a limb or a loss of all muscle tone leading to a slumping to the ground. When these attacks are extremely brief they are known as "drop attacks".

Unclassified Epileptic Seizures. This category includes all seizures which cannot be classified because of inadequate or incomplete data.

E. Syndromes of Epilepsy

As it has been pointed out (LUND 1980), "during the past 2–3 decades epileptological studies have led to the recognition of a number of syndromes of epilepsy which have gradually become defined on the basis of clinical observation as regards type of seizure, age of onset, electroencephalographic abnormalities and prognosis. These syndromes are to a great extent internationally accepted, and their terminology is used in daily informal communications between colleagues and as diagnostic entries on hospital records. They are also to some extent related to the effect of certain of the anticonvulsive drugs. The individual syndromes have been the subject of controlled clinical trials and other investigations which have been reported in the form of papers or even monographs."

The characteristics EEG findings and the more or less specific treatment for each syndrome are to be found in Chap. 2 and 27 of this volume.

F. Age-Related Syndromes

I. Neonatal Convulsions (Neonatal Seizures)

These comprise all epileptic manifestations during the first 10 days of life. Polymorphism and topographic as well as temporal variability characterize these seizures. They occur more often with multifocal than with generalized jerks but can also involve a general or local increase in tone, alternating hemiclonic jerks, or more subtle phenomena such as yawning, lip-smacking or cycling movements; or can be manifested merely in the form of apnoic episodes, eye-rolling, blinking and general hypotension, and lack of responsiveness. Such seizures occur in 5–14 in every 1,000 neonates (BURKE 1954; WOODBURY 1977, FORFAR et al. 1972; KEEN and LEE 1973; DENNIS 1978). Frequent causes are ischemic or hemorrhagic brain lesions and the metabolic disorders hypoglycemia and hypomagnesemia. Rarer causes are malformations and infections of the CNS. Familial occurrence appears to be very rare (BJERRE and CORELIUS 1968; QUATTLEBAUM 1979). There seems to be no genetic relationship with epilepsy (LIPINSKI 1982).

In the majority of cases the seizures do not recur. In many cases, however, the prognosis is clouded by the underlying brain damage. About one-fourth of the children affected die early. Of the surviving children about one-half remain retarded in their development. In about one-fourth chronic epilepsy develops, not infrequently in the form of infantile spasms (West's syndrome) or myoclonic-astatic seizures (Lennox-syndrome) (DENNIS 1978; KUROMORI et al. 1976; LOMBROSO 1974; NOLTE and BANTZ 1977; RAUTENSTRAUCH and BRUNNER 1980; SCHULTE 1966; LAGENSTEIN 1980).

II. Febrile Convulsions

Febrile convulsions are solitary infantile seizures (*kindliche Gelegenheitskrämpfe*) which occur in about 3%–4% of all children (33/1,000 according to HAUSER and KURLAND 1975) usually between the ages of 9 and 20 months and are seldom seen after the 5th year of life. They are usually generalized tonic-clonic or generalized tonic convulsions, and rarely focal seizures (MATTHES 1977). The seizures are elicited by banal catarrhal infections, in which the rapidity of the temperature increase at the beginning of the infection appears to be the significant factor rather than the actual height of the temperature (MATTHES 1977). Twenty-five to fifty percent of affected children have one or more relapses and 2%–3% develop chronic epilepsy either immediately or after some time (TSUBOI and ENDO 1977; TSUBOI and YAMAMURA 1978; NELSON and ELLENBERG 1976, 1978; LENNOX-BUCHTHAL 1973; ANNEGERS et al. 1979; ELLENBERG and NELSON 1980). Development into or occurrence of epilepsy is more likely in the presence of the following factors: familial occurrence of epilepsy, previous cerebral lesions, manifestation before the 4th months or after the 5th year, focal nature of seizures, duration greater than 30 min (*crise prolongée* or febrile status convulsivus), and frequent repetition of febrile convulsions (ANNEGERS et al. 1979; DOOSE et al. 1966; NELSON and ELLENBERG 1976, 1978). If the above factors are present complex febrile convulsions are said to occur.

Etiologically, multifactorial (TSUBOI 1977 a) or dominant inheritance with incomplete manifestation is assumed (LENNOX-BUCHTHAL 1973) – in 25% of the cases a familial disposition to febrile convulsions is found (LENNOX-BUCHTHAL 1973). There is also, however, a genetic relationship to epilepsy with generalized seizures. Children of parents with generalized epilepsy are more susceptible to febrile convulsions than children of parents with focal epilepsy (BECK-MANNAGETTA et al. 1982).

Prophylactic treatment with antiepileptic drugs can be considered in the case of complex febrile convulsions (FISHMAN 1980). In the case of fever, however, direct prophylaxis is also possible in the form of temperature reduction and preventive diazepam clysma.

III. Epilepsy with Infantile Spasms (West Syndrome, Infantile Spasms, Epilepsy with Propulsive Petit Mal)

West syndrome describes a triad occurring in babies and infants comprising epileptic seizures mainly involving short flexion spasms, retarded development, and a characteristic EEG pattern known as hypsarrhythmia (GIBBS and GIBBS 1952).

The seizures begin with a sudden bilateral symmetric muscle contraction which is either very short – as in the case of the more frequent lightning seizures – or lasts for a few seconds – as in the rarer salaam convulsions. They can occur in global form with generalized seizures or in partial form with variants limited to head movements and eye movements. The generalized seizures occur mostly as flexion spasms, less often as extension spasms, and not infrequently as combined flexion-extension spasms (JANZ and MATTHES 1955; JEAVONS and BOWER 1974; GASTAUT et al. 1964; KELLAWAY et al. 1979). In the case of flexion spasms the head, trunk, and legs are flexed, likewise the arms which are either adducted or abducted. On account of the predominant forward-bent position, seizures of this type are also called salaam convulsions (CLARKE 1841 cited by WEST 1941) or propulsive convulsions (ABRAHAMSON 1922; JANZ and MATTHES 1955). Partial variants are so-called head-nodding spells, in which only the head is jerked forward, and attacks of blinking or nystagmic bulbus movements (HORITA et al. 1977). During or shortly after the seizures the child often cries out as though he or she has had a fright, or sometimes only a short whimper is heard.

Usually several seizures occur per day, often occurring after awakening in series of 5–20 seizures which can accumulate to a status epilepticus. Sooner or later longer-lasting generalized tonic or clonic seizures (grand mal) can also occur, usually in sleep (JANZ and MATTHES 1955).

The EEG shows a pattern described and depicted in Fig. 11, Chap. 2, this volume and known as "hypsarrhythmia" (GIBBS and GIBBS 1952).

The seizures can begin between the 3rd week and the 3rd year of life, but onset is usually between the 3rd and 8th months of life with a peak at the age of 6 months (JANZ 1969; LACY and PENRY 1976).

It is assumed that in about one-half of the children the seizures disappear within 2 years and that in the remainder they do not generally persist for longer than 4 years (LACY and PENRY 1976). According to the only follow-up of cases not affected by modern treatment methods, after 4 years 11% of the children had died and only 20% had become free of seizures. After 10 years 23% had died and only 13% were free of seizures (JANZ and MATTHES 1955). Development into epilepsy with myoclonic astatic seizures is not infrequent (KRUSE 1968, OHTAHARA 1978), but progression to epilepsy with pyknoleptic absences is rare (RABE 1961).

The illness affects mainly boys. Most studies show a predominance of boys over girls in a ratio of about 60% : 40% (JANZ and MATTHES 1955; LACY and PENRY 1976; JEAVONS et al. 1973). In only a third of the cases is the development of the children from birth to onset of the seizures unremarkable, while all others already show signs of retarded development prior to onset (JANZ and AKOS 1967). About 80% of the children show more or less pronounced mental retardation in the course of the illness. About 70% also show neurological disturbances in the form of cerebral palsies, less often athetosis and ataxias (LACY and PENRY 1976).

The etiology is not uniform. In only a minority of the cases can no etiologically relevant factors be found. Very often these are congenital illnesses such as phacomatoses, fetal infections, connatal metabolic disorders, and congenital malformations or functional disturbances such as microcephaly, ocular symptoms, and callosal agenesis. Factors found relatively frequently are premature delivery and low birth weight (LACY and PENRY 1976). Postnatal circumstances probably have only the role of realization factors (JANZ 1969). We assume on the basis of a systematic study that the common pathogenetic factor is to be found in a maturation arrest of genetic or exogenous origin which affects the organism between the 4th week and the 4th month of the fetal period (JANZ and AKOS 1967). This view has not remained undisputed (JELLINGER 1970), but has been confirmed in more recent pathological-anatomical investigations (MEENCKE and GERHARD 1984).

In apparent contradiction to the assumption of a predominantly exogenous etiology the heritability is relatively high. The incidence of epileptic seizures in the family is given as 7%–25% (LACY and PENRY 1976; JANZ and AKOS 1967; JANZ and MATTHES 1955; DOOSE 1964a). Homologous cases in the family (LACY and PENRY 1976), in siblings (JANZ 1969), and in monozygotic twins (MUNDE 1969) have also been observed.

Nosologically closely related to West syndrome is the rare *Aicardi syndrome* (AICARDI et al. 1969), a combination of infantile spasms with cerebral malformations (agenesis of the corpus callosum, porencephalia, cortical heterotopia), malformations of the eyes (chorioretinopathy, coloboma), and vertebral anomalies, which begins in the first months of life and has hitherto only been observed in girls. The Aicardi syndrome has a characteristic EEG pattern which consists of multifocal epileptiform abnormalities occurring on a burst-suppression pattern showing complete asynchrony between the two hemispheres (DENNIS and BOWER 1972; RENIER et al. 1973; JEAVONS and BOWER 1974; KARCH et al. 1980; FARIELLO et al. 1977).

So-called early *infantile epileptic encephalopathy with suppression-burst* (OHTAHARA 1978), a combination of infantile spasms which begin very early – before the 3rd month – and severe psychomotor retardation, a poor prognosis, and a characteristic EEG pattern which in time develops into hypsarrhythmia, appears to be closely related to this syndrome (OHTAHARA et al. 1976, YAMATOGI and OHTAHARA 1981).

IV. Epilepsy with Myoclonic-Astatic Seizures (Lennox-Gastaut Syndrome)

The Lennox or Lennox-Gastaut syndrome is an epileptic syndrome beginning in early childhood and characterized by certain types of generalized seizures, signs of mental retardation, and slow variants of the spike-wave pattern in the EEG. A combination of astatic seizures, generalized tonic convulsions, and absences which can be accompanied by generalized tonic-clonic seizures with no particular relationship to the sleeping-waking cycle is typical of this syndrome. In the case of the astatic seizures the children can, without losing consciousness and without perceptible jerks, suddenly fall down and immediately get up again. Sometimes, however, sudden violent jerks through all their limbs throw them to the ground. In milder forms there is only a short throwing up of the arms and a short buckling of the knees or abrupt head nods (nodding spells). During the extremely short absences there is a scarcely perceptible myoclonus of the eyelids and/or arms. The tonic seizures are of short duration, are often accompanied by a cry, and are either generalized or occur in abortive form restricted to the shoulders and face. The tonic seizures can occur only in sleep. Tonic seizures occurring during the day can also lead to a fall and are often followed by a postparoxysmal impairment of consciousness during which oral automatisms occur – "tonic-psychomotor seizures" (STENZEL and PANTELI 1982). Usually several types of seizure occur in one and the same patient (AICARDI 1973; CHEVRIE and AICARDI 1972; CAPELLA et al. 1972; BLUME et al. 1973; BEAUMANOIR et al. 1968; DOOSE 1964b; DOOSE et al. 1970; GASTAUT et al. 1966; KRUSE 1968; LAGENSTEIN 1980; LOISEAU et al. 1974; NIEDERMEYER 1969; OLLER-DAURELLA 1972; SCHNEIDER et al. 1970; SOREL 1964).

Several seizures occur in a day at intervals of days or weeks. They tend to occur in series and in the form of a status epilepticus. Here status can occur with more or less violent jactitations reminiscent of chorea as well as apathetic states in which only an occasional nodding of the head or buckling of the body are suggestive of seizures (KRUSE 1968).

Electroencephalographically all variants of the spike-wave complex with a frequency of less than three per second are characteristic (see Fig. 10, Chap. 2, this volume).

The manifestation age ranges from the 9th month to the 9th year but is usually between the 2nd and 4th years with a maximum in the 4th year. Onset in the 2nd decade has not infrequently been observed (NIEDERMEYER 1969; LIPINSKI 1977; OSAWA et al. 1976; STENZEL 1979; SENGOKU et al. 1976; HIGANO and OHTAKA 1976; JANZ 1969; SOREL 1964). However, such late-onset astatic seizures can also occur in addition to already existing epilepsy which has begun with pyknoleptic absences and awakening grand mal, with psychomotor seizures and grand mal during sleep, or grand mal which is randomly distributed (LIPINSKI 1977).

In a third of the cases psychomotor development is retarded before the onset of seizures and in about half of the cases it becomes impaired to a greater or lesser degree in the course of the illness (KRUSE 1968). As regards the nature and frequency of the seizures, the extent of psychic impairment, and the degree of therapeutic amenability, the course of the illness is very variable. The prognosis cannot, however, be considered generally unfavorable as a third of cases become seizure free after 4 years (KRUSE 1968). While transition from West syndrome to Lennox syndrome is not unusual (YAMATOGI and OHTAHARA 1981), transitions from Lennox syndrome to Friedmann syndrome appear to be the exception (JANZ 1969; KRUSE 1968; LAGENSTEIN 1977; OLLER-DAURELLA 1976; RABE 1961).

From the etiological point of view, too, the Lennox syndrome comes between West's syndrome and the Friedmann syndrome. In about one-third of the cases no etiological factors can be found. The circumstances to which the syndrome is attributed include prenatal, perinatal, and postnatal damage (JANZ 1969; SCHNEIDER et al. 1965; DOOSE et al. 1970; CAPELLA et al. 1972; CHEVRIE and AICARDI 1972; BLUME et al. 1973).

Familial occurrence of epilepsy or solitary epileptic seizures is found in 12.8%–27% of cases (BLUME et al. 1973; BEAUMANOIR et al. 1968; KRUSE 1968; SCHNEIDER et al. 1970). Reports of homologous illnesses in siblings are rare (DOOSE 1964 b; DOOSE et al. 1969; KRUSE 1968).

The distinction between primary and secondary or generalized and multifocal forms is justified less by the pathological-anatomical findings available to date (MEENCKE 1984; TCHICALOFF et al. 1974; VIANI et al. 1977) than by the expectation of prognostic and perhaps also genetic differences (BEAUMANOIR et al. 1968; DOOSE 1964 b, c; DOOSE et al. 1970; LAGENSTEIN 1977, 1980; GASTAUT et al. 1973).

The following hitherto not clearly defined subentities are closely related to the Lennox syndrome: *epilepsy with infantile myoclonic seizures* or *myoclonic epilepsy of childhood* (AICARDI and CHEVRIE 1971; LOISEAU et al. 1974; JEAVONS 1977) and *epilepsy with infantile or "atypical" absences* (RABENDING et al. 1981; JACOBI 1979; GASTAUT et al. 1974).

V. Epilepsy with Frequent Absences (Friedmann Syndrome, Pyknolepsy)

When FRIEDMANN (1906, 1912, 1915) originally described the syndrome of frequent minor seizures in children he understood it to be a nonepileptic paroxysmal illness in the belief that it had generally cleared by puberty and did not involve personality changes. Since it has become known that major seizures often follow (ROSENTHAL 1935) and that the absences have a characteristic EEG pattern and a spike-wave complex of three per second (GIBBS et al. 1935; JUNG 1939; see also Fig. 7, Chap. 2, this volume), the Friedmann syndrome (DALBY 1969) is considered a definite epileptic syndrome.

The absences begin and end suddenly, i.e., an aura does not precede the abruptly beginning absence attack; the seizure usually lasts less than 10 s and mental clarity returns instantly at the end of the seizure. During the absences there are usually mild motor manifestations in the form of upward (retropulsive petit mal) (JANZ 1955) and less often sideward movements of the eyes and head, blinking, slight jerking of the arms, or, if the absences last longer, also mild automatisms. They recur several times a day, can become very frequent – thence the term "pyknoleptic" – and can accumulate to a series or to a status ("petit mal status" or "absence status") which can last for hours or days.

This type of epilepsy manifests itself between 4 and 14 years of age. Three-fourths of all cases begin between the 5th and 11th years, with a peak in the 7th and 8th years (JANZ 1969). In a minority of cases the onset of absences is preceded by major seizures (DALBY 1969; JANZ 1969). These are seldom neonatal seizures but more often febrile convulsions or other types of solitary grand mal. Girls are affected more often than boys in a ratio of 60:40 (JANZ 1969; BAMBERGER and MATTHES 1959).

Spontaneously 16%–36% become seizure free, in 31%–33% the minor seizures remain but their frequency decreases, and in 32%–53% major seizures ensue, occurring predominantly (88%) after awakening in the form of awakening epilepsy (JANZ 1969). There have recently been reports of both a worse (OLLER-DAURELLA and OLLER 1977) and – under therapy however – a distinctly better (SATO et al. 1977) prognosis than hitherto assumed.

Etiologically pyknolepsy is considered the prototype of primary (idiopathic) epilepsy. In 4%–14% (DALBY 1969; JANZ 1969) the history shows evidence of exogenous, especially perinatal, lesions (COURJON et al. 1959; DALBY 1969; DOOSE et al. 1965), which are of pathoplastic rather than etiological significance.

Family and sibling studies have shown this form of epilepsy to have a hereditary basis although the type of heredity is still under discussion (METRAKOS and METRAKOS 1961; DOOSE et al. 1967; NEWMARK and PENRY 1980).

Between the syndrome of pyknoleptic absences and the syndrome of juvenile myoclonic jerks (impulsive petit mal) lies a further form of age-related minor seizures which is characterized clinically by *nonpyknoleptic or nonfrequent absences* and electroencephalographically by rapid spike-wave complexes (JANZ 1969). In this syndrome, also known as *juvenile absence epilepsy* (DOOSE et al. 1965), usually only short simple absences occur which recur not with pyknoleptic frequency but in periodic clusters (cycloleptically) or in a spanioleptic manner (singly). In the majority of cases age manifestation is between 10 and 14 years of age (JANZ 1969). The difference between the syndrome of juvenile absences and epilepsy with impulsive petit mal, which is not infrequently also accompanied by simple absences, lies clinically in the absence of myoclonic jerks and electroencephalographically in the absence of typical multispike-wave complexes. Features which it shares with the preceding and following syndromes are the frequent combination with awakening grand mal, a high heritability, and the rarity of etiologically relevant noxae.

VI. Epilepsy with Juvenile Myoclonic Jerks (Herpin-Janz Syndrome, Epilepsy with Impulsive Petit Mal, Juvenile Myoclonic Epilepsy)

This is a form of epilepsy beginning in youth and characterized by abrupt jerks through the shoulders and arms occurring mainly on awakening, in combination with awakening grand mal, frequent familial occurrence, absence of exogenous etiological factors, and a multispike-wave EEG pattern (JANZ and CHRISTIAN 1957; JANZ 1969; SIMONSEN et al. 1976; LUND et al. 1976; ENVILE-BACSAL and DELGADO-ESCUETA 1981; TSUBOI 1977b).

The impulses or impulsive jerks through the arms and shoulders can be mild or violent, can occur singly or several times in succession, or can increase to a volley or a genuine status of arrhythmic jerks (impulsive petit mal status) (GRÜNBERG and HELMCHEN 1969; JANZ and CHRISTIAN 1957). It is not uncommon for short simple absences to occur in addition. The minor and the major seizures occur mainly after waking and are precipitated by lack of sleep and alcohol excess. On account of a neurotic instability of character, patients with jerks of the impulsive petit mal tend to have an irregular life-style which can impair compliance (LUND et al. 1976; VÖLZKE et al. 1981).

An example of the characteristic multispike-wave EEG pattern is shown in Fig. 8, Chap. 2, this volume. From the electroencephalographic point of view the syndrome must be further extended to include pure grand mal epilepsies with subclinical multispike-wave complexes which are as a rule also awakening epilepsies.

The predilection age is between the 14th and 18th years of life with a broad span between the 9th and 27th year (JANZ 1969).

Cases in which only jerks occur for decades appear to be rare. In the course of the illness major seizures usually soon occur. In a third of the cases the syndrome begins with major seizures.

Etiologically the frequency of familial occurrence is striking as are the not infrequent reports of homologous cases in families (JANZ 1969; TSUBOI 1977b). Family studies indicate a genetic disposition of probably polygenic type (TSUBOI 1977b).

VII. Awakening Epilepsy (Epilepsy with Nonfocal Grand Mal)

According to their connection with the sleeping-waking cycle grand mal epilepsies can be divided into awakening epilepsy, sleep epilepsy, and random epilepsy. In the clinical, pathophysiological, and therapeutic respect these forms differ so distinctly from each other that at least in the case of awakening epilepsy we can describe a syndrome in its own right (JANZ 1953, 1962, 1969, 1974).

The grand mal seizures occur mainly after awakening and occasionally, sometimes also mainly, "around going home time." They usually begin between 10 and 25 years of age whereas sleep epilepsy and random epilepsy show no age predilection. Awakening epilepsies are usually idiopathic epilepsies while sleep epilepsies are symptomatic epilepsies in one-fourth of the cases and random epilepsies in over one-half of the cases. If they do not occur in pure form but combined with minor seizures, these usually take the form of frequent pyknoleptic or nonfrequent absences and/or impulsive jerks, whereas combined sleep epilepsy is mainly associated with complex focal seizures and combined random epilepsy mainly with simple focal seizures.

In its course awakening epilepsy can evolve into sleep epilepsy or random epilepsy, but sleep or random epilepsy never develops into awakening epilepsy. The seizures in awakening epilepsy are often precipitated by exogenous circumstances (sleep withdrawal, alcohol, photosensitivity), which have less significance in the other forms.

Substantiated experience indicates that the psychic and sleep-waking behavior of patients with awakening epilepsy differs clearly from that of patients with the other forms (JANZ 1969, 1974).

According to the EEG, awakening epilepsies are primary generalized epilepsies while in the other two forms focal slow waves and discharges frequently suggest classification as focal epilepsy (JANZ 1969, 1974; KITAGAWA 1975; TSUBOI and CHRISTIAN 1976).

VIII. Benign Focal Epilepsy of Childhood [Benign Epilepsy of Children with Rolandic (Centrotemporal) Foci]

This is the only age-related form of epilepsy which involves focal and not generalized seizures. Further characteristics of this syndrome are the occurrence of the seizures mainly in sleep, unilateral centrotemporal sharp-wave focus in the EEG, and favorable prognosis (BANCAUD et al. 1958; BEAUSSART 1972; BLOM et al. 1972; LERMAN and KIVITY 1975; LIPINSKI 1980; LOISEAU and BEAUSSART 1973).

Mainly short, unilateral, simple, brachiofacial focal seizures with paraesthesia and/or jerks; tonic hemifacial seizures with hypersalivation and speech arrest; and masticatory seizures, hemi-grand mal, and grand mal with focal onset occur. The seizures often recur only in sleep, less often also or only during waking. As a rule only a few seizures occur but there are cases with several seizures daily.

The manifestation age ranges from 9 months to 12 years, with predilection between 7 and 10 years. The syndrome affects boys more often than girls.

The EEG is characterized by an isomorphous centrotemporal sharp-wave focus of high amplitude near the fissure of Rolando (see Fig. 4, Chap. 2, this volume). It is possible for the focus to change sides. As a rule no etiological factors can be detected. The autosomal dominant mode of inheritance has been discussed.

Seizures and focus disappear completely at puberty.

G. Age-Unrelated Epilepsy Syndromes

I. Epilepsies with Complex Focal (Psychomotor) Seizures (Temporal, Rhinencephalic, Limbic Epilepsy)

The term temporal epilepsy is generally taken to mean epilepsy with complex focal seizures. There are, however, two reasons why the two terms cannot be regarded as completely synonymous:

1. There are cases where grand mal seizures are the additional or only manifestation of temporal epilepsy. Then they are, however, as a rule preceded by specifically temporal seizure symptoms.
2. Psychomotor or complex focal seizures can in rare cases also stem from extratemporal foci (LUDWIG et al. 1975; SCHNEIDER et al. 1965; GEIER et al. 1976), whose discharges are projected into temporal regions.

The diagnosis "temporal epilepsy" must therefore be supplemented by the type of seizure and the diagnosis "complex focal seizures" by the exact localization of the lesions.

The lateral sections of the temporal lobe belong to the neocortex and the mediobasal portions to the paleocortex or the rhinencephalon, which is functionally related to the entire limbic system. Thus with regard to localization we should distinguish two forms of temporal epilepsy, a neocortical and a paleocortical (rhinencephalic, limbic) form.

The neocortical form is relatively rare. It originates from discharges of the four temporal gyri with the exception of the temporal pole. The predominant seizure symptoms are acoustic, visual, vestibular, and – over the dominant hemisphere – dysphasic auras. Dreamy states are also related to the temporal neocortex with the exception of the specific auditory and vestibular projection areas and the speech region. Temporolateral seizures appear to be accompanied less often by disturbed consciousness and by postictal cloudy states than rhinencephalic seizures and more often by adversive automatisms.

The paleocortical form is the more frequent. It arises from discharges in the uncinatus region (JACKSON and COLMAN 1898) or the pararhinal region (GASTAUT 1961). (With regard to the EEG, see Figs. 2, 6, 12, 13, 16, Chap. 2, this volume.) The uncinatus region encompasses the nucleus amygdalae, the pars uncinata of the gyrus hippocampi, and the anterior insular and periinsular regions of the temporal lobe, perhaps also the hippocampus and the area entorhinalis. The pararhinal region additionally includes the substantia perforata anterior and the posterior portions of the gyri orbitales. The clinical symptoms are characterized by epigastric, olfactory, and gustatory auras, by stereotype oral automatisms, and by vegetative symptoms. The seizures are as a rule associated with disturbances of consciousness and terminate in postictal cloudy states with slow reorientation.

Complex focal seizures as a rule recur in a cycloleptic manner (in periodic clusters): After seizure-free intervals of days to weeks several seizures or series of seizures occur in the course of a few days. There are undoubtedly also states which can be considered as status epilepticus of complex focal seizures, in which seizures or seizure fragments follow each other continuously or discontinuously over a prolonged period (GASTAUT et al. 1956; KARBOWSKI 1980; WOLF 1970). The clinical spectrum ranges from phenomena which can be termed "aura continua"

(SCOTT and MASLAND 1953; WOLF 1982), through so-called epileptic delirium or epileptic cloudy states (PASSOUANT et al. 1957, PENFIELD and JASPER 1954) to frequent seizures with unremarkable behavior in the intervening periods (JANZ 1969).

The manifestation age shows no predilection. In our patient sample 29% had become ill in the 1st decade of life; in 50% seizures began after the 20th year of life (JANZ 1969).

With regard to the course we can distinguish between a primary and a secondary form. We talk of a primary form when it begins with complex focal seizures and of a secondary form when the onset of complex focal seizures is preceded by seizures of a different type. Grand mal seizures in combination with complex focal seizures usually (55%) occur in the form of sleep epilepsy, often (30%) in the form of random epilepsy, and only relatively seldom (15%) in the form of awakening epilepsy (JANZ 1969).

Etiologically, definable causes were known in 27% of the cases in our patient sample and not known in 73%. The most frequent causes were pre- and perinatal brain lesions (7.4%) and traumatic brain lesions (6.6%); these are followed by cerebral tumors (4.6%), brain infections (2.7%), and cerebrovascular diseases (0.9%). When the onset is in the 1st decade of life pre- and perinatal brain lesions are the most frequent causes while brain injuries predominate in the 3rd decade. In the 3rd and 4th decades brain injuries compete with brain tumors and the latter predominate in the 6th decade (JANZ 1969).

The hereditary occurrence of epilepy in the family is only one-half to one-third of that in epilepsies with generalized seizures. It is worth noting that it is higher in children and institutionalized patients than in a neurological patient sample (JANZ 1969). Twin studies have shown a concordance of 38.5% in monozygotic twins and a concordance of 6% in dizygotic twins (LENNOX 1960). In the literature there are reports of a number of homologous cases in siblings and also in the ascending line (BARSLUND and DANIELSEN 1963; ANDERMANN and METRAKOS 1969; BRAY and WISER 1965; DALY and BICKFORD 1951; GIBSON 1959/60; JENSEN 1975; LENNOX 1960; MATTHES 1961; NEWMARK and PENRY 1980; RODIN and WHELAN 1960).

II. Epilepsies with Simple Focal Seizures (Neocortical Epilepsy, Epilepsy with Jacksonian Seizures, Adversive Seizures, Sensory Auras, Sensory Seizures)

Simple focal seizures begin with symptoms which reflect the functions of circumscribed cortical areas. Thus seizures of the central region begin with somatomotor or somatosensory symptoms; seizures of the projection areas for the specific senses with visual (optic), auditory (acoustic), or vertiginous sensations; and seizures of the dorsomedial and dorsolateral areas of the frontal lobe with postural changes and turning movements. Seizures of the speech region lead to dysphasic symptoms while seizures with speech disturbance (vocalization or arrest of speech) are of unspecific location. Whether seizures associated only with autonomic symptoms exist is questionable, as is their localizational correlate.

Common to all simple focal seizures is that consciousness is initially not impaired, which is why the patients are able to describe the nature of the focal symptoms from their own experience. Only when the discharge becomes secondarily generalized or when generalized convulsions occur is consciousness extinguished. The term simple focal seizures is not completely identical with the term neocortical seizures because although voluntary motor activity and the sensations of the "higher" senses are represented by the neocortex, sensations of the "lower" senses, such as epigastric, olfactory, and gustatory sensations, are represented by the rhinencephalon, which belongs to the paleocortex, or by the limbic structures of the insular and parainsular regions and of the uncus region.

As long as the seizures are only manifested in local symptoms we speak of motor, sensorimotor, or sensory Jacksonian seizures, contralateral (mostly) or ipsilateral (rarely) versive seizures, sensory seizures (with optic, acoustic, vertiginous sensations), or dysphasic seizures. Simple focal seizures can develop into generalized tonic-clonic seizures. They can, however, particularly when they are associated with sensations of the "lower" senses, with complex hallucinations, and/or with a dreamy state, also develop into complex focal seizures. Finally there are also focal seizures which begin with simple symptoms and then progress via complex symptoms to generalized tonic-clonic convulsions. Focal seizures can thus remain focal, combine with grand mal seizures of focal onset, or only go along with focal grand mal seizures.

Simple focal seizures can also occur in series or accumulate to a status. A status epilepticus of versive seizures is not infrequent but has not been described as such probably because in the case of such events focal grand mal seizures predominate and are succeeded in the subsequent course by versive seizures which no longer generalize. A status of sensory seizures has often been described under the term aura continua (SCOTT and MASLAND 1953; WOLF 1982; HELMCHEN et al. 1969). A status of focal-motor seizures is also known as epilepsia partialis continua (Kojewnikow) (BAMBERGER and MATTHES 1959; JANZ 1969; JUUL-JENSEN and DENNY-BROWN 1966; BAROLIN et al. 1976; LÖHLER and PETERS 1974; THOMAS et al. 1977). By this we understand clonic jerks in a limited area occurring more or less continously over a prolonged period without impairment of consciousness. The state can occur in isolation but is frequently accompanied by Jacksonian seizures or by grand mal seizures which precede, interrupt, or follow it (for EEG see Fig. 15c, Chap. 2, this volume). Speech disturbances of prolonged duration with epileptic discharges in the EEG above the temporal region of the dominant hemisphere have also been described as a status of dysphasic or aphasic seizures (GERSTLE DE PASQUET et al. 1976; HAMILTON and MATTHEWS 1979).

Epilepsies with simple focal seizures usually begin in adulthood. In our patient sample only 12.5% had started in the 1st decade of life; in 73% of the cases the seizures did not begin until after 20 years of age and in 21% not until after 50 years (JANZ 1969).

As regards the course, primary forms (beginning with simple focal seizures) predominate by far over the secondary forms (beginning with focal grand mal seizures). Primary forms are caused by tumors in half the cases and secondary forms in only a fifth of the cases. Grand mal seizures in epilepsies with simple focal seizures of neocortical origin are unrelated to the time of day in half of the cases; in over a third of the cases they occur mainly in sleep and only relatively seldom mainly after waking (JANZ 1969).

Etiologically, epilepsies with simple focal seizures of neocortical origin are mainly symptomatic. But in our sample, too, the cause remains unknown in 29% of the cases. The most frequent cause is brain tumor (34%), followed by traumatic (15%), pre- and perinatal (9%), inflammatory (3%), vascular (3%), and less commonly (7%) brain lesions. Pre- and perinatal brain lesions predominate in the 1st decade of life and traumatic brain lesions in the 2nd and 3rd decades; from puberty onward brain tumors increase gradually and go into the lead from the 4th decade on, while cerebrovascular diseases retain their subordinate role even in advanced years (JANZ 1969).

III. Status Epilepticus

According to the revised seizure classification the term "status epilepticus is used whenever a seizure persists for a sufficient length of time or is repeated frequently enough that recovery between attacks does not occur" (DREIFUSS 1981). Within generalized status epilepticus, GASTAUT (1982) distinguishes between convulsive and nonconvulsive forms. He classifies as convulsive forms the historic "grand mal status", which can be generalized from the beginning or can have a focal onset; a status of generalized tonic or generalized clonic seizures; and a status of massive bilateral myoclonia, which is further subdivided into that occurring in primary generalized epilepsy and that occurring in severe subacute or acute encephalopathies. As nonconvulsive generalized status forms he classifies the absence status, which he again subdivides into that with typical and that with atypical absences, and a status of atonic seizures. The forms of a focal status epilepticus such as the somatomotor form of epilepsia partialis continua (Kojewnikow), the somatosensory form of aura continua, and the possibility of a status with dysphasic seizures have already been mentioned in connection with the syndrome of simple focal seizures and the status psychomotoricus in connection with the syndrome of complex focal seizures.

A status epilepticus convulsivus or grand mal status is characterized by grand mal seizures which follow each other at short intervals usually of less than 1 h without the patient regaining clear consciousness in between (HEINTEL 1972; JANZ 1969). Mortality even in recent years has still been 2.5%–25% (AMINOFF and SIMON 1980; HEINTEL 1972; JANZ and KAUTZ 1964; KAS and ORSZAGH 1976; KETZ and MEIER 1979; WHITTY and TAYLOR 1949; ROWAN and SCOTT 1970). However, death seldom occurs during the status but usually in the postparoxysmal coma, mainly as a result of complications of the respiratory tract (HEINTEL 1972). The morbidity rate of a grand mal status in epilepsy is given as 1%–10% (HEINTEL 1972; HUNTER 1959/60; JANZ 1961; LENNOX 1960). The etiology of grand mal status is more often known than unknown (JANZ 1982). Among the specific causes brain trauma, brain tumor, and encephalitis are more frequent than expected; vascular lesions and perinatal brain damage are not.

Among brain tumors astrocytomas and among brain traumas open head injuries show a significant predisposition to grand mal status (HEINTEL 1972). In epilepsies of unknown origin a grand mal status is relatively rare; its occurrence presupposes a long-standing course, in generalized epilepsy even longer than in focal epilepsy; it never marks the beginning of an idiopathic epilepsy (HEINTEL 1972; JANZ 1961, 1982; HEYCOP TEN HAM et al. 1967). The semiological differentiation between a status as an isolated, an initial, or an intercurrent event can be of help in differential diagnosis insofar as an isolated and an initial status epilepticus almost always have an exogenous cause. The fact that a status epilepticus in cryptogenic epilepsies does not occur until after a long duration of the illness, on average 13 (JANZ 1961) to 15.5 (HEINTEL 1972) years, indicates that in cryptogenic epilepsies too a morphological brain lesion is the prerequisite for a status.

In many cases a grand mal status appears to be a symptom of diffuse brain damage. When it is based on a circumscribed lesion it is mostly a unilateral lesion of the frontal lobes (JANZ 1964, 1982). Among the manifold circumstances which can be identified as precipiting factors, errors in medication and intercurrent infections are the most frequent (AMINOFF and SIMON 1980; HUNTER 1959/1960, KAS and ORSZAGH 1976; ROWAN and SCOTT 1970; JANZ 1982).

IV. Syndromes of Seizures Elicited by Sensory Stimuli (So-called Reflex Epilepsies)

Seizures occurring from time to time or regularly in comparable circumstances have previously been termed reflex epilepsies. This term is, however, clinically diffuse, etiologically meaningless, and pathophysiologically dubious. It is clinically diffuse because the precipitating circumstances and the nature of the seizures are very varied. The circumstances range from definable exteroceptive to indefinable interoceptive stimuli, biological constellations, and psychic situations. The clinical phenomena also include nonepileptic paroxysms such as syncopal and extrapyramidal seizures. The term has no etiological meaning because precipitating circumstances are not causes. Also, the assumption that the elicitation of the seizures takes place in the same manner as a reflex is physiologically inadequate as the conditions of a reflex arc have never been shown to exist. Moreover, the epileptic seizures precipitated by stimuli are always the consequence of self-supporting afterdischarges whose intensity and duration are not strictly dependent on the stimulus (JASPER 1954). Finally, as sensory stimuli can also inhibit seizures, in such cases it is preferable to speak of sensory precipitation or inhibition (BICKFORD 1954; BICKFORD and KLASS 1969; PENFIELD and JASPER 1954).

According to the type of precipitation we distinguish among others between tactile (haptogenic), optic (photogenic), and acoustic (musicogenic) forms and forms precipitated particularly by reading, by movements, and by being startled.

The seizures elicited by tactile stimuli are usually somatomotor and somatosensory cortical seizures (GOLDIE and GREEN 1959; JANZ 1969; KREIS 1968; PENFIELD and JASPER 1954; SCOLLO-LAVIZZARI and HESS 1967; SERVIT 1962; VIZIOLI 1962).

That sensory seizures can also be precipitated by sensory stimuli is shown by the example of precipitation of optic auras by sudden alternation of light and dark (JANZ 1969; PENFIELD and JASPER 1954), of acoustic auras by acoustic stimuli (CRITCHLEY 1935; JANZ 1969), and of vestibular auras by vestibulogenic stimuli (BEHRMANN and WYKE 1958).

We speak of *photogenic epilepsy* when epileptic seizures are precipitated by intermittent light stimuli. Occasionally a look into the sun will suffice (FRIEDMANN 1912; RADOVICI et al. 1932; SCHRÖDER 1913), but usually blinking or some other alternation from light to dark is necessary to elicit seizures in the patients with the appropriate disposition (BICKFORD and KLASS 1969; JEAVONS and HARDING 1975; KLASS 1976; NEWMARK and PENRY 1979; RABENDING and KLEPEL 1978). Clinically we usually find generalized primary epilepsies with awakening grand mal, pyknoleptic absences, or jerks of the impulsive petit mal type. Photogenic epilepsy or the so-called photosensitive seizures (RABENDING et al. 1981) are a special case of so-called *photosensitive epilepsy*, i.e., epilepsies with photosensitivity (JEAVONS and HARDING 1975). Photosensitivity is the ability of the brain to respond to intermittent light stimuli (photostimulation) with hypersynchronous discharges which appear in the EEG in the form of mostly bilateral spike and slow-wave complexes either limited to the occipital and temporal regions or generalized (see Fig. 14, Chap. 2, this volume). Photosensitivity is a genetically determined characteristic which is distinctly age related, with maximum penetrance between the 5th and the 15th year of life and is mostly found in girls.

Precipitation of seizures by patterns (pattern-sensitive epilepsy) is considered a rare subform of so-called photosensitive epilepsy. The seizures are generally elicited by looking at patterns or pictures with sharp contours. Usually absences or generalized tonic-clonic seizures occur (BICKFORD et al. 1953; BICKFORD and KLASS 1969; CHATRIAN et al. 1970a, b; DREYER 1972; WILKINS et al. 1979) but rarely focal seizures (MEYER and MEYER-WAHL 1975).

We speak of *musicogenic epilepsy* when epileptic seizures occur only or with a certain regularity when listening to music. The first such case was described by MERZHEEVSKY in 1884 (cited by CRITCHLEY 1937). Some degree of fame was attained by the case observed by NIKITIN (1935) of a singer in whom seizures occurred only when he listened to or sang a certain aria and later even when he merely thought of it. Some patients, as in the case described by NIKITIN (1935), react only to a certain melody and others to a particular type of music, which is as a rule sentimental in character. It is undoubtedly the emotion elicited by the music which is decisive in precipitating the seizures, provided "the gun was loaded" (CRITCHLEY 1937, 1942). Clinically we find psychomotor or grand mal seizures, electroencephalographically practically always temporal epilepsy (BASH and BASH-LIECHTI 1959; DALY and BARRY 1957; JANZ 1969; JOYNT and GREEN 1962; POSKANZER et al. 1962; TITECA 1965; TOIVAKKA and LEHTINEN 1965; WEBER 1956).

Audiogenic epilepsy in the strict sense is the constitutional ability of certain strains of mice and rats to respond to loud sounds with epileptiform seizures. This characteristic is used specifically for testing the anticonvulsant action of drugs (COLLINS and FULLER 1968; FULLER and COLLINS 1968; HERBERG et al. 1969; SCHLESINGER et al. 1968). In man seizures elicited by simple sounds or noises – apart from startle seizures – have not been demonstrated.

Vestibulogenic epilepsy in the sense of seizures repeatedly elicited by vestibular stimuli also appears to be the exception in man (BEHRMANN and WYKE 1958; ORBAN and LANG 1963).

"Seizures elicited by movement" are not a clinically uniform syndrome. Under this heading numerous observations have been reported of fits of unilateral and bilateral tonic convulsions and/or athetotic and choreatic movements without impairment of consciousness which are of short duration, recur frequently, and are elicited by sudden active movements or postural changes, occasionally also by being startled. On the basis of our own experience we share the opinion of PEREZ-BORJA et al. (1967), that at least two syndromes must be distinguished: (1) An extrapyramidal-motor syndrome mostly occurring at school age, also showing familial occurrence and manifested paroxysmally in predominantly unilateral dystonic but also choreo-athetoid movements which lead to bizarre postures and are not accompanied by impairment of consciousness (FUCHS and JUNKERS 1973; HISHIKAWA et al. 1973). (2) An age-unrelated focal epileptic syndrome mostly associated with unilateral tonic seizures which can develop into complex focal or generalized tonic-clonic seizures and presumably originates in the supplementary-motor region (FALCONER et al. 1963; PENFIELD and JASPER 1954; JANZ 1969; KENNEDY 1959; OLLER-DAURELLA and DINI 1970).

Seizures elicited by being startled also lack clinical uniformity. Although both are precipitated by surprising tactile or accoustic stimuli we distinguish between (1) a pathologically exaggerated startle reaction (hyperexplexia, *synkinesie-sursaut*) (GASTAUT and VILLENEUVE 1967) in children with infantile hemiparesis or diplegia in the form of short unilateral or bilateral tonic cramps or clonic jerks and (2) epileptic seizures elicited by startle (startle epilepsy) such as not infrequently occur in infantile spasms and in myoclonic astatic or tonic seizures (ALAJOUANINE and GASTAUT 1955).

Seizures precipitated by reading (reading epilepsy) are a clearly defined epileptic syndrome (MEYER and WOLF 1973; GILLIGAN 1969; BROOKS and JIRAUCH 1971) since it was first described by BICKFORD (1954). After reading for a short or longer period the patients experience a feeling of tension in the masticatory muscles and in the lips, occasionally also clonic jerks in the jaw, tongue, and throat muscles. If the reading is not then interrupted a major epileptic seizure inevitably occurs. Photostimulation has no provoking effect. Reflex action to proprioceptive impulses from speech muscles or the eyes, a subvariety of photosensitive epilepsy, a multifactorial mechanism combining all these, and psychological factors such as attention, emotional, and conditioned responses have been suggested. Most interesting is that the mechanism of precipitation seems closely related to the processes of decoding of words as optic entities into its acoustic speech motor counterpart (WOLF 1978). In several cases, homologous cases in the family have been demonstrated (DALY and FORSTER 1975, LASATER 1962; MATTHEWS and WRIGHT 1967).

References

Abrahamson I (1922) Diskussion. Neurol. Soc. of New York, 6. 6. 1922. J Nerv Ment Dis 56:355

Aicardi J (1973) The problem of the Lennox-syndrome. Develop. Med Child Neurol 15:77–81

Aicardi J, Chevrie J-J (1971) Myoclonic epilepsies of childhood. Neuropädiatrie 3:177–190

Aicardi J, Chevrie JJ, Rousselie F (1969) Le syndrome spasmes en flexion agénésie calleuse, anomalies chorio-rétiniennes. Arch Fr Pediatr 26:1103–1120

Alajouanine Th, Gastaut H (1955) La syncinesie-sursaut et l'épilepsie-sursaut à declenchement sensoriel ou sensitif inopiné, part 1 (Les faits anatomo-cliniques, 15 observations). Rev Neurol 93:29–41

Aminoff MJ, Simon RP (1980) Status epilepticus, clinical features and consequences in 98 patients. Am J Med 69:657–666

Andermann E, Metrakos JD (1969) EEG studies of relatives of probands with focal epilepsy who have been treated surgically. Epilepsia 10:415–420

Annegers JF, Hauser WA, Elveback LR, Kurland LT (1979) The risk of epilepsy following febrile convulsions. Neurology 29:297–303

Bamberger Ph, Matthes A (1959) Anfälle im Kindesalter. Karger, Basel

Bancaud J, Colomb D, Dell MB (1958) Les pointes rolandiques: un symptom E.E.G. propre á l'enfant. Rev Neurol 99:206–209

Barolin GS, Scholz H, Breitfellner G, Widder W (1976) Epilepsia partialis continua Kojevnikov – 7 Fälle. Nervenarzt 47:609–613

Barslund I, Danielsen J (1963) Temporal epilepsy in monozygotic twins. Epilepsia 4:138–150

Bash KW, Bash-Liechti J (1959) Die Psychotherapie eines Falles von musikogener Epilepsie. Schweiz Arch Neurol Psychiatr 83:196–221

Beaumanoir A, Martin F, Panagopoulos M, Mundler F (1968) Lennox-syndrome. A longterm study of thirty cases. Schweiz Arch Neurol Neurochir Psychiatr 102:31–62

Beaussart M (1972) Benign epilepsy of children with (centro-temporal) foci. Epilepsia 13:795–811

Beck-Mannagetta G, Janz D, Lipinski CG (1982) Febrile convulsions in children of epileptic parents: a retrospective study. In: Janz D, Bossi L, Dam M, Helge H, Richens A, Schmidt D (eds) Epilepsy, pregnancy and the child. Raven, New York, pp 521–526

Behrmann S, Wyke BD (1958) Vestibulogenic seizures. A consideration of vertiginous seizures, with particular reference to convulsions produced by stimulation of labyrinthine receptors. Brain 81:529–541

Bickford RG (1954) Sensory precipitation of seizures. J Mich Med Soc 53:1018–1020

Bickford RG, Klass DW (1969) Sensory precipitation and reflex mechanisms. In: Jasper HH, Ward AA, Pope A (eds) Basic mechanisms of the epilepsies. Little Brown, Boston

Bickford RG, Daly F, Keith HM (1953) Convulsive effects of light stimulation in children. Am J Dis Child 86:170–183

Bjerre I, Corelius E (1968) Benign familial neonatal convulsions. Acta Pediatr Scand 57:557–561

Blom S, Heijbel J. Bergfass JG (1972) Benign epilepsy of children with centrotemporal EEG-foci. Prevalence and follow-up study of 40 patients. Epilepsia 13:609–619

Blume WT, David R, Gomez M (1973) Generalized sharp-and-slow-wave-complexes. Associated features and longterm follow-up. Brain 96:289–306

Bray PF, Wiser WC (1965) The relation of focal to diffuse epileptiform discharge in genetic epilepsy. Arch Neurol 13:223–237

Brooks I, Jirauch PM (1971) Primary reading epilepsy: a misnomer. Arch Neurol 25:97–104

Burke JB (1954) The prognostic significance of neonatal convulsions. Arch Dis Child 29:342–345

Capella L et al. (1972) Contributo su alcuni aspetta della sindrome di Lennox (Casistica di 100 casi). Riv Neurol 42:530–536

Chatrian GE, Lettich E, Miller LH, Green JR (1970 a) Pattern-sensitive epilepsy. Part 1: an electrographic study of its mechanisms. Epilepsia 11:125–149

Chatrian GE, Lettich E, Miller LH, Green JR, Kupfer C (1970 b) Pattern-sensitive epilepsy. Part 2: clinical changes, tests of responsiveness and motor output, alterations of evoked potentials and therapeutic measures. Epilepsia 11:151–162

Chevrie J-J, Aicardi J (1972) Childhood epileptic encephalopathy with slow spike-wave. A statistical study of 80 cases. Epilepsia 13:259–271

Collins RL, Fuller JL (1968) Audiogenic seizure prone (asp.): a gene affecting behavior in linkage group VIII of the mouse. Science 162:1137–1139
Courjon J, Favel P, Lang M, Miribel J, Rouves L (1959) L'évolution du petit mal rebelle de l'enfant. Congr. de Pédiátrie de Langue franc., vol. IV, Montpellier, p 240
Critchley M (1935) Über Reflex-Epilepsie. Schweiz Arch Neurol Psychiatr 35:256
Critchley M (1937) Musicogenic epilepsy. Brain 60:13–37
Critchley M (1942) Two cases of musicogenic epilepsy. J R Nav Med Serv 28:182–184
Dalby MA (1969) Epilepsy and 3 per second spike and wave rhythms. A clinical, electroencephalographic and prognostic analysis of 346 patients. Munksgaard, Copenhagen
Daly D, Barry MJ (1957) Musicogenic epilepsy. Psychosom Med 19:399–408
Daly D, Bickford RG (1951) Electroencephalographic studies of identical twins with photo-epilepsy. Electroencephalogr Clin Neurophysiol 3:245–249
Daly RF, Forster FM (1975) Inheritance of reading epilepsy. Neurology 25:1051–1054
Dennis J (1978) Neonatal convulsions: aetiology, late neonatal status, and long-term outcome. Develop Med Child Neurol 20:143–158
Dennis J, Bower BD (1972) The Aicardi syndrome. Develop Med Child Neurol 14:382–390
Doose H (1964a) Zur Nosologie der Blitz-Nick-Salaam-Krämpfe. Arch Psychiatr Nervenkr 206:28–48
Doose H (1964b) Das akinetische Petit mal. I. Das klinische und elektroencephalographische Bild der akinetischen Anfälle. Arch Psychiatr Nervenkr 205:625–636
Doose H (1964c) Das akinetische Petit mal. II. Verlaufsformen und Beziehungen zu den Blitz-Nick-Salaam-Krämpfen und den Absencen. Arch Psychiatr Nervenkr 205:637–654
Doose H, Völzke E, Scheffner D (1965) Verlaufsformen kindlicher Epilepsien mit Spike-wave-Absencen. Arch Psychiatr Nervenkr 207:394–415
Doose H, Petersen CE, Völzke E, Herzberger E (1966a) Fieberkrämpfe und Epilepsie. I. Ätiologie, klinisches Bild und Verlauf der sogenannten Infekt- oder Fieberkrämpfe. Arch Psychiatr Nervenkr 208–400–412
Doose H, Völzke H, Petersen CE, Herzberger E (1966b) Fieberkrämpfe und Epilepsie. II. Elektroencephalographische Verlaufsuntersuchungen bei sogenannten Fieber- oder Infektkrämpfen. Arch Psychiatr Nervenkr 208:413–432
Doose H, Völzke E (1967) Elektroencephalographische Untersuchungen über die Genetik zentrencephaler Epilepsien. Z Kinderheilkd 101:242–257
Doose H, Gerken H, Hien-Völpel KF, Völzke E (1969) Genetics of photosensitive epilepsy. Neuropädiatrie 1:56–63
Doose H, Gerken H, Leonhardt R, Völzke E, Völz C (1970) Centrencephalic myoclonic-astatic petit mal. Clinical and genetic investigations. Neuropädiatrie 2:59–78
Dreifuss FE (1981) Proposal for revised clinical and electroencephalographic classification of epileptic seizures. Epilepsia 22:489–501
Dreyer R (1972) Mustersehen als Provokationsmittel zur Auslösung epileptischer Phänomene. Arch Psychiatr Nervenkr 216:58–69
Ellenberg JH, Nelson KB (1980) Sample selection and the natural history of disease. Studies of febrile seizures. JAMA 243:1337–1340
Enrile-Bacsal F, Delgado-Escueta AV (1981) Generalized epilepsy with myoclonia during adolescence: the impulsive petit mal syndrome of Janz. In: Epilepsy International Congress 1981 Kyoto, Epilepsy International, p 241 (abstract)
Falconer MA, Driver MV, Serafetinides EA (1963) Seizures induced by movement: report of a case relieved by operation. J Neurol Neurosurg Psychiatr 26:300–307
Fariello RG, Chun RWM, Doro JM, Prichard JS (1977) EEG recognition of Aicardi's syndrome. Arch Neurol 34:563–566
Fishman MA (1980) Commentary: the consensus development conference on febrile seizures. J Pediatr 97:933–934
Forfar JO et al. (1972) Early infantile convulsions and later epilepsy. In: Parsonage MJ (ed) Prevention of epilepsy and its consequences. International Bureau for Epilepsy, London, pp 38–43
Friedmann M (1960) Über die nichtepileptischen Absencen oder kurzen narkoleptischen Anfälle. Dtsch Z Nervenheilkd 30:462–492

Friedmann M (1912) Zur Kenntnis der gehäuften nichtepileptischen Absencen im Kindesalter. Z Ges Neurol Psychiatr 9:245–267
Friedmann M (1915) Zur Auffassung der gehäuften kleinen Anfälle. Monatsschr Psychiatr Neurol 38:76–97
Friis ML, Lund M (1974) Stress convulsions. Arch Neurol 30:155–159
Fuchs U, Junkers B (1973) Über choreoathetotische Anfälle. Nervenarzt 44:300–303
Fuller JL, Collins RL (1968) Mice unilaterally sensitized for audiogenic seizures. Science 12:1295
Gastaut H (1961) Note sur l'importance pathologique de la région pararhinale. In: Gastaut H, Lammers HJ (eds) Anatomie du rhinencéphale, vol I. Masson, Paris
Gastaut H (1970) Clinical and electroencephalographical classification of epileptic seizures. Epilepsia 11:102–113
Gastaut H (1973) Evolution clinique et pronostic du syndrome de Lennox-Gastaut. In: Evolution and prognosis of epilepsies. Italseber, Milano, pp 133–154
Gastaut H (1982) Classification of status epilepticus. In: Escueta-Delgado T, Wasterlain CG (eds) Status epilepticus. Raven, New York, pp 15–35
Gastaut H, Villeneuve A (1967) The startle disease or hyperexplexia. Pathological surprise reaction. J Neurol Sci 5:523–542
Gastaut H, Roger J, Roger A (1956) Sur la signification de certaines fugues épileptiques. A propos d'une observation électroclinique d'état de mal temporal. Rev Neurol 94:298–301
Gastaut H, Roger J, Soulayrol R, Pinsard N (1964) L'encephalopathie myoclonique infantile avec hypsarythmie (Syndrome de West). Masson, Paris
Gastaut H, Roger J, Soulayrol R, Salamon G, Régis H, Lob H (1965) Encéphalopathie myoclonique infantile avec hypsarhythmia (syndrome de West) et sclérose tubéreuse de Bourneville. J Neurol Sci 2:140–160
Gastaut H, Roger J, Soulayrol R, Tassinari CA, Régis H, Dravet C (1966) Childhood epileptic encephalopathy with diffuse slow spike-waves (otherwise known as "petit mal variant") or Lennox-syndrome. Epilepsia 7:139–176
Gastaut H, Broughton R, Roger J, Tassinari CA (1974) Generalized nonconvulsive seizures without local onset. In: Magnus O, Lorentz de Haas AM (eds) The epilepsies. North Holland, Amsterdam, pp 130–144 (Handbook of clinical neurology, vol 15)
Geier S, Bancaud J, Tailairach J, Bonis A, Engelvin M, Hossard-Bouchand H (1976) Automatisms during frontal lobe epileptic seizures. Brain 99:447–458
Gerstle de Pasquet E, Gaudin E, Bianchi A, De Mendilaharsu S (1976) Prolonged and monosymptomatic dysphasic status epilepticus. Neurology 26:244–247
Gibbs FA, Gibbs EL (1952) Atlas of electroencephalography. Addison-Wesley, Cambridge, Mass
Gibbs FA, Davis H, Lennox WG (1935) The electroencephalogram in epilepsy and in conditions of impaired consciousness. Arch Neurol Psychiatr 34:1133–1148
Gibson WC (1959/60) Temporal lobe epilepsy in two sisters. Epilepsia 1:316–324
Gilligan BS (1969) Primary reading epilepsy. Med J Aust 56:1025–1028
Goldie L, Green JM (1959) A study of the psychological factors in a case of sensory reflex epilepsy. Brain 82:505–524
Gowers WE (1901) Epilepsy and other chronic convulsive diseases. Their causes, symptoms and treatment, 2nd edn. Churchill, London
Grünberg F, Helmchen H (1969) Impulsiv-Petit mal-Status und paranoide Psychose. Nervenarzt 40:381–385
Hamilton NG, Matthews T (1979) Aphasia: the sole manifestation of focal status epilepticus. Neurology 29:745–748
Hauser WA, Kurland LT (1975) The epidemiology of epilepsy in Rochester, Minnesota, 1935 through 1967. Epilepsia 16:1–66
Heintel H (1972) Der Status epilepticus. Seine Ätiologie, Klinik und Mortalität. Fischer, Stuttgart
Helmchen H, Hoffmann I, Kanowski S (1969) Dämmerzustand oder Status fokaler sensorischer Anfälle. Nervenarzt 40:389–392

Herberg LJ, Tress KH, Blundell JE (1969) Raising the threshold in experimental epilepsy by hypothalamic and septal stimulation and by audiogenic seizur. Brain 92:313–328
Heycop ten Ham W van, Kuijer A, Lorentz de Haas M (1967) Recherches sur la génèse de l'état de mal épileptique. In: Gastaut H, Roger J, Lob H (eds) Les états de mal epileptiques. Masson, Paris
Higano H, Ohtaka T (1976) The electroencephalographic study on adult-type Lennox-Gastaut syndrome. Folia Psychiatr Neurol Jpn 30:315–324
Hishikawa Y, Furuya F, Yamamoto J, Nanno H (1973) Dystonic seizures induced by movement. Arch Psychiatr Nervenkr 217:113–138
Horita H, Hoashi E, Okuyama Y (1977) The studies of the attacks of abnormal eye movement in a case of infantile spasms. Folia Psychiat Neurol Jpn 31:393–402
Hunter RA (1959/1960) Status epilepticus. History, incidence and problems. Epilepsia 1:162–188
Jackson JH (1931) On the anatomical, physiological, and pathological investigation of epilepsies. In: Selected writings of John Hughlings Jackson, vol I. Hodder & Stoughton, London, p 94
Jackson JH, Colman S (1898) Case of epilepsy with tasting movements and "dreamy state" – very small patch of softening in the left uncinate gyrus. In: Selected writings of John Hughlings Jackson, vol I. Hodder & Stoughton, London, pp 458–463
Jacobi G (1979) Epilepsien mit atypischen Absencen. Klinik und EEG. In: Doose H, Kruse R, Lipinski Ch, Scheffner D, Weinmann HM (eds) Beiträge zur Klassifikation und medikamentösen Therapie epileptischer Anfälle. Desitin-Werk, Hamburg, pp 33–36
Janz D (1953) „Aufwach"-Epilepsie (als Ausdruck einer den „Nacht" oder „Schlaf"-Epilepsien gegenüberzustellenden Verlaufsform epileptischer Erkrankungen). Arch Psychiatr Nervenkr 191:73–98
Janz D (1955) Die klinische Stellung der Pyknolepsie. Dtsch Med Wochenschr 80:1392–1394, 1399–1400
Janz D (1961) Conditions and causes of status epilepticus. Epilepsia 2:170–177
Janz D (1962) The grand mal epilepsies and the sleeping waking cycle. Epilepsia 3:69–109
Janz D (1964) Status epilepticus and frontal lobe lesions. J Neurol Sci 1:446–457
Janz D (1969) Die Epilepsien. Spezielle Pathologie und Therapie. Thieme, Stuttgart
Janz D (1973) DFG-Denkschrift „Epilepsie". Boldt, Boppard
Janz D (1974) Epilepsy and the sleeping-waking cycle. In: Magnus O, Lorentz de Haas AM (eds) The epilepsies. North Holland, Amsterdam, pp 457–490. (Handbook of clinical neurology, vol 15)
Janz D (1982) Aetiology of convulsive status epilepticus. In: Escueta-Delgado T, Wasterlain CG (eds) Status epilepticus. Raven, New York, pp 47–54
Janz D, Akos R (1967) Über die Rolle pränataler Faktoren bei der Propulsiv-Petit mal-Epilepsie (West-Syndrom). J Neurol Sci 4:401–415
Janz D, Christian W (1957) Impulsiv-Petit mal. Dtsch Z Nervenheilkd 176:346–386
Janz D, Kautz D (1964) Aetiology and treatment of status epilepticus. German Med Mthly 9:451–459
Janz D, Matthes A (1955) Die Propulsiv-Petit-Mal-Epilepsie. Klinik und Verlauf der sog. Blitz-, Nick- und Salaamkrämpfe. Karger, Basel
Jasper H (1954) Electroencephalography. In: Penfield W, Jasper H (eds) Epilepsy and the functional anatomy of the human brain. Little Brown, Boston
Jeavons PM (1977) Nosological problems of myoclonic epilepsies in childhood and adolescence. Develop Med Child Neurol 19:3–8
Jeavons PM, Bower BD (1974) Infantile spasms. In: Magnus O, Lorentz de Haas AM (eds) The epilepsies. North Holland, Amsterdam, pp 219–234. (Handbook of clinical neurology, vol 15)
Jeavons PM, Harding GFA (1975) Photosensitive epilepsy. Heinemann, London
Jeavons PM, Bower BD, Dimitrakoudi M (1973) Longterm prognosis of 150 cases of "West-Syndrome". Epilepsia 14:153–164
Jellinger K (1970) Neuropathological aspects of hypsarrhythmia. Neuropädiatrie 1:277–294

Jensen J (1975) Genetic factors in temporal lobe epilepsy. Acta Neurol Scand 52:381–394
Joynt RF, Green D (1962) Musicogenic epilepsy. JAMA 179:501–504
Jung R (1939) Über vegetative Reaktionen und Hemmungswirkung von Sinnesreizen im kleinen epileptischen Anfall. Nervenarzt 12:169–185
Juul-Jensen P, Denny-Brown D (1966) Epilepsia partialis continua. A clinical, electroencephalographic, and neuropathological study of nine cases. Arch Neurol 15:563–578
Karbowski K (1980) Status psychomotoricus. Klinische und elektroencephalographische Aspekte. In: Karbowski K (ed) Status psychomotoricus. Huber, Bern, pp 39–72
Karch D et al. (1980) BNS-Krämpfe und Aicardi-Syndrom. Monatsschr Kinderheilkd 128:378–379
Kas S, Orszagh J (1976) Clinical study of status epilepticus: review of 111 statuses. Acta Univ Carol [Med] (Praha) 22:133–178
Keen JH, Lee D (1973) Sequelae of neonatal convulsions. Arch Dis Child 48:542–546
Kellaway P et al. (1979) Precise characterization and quantification of infantile spasms. Ann Neurol 6:214–218
Kennedy WA (1959) Clinical and electroencephalic aspects of epileptogenic lesions of the medial surface and superior border of the cerebral hemisphere. Brain 82:147–161
Ketz E, Meier HR (1979) Verlauf- und prognosebestimmende Faktoren beim Grand mal-Status. Aktuel Neurol 6:233–239
Kitagawa T (1975) Clinical and EEG studies on 500 patients with grand mal epilepsy (an investigation of the sleeping-waking cycle) In: Hara T, Wada T (eds) Circadian rhythm and epilepsy. Japanese Branch of the ILAE, Tokyo
Klass DW (1976) Sensory stimulation. In: Rémond A (ed) Handbook of electroencephalography and clinical neurophysiology, vol 3, part D. Elsevier, Amsterdam
Kreis A (1968) Reflexepilepsie. Schweiz Arch Neurol Neurochir Psychiatr 101:41–59
Kruse R (1968) Das myoklonisch-astatische Petit mal. Springer, Berlin Heidelberg New York
Kuromori N et al. (1976) A prospective study of epilepsy following neonatal convulsions. Folia Psychiatr Neurol Jpn 30:379–388
Lacy JR, Penry JK (1976) Infantile spasms. Raven, New York
Lagenstein I (1980) Das myoklonisch-astatische Petit mal und seine Verlaufsformen, eine klinische und elektroenzephalographische Verlaufsstudie an 95 Patienten. Fortschr Med 98:573–579
Lasater GM (1962) Reading epilepsy. Arch Neurol 6:492–495
Lennox WG (1945) The petit mal epilepsies; their treatment with Tridione. JAMA 129:1069–1974
Lennox WG (1960) Epilepsy and related disorders. Little Brown, Boston
Lennox-Buchthal M (1973) Febrile convulsions. A reappraisal. Electroencephalogr Clin Neurophysiol [Suppl] 32:1–138
Lerman P, Kivity S (1975) Benign focal epilepsy in childhood. A follow-up study of 100 recovered patients. Arch Neurol 32:261–264
Lipinski ChG (1977) Epilepsies with astatic seizures of late onset. Epilepsia 18:13–20
Lipinski ChG (1980) Die benigne Epilepsie im Kindesalter mit Rolando-Sharp-Wave-Focus. Nervenarzt 51:579–581
Lipinski ChG (1982) Incidence and prognosis of neonatal seizures in offspring of epileptic parents. In: Janz D, Bossi L, Dam M, Helge H, Richens A, Schmidt D (eds) Epilepsy, pregnancy and the child. Raven, New York, pp 515–520
Löhler J, Peters UH (1974) Epilepsia partialis continua (Koźevnikov-Epilepsie). Fortschr Neurol Psychiatr 42:165–212
Loiseau P, Beaussart M (1973) The seizures of benign childhood epilepsy with rolandic paroxysmal discharges. Epilepsia 14:381–389
Loiseau P, Legroux M, Grimond P, du Pasquier P, Henry P (1974) Taxometric classification of myoclonic epilepsies. Epilepsia 15:1–11
Lombroso CT (1974) Seizures in the newborn period. In: Magnus O, Lorentz de Haas AM (eds) The epilepsies. North Holland, Amsterdam. pp 189–234 (Handbook of clinical neurology, vol 15)

Ludwig B, Ajmone Marsan C, Van Buren J (1975) Cerebral seizures of probably orbitofrontal origin. Epilepsia 16:141–158
Lund M (1980) Some remarks by the Danish society on classification of seizures versus a classification according to type of epileptic syndromes. Letter to the International League Against Epilepsy
Lund M, Reintoft H, Simonsen N (1976) Eine kontrollierte soziologische und psychologische Untersuchung von Patienten mit juveniler myoklonischer Epilepsie. Nervenarzt 47:708–712
Matthes A (1961) Die psychomotorische Epilepsie im Kindesalter. III. Mitteilung. Z Kinderheilkd 85:668–685
Matthes A (1977) Epilepsie. Diagnostik und Therapie für Klinik und Praxis, 3 edn. Thieme, Stuttgart
Matthews WB, Wright FK (1967) Hereditary primary reading epilepsy. Neurology (Minneap) 17:919–921
Meencke HJ, Gerhard C (1984) Morphological aspects of etiology and clinical course of infantile spasms-Neuropediatrics
Merlis JK (1970) Proposal for an international classification of the epilepsies. Epilepsia 11:114–119
Metrakos K, Metrakos JD (1961) Genetics of convulsive disorders. II. Genetics and electroencephalographic studies in centrencephalic epilepsy. Neurology (Minneap) 11:474–483
Meyer JG, Meyer-Wahl L (1975) Über die fokale Entstehung der durch Mustersehen ausgelösten epileptischen Anfälle (pattern-sensitive epilepsy). Nervenarzt 46:24–30
Meyer JG, Wolf P (1973) Über primäre Leseepilepsie. Nervenarzt 44:155–160
Munde B (1969) Verlauf eines BNS-Anfallsleidens bei eineiigen Zwillingen. Arch Kinderheilkd 179:66–72
Nelson KB, Ellenberg JH (1976) Predictors of epilepsy in children who have experienced febrile seizures. N Engl J Med 295:1029–1033
Nelson KB, Ellenberg JH (1978) Prognosis in children with febrile seizures. Pediatrics 61:720–727
Newmark ME, Penry JK (1979) Photosensitivity and epilepsy: a review. Raven, New York
Newmark ME, Penry JK (1980) Genetics of epilepsy. Raven, New York
Niedermeyer E (1969) The Lennox-Gastaut syndrome: a severe type of childhood epilepsy. A statistical study of 80 cases. Dtsch Z Nervenheilkd 195:263–282
Nikitin MP (1935) Zur Psychogenese der epileptischen Anfälle. Nervenarzt 8:66–69
Nolte R, Bantz B (1977) Neuropsychologische Befunde bei im Vorschulalter nachuntersuchten Kindern mit Krämpfen in der Neugeborenenperiode. Monatsschr Kinderheilkd 125:392–393
Ohtahara S (1978) Clinico-electrical delineation of epileptic encephalopathies in childhood. Asian Med J 21:499–509
Ohtahara S, Ishida T, Oka E, Yamatogi Y, Inoue H (1976) On the specific age-dependent epileptic syndrome: the early-infantile epileptic encephalopathy with suppression-burst. Brain and Development 8:270–280
Oller-Daurella L (1972) Sindrome de Lennox-Gastaut. Arch Neuro-Psiquiatr 30:271–287
Oller-Daurella L (1976) Las fronteras entre el „Petit mal" y el sindrome de Lennox-Gastaut. Rev Oto-Neuro-Oftalm 34:27–44
Oller-Daurella L, Dini J (1970) Las crisis epilepticas desencadenadas por movimientos voluntarios. Diagnóstico diferencial con la coreoatetosis paroxistica y discusión de su posible relación con la epilepsia-sobresalto. Med Clíni (Barc) 54:189–198
Oller-Daurella L, Oller L (1977) El prognóstico del petit mal. Evolución de 147 casos de epilepsia iniciada por ausencias tipicas. Rev Esp Pediatr 33:3–22
Orban L, Lang J (1963) The pathogenesis of vestibulogenic epilepsy. Psychiatr Neurol 146:193–198
Osawa T et al. (1976) Slow spike-wave discharges in elder patients. Folia Psychiatr Neurol Jpn 30:331–341

Passouant P, Duc N, Cadilhac J, Minvielle J (1957) Accès confusionel de longue durée et décharge epileptique temporal au cours de l'évolution d'une paralysie générale. Rev Neurol 96:329–332
Penfield W, Jasper H (1954) Epilepsy and the functional anatomy of the human brain. Little Brown, Boston
Perez-Borja C, Tassinari AC, Swanson AG (1967) Paroxysmal choreoathetosis and seizure induced by movement (reflex epilepsy). Epilepsia 8:260–270
Poskanzer DC, Brown AE, Miller H (1962) Musicogenic epilepsy caused only by a discrete frequency band of church bells. Brain 85:77–92
Quattlebaum TG (1979) Benign familial convulsions in the neonatal period and early infancy. Paediatrics 95:257–259
Rabe F (1961) Zum Wechsel des Anfallscharakters epileptischer Anfälle Dtsch Z Nervenheilkd 182–201
Rabending G, Klepel H (1978) Die Fotostimulation als Aktivierungsmethode in der Elektroencephalographie. Fischer, Jena
Rabending G, Jährig K, Fischer W (1981) Epilepsien. Leitfaden für die Praxis. Thieme, Leipzig
Radovici A, Misirliou V, Gluckmann M (1932) Epilepsie réflexe provoquée par excitations optiques des rayons solaires. Rev Neurol 1:1305–1308
Rautenstrauch T, Brunner B (1980) Ätiologie und Prognose von Neugeborenenkrämpfen. Pädiatr Praxis 23:361–370
Renier W (1973) Agenesis of the corpus callosum, chorioretinopathy and infantile spasms (Aicardi syndrome). Psychiatr Neurol Neurochir 76:39–45
Rodin EA, Whelan JL (1960) Familial occurrence of focal electroencephalographic abnormalities. Neurology (Minneap) 10:542–545
Rosenthal C (1935) Die gehäuften kleinen Anfälle des Kindesalters (Pyknolepsie). Erg Innere Med Kinderheilkd 48:77–124
Rowan AJ, Scott DF (1970) Major status epilepticus. A series of 42 patients. Acta Neurol Scand 46:573–584
Sato S, Dreifuss FE, Penry JK (1977) Prognosis factors in absence seizures. Neurology (Minneap) 26:788–796
Schlesinger K, Boggon WO, Griek BJ (1968) Pharmacogenetic correlates of pentylentetrazol and electroconvulsive seizure thresholds in mice. Psychopharmacology 13: 181–188
Schneider H, Vasella F, Karbowski K (1970) The Lennox-syndrome. A clinical study of 40 children Eur Neurol 4:289–300
Schneider RC, Crosby EC, Farhat SM (1965) Extratemporal lesions triggering the temporal lobe syndrome. J Neurosurg 22:246–263
Schröder P (1913) Über Narkolepsie. Allg Z Psychiatr 70:631; Neurol Zbl 32:598
Schulte F (1966) Neonatal convulsions and their relation to epilepsy in early childhood. Develop Med Child Neurol 8:381–392
Scollo-Lavizzari G, Hess R (1967) Sensory precipitation of epileptic seizures. Report on two unusual cases. Epilepsia 8:157–161
Scott JS, Masland RL (1953) Occurrence of "continuous symptoms" in epilepsy patients. Neurology (Minneap) 3:297–301
Sengoku A, Kawai I, Hojo H (1976) On the Lennox syndrome with the onset in puberty. Folia Psychiatr Neurol Jpn 30:325–330
Servit Z (1962) The application of the reflex theory in the interpretation of the clinical picture, genesis, and treatment of epilepsy. Epilepsia 3:209–228
Simonsen N, Møllgaard V, Lund M (1976) A controlled clinical and electroencephalographic study of myoclonic epilepsy (Impulsiv-Petit-Mal): preliminary report. In: Janz D (ed) Epileptology. Proceedings of the seventh international symposium on epilepsy. Thieme, Stuttgart, pp 41–48
Sorel L (1964) L'épilepsie myokinetiqué grave de la première enfance avec pointe-onde lent (petit mal variant) et son traitement. Rev Neurol 110:215–223

Stenzel E (1979) Myoklonisch-astatische Anfälle des Jugendlichen- und Erwachsenenalters. In: Doose H, Kruse R, Lipinski Ch, Scheffner D, Weinmann HM (eds) Beiträge zur Klassifikation und medikamentösen Therapie epileptischer Anfälle. Desitin-Werk, Hamburg
Stenzel E, Panteli C (1982) Lennox-Gastaut-Syndrom des 2. Lebensjahrzehnts. In Remschmidt H, Rentz R, Jungmann J (eds). Epilepsie 1981. Thieme, Stuttgart New York
Tchicaloff M, Déruaz JP, Rabinowicz I (1974) Klinisch-anatomische Untersuchungen bei zwei Kindern mit myoklonisch-astatischem Petit mal. Z EEG-EMG 5:114–122
Thomas JE, Reagan TJ, Klass DW (1977) Epilepsia partialis continua. A review of 32 cases. Arch Neurol 34:266–275
Titeca J (1965) L'épilepsie musicogénique. Revue générale á propos d'un cas personel suivi pendant 14 ans. Acta Neurol Belg 65:598
Toivakka E, Lehtinen LOJ (1965) Musicogenic epilepsy. A case report. Acta Neurol Scand 41 [Suppl] 13:529–533
Tsuboi T (1977 a) Genetic aspects of febrile convulsions. Hum Genet 38:169–173
Tsuboi T (1977 b) Primary generalized epilepsy with sporadic myoclonias of myoclonic petit mal type. A clinical, electroencephalographic, statistical and genetic study of 399 probands. Thieme, Stuttgart
Tsuboi T, Christian W (1976) A clinical, electroencephalographic and statistical study on epilepsies. Neurology series. Springer, Berlin Heidelberg New York
Tsuboi T, Endo Sh (1977) Febrile convulsions followed by nonfebrile convulsions. A clinical, electroencephalographic and follow-up study. Neuropädiatrie 8:209–223
Tsuboi T, Yamamura K (1978) Febrile convulsions followed by nonfebrile convulsions. Analysis based on a maximum likelihood method and discriminant function. Neuropädiatrie 9:103–108
US Department of Health, Education and Welfare (1977) Plan for nationwide action on epilepsy. D.H.E.W. Publication No (NIH) 78–276, vol I, pp 1–249; vol IV, pp 1–234
Viani F, Strada GP, Riboldi A, Riboldi A, Manghi E, Rossotti V, Allegranza A (1977) Aspetti neuropatologici della sindrome di Lennox-Gastaut: Considerazoni su tre casi. Riv Neurol 47:1–40
Vizioli R (1962) The problem of human reflex epilepsy and the possible role of masked epileptogenic factors. Epilepsia 3:293–302
Völzke E, Reinicke U, Doose H (1981) Impulsive (myoclonic) petit mal treatment with valproate. Abstracts, XIIIth Epilepsy Internat. Symp. Kyoto, p 241
Weber R (1956) Musikogene Epilepsie. Nervenarzt 27:337–340
West WJ (1841) On a peculiar form of infantile convulsions. Lancet I:724
Whitty CWM, Taylor M (1949) Treatment of status epilepticus. Lancet II:591–594
Wilkins AJ, Darby CE, Binnie CD (1979) Neurophysiological aspects of pattern sensitive epilepsy. Brain 102:1–25
Wolf P (1970) Zur Klinik und Psychopathologie des Status psychomotoricus. Nervenarzt 41:603–610
Wolf P (1978) Reading epilepsy. Evidence for a cognitive factor in seizure precipitation. In: Meinardi H, Rowan AJ (eds) Advances in epileptology 1977. Swets and Zeitlinger, Amsterdam, pp 85–90
Wolf P (1982) Abwandlungen subjektiver Anfallssymptome (Auren) im Status fokaler sensorischer Anfälle (Aura continua). In: Remschmidt H, Rentz R, Jungmann J (eds) Epilepsie 1981. Thieme, Stuttgart.
Woodbury LA (1977) A brief consideration of the prognosis of epilepsy. In: U.S. Department of Health, Education and Welfare, D.H.E.W.Publication No (NIH) 78–276 (ed) Plan for nationwide action on epilepsy, vol IV, pp 3–23
Yamatogi Y, Ohtahara S (1981) Age-dependent epileptic encephalopathy: a longitudinal study. Folia Psychiatr Neurol 35:321–332
Zielinski JJ (1974) Epileptics not in treatment. Epilepsia 16:203–210

CHAPTER 2

Electroencephalography

R. Hess

A. Introduction

Electroencephalography in the widest sense of the word means measuring and recording the bioelectrical potential changes of the brain, from animal experimentation to the auxiliary methods of neurology, i.e., the routine tests given to patients suspected of suffering from pathological cerebral conditions. For the physician as well as for the general public the word has this latter restricted meaning, and it is in this sense that it will be used in this chapter.

Direct recording from the cerebral cortex is called *electrocorticography* (ECoG). The activity of deep-lying structures can be examined by depth electrodes; if this is performed under stereotactic conditions, it is called *stereoelectroencephalography* (SEEG). These procedures, the use of which is restricted to neurosurgical units, will be dealt with briefly at the end of this chapter.

The clinical EEG has the advantages of being innocuous and easily performed over almost any length of time. It reflects, however, one facet of the brain's functions only and is far from conveying an image of the subtle and intricate integration of information and organization of outgoing commands, which is the function of the cerebral cortex. The prominent potential changes in the normal EEG are rather a correlate of the resting state, in which excitability oscillates around an optimal level. Otherwise, the EEG is a fairly accurate indicator of the level of alertness and of the depth or stage of sleep. It does also show certain deviations from the normal state, which is its raison d'être.

Pathological changes represent disturbances of cortical function, but these changes must be gross and extended to be picked up through the scalp, skull, and cerebrospinal fluid by the recording electrodes. It has been calculated that potentials must change synchronously and in the same spatial orientation over a cortical area of several square centimeters in order to sum sufficiently to appear on the conventional EEG (Cooper et al. 1965). It is obvious that even substantial abnormalities in deep-lying cerebral structures, including mesial and basal surfaces of the hemispheres, must in many cases remain undetected. Basically, this limitation also applies to epileptic dysfunction, a great part of which never reaches the surface (cf. SEEG). The propensity of epileptic discharges to spread and drive activity of remote cerebral structures is apt to lessen the handicap to some extent.

The distinguishing features of the EEG – the often spectacular transient wave forms and complexes and their spatial distribution – were empirically correlated to clinical seizure types in the pioneer years (Gibbs et al. 1938). In the meantime, as clinical experience and animal experimentation have supplied us with a wealth of information about the underlying aberrant neurophysiological functions and as the role of transmitters in the various cerebral systems becomes increasingly obvious, we have had to gradually adapt and specify our concepts about epilepsy. Along with this evolution, many details of EEG interpretation have shifted in their significance, but the principal electroclinical correlations have remained remarkably valid.

B. Main Forms of Epileptiform Patterns

Generally, the mark of epilepsy is the presence of paroxysmal potential changes, which clearly stand out against the background activity by their different parameters: Most cases show a sudden rise of amplitudes, but also changes in frequency and wave forms, single or in combination. The best known and most common are short transients, which are termed "spikes" if of less than 70 ms in duration and "sharp waves" if longer. No such clear-cut contrast exists of course in their biological meaning, but it may be assumed that shorter transients are picked up directly from restricted superficial areas, whereas blunt sharp waves are the result of nervous conduction at slightly different velocities (temporal dispersion: JASPER 1949) or of recruitment of spikes over a wider area with different synaptic delays.

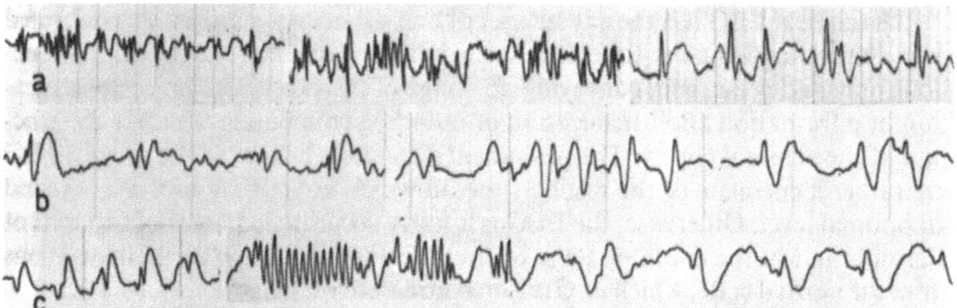

Fig. 1. Various forms of intercritical paroxysmal patterns, taken from different EEG records. *a*, spikes; *b*, spike wave complexes (*left*) and sharp wave complexes; *c*, train of spikes (*center*) passing over into repetitive sharp wave complexes, some with unobtrusive faster components; *d*, section out of a record, with bipolar leads showing the right anterior temporal epileptogenic area. Note phase reversal of the highest sharp waves near the anterior electrode; smaller spikes are seen close to the mid-temporal electrode

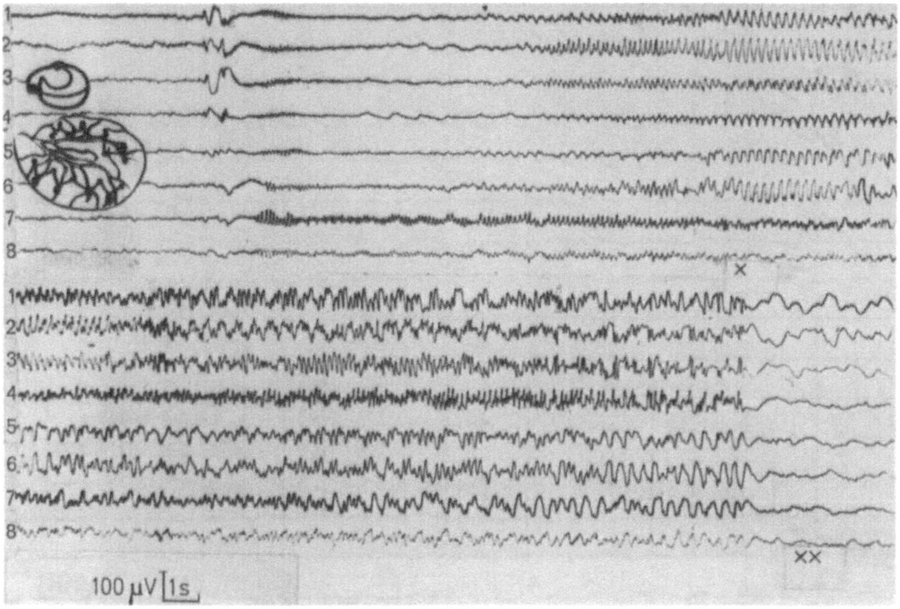

Fig. 2. Short seizure recorded from the cortex in a case of right temporal epilepsy, operated on under local anesthesia. *Channels 1–4*, T1 from the temporal pole to the posterior temporal; *Channels 5–8*, above the Sylvian fissure. The *bottom half of the figure* ist the immediate continuation. Note the initial paroxysmal complex in the temporal lobe. Subsequent fast activity spreads rapidly, slows down, and increases in amplitude. The *bottom half* shows further slowing and an abrupt end of the seizure. *x*, no response to call; *xx*, responsive again

These rapid deflections are as a rule of negative sign (in reference recording, the pen goes upward, in bipolar recording the pens of the two adjoining channels move toward each other). Pure monophasic spikes and sharp waves represent the simplest but not the most common type: More often they are multiphasic and followed by a slow wave which is thought to be the sign of an inhibitory influence (hyperpolarization) terminating the paroxysmal discharge. Such "spike-wave complexes," single or groups of spikes, sharp waves, etc., which do not usually last longer than ½–1 s, are called *interictal* or *intercritical* (Fig. 1).

If the inhibition fails and paroxysmal activity goes on, it develops into a (*critical*) seizure discharge, i.e., into longer-lasting pathological overactivity, as it is often seen during clinical attacks. Basic features are: onset with low-voltage fast activity, gradually growing higher and slowing down, at the same time spreading over wider areas. When the frequency reaches the θ-band (4–7/s) the regular trains are broken up and interrupted by slow waves, thus forming a rhythm of alternating fast and slow waves, which also tends to slow down to 2–3/s. The end is fairly abrupt in most cases (taken as evidence of an inhibitory effect; Fig. 2). Subsequent flattening of the record is possible, followed by irregular slow waves, possibly due to metabolic exhaustion.

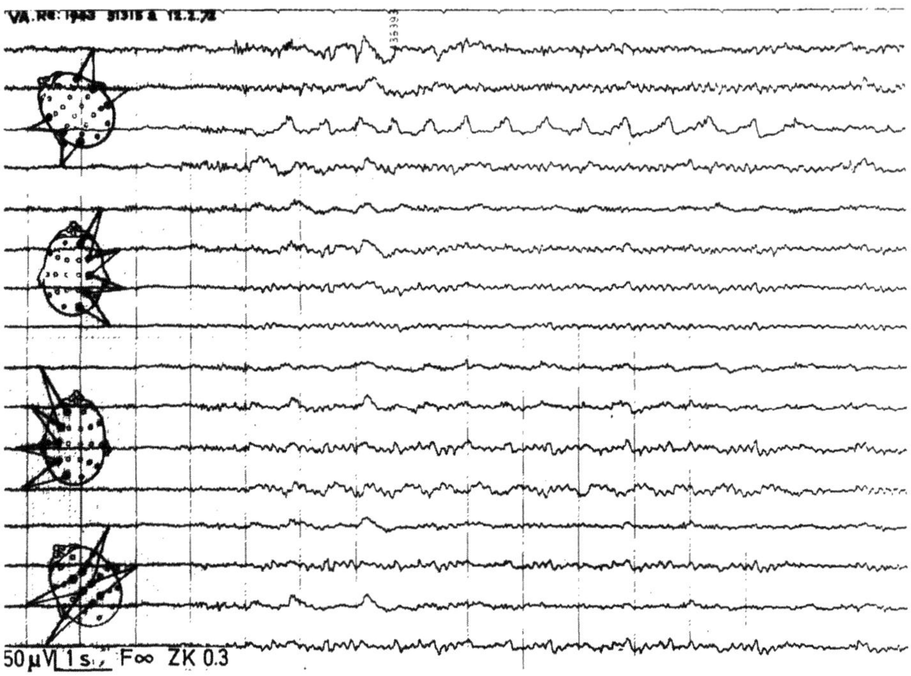

Fig. 3. Subclinical discharge, consisting essentially of a train of 1.5/s sawtooth-shaped waves, best seen in the left temporal leads but spreading to the parietal region. This spatial distribution permits us to conclude that there is a deep origin in the left posterior quadrant. The form of the rhythmic waves suggests that they are distant effects of repetitive sharp waves (bilateral frontal single slow waves are *K*-complexes in a light sleep stage)

The above description is a simplification, because it is rarely encountered in practice in such a regular succession of phases. The discharge patterns may mix, may vary from one place to another (most clearly observed in the ECoG; Fig. 15), or may change back to earlier phases, etc. As not more than one-fifth of the cortex lies close to the convexity, the initial phases may be lacking or only part of the seizure activity may reach the scalp EEG, often in the form of indirectly induced changes, as rhythmical slow waves, repetitive single sharp waves, or irregular fast activity (Figs. 3, 16). Occasionally, the EEG fails altogether to reflect the clinical attack.

If the whole sequence of a bioelectrical seizure is recorded, its different phases correlate grossly with the *clinical signs*: the low-voltage fast activity with the aura, the regular rhythms of increasing voltage and shifting from the β- through the α- to the θ-band with the tonic muscle contraction (in the case of a motor attack), the interrupted multiple spike-slow wave rhythm with the clonic phase. The flattening may correspond to a postparoxysmal palsy.

It is particularly in short, aborted, or atypical seizure discharges that no overt clinical signs can be observed. This is then called a *subclinical discharge* (Fig. 3).

On the other hand, excessive epileptic activity may exceptionally last for hours or days, either in the form of repeated complete seizures in rapid succession (correlated to an epileptic status) or as paroxysmal complexes occurring more or less continuously in a restricted area: The clinical equivalent is epilepsia partialis continua, aura continua, or sometimes none (Fig. 15c, e).

It must be realized of course that the boundaries between the described categories are fluid and that the patterns as recorded in the clinical EEG are an incomplete reflection of what is going on at depth, where long-lasting discharges may occur when the surface is reached by intercritical paroxysmal outbursts only. Although ictal discharges are of the highest diagnostic value, the interictal ones are of much higher incidence and, insofar as they can be specific for certain types of epilepsy, essentially they account for the clinical value of the EEG.

Paroxysmal patterns exist in almost numberless variations, but some are more common than others and an overall division, corresponding to that of the clinical seizures, suggests itself: In the first place *focal* patterns must be distinguished from *bilateral* or *generalized* ones.

C. Focal Epileptiform Activity

Focal epileptiform activity corresponds most closely to the general description (Sect. B) when originating in the superficial cortex of the convexity; it then correlates with *neocortical partial seizures* (Fig. 1a). Focal spikes and sharp waves usually indicate the presence of a localized lesion and are known to develop in its borderline area. Higher amplitudes, faster spikes, more complex bursts, and seizure discharges are generally most significant, both for indicating susceptibility to epileptic seizures and for the location of the underlying lesion. Simple paroxysmal transients are less reliable, particularly so in the older and the youngest age groups. In elderly people monophasic sharp waves are commonly seen in the temporal regions, assumably as a consequence of inadequate vascular supply. This does not as a rule imply the danger of epileptic seizures, nor has it, in the case of an expansive lesion, any localizing value (VAN DER DRIFT and MAGNUS 1961). In small children, on the other hand, especially around the age of 4 years, occipital focal sharp waves are not usually evidence of a local lesion but rather of a general hyperexcitable state, with or without clinical signs of epilepsy. They are also observed in children with impaired eyesight (LAIRY et al. 1964). In children of school age such sharp waves are most often localized in the centroparietal region. Many of these children do not suffer from clinical epilepsy; those who do may have focal seizures (mainly nocturnal), but corresponding structural lesions are rarely found and the prognosis is favorable (Fig. 4; BEAUSSART et al. 1970; GASTAUT 1952; LOISEAU et al. 1967).

Epileptic discharges originating at some depth but still reaching the cortex may have special features. Apart from the sharp waves being broader, they also tend to recede behind the accompanying slow waves. Often a paroxysmal component consisting of a rapid positive deflection in the θ-band is locked to a large negative slower wave; occasional preceding small negative sharp waves confirm the epileptic implication (Fig. 1c). Even a train of slow rhythms without sharper com-

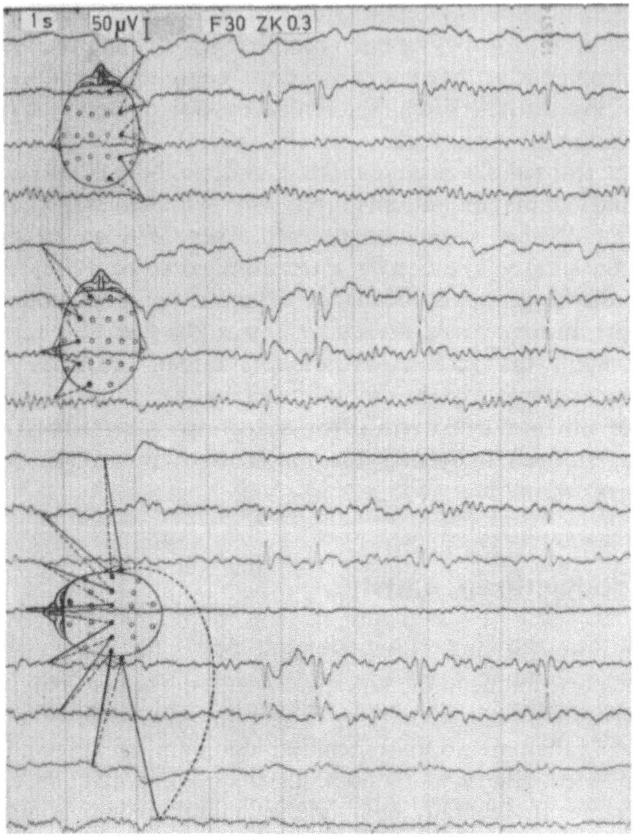

Fig. 4. Rolandic sharp waves in a boy of 14 suffering from benign epilepsy with focal features. Primary focus in the left central region; mirror focus *on the right* with incomplete phase reversal, owing to synchronous occurrence over the posterior half of the hemisphere

ponents may represent indirect evidence of epileptic activity at a distance (Fig. 3). If such changes are clearly separated from the rest of the record with well-defined onset and end, their epileptic nature is reliable and they represent a common form of *"subclinical focal attacks."*

A special constellation with deep-lying epileptogenic areas is represented by the group of *limbic epilepsies*, the clinical expression of which is complex partial or psychomotor seizures in their various forms. The amygdala and hippocampus are mainly involved, but the other limbic structures as well as the temporal neocortex usually play a role (cf. paragraph on SEEG). In the scalp EEG, the great majority of intercritical paroxysmal graphoelements consist of anterior temporal sharp waves (Fig. 1 d). They are often found on both sides, simultaneously (cf. mirror foci) or independently. Other secondary foci may be situated in the posterior temporal area (often less conspicuous).

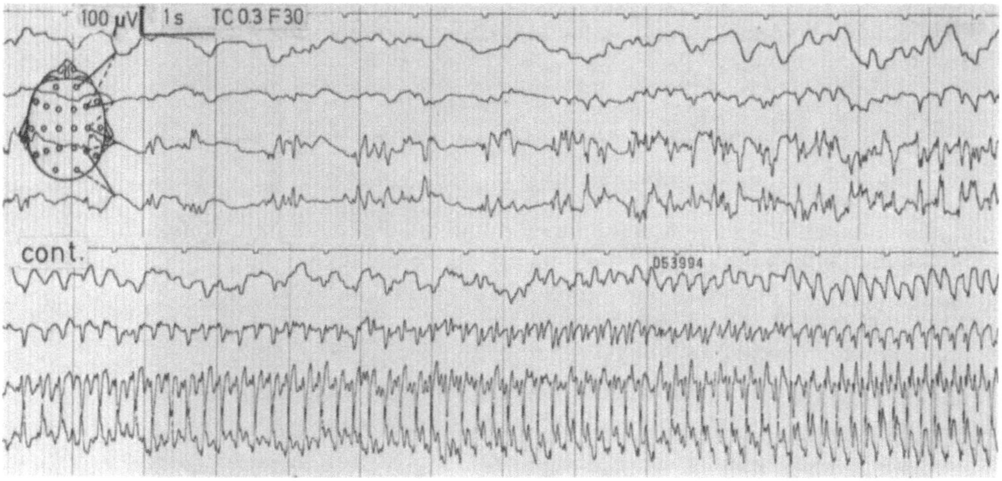

Fig. 5. Focal motor epileptic status (left arm) after cardiac surgery. Section shows four channels leading from the right hemisphere. *Top*, "semicritical" onset with increasing incidence of irregular spikes. *Bottom* (*immediate continuation*), rhythmic discharge with wider spread (tonic phase)

Ictal discharges in neocortical focal seizures are in accordance with the general description (Sect. B), supplemented by specifications concerning spatial distribution: They start in a defined area, spread within seconds over the involved cerebral lobe and further (Fig. 5). If it has not already aborted, the excessive activity reaches the contralateral hemisphere usually in the late tonic phase (coinciding with the loss of consciousness), and eventually the whole of the convexity, when the clinical attack becomes generalized. In small children the seizure discharges may also remain restricted to one hemisphere, continue status-like for a long period, and leave in their wake severe depression of all activity or slowing. This corresponds to clinical hemiconvulsions with subsequent hemiparesis.

In *limbic seizures*, ictal discharges occur in many different variations. Fairly common is an initial flattening of the record, either in a restricted area (effect of circumfocal inhibition? PRINCE and WILDER 1967) or generalized (arousal effect owing to aura?) Thereafter, the most common concomitant of the psychomotor seizure consists of bilateral slow rhythms, which are most pronounced in the parasagittal frontal regions, but often more marked over one temporal lobe, where furthermore faster rhythms or repetitive sharp waves may prevail (Fig. 6). It is, however, not uncommon that limbic seizures are reflected on the surface EEG by minor and equivocal abnormalities only; on occasions the EEG remains virtually unchanged (Fig. 16).

Multiple epileptogenic foci are not rare, particularly in children, often with extended or multiple lesions (GIBBS and GIBBS 1964). Still more frequently seen are secondary foci, most often in the homologous area of the primary ones: so-called *mirror foci*. They are common at the age-dependent predilection sites, namely occipital in small children, centroparietal in schoolchildren (Fig. 4), and anterior

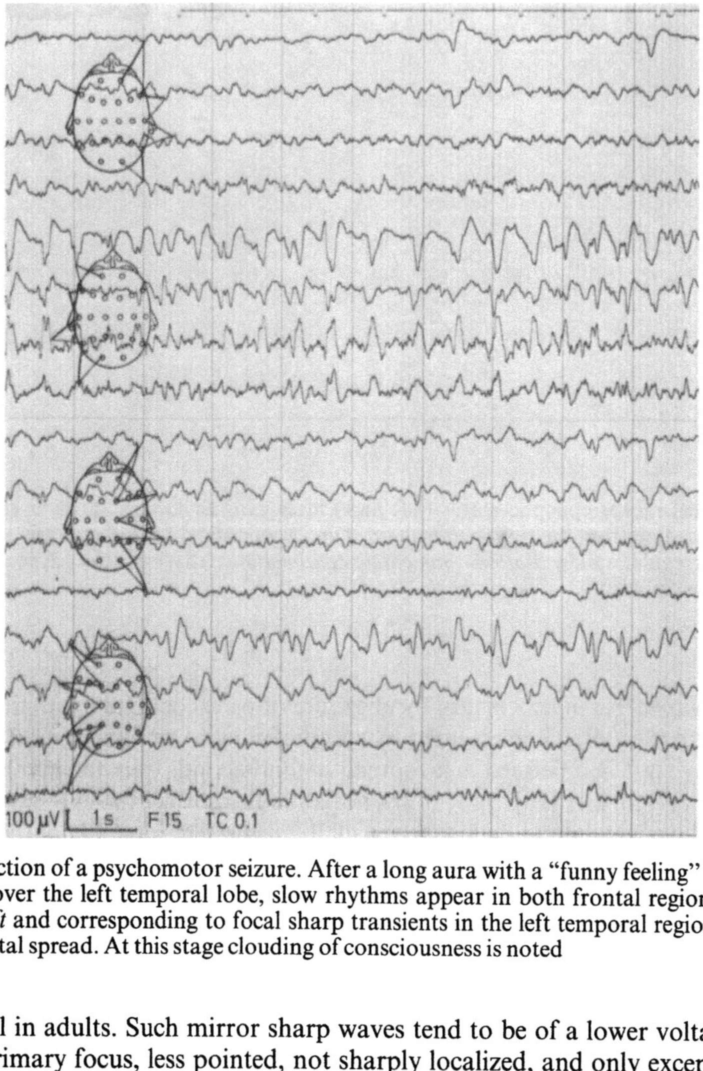

Fig. 6. Section of a psychomotor seizure. After a long aura with a "funny feeling" and focal slowing over the left temporal lobe, slow rhythms appear in both frontal regions, higher *on the left* and corresponding to focal sharp transients in the left temporal region, in part with frontal spread. At this stage clouding of consciousness is noted

temporal in adults. Such mirror sharp waves tend to be of a lower voltage than in the primary focus, less pointed, not sharply localized, and only exceptionally showing a measurable delay. In temporal foci especially, such differences are often missing and sharp wave complexes occur independently on both sides. There is some evidence that a pure mirror focus, which reflects the commissural propagation, is transformed by the chronic bombardment into an independent focus, including local structural changes (Morell 1960). It is interesting to note that ictal discharges are not transmitted in a similar form to the homologous area: If they do reach the contralateral hemisphere it is in the context of a more extended seizure.

D. Bilateral Epileptiform Patterns

Bilateral epileptiform patterns correlate broadly with the generalized epilepsies. *Bilateral synchrony,* often used for definition, is true only as a first approxima-

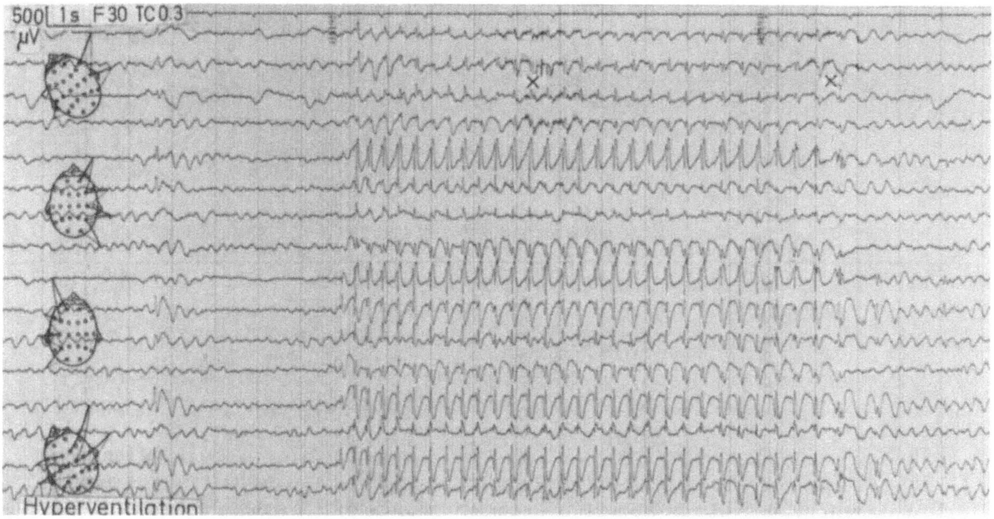

Fig. 7. Juvenile petit mal. Induced by hyperventilation, a short spike wave complex is followed by a long train of regular, symmetrical alternating spikes and slow waves at a frequency of 3/s at the onset, 2/s at the end, tapering off within 1 s. Muscle potentials in temporal leads (x) are connected to clinical expression of absence

tion, since accurate measurements show that one or other hemisphere may be leading by milliseconds (GOTMAN 1981). All forms of paroxysmal potential changes may occur bilaterally, but the majority consist of spikes or sharp waves and slow waves, in varying combinations. Series of spikes with few or no slow components are rather rare, as are paroxysmal bilateral slow waves alone; much more common is a fairly regular alternation of slow and fast waves, which is interpreted as sustained hyperactivity interrupted by inhibition (JUNG 1949; GLOOR 1979). The typical patterns are commonly called "spikes and waves" (abbreviated SAW or SW). They are characterized by a more or less sudden onset, often with a short buildup of slowing θ-waves, sometimes asymmetrical at the beginning, and thereafter by regular trains of 3.5–3/s rhythms, gradually slowing to 2.5–2/s. The amplitude is highest in the parasagittal frontal regions. Regularly locked to the rhythmic slow waves are high-voltage spikes, often multiphasic and usually symmetrical, occasionally with a temporal maximum on one or both sides. These spikes are most marked as a rule in the early phase, then diminish in amplitude; sometimes they alternate, every second one being smaller. The end is usually abrupt, and less commonly the slow rhythms taper off (Fig. 7; cf. JASPER and DROOGLEEVER-FORTUYN 1947).

The spectacular trains of periodical 3/s spikes and waves represent a special case with fairly well-defined *clinical implications*: In the first place, this pattern affords almost certain evidence of the presence of overt epilepsy (SILVERMAN 1954), in particular of the "centrencephalic" form, which means a notable hereditary factor and a negligible risk of a gross organic lesion, although exogenic causal factors – mostly perinatal – may play a role (LENNOX 1960). Runs lasting more

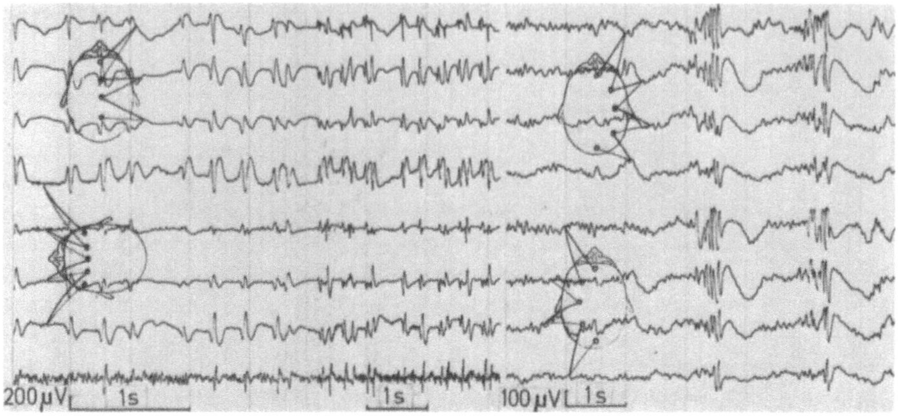

Fig. 8. Juvenile myoclonic epilepsy. *Left*, myoclonic status with irregular jerking of the neck muscles. *The lowermost channel* records the electromyogram from the left musculus sternocleidomastoideus. Note the approximate correspondence of EEG sharp waves and EMG spikes. *Right*, same child in the interval: bilateral multiple spike waves, usually coinciding with jerks of the upper extremities

than a few seconds are generally associated with a clinical "absence," which may range from the slightest impairment of mental function to a full-blown petit mal with twitching of eyes and head at the rhythm of the SW complexes. Unobtrusive automatisms are common especially in longer runs. Short bursts of 1–3 s are usually subclinical; the boundaries are fluid.

Spikes and waves can occasionally occur in a status-like form for long periods, either as closly spaced absences (accompanied by an undulating level of consciousness: absence status) or more continually in a somewhat distorted form [accompanied by varying degrees of impaired mental functions: petit-mal stupor (NIEDERMEYER and KALIFEH 1965)].

Typical spikes and waves are definitely *age linked*, insofar as they are most commonly seen in schoolchildren, hardly ever before the age of 3 years, and gradually less after adolescence, although cases of patients 60 years and older with spikes and waves are occasionally met with (METRAKOS and METRAKOS 1961).

Far more common in adult patients are shorter and more irregular bursts as intercritical signs of "centrencephalic" epilepsy, and as signs of pure grand mal epilepsy, into which the petit mal of childhood often develops (see Chap. 1, this volume, Sect. F.VI.). Myoclonic jerks are as a rule associated with a paroxysmal burst of high-voltage spikes, followed by one or several slow waves ("multiple spikes and waves"). They are not, however, pathognomonic for myoclonus epilepsy (Fig. 8).

The *critical activity* during grand mal (GM) attacks is as described for the focal seizures, but bilateral from the beginning or nearly so. The preliminary, initiating increasing fast activity starts mainly over the frontal lobes. A paroxysmal

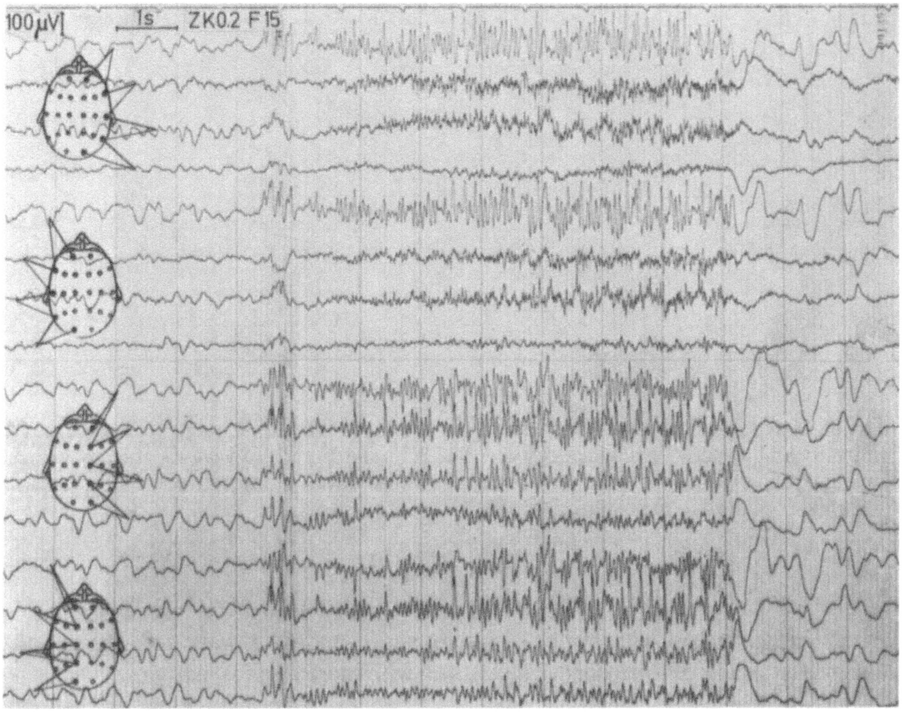

Fig. 9. Youth in a status of tonic extension seizures. The EEG shows a short attack of "grand mal" type: onset with a group of high-voltage spikes, subsiding for a fraction of a second, resuming with low amplitudes which rapidly increase, and terminated by a large slow wave. Bifrontal maximum throughout. Superimposed muscle artifact in temporal leads

spike wave complex may precede by one or a few seconds. During a full-blown seizure the record is usually marred by a massive artefact (Fig. 9).

In *children*, generalized epilepsy often manifests itself in *age-specific forms*: in toddlers up to preschool age a syndrome named after *Lennox* and *Gastaut* (cf. GASTAUT et al. 1966; Chap. 1, this volume). The EEG correlate, intercritical and during the absences, is a pattern called slow spikes and waves, consisting of alternating sharp and slow waves at 2–2½/s. Spatial distribution is bilateral, sometimes asymmetrical, the amplitude maximum is frontal, and onset and end are rather gradual (Fig. 10). Other forms of attacks may show different critical activity, often a series of spikes or a short interruption of the ongoing slow spike-and-wave activity.

In *infants* of 6–18 months, or occasionally older, the *West* syndrome occurs, consisting of short flexion spasms along with mental deterioration. The EEG shows the pattern called *"hypsarrhythmia"* (GIBBS and GIBBS 1952), which is composed of multifocal spikes and sharp waves on a background of high-voltage generalized slow activity (Fig. 11). The typical massive flexion spasms are accom-

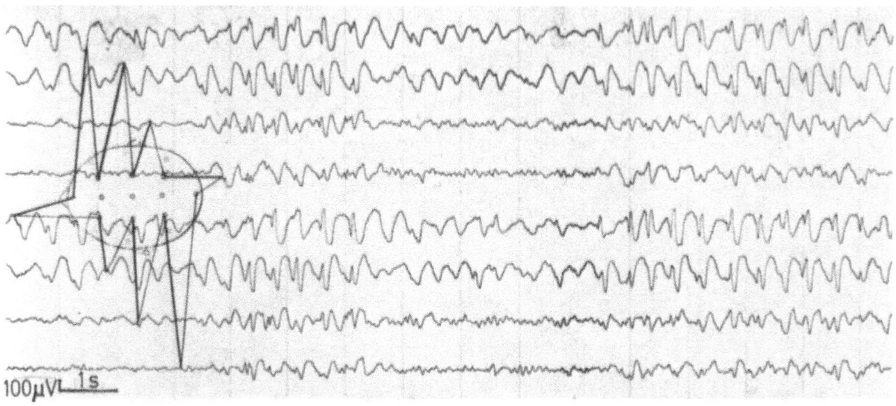

Fig. 10. Sharp and slow waves ("spike-and-wave variant") in a child of 10 years with mental infirmity and episodic behavior disorder. The 2.5/s sharp-and-slow waves gradually develop out of and change back into pure or notched slow waves, along with some alpha activity – normal for the age – in posterior aspects

panied either by more prominent bilateral sharp-and-slow wave complexes or by a short flattening of the record, often along with increased fast activity.

In *newborn* babies, in which, apart from generalized convulsions, focal attacks of varying localization are typical, multiple independent foci of spikes and sharp waves represent the intercritical patterns. During the seizures, strictly localized discharges are seen in the appropriate area, which may also shift from one place to another (DREYFUSS-BRISAC and MONOD 1964).

It thus appears that age-specific bilateral epileptic patterns are irregular and diffuse in the youngest age group and become more organized in time and space as the brain develops toward maturity. After adolescence, the tendency of paroxysmal patterns to spread over wider areas seems to decrease, and with increasing age they become infrequent, even when clinical attacks persist.

E. Activation Procedures

A noncontributive EEG is a nuisance, particularly in otherwise unclear cases. Various methods are used to coax more information out of the reticent brain. *Sphenoidal* or *pharyngeal leads* occasionally produce evidence of a spike focus restricted to the basal part of the temporal pole (Fig. 12). These procedures can also be used in conjunction with true activation methods:

Hyperventilation, easy to perform in patients able to cooperate, has found widest application. The changes in blood gas concentration thus induced facilitate excessive synchronization and markedly increase the incidence of spike-and-wave discharges in particular (Fig. 7). Inasmuch as overbreathing also involves some physical strain, a certain arousal effect counteracts the activating influences; they

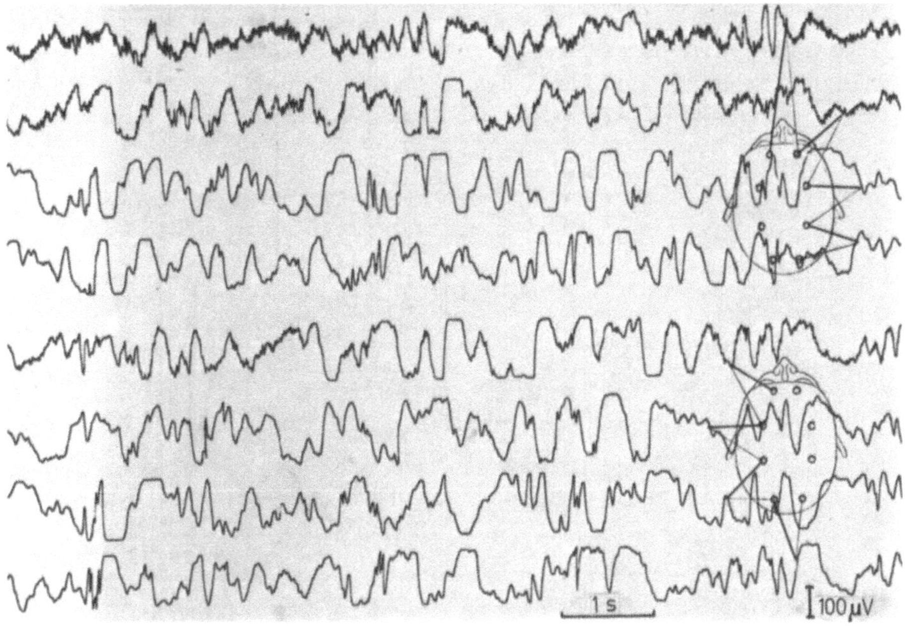

Fig. 11. Hypsarrhythmia in an infant with malignant flexion spasms. The main features are multifocal spikes and sharp waves on a background of high-voltage irregular generalized slow activity

may prevail subsequently, when the effort ceases and a degree of drowsiness follows. This is when focal epilepsies often become manifest.

Lowering the level of alertness is a most effective facilitating factor for epileptic disturbances, especially so in temporal foci. *Sleep records* were first advocated by GIBBS and GIBBS (1947) and they are now in general use (MATTSON et al. 1965; Fig. 13). *Sleep deprivation* is a useful means of obtaining a sleep EEG, and furthermore it is in itself an activating factor (PRATT et al. 1968).

Photic stimulation acts in a different way (WALTER and WALTER 1949; BICKFORD et al. 1969): Series of short light flashes lead to a massive increase of visual afferences. Inasmuch as rhythmicity and a frequency of between 10 and 20/s are important prerequisites for an activating effect, it is obvious that a resonating mechanism is involved. More or less generalized paroxysmal outbursts are often induced. Their diagnostic significance is highest if they become self-sustained when stimulation is discontinued. Sometimes they take the form of spike-wave discharges with or without clinical signs. Positive effects are essentially restricted to generalized (centrencephalic) epilepsies, with rare exceptions (Fig. 14).

Pharmocological activation – application of convulsant agents, usually by intraveneous injection – is the easiest way to produce epileptiform EEG changes, even in healthy people; its vast application in earlier times led to many false-positive results and the proposed "seizure threshold" was an unreliable measure.

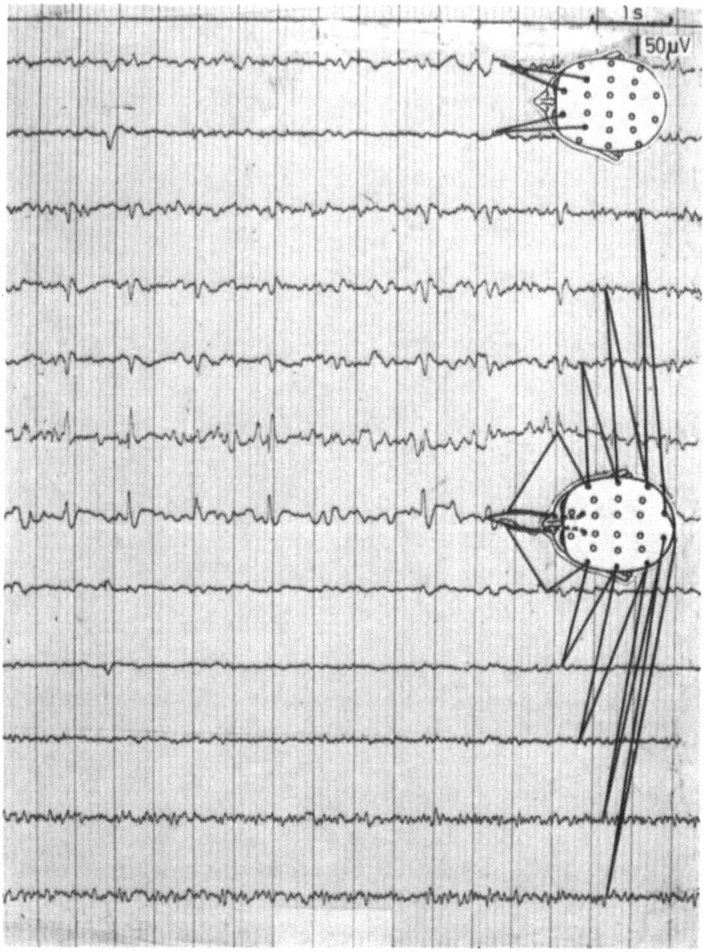

Fig. 12. Temporal epilepsy examined with pharyngeal electrodes, inserted through the nose into the nasopharyngeal cavity. Many sharp waves show highest amplitudes at the frontotemporal convexity, whereas a few fine spikes are picked up from the mediobasal surface of the temporal pole only

While the method is unsuitable for distinguishing epileptics from nonepileptics, it can still be used to demonstrate a focus in a case of established epilepsy but of undetermined nature. This is of special importance if surgical therapy is considered in a drug-resistant patient.

The most *natural way* of increasing positive EEG results should be to take the record at the time when experience shows that attacks are most likely to occur. In women the menstrual cycle may give a lead. For practical reasons, the EEG cannot always be carried out at the desired time, and the attempt to "catch a seizure" is all too often unsuccessful, except when many repeats are possible. This is decidedly the *most innocuous* method to get more positive results.

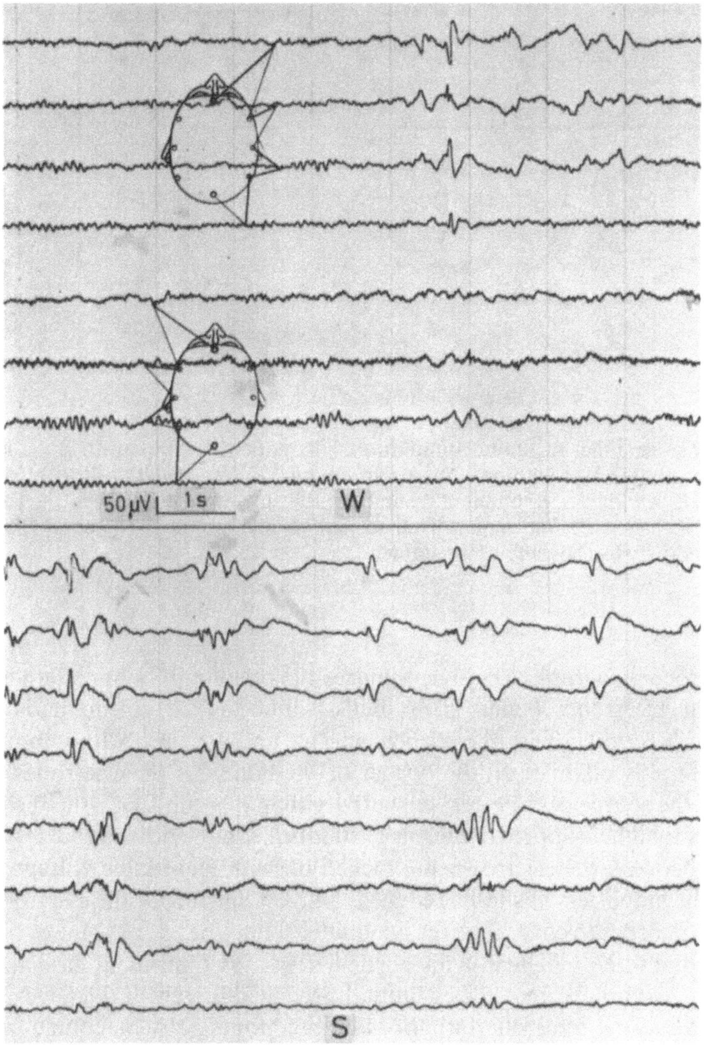

Fig. 13. Right frontotemporal spike complex in a waking record (*w*). In light sleep (*s*), epileptiform activity is enhanced and paroxysmal complexes appear *on the left side*, presumably induced by the epileptiform activity and with a short delay with respect to the primary focus

F. Electrocorticography and Depth-recording

While conventional EEG is a routine method, *electrocorticography* (direct recording from the cortical surface) and *recording from depth* with multicontact needle electrodes are invasive methods reserved for neurosurgical units. They are subject to strict medical indications and are almost exclusively used for detailed delimination of epileptogenic areas with the aim of their possible surgical removal (PENFIELD and JASPER 1954).

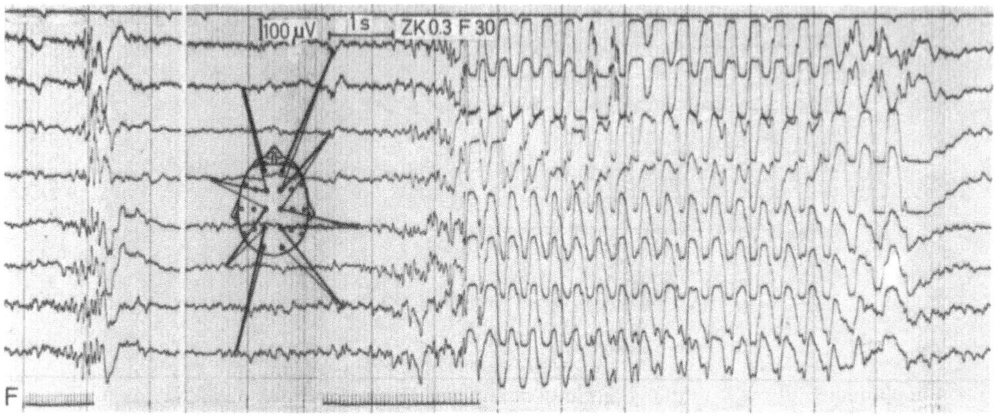

Fig. 14. Positive effect of photic stimulation. The patient is exposed to short bright light flashes (monitored by a photocell *in the bottom line, F*). *On the left* a short burst of generalized spikes is induced, terminated by an occipital slow wave (the one in the frontal leads is an eye artifact). *On the right* a train of spikes and waves is triggered: the excessive neuronal activity has become self-sustained

Electrocorticography (ECoG) requires the opening of a bone flap and of the dura. The electrodes (small silver balls, saline-soaked cotton pads, etc.) are brought into contact with the cortical surface and are fixed with a mounting device, preferably clamped to the border of the bone. As the electrodes are much closer to the source of the electrical activity than in scalp EEG, the recorded amplitudes are higher (approximately a 1 : 10 ratio). On the other hand, less potential changes between the electrodes are picked up with recordable voltage, since the gain of the amplifiers has to be reduced. Narrow spacing of the electrodes is thus required, in order to cover the area adequately (Fig. 15).

Epileptic activity in deep-lying cortical areas – in fissures, at basal and medial surfaces – cannot be recognized initially by ECoG. It will, however, show up when, after a first removal of abnormally functioning cortex, control recordings are made from the remaining structures. It is also possible to complement the ECoG by *depth electrodes*, particularly in cases where the surface record is of little localizing significance. Although such depth probes can cover but a few points, the most important ones are often known in advance; they comprise almost invariably the amygdala and hippocampus.

The success rate of surgical therapy based on this diagnostic procedure is moderate. The main drawback lies in the failure of obtaining accurate direct recordings from brain areas other than those made accessible by the craniotomy. Better results can be expected by multiple depth recordings prior to surgery; it should in most cases include both mediobasal temporal structures.

The most systematic approach under strict stereotactic conditions has been introducted by BANCAUD and TALAIRACH (1965) and is called *stereoelectroencephalography (SEEG)*. The procedure is expensive and time consuming, but remarkably successful. Multicontact electrodes are inserted (through small burr

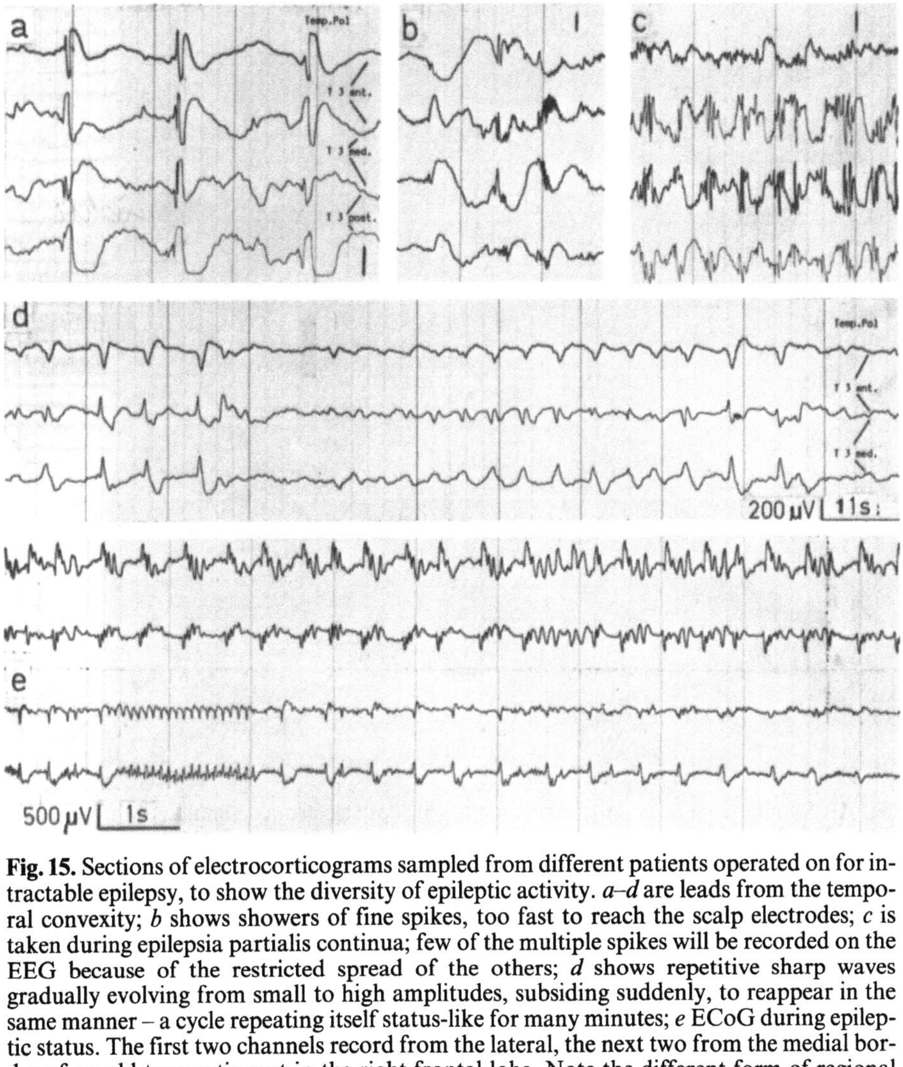

Fig. 15. Sections of electrocorticograms sampled from different patients operated on for intractable epilepsy, to show the diversity of epileptic activity. *a–d* are leads from the temporal convexity; *b* shows showers of fine spikes, too fast to reach the scalp electrodes; *c* is taken during epilepsia partialis continua; few of the multiple spikes will be recorded on the EEG because of the restricted spread of the others; *d* shows repetitive sharp waves gradually evolving from small to high amplitudes, subsiding suddenly, to reappear in the same manner – a cycle repeating itself status-like for many minutes; *e* ECoG during epileptic status. The first two channels record from the lateral, the next two from the medial border of an old traumatic cyst in the right frontal lobe. Note the different form of regional epileptic activity

holes) into the brain at the presumed main sites of epileptic activity, and it can thus be demonstrated that – in the selection of cases in which these procedures are indicated – the major part of the abnormalities picked up at depth are not reflected in the simultaneously recorded scalp EEG (Wieser 1981). It takes massive discharges spreading over wide areas or many electrode contacts to show up in a discernible form over the scalp (Fig. 16).

The epileptiform patterns as sampled from individual deep-electrode sites present a spectacular variety of forms from single spikes to multifarious complex-

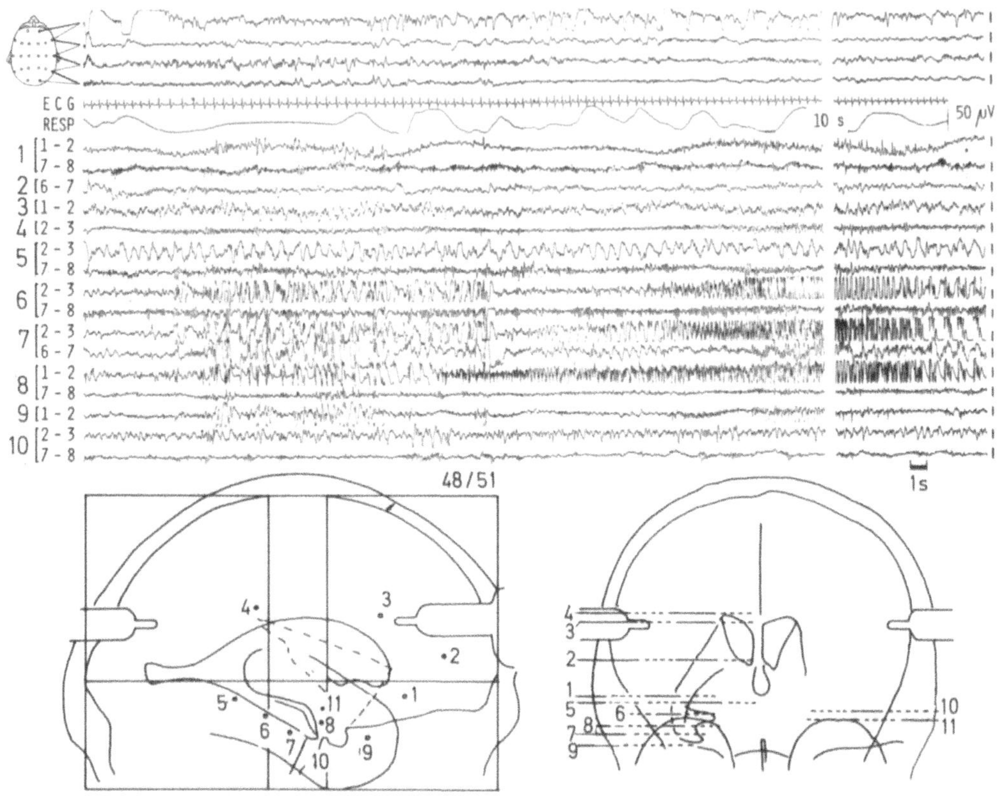

Fig. 16. Spontaneous short seizure recorded with depth electrodes, simultaneously with surface EEG (only four temporal leads represented). *Large figures* refer to composite needle electrodes, *small figures* to individual contacts: *1* at the tip, *7* and *8* close to the surface. After a widespread semi-ictal prelude, partially represented on the posterior temporal EEG, a focal discharge starts in the right nucleus amygdalae (*8/1–2*), spreading to the anterior hippocampus (*7/2–3*) and to the parahippocampal gyrus (*6/2–3*). The patient announces epigastric aura; pallor, anxious behaviour, and pupillary dilatation are observed. Note the change of heart rate and respiratory arrest (*channels 5 and 6*). The surface EEG fails to reflect the excessive discharges. After 10 s (the record of this epoch is left out), the epileptic activity becomes intermittent. At this stage, the surface EEG again shows some posterior temporal abnormality, without patterns specific to epilepsy, however. (Courtesy of PD Dr. H. G. Wieser)

es and long-lasting intermittent or continuous discharges, in most cases without overt signs of a seizure, but sometimes associated with symptoms which otherwise might not be suspected to have epileptic connotations. It is only when excessive discharges spread to a number of other sites that clinical signs of a seizure manifest themselves. If they correspond to the patients' habitual attacks, the approximate area of origin – the *real epileptogenic focus* – is established; it is not necessarily that of maximal *interictal* activity (BANCAUD and TALAIRACH 1970). While this is the main objective of the procedure, the way of seizure spread may also be conjectured, and secondary foci (common in homologous regions of the primarily involved limbic structures) and their importance for triggering and maintaining the ictal event can often be recognized.

From this information the epileptologist assesses the feasibility, likely benefits, and possible risks of surgical intervention. In cases with multiple epileptic foci, where seizures start from more than one site, or where the main point of origin is situated in a cortical area of high value, surgery must be dismissed. Other patients, however, stand a much better chance than with conventional procedures: the epileptogenic cortex can be removed with minimal damage to the rest of the brain, especially if microsurgical methods are used.

Important as systematic investigations with depth electrodes are for the handling of severe reticent epilepsies, their *theoretical contributions* must not be overlooked. Their impact on epileptology has been considerable, and more insight into the nature of the condition is to be expected. There are reasons to believe that depth-recording will help toward a better understanding of surface EEG.

References

Bancaud J, Talairach J (1970) L'électroencéphalographie de profondeur. Epilepsy Mod Probl Pharmacopsychiatry 4:29–41

Bancaud J, Talairach J, Bonis A, Schaub C, Szikla G, Morel P, Bordas-Ferrer M (1965) La stéréo-electroencéphalographie dans l'épilepsie. Masson, Paris

Beaussart M, Beaussart-Boulenge L, Mahieu N (1970) L'épilespie avec paroxysms E.E.G. rolandiques. Le concours médical 7:2195–2212

Bickford RG, Klass DW (1969) Sensory precipitation and reflex mechanisms. In: Jasper HH, Ward AA, Pope A (eds) Basic mechanisms of the epilepsies. Churchill, London, pp 543–564

Cooper R, Winter AL, Crow HJ, Walter WG (1965) Comparison of subcortical, cortical and scalp activity using chronically indwelling electrodes in man. Electroencephalogr Clin Neurophysiol 18:217–228

Dreyfus-Brisac C, Monod N (1964) Electroclinical studies of status epilepticus and convulsions in the new-born. In: Kellaway P, Petersen I (eds) Neurologic and electroencephalographic correlative studies in infancy. Grune and Stratton, New York, pp 250–272

Gastaut Y (1952) Un élément déroutant de la séméilogie électroencéphalographique: les pointes prérolandiques sans signification focale. Rev Neurol 87:488–490

Gastaut H, Roger J, Soulayrol R, Tassinari CA, Régis H, Dravet C, Bernard R, Pinsard N, Saint-Jean M (1966) Childhood epileptic encephalopathy with diffuse slow spike-waves (otherwise known as "petit mal variant") or Lennox syndrome. Epilepsia 7:139–179

Gibbs EL, Gibbs FA (1947) Diagnostic and localizing value of electroencephalographic studies in sleep. Res Publ Assoc Nerv Ment Dis 26:366–376

Gibbs FA, Gibbs EL (1952) Atlas of electroencephalography, vol II. Addison-Wesley, Cambridge, Mass, pp 24–30

Gibbs FA, Gibbs EL, Lennox WG (1938) Cerebral dysrhythmias of epilepsy. Arch Neurol Psychiatr 39:298–314

Gloor P (1979) Generalized epilepsy with spike-and-wave discharge: a reinterpretation of its electrographic and clinical manifestations. Epilepsia 20:571–588

Gotman J (1981) Interhemispheric relations during bilateral spike-and-wave acitivity. Epilepsia 22:453–466

Jasper HH (1949) Electrical signs of epileptic discharge. Electroencephalogr Clin Neurophysiol 1:11–18

Jasper HH, Droogleever-Fortuyn J (1947) Experimental studies on the functional anatomy of Petit Mal epilepsy. Res Publ Assoc Nerv Ment Dis 26:272–298
Jung R (1949) Hirnelektrische Untersuchungen über den Elektrokrampf: Die Erregungsabläufe in corticalen und subcorticalen Hirnregionen bei Katze und Hund. Arch Psychiatr Nervenkr 183:206–244
Lairy GC, Harrison A, Leger EM (1964) Foyers EEG bi-occipitaux asynchrones de pointes chez l'enfant mal voyant et aveugle d'âge scolaire. Rev Neurol 111:351–353
Lennox WG (1960) Epilepsy and related disorders. Little Brown, Boston
Loiseau P, Cohadon F, Mortureux Y (1967) A propos d'une forme singulière d'épilepsie de l'enfant. Rev Neurol 116:244–248
Mattson RH, Pratt KL, Calverly JR (1965) Electroencephalograms of epileptics following sleep deprivation. Arch Neurol 13:310–315
Metrakos K, Metrakos JD (1961) Genetics of convulsive disorders. II Genetic and electroencephalographic studies in centrencephalic epilepsy. Neurology (Minneap) 11:474–483
Morell F (1960) Secondary epileptogenic lesions. Epilepsia 1:538–560
Niedermeyer E, Kalifeh R (1965) Petit mal status ("spike-wave stupor"): an electroclinical appraisal. Epilepsia 6:250–262
Penfield W, Jasper HH (1954) Epilepsy and the functional anatomy of the brain. Little Brown, Boston, pp 692–738
Pratt KL, Mattson RH, Weiker NJ, Williams R (1968) EEG activation of epileptics following sleep derivation: a prospective study of 114 cases. Electroencephalogr Clin Neurophysiol 24:11–15
Prince DA, Wilder BJ (1967) Control mechanisms in cortical epileptogenic foci. Arch Neurol 16:194–202
Silverman D (1954) Clinical correlates of the spike-wave complex. Electroencephalogr Clin Neurophysiol 6:671–673
Van der Drift JHA, Magnus O (1961) The value of the EEG in the differential diagnosis of cases with cerebral lesions. Electroencephalogr Clin Neurophysiol [Suppl] 19:183–196
Walter VJ, Walter GW (1949) The central effects of rhythmic sensory stimulation. Electroencephalogr Clin Neurophysiol 1:57–86
Wieser HG (1981) Stereo-Elektroencephalographisches Korrelat motorischer Anfälle. Z EEG EMG 12:1–13

CHAPTER 3

Epilepsy in Animals

T. A. HOLLIDAY

A. Introduction

The similarity of certain animal diseases to human epilepsy has been recognized for at least 300 years. In the seventeenth century Paracelsus said that epilepsy "exists not only in man but in all living creatures." Paracelsus also recognized the disease could be inherited and, in stating that "some species of animals suffer the disease by heredity," has permitted us to deduce that he believed some species might suffer diseases now termed "acquired epilepsy" (for Paracelsus' quotations, see LENNOX and LENNOX 1960).

Epilepsy of animals will be defined here as any of several brain disorders which cause recurrent seizures that are accompanied by characteristic paroxysmal EEG events. This definition includes those seizure disorders caused by genetically determined primary brain dysfunction (inherited epilepsy) and those brain diseases that, although once active, have run their course and have become inactive but have left the brain in a seizure-prone state (acquired epilepsy). Excluded from this definition are genetically determined intracranial disorders that cause seizures simply as one manifestation of a spectrum of clinical signs and structural changes; also excluded, regardless of chronicity, are acquired disorders that cause seizures as a part of progressive, brain-destructive processes.

In the centuries since Paracelsus, many recurrent seizure disorders of animals have been likened to human epilepsy. Designation of these conditions as epileptic often has been based entirely or almost entirely on observations of recurrent seizures. In the light of our present-day understanding of epilepsy and modern technological analysis, some of these conditions do not fulfill the requirements of a definition of epilepsy such as that given above; nevertheless a substantial number of diseases of animals, either inherited or acquired, meet those criteria and warrant designation as epilepsy.

B. Acquired Epilepsies in Animals

The ease with which chronic epileptogenic foci can be induced experimentally (WARD 1972; LEWIN 1972) suggests a rather high level of susceptibility to acquired epilepsy in some animals, and the existence of naturally occurring acquired epilepsy in animals is alluded to by many authors in the veterinary literature (DE-LAHUNTA 1977; HOERLEIN 1978; HOLLIDAY et al. 1970; PALMER 1976). Nevertheless, there are few reports of systematic investigations of its incidence and causes, or of its clinical, EEG, or pathological manifestations in animals. Outstanding among those available are the reports by GASTAUT et al. (1958 a), who studied 19 dogs including some that probably had acquired epilepsy. Also, there is a report by VAN BOGAERT (1973) on clinical and pathological observations of seizure disorders in 212 captive subhuman primates from a zoological garden, some of which had focal seizures, suggesting acquired epilepsy. (Interestingly, in the latter report, the author also mentions observing baboons with myoclonic seizures.) Unfortunately, none of the existing reports permits adequate characterization of acquired epilepsies in any animal species. From the available information and from the author's personal experience, it appears that naturally occurring acquired epilepsies occur in such an unpredictable fashion that they are not useful for the study of underlying pathophysiological mechanisms or pharmacological characteristics. However, it seems possible that systematic studies of the epizootiology of acquired epilepsies in animals might be of value, particularly if the investigations were focused on species that live in close association with man in many societies (e.g., dog).

Because of the scarcity of information available, acquired epilepsies in animals are not discussed further here.

C. Inherited Epilepsies in Animals

Inherited epilepsies have been described in a large number of vertebrates, encompassing one primate species, dogs, domestic fowl, several rodent species, swine, and cattle. The large number of species and the extensive literature on some of them necessitate limiting this review to only a few; thus only the epilepsies of the baboon, dog, Mongolian gerbil, and domestic fowl will be discussed here.

The reader is referred to other sources for information on the conditions of mice (HARE and HARE 1979; NOEBELS 1979; SEYFRIED 1979), rats (CONSROE et al. 1979), rabbits (ANTONITIS et al. 1954; HOHENBOKEN and NELLHAUS 1970; NACHTSHEIM 1939; NELLHAUS 1958), and Syrian hamsters (YOON et al. 1976); and the review of audiogenic seizures by COLLINS (1972); other useful sources are CONSROE and EDMONDS (1979) and NEWMARKET and PENRY (1980). The disorders that have been reported in swine (SAUNDERS 1952), Brown Swiss cattle (ATKESON et al. 1944), and Swedish Red cattle (ISAKSSON 1943) lack adequate pathological, biochemical, or EEG evidence for epilepsy and are not discussed here.

This review attempts to provide an overview of the inherited epilepsies of the baboon, dog, Mongolian gerbil, and domestic fowl because of the promise they hold for future contributions to our understanding of basic mechanisms of epilepsy and its causes, prevention, and treatment in man.

The available neurochemical, neuropharmacological, and biochemical information on these conditions is presented elsewhere in this volume and therefore is not discussed here except for some data on the epilepsies of dogs and chickens.

I. Photomyoclonic Seizures in the Baboon (*Papio papio*)

1. Introduction

A photomyoclonic syndrome in *Papio papio* was first reported by KILLAM et al. (1966 b). Extensively studied since that time, this genetically determined trait has proven to be extremely valuable because of its many similarities to human epilepsies.

2. Electroencephalographic and Clinical Characteristics

Intermittent light stimulation (ILS) of affected *P. papio* at 25 Hz elicits "following" responses in the occipital cortex, with spikes, spike waves, and polyspike waves appearing suddenly as bifrontal discharges; the discharges spread to involve the entire cortex, internal capsule, pons, and brain stem and finally include other deep structures. The step-by-step involvement of structures suggests an organized progression rather than simply a randomly spreading generalized paroxysm (KILLAM et al. 1969; FISCHER-WILLIAMS et al. 1968). A relative electrographic independence of the frontal and occipital cortex may be observed, with the ILS "following" response occuring in occipital regions at the time a seizure discharge has begun in the frontorolandic regions; the occipital cortex may become incorporated in the paroxysmal activity later. Somewhat analogously, paroxysmal activity in the rhinencephalon tends to occur later than in other deep structures and consists of higher voltage more irregular multiple spikes without spike-wave complexes; these persist independently after discharges in other structures have ceased (FISCHER-WILLIAMS et al. 1968).

Within a few seconds after the EEG discharges, clinical manifestations appear, beginning with small, regular, rapid, bilateral clonic movements in the eyelids and periocular muscles. As the electrographic paroxysms increase, the clonic movements spread to the face and neck. There may be intense isolated jerks of the head, groups of clonic jerks of the body, tonic spasms of the facial muscles, and generalized clonic jerks with flexion of the head and upper body and tonic extension of the legs; these may be followed by generalized clonus. Clinical signs lessen as the EEG paroxysms subside (KILLIAM 1979; KILLIAM et al. 1967a; FISCHER-WILLIAMS et al. 1968). If ILS is interrupted within a few seconds after EEG or clinical signs appear, the latter disappear immediately. Interruption of ILS 5–10 s after generalized body movements have begun may either end the seizure, or a "self-sustained" seizure may result. The latter may vary in severity from clonic jerking to generalized clonus followed by generalized tonus and gradually diminishing clonic jerks (KILLAM 1979; KILLIAM et al. 1967a).

In animals which respond to 25-Hz ILS with maximal seizure patterns, the visual evoked responses (VER) to low frequency (1–5 Hz ILS) differ from less-sensitive subjects. In less-sensitive animals, there is no difference in the form of VERs elicited with the eyes open or closed, and the VERs are found only in occipital regions. VERs recorded from sensitive animals when the eyes are open are similar to those of nonsensitive animals, but when VERs are recorded with the eyes closed there are short latency responses in the frontal regions, longer latency responses from parietal regions, and increased amplitude in the occipital regions (KILLAM et al. 1967b, 1969; MELDRUM et al. 1970). In these respects, the VERs of photosensitive baboons resemble their human counterparts; they differ, however, in that the most effective rate of ILS in *P. papio* is about 25 Hz whereas in man 14–17 Hz is more effective.

Seizure responses have not been observed in animals under 5 months of age (BALZAMO et al. 1975) or 7.5 months of age (KILLAM 1979), and severity increases with age until stabilizing at 2–3 years of age (KILLAM 1979).

The animals are affected to varying degrees, with ILS responses falling into three categories: consistently maximal responses, responses varying from eye clonus to a maximal seizure, and responses rarely proceeding beyond eye clonus. The phenomenon does not appear to be some sort of exaggerated proprioceptive reflex because the EEG events precede the motor events and the complete EEG sequence can be recorded from curarized animals (FISCHER-WILLIAMS et al. 1968).

ILS is not the only effective provocative agent in *P. papio*. Hyperventilation, overexercise, and the stresses of capture, restraint, or heat and humidity can induce seizures or render them more severe (BALZAMO et al. 1975; KILLAM 1979; KILLAM et al. 1967a). Also, even in the absence of light, EEG paroxysms occur during sleep; they appear in association with spindles or as isolated phenomena and are more frequent during rapid eye movement sleep (KILLAM et al. 1967a, 1969). Further, the threshold for convulsant effects of pentylenetetrazol is much lower in affected individuals and the response to ILS may be minimal before administration of chlorpromazine, and yet maximal seizures can be elicited by ILS after chlorpromazine; the enhanced sensitivity remains for 5–7 days after a single dose (KILLAM et al. 1967a, 1969).

3. Inheritance

The incidence of ILS susceptibility in *P. papio* populations varies with their geographical origin, being lower in groups in eastern Senegal and highest (above 70%) in those from the Casamance area of Senegal (KILLAM 1979; KILLAM et al. 1969; NAQUET and MELDRUM 1972; KITSIKIS et al. 1970; BALZAMO et al. 1975). ILS sensitivity was found in 7 of 12 *P. papio* that were of unknown origin but were members of a colony that had been resident in a zoo for 20 years (KILLAM et al. 1967a). The incidence of ILS sensitivity in other *Papio* species (*P. hamadryas, P. anubis, P. cynocephalus, P. nes*) is very low and is generally less than 10% (KILLAM et al. 1967c, 1967; KITSIKIS et al. 1970). In studies of other subhuman primates, including members of ten species from seven genera, the incidence of sensitivity to ILS has been equally low (KILLAM et al. 1966a, 1969; STARK et al. 1968; RHODES et al. 1969; NAQUET et al. 1967; WADA et al. 1972; NAQUET and MELDRUM 1972).

These data suggest that sensitivity to ILS is not a characteristic of genus or species but is a unique feature of *P. papio* from the Casamance area. Genetic transmission of this characteristic seems clear but the exact mode of inheritance has not been defined. No definite sex linkage has been shown (KILLAM 1979), although BALZAMO et al. (1975) noted a tendency for a higher incidence of ILS sensitivity in young females than in young males. It has been pointed out that nongenetic factors might influence the variations in light sensitivity that are seen in *P. papio* (BALZAMO et al. 1975).

4. Pathology

Very little information has been published regarding pathological changes in epileptic *P. papio*. In an early report, no abnormalities were found in the brains of 15 animals (KILLAM 1969 p 237) and, in subsequent studies, no lesions have been found (K. F. KILLAM 1982, personal communication).

5. Remarks

Some of the most valuable uses of *P. papio* as a model of human seizure disorders result from the position of this animal high on the phylogenetic scale relative to other spontaneously epileptic animals. The comparatively large body size, long life span, and high intelligence of this subhuman primate permit experiments to be designed to detect some of the more subtle effects of the disease itself or of drugs used to treat it. Thus, studies of *P. papio* born and reared in the laboratory have revealed differences in learning ability and emotionality in untreated affected individuals (WEINBERGER and KILLAM 1979). These seem to parallel the behavior and intellectual performance of some human epileptics and have offered the opportunity to study this particular type of correlate of epilepsy in an experimental context more similar to that of human epilepsy than is found in other experimental inherited epilepsies. Also, in epileptic baboons the behavioral effects of anticonvulsant drugs can be studied, in order to discern the "behavioral price" (KILLAM 1979) of seizure control; finally, the summated effects of the disease and its various treatments on this subhuman primate can be studied (PAULE and KILLAM 1979; STANTON et al. 1977; WEINBERGER and KILLAM 1978).

Photomyoclonic epilepsy in *P. papio* provides a reproducible model of the analogous human syndrome. It permits study of pathophysiology of seizures, special opportunities for testing anticonvulsant drugs, and excellent possibilities for studying the effects of the disease and its treatment in an animal that is relatively close to man on the phylogenetic scale.

II. Inherited Epilepsy in Dogs

1. Introduction

There is evidence for genetic transmission of epilepsy in beagle dogs and in Horak's breed of laboratory dogs. These conditions have been well characterized by researchers in the United States and Europe and, at this time, the data suggest that these may be two different forms of the disease because of apparent differences in the mode of inheritance and because of differences in the manner in which seizures can be induced (Sect. C.II.2.c, C.II.3.c).

In addition, many veterinarians in North America, Western Europe, and Great Britain have concluded that epilepsy occurs in certain other breeds of dogs simply on the basis of the frequency with which the disease is encountered in these breeds as compared with the dog population at large; evidence tending to confirm that impression, for some breeds at least, is presented in Sect. C.II.4.

2. Inherited Epilepsy in Beagle Dogs

a) Introduction

Several colonies containing large numbers of Beagle dogs were formed in the United States during the 1960s for the purpose of producing dogs for use in research. Shortly after these colonies were established it became apparent that a rather high proportion of colony-reared dogs were afflicted with recurrent seizure disorders. Early publications on the subject recognized the existence of the problem (KOESTNER and REHFELD 1968; REDMAN and WEIR 1969) and began its genetic (BIELFELT et al. 1971), pathological (HOLLAND et al. 1970), and electroencephalographic characterization (REDMAN et al. 1972; CUNNINGHAM 1971). Subsequently, there have been further descriptions of clinical and EEG characteristics of the syndrome and studies of the pathology, biochemistry, neurochemistry, and pharmacology.

b) Electroencephalographic and Clinical Characteristics

Seizures are reported to begin at about 1–4 years of age (KOESTNER and REHFELD 1968; BIELFELT et al. 1971). CUNNINGHAM (1971) observed seizures and EEG paroxysms in beagle dogs less than 1 year of age; however, his dogs were progeny of epileptic × epileptic matings which might have concentrated gene(s) influencing age of onset.

Both generalized seizures and brief episodes limited to ataxia, jaw movements, salivation, pupillary dilatation, and staring have been noted (WIEDERHOLT 1974; BIELFELT et al. 1971). At least outwardly, the latter appear to be partial seizures similar to the "psychomotor seizures" of dogs described by GASTAUT et al. (1958 a, b).

Partial seizures sometimes occur without sequellae and sometimes are followed by generalized seizures. It is not clear, from available reports, whether generalized seizures occur without prodromal signs or whether some such signs occur at the onset of every generalized seizure. The generalized paroxysms consist of generalized, symmetrical, clonic-tonic contractions of the axial and appendicular muscles, with opisthotonus, salivation, and apparent unconsciousness (BIELFELT et al. 1971; KOESTNER and REHFELD 1968; CUNNINGHAM 1971; REDMAN and WEIR 1969; REDMAN et al. 1972). Generalized seizures persist for only a few moments and usually are followed by a period of walking or running movements of the legs that lasts several minutes. This, in turn, is followed by a period of quietness, after which the animal arises and may be ataxic and appear dazed for a brief period or may seem outwardly normal (CUNNINGHAM 1971; EDMONDS et al. 1979).

Either partial or generalized seizures occur at seemingly random intervals, often with interictal periods of a month or more (KOESTNER and REHFELD 1968; BIELFELT et al. 1971). The animals usually are not maintained under continuous observation; therefore, some seizures probably are not observed (BIELFELT et al. 1971).

Neither clinical signs nor EEG paroxysms can be provoked in epileptic beagle dogs with ILS (REDMAN et al. 1972; WIEDERHOLT 1974; KOESTNER and REHFELD 1968) and, to date, no regularly effective stimulus for seizures has been found except pentylenetetrazol (PTZ) and maximal electric shock (REDMAN et al. 1972; WIEDERHOLT 1974; EDMONDS et al. 1978).

The convulsion threshold for PTZ has been reported to be lower in epileptic beagle dogs (WIEDERHOLT 1974; REDMAN et al. 1972; EDMONDS et al. 1978); however, CUNNINGHAM (1971) and EDMONDS et al. (1979, unpublished data) reported no significant differences in this characteristic.

Systematic EEG studies using chronically implanted cortical and depth electrodes have been reported by WIEDERHOLT (1974) and CUNNINGHAM (1971). WIEDERHOLT (1974) reported that during interictal periods bilateral spike discharges occurred independently in the temporal cortex, amygdala, and hippocampus and less often from central or rostral cortical areas. WIEDERHOLT (1974) did not report EEG observations during spontaneous seizures because of the unpredictability of seizure occurrence, but did describe EEG changes after PTZ, methohexital, and thiopental administration. PTZ infusion at first caused myoclonic jerks and generalized spike discharges; as the PTZ infusion was continued, 15- to 20-Hz waves appeared in the temporal regions, amygdala, hippocampus, and frontal and central cortical areas. This activity rapidly spread to all areas, and a generalized seizure occurred. High-frequency acitivity (300–500 Hz) occurred in the pontine and tegmental reticular formation for a few seconds before the generalized seizure discharge. Methohexital and thiopental activated spike discharges in a somewhat similar manner (WIEDERHOLT 1974).

CUNNINGHAM (1971) also could not record during spontaneous seizures; his results were similar to those of WIEDERHOLT (1974).

c) Inheritance

BIELFELT et al. (1971) reported that "maximal" seizures occurred in 5.7% of 1,200 beagle dogs in the colony at Albuquerque. The incidence in offspring of an epileptic male was 15.3%. Male offspring were affected approximately five times as often as females. A two-locus inheritance with a suppressor gene located on the X chromosome has been postulated as a probable mode of inheritance (BIELFELT et al. 1971), but this hypothesis has not been verified by appropriate trial matings. In CUNNINGHAM'S (1971) studies two epileptic beagle dog females and an epileptic Siberian Husky female were mated to an epileptic beagle dog male; within the 1st year of life, 5 of 13 pups had developed recurrent seizures and another 4 had spike complexes in their EEGs; all pups that had seizures developed EEG abnormalities before clinical seizures were observed. Neither clinical seizures nor EEG abnormalities occurred in control animals; the sex of the affected F_1 animals was not reported (CUNNINGHAM 1971). These reports seem to establish that epilepsy in the beagle dog is transmitted genetically. More work is necessary to determine the precise inheritance.

d) Pathology

KOESTNER and REHFELD (1968) and EDMONDS et al. (1979) reported that blood chemistry studies of epileptic beagle dogs did not reveal evidence for extracranial metabolic diseases that might cause seizures.

At necropsy of three dogs, polysaccharide-rich, diastase-resistant intracytoplasmic inclusions resembling Lafora bodies (LB) were found in the thalamus, caudate, and dentate nuclei by HEGREBERG and PADGETT (1976), who noted also the presence of periodic acid-Schiff positive material in reticuloendothelial cells of the liver, spleen, and lymph nodes. Other lesions found in the brains of these dogs probably were associated with their terminal status epilepticus. These workers called attention to the similarity of the clinical and pathological changes in epileptic beagle dogs to Lafora's disease (progressive myoclonic epilepsy) of man (HEGREBERG and PADGETT 1976).

However, the relationship of LB to the seizures in these dogs is uncertain since LB have been observed in the brains of normal dogs, even in areas believed to be intimately related to seizure physiology (HOLLAND et al. 1970; MACKENZIE and JOHNSON 1976; NEWBERNE et al. 1960; SUZUKI et al. 1979a, b). These observations indicate that the presence of LB in the dog brain, even in structures intimately related to seizure physiology, is not sufficient to produce seizures; if LB are related to seizures in dogs then some additional factor(s) must be necessary for seizures to occur.

e) Biochemistry

VAN GELDER et al. (1980) reported that amino acid profiles of serum, CSF, and parietal cerebral cortex biopsies from epileptic and seizure-free sibling beagle dogs did not differ in absolute amounts. When the amounts were expressed as percent ages of total free amino acids, ten significant correlations between pairs of amino acids were found in the epileptic dogs but only one such correlation was found in the normal dogs. Seven of the ten correlated amino acids involved glutamate or taurine, and those amino acids which were correlated (taurine, glycine, glutamine, glutamate, alanine) all use sodium-dependent membrane transport processes (VAN GELDER et al. 1980). The sum of aspartate, glutamate, and glycine in serum of epileptic beagle dogs was lower than that of controls, but no differences in the concentration of these substances in brain or CSF were found (VAN GELDER et al. 1980). The authors suggested their data might indicate that epileptic beagle dogs had a diminished capacity for sodium-dependent high-affinity renal transport of acidic and certain small amino acids. On the basis of the report by BULANOVA (1957, cited by VAN GELDER et al. 1980) of lowered serum glutamate in dogs with "reflex" epilepsy, their own findings, and considerations of sodium-dependent transport systems, they suggested that sodium-dependent amino acid transport systems and central mechanisms of sodium homeostasis might be implicated in the pathogenesis of "idiopathic" canine epilepsy (VAN GELDER et al. 1980).

3. Inherited Epilepsy in Horak's Laboratory Dogs

a) Introduction

MARTINEK and HORAK (1970) reported that seizures could be induced in some individuals of Horak's breed of laboratory dogs by conditions that produce emotional excitement or fright. Subsequently it has been determined that the trait is inherited, and some of its characteristics have been described.

b) Electroencephalographic and Clinical Characteristics

Emotionally stressful circumstances tended to elicit seizures. Placing the animal in a completely empty room was found to be an effective means of producing seizures and one which could be standardized (MARTINEK and HORAK 1970); seizures did not develop if a person in whom the dog seemed to have confidence was present in the room (MARTINEK and DAHME 1977).

Two types of seizures were described, "minor seizures" and "generalized convulsive (grand mal) seizures" (MARTINEK and HORAK 1970). Most of the dogs had minor seizures for a period of time before major seizures were observed. In animals not selectively bred for the trait the mean age of onset of observed minor seizures was 662 days. The mean age of onset of generalized seizures in six dogs was 808 days; the mean interval between onset of minor seizures and onset of generalized seizures was 151 days. Interestingly, once a generalized seizure was observed a minor seizure was never again recorded (MARTINEK and HORAK 1970). Except for animals selectively bred for the trait, no convulsive attacks were observed in "prepuberal" dogs (MARTINEK and HORAK 1970).

Minor seizures began with characteristic masticatory movements of the tongue and jaw which resembled those of an animal attempting to chew food or to expel an object from its mouth. These low-frequency movements occurred while the animal was standing or walking and were accompanied by increased salivation. The duration of these episodes was not more than "a few dozen seconds"; occasionally the episodes terminated in vertical head jerks (MARTINEK and HORAK 1970).

The generalized seizures usually began with the dog standing rigidly with its head bent down, after which chewing movements began that quickly evolved into "convulsions of the masticatory muscles." The latter led to a period when the mouth was held wide open (tonically) while the head was held back in opisthotonus and turned to one side or the other. Soon the animal sat on the floor and began to turn its body in the direction of the head. At this time one foreleg might be held flexed and undergo clonic movements; if this occurred, it was always in the foreleg opposite the direction in which the head was turned. The animal then lost its balance and fell to the floor where clonic-tonic movements began. These movements did not occur in clearly separable phases but were intermingled, with one or the other predominating; in rare cases tonus was absent, and frequently tonus might occur in one limb and clonus in the opposite limb. Clonic convulsions began in the rear limbs and were accompanied by whirling movements of the tail. When the animal first fell to the ground the spine was curved with the head pointing forward or bent toward the forelimbs ("emprosthotonus") with the mouth still widely opened; as the clonic-tonic movements progressed the posture gradually changed to opisthotonus and the mouth became partly closed. Also, during the clonic-tonic phase, snarling movements occurred in the facial muscles and there was salivation and urination; defecation was not observed. The mean duration of the clonic-tonic phase was 64 s (MARTINEK and HORAK 1970).

Following the clonic-tonic phase a period of "automatisms" appeared. During this period there were coordinated movements of the limbs; these occurred at a rate approximating that of a trotting animal. The movements became weaker and weaker until the animal finally attempted to arise or, in some animals, until it finally lay motionless. The mean duration of the entire seizure, from onset until the animal first attempted to rise, was 140 s (MARTINEK and HORAK 1970).

Seizures could be elicited only during so-called periods of crisis, usually not more often than every 1–2 weeks, and usually could not be elicited during the intervening periods (MARTINEK and DAHME 1977).

Electroencephalographic studies of these dogs are not yet available.

c) Inheritance

MARTINEK and HORAK (1970), MARTINEK and DAHME (1977), and MARTINEK (1980) have published pedigrees of epileptic Horak's dogs which strongly suggest the trait is inherited by a simple recessive mode. Males and females are affected in approximately equal numbers, indicating that sex-linked suppressors do not affect expression of the gene as has been suggested for epileptic beagle does (BIELFELT et al. 1971).

d) Pathology

Detailed studies of the brains of six of the dogs revealed no evidence of neuropathological lesions that appeared to be related to the genesis of the seizures; interestingly, none of the cellular changes often believed to result from seizures were found (MARTINEK and DAHME 1977).

4. Epilepsy in Other Breeds of Dogs

a) Introduction

The frequency with which epilepsy has been encountered in certain breeds of dogs has led many veterinarians to believe that genetically transmitted epilepsy occurs in numerous breeds. In most of these, however, the evidence for inheritance must be regarded as anecdotal. Data in support of inheritance has been adduced only for epilepsy of German Shepherd, (British Alsatian) dogs, Belgian (Tervueren) Shepherd dogs, and dogs of the Keeshond breed [a paper with evidence regarding genetic transmission of epilepsy in Collie dogs by URBICH (1973) was not available to the author in time for review; the following remarks refer only to the above breeds].

b) Clinical, Electroencephalographic, and Pathological Characteristics

Aside from the evidence for inheritance in these breeds, very little has been done to characterize their seizure disorders. Seizures are described as generalized clonic-tonic with opisthotonus, salivation, urination, defecation, and apparent unconsciousness. In one paper, convulsions in German Shepherd (British Alsatian) dogs are described as beginning with contractions of the masticatory and facial muscles similar to those described in the seizures of beagle dogs and Horak's dogs (BARKER 1973). This has not been reported by other authors; therefore, it is not certain that this typpe of onset occurs in all breeds or occurs only in dogs of the above breeds.

The seizures of dogs of these breeds tend to occur in clusters of 2–30 or more in 1-, 2-, or 3-day periods at intervals of several weeks. No explanation for this periodicity is available, nor have any reliable seizure-inducing stimuli been reported.

EEGs recorded during interictal periods are usually stated to be normal. No systematic studies of ictal EEGs have been reported.

No systematic search for pathological changes has been reported except for that of PALMER (1972), who examined necropsy material from 40 dogs that had had "fits," including 12 dogs classified as having had "idiopathic" epilepsy; no lesions were found in the latter group, which contained seven beagle dogs. Routine gross and microscopic examination of epileptic dogs of these breeds at the author's institution has failed to reveal lesions in the nervous system that seemed causally related to seizures (personal observation).

c) Inheritance of Epilepsy in German Shepherd (British Alsatian) Dogs, Belgian (Tervueren) Shepherd Dogs, and Dogs of the Keeshond Breed

Numerous references in the literature, based on the frequency with which veterinarians encountered seizure disorders in the breed, led FALCO et al. (1974) to analyze the pedigrees of 289 German Shepherd dogs, 68 of which had had seizures prior to the study. The authors concluded that their data made it appropriate to say that dogs of this breed inherited a "liability to seizures." The data indicated also that males were more at risk than females by a ratio of 3.6:1, and the authors concluded that this more likely reflected sex modification of the trait rather than sex linkage (FALCO et al. 1975). Their conclusions on inheritance of the trait were based largely on high coefficients of inbreeding and the frequent appearance of a common ancestor (their dog 18) in the pedigrees of affected probands in the population they studied. Since the population apparently was drawn entirely from Great Britain, the trait might not exist in the breed in other nations. However, in the United States at least, the breed is widely believed by veterinarians to have a hereditary epilepsy because of the frequency with which they encounter recurrent generalized seizure disorders in German Shepherd dogs (DE LAHUNTA 1977; CHRISMAN 1982).

VAN DER VELDEN (1968) reported a pedigree analysis of 216 dogs of the Tervueren variety of Belgian Shepherd dogs in the Netherlands. The results suggested that an inherited tendency for seizures existed among the dogs in the study. No information about sex differences in expression of the trait was mentioned in the text; however, in the pedigree chart published with the paper, males and females appear with approximately equal frequency among the dogs for which information was available.

The view that a genetically transmitted tendency for seizures exists in dogs of the Keeshond breed was suggested by CROFT and STOCKMAN (1964) and CROFT (1968). This was followed by a pedigree analysis and EEG study of 321 dogs and pedigree analysis of an additional 108 which failed to confirm genetic transmission of the trait but did leave open that possibility of a familial nature for it (WALLACE 1975).

5. Remarks

The partial seizures of epileptic beagle dogs and Horak's dogs consist largely of masticatory movements of the lips, jaws, and tongue. The generalized seizures of these breeds and also those of epileptic German Shepherd dogs are reported to begin with the same movements (BARKER 1973; EDMONDS et al. 1979; MARTINEK and HORAK 1970; WIEDERHOLT 1974). As noted earlier, it has not been established that this is a characteristic of generalized seizures iin all breeds of dogs; however, PARRY (1949) described masticatory movements as typical events in *"grand mal"* seizures of dogs, and similar movements were observed by GASTAUT et al. (1958 a, b). The presence of these masticatory movements in some canine seizures has led to a likening of canine epilepsy to human psychomotor epilepsy (GASTAUT et al. 1958a, b). However, these movements need not be accompanied by complex behavioral manifestations but can occur separately and independently, as in beagle dogs and Horak's dogs; therefore, it seems incorrect to regard them necessarily as "psychomotor" manifestations. As noted above, seizure discharges were widespread in the cortex of epileptic beagle dogs, involving areas in addition to those related to psychomotor seizures (WIEDERHOLT 1974), and it seems reasonable that the temporal pole and hippocampal discharges which were observed were simply reflections of a widespread cortical hyperexcitability, as suggested by WIEDERHOLT (1974). As an alternative explanation, it seems possible that the regular appearance of masticatory movements might occur early in the generalized seizures of these various types of canine epilepsy as a manifestation of the wide cortical representation of mouth and jaw movements in the canine cortex (BREAZILE and THOMPSON 1967; WOOLSEY 1933) as first suggested by PARRY (1949).

The ease of inducing seizures and the lack of sex differences in the incidence of epilepsy in Horak's dogs (MARTINEK and HORAK 1970; MARTINEK and DAHME 1977; MARTINEK 1980) suggest that the disease might be governed by a different gene(s) than that which causes epilepsy in beagle dogs (BIELFELT et al. 1971). Different genes might determine the inheritance of epilepsies of dogs in a manner analogous to that in mice, where evidence indicates that single gene defects at one of multiple chromosomal loci can cause similar epileptic patterns (NOEBELS 1979). Alternately, at least with regard to sex differences in the frequency of epilepsy, there might be absence, in Horak's dogs, of the X-chromosome suppressor genes that are believed to modify the expression of epilepsy in beagle dogs (BIELFELT et al. 1971).

III. Inherited Epilepsy in Mongolian Gerbils (*Meriones unguiculatus*)

1. Introduction

A seizure disorder of Mongolian gerbils (*Meriones unguiculatus*) was first reported by THIESSEN et al. (1968), who recognized the trait in animals in their laboratory at the University of Texas. Later studies of the disorder have described its clinical and electrographic characteristics, and neurochemical and pharmacological studies have been reported.

2. Electroencephalographic and Clinical Characteristics

Seizures in gerbils occur in response to stimulation and this has led to designation of the disorder as a "reflex epilepsy." The type of stimulus seems to be unimportant, the primary or essential requirements being simply that the stimulus be of sufficient intensity and that it be novel (THIESSEN et al. 1968; LOSKOTA et al. 1974). Effective stimuli include handling, cage cleaning, bright lights, exposure to activity wheels or visual cliffs, and placing in unfamiliar cages (THIESSEN et al. 1968; LOSKOTA et al. 1974). Animals that are caged singly have more seizures than animals maintained in groups of eight (PETTIJOHN 1978). The animals show habituation and refractoriness to the stimuli, as might be expected in a "reflex epilepsy" (LOSKOTA et al. 1972, 1974; THIESSEN et al. 1968).

The mean age of onset of seizures in a colony where breeding stock had been selected for seizures was 54 ± 3 days (males 57 ± 3 and females 47 ± 3 days); the sex difference was not significant (LOSKOTA et al. 1974).

The clinical signs vary in severity from very slight to severe. LOSKOTA et al. (1974) described seven levels of severity, varying from grade 0, no seizures, to grade 5, severe clonic-tonic seizures, and grade 6, clonic-tonic seizures ending fatally (during the course of their study three of their animals died while in seizures). Grade 1 seizures consisted of movements of the vibrissae and flattening the pinnae against the head. During grade 2 seizures these events occured and the animal also stopped moving about the cage. In grade 3 seizures myoclonic jerks were superimposed on the previously described movements, after which the animal remained quiescent for a while and then suddenly resumed normal motor activity. Grade 4 seizures began as in the lower grades but progressed to opisthotonus while standing with the pelvic limbs splayed and the forelegs jerking, causing the animal to jump vertically; this was followed by tonic extension of all legs and then by a quiescent period. In grade 5 seizures, following a period of opisthotonus, the animal began torsion movements of the body and, after falling down, rapidly righted itself and stood on the floor in tonic extensor rigidity. Thereafter it slowly regained normal locomotion while undergoing incoordination, salivation, and various behavioral abnormalities. Some seizures were preceded by rapid thumping of the hind limbs and some animals would vocalize before falling or during myoclonus. Defecation and urination were common during seizures (LOSKOTA et al. 1974).

Using a transducer and recorder, LOSKOTA et al. (1974) were able to quantitate the motor activity of epileptic gerbils and correlate that data with the characteristic phases of the seizures. They found that seizure patterns varied among individuals but tended to remain fairly constant and predictable within individual animals (LOSKOTA et al. 1972; LOSKOTA and LOMAX 1975). The mean latency of seizures varied with the severity from 22.5 ± 4.1 s for grade 1 to 35.2 ± 5.3 s for grade 5. Duration varied from 9.4 ± 1.1 s in grade 1 to 286.6 ± 5.5 s in grade 5 (LOSKOTA et al. 1974).

LOSKOTA and LOMAX (1975) recorded EEGs from epileptic gerbils using chronically implanted dural and depth electrodes. During mild seizures there were localized EEG bursts. With generalized myoclonus and the subsequent behavioral depression there were equivalent EEG changes including high-amplitude electrographic bursts during myoclonic jerking. At the time of severe seizures accompanied by unique postural movements, which the authors likened to automatisms, there was high-voltage activity in many leads and spikes or spike-wave complexes in the hippocampus. Severe clonic-tonic seizures were accompanied by continuous high-frequency activity in all leads. Some ictal EEG paroxysms of epileptic gerbils had focal onset in parietal derivations (LOSKOTA and LOMAX 1975; SUZUKI and NAKAMOTO 1978). LOSKOTA and LOMAX (1975) suggested this might be related to the stimulus-bound nature of the seizures. Interictal paroxysmal EEG activity was observed in these investigations (LOSKOTA and LOMAX

1975; SUZUKI and NAKAMOTO 1978), which might reflect the existence of self-sustaining foci or, as suggested by LOSKOTA and LOMAX (1975), this might be a reflection of an unstable neuronal population that is readily affected by the precipitating environmental stimuli.

3. Inheritance

Epileptic gerbils have been produced by selective mating of seizure-sensitive animals and as high as 97% of the progeny have had seizures by 6 months of age (LOSKOTA et al. 1974; THIESSEN et al. 1968). Gerbils selected for seizure resistance and maintained in the same colonies do not develop seizures (LOSKOTA et al. 1974). Despite these strong indications of genetic transmission of the trait, the exact mode of inheritance apparently has not been determined.

4. Pathology

Both gross and microscopic changes have been observed in the brains of epileptic gerbils. In seizure-sensitive gerbils, SCHONFELD and GLICK (1979) found the left and right rostral cerebral arteries maintained separate courses to the frontal lobes of the cerebrum. In seizure-resistant subjects, these arteries united before passing between the cerebral hemispheres, which were supplied by branches of the single artery formed by the union. The anomaly was found in a majority (80%) but not in all seizure-sensitive gerbils, and a direct relationship, if any, to the pathogenesis of seizures was not evident. The same anomaly has been reported in gerbils that developed brain infarction after unilateral carotid artery ligation (LEVINE and SOHN 1969).

Using microscopic and submicroscopic methods, PAUL et al. (1981) reported that seizure-sensitive and seizure-resistant gerbils differed in presynaptic and in postsynaptic structures of cells in areas CA3 and CA4 of the hippocampus. CA3 and CA4 cells of seizure-sensitive gerbils had significantly fewer dendritic spines per unit length of dendrite, but the neocortical cells did not differ from seizure-resistant gerbils in this respect. Also, in seizure-sensitive gerbils, the area of mossy tuft containing synaptic vesicles was greater in axons and axon collaterals projecting from dentate granule cells into hippocampal CA3 and CA4 areas (stratum oriens and stratum pyramidale), and the area of mossy tuft occupied by spines was smaller (PAUL et al. 1978). These authors pointed out the similarity of these changes to those found in chronic irritative foci (WESTRUM et al. (1964), epileptic human temporal lobe (SCHEIBEL et al. 1974), and isolated cortical slabs (RUTLEDGE 1978). PAUL et al. (1981) noted that, in the circumstances where these changes had been observed previously, exogenous agents, chronic scarring, or long-term surgical manipulation might have contributed to their development, whereas these conditions could not apply to the epileptic gerbil. Their data did not reveal whether the decreased number of spines occurred over the entire neuron or whether it occurred only in certain strata; they suggested the latter might be of great importance in explaining episodic phenomena such as seizures (PAUL et al. 1981).

5. Remarks

The low cost and ready reproducibility of the epileptic gerbil lend it great appeal as a model for epilepsy research. It should have great value for studies of biochemistry and pathophysiology because of the above features and also because of the ease of production of seizures. At the same time, the latter characteristic places sharp limits on the use of this animal for certain types of investigations, in particular, the screening of potential antiepileptic drugs. The results of the pharmacokinetic studies by FREY et al. (1981) emphasize the need for drug efficacy trials to be based upon precise knowledge of the metabolism of the drugs being tested in the species used for the test.

IV. Inherited Epilepsy in Domestic Fowl

1. Introduction

At least two inherited paroxysmal disorders of the central nervous system of the domestic fowl have been reported. One of these, so-called "paroxysm," caused seizures in response to sudden auditory or visual stimuli. Inherited as a sex-linked trait, affected individuals all died by the age of 15 weeks, a characteristic which might limit the usefulness of these animals for study of epilepsy (COLE 1961).

A second mutation that caused spontaneous convulsions was first reported by CRAWFORD (1969, 1970). This condition, designated "epi," was first observed in chickens of the Fayoumi breed but was later introduced into chickens of other breeds (CRAWFORD 1970).

2. Electroencephalographic and Clinical Characteristics

Seizures can be initiated on the day of hatching or later by stimuli which induce vigorous muscular exertion and by rhythmical auditory stimuli (beating on the wire cages), by combined rhythmical auditory and photic stimulation, or by ILS alone (CRAWFORD 1970; JOHNSON et al. 1979). Affected chicks are highly susceptible to ILS at 14 Hz; heterozygous chicks are clinically normal and are unaffected by ILS.

Seizures induced by all stimuli follow the same general course; however, the timing of events in the seizures can be determined most precisely if ILS is used. After 12–20 s of 14-Hz ILS, affected chickens appear to show increased alertness and then dorsiflexion and rotation of the head and neck (apparently analogous to the opisthotonus of seizures in other species). In 5–7 s the chickens lose control of postural muscles of the legs and assume a sitting position with wings extended and directed downward. After a few seconds in this position, running movements of the legs and flapping movements of the wings begin and the violence of these movements causes the chicken to fall and roll about the cage. This phase of the seizure continues for 25–30 s and is followed by a period of apparent postictal depression and disorientation. CRAWFORD (1970) reported that, in seizures induced by various stimuli, the period of apparent increased alertness at the onset of the seizure was accompanied sometimes by vocalization and violent pecking motions; during the immediate postictal period, a variable period of apparent coma occurred after which the bird appeared to be totally blind or, at least, refractory to visual stimuli.

The interictal EEG of epileptic chickens has a high-amplitude, slow wave pattern. During ILS the interictal background rhythms are replaced by "following" waves at the ILS rate. These develop into high-voltage spikes and, at that time, clinical manifestations appear (CRICHLOW and CRAWFORD 1974; JOHNSON et al. 1979).

3. Inheritance

This form of epilepsy of the fowl is inherited as an autosomal recessive. Some chicks of affected parents are clinically normal and somewhat fewer chicks from matings of heterozygous parents are affected, indicating that the gene has incomplete penetrance (CRAWFORD 1970). Test matings made to determine the location of the mutation on the domestic fowl linkage map were unsuccessful (CRAWFORD 1970). The trait was observed first in chickens of the Fayoumi breed but was introduced later into chickens of other breeds (CRAWFORD 1970), and a crossbred "synthetic" population has been maintained for experimental purposes (JOHNSON et al. 1979). Affected chickens have a higher than normal early post-hatching mortality because they are slower to adapt to cage rearing; once adapted, the life span of affected individuals is said to be normal (JOHNSON et al. 1979).

4. Pathology

At this time there are no reports of gross or microscopic studies of the brains of epileptic fowl.

5. Neurochemistry and Neuropharmacology

Neurochemical studies of the brains of epileptic fowl have included determinations of the concentrations of monoamines, acetylcholinesterase, and choline-acetyltransferase.

Epileptic chickens had lower concentrations of 5-hydroxytryptamine (5-HT) and of dopamine (DA) in their cerebral hemispheres than did normal (heterozygous) chickens, but norepinephrine (NE) levels were higher; no significant differences were found in the concentrations of these substances in the optic "lobes" (tectum), brain stem, or cerebellum (JOHNSON et al. 1979, 1981). In acute experiments, elevation of 5-HT in the cerebral hemispheres, produced by administering tryptophan and phenelzine, did not reduce seizure susceptibility. Similarly, no change in seizure susceptibility occurred after DA concentrations were increased by administration of L-dopa. Administration of the alpha-adrenergic blocking agents phenoxybenzamine and phentolamine, or administration of the beta-adrenergic blocker propanolol, did not affect seizure susceptibility (JOHNSON et al. 1979, 1981). These data suggest that the differences in concentrations of these substances in the cerebral hemispheres of epileptic versus normal chickens are not related to the generation of their seizures.

Epileptic chickens were found to have higher acetylcholinesterase and lower choline-acetyltransferase activities; a relationship of these data to the pathophysiology of the seizures has not been established (JOHNSON et al. 1979).

6. Remarks

The domestic fowl, normal or epileptic, has low initial and low maintenance costs, and large numbers of genetically defined subjects can be produced with relative ease. The results of the investigations described above suggest that the fortuitous occurrence of an epileptic mutant in the domestic fowl has indeed provided researchers with an extremely valuable means for large-scale testing of antiepileptic drugs. It seems likely that other uses will be found for this unique model of epilepsy in the future.

D. Concluding Remarks

The inherited epilepsies discussed above occur in species that are widely separated phylogenetically. Despite the divergence of species there are similarities in the clinical mainfestations of their epilepsies. Movements of the facial, masticatory, or lingual muscles, movements of the eyelids or pinnae, or movements of the head appear early in their seizures; if the seizures do not stop at this point, involvement of the major postural muscles occurs, with rapid progression from cranial to caudal parts of the body. These similarities suggest similarities in basic pathophysiological mechanisms. The differences in details of the seizures may well arise from differences in relative development of parts of the nervous system that are important in the generation of clinical signs of seizures. For example, the development of the limbic system relative to that of the neocortex, or even a more limited area such as the sensorimotor cortex, might be important in determining the predominant clinical signs during the onset of seizures. Differences in threshold of specific areas or in precise time of their involvement in the spread of the seizure discharge also might be important determinants of the order of appearance of clinical signs. Audiogenic seizures of one strain of rats have been reported to begin with facial myoclonus (KRUSHINSKY et al. 1970); however, it is more typical for audiogenic seizures of both rats and mice to begin with a burst of wild running (CONSROE et al. 1979; SEYFRIED 1979), suggesting the possibility of marked differences in the pathophysiology of seizures in these species. Nevertheless, it appears possible that the differences in clinical characteristics and in electrographic spread of the seizures in all these widely divergent species might be explained to a great extent on the basis of neuroanatomical or neurophysiological differences that need not reflect differences in basic pathophysiological mechanisms. If this is, in fact, true then each of the available animal "models" has value as an experimental tool, a value that is based primarily on its usefulness for answering the particular questions at hand rather than on the similarity of details of its clinical or electrographic characteristics to those of epilepsies in any other species, including man.

One of the most important potential uses of experimental animals with inherited epilepsy is in the testing of new drugs for antiepileptic potency. Determination of the responsiveness of the seizures of each of the species to drugs having known efficacy against the major types of human epilepsies, as exemplified by the work of DAVIS et al. (1978a, b) and JOHNSON et al. (1979) with the fowl, might be helpful in establishing a specific type of epilepsy for which each experimental animal is most suited for drug testing. In this regard, the work of FREY et al. (1981)

illustrates the need for pharmacokinetic studies in a test species as a basis for accurate assessment of the efficacy of drugs being tested.

The low inital and maintenance costs of the small rodents and domestic fowl and the ease with which their seizures can be initiated make these species appear to be valuable for large-scale testing of new drugs. The present need to initiate seizures in epileptic beagle dogs by the use of PTZ or electroshock would seem to limit their usefulness for drug testing; however, this limitation does not apply to epileptic Horak's dogs. The costs of producing and maintaining dogs in the numbers necessary for drug testing would seem to restrict sharply the usefulness of either of the canine models. As noted earlier, the epileptic baboon offers unique opportunities for testing the more subtle effects of drugs on behavior in an experimental paradigm that might permit more accurate prediction of drug effects in man.

The ultrastructural changes in CA3 and CA4 hippocampal neurons of epileptic gerbils (PAUL et al. 1981) constitute the first report of this sort in an inherited epilepsy. Confirmation of this work and the demonstration of similar changes in the gerbil or in other species prior to or coinciding with the onset of seizures could be of great significance in the understanding of seizure pathophysiology. Future studies of these or other structural or functional abnormalities in animals with inherited epilepsy should help to identify those cellular characteristics common to all of them and hence those that might most accurately reflect the basic alterations that lead to the production of seizures in all species, including man.

References

Antonitis JJ, Carary DD, Sawin EB, Cohen CJ (1954) Sound-induced seizures in rabbits. J Hered 45:279–284

Atkeson FW, Ibsen A, Eldridge E (1944) Inheritance of an epileptic type character in Brown Swiss cattle. J Hered 35:45–48

Balzamo E, Bert J, Menini CH, Naquet R (1975) Excessive light sensitivity in *Papio papio*: its variation with age, sex and geographic origin. Epilepsia 16:269–276

Barker J (1973) Epilepsy in the dog, a comparative approach. J Small Anim Pract 14:281–289

Bielfelt SW, Redman HC, McClellan RO (1971) Sire- and sex-related differences in rates of epileptiform seizures in a purebred beagle dog colony. Am J Vet Res 32:2039–2048

Breazile JE, Thompson WD (1967) Motor cortex of the dog. Am J Vet Res 28:1483

Chrisman CL (1982) Problems in small animal neurology. Lea and Febiger, Philadelphia

Cole RK (1961) Paroxysm – a sex-linked lethal of the fowl. J Hered 52:46–52

Collins RL (1972) Audiogenic seizures. In: Purpura DP, Penry JK, Tower DB, Woodbury DM, Walter RD (eds) Experimental models of epilepsy. Raven, New York

Consroe P, Edmonds HL (1979) Genetic animal models of epilepsy. Fed Proc 38:2397–2398

Consroe P, Picchioni H, Chin L (1979) Audiogenic seizure susceptible rats. Fed Proc 38:2411–2416

Crawford RD (1969) A new mutant causing epileptic seizures in domestic fowl. Poulty Sci 48:1799

Crawford RD (1970) Epileptic seizures in domestic fowl. J Hered 61:185–188

Crichlow EC, Crawford RD (1974) Epileptiform seizures in domestic fowl II. Intermittent light stimulation and the electroencephalogram. Can J Physiol Pharmacol 52:424–429

Croft PG (1968) The use of the electro-encephalograph in the detection of epilepsy as a hereditary condition in the dog. Vet Rec 80:712–713

Croft PG, Stockman MJR (1964) Inherited defects in dogs. Vet Rec 76:260–261

Cunningham JG (1971) Some clinical, electrographic, developmental, and neurophysiological aspects of canine epilepsy. PhD Thesis, University of California, Davis

Davis HL, Johnson DD, Crawford RD (1978 a) Epileptiform seizures in domestic fowl. VII. Plasma phenytoin concentration and anticonvulsant activity. Can J Physiol Pharmacol 56:310–315

Davis HL, Johnson DD, Crawford RD (1978 b) Epileptiform seizures in domestic fowl. IX. Implications of the absence of anticonvulsant activity of ethosuximide in a pharmacological model of epilepsy. Can J Physiol Pharmacol 56:893–896

deLahunta A (1977) Veterinary neuroanatomy and clinical neurology. Saunders, Philadelphia

Edmonds HL Jr, Bellin SI, Chen FC, Hegreberg GA (1978) Anticonvulsant properties of ropizine in epileptic and nonepileptic beagle dogs. Epilepsia 19:139–146

Edmonds HL, Hegreberg GA, van Gelder NM, Sylvester DM, Clemmons RM, Chatburn CG (1979) Spontaneous convulsions in beagle dogs. Fed Proc 38:2424–2428

Falco MJ, Barker J, Wallace ME (1974) The genetics of epilepsy in the British Alsatian. J Small Anim Pract 15:685–692

Fischer-Williams M, Poncet M, Riche D, Naquet R (1968) Light-induced epilepsy in the baboon, *Papio papio:* cortical and depth recordings. EEG Clin Neurophysiol 25:557–569

Frey H-H, Löscher W, Reiche R, Schultz D (1981) Pharmacology of antiepileptic drugs in the gerbil 1. Pharmacokinetics, Neuropharmacol 20:769–771

Gastaut H, Berard-Badier M, Darraspen M, Van Bogaert L (1958 a) Anatomic and clinical study of 19 epileptic dogs. In: Baldwin M, Bailey P (eds) Temporal lobe epilepsy. Thomas, Springfield

Gastaut H, Toga M, Naquet R (1958 b) Clinical, electrographical and anatomical study of epilepsy induced in dogs by the ingestion of agenized proteins. In: Baldwin M, Bailey P (eds) Temporal lobe epilepsy. Thomas, Springfield

Hare JE, Hare AS (1979) Epileptiform mice: a new neurological mutant. J Hered 70:417–420

Harriman AE (1978) "Spontaneous" seizing in open-field tests by Mongolian gerbils fed magnesium at different rates. Percept Mot Skills 47:1031–1035

Hegreberg GA, Padgett GA (1976) Inherited progressive epilepsy of the dog with comparisons to Lafora's disease of man. Fed Proc 35:1202–1205

Hoerlein F (1978) Canine neurology. Diagnosis and treatment. Saunders, Philadelphia

Hohenboken WD, Nellhaus G (1970) Inheritance of audiogenic seizures in the rabbit. J Hered 61:107–112

Holland JM, Davis WC, Prieur DJ, Collins GH (1970) Lafora's disease in the dog. Am J Pathol 58:509–529

Holliday TA, Cunningham JG, Gutnick MJ (1970) Comparative clinical and electroencephalographic studies of canine epilepsy. Epilepsia 11:281–292

Isaksson A (1943) Genuin epilepsi hos not-kreatur (Genuine epilepsy in cattle). Skand Vet Tidskr 33:1–27

Johnson DD, Davis HL, Crawford RD (1979) Pharmacological and biochemical studies in epileptic fowl. Fed Proc 38:2417–2423

Johnson DD, Jaju AT, Ness L, Richardson JS, Crawford RD (1981) Brain norepinephrine, dopamine and 5-hydroxytryptamine concentration abnormalities and their role in the high seizure susceptibility of epileptic chickens. Can J Physiol Pharmacol 59:144–149

Kaplan H, Miezejeski C (1972) Development of seizures in the Mongolian gerbil (*Meriones unguiculatus*). J Comp Physiol Psychol 81:267–273

Killam EK (1979) Photomyoclonic seizures in the baboon, *Papio papio*. Fed Proc 38:2429–2433

Killam KF, Killam EK, Naquet R (1966a) Études pharmacologique realisées chez des signes présentant une activité EEG paroxystique particulière à la stimulation lumineuse intermittente. J Physiol (Paris) 58:543–544

Killam KF, Killam EK, Naquet R (1966 b) Mise en évidence chez certains singes d'un syndrôme photomyoclonique. CR Acad Sci [D] (Paris) 262:1010–1012

Killam KF, Naquet R, Bert J (1966c) Paroxysmal responses to intermittent light stimulation in a population of baboons (*Papio papio*). Epilepsia 7:215–219
Killam KF, Killam EK, Naquet R (1967a) An animal model of light sensitive epilepsy. EEG Clin Neurophysiol 22:497–513
Killam KF, Killam EK, Naquet R (1967b) Evoked potential studies in response to light in the baboon (*Papio papio*). EEG Clin Neurophysiol [Suppl] 26:108–113
Killam EK, Stark LG, Killam KF (1967c) Photic stimulation in three species of baboon. Life Sci 6:1569–1574
Killam KF, Joy RM, Killam EK, Stark LG (1969) Genetic models of epilepsy with special reference to the syndrome of *Papio papio*. Epilepsia 10:229–238
Kitsikis A, Dimov S, Dubouch P, Pons C, Naquet R (1970) Etude de la photosensibilité du *Papio anubis*, du *Papio cynocephalus* et de *Papio nes* de leur croisement. Rev Neurol (Paris) 121:366–367
Koestner A, Rehfeld CE (1968) Idiopathic epilepsy in a beagle colony. Argonne Nat Lab Rec, p 178–179
Krushinsky LV, Molodkina LN, Fless DA, Dobrokhotora LP, Steshenko AP, Semiokhina AF, Zorina ZA, Romanova LG (1970) The functional state of the brain during sonic stimulation. In: Welch BL, Welch AS (eds) Physiological effects of noise. Plenum, New York, p 159
Lee KE (1973) Studies of behavioral and physiological bases of genetically controlled epileptiform seizures in domestic fowl. PhD thesis, University of Saskatchewan, Saskatoon, Saskatchewan
Lennox WG, Lennox MA (1960) Epilepsy and related disorders, vol I. Little Brown, Boston, p 3
Levine S, Sohn D (1969) Cerebral ischemia in infant and adult gerbils. Arch Pathol 87:315–317
Lewin E (1972) The production of epileptogenic cortical foci in experimental animals by freezing. In: Purpura DP, Penry JK, Tower DB, Woodbury DM, Walter RD (eds) Experimental models of epilepsy. Raven, New York, p 37
Loskota WJ, Lomax P (1975) The mongolian gerbil (*Meriones unguiculatus*) as a model for the study of the epilepsies: EEG records of seizures. EEG Clin Neurophysiol 38:597–604
Loskota WJ, Lomax P, Rich ST (1972) The gerbil as a model for the study of epilepsy: seizure habituation and seizure patterns. Proc West Pharmacol Soc 15:189–194
Loskota WJ, Lomax P, Rich ST (1974) The gerbil as a model for the study of epilepsy seizure patterns and ontogenesis. Epilepsia 15:109–119
Martinek Z (1980) Genetische bedingte Epilepsie bei Hunden. Kleintierpraxis 25:44–46
Martinek Z, Dahme E (1977) Spontaneous epilepsy in dogs: long-term studies on a group of genetically related animals. Zentralbl Veterinärmed 24A:353–371
Martinek Z, Horak F (1970) Development of so-called "genuine" epileptic seizures in dogs during emotional excitement. Physiol Bohemoslov 19:185–195
Meldrum BS, Balzamo E, Gadea M, Naquet R (1970a) Photic and drug induced epilepsy in the baboon (*Papio papio*); the effects of isoniazid, thiosemicarbazide, pyridoxine and amino-oxyacetic acid. EEG Clin Neurophysiol 29:333–347
Meldrum BS, Naquet R, Balzamo E (1970b) Effects of atropine and eserine on the electroencephalogram, on behavior and on light-induced epilepsy in the adolescent baboon, *Papio papio*. EEG Clin Neurophysiol 28:449–458
Nachtsheim H (1939) Krampfbereitschaft und Genotypus. Z Menschliche Vererbungs- und Konstitutionslehre 22:791–810
Naquet R, Meldrum BS (1972) Photogenic seizures in the baboon. In: Purpura DP, Penry JK, Tower DB, Woodbury DM, Walter RD (eds) Experimental models of epilepsy. Raven, New York, p 374–406
Naquet R, Menini CH (1972) La photosensibilité excessive du *Papio papio*: approaches neurophysiologiques et pharamacologiques de ses mechanismes. Electroencephalogr Clin Neurophysiol [Suppl] 31:13–26
Naquet R, Killam KF, Rhodes JM (1967) Flicker stimulation with chimpanzees. Life Sci 6:1575–1578

Nellhaus G (1958) Experimental epilepsy in rabbits: development of a strain susceptible to audiogenic seizures. Am J Physiol 193:567–572

Newberne JW, Robinson VB, Estil L, Brinkman DC (1960) Granular structures in brains of apparently normal dogs. Amer J Vet Res 21:782–786

Newmarket ME, Penry JK (1980) Genetics of epilepsy. Raven, New York

Noebels JL (1979) Analysis of inherited epilepsy using single locus mutations in mice. Fed Proc 38:2405–2410

Palmer AC (1972) Pathological changes in the brain associated with fits in dogs. Vet Rec 90:167–173

Palmer AC (1976) Introduction to animal neurology, 2nd edn. Blackwell, Oxford

Parry HB (1949) Epileptic states in the dog, with special reference to canine hysteria. Vet Rec 61:23–31

Paul LA, Fried I, Watanabe K, Forsythe AB, Scheibel AB (1981) Structural correlates of seizure behavior in the Mongolian gerbil. Science 213:924–926

Paule M, Killam EK (1979) Disruption of learing performance by chronic ethosuximide administration in the baboon. Fed Proc 38:862

Pettijohn TF (1978) Influence of social group size on seizure frequency in Mongolian gerbils. J Gen Psychol 99:149–150

Redman HC, Weir JE (1969) Detection of naturally occurring neurologic disorders of beagle dogs by electroencephalography. Am J Vet Res 30:2075–2082

Redman HC, Hogan JE, Wilson GL (1972) Effect of intermittent light stimulation singly and combined with pentylenetetrazol on the electroencephalogram and clinical response of the beagle dog. Am J Vet Res 33:677–685

Robinson DG (1968) Animals suited to epileptic research. Science News 93:16–18

Rutledge LT (1978) The effects of denervation and stimulation upon synaptic ultrastructure. J Comp Neurol 178:117–128

Saunders LZ (1952) A check list of hereditary and familial diseases of the central nervous system in domestic animals. Cornell Vet 42:592–600

Scheibel ME, Crandall PH, Scheibel AB (1974) The hippocampal-dentate complex in temporal lobe epilepsy. Epilepsia 15:55–80

Schonfeld AR, Glick SD (1978) Effect of handling-induced seizures on passive avoidance learning in the Mongolian gerbil (*Meriones unguiculatus*). Behav Biol 24:101–106

Schonfeld AR, Glick SD (1979) Cerebrovascular abnormalities associated with seizure susceptibility in the Mongolian gerbil. Brain Res 173:147–151

Seyfried TN (1979) Audiogenic seizures in mice. Fed Proc 38:2399–2404

Stanton D, Paule M, Weinberger SB (1977) Disruption of learning performance by chronic chlorpromazine administration in the baboon. Pharmacologist 19:228

Stark LG, Joy RM, Hance AJ, Killam KF (1968) Further studies of photic stimulation in subhuman primates. Life Sci 7:1037–1039

Suzuki J, Nakamoto Y (1978) Sensory precipitating epilepsy focus in El mice and Mongolian gerbils. Folia Psychiatr Neurol Jpn 32:349–350

Suzuki Y, Ohta K, Suu S (1979a) Correlative studies of axonal spheroids and Lafora-like bodies in aged dogs. Acta Neuropathol (Berlin) 48:77–81

Suzuki Y, Kamiya S, Ohta K, Suu S (1979b) Lafora-like bodies in a cat. Case report suggestive of glycogen metabolism disturbances. Acta Neuropathol (Berlin) 48:55–58

Thiessen DD, Lindzey G, Friend HC (1968) Spontaneous seizures in the Mongolian gerbil (*Meriones unguiculatus*). Psychon Sci 11:227–228

Urbich R (1973) Ätiologie, Klinik und Genetik der epileptischen Anfälle beim Hund unter besonderer Berücksichtigung der epileptiformen Krämpfe beim Collie. Beitr Erbpathol Zuchthyg 5:171–174

Van Bogaert L (1973) De l'epilepsie spontanee des singes en captivite. Schweiz Arch Neurol Neurochir Psych 112:329–339

Van der Velden NA (1968) Fits in Tervueren shepherd dogs: a presumed hereditary trait. J Small Anim Pract 9:63–70

Van Gelder NM, Edmonds HL, Hegreberg GA, Chatburn CC, Clemmons RM, Sylvester DM (1980) Amino acid changes in a genetic strain of epileptic beagle dogs. J Neurochem 35:1087–1091

Wada JA, Naquet R (1972) Proceedings: examination of neural mechanism involved in photogenic seizure susceptibility in epileptic Senegalese baboon: *Papio papio*. Epilepsia 32:344–345
Wada JA, Terao A, Booker HC (1972) Longitudinal correlative analysis of epileptic baboon, *Papio papio*. Neurology 22:1272–1285
Wallace ME (1975) Keeshonds: a genetic study of epilepsy and EEG readings. J Small Anim Pract 16:1–10
Ward AA (1972) Topical convulsant metals. In: Purpura DP, Penry JK, Tower DB, Woodbury DM, Walter RD (eds) Experimental models of epilepsy. Raven, New York, p 13
Weinberger SB, Killam EK (1978) Alterations in learning performace in the seizure prone baboon: effects of elicited seizures and chronic treatment with diazepam and phenobarbital. Epilepsia 19:301–316
Weinberger SB, Killam EK (1979) Learning and behavioral abnormalities in the seizure prone baboon. Biol Psychiatry 14:525
Westrum LE, White LE, Ward AA (1964) Morphology of the experimental epileptic focus. J Neurosurg 21:1033–1046
Wiederholt WC (1974) Electrophysiologic analysis of epileptic beagles. Neurology 24:149–155
Woolsey CN (1933) Postural relations of the frontal and motor cortex of the dog. Brain 56:353–370
Yoon CH, Peterson JS, Corrow D (1976) Spontaneous seizures: a new mutation in Syrian golden hamsters. J Hered 67:115–116

Pathophysiology of Seizure Disorders

CHAPTER 4

Intermediary Metabolism

B. E. DWYER and C. G. WASTERLAIN

A. Introduction

Metabolism can be divided, for convenience, into anabolism, the enzymatic synthesis of macromolecules from simple precursors, and catabolism, the degradation of precursor molecules of either intra- or extracellular origin to simple organic molecules and waste products. Examples of the former are lipid, protein, and nucleic acid synthesis and of the latter proteolysis, glycogenolysis, and the energy-producing reactions of glycolysis and the mitochondrial respiratory chain. Intermediary metabolism encompasses the compounds which are intermediates in the processes and the regulatory mechanism which maintain their homeostasis. These reactions serve to ensure there is adequate energy in the form of ATP for production of essential cell substances (structural macromolecules, enzymes, and neurotransmitters), uninterrupted operation of essential cell processes (maintenance of ionic concentration gradients), and elimination of metabolic waste products (ammonia fixation).

Seizures place a tremendous strain on the ability of brain to maintain homeostasis. Anabolic processes are halted (VESCO and GIUDITTA 1968; COTMAN et al. 1971; WASTERLAIN 1974a, 1977; DWYER et al. 1982) presumably so that energy may be used for essential cell functions. In spite of this, prolonged seizures are known to damage brain cells. This chapter will review the effects of seizures on intermediary metabolism and the possible link between metabolic imbalance and mechanisms of cell injury.

B. Brain Energy Reserves and the Cell Redox Potential

I. Cerebral Energy Use During Seizures

Epileptic seizures place one of the most severe energy demands known on brain tissue. ATP utilization has been estimated to increase from three to five times during the seizure discharge (SACKTOR et al. 1966; KING et al. 1967; COLLINS et al. 1970; FERRENDELLI and MCDOUGAL 1971 a). Repeated membrane depolarization by seizure discharge requires substantial energy expenditure to restore ion gradients.

Single seizures induced by a variety of convulsants reduce brain high-energy phosphates (Table 1). Energy depletion is found shortly after seizure onset when electroconvulsive shock (ECS) (KING et al. 1967; COLLINS et al. 1970; FERRENDELLI and MCDOUGAL 1971 a; MCCANDLESS et al. 1979), sound (FERRENDELLI and

Table 1. Effect of single seizures on brain high-energy phophate compounds in freely convulsing animals

Species	Convulsant	ATP[a]	Phospho-creatine[a]	Literature source
Mouse, 10 days old	Flurothyl	85	50 (30 s)[b]	SACKTOR et al.
Cerebral hemisphere	(Indoklon)			(1966)
	40 μl/Liter air	80	47 (60 s)	
Mouse, adult	Maximal ECS	71	24 (3 s)	KING et al.
Cerebral cortex		14	6 (20 s)	(1967)
Mouse, adult	ECS	59	26 (4 s)	COLLINS et al.
Cerebral hemisphere		43	22 (10 s)	(1970)
Mouse, 20 g	DL-Methionine			FOLBERGROVA
Cerebral cortex	sulfoximine	NS	NS	et al. (1969)
Cerebellum	(300 mg/kg,	NS	NS	
Subcortical forebrain	I.P.)	NS	NS	
Mouse, 21–28 days	ECS			FERRENDELLI
Cerebral cortex		78	30 (5 s)	and
		44	12 (17 s)	McDOUGAL
Thalamus		70	41 (5 s)	(1971a)
		39	18 (17 s)	
Cerebellum		75	38 (5 s)	
		45,51	8 (17 s)	
Mouse, 21–28 days	Sound			FERRENDELLI
Cerebral cortex		NS	NS	and
Thalamus		82	55 (3.5 s)	McDOUGAL
Cerebellum		NS	80 (3.5 s)	(1971b)
		91	51 (20 s)	
Mouse, 5 weeks	DL-Homocys-	14	60 (during	FOLBERGROVA
Cerebral cortex	teine		first	(1974)
	Thiolactone HCl		clonic sei-	
	(5.5 mmol/kg,		zure)	
	IP)			
Mouse, 25–29 g	ECS			McCANDLESS
Cerebellum				et al. (1979)
Molecular layer		41	13 (10 s)	
Purkinje cell-rich layer		48	17 (10 s)	
Granular layer				
White matter		42	17 10 s)	
		67	NS (10 s)	

NS, differences not statistically significant
[a] Results expressed as a percentage of control; control = 100
[b] Time after seizure onset that the animal was killed

McDOUGAL 1971 b), and homocysteine were employed as convulsive stimuli, but not after seizures induced by methionine sulfoximine (FOLBERGROVA et al. 1969). Most of the reduction of high-energy phosphate compounds could be prevented by paralyzing animals and ventilating them with oxygen during the seizures (Table 2). This is also true during prolonged, continuous seizures (status epilep-

Table 2. Effect of single seizures on brain high-energy phophate compounds in paralyzed and oxygenated animals

Species	Convulsant	ATP[a]	Phospho-creatine[a]	Literature source
Mouse, adult Cerebral hemi-sphere	ECS	NS	NS	COLLINS et al. (1970)
Cat, adult Cerebral cortex	Flurothyl (0.05 ml/kg)	88 92	86 (10 s)[b] 76 (30 s)	HOWSE et al. (1974)
Mouse, adult Cerebral hemi-sphere	ECS	NS	NS (10 s)	DUFFY et al. (1975)
Mouse, adult Forebrain	Flurothyl (20 µl)	85	51 (10 s)	DUFFY et al. (1975)
Cerebellum		78	41 (10 s)	DUFFY et al. (1975)
Brain stem		NS	NS	DUFFY et al. (1975)
Mouse, adult Cerebral hemi-sphere	Pentylenetetrazol (150 mg/kg, I.P.)	NS 96	NS (20 s) 81 (45 s)	DUFFY et al. (1975)
Rat, adult Cerebral cortex	ECS Pentylenetetrazol (120 ml/kg i.a.)	96 60	84 (10 s) 70 (60 s)	DUFFY et al. (1975)

NS, differences not statistically significant
[a] Results expressed as a percentage of control; control = 100
[b] Time after seizure onset that the animal was killed

ticus) when animals are paralyzed and oxygenated (Table 3). The energy charge potential[1] was reduced by a small but significant extent after seizures induced by ECS, pentylenetetrazol (PTZ), flurothyl, or bicuculline (BCC) (DUFFY et al. 1975; CHAPMAN et al. 1977; HOWSE 1979; FOLBERGROVA et al. 1981). ATP in rat cerebral cortex falls within 1 min (CHAPMAN et al. 1977), but following this initial reduction it is maintained close to control values until seizures become self-sustaining in the absence of convulsive stimuli.

1 The energy charge potential (ECP) as defined by ATKINSON (1968) is given by the equation:

$$ECP = \frac{[ATP] + 1/2\,[ADP]}{[ATP] + [ADP] + [AMP]}$$

and is a measure of the availability of high-energy phosphate bonds for performing cell work

Table 3. Effect of status epilepticus on brain high-energy phosphate compounds in paralyzed and oxygenated animals

Species	Convulsant	ATP[a]	Phosphocreatine[a]	Literature source
Mouse, adult Cerebral hemisphere	5 ECS[b]	95	NS (10 s)[c]	DUFFY et al. (1975)
	10 ECS	97	NS (10 s)	
	25 ECS (status)	89	64 (10 s)	
Mouse, adult Cerebral hemisphere	5-Flurothyl[b] (20 µl)	91	66 (10 s)	DUFFY et al. (1975)
	10-Flurothyl	84	43 (10 s)	
	20-Flurothyl (status)	65	41 (10 s)	
Mouse, adult Cerebellum	5-Flurothyl[b]	90	67 (10 s)	DUFFY et al. (1975)
	10-Flurothyl	90	67 (10 s)	
	20-Flurothyl (status)	90	NS (10 s)	
Mouse, adult Cerebral hemisphere	Pentylenetetrazol (150 mg/kg, I.P.)	89	59 (5 min)	DUFFY et al. (1975)
Rat, adult Cerebral cortex	Bicuculline (1.2 mg/kg, I.V.)	91	50 (30 s)	CHAPMAN et al. (1977)
		91	65 (5 min)	
		NS	55 (120 min)	
Cat, adult Cerebral cortex	Pentylenetetrazol (120 mg/kg, I.P.)	88	67 (30 min)	HOWSE (1979)
		94	59 (60 min)	
		87	63 (120 min)	
Cat, adult Cerebral cortex	Pentylenetetrazol (120 mg/kg, I.P.)	91	48 (60 min)	HOWSE (1979)
		91	46 (120 min)	
Rat, adult Cerebral cortex	Bicuculline (1.2 mg/kg, I.V.)	93	71 (20 min)	FOLBERGROVA et al. (1981)
		89	58 (120 min)	
Hippocampus		90	76 (20 min)	
		89	77 (120 min)	
Rat, adult Cerebellum	Bicuculline	95	85 (20 min)	FOLBERGROVA et al. (1981)
		NS	NS (120 min)	

NS, differences not statistically significant
[a] Results expressed as a percentage of control; control = 100
[b] ECS and flurothyl seizures given at 2-min intervals
[c] Time after last seizure that the animal was killed

From these data we can conclude that gross energy failure in brain, resulting from the increased energy demand of seizure activity, can be prevented when convulsive activity is prevented by paralysis and when adequate cerebral oxygenation is maintained. Presumably in the adult brain ATP production by oxidative phosphorylation can increase sufficiently to meet increased demands for ATP utilization.

Table 4. The effect of status epilepticus on brain glucose, glycogen, lactate, and pyruvate

Species	Convulsant	Glucose	Glycogen[a]	Lactate[a]	Pyruvate[a]	Lactate[a] / Pyruvate	Literature source
Rat, adult Cerebral cortex	Bicuculline (1.2 mg/kg I.V.)	83	NS	286	139	203 (30 s)[b]	Chapman et al. (1977)
		50	54	574	184	310 (60 min)	Chapman et al. (1977)
		32	NS	718	184	386 (120 min)	Chapman et al. (1977)
Rat, adult Cerebral cortex	Pentylenetetrazol (120 mg/kg, i.a.)	27	NM	266	103	259 (60 min)	Howse (1979)
		18	NM	219	64	341 (120 min)	
Cat, adult Cerebral cortex	Pentylenetetrazol (120 mg/kg, i.a.)	NS	NM	621	149	417 (60 min)	Howse (1979)
		60	NM	570	225	342 (120 min)	
Rat, adult Cerebral	Bicuculline (1.2 mg/kg, I.V.)	60	18	398	179	222 (20 min)	Folbergrova et al. (1981)
		27	29	283	157	170 (120 min)	
Hippocampus	Bicuculline (1.2 mg/kg, I.V.)	51	15	484	171	290 (20 min)	Folbergrova et al. (1981)
		27	54	250	135	194 (120 min)	
Cerebellar cortex	Bicuculline (1.2 mg/kg, I.V.)	NS	18	448	206	220 (20 min)	Folbergrova et al. (1981)
		56	75	155	126	125 (120 min)	

NS, differences not statistically significant
NM, not measured

[a] Percentage of control; control = 100
[b] Time after seizure onset that the animal was killed

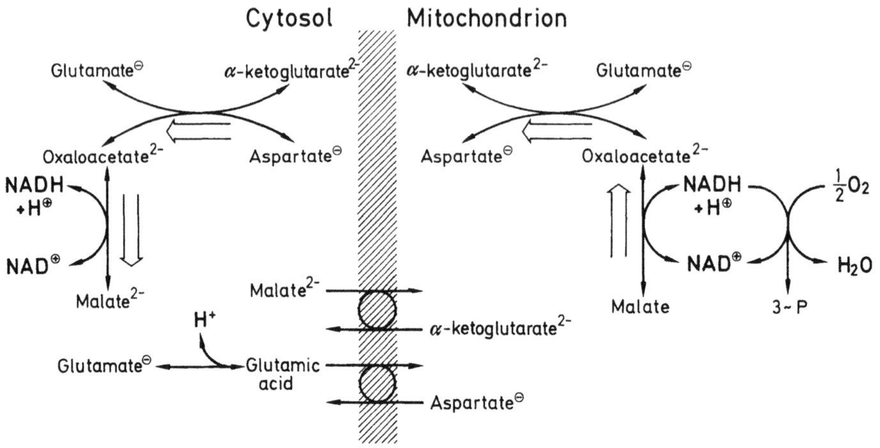

Fig. 1. The malate aspartate shuttle of electrons. NADH generated in the cytosol cannot penetrate the mitochondrial membrane. The accumulation of NADH will shift the equilibrium of cytosolic malate dehydrogenase in favor of malate formation from oxaloacetate. Malate can penetrate the mitochondrial membrane, where it is oxidized in the mitochondrial matrix-forming NADH, which can be utilized by electron transport chain enzymes in the production of ATP (McGilvery 1979)

II. Brain Redox Potential and Lactic Acidosis

Seizures result in a nonhypoxic lactic acidosis in brain. The cytoplasmic redox potential ($NADH/NAD^+$) becomes more reduced. Lactate and pyruvate are elevated in brain; the ratio of lactate to pyruvate is increased despite adequate oxygenation (Table 4).

Howse and Duffy (1975) suggested that the redox potential may be regulated in part by the energy charge potential similar to a system proposed for liver (Krebs and Veech 1970; Stubbs et al. 1972). However, the possibility that during seizures the increased cytoplasmic ratio of $NADH/NAD^+$ could result from impaired or saturated transport of NADH-reducing equivalents into the mitochondria (e.g., via the malate-aspartate shuttle shown in Fig. 1) could not be excluded. Nicotinamide adenine dinucleotide takes part in many intracellular reactions. Among the most conspicuous are those catalyzed by ($NADH$-NAD^+)-linked dehydrogenases which produce NADH that is subsequently oxidized by components of the mitochondrial electron transport chain.

A shift toward a more reduced cell cytoplasm during seizures would presumably ensure that adequate NADH was available for supporting maximal rates of oxidative phosphorylation. On the other hand, elevation of the $NADH/NAD^+$) ratio would shift the equilibrium of the lactate dehydrogenase reaction [Eq. (1)] in favor of lactate production.

$$\text{Pyruvate} + \text{NADH} + \text{H}^+ \rightarrow \text{lactate} + \text{NAD}^+ \tag{1}$$

While it appears that H^+ is consumed in this reaction, the overall stoichiometry for the formation of lactate from glucose [Eq. (2)] makes it clear why anaerobic glycolysis is accompanied by acidosis.

$$\text{Glucose} \rightarrow 2(\text{lactate})^- + 2H^+ \qquad (2)$$

High levels of intracellular lactic acid are thought to cause brain-cell damage (MYERS 1977; DECOURTEN et al. 1981). It is possible that the cytoplasmic redox shift is balanced so that adequate amounts of NADH are available to support increased rates of oxidative phosphorylation, while at the same time lactic acid production is held below a rate which would result in a lethal cellular lactic acidosis.

C. Seizures and Glycolytic Flux

The adult brain is an obligate glucose user. Since brain glucose and glycogen stores are limited and can only support cerebral metabolism for a very short time, proper cerebral function requires continuous transport of glucose from blood to brain.

Rates of cerebral glucose utilization increase severalfold during seizures (BORGSTROM et al. 1976; HAWKINS et al. 1979). Single seizures in freely convulsing animals rapidly reduce brain glucose and glycogen and result in a marked elevation of lactate. Paralysis and oxygenation can prevent the initial reduction of glucose and glycogen after one ECS but not the elevation of lactate in brain (DUFFY et al. 1975). These authors did find glucose and glycogen reduction in mouse forebrain 10 s after onset of a flurothyl-induced seizure. This difference may reflect the severity of seizure discharge as ATP and phosphocreatine were reduced by the latter treatment but not by the former. The conclusion to be drawn is that seizures result in increased glycolytic flux which initially is more rapid than glucose transport from blood to brain. As seizures are more prolonged brain glucose progressively falls (see Table 4). It is possible that a new balance is never achieved in brain regions like the cortex and hippocampus, which are known to have high rates of glucose utilization during seizures (HAWKINS et al. 1979). In this case transport of glucose from blood to brain may become rate limiting for glucose utilization, and late in the course of status epilepticus could result in brain glucose depletion (FOLBERGROVA et al. 1981). While transport limitation and brain glucose depletion have been demonstrated in normoglycemic neonates during status epilepticus (WASTERLAIN and DUFFY 1976; DWYER and WASTERLAIN 1981; WASTERLAIN and DWYER 1982), this is a recent concept for the adult brain.

I. Regulation of Glycolysis: Phosphofructokinase

When transport of glucose from blood to brain is not the rate-limiting step for glucose utilization, regulation of glycolytic flux is exerted primarily at the level of phosphofructokinase (PFK), while hexokinase and possibly pyruvate kinase serve in a lesser role (LOWRY and PASSONNEAU 1964).

Seizures reduce glucose 6-phosphate (G6P) and fructose 6-phosphate (F6P) in brain. Where hypoxemia was prevented by paralysis and oxygenation, similar changes were found within 1 min of the onset of seizures (Fig. 2). After several

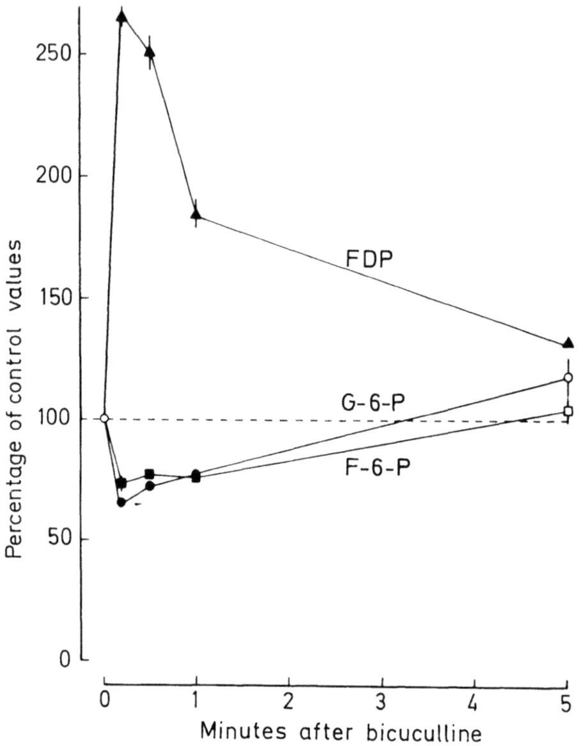

Fig. 2. Changes in fructose-6-phospate, glucose-6-phosphate, and fructose 1,6-diphosphate of cerebral cortex tissue during the first 5 min of BCC-induced seizures in rats. The values are given as percentages of controls. *Filled symbols* indicate statistically significant changes ($P < 0.05$) (CHAPMAN et al. 1977)

minutes levels of G6P, F6P and fructose diphosphate (FDP) approached control values, suggesting hexokinase and possibly pyruvate kinase were also activated. Phosphofructokinase stimulation probably results from a combination of the effects of increased amounts of 5′-AMP, 3′,5′-cyclic AMP, inorganic phosphate ion, FDP, and NH_4, which stimulate the enzyme, and reduced levels of ATP, which release the enzyme from inhibition (MAKER et al. 1976).

II. Hexokinase

Hexokinase may be regulated by the distribution of enzyme between the free and mitochondrial bound forms, the latter being more active (WILSON 1968). During times of energy need (reduced ratio of intracellular ATP/ADP) the bound state is favored (KNULL et al. 1973). This form of the enzyme from calf brain has a lower K_m for ATP (FROMM and ZEWE 1962; COPLEY and FROMM 1967) and is less sensitive to product inhibition by G6P (TUTTLE and WILSON 1970). Inorganic phosphate may partially release the enzyme from inhibition by G6P. Seizures which reduce ATP and G6P and elevate inorganic phosphate favor activation of hexokinase and increased glucose flux through this control point.

III. Pyruvate Kinase

Pyruvate kinase (PK) catalyzes the formation of pyruvate from phosphoenolpyruvate, forming ATP in the process. PK may also be a glycolytic control point. It is presumed that flux of triosephosphates through this enzyme is increased during seizures, based on the fact that the overall glycolytic rate is accelerated (CHAPMAN et al. 1977). Possibly the brain enzyme is activated by FDP, which relieves inhibition by ATP (MCGILVERY 1979), although this would not be the case after several minutes when levels of FDP approach control values. The pyruvate thus formed can then diffuse into the mitochondrial compartment, where it is converted via pyruvate dehydrogenase to acetyl coenzyme A (CoA), which then enters the citric acid cycle.

D. The Citric Acid Cycle and Epileptic Seizures

I. Energy Metabolism

The citric acid cycle (CAC) provides the means by which acetylCoA derived from glucose, fatty acid, or amino acid catabolism can be oxidized to CO_2 and H_2O via (NAD^+)-linked dehydrogenase enzymes in the mitochondria (Fig. 3). NADH is oxidized by mitochondrial respiratory chain enzymes to produce ATP. In paralyzed and oxygenated rats seizures result in the elevation of most CAC intermediates, with the exception of transient reductions in the levels of α-ketoglutarate and oxaloacetate immediately after seizure onset (HOWSE and DUFFY 1975; CHAPMAN et al. 1977). The expanded size of the pool of CAC intermediates is suggestive of increased CAC activity, but the exact magnitude of the increase is not known. However, CAC activity appears adequate since energy failure is not found to occur in these animals.

II. Amino Acid Metabolism

Intracellular pools of citric acid cycle intermediates and amino acids are linked enzymatically so the CAC is also involved in the regulation of amino acid and ammonia metabolism in the brain (Fig. 3).

Brain glutamate falls early after the onset of convulsive seizures (WHISLER et al. 1968; NAHORSKI et al. 1970) although not after one electroshock in paralyzed and oxygenated rats (HOWSE and DUFFY 1975). Alpha-ketoglutarate also falls after the onset of convulsive seizures in mice (KING et al. 1973) and in the cortex of paralyzed and oxygenated rats (HOWSE and DUFFY 1975; CHAPMAN et al. 1977), although the difference in the study of HOWSE and DUFFY did not reach statistical significance. It is probable that ictal energy demands increased flux through the citric acid cycle, reducing levels of α-ketoglutarate. Alpha-ketoglutarate can be replaced via conversion of glutamate by amino acid transaminase reactions.

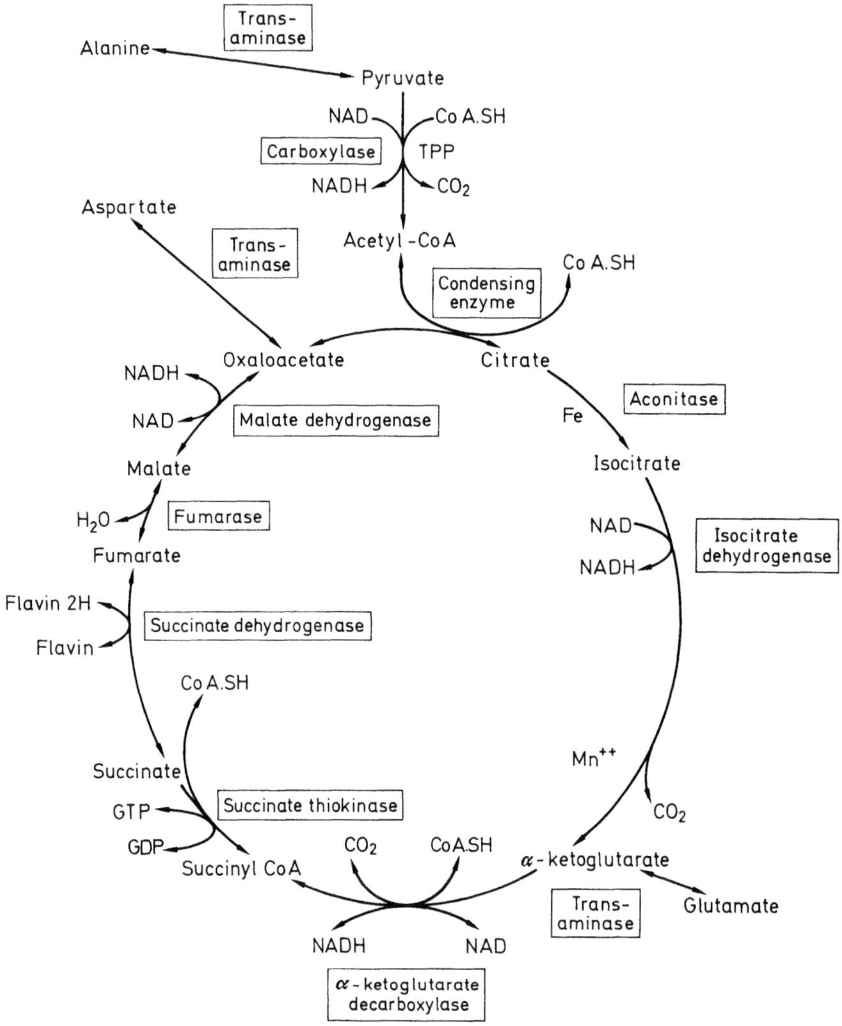

Fig. 3. Citric acid cycle. AcetylCoA which enters the citric acid cycle by condensing with oxaloacetate to form citrate can be derived from glucose, fatty acid, or amino acid catabolism. Amino acid metabolism is linked with the citric acid cycle via transaminase reactions shown in the figure. Glutamate which can be derived from α-ketoglutarate via transamination can be used for the production of gamma-aminobutyric acid (GABA) or for removal of NA_4^+ via the glutamine synthetase reaction (MAKER and LEHRER 1972)

The equilibrium constant for such reactions is close to 1.0 so that they are freely reversible. The relatively large brain content of glutamate measured by CHAPMAN et al. (1977) (12.74 ± 0.14 μmol/g), the relatively low concentration of α-ketoglutarate (0.159 ± 0.006 μmol/g), and the magnitude of the reduction of α-ketoglutarate in the 1st min after seizures (approximately 0.05–0.06 μmol/g) precludes a significant reduction in glutamate being measured by these authors. A similar argument may be made for aspartic acid. Oxaloacetate appears to fall immediately after seizures begin (CHAPMAN et al. 1977; HOWSE and DUFFY 1975).

NAHORSKI et al. (1970) found a small decrease in aspartate during the tonic phase of a pentylenetetrazol seizure while no reduction was found up to 3 min after the onset of flurothyl seizures (SACKTOR et al. 1966) or 10 s after electroshock (DUFFY et al. 1975). CHAPMAN et al. (1977) found a small but significant fall in aspartate at 1 min of BCC seizures. Thus we speculate that the initial seizure-induced fall in oxaloacetate is followed by increased conversion of aspartate into oxaloacetate via transamination. Since the normal brain concentration of aspartate is high (3.60 ± 0.08 µmol/g) and that of oxaloacetate low [0.0072 µmol/g reduced to 0.0044 10 s after electroshock (HOWSE and DUFFY 1975)], the precision with which aspartate was measured would preclude finding a significant difference.

III. Ammonia Metabolism

In paralyzed and oxygenated rats brain NH_4 increases immediately after onset of BCC seizures and then reaches a plateau after about 5 min (CHAPMAN et al. 1977). Between 5 and 20 min brain glutamate and aspartate begin to fall while glutamine and alanine increase. Glutamate is utilized as a substrate for glutamine synthetase, which catalyzes the ATP-dependent formation of glutamine, as well as for gamma-aminobutyric acid (GABA) production. Glutamate can be replenished via the CAC (and hence from glucose) by transamination of aspartate with α-ketoglutarate. This may account in part for the steady fall in brain aspartate as the duration of seizures increases, although formation of asparagine to detoxify NH_4 may also be occurring. The marked increase in alanine undoubtedly reflects increased transamination of pyruvate. When rats are similarly treated except for being deprived of food for 24 h prior to administration of seizures a striking result is failure to "fix" NH_4. Thus at 5 min after seizure onset brain NH_4 was severalfold higher in starved than in well-fed counterparts. As the seizure duration lengthened NH_4^+ continued to increase while glutamine was unchanged and the elevation of alanine was not sustained as it was in well-fed rats. Furthermore, glutamate was reduced to a greater extent and aspartate was elevated (BLENNOW et al. 1979). The reason for reduced glutamine synthesis is not known, but it is an ATP-dependent reaction and the energy charge potential in brains of starved rats was lower than in well-fed counterparts. Reduced formation of alanine probably reflects reduced levels of pyruvate possibly as a result of reduced glucose transport into brain as blood glucose falls. Glutamate may fall as a result of consumption following transamination to α-ketoglutarate, and aspartate may increase as a result of transamination of oxaloacetate with glutamate. This could conceivably provide a shunt mechanism by which glutamate can be introduced into the CAC at the level of α-ketoglutarate (α-KG) and exit at the level of oxaloacetate. From this shunt (Fig. 3) 1 mol NADH capable of generating 3 mol ATP is produced per mole of glutamate entering the CAC at the level of α-KG, and 1 mol GTP is produced by substrate level phosphorylation during the hydrolysis of succinyl CoA to succinate. Such a mechanism may provide an additional source of ATP when blood and brain glucose levels can only marginally support ATP production.

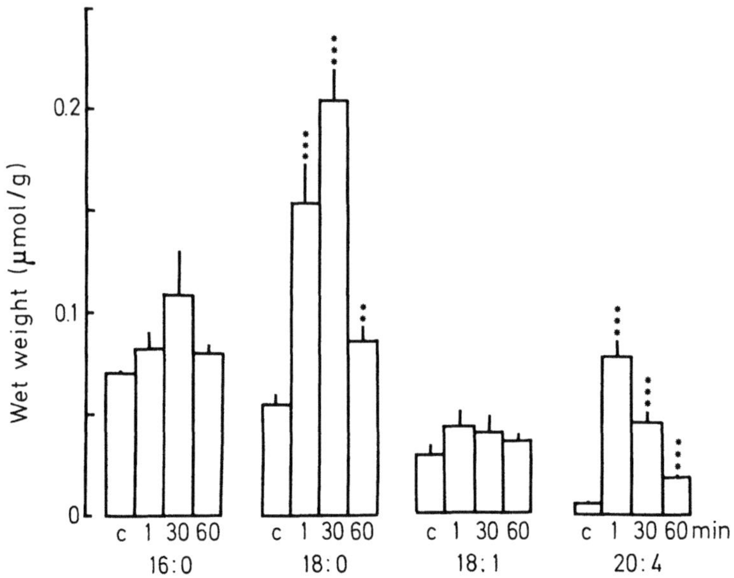

Fig. 4. Changes in the cerebral cortex concentrations of some free fatty acids during BCC-induced status epilepticus of 1-, 30-, and 60-min duration. The values are means ±SE in µmol/g wet weight for groups of six animals. *C*, control. **, $P<0.01$; ***, $P<0.001$ (CHAPMAN et al. 1980)

E. Free Fatty Acid Metabolism

Following ECS and PTZ seizures, free fatty acids are found to accumulate both in freely seizing animals (BAZAN 1976; MARION and WOLFE 1978) and in paralyzed and oxygenated rats within 1 min after BCC seizures (CHAPMAN et al. 1977, 1980; Fig. 4). Levels of arachidonic acid were highest at 1 min after seizure onset, but were significantly elevated at 30 and 60 min also (CHAPMAN et al. 1980). Arachidonic acid can be metabolized to prostaglandins and leukotrienes, which may play a role in epileptic brain damage (SIESJO 1981).

F. Metabolic Mechanisms of Neuronal-Cell Damage During Status Epilepticus

I. Role of Extracerebral Factors

Single seizures in adults are not associated with brain damage. The probable explanation is that, while energy reserves are severely reduced, it is a transient phenomenon, and shortly after the seizure discharge energy reserves are restored. However, the situation is entirely different when seizures become continuous. Both brain damage and death are common occurrences during uncontrolled status epilepticus (MELDRUM and HORTON 1973; MELDRUM and BRIERLEY 1973). Death often follows from cardiac arrhythmias most likely resulting from the combination of hypoxemia and intense vagal and sympathetic discharges. Lactic acidosis, arterial hypotension, CO_2 retention, and hyperthermia may also contribute to brain damage and mortality. In such instances, failure to maintain adequate oxygenation of cerebral tissue may lead to gross energy failure and cell damage evident to the histopathologist as ischemic cell change (SCHOLTZ 1959; NORMAN 1964; MELDRUM and BRIERLEY 1973; CORSELLIS 1982). Since most deaths in uncontrolled status epilepticus ensue from systemic factors, immediate therapeutic measures during human status epilepticus are aimed at providing adequate oxygenation, preventing muscular convulsions, and supporting cardiovascular function.

II. Role of Sustained Cell Firing

It is now becoming clear that, while brain damage is more severe and widespread in freely seizing animals (MELDRUM and BRIERLEY 1973), it is also evident in key neuronal populations when the systemic effects of seizure activity are prevented and adequate cerebral blood flow and oxygenation is maintained (MELDRUM et al. 1973; BLENNOW et al. 1978; SODERFELDT et al. 1981).

It is of immediate clinical importance to ascertain the mechanisms of neuronal-cell damage during EEG seizures when cardiovascular and respiratory function is maintained. It is often the case where epileptiform activity is obvious in the EEG while convulsive activity is absent as for example in neonates on respirators or when seizures are continuous but not life threatening as in some cases of complex partial status epilepticus. In such instances, aggressive treatment to prevent prolonged epileptiform activity and the resulting brain damage may be warranted.

After BCC-induced status epilepticus in paralyzed and oxygenated rats, neuronal-cell damage is found extensively in pyramidal cells of the hippocampus and layer 3 of the cerebral cortex and to a lesser extent in the thalamus and striatum (MELDRUM et al. 1973; BLENNOW et al. 1978; SODERFELDT et al. 1981). Purkinje cells in the cerebellum are spared during seizures when animals are paralyzed and oxygenated. Status spongiosis has been described in the cerebral cortex after 1 and 2 h of seizures, and is found predominantly in cortical layer 3 (SODERFELDT et al. 1981). The severity increased with increasing seizure duration.

III. Role of Energy Failure

Seizures are characterized by dramatic increases in cerebral metabolism and, consequently, energy failure would seem an attractive hypothesis to explain neuronal damage. Available evidence suggests that this explains why brain damage develops so quickly during convulsive seizures, with their accompanying anoxemia, lactic acidosis, shock, and failure of cerebral blood flow. Massive cerebral energy failure develops (KING et al. 1967). Initially, increased blood pressure assures increased blood flow, as autoregulation is abolished (PLUM et al. 1974). However, severe lactic acidosis results from the convulsive activity (WASTERLAIN 1974b). It leads to arterial hypotension and to a fall in cerebral blood flow no longer protected by autoregulation (WASTERLAIN 1980). This increases further the oxygen debt and the brain's energy debt, a situation partially reversed by correction of the lactic acidosis (WASTERLAIN 1974b, 1980). However, energy failure cannot explain the neuronal necrosis observed in animals paralyzed and ventilated with oxygen (SODERFELDT et al. 1981). Seizures result in a two- to threefold elevation in the cerebral metabolic rate of glucose and oxygen consumption (CHAPMAN et al. 1975; MELDRUM and NILSSON 1976; BORGSTROM et al. 1976; SIESJO and ABDUL-RAHMAN 1979; HAWKINS et al. 1979). Parallel increases in cerebral blood flow accompany elevated rates of glucose utilization. SIESJO (1982) postulated that a mismatch between blood flow and metabolic rate may result in local energy failure, and indeed has shown that while metabolic rate of glucose utilization remains elevated in cortex and hippocampus, local cerebral blood flow falls between 20 and 120 min. HOWSE (1981) showed cell damage in the area of highest metabolic activation such as substantia nigra. However, it is clear that energy charge potential is upheld in these regions even at 120 min (FOLBERGROVA et al. 1981) when extensive histopathological evidence for cell damage is evident (SODERFELDT et al. 1981). Furthermore, it is known from experimental hypoglycemia that energy failure does not always lead to cell damage (AGARDH et al. 1981; AGARDH and SIESJO 1981).

If energy failure is not a cause of brain damage, then the answer may lie in the metabolic response of cells to elevated rates of energy metabolism required to sustain massive neuronal discharges.

IV. Lactic Acidosis

Accumulation of lactic acid in cells has long been held to be an important factor in brain damage from perinatal anoxic-ischemic insults (MYERS 1977).

Several studies show that elevated blood glucose increases mortality from cerebral ischemia in rat (SIEMKOWICZ and HANSEN 1978; SIEMKOWICZ 1981) and that recovery of cerebral blood flow, glucose utilization, and cerebral metabolites in cat brain after a period of ischemia was poor if blood glucose was elevated by glucose pretreatment (GINSBERG et al. 1980; WELSH et al. 1980). These results have been confirmed in rat brain where tissue damage following ischemia was correlated with the degree of tissue lactic acidosis (REHNCRONA et al. 1981; KALIMO et al. 1981a, b). Levels of lactic acid associated with ischemic cell damage are well in excess of 20 μmol/g. Such high levels are not found during status epilepticus as long as cerebral perfusion and oxygenation are adequate so that tissue lactic acidosis is not a likely cause of seizure-induced brain damage. This is particularly true in the neonate, where lactate is easily transported from brain to blood by the lactate carrier, abundant in the blood-brain barrier of suckling animals.

V. Calcium "Cytotoxicity"

MELDRUM (1982) and SIESJO (1981) recently proposed a mechanism by which abormally large entry of calcium into selectively vulnerable cells during seizures would lead to cell death. Calcium has previously been implicated in heart and liver cytotoxicity (WROGEMANN and PENA 1976; SCHANNE et al. 1979).

Sustained entry of Ca^{2+} into neurons can occur as a result of burst firing in these neurons associated with a paroxysmal depolarization shift in membrane potential during epileptic seizures (SCHWARTZKROIN and WYLER 1979). When the ability of the cell to maintain low intracellular Ca^{2+} levels is exceeded, it has been postulated that accumulation of Ca^{2+} results in swollen and possibly damaged mitochondria (although actual damage in isolated mitochondria has never been demonstrated) and in activation of intracellular lipases and proteases which leads to ischemic cell change and neuronal death. It is not clear whether or how energy failure intervenes in this process as a result of mitochondrial Ca^{2+} accumulation and concomitant swelling. One attractive aspect of this hypothesis is that it suggests a reason why cerebellar Purkinje cells are not damaged during prolonged seizures when animals are paralyzed and oxygenated. It is suggested that burst firing in neurons, which enhances Ca^{2+} influx, requires an excitatory input. Burst firing in cerebellar Purkinje cells, which can be induced by excitatory afferent stimulation resulting from peripheral motor activity, is absent in paralyzed animals and so is Purkinje-cell damage. Aspects of this hypothesis are testable. Presumably drugs which limit intracellular Ca^{2+} accumulation should reduce seizure-related brain damage. Secondly, stimulation of Purkinje-cell afferents, which cause burst firing in this cell population (and presumably Ca^{2+} influx as well), may be expected to result in cerebellar Purkinje-cell damage during prolonged seizures in paralyzed and oxygenated rats.

A primary role for Ca^{2+} ion has also been envisioned by SIESJO (1981, 1983). Increased intracellular Ca^{2+} resulting from the repetitive seizure discharge would overwhelm cell mechanisms which sequester Ca in the cell or extrude it to the extracellular space. These processes divert respiratory energy which would otherwise be utilized for ATP production. Increased intracellular Ca^{2+} activates various hydrolases, including phospholipase A_2, resulting in accumulation of free fatty acids including a manyfold increase in arachidonic acid (BAZAN 1976; CHAPMAN et al. 1980). Increased extracellular K^+ released from neurons during the seizure is taken up into the glia. This and the free fatty acid accumulation may contribute to the swelling of astrocyte processes observed during sustained seizures (SODERFELDT et al. 1981). Since K^+ uptake into astrocytes is O_2 dependent, this and astrocyte swelling may further impede delivery of energy substrate to neurons. Lastly, the increased accumulation of arachidonic acid in the presence of O_2 may result in the formation of prostaglandins and leukotrienes (via cyclooxygenase and lipoxygenase, respectively) possibly contributing to microcirculatory problems and to the formation of cell-damaging free radicals.

Purkinje cells have a high Ca^{2+} conductance, and, like MELDRUM (1981), SIESJO (1981) makes the assumption that the voltage-dependent Ca^{2+} influx in these cerebellar Purkinje cells is only moderate, sparing them from damage. Reduced accumulation of free fatty acids in the cerebellum during seizures (SIESJO 1982) may also contribute to the sparing effect. This exciting hypothesis, however, does not explain all the available data. The well-documented finding that energy failure does not occur during seizures would argue against the proposition that ion pumping or edema may impede substrate supply and neuronal energy metabolism. Direct evidence for damaging free radical formation during seizures is lacking at present and would hardly explain why brain damage is accelerated by anoxia, which reduces free radical formation.

G. Epileptic Seizures in the Neonate

The neonatal brain is physiologically quite different from that of the adult. Current evidence indicates that it is in some ways protected from the damaging effects of seizures but in other ways is more vulnerable. Possibly the most important factor protecting the neonate's brain is that cerebral metabolic rate and energy requirements are low, possibly 1/10–1/20 of that of the adult's brain. However, epileptic seizures can elevate cerebral metabolic rate nearly fourfold in the neonate's brain (WASTERLAIN and DWYER 1982), and this relative increase is similar to what is found in the adult brain (CHAPMAN et al. 1975; BORGSTROM et al. 1976; MELDRUM and NELSON 1976; ABDUL-RAHMAN et al. 1979) even if the absolute metabolic rate is relatively low. A second protective factor in the newborn is the presence in the blood-brain barrier of large amounts of lactate carrier (CREMER et al. 1976, 1979) so that lactate produced in brain easily escapes into blood as long as circulation to the brain is maintained. Lactate concentrations in brain during neonatal seizures have never been found to reach levels associated with cell damage (WASTERLAIN and DUFFY 1976, WASTERLAIN and DWYER 1982).

Several factors, however, place the neonatal brain at great risk during seizures: first, its supply of glucose is more precarious than that in the adult. Second, protein synthesis and growth, two energy-intensive processes that are easily compromised by metabolic stress, are a necessity for its harmonious development.

I. Mobilization of Glycogen Reserves

Glycogen reserves in the neonate are as great as in the adult (VANNUCCI and VANNUCCI 1980). They can sustain cerebral energy demands for significantly longer periods during hypoxic episodes and seizures. The ability to mobilize glycogen reserves in the neonatal brain may be less than in the adult owing to lower levels of phosphorylase and phosphoglucomutase (VANNUCCI and VANNUCCI 1980; SHAPIRO and WERTHEIMER 1943) and during seizures owing to a lower accumulation of cyclic adenosine monophosphate (cAMP) (WASTERLAIN 1978) necessary for activation of a protein kinase to transform phosphorylase B to phosphorylase A, which is active in glycogenolysis. In spite of this slow mobilization, glycogen is able to provide significant amounts of substrate for meeting cerebral energy requirements (VANNUCCI and VANNUCCI 1980; WASTERLAIN and DWYER 1982). When seizures are prolonged, however, they may be insufficient and brain glucose can rapidly become depleted in the neonate.

II. Limited Transport Capacity of the Blood-brain Barrier

The problem lies in the low capacity for glucose transport across the immature blood-brain barrier. Its maximal rate has been estimated at one-fifth the rate of the adult (MOORE et al. 1971). On the other hand, glycolytic rates can be relatively high (Table 5). Thus in spite of normal or elevated blood glucose levels, brain glucose rapidly falls after onset of seizures in newborn rats, rabbits, and marmosets (WASTERLAIN and DUFFY 1976; WASTERLAIN and DWYER 1982), possibly reaching levels which are rate limiting for brain hexokinase and hence energy production.

Table 5. Cerebral energy balance during neonatal seizures

Blood (Glucose	27 mg-%	90 mg-%	200 mg-%
Max. rate of glycolysis (nmol ~ P/kg/min)[a]	0.69	0.69	0.69
Max. rate of glucose transport (nmol/kg/min)	0.072	0.168	0.24
Max. rate of glycolysis from glucose transported across the blood-brain barrier (nmol ~ P/kg)	0.144	0.336	0.48
Energy reserves (nmol ~ P/kg)	24	24	24
Max. rate of reserve mobilization (nmol ~ P/kg)	0.37	0.37	0.37
Energy balance			
Calculated	− 0.176	+ 0.016	+ 0.160
Measured	Negative	– − 0.028	Positive
(nmol ~ P/kg/min)			

[a] ~, high-energy phosphate bonds

Table 6. Blood glucose concentration and transport across the blood-brain barrier

$V = \frac{V_{max} \times (S)}{K_m + (S)}$	$K_m = \mathrm{m}M$
Blood (glucose)	(Transport rate)
27 mg% = 1.8 mM	18% V_{max} = 0.07 mmol/kg/min
90 mg% = 5 mM	42% V_{max} = 0.17 mmol/kg/min
200 mg% = 11 mM	61% V_{max} = 0.24 mmol/kg/min

The healthy, suckling neonate's brain may attain as much as one-third of its energy from ketone bodies, which cannot be utilized in anoxic states (such as convulsive seizures) because molecular oxygen is needed to regenerate NAD^+ from NADH. This increases the brain's reliance on glucose during seizures and anoxia, and makes glucose supply even more critical.

Since the K_m for glucose transport into brain is about 7 mM, the carrier is less than half saturated at physiological blood glucose concentrations (5 mM). Increasing blood glucose levels can increase transport of glucose from blood to brain as shown in Table 6 and prevent brain glucose depletion in neonatal rats, rabbits, and marmosets during seizures (Fig. 5). Thus glucose supplements may offer a strategy to protect the brain of human neonates during seizures. The role of glucose supplements in maintaining adequate cerebral energy supplies during seizures has been extensively discussed elsewhere (WASTERLAIN and DWYER 1982).

It should be kept in mind that other factors may play a role in normal brain development. Thus seizures during the neonatal period, even where not causing cell loss (WASTERLAIN 1976), may contribute to brain damage by inhibiting cell growth (JORGENSEN et al. 1980; DWYER and WASTERLAIN 1982) and brain pro-

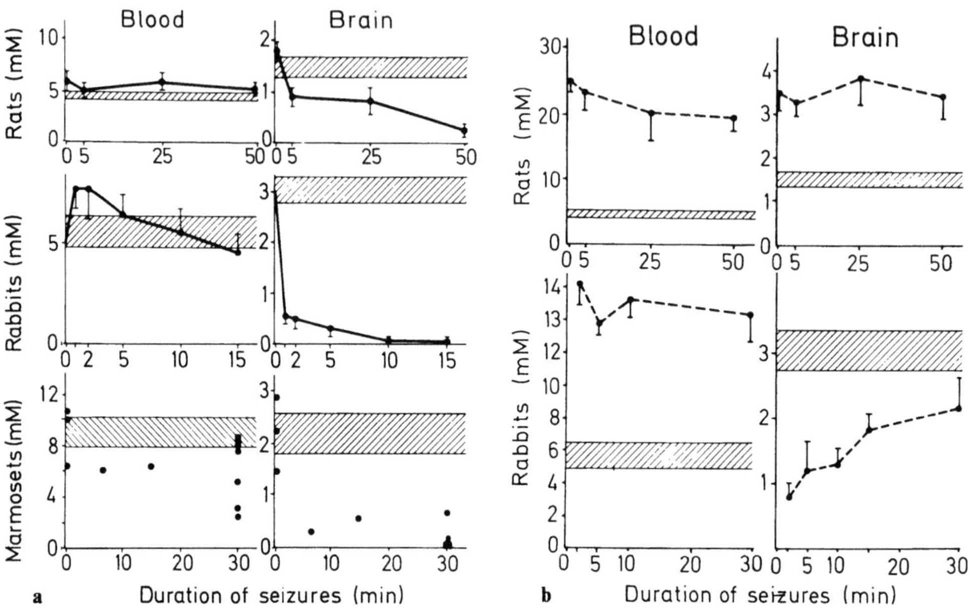

Fig. 5 a, b. Blood and brain glucose concentration during status epilepticus in the newborn. Epileptic seizures were induced in 4-day-old rats by exposure to the volatile convulsant flurothyl and in 1-day-old rabbits and 5-day-old marmoset monkeys with BCC. The results shown in **a** were obtained from animals which were pretreated with isotonic saline 30 min prior to seizure activity (rats: 10% of body weight, i.p.; rabbits: 5% of body weight s.c.). Marmosets were not pretreated before seizures. **b** shows the effects of seizures on blood and brain glucose in rats and rabbits which had been pretreated with isotonic glucose 30 min before seizures were induced (rats: 10% of body weight, i.p.; rabbits: 5% of body weight, s.c.). The *Hatched areas* represent the mean ± SE of untreated controls

tein synthesis (DWYER and WASTERLAIN 1980) or by disrupting the chronology of numerous processes whose close coordination is required for proper development of the nervous system.

Acknowledgement. This work was supported by research grant # NS 13515 from NINCDS and the Research Service of the Veterans Administration.

References

Agardh CD, Siesjo BK (1981) Hypoglycemic brain injury: phospholipids, free fatty acids, and cyclic nucleotides in the cerebellum of the rat after 30 and 60 minutes of severe insulin-induced hypoglycemia. J Cereb Blood Flow Metabol 1:267–275

Agardh CD, Kalino H, Olsson Y, Siesjo BK (1981) Hypoglycemic brain injury: metabolic and structural findings in rat cerebellar cortex during profound insulin induced hypoglycemia and in the recovery period following glucose administration. J Cereb Blood Flow Metabol 1:71–84

Atkinson DE (1968) The energy charge of the adenylate pool as a regulatory parameter. Interaction with biofeedback modifiers. Biochemistry 7:4030–4034

Bazan NG (1976) Free arachidonic acid and other lipids in the nervous system during early ischemia and after electroshock. In: Porcellati G, Amaducci L, Galli C (eds) Function and metabolism of phospholipids in the central and peripheral nervous system. Adv Exp Med Biol 72:317–335

Blennow G, Brierley JB, Meldrum BS; Siesjo BK (1978) Epileptic brain damage. The role of systemic factors that modify cerebral energy metabolism. Brain 101:687–700

Blennow G, Folbergrova J, Nilsson B, Siesjo BK (1979) Effects of bicuculline-induced seizures on cerebral metabolism and circulation of rats rendered hypoglycemic by starvation. Ann Neurol 5:139–151

Borgstrom L, Chapman AG, Siesjo BK (1976) Glucose consumption in the cerebral cortex of rat during bicuculline-induced status epilepticus. J Neurochem 27:971–973

Carl JL, King LJ (1970) Hexose and pentose phosphates in brain during convulsions. J Neurochem 17:293–295

Chapman AG, Meldrum BS, Siesjo BK (1975) Cerebral blood flow and cerebral metabolic rate during prolonged epileptic seizures in rats. J Physiol (Lond) 254:61–62P

Chapman AG, Meldrum BS, Siesjo BK (1977) Cerebral metabolic changes during prolonged epileptic seizures in rats. J Neurochem 28:1025–1035

Chapman A, Ingvar M, Siesjo BK (1980) Free fatty acids in the brain in bicuculline-induced status epilepticus. Acta Physiol Scand 110:335–336

Collins RC, Posner JB, Plum F (1970) Cerebral energy metabolism during electroshock seizures in mice. Am J Physiol 218:943–950

Copley M, Fromm HJ (1967) Kinetic studies of the brain hexokinase reaction. A reinvestigation with the solubilized bovine enzyme. Biochemistry 6:3503–3509

Corsellis JAN (1983) Neuropathology of status epilepticus. In: Delgado-Escueta AV, Wasterlain C, Treiman D, Porter R (eds) States epilepticus. Raven, New York

Cotman CW, Banker G, Zornetzer SF, McGaugh JL (1971) Electroshock effects on brain protein synthesis: relation to brain seizures and retrograde amnesia. Science 173:454–456

Cremer JE, Braun LD, Oldendorf WH (1976) Changes during development in transport processes of the blood-brain barrier. Biochim Biophys Acta 448:633–637

Cremer JE, Cunningham VJ, Pardridge WM, Braun LD, Oldendorf WH (1979) Kinetics of blood-brain barrier transport of pyruvate, lactate and glucose in suckling, weanling, and adult rat. J Neurochem 33:439–445

De Courten GM, Myers RE, Yamaguchi S (1981) Serum glucose concentration as determiner of brain pathologic response to marked hypoxia with hypotension. Neurology 31:131

Duffy TE, Howse DC, Plum F (1975) Cerebral energy metabolism during experimental status epilepticus. J Neurochem 24:95–934

Dwyer BE, Wasterlain CG (1980) Regulation of the first step of the initiation of brain protein synthesis by guanosine diphosphate. J Neurochem 34:1639–1647

Dwyer BE, Wasterlain CG (1981) Prolonged seizures deplete brain glucose in normoglycemic neonates. Neurology 31:162

Dwyer BE, Wasterlain CG (1982) Electroconvulsive seizures selectively impair myelin accumulation in the immature rat. Exp Neurol 78:616–628

Dwyer BE, Donatoni P, Wasterlain CG (1982) The effect of status epilepticus on local rates of brain protein synthesis. Trans Am Soc Neurochem 12:115

Ferrendelli JA, McDougal DB Jr (1971 a) The effect of audiogenic seizures on regional CNS energy reserves, glycolysis and citric acid cycle flux. J Neurochem 18:1207–1220

Ferrendelli JA, McDougal DB Jr (1971 b) The effect of electroshock on regional CNS energy reserves in mice. J Neurochem 18:1197–1205

Folbergrova J (1974) Energy metabolism of mouse cerebral cortex during homocysteine convulsions. Brain Res 81:443–454

Folbergrova J, Passonneau JV, Lowry OH, Schulz DW (1969) Glycogen, ammonia and related metabolites in the brain during seizures evoked by methionine sulphoximine. J Neurochem 16:191–203

Folbergrova J, Ingvar M, Siesjo BK (1981) Metabolic changes in cerebral cortex, hippocampus, and cerebellum during sustained bicuculline-induced seizures. J Neurochem 37:1228–1238

Fromm HJ, Zewe V (1962) Kinetic studies of the brain hexokinase reaction. J Biol Chem 237:1661–1667

Ginsberg MD, Welsh FA, Budd WW (1980) Deleterious effect of glucose pretreatment on recovery from diffuse cerebral ischemia in the cat. I. Local cerebral blood flow and glucose utilization. Stroke 11:347–354

Hawkins R, Hass WK, Ransohoff J (1979) Measurement of regional brain glucose utilization in vivo using [2-^{14}C] glucose. Stroke 10:690–703

Howse DCN (1979) Metabolic responses to status epilepticus in the rat, cat and mouse. Can J Physiol Pharmacol 57:205–212

Howse DCN (1983) Cerebral energy metabolism during experimental status eplilepticus. In: Delgado-Escueta AV, Wasterlain C, Treiman D, Porter R (eds) Status epilepticus. Raven, New York

Howse DC, Duffy TE (1975) Control of the redox state of the pyridine nucleotides in the rat cerebral cortex. Effect of electroshock-induced seizures. J Neurochem 24:935–940

Howse DC, Caronna JJ, Duffy TE, Plum F (1974) Cerebral energy metabolism, pH and blood flow during seizures in the cat. Am J Physiol 227:1444–1451

Jorgensen OS, Dwyer BE, Wasterlain CG (1980) Synaptic proteins after electroconvulsive seizures in immature rats. J Neurochem 35:1235–1237

Kalimo H, Rehncrona S, Soderfeldt B (1981 a) the role of lactic acidosis in the ischemic nerve cell injury. Acta Neuropathol (Berl) [Suppl] 7:20–22

Kalimo H, Rehncrona S, Soderfeldt B, Olsson Y, Siesjo BK (1981 a) Brain lactic acidosis and ischemic cell damage: 2. Histopathology. J Cereb Blood Flow Metabol 1:313–327

Kalimo H, Rehncrona S, Soderfeldt B (1981 b) The role of lactic acidosis in the ischemic nerve cell injury. Acta Neuropathol [Suppl VII]:20–22

King LJ, Carl JL, Lao L (1973) Carbohydrate metabolism in brain during convulsions and its modification by phenobarbitone. J Neurochem 20:477–485

King LJ, Lowry OH, Passonneau J, Venson V (1967) Effects of convulsants on energy reserves in the cerebral cortex. J Neurochem 14:599–611

Knull HR, Taylor WF, Wells WW (1973) Effects of energy metabolism on in vivo distribution of hexokinase in brain. J Biol Chem 248:5414–5417

Krebs HA, Veech RL (1970) Regulation of the redox state of the pyridine nucleotide in rat liver in pyridine nucleotide-dependent dehydrogenases. In:Sund H (ed) Pyridine nucleotide dependent dehydrogenases. Springer, Berlin Heidelberg New York, pp 413–434

Lowry OH, Passonneau JV (1964) The relationship between substrate and enzymes of glycolysis in brain. J Biol Chem 239:31–42

Maker HS, Lehrer GM (1972) Carbohydrate chemistry in the brain. In: Albers RW, Siegel GJ, Katzman R, Agranoff BW (eds) Basic neurochemistry. Little Brown, Boston

Maker HS, Clarke DD, Lajtha A (1976) Intermediary metabolism of carbohydrates and amino acids. In: Siegel GJ, Albers RW, Katzman R, Agranoff BW (eds) Basic neurochemistry. Little Brown, Boston, pp 279–307

Marion J, Wolfe LS (1978) Increase in vivo of unesterified fatty acids prostaglandin $F_{2\alpha}$ but not thromboxane B_2 in rat brain during drug induced convulsions. Prostaglandins 16:99–110

McCandless DW, Feussner GK, Lust WD, Passonneau JV (1979) Metabolite levels in brain following experimental seizures: the effects of maximal electroshock and phenytoin in cerebellar layers. J Neurochem 32:743–753

McGilvery RW (1979) In: Biochemistry. A functional approach. Saunders, Philadelphia, p 719

Meldrum BS (1983) Metabolic factors during prolonged seizures and their relation to nerve cell death. In: Delgado-Escueta AV, Wasterlain C, Treiman D, Porter R (eds) Status epilepticus. Raven, New York

Meldrum BS, Brierley JB (1973) Prolonged epileptic seizures in primates. Ischemic cell change and its relation to ictal physiological events. Arch Neurol 28:10–17

Meldrum BS, Horton RW (1973) Physiology of status epilepticus in primates. Arch Neurol 28:1–9

Meldrum BS, Nilsson B (1976) Cerebral blood flow and metabolic rate early and late in prolonged epileptic seizures induced in rats by bicuculline. Brain 99:523–542

Meldrum BS, Vigoroux RA, Brierley JB (1973) Systemic factors and epileptic brain damage. Prolonged seizures in paralyzed, artificially ventilated baboons. Arch Neurol 29:82–87
Moore TJ, Lione AP, Regen DM, Tarpley HL, Raines PL (1971) Brain glucose metabolism in the newborn rat. Am J Physiol 221:1746–1753
Myers RE (1977) Experimental models of perinatal brain damage: relevance to human pathology. In: Intrauterine asphyxia in the developing fetal brain. Gluck L (ed) Yearbook Medical, Chicago, pp 37–97
Nahorski SR, Roberts DJ, Stewart GG (1970) Some neurochemical aspects of pentamethylenetetrazole convulsive activity in rat brain. J Neurochem 17:621–631
Norman RM (1964) The neuropathology of status epilepticus. Med Sci Law 4:46–51
Plum F, Howse DC, Duffy TE (1974) Metabolic effects of seizures in brain dysfunction in metabolic disorders. Plum F (ed) Res Publ Assoc Nerv Ment Dis 53:141–157
Rehncrona S, Rosen I, Seisjo BK (1981) Brain lactic acidosis and ischemic cell damage: 1. Biochemistry and neurophysiology. J Cereb Blood Flow Metabol 1:297–311
Sacktor B, Wilson JE, Tiekert CG (1966) Regulation of glycolysis in brain, in situ, during convulsions. J Biol Chem 241:5071–5075
Schanne FAX, Kane AB, Young EE, Farber JL (1979) Calcium dependence of toxic cell death: a final common pathway. Science 206:700–702
Scholtz W (1959) The contribution of patho-anatomical research to the problem of epilepsy. Epilepsia 1:36–55
Schwartzkroin PA, Wyler AR (1979) Mechanisms underlying epileptiform burst discharges. Ann Neurol 7:95–107
Shapiro B, Wertheimer E (1943) Phosphorolysis and synthesis of glycogen in animal tissues. Biochem J 37:397–403
Siesjo BK (1981) Cell damage in the brain: a speculative synthesis. J Cereb Blood Flow Metabol 1:155–185
Siesjo BK (1983) Local cerebral circulation and metabolism in bicuculline-induced status epilepticus: relevance for development of cell damage. In: Dalgado-Escueta AV, Wasterlain C, Treiman D, Porter R (eds) Status epilepticus. Raven
Siesjo BK, Abdul-Rahman A (1979) A metabolic basis for the selective vulnerability of neurons in status epilepticus. Acta Physiol Scand 106:377–378
Siemkowicz E (1981) Hyperglycemia in the reperfusion period hampers recovery from cerebral ischemia. Acta Neurol Scand 64:207–216
Siemkowicz E, Hansen AJ (1978) Clinical restitution following cerebral ischemia in hypo-, normo- and hyperglycemica rats. Acta Neurol Scand 58:1–8
Soderfeldt B, Kalino H, Olsson Y, Siesjo BK (1981) Pathogenesis of brain lesions caused by experimental epilepsy. Light and electronmicroscopic changes in the rat cerebral cortex following bicuculline induced status epilepticus. Acta Neuropathol (Berl) 54:219–231
Stubbs M, Veech RL, Krebs HA (1972) Control of the redox state of the nicotinamide-adenine dinucleotide couple in rat liver cytoplasm. Biochem J 126:59–65
Tuttle JB, Wilson JE (1970) Rat brain hexokinase: a kinetic comparison of soluble and particulate forms. Biochim Biophys Acta 212:185–188
Vannucci SJ, Vannucci RC (1980) Glycogen metabolism in neonatal rat brain during anoxia and recovery. J Neurochem 34:1100–1105
Vesco C, Giuditta A (1968) Disaggregation of brain polysomes induced by electroconvulsive treatment. J Neurochem 15:81–85
Wasterlain CG (1974a) Inhibition of cerebral protein synthesis by epileptic seizures without motor manifestations. Neurology 14:175–180
Wasterlain CG (1974b) Mortality and morbidity from serial seizures. An experimental study. Epilepsia 15:155–176
Wasterlain CG (1976) Effects of neonatal status epilepticus on rat brain development. Neurology 26:975–986
Wasterlain CG (1977) Effects of epileptic seizures on brain ribosomes: mechanism and relationship to cerebral energy metabolism. J Neurochem 29:707–716
Wasterlain CG (1978) Neonatal seizures and brain growth. Neuropädiatrie 9:213–228

Wasterlain CG, Duffy TE (1976) Status epilepticus in immature rats. Arch Neurol 33:821–827
Wasterlain CG, Dwyer BE (1983) Brain metabolism during prolonged seizures in the neonate. In: Status epilepticus. Delgado-Escueta AV, Wasterlain C, Treiman D, Porter R (eds). Raven, New York
Wasterlain CG, Graham SL (1980) Loss of autoregulation of cerebral blood flow: an asset during single seizures, a liability during status epilepticus. Ann Neurol 8:94
Welsh FA, Ginsberg MD, Rieder W, Budd WW (1980) Deleterious effect of glucose pretreatment on recovery from diffuse cerebral ischemia in the cat. II. Regional metabolite levels. Stroke 11:355–363
Whisler KE, Tews JK, Stone WE (1968) Cerebral amino acids and lipids in drug-induced status epilepticus. J Neurochem 15:315–320
Wilson JE (1968) Brain hexokinase. A proposed relation between soluble-particulate distribution and activity in vivo. J Biol Chem 243:3640–3647
Wrogemann K, Pena SDJ (1976) Mitochondrial calcium overload: a general mechanism for cell-necrosis in muscle diseases. Lancet 1:672–674

CHAPTER 5

Monoamines and the Pathophysiology of Seizure Disorders

E. PRZEGALIŃSKI

A. Introduction

One of the ways of understanding the pathophysiology of seizure disorders is by learning about the effects of the various factors that modulate susceptibility to seizures in experimental conditions. Obviously, neurochemical factors come into prominence here, and among them neuromediators attract especial interest. In this chapter, some of these will be reviewed, namely the monoamines, i.e., the catecholamines (noradrenaline and dopamine) serotonin (5-hydroxytrytamine), and histamine.

Interest in the role of the central monoamines in seizures dates back to the discovery of CHEN et al. (1954), who found that reserpine lowers the seizure threshold to various seizure-provoking agents [electrical current, pentylenetetrazol (PTZ), caffeine], and to the subsequent discovery by others that this drug also lowers the levels of catecholamines and 5-hydroxytrytamine (5-HT) in brain. Since then, with an increasing number of new drugs and substances which modulate the activity of the central monoaminergic systems and with the introduction of new experimental models, this problem has become the subject of numerous publications and of several reviews (e.g., BOGGAN 1973; LOVELL 1971; MAYNERT 1969; MAYNERT et al. 1975).

There are many experimental approaches to the study of the role of brain monoamines in seizures. The most common method used is based on pharmacological intervention in the function of a monoaminergic system and subsequent observation of how this affects seizures induced by various agents. With other methods, susceptibility to seizures is determined in animals which are known to differ with respect to the level and turnover rate of monoamines; or, conversely, the levels and turnover rate of monoamines are determined in animals with different susceptibilities to seizures. The present review is based mainly on results obtained with the above-outlined experimental procedures; it will not, however, deal with studies on the effect of compounds modulating monoaminergic system in the action of antiepileptic drugs, or the effect of the latter on the disposition of brain monoamines, because this type of study is more suitable for assessing the role of neuromediators in the mechanism of action of antiepileptics than for studying the actual phenomenon of seizures.

Pharmacological intervention in the function of monoaminergic systems is based on the employment of drugs or substances which affect neurotransmission; this is regarded as a process of the release of neurotransmitter from the nerve terminals into the synaptic cleft and its subsequent interaction with postsynaptic receptors. In this way, substances that decrease or increase the concentration of a neuromediator at the receptor inhibit or facilitate neurotransmission, respectively. The use of drugs which directly stimulate (agonist) or block (antagonist) postsynaptic receptors is another way in which neurotransmission can be affected.

Within the catecholaminergic system, neurotransmission can be inhibited with compounds that prevent storage [reserpine, tetrabenazine, 2-hydroxy-2-ethyl-3-isobutyl-9,10-dimethoxy-1,2,3,4,6,7-hexahydro-11b*H*-benzoquinolizine (Ro 4-1284)], inhibit synthesis [the inhibitor of tyrosine hydroxylase – α-methyl-*p*-tyrosine (α-MT); inhibitors of aromatic L-amino acid decarboxylase – α-methyl-*m*-tyrosine (α-MMT), α-methyl-3,4-dihydroxyphenylalanine (α-methyl-DOPA), and others; inhibitors of DA-β-hydroxylase – disulfiram, diethyldithiocarbamate (DDC), (bis(4-methyl-1-homopiperazinylthiocarbonyl)disulfide) (Fla-63)], damage catecholaminergic nerve terminals [6-hydroxydopamine (6-OHDA), 6-hydroxy-DOPA (6-OHDOPA)], or block postsynaptic NA receptors (e.g., phenoxybenzamine, phentolamine – blockers of α-adrenoceptors) propranolol – (a blocker of β-adrenoceptors) or DA receptors (neuroleptics, i.e., haloperidol, pimozide). The facilitation of catecholaminergic transmission results from the action of inhibitors of enzymatic degradation of catecholamines [inhibitors of monoamine oxidase (MAO) or catechol-*O*-methyl transferase]; precursor (DOPA); releasers (e.g., amphetamine); inhibitors of uptake (imipramine, desmethylimipramine, cocaine); agonists of NA (e.g., clonidine) or DA receptors (e.g., apomorphine); and the amines (NA and DA) themselves. The amines, as well as 6-OHDA, must be administered intracerebroventricularly (i.c.v.) or intracisternally because of the impermeability of the blood-brain barrier.

The inhibition of neurotransmission within the 5-HT system is brought about most often with *p*-chlorophenylalanine (PCPA), which is an inhibitor of tryptophan hydroxylase; 5,6-dihydroxytryptamine (5,6-DHT) or 5,7-dihydroxytryptamine (5,7-DHT), both of which cause damage to 5-HT nerve terminals; and 5-HT receptor blockers (cyproheptadine, methysergide, metergoline). To facilitate 5-HT transmission, precursors [tryptophan, 5-hydroxytryptophan (5-HTP)], releasers (e.g., fenfluramine, *p*-chloroamphetamine), inhibitors of the reuptake (e.g., fluoxetine), 5-HT receptor agonists [lysergic acid diethylamide (LSD), quipazine, *m*-chlorophenyl-piperazine], or 5-HT itself (i.c.v. or intracisternally) are used.

When analyzing the results of investigations with the above-listed compounds and drugs used as pharmacological tools their limitations should be borne in mind. For instance, the majority of substances which interfere with catecholaminergic transmission simultaneously affect the NA and DA system. Moreover, some substances (storage inhibitors, inhibitors of aromatic L-amino acid decarboxylase, MAO inhibitors, some reuptake inhibitors, e.g., imipramine) also modify the 5-HT system; DOPA can be decarboxylated not only in catecholaminergic but also in 5-HT neurons and can subsequently release 5-HT (in analogy with the effct of DOPA, 5-HTP may release catecholamines). Only inhibitors of DA-β-hydroxylase (which selectively lower levels of NA), some uptake inhibitors (e.g., desmethylimipramine), and agonists and antagonists of catecholamine receptors may be regarded as relatively specific pharmacological tools. Among the compounds affecting the serotonergic system a number of 5-HT antagonists also have cholinolytic and antihistaminic activities.

The inhibition or facilitation of neurotransmission may also be obtained with electrical lesions or electrical stimulation of cell bodies of neurons which produce a neuromediator (the locus ceruleus for NA, the substantia nigra for DA, and the raphe nuclei for 5-HT).

The second component in the study of the role of central monoamines in convulsive phenomena is the assessment of susceptibility to seizures. For this purpose seizures are evoked in laboratory animals by various agents (electrical current, chemical compounds, sound, light, etc.). Moreover, some experimental models are used in forms which enable separate components of convulsive behavior (clonus, tonus) or involvement of particular brain structures (e.g., amygdaloid kindling) to be assessed. Since many data indicate that the involvement of central monoamines in susceptibility to seizures may depend on a particular agent evoking seizures or on the type of seizures evoked, the problem of the involvement of central monoamines in susceptibility to seizures will be discussed here seperately with reference to each experimental model.

B. Catecholamines

I. Electrically Induced Seizures

1. Minimal Electroshock Seizure Threshold (EST)

a) Low-Frequency EST

In mice, depletion of brain catecholamines does not influence susceptibility to seizures in this model. CHEN et al. (1954) reported a decrease in the seizure threshold after the administration of reserpine, but they used a high dose of the drug (8 mg/kg). Other authors (BUTERBAUGH and LONDON 1977; YEOH and WOLF 1968) administered reserpine at lower doses (2–2.5 mg/kg), but still high enough to produce a severe depletion of brain catecholamines (and 5-HT), and found it to be ineffective. Moreover, the lack of effect was shown after the administration of other depletors of catecholamines, i.e., α-MMT (YEOH and WOLF 1968) and α-MT (BUTERBAUGH and LONDON 1977).

On the other hand, the α-1 adrenoceptor antagonist phenoxybenzamine was found to decrease the seizure threshold in mice (YEOH and WOLF 1968), but the specificity of this effect is doubtful as it was shown only for a very high dose of the drug (37 mg/kg) and since it could not be demonstrated in animals depleted of brain catecholamines by reserpine or α-MMT. Actually, if the effect of phenoxybenzamine depended on α-1 blockade, then catecholamine depletors should rather potentiate it. The same authors also reported alterations in the seizure threshold after the administration of drugs acting on the β-receptor. They found a decrease in the threshold after the administration of β-receptor agonist isoprenaline and an increase after β-receptor antagonists (propranolol and pronethalol). But again, these effects were shown after very high doses of the drugs and the effects induced by isoprenaline and pronethalol – but not by propranolol – were antagonized by reserpine or α-MMT. Moreover, isoprenaline – like other drugs in their experiments – was given systemically, so its effect, because of poor penetration into the brain, may originate mainly from the periphery.

GERALD and RIFFEE (1973) studied the effects of *d*- and *l*-amphetamine. Both isomers, given at a high dose of 15 mg/kg, decreased the seizure threshold, and since *d*-amphetamine was only about twice as active as the *l*-isomer, the authors suggested that the dopaminergic rather than the noradrenergic mechanism is involved.

In the light of all the data presented above the participation of central catecholamines in the low-frequency EST seems doubtful. The deficit in brain catecholamines is of no importance, whereas those few positive effects observed after noradrenergic agonists and antagonists do not seem to be sufficiently specific. The hypothesis of the involvement of the dopaminergic system (GERALD and RIFFEE 1973) should be verified by more specific means.

b) High-Frequency EST

The impairment of catecholaminergic transmission decreases the seizure threshold in mice and rats. This was shown not only after reserpine (AZZARO et al. 1972; BUTERBAUGH and LONDON 1977; PICCHIONI et al. 1962; WENGER et al. 1973) and tetrabenazine (AZZARO et al. 1972), which deplete both catecholamines and 5-HT, but also after α-MT (BUTERBAUGH 1978; BUTERBAUGH and LONDON 1977) or intracisternally administered 6-OHDA (BROWNING and MAYNERT 1978 b), which reduce brain levels of NA and DA and leave the concentration of brain 5-HT unchanged. Although time-response studies have shown a lack of correlation between reserpine- or tetrabenazine-induced increase in susceptibility to seizures and the depletion of brain catecholamines produced by these drugs (AZZARO et al. 1972; PICCHIONI et al. 1962), there is some evidence that their pharmacological effect may depend on the deficit of central NA and/or DA. Thus, AZZARO et al. (1972) found that DOPA given alone or in combination with a MAO inhibitor antagonized the reserpine-induced decrease in the threshold, and AZZARO et al. (1972) and WENGER et al. (1973) reported that inhibitors of catecholamine synthesis (α-MT and disulfiram) prolong this effect of reserpine. The finding that the inhibitor of DA-β-hydroxylase disulfiram produces the same effect as does the inhibitor of tyrosine hydroxylase α-MT may indicate the importance of NA but not DA.

On the other hand there are some data which are not in line with the above results. PICCHIONI et al. (1962) found that the MAO inhibitor iproniazid did not influence the minimal seizure threshold in rats at a time when maximum increase in the brain levels of NA and 5-HT (DA not measured) occurred and when the threshold for maximal seizures was enhanced. Moreover, BROWNING and MAYNERT (1978 a) reported that i.c.v. injection of NA or DA in rats produced the same effect as catecholamine depletors, i.e., they decreased the threshold. However, this effect of NA and DA was accompanied by the decrease in body temperature and was not demonstrated in animals sufficiently supplied with external heat to prevent hypothermia.

It should also be added that among the several β-adrenoceptor antagonists studied (JAEGER et al. 1979; Madan and BARAR 1974) only one D-(−)-1-(4-nitrophenyl)-2-isopropylaminomethanol (D(−)INPEA) was shown to increase susceptibility to seizures (MADAN and BARAR 1974).

Thus, most of the data indicate that brain catecholamines – and most probably NA – play an inhibitory role in the control of susceptibility to minimal seizures induced by high-frequency electroshock, and that β-adrenoceptors are not involved in this function.

2. Maximal Electroshock Seizures

A large body of evidence indicates that central catecholamines are attenuators of maximal seizures induced by electroshock; most of this evidence is based on changes in the threshold for these seizures after pharmacological modification of catecholaminergic activity.

Thus, drugs which deplete the brain of catecholamines lower the threshold, i.e., they increase susceptibility to seizures in mice and rats (Table 1). Such an effect has been reported not only after reserpine, tetrabenazine, and Ro 4-1284, which additionally decrease the concentration of brain 5-HT, but also after drugs which leave the level of indoleamine unchanged. They include guanethidine, inhibitors of catecholamine synthesis (α-MT and a number of DA-β-hydroxylase inhibitors) and a catecholamine neurotoxin (6-OHDA). The latter drug increases susceptibility to seizures not only after i.c.v. injection but also after its systemic administration to newborn rats (prior to the full development of the blood-brain barrier) with the measurement of susceptibility during their adult lives (OSUIDE and WAMBEBE 1979). Furthermore, the decrease in seizure threshold was also found by some authors after α-adrenoceptor blocking agents and DA antagonists, whereas several β-adrenoceptor blockers were found to produce the opposite effect, which was manifested as an increase in the threshold as well as a virtual anticonvulsant action. However, strong evidence has been presented that the effects of the latter drugs are not related to β-blockade (JAEGER et al. 1979; MADAN and BARAR 1974; MURMANN et al. 1966). It should also be underlined that the absence of changes in susceptibility to seizures reported after the other two catecholamine (and 5-HT) depletors (α-MMT and α-methyl-DOPA) probably depends on the formation of their catabolites, which may act as false neurotransmitters at catecholaminergic receptors.

On the other hand, the pharmacologically induced enhancement of catecholaminergic function (Table 2) obtained by the inhibition of catecholamine catabolism (MAO inhibitors), treatment with their precursor (DOPA), their release (amphetamines), or the inhibition of NA uptake (imipramine, cocaine) leads in most cases to decrease in susceptibility to seizures. A similar effect was reported after administration of the DA receptor agonists piribedil and apomorphine, though the effect of the latter drug in mice is questionable. In contrast, another DA agonist amantadine and i.c.v.-administered DA or NA produced the opposite effect, i.e., they increased susceptibility. As to the specificity of these results the following reservations, however, should be made: (1) DOPA-induced increase in the threshold in mice was antagonized neither by the α-adrenoceptor antagonist phentolamine nor by neuroleptics, and 5-HT release was suggested to be responsible for this effect of DOPA (KLEINROK et al. 1978); (2) the effects of imipramine and cocaine do not depend on NA uptake inhibition as desmethylimipramine, another inhibitor of the amine uptake, was ineffective (Table 2); and (3) a

Table 1. The effects of drugs reducing catecholaminergic activity in susceptibility to maximal electroshock seizures in mice (M) and rats (R)

Drug	Susceptibility to seizures (animal species)	References
Reserpine	Increase (M)	Buterbaugh and London (1977), Chen et al. (1954, 1968a, b), Chow and Hendley (1959), Jenney (1954), Jenney and Pfeifer (1956), Przegaliński (1976a), Rudzik and Johnson (1970)
	Increase (R)	Gray and Rauh (1971), Jobe et al. (1974), Picchioni et al. (1962), Prockop et al. (1959), Przegaliński (1976b), Rudzik and Johnson (1970)
Tetrabenazine	Increase (M)	Chen et al. (1968b)
Ro 4-1284	Increase (R)	Jobe et al. (1974), Stull et al. (1973, 1977)
Guanethidine	Increase (R)	Pfeifer et al. (1964)
α-MT	Increase (M)	Buterbaugh and London (1977), Chen et al. (1968a, b), Kilian and Frey (1973), Rudzik and Johnson (1970)
	No effect (M)	Gray and Rauh (1971), Przegaliński (1976a), Roussinov et al. (1976)
	Increase (R)	Kilian and Frey (1973), Przegaliński (1976b), Rudzik and Johnson (1970)
	No effect (R)	Gray and Rauh (1971)
α-MMT	No effect (M)	Chen et al. (1968b)
α-Methyl-DOPA	No effect (M)	Chen et al. (1968b)
6-OHDA (i.c.v. or intracisternally)	Increase (M)	Fukuda et al. (1975)
	Increase (R)	Browning and Maynert (1978b), London and Buterbaugh (1978), Quattrone and Samanin (1977), Quattrone et al. (1978)
DA-β-hydroxylase inhibitors	Increase (M)	Chen et al. (1968b), Kilian and Frey (1973), Rudzik and Johnson (1970), Roussinov et al. (1976)
	Increase (R)	Kilian and Frey (1973), Rudzik and Johnson (1970)
α-Blockers	Increase (M)	Chen et al. (1968b), Kilian and Frey (1973)
	No effect (M)	Gray and Rauh (1974)
β-Blockers	Decrease (M)	Chen et al. (1968b), Leszkovszky and Tardos (1965), Madan and Barar (1974), Mennear and Rudzik (1968), Murmann et al. (1966)
	No effect (M)	Chen et al. (1968b), Gray and Rauh (1974), Kilian and Frey (1973), Murmann et al. (1966)
	Decrease (R)	Jaeger et al. (1979), Leszkovszky and Tardos (1965)
DA antagonists (neuroleptics)	Increase (M)	Chen et al. (1968b), Kleinrok et al. (1978)
No effect (M)	E_{max}	György (1979), Kilian and Frey (1973), Kleinrok et al. (1978)

Table 2. The effects of drugs enhancing catecholaminergic activity in susceptibility to maximal electroshock seizure in mice (M) or rats (R)

Drug	Susceptibility to seizures (animal species)	References
MAO inhibitors	Decrease or no effect (M)	CHEN et al. (1968a, b), CHOW and HENDLEY (1959), P'AN et al. (1961), RUDZIK and JOHNSON (1970)
	Decrease (R)	PICCHIONI et al. (1962), P'AN et al. (1961), PROCKOP et al. (1959)
DOPA[a]	Decrease (M)	CHEN et al. (1968b,), KILIAN and FREY (1973), KLEINROK et al. (1978), KCKENZIE and SOROKO (1972, 1973), RUDZIK and JOHNSON (1970)
	Decrease (R)	KILIAN and FREY (1973), MCKENZIE and SOROKO (1972)
NA (i.c.v.)	Increase (R)	BROWNING and MAYNERT (1978a)
DA (i.c.v.)	Increase (R)	BROWNING and MAYNERT (1978a)
Amphetamine	Decrease (M)	FREY (1964), KILIAN and FREY (1973), KLEINROK et al. (1978), MCKENZIE and SOROKO (1972), RUDZIK and JOHNSON (1970)
	Decrease (R)	RUDZIK and JOHNSON (1970), KCKENZIE and SOROKO (1972)
N-Methylamphetamine	Decrease (M)	RUDZIK and JOHNSON (1970)
	Decrease (R)	RUDZIK and JOHNSON (1970)
Imipramine	Decrease (M)	CHEN et al. (1968a, b), CHOW and HENDLEY (1959)
Desmethylimipramine	No effect (M)	CHEN et al. (1968a)
Cocaine	Decrease (M)	CHEN et al. (1968a)
Apomorphine	No effect (M)	KLEINROK et al. (1978), MCKENZIE and SOROKO (1972)
	Decrease (M)	GYÖRGY (1979)
	Decrease (R)	MCKENZIE and SOROKO (1972)
Piribedil	Decrease (M)	GYÖRGY (1979)
Amantadine	Increase (M)	KLEINROK et al. (1978)

[a] In some experiments mice pretreated with MAO inhibitors were used

rather unexpected increase in susceptibility to seizures induced in mice by amantadine was not prevented by DA antagonists (KLEINROK et al. 1978), and the same effect produced by i.c.v.-administered DA or NA in rats was attributed to the hypothermic action of these amines (BROWNING and MAYNERT 1978 a).

Further evidence indicating the involvement of catecholamines originates from experiments in which a reserpine-, tetrabenazine-, Ro 4-1284-, or α-MT-induced increase in susceptibility to seizures was reversed if brain catecholamines were restored by MAO inhibitors (CHEN et al. 1968a, b; CHOW and HENDLEY 1959; PICCHIONI et al. 1962; STULL et al. 1977) or by DOPA given alone, in combination with an MAO inhibitor, or with an inhibitor of extracerebral aromatic L-amino acid decarboxylase (CHEN et al. 1968b; JOBE et al. 1974; STULL et al. 1977). Furthermore, the effects of reserpine and tetrabenazine were also antagonized by amphetamines (RUDZIK and JOHNSON 1970) and by NA uptake inhibitors including desmethylimipramine (CHEN et al. 1968a, b).

Similar conclusions may also be drawn from the papers of SCHLESINGER et al. (1968b) and SCUDDER et al. (1966), who studied susceptibility to seizures in several strains of mice with different levels of brain monoamines and found it to be raised in strains with low concentrations of catecholamines (and 5-HT), and from the results reported by GOLDBERG et al. (1975), who have shown increased susceptibility to seizures in spontaneously hypertensive rats which have a slow turnover rate of brain NA and DA.

On the other hand, when depletors of central monoamines were studied in spontaneously nonextensor rats, restoration of hind limb tonic extension (a criterion for maximal seizures) was found after administration of reserpine (BUTERBAUGH 1978; KOSLOW and ROTH 1971) but not after administration of α-MT (BUTERBAUGH 1978), and this is the only finding against the participation of catecholamines.

On the basis of all the above-cited data it is, however, difficult to differentiate the importance of NA and DA, as most treatments used in pharmacological experiments affect both amines. Nevertheless, the increase in susceptibility to seizures after the administration of DA-β-hydroxylase inhibitors and the decrease after the administration of NA uptake inhibitors, which also antagonize the effects of reserpine and tetrabenazine, suggest the involvement of NA, whereas the increase in the convulsive threshold after apomorphine and piribedil (antagonized by haloperidol – GYÖRGY 1979) and the opposite effect of most DA antagonists may indicate the involvement of DA.

Other data, however, seem to indicate the importance of NA and exclude the participation of DA. They are: (1) The antagonism of the anticonvulsant action of DOPA (in mice pretreated with an MAO inhibitor) by an inhibitor of DA-β-hydroxylase (MCKENZIE and SOROKO 1973); (2) the increase in susceptibility to seizures in rats with a selective depletion of brain NA by benztropine + 6-OHDA treatment (SIMONTON and BROWNING 1977) but not with a selective reduction of brain DA concentration by a desmethylimipramine- or protriptyline-6-OHDA combination (QUATTRONE et al. 1978; SIMONTON and BROWNING 1977); and (3) increased susceptibility to seizures in rats with a selective depletion of forebrain NA (after a microinjection of 6-OHDA into NA fibers in the mesencephalon) but not with a selective DA depletion after a microinjection of 6-OHDA into the nigrostriatal bundle (MASON and CORCORAN 1979b). Interestingly, depletion of forebrain NA induces only a prolongation of maximal seizures, whereas the decrease in the threshold was shown by the same authors (MASON and CORCORAN 1979a) after a selective depletion of spinal cord NA.

On the other hand, an amphetamine-induced decrease in susceptibility to seizures in mice was antagonized by phentolamine as well as by several DA antagonists (KLEINROK et al. 1978). The reversal of Ro 4-1284-induced increase in the susceptibility in rats by DOPA (+ an MAO inhibitor) was not antagonized by pimozide or by an inhibitor of DA-β-hydroxylase alone but was completely abolished by their combined administration (JOBE et al. 1974). Moreover, the abovementioned effect of Ro 4-1284 in rats was antagonized not only by i.c.v.-administered NA (STULL et al. 1977), but also by apomorphine or i.c.v.-injected DA (STULL et al. 1973, 1977). In addition, these effects of apomorphine and DA were blocked by pimozide (STULL et al. 1973). Therefore, it may be concluded from these studies that both NA and DA are involved. It is relevant to add that pharmacological data suggest the involvement of DA (DE SCHAEPDRYVER et al. 1962) or both NA and DA (BILLIET et al. 1970) in susceptibility to maximal seizures also in rabbits.

3. Amygdaloid Kindling

The repeated electrical stimulation of different brain structures with a stimulus which is initially subconvulsive produces EEG seizure responses and behavioral (clonic) convulsions in rats, rabbits, and other species, and this phenomenon is called "kindling." Among the brain structures, the limbic system seems to be the most sensitive. Hence amygdaloid kindling in rats was used by several authors to study the role of brain catecholamines – and other neurotransmitters – in this model of epileptogenesis.

ARNOLD et al. (1973) were the first to find that rats treated with 6-OHDA (i.c.v.) or reserpine required fewer stimulations to induce motor seizures than nontreated control animals, and they suggested that this effect results from the depletion of central catecholamines. The influence of i.c.v.-administered 6-OHDA was also studied by CORCORAN et al. (1974), who reported the facilitation of seizure development in animals treated with an MAO inhibitor and 6-OHDA (a substantial depletion of both NA and DA) but not with 6-OHDA alone (the preferential depletion of NA). Therefore, they supposed that the destruction of either catecholaminergic or only dopaminergic neurons is responsible for this effect.

However, further studies with 6-OHDA or other drugs affecting catecholaminergic transmission indicate that NA is more important. Thus, MCINTYRE et al. (1979) have shown that the depletion of both NA and DA after 6-OHDA (i.c.v.) but not of DA alone (desmethylimipramine + 6-OHDA) facilitates the development of behavioral convulsions. Furthermore, a similar effect was found when 6-OHDA was injected into the bilateral trajectories of the NA-ascending fibers, selectively depleting forebrain NA (CORCORAN and MASON 1980; MOHR and CORCORAN 1981), but not when forebrain DA was selectively depleted as the result of a 6-OHDA injection into the ascending DA fibers in the mesencephalon (CORCORAN and MASON 1980). It was also reported that fewer stimulations were necessary to evoke seizures in rats treated with α-MT or disulfiram during the kindling procedure (CALLAGHAN and SCHWARK 1979). A similar effect was shown by these authors after the administration of propranolol, whereas phenoxybenzamine, clonidine, pimozide, and apomorphine were inactive in their study. Interestingly, they also found that amygdaloid kindling decreases the NA level in several brain structures, leaving the DA concentration unchanged. All these results confirm the importance of NA but not DA. Additionally, they indicate the involvement of β- rather than α-receptors in this phenomenon.

It should also be added that the impairment of NA transmission not only facilitates the development of behavioral seizures but also enhances EEG responses, increasing the duration of afterdischarges, leaving only the first of them intact (CALLAGHAN and SCHWARK 1979; CORCORAN et al. 1974; CORCORAN and MASON 1980; MOHR and CORCORAN 1981). The latter finding and the lack of influence of drugs reducing NA activity on the afterdischarge threshold (ARNOLD et al. 1973; CORCORAN and MASON 1980; MOHR and CORCORAN 1981) suggest that the facilitation of kindling observed under such experimental conditions is a result of disinhibition of the spread of epileptiform activity and not of an increase in epileptogenicity of the stimulated brain structure (amygdala). In other words under physiological conditions NA would be a neurotransmitter playing an inhibitory role in the propagation of seizure activity during kindling.

In all the above-cited studies the development of seizures was investigated when drugs used to modify the catecholaminergic function were given before the start or during the kindling procedure. However, there are also some data on the effect of these drugs in kindled rats with fully developed behavioral convulsions. Reserpine was shown to potentiate them (ARNOLD et al. 1973; CORCORAN et al. 1974), clonidine and propranolol were found to have an anticonvulsant effect (ASHTON et al. 1980), whereas α-MT, phenoxybenzamine, haloperidol, and apomorphine were reported as inactive (ASHTON et al. 1980; CORCORAN et al. 1974; MCINTYRE et al. 1979). So, the picture is unclear, especially since the effect of propranolol was suggested to be unspecific and clonidine, used as an NA agonist, could at the effective dose (0.16 mg/kg) stimulate the α-2 receptor and actually decrease NA activity, producing at the same time an effect opposite to that of reserpine. These results suggest that a quite different, or more, neurotransmitter system(s) may be involved in the expression of kindled seizures than in their development. However, further studies are necessary to elucidate this problem.

II. Seizures Induced by Chemical Agents

1. Pentylenetetrazol

a) Clonic Convulsions

In spite of the large amount of research carried out no clear conclusion can be drawn as to the role of catecholamines in pentylenetetrazol (PTZ)-induced clonic convulsions in mice. As shown in Table 3, there is no correlation between pharmacologically changed catecholaminergic activity and susceptibility to PTZ-induced seizures. Even if some particular drugs are taken into consideration (e.g., reserpine or a low dose of amphetamine), different results (decrease or increase in susceptibility to seizures or no effect) were reported.

The reasons for these discrepancies are not completely clear. Some of them may result from the different strains of mice used in experiments as, for example, GERALD and RIFFEE (1973) using ICR mice found no effect, whereas using CD-1 mice in another study they (RIFFEE and GERALD 1976) found a decrease in susceptibility to seizures after a low dose of amphetamine. Other discrepancies may de-

Table 3. The effects of drugs affecting catecholaminergic activity in PTZ-induced clonic convulsions in mice

Drug	Susceptibility to seizures	References
Drugs reducing catecholaminergic activity		
Reserpine	Increase	CHIMOTE and MOGHE (1977), LITTLE and CONRAD (1960), PRZEGALIŃSKI (1975)
	No effect	CHEN and BOHNER (1956, 1961), CHEN et al. (1954), KOBINGER (1958b)
	Decrease	GERALD and GUPTA (1977)
α-MT	Increase	KILIAN and FREY (1973)
	No effect	GERALD and GUPTA (1977)
6-OHDA (i.c.v.)	No effect	OISHI et al. (1979b)
6-OHDOPA	Decrease	GERALD and GUPTA (1977)
DA-β-hydroxylase inhibitors	Increase	CHIMOTE and MOGHE (1977), KILIAN and FREY (1973)
	No effect	GERALD and GUPTA (1977)
α-Blockers	No effect	RIFFEE and GERALD (1976), KILIAN and FREY (1973)
	Decrease	OISHI et al. (1979b)
β-Blockers	Increase	KILIAN and FREY (1973)
	No effect	RIFFEE and GERALD (1976)
DA antagonists (neuroleptics)	No effect	KILIAN and FREY (1973), PRZEGALIŃSKI (1975), RIFFEE and GERALD (1976)
	Decrease	CHIMOTE and MOGHE (1977)
Drugs enhancing catecholaminergic activity		
MAO inhibitors	No effect	KLEINROK et al. (1977), KOBINGER (1958b), PRZEGALIŃSKI (1975)
DOPA[a]	Decrease	KILIAN and FREY (1973), KOBINGER (1958b)
Amphetamine (low dose)[b]	Decrease	GERALD und GUPTA (1977), KILIAN and FREY (1973), RIFFEE and GERALD (1976, 1977)
	No effect	GERALD and RIFFEE (1973), WOLF and STOCK (1966)
	Increase	WOLF et al. (1969)
Amphetamine (high dose)[c]	Increase	GERALD and GUPTA (1977), GERALD and RIFFEE (1973), RIFFEE and GERALD (1976, 1977), WOLF et al. (1969), WOLF and STOCK (1966)
Clonidine	Increase or no effect	OISHI et al. (1979b)

[a] In some experiments mice pretreated with MAO inhibitors were used
[b] Refers to 2–5 mg/kg *d*-amphetamine
[c] Refers to 8–16 mg/kg *d*-amphetamine

pend on the experimental procedure used. For example, OISHI et al. (1979 b) have shown that clonidine was ineffective if the PTZ seizure threshold was measured, whereas the drug enhanced the incidence of generalized clonic convulsions after the injection of a fixed dose of PTZ.

It is also noteworthy that some results presented by the same authors even in the same report seem to lead to opposite conclusions. Thus, GERALD and GUPTA (1977) found that the decrease in susceptibility to seizures induced by a low dose of amphetamine was antagonized by reserpine, α-MT, 6-OHDOPA, or an inhibitor of DA-β-hydroxylase; this suggests the inhibitory role of catecholamines or NA. On the other hand, they also showed that the increase in susceptibility after a high dose of amphetamine – though not antagonized by any of the above-mentioned drugs – was prevented by the combined treatment with reserpine and α-MT; this indicates rather a facilitatory effect of catecholamines.

These and other facts indicate that, as far as clonic convulsions in mice are concerned, the interaction between PTZ and the drugs which affect catecholaminergic transmission cannot be explained by alteration in catecholaminergic activity.

Much less study was carried out on rats. SPENCER and TURNER (1969) reported the potentiation of PTZ clonic convulsions in this species by amphetamine and antagonism of this effect by α-MT but not DDC. Therefore they suggested that DA is responsible for the amphetamine effect. However, as neither α-MT nor DDC influenced susceptibility to seizures in animals treated with PTZ only, the facilitatory function of DA (or NA) seems dubious. Other studies unanimously indicate the inhibitory role of NA. Thus, KILIAN and FREY (1973) have shown a decrease in the PTZ threshold not only after α-MT but also after DA-β-hydroxylase inhibitors. BHATTACHARYA et al. (1978) reported an increase in susceptibility to seizures after the administration of reserpine, α-MT, and DDC and inhibition of the seizures after the administration of DOPA, with the effect of the latter drug being antagonized by DDC. Moreover, they also found some tendency for susceptibility to increase after administration of the α-adrenoceptor antagonist phenoxybenzamine and administration of the β-adrenoceptor blocker propranolol but not after administration of the DA antagonist haloperidol. OISHI et al. (1979 a) studied the correlation between susceptibility to the PTZ convulsions and changes in NA contents of different brain regions, and suggested the inhibitory role of brain stem NA. They found a decrease in the PTZ threshold in adult rats after i.c.v.-administered 6-OHDA, which produced the depletion of NA in several brain structures (including the brain stem) and of DA in the striatum. On the other hand, when 6-OHDA was given by the same route to 8-day-old animals and the PTZ challenge was carried out 14–18 weeks after birth, no effect on susceptibility to seizures was shown. In these animals the level of NA was decreased in all examined structures except the brain stem (where it was elevated), and striatal DA was profoundly depleted. Moreover, the lack of an effect on susceptibility was also shown after microinjections of 6-OHDA into the dorsal or ventral NA bundle which were accompanied by the depletion of NA in the cortex and hypothalamus but not in the brain stem. In this context it is interesting to underline that the 6-OHDA-induced depletion of cerebellar or spinal NA does not affect clonic convulsions produced by PTZ in rats (MASON and CORCORAN 1979a).

b) Tonic Convulsions

Similarly to clonic convulsions, the participation of central catecholamines in PTZ-induced tonic seizures in mice is also doubtful. On the one hand – as can be seen in Table 4 – the increase in susceptibility to seizures was found not only in animals depleted of brain catecholamines and 5-HT (reserpine, tetrabenazine) but also in those with only the catecholamine level decreased (prenylamine, 6-OHDA i.c.v.) or even with selective depletion of NA (guanethidine). Furthermore, the effects of reserpine, tetrabenazine, prenylamine, and guanethidine were reversed if brain catecholamines were restored by MAO inhibitors (CHEN and BOHNER 1961; KOBINGER 1958b; LESSIN and PARKES 1959; PFEIFER and GALAMBOS 1967a) and that of reserpine was additionally antagonized by DOPA (+ an MAO inhibitor), NA uptake inhibitors (imipramine and cocaine), and i.c.v.-administered NA or DA (CHEN and BOHNER 1961; JONES and ROBERTS 1968). It should also be added that mice of a strain characterized by a low concentration of catecholamines (and 5-HT) in the brain are more susceptible to PTZ seizures than those with a higher level of the monoamines (SCHLESINGER et al. 1968b).

On the other hand, depletion of brain catecholamines by α-MMT, α-methyl-DOPA, α-MT, and some DA-β-hydroxylase inhibitors had no effect on the PTZ threshold. Inasmuch as the depletion of catecholamines induced by α-MMT and α-methyl-DOPA may be counteracted by the catabolites of these depletors (see Sect. B.I.2), the lack of an effect of α-MT and some DA-β-hydroxylase inhibitors is strong evidence against the involvement of cerebral catecholamines. Data on catecholaminergic antagonists are also controversial. A low dose of the α-adrenoceptor blocker phentolamine (1 mg/kg) was found inactive, whereas a higher dose of the drug (10 mg/kg) increased the PTZ threshold. Since this effect did not appear in mice pretreated with 6-OHDA (i.c.v.), OISHI et al. (1979b) suggested that it results from the blockade of presynaptic α-2 receptors and from the increased release of NA. The DA antagonist haloperidol is ineffective whereas β-blockers produce different effects including the decrease in the PTZ threshold after a low dose of propranolol (KILIAN and FREY 1973) and virtual anticonvulsant action after higher doses of propranolol and pronethalol (MURMANN et al. 1966). The latter effect does not seem to be specific, however, as other β-antagonists do not share this property (MADAN and BARAR 1974; MURMANN et al. 1966).

Regarding the drugs which enhance catecholaminergic activity (Table 4), both DOPA and MAO inhibitors produce different effects, including a rather unexpected increase in susceptibility to seizures. However, such an effect was found for some MAO inhibitors shortly after their injection and it seems to be unrelated to the increase in brain monoamines (SPOERLEIN and ELLMAN 1961). The effect of DOPA was shown after a very high dose (500 mg/kg), which, not being antagonized by haloperidol, enables at least the participation of DA to be excluded (LAZAROVA and ROUSSINOV 1978). In other studies the MAO inhibitors and DOPA were either ineffective or decreased susceptibility. A decrease in susceptibility was also reported after i.c.v. administration of DA but not NA. However, the inhibitory function of DA seems doubtful as apomorphine was inactive whereas an-

Table 4. The effects of drugs affecting catecholaminergic activity on PTZ-induced tonic convulsions in mice

Drug	Susceptibility to seizures	References
Drugs reducing catecholaminergic activity		
Reserpine	Increase	CHEN et al. (1954), CHEN and BOHNER (1956), KOBINGER (1958a, b), LESSIN and PARKES (1959)
Tetrabenazine	Increase	LESSIN and PARKES (1959)
Prenylamine	Increase	PFEIFER and GALAMBOS (1967a)
Guanethidine	Increase	PFEIFER and GALAMBOS (1967a)
α-MT	No effect	KILIAN and FREY (1973), ROUSSINOV et al. (1976), RUDZIK and JOHNSON (1970)
α-MMT	No effect	PFEIFER and GALAMBOS (1967a, b)
α-Methyl-DOPA	No effect	PFEIFER and GALAMBOS (1965)
6-OHDA (i.c.v.)	Increase	OISHI et al. (1979b)
DA-β-hydroxylase inhibitors	Increase or no effect	KILIAN and FREY 1973) MAJ and VETULANI (1970), ROUSSINOV et al. (1976), RUDZIK and JOHNSON (1970)
Phentolamine	No effect	KILIAN and FREY (1973)
	Decrease	OISHI et al. (1979b)
β-Blockers	Different effects [a]	KILIAN and FREY (1973), MADAN and BARAR (1974), MURMANN et al. (1966)
Haloperidol	No effect	KILIAN and FREY (1973), LAZAROVA and ROUSSINOV (1978)
Drugs enhancing catecholaminergic activity		
MAO inhibitors	Different effects [a]	KLEINROK et al. (1977), KOBINGER (1958b), LESSIN and PARKES (1959), PFEIFER and GALAMBOS (1967a), PROCKOP et al. (1959), SPOERLEIN and ELLMAN (1961)
DOPA [b]	Different effects [a]	KILIAN and FREY (1973), KOBINGER (1958b), LAZAROVA and ROUSSINOV (1978), LESSIN and PARKES (1959), RUDZIK and JOHNSON (1970)
NA (i.c.v.)	No effect	JONES and ROBERTS (1968)
DA (i.c.v.)	Decrease	JONES and ROBERTS (1968), ROUSSINOV and LAZAROVA (1978)
Amphetamine (low dose) [c]	No effect	GERALD and RIFFEE (1973), KILIAN and FREY (1973), RUDZIK and JOHNSON (1970)
	Increase	LAZAROVA and ROUSSINOV (1978)
Amphetamine (high dose)	No effect	RUDZIK and JOHNSON (1970)
	Decrease	GERALD and RIFFEE (1973)
Apomorphine	No effect	LAZAROVA and ROUSSINOV (1978)
Amantadine	Increase	LAZAROVA and ROUSSINOV (1978)
Clonidine	Increase	OISHI et al. (1979b)

[a] Increase, decrease, or no effect. [b] In some experiments mice pretreated with MAO inhibitors or with an inhibitor of extracerebral aromatic L-amino acid decarboxylase were used. [c] Refers to 1–5 mg/kg *d*-amphetamine. [d] Refers to 10–25 mg/kg *d*-amphetamine

other DA agonist, amantadine, even facilitated PTZ-induced tonic convulsions. The latter effect, however, is rather unspecific since it was not prevented by haloperidol (LAZAROVA and ROUSSINOV 1978). Results obtained with amphetamine are too variable to be useful for any conclusion whereas the increase in susceptibility to seizures after the NA agonist clonidine was suggested to be a result of the stimulation of presynaptic α-2 receptors and of the inhibition of NA release (OISHI et al. 1979 b). The prevention of this effect by phentolamine was considered as evidence. However, the effect of clonidine was still present in 6-OHDA-pretreated mice when the presynapic parts of NA synapses were destroyed.

In rats, there is some evidence indicating the inhibitory role of NA. Although DE LA TORRE and MULLAN (1970) found that neither α-MT nor the DA-β-hydroxylase inhibitor disulfiram affect susceptibility to PTZ-induced seizures, only the inhibitory and not the proconvulsant effect could be detected in their experiment – at least if tonic convulsions are taken into consideration. On the other hand, an increase in susceptibility was reported after administration of reserpine (EICHBAUM and YASAKA 1973; PFEIFER and GALAMBOS 1965) as well as after i.c.v.-administered 6-OHDA (CORCORAN et al. 1973, 1974). Moreover, the same effect was shown in rats with selective depletion of forebrain NA induced by the microinjection of 6-OHDA into ascending noradrenergic pathways (MASON and CORCORAN 1978, 1979 b).

As to the involvement of DA, FARIELLO and HORNYKIEWICZ (1979) studied the PTZ threshold after electrolytic lesions of the substantia nigra. They found a decrease in the threshold 12 h after the lesion when striatal DA and its metabolites were augmented and a considerable increase in the threshold at a time when striatal DA and its metabolites were reduced. This suggests the facilitatory role of the amine. In line with this conclusion the increase in susceptibility to PTZ was also reported after DOPA, amphetamine, and amantadine (LAZAROVA and ROUSSINOV 1978; SAFTA et al. 1976), though the effect of the latter drug was suggested to be unspecific (SAFTA et al. 1976). In contrast neither the selective depletion of striatal DA after a microinjection of 6-OHDA into the nigrostriatal bundle (MASON and CORCORAN 1979 b) nor apomorphine and haloperidol (LAZAROVA and ROUSSINOV 1978) modify susceptibility to PTZ-induced tonic convulsions in rats.

2. Other Chemical Agents

There is some evidence that brain catecholamines may play a role in the convulsions produced by other chemicals. As it was reported that not only reserpine, α-MT, and α-methyl-DOPA but also DA-β-hydroxylase inhibitors increase susceptibility to caffeine- (CHEN and BOHNER 1956, 1961; CHEN et al. 1954; RUDZIK and JOHNSON 1970), bemegride- (CHIMOTE and MOGHE 1977; RUDZIK and JOHNSON 1970), and procaine-induced seizures (CHIMOTE and MOGHE 1977), NA was suggested to be an attenuator of the convulsions induced by these drugs. The inhibitory role of the amine was also suggested in bicuculline-evoked convulsions as α-blockers potentiated them and antagonized the anticonvulsant effect of neuroleptics (WORMS and LLOYD 1979). Some other reports indicate that brain catecholamines also participate in hexafluorodiethyl ether- or morphine-induced seizures

(AYHAN 1976; BROWNING and MAYNERT 1978 b; TRUITT and EBERSBERGER 1962); however, it is not clear whether NA or DA is involved.

On the other hand central catecholamines do not seem to be involved in convulsions produced by strychnine (CHEN and BOHNER 1956, 1961; CHEN et al. 1954; EICHBAUM and YASAKA 1973; PROCKOP et al. 1959) or cocaine (MASON and CORCORAN 1979 b).

III. Reflex Epilepsy Models

1. Audiogenic Seizures

Most studies on the role of catecholamines in audiogenic seizures were carried out on susceptible strains of mice. These studies have shown that substances which lower the catecholamine level in the brain (reserpine, tetrabenazine, Ro 4-1284, α-MT, 6-OHDA) increase susceptibility to seizures (ALEXANDER and KOPELOFF 1976; BOGGAN and SEIDEN 1971; LEHMANN 1968, 1977; SCHLESINGER et al. 1968 a, 1970), whereas drugs which increase brain catecholamine concentrations (DOPA, MAO inhibitors, pyrogallol) bring about the opposite effect, that is, they inhibit audiogenic convulsions (ALEXANDER and KOPELOFF 1976; BOGGAN and SEIDEN 1971; BOGGAN et al. 1971; KELLOGG 1976; LEHMANN 1967; SCHLESINGER et al. 1968 a, 1970, 1975). The above data do not permit the differentiation of the roles of NA and DA, because all these substances affect the level of both catecholamines, and most of them also affect the 5-HT level. A similar limitation, in this respect, is seen in a study of COLEMAN and SCHLESINGER (1965), who found increased susceptibility to seizures in mice maintained on a diet with pyridoxine deficiency, since the vitamin is a cofactor in the synthesis of both catecholamines and also of other neurotransmitters (5-HT, γ-aminobutyric acid).

There exists, however, a large body of additional data which discusses separately the involvement of NA and DA. Time-response studies in mice treated with reserpine, α-MT, and MAO inhibitors have shown some correlation between the endogenous level of brain NA (and also 5-HT) and susceptibility to audiogenic seizures (SCHLESINGER et al. 1970). The relationship was not perfect, however, and the authors did not measure the concentration of DA. LEHMANN (1977) reported that the i.c.v. administration of 6-OHDA increases susceptibility to seizures in such a way that it transforms clonic seizures into tonic convulsions in a clonic mouse strain. This effect did not appear, however, if 6-OHDA-induced depletion of brain NA – but not DA – was effectively prevented by a pretreatment with desmethylimipramine. It should be added here that not only central but also peripheral NA may be of some inportance for the nature of the audiogenic seizure response, as ALEXANDER and KOPELOFF (1978) and LEHMANN (1977) found that systematically injected 6-OHDA increases the number of lethal seizures in mice which before the treatment had responded with tonic convulsions.

In line with the above results SCHLESINGER et al. (1969) found that an intracranial injection of NA reduced the incidence of lethal seizures. Moreover, some NA receptor agonists (clonidine, oxymetazoline, UK 14,304) have been reported to antagonize audiogenic seizures (HORTON et al. 1980; KELLOGG 1976). However, these agonists preferentially stimulate α-2 receptors and therefore the reduction rather than activation of NA transmission can be expected under their influence.

Furthermore, the anticonvulsant effect of these agonists was blocked by α-2 antagonists (yohimbine, piperoxan, phentolamine) but not by the α-1 antagonist phenoxybenzamine (HORTON et al. 1980). The latter drug was, however, given in too small a dose (5 mg/kg) to exclude completely the involvement of α-1 receptors. Neither of the above-mentioned α-2 and α-1 antagonists showed their own action in audiogenic seizures, though since the almost maximum effect was observed in control groups only antagonistic action could be demonstrated in this experiment (HORTON et al. 1980).

The anticonvulsant effect of the β-adrenoceptor antagonist propranolol has been described by ANLEZARK et al. (1979). However, this effect seems to be unrelated to β-blockade since (−) and (+) enantiomers of the drug acted with similar potency, whereas the (−) enantiomer is 10–100 times stronger as a β-antagonist.

Other arguments supporting the role of NA come from studies in which a correlation between susceptibility to audiogenic seizures and the level or metabolism of the amine was sought in various strains of mice. Thus, SCHLESINGER et al. (1965) compared three strains of mice (DBA/2J, B6D2F1, C57BL/6J) and showed that DBA/2J mice demonstrated greatest susceptibility to seizures and the lowest level of NA (and also of 5-HT) in the brain whereas C57BL/6J mice, which were resistant to audiogenic seizures, had a significantly higher concentration of brain NA (and 5-HT). Similar results were reported by KELLOGG (1971, 1976), who found a lower NA level in the forebrain and hindbrain and reduced MAO activity in the whole brain of DBA/2J mice in comparison to C57BL/6J ones. Other authors described the lower activity of catechol-*O*-methyl transferase, but not of MAO, in the brain of the susceptible strain of mice (SCHLESINGER et al. 1975). The above differences pertaining to the NA level as well as catechol-*O*-methyl transferase and MAO activity were most conspicuous in 21-day-old mice, which is the age when DBA/2J mice showed the greatest susceptibility to seizures. On the other hand MCGEER et al. (1969) found no difference in the brain NA concentration between DBA/2J and C57BL/6J mice. However, these authors performed their study on 6-week-old animals, which is the age when – according to SCHLESINGER et al. (1965) – DBA/2J mice are almost nonresponsive to audiogenic shock.

As to the role of DA in mice, the most important finding is that several agonists of DA receptors (apomorphine, *N*-*n*-propyl-norapomorphine, bromocryptine, ergometrine, ergocornine, piribedil) decrease susceptibility to seizures (ANLEZARK and MELDRUM 1975; ANLEZARK et al. 1976, 1978; ASHTON et al. 1976; KELLOGG 1976) and that this effect is blocked by the neuroleptic agent haloperidol (ANLEZARK et al. 1976). Further evidence has been reported by BOGGAN and SEIDEN (1971), who found that DOPA antagonizes audiogenic seizures and reverses the reserpine-induced increase in susceptibility to seizures. Both effects were better correlated with the increase in brain DA than NA concentrations. On the other hand, LEHMANN (1977) could not demonstrate any changes in seizures reactivity in clonic and tonic strains of mice after central DA depletion (desmethylimipramine + 6-OHDA i.c.v.), and PLOTNIKOFF (1960) reported that – depending on the strain of mice used – the DA antagonist chlorpromazine had either no effect or antagonized audiogenic seizures. Moreover, no significant differences in brain DA levels were found when mice susceptible to audiogenic seizures and nonsensitive mice were compared (KELLOGG 1976; MCGEER et al. 1969).

Considering the role of catecholamines there are relatively few data from studies performed on rats. JOBE et al. (1973 b, c) showed the increase in susceptibility to audiogenic seizures after administration of Ro 4-1284. This effect was better correlated with the depletion of brain NA than DA and was potentiated not only by α-MT but also by DDC. The same authors also found that imipramine, which by itself shows anticonvulsant action, antagonized the Ro 4-1284-induced increase in susceptibility to seizures and the depletion of brain NA but not DA. They also demonstrated a marked intensification of audiogenic seizures after i.c.v. administration of reserpine and after combined treatment with α-MT and α-MMT, or α-MT and lithium carbonate. Also in these experiments the pharmacological effect was better correlated with the depletion of brain NA than DA. A weak point of these studies that should be underlined is that α-MT, given alone, had no influence on audiogenic seizures although it lowered brain NA and DA levels considerably. On the other hand, the lack of the influence of DDC should be associated with the experimental conditions used (dose, treatment time) where this inhibitor of NA synthesis did not change the level of that amine.

The results of studies where 6-OHDA was used also suggest the involvement of NA rather than DA. BOURN et al. (1972, 1978) found an increase in convulsive seizure intensity after its i.c.v. administration. This effect was strongly antagonized by pretreatment with desmethylimipramine, which at the same time prevented the depletion of brain NA but not DA. The same authors (BOURN et al. 1977) administered 6-OHDA also systemically to newborn rats and found that at an age of 60 days these animals were more susceptible to audiogenic seizures and had a much lower concentration of NA, and not DA, in some brain structures. The results of JERLICZ et al. (1978 b), who described the increase in susceptibility to seizures in rats with bilateral lesions of the locus ceruleus, should also be regarded as important evidence for the involvement of brain NA. On the other hand, it should be mentioned that MCGEER et al. (1969) compared the levels of tyrosine, NA, and DA and the activity of tyrosine hydroxylase in the brain of rats susceptible and not susceptible to audiogenic seizures and found no significant differences.

2. Photogenic Seizures

The intermittent light stimulation induces a paroxysmal myoclonic response and paroxysmal EEG activity in the Senegalese baboon, *Papio papio*, and studies in recent years have shown that this reaction is modified by many substances affecting brain catecholamines. The results of those studies are, however, too remotely related to be used here to draw a definite conclusion pertaining to the role of NA or DA. The interpretation of some of those results is also made difficult by the absence of appropriate biochemical data (brain levels of NA and DA) in this species, especially after administration of substances which are assumed to be able to modify the levels of those amines. Therefore – in contrast to studies performed on other species (mice, rats) – it is difficult to assess whether suitable experimental conditions (dose, treatment time, etc.) were chosen for such drugs as reserpine, α-MT, DOPA, and MAO inhibitors.

The depletion of brain catecholamines seems to have no influence, as α-MT was shown to be ineffective (BALZAMO and MELDRUM 1972; MELDRUM and BALZAMO 1971). These authors (BALZAMO and MELDRUM 1972) also did not demonstrate the effect of reserpine, although others (ALTSHULER et al. 1976) have reported its inhibitory or proconvulsant effect after acute or chronic treatments, respectively. On the other hand, the increased availability of catecholamines at their receptors seems to produce an anticonvulsant effect. This was shown after the MAO inhibitor tranylcypromine (BALZAMO and MELDRUM 1972; MELDRUM et al. 1972) and – most interesting – after i.c.v. administration of NA or adrenaline (ALTSHULER et al. 1976). However, NA uptake inhibitors (imipramine, desmethylimipramine, maprotiline) are inactive or even enhance photically induced seizures (KILLAM 1976; TRIMBLE et al. 1977).

Several DA receptor agonists (apomorphine, *N*-*n*-propylnorapomorphine, piribedil, ergometrine, ergocornine, bromocryptine) decrease susceptibility to seizures (ANLEZARK and MELDRUM 1978; ASHTON et al. 1976; MELDRUM et al. 1975). A similar effect has been found after administration of amphetamine (KILLAM 1976), the DA and NA uptake inhibitor nomifensine (TRIMBLE et al. 1977), and DOPA. The latter drug, however, was only effective when given together with an MAO inhibitor (MELDRUM et al. 1972) and not alone (ALTSHULER et al. 1976; BALZAMO and MELDRUM 1972; MELDRUM et al. 1972). In line with the above results the DA receptor antagonists (haloperidol, pimozide) enhanced reactivity to photic stimulation though the effect was limited to only paroxysmal EEG activity whereas the myoclonic response remained unchanged (MELDRUM et al. 1975). The conclusion which could be proposed in this situation, that DA plays a central inhibitory role in the photosensitive baboons *Papio papio,* was recently weakened when ALTSHULER et al (1976) showed that i.c.v. administration of DA did not affect the photomyoclonic syndrome.

IV. Other Models of Epilepsy

Recently, there have appeared some reports on the effect of drugs affecting central catecholamines in convulsions or the EEG pattern in some other models of epilepsy. Thus, COX and LOMAX (1976) studied handling-induced seizures in Mongolian gerbils of the strain (WJL/UC) susceptible to seizures. They suggested an inhibitory role of central NA and DA since D,L-*threo*-dihydroxyphenylserine (an immediate precursor of NA) and apomorphine exerted an anticonvulsant action. Admittedly they also found an anticonvulsant effect of two depletors of catecholamines (α-MMT and DDC), but both drugs were administered in doses producing serious sedation so their unspecific effect cannot be excluded. Moreover, the authors suggested that the anticonvulsant effect of DDC depends on the increase of central DA, though the brain level of the amine was not measured. Results supporting the involvement of DA were also reported by SCHONFELD and GLICK (1980), who described an anticonvulsant effect of amphetamine and apomorphine and an increase in susceptibility to seizures after administration of haloperidol. On the other hand, they found no effect of α-MT, but in this experiment an almost maximal seizure score was observed in the control group so an increase in susceptibility to seizures could not be demonstrated.

In rats with cobalt-induced epilepsy DOW et al. (1974) reported that several dopaminergic drugs (amphetamine, apomorphine, ergocornine) suppressed epileptiform activity in EEG recordings. Furthermore, they found that this effect was reduced by the DA antagonist spiroperidol, which itself exacerbated cobalt-induced discharges. Similarly, SCUVEE-MOREAU et al. (1977) found an antagonistic effect of DOPA in rats pretreated with an inhibitor of extracerebral aromatic L-amino acid decarboxylase. ALTAMURA et al. (1978) measured the activities of tyrosine hydroxylase, aromatic L-amino acid decarboxylase, and other neurotransmitter-synthesizing enzymes in some brain areas of rats with cobalt-induced epilepsy and found a significant reduction in the cortex. The reduction, however, was not correlated with the development of EEG epileptic manifestations, and the authors suggested that it depends on nerve degeneration produced by the experimental lesion.

KOBAYASHI et al. (1976) studied the involvement of catecholamines in the penicillin-induced epileptic focus of the cat cerebral cortex. Levels of NA and DA were significantly lower in the focus during the first and second – but not during the third – stage of propagation. On the other hand, only DOPA and DA – but not NA – inhibited the penicillin-induced spike discharges after topical application. Moreover, DOPA was also effective after systemic administration.

C. Serotonin

I. Electrically Induced Seizures

1. Minimal EST

a) Low-Frequency EST

Neither the depletion of brain monoamines (including 5-HT) after reserpine (Sect. B.I.1.a) nor the selective inhibition of 5-HT synthesis by means of *p*-chlorophenylalanine (PCPA) (BUTERBAUGH and LONDON 1977) modify susceptibility to seizures in this model in mice. Other data are not available. Though the involvement of the serotonergic system seems to be questionable, other studies are necessary.

b) High-Frequency EST

The selective depletion of brain 5-HT by PCPA was shown to have no effect in rats (BUTERBAUGH 1978) and to decrease the threshold (BUTERBAUGH and LONDON 1977) or have no effect (AZZARO et al. 1972) in mice. Rather unexpectedly, a decrease in the threshold was also found after an i.c.v. injection of 5-HT in rats, but this effect was attributed to the hypothermic action of the amine (BROWNING and MAYNERT 1978a).

On the other hand, the reserpine-induced increase of susceptibility to seizures in mice was prolonged by PCPA (AZZARO et al. 1972; WENGER et al. 1973) and partially antagonized by 5-HTP given alone or in combination with an MAO inhibitor (AZZARO et al. 1972).

On the basis of these data the involvement of central 5-HT in the control of susceptibility to minimal electroshock seizure, but only in mice, cannot be excluded. The amine might be an attenuator of the seizures.

2. Maximal Electroshock Seizures

As shown in Table 5 drugs which reduce the brain level or turnover of 5-HT increase susceptibility to seizures in mice, i.e., they decrease the threshold for maximal convulsions. This effect was found by most authors after administration of PCPA and also after subacute treatment with *p*-chloroamphetamine. On the other hand, data on 5-HT antagonists, which could be expected to produce similar effects, are not so unequivocal. KILIAN and FREY (1973) reported an increase in susceptibility after administration of cyproheptadine whereas PRZEGALIŃSKI (1976a) found no effect for cyproheptadine and methysergide and even a decrease in susceptibility after administration of danitracen. The latter drug, however, increased seizure threshold only when given at a high dose so the specificity of this effect may be questioned.

Among the drugs which induce serotonergic activation in mice (Table 5) *p*-chloroamphetamine and *p*-chloro-*N*-methylamphetamine (5-HT releasers) have been shown to decrease susceptibility. Some authors found a similar effect after 5-HTP whereas others reported that this precursor of 5-HT had no influence. Another 5-HT precursor tryptophan and 5-HT receptor agonist LSD were found to be inactive. It should be emphasized, however, that (a) the negative results of RUDZIK and JOHNSON (1970) were undoubtedly connected with the too small dose of 5-HTP (10 mg/kg) used in their experiment, (b) the 5-HTP-induced decrease in susceptibility is easier to demonstrate in mice pretreated with MAO inhibitors (CHEN et al. 1968b; PRZEGALIŃSKI 1976a) or especially with the monoamine uptake inhibitor imipramine (CHEN et al. 1968a), and (c) 5-HTP (+ MAO inhibitor) abolishes the increase in the susceptibility induced by reserpine (CHEN et al. 1968b).

It is also noteworthy that when several strains of mice with different brain levels of catecholamines and 5-HT were compared, those with low concentrations of the monoamines were more susceptible to maximal electroshock convulsions (SCHLESINGER et al. 1968b; SCUDDER et al. 1966). Moreover, 5-HTP decreased susceptibility in these animals (SCHLESINGER et al. 1968b).

Only few data suggest the involvement of 5-HT in rats (Table 5). They include a decrease in maximal seizure threshold found by several authors after the inhibition of 5-HT synthesis with PCPA, an increase in the threshold after 5-HTP and – as reported by PROCKOP et al. (1959) – anticonvulsant effect of the 5-HT precursor in animals pretreated with an MAO inhibitor. Although 5,6-DHT (i.c.v.) produced an effect similar to PCPA, the depletion of brain 5-HT by means of another 5-HT neurotoxin 5,7-DHT (i.c.v. or intracisternally) was shown to be ineffective. Moreover, only one 5-HT antagonist, methysergide, increased susceptibility to seizures whereas several others (cyproheptadine, metergoline, danitracen) were inactive. As to the direct or indirect 5-HT receptor agonists only fenfluramine was shown to decrease susceptibility, whereas *p*-chloroamphetamine, *p*-chloro-*N*-methylamphetamine, quipazine, and *m*-chlorophenylpiperazine were ineffective. Furthermore, the effect of fenfluramine was not antagonized by metergoline (CRUNELLI et al. 1979).

Other evidence against the involvement of 5-HT in susceptibility to maximal seizures in rats is as follows: (a) 5-HTP given alone (LONDON and BUTERBAUGH 1978) or in combination with an inhibitor of peripheral aromatic L-amino acid

Table 5. The effects of drugs affecting serotonergic activity in susceptibility to maximal electroshock seizures in mice (M) and rats) (R)

Drug	Susceptibility to seizures (animal species)	References
Drugs reducing serotonergic activity		
PCPA	Increase (M)	BUTERBAUGH and LONDON (1977), CHEN et al. (1968a), GRAY and RAUH (1971), KILIAN and FREY (1973), PRZEGALIŃSKI (1976a)
	No effect (M)	RUDZIK and JOHNSON (1970)
	Increase (R)	CRUNELLI et al. (1979), GRAY and RAUH (1971), KILIAN and FREY (1973), KOE and WEISSMAN (1968), PRZEGALIŃSKI (1976b), RUDZIK and JOHNSON (1970)
5,6-DHT (i.c.v.)	Increase (R)	PRZEGALIŃSKI (1976b)
5,7-DHT (i.c.v. or intracisternally)	No effect (R)	CRUNELLI et al. (1979), LONDON and BUTERBAUGH (1978)
p-Chloroamphetamine (subacute)	Increase (M)	KILIAN and FREY (1973)
Cyproheptadine	Increase (M)	KILIAN and FREY (1973)
	No effect (M)	PRZEGALIŃSKI (1976a)
	No effect (R)	PRZEGALIŃSKI (1976b)
Methysergide	No effect (M)	PRZEGALIŃSKI (1976a)
	Increase (R)	PRZEGALIŃSKI (1976b)
Metergoline	No effect (R)	CRUNELLI et al. (1979)
Danitracen (WA-335-BS)	Decrease (M)	PRZEGALIŃSKI (1976a)
	No effect (R)	PRZEGALINSKI (1976b)
Drugs enhancing serotonergic activity		
Tryptophan	No effect (M)	PRZEGALIŃSKI (1976a)
5-HTP	Decrease (M)	CHEN et al. (1968b), KILIAN and FREY (1973), PRZEGALIŃSKI (1976a)
	No effect (M)	CHEN et al. (1968a), RUDZIK and JOHNSON (1970)
	Decrease (R)	KILIAN and FREY (1973), PRZEGALIŃSKI (1976b)
5-HT (i.c.v.)	Increase (R)	BROWNING and MAYNERT (1978a)
p-Chloroamphetamine	Decrease (M)	KILIAN and FREY (1973), RUDZIK and JOHNSON (1970)
	No effect (R)	RUDZIK and JOHNSON (1970)
p-Chloro-*N*-methylamphetamine	Decrease (M)	RUDZIK and JOHNSON (1970)
	No effect (R)	RUDZIK and JOHNSON (1970)
Fenfluramine	Decrease (R)	CRUNELLI et al. (1979)
LSD	No effect (M)	PRZEGALIŃSKI (1976a)
Quipazine	No effect (R)	GRUNELLI et al. (1979)
m-Chlorophenylpiperazine	No effect (R)	GRUNELLI et al. (1979)

decarboxylase (JOBE et al. 1974) does not antagonize the tetrabenazine- or reserpine-induced increase in susceptibility to seizures, (b) neither electrolytic and 5,7-DHT-induced lesions of the dorsal raphe nucleus (CRUNELLI et al. 1979) nor electrolytic lesions of the nucleus raphe medianus (QUATTRONE et al. 1978) affect the maximal seizure threshold, and (c) 5,6-DHT injected into the spinal cord does not change the threshold (CRUNELLI et al. 1979).

Interesting studies have been performed by BUTERBAUGH (1978) on rats classified by maximal electroshock stimulation as extensors or nonextensors. The authors showed that the enhancement of serotonergic function by means of 5-HTP, *p*-chloroamphetamine, fenfluramine, fluoxetine, or 5-methoxy-*N,N*-dimethyltryptamine prevents hind limb extension in extensor rats, whereas the reduction of serotonergic activity by means of reserpine, PCPA, or subacute treatment with *p*-chloroamphetamine restores hind limb extension in nonextensor rats. Moreover, the effects of *p*-chloroamphetamine, fenfluramine, and fluoxetine in extensors were antagonized by PCPA. In contrast to these results, however, 5-HT receptor antagonists (cyproheptadine and methysergide) did not induce effects similar to 5-HT depletors in nonextensors and behaved like 5-HT agonists (i.e., they prevented hindlimb extension) in extensors.

Altogether 5-HT does not seem to participate in the control of maximal electroshock seizures in rats, while its inhibitory function in mice canot be excluded.

3. Amygdaloid Kindling

There are only a few reports on the participation of 5-HT in the development of seizures kindled from the amygdala. RACINE and COSCINA (1979) studied the effect of PCPA and midbrain raphe lesions in rats. They have shown that lesions of both dorsal and median raphe nuclei facilitate seizure development as fewer stimulations were required to evoke behavioral convulsions. At the same time no effect on the afterdischarge duration but a decrease in the afterdischarge threshold was observed. These results could indicate that 5-HT inhibits the propagation of epileptiform activity and – possibly – the epileptogenicity of the amygdala. On the other hand, however, the same authors – though using a different kindling procedure – found that PCPA delayed rather than facilitated the development of motor seizures without any effect on afterdischarge duration. Furthermore, a similar effect of PCPA (with some decrease in afterdischarge duration) and no effect for 5-HTP (plus an inhibitor of extracerebral aromatic L-amino acid decarboxylase) were shown in rabbits chronically treated with these drugs during kindling (LAZAROVA et al. 1981; STACH et al. 1981). The reason for these conflicting data is not clear. It should be emphasized, however, that the anticonvulsant effect of PCPA has been reported by some authors in another model of epilepsy (see Sect. C.III.1) – though RACINE and COSCINA (1979) have shown the potentiation of the convulsions kindled from the cortex by the drug – and that midbrain raphe lesions in the study of the latter authors also produced some damage outside the raphe nuclei and therefore the destruction of other than 5-HT system(s) could not be excluded. This makes it somewhat harder to draw unequivocal conclusions and further studies are necessary.

The role of 5-HT in relation to already developed kindled seizures is also not clear. In this model drugs or other treatments used to affect the serotonergic system were given acutely when full behavioral convulsions were established. Thus, KOVACS and ZOLL (1974) reported that electrical stimulation of the median raphe nucleus decreased the intensity of kindled seizures in rats. In contrast, ASHTON et al. (1980), using the same animal species, have shown the potentiation (prolongation in duration) of the seizures after administration of 5-HTP (plus an inhibitor of extracerebral aromatic L-amino acid decarboxylase) and inhibition (reduction in duration) after administration of the 5-HT receptor antagonists metergoline and mianserine. However, the effective doses of these antagonists were very high (20 and 40 mg/kg, respectively) so their effect could be unspecific. SIEGEL and MURPHY (1979) performed their experiments on cats and found a strong inhibitory effect (increase in the threshold current to produce seizures) after electrical stimulation of the nucleus raphe dorsalis and after treatment with the selective inhibitor of 5-HT uptake fluoxetine. On the other hand, *p*-chloroamphetamine (administered in such a way that depletion of the central 5-HT could be expected) was inactive. In rabbits, 5-HTP (plus an inhibitor of peripheral aromatic L-amino acid decarboxylase) and another 5-HT uptake inhibitor femoxetine, but not the 5-HT receptor agonist quipazine, were shown to increase the duration (but not intensity) of kindled convulsions, whereas PCPA and the 5-HT receptor blocker cyproheptadine reduced the duration and intensity (PCPA only) of the convulsions (STACH et al. 1981). From all these data it can be seen that electrical stimulation of the raphe nuclei antagonizes kindled seizures; this would indicate an inhibitory function of 5-HT. On the contrary, pharmacological data – especially from rats and rabbits – lead toward the opposite conclusion. A possible explanation is that pharmacological intervention induces alterations in the 5-HT neurotransmission of the whole brain whereas the stimulation of the raphe nuclei release 5-HT only in target structures, i.e., structures receiving serotonergic input from the respective raphe nucleus.

II. Seizures Induced by Pentylenetetrazol

a) Clonic Convulsions

Regarding the involvement of 5-HT in PTZ-induced clonic convulsions, there seems to be a species-related difference between mice and rats.

Participation of this amine in mice seems to be dubious. In some studies PCPA has been found to decrease the PTZ seizure threshold (CHIMOTE and MOGHE 1977; PRZEGALIŃSKI 1975), whereas it is increased by tryptophan (CHIMOTE and MOGHE 1977), 5-HTP (KILIAN and FREY 1973), *p*-chloroamphetamine (KILIAN and FREY 1973), and the combination of an MAO inhibitor with the 5-HT agonist 5-methoxytryptamine (KLEINROK et al. 1977). However, other data do not confirm these findings. Thus, KILIAN and FREY (1973) and KLEINROK et al. (1977) found PCPA to be inactive, and KLEINROK et al. (1977), KOBINGER (1958b), and PRZEGALIŃSKI (1975) found no effect for 5-HTP. Moreover, the lack of an effect was shown after *p*-chloroamphetamine given subacutely as well as after fenfluramine and several 5-HT antagonists (KILIAN and FREY 1973; KLEINROK et al. 1977; PRZEGALIŃSKI 1975).

On the other hand, most data indicate the importance of 5-HT in rats. An increase in susceptibility to seizures was shown in this species after the depletion of brain 5-HT by PCPA (ALEXANDER and KOPELOFF 1970; BHATTACHARYA et al. 1978; KILIAN and FREY 1973) or by i.c.v.-administered 5,6-DHT (BHATTACHARYA et al. 1978) as well as after 5-HT receptor blockade with methysergide (BHATTACHARYA et al. 1978), whereas the opposite effect, i.e., decrease in susceptibility, was found after administration of 5-HTP (BHATTACHARYA et al. 1978; KILIAN and FREY 1973). It should be added, however, that there is also one report (SPENCER and TURNER 1969) indicating a lack of effect with PCPA.

b) Tonic Convulsions

A similar species-related difference also seem to exist when the role of 5-HT in PTZ-induced tonic convulsions is considered.

In mice some controversial data have been reported and no explicit conclusion is possible. For example, PCPA was found to increase susceptibility to seizures (KILIAN and FREY 1973; LAZAROVA et al. 1980; RUDZIK and JOHNSON 1970) or to be without effect (KLEINROK et al. 1977; KOSTOWSKI et al. 1978). The lack of effect has also been reported after administration of metergoline and methysergide (KLEINROK et al. 1977; KOSTOWSKI et al. 1978), whereas another 5-HT receptor antagonist, cyproheptadine, was shown to increase susceptibility (KILIAN and FREY 1973; KOSTOWSKI et al. 1978) or to be ineffective (KLEINROK et al. 1977). As to the drugs which increase serotonergic activity, KILIAN and FREY (1973) found 5-HTP to be inactive, whereas several other authors reported a decrease in susceptibility to seizures after the 5-HT precursor given alone or in combination with MAO inhibitors (KLEINROK et al. 1977; KOBINGER 1958b; KOSTOWSKI et al. 1978; LAZAROVA et al. 1980; LESSIN and PARKES 1959; RUDZIK and JOHNSON 1970). A decrease in susceptibility has also been reported after administration of *p*-chloroamphetamine and *p*-chloro-*N*-methylamphetamine (KILIAN and FREY 1973; PFEIFER and GALAMBOS 1967b; RUDZIK and JOHNSON 1970), but not after administration of another 5-HT-releasing agent, fenfluramine, or after administration of the direct 5-HT receptor agonist 5-methoxytryptamine – the latter given together with an MAO inhibitor (KLEINROK et al. 1977). On the other hand, 5-HTP, *p*-chloroamphetamine, and LSD have been shown to antagonize the reserpine-induced facilitation of tonic convulsions evoked by PTZ (CHEN and BOHNER 1961; LESSIN and PARKES 1959; PFEIFER and GALAMBOS 1967b).

Though only a few studies have been performed on rats, their results seem to indicate the inhibitory role of 5-HT in this species. Such a conclusion is supported by the facilitation of tonic convulsions after administration of PCPA (DE LA TORRE and MULLAN 1970; DE LA TORRE et al. 1970; LAZAROVA et al. 1981) and by their inhibition after administration of *p*-chloroamphetamine (PFEIFER and GALAMBOS 1967b) or 5-HTP, but only if given to animals pretreated with an inhibitor of extracerebral aromatic L-amino acid decarboxylase (DE LA TORRE and MULLAN 1970; DE LA TORRE et al. 1970).

III. Reflex Epilepsy Models

1. Audiogenic Seizures

According to SCHLESINGER et al. (1965), seizure-prone DBA/2J mice have a lower level of brain 5-HT (and also NA) than seizure-resistant C57BL/6J mice. Moreover, the most pronounced difference was found at 21 days of age, which corresponds to the time of maximal susceptibility to seizures in DBA/2J mice. These results were confirmed by KELLOGG (1971, 1976), who compared the same strains of mice and suggested that DBA/2J mice possess a markedly inefficient 5-HT system. The author found that they have not only a lower endogenous 5-HT level, but also – probably as a compensatory mechanism – a faster rate of 5-HT synthesis (measured in the whole brain as 5-HT accumulation or 5-hydroxyindoleacetic acid disappearance after MAO inhibition or in the hindbrain as 5-HTP accumulation after inhibition of central aromatic L-amino acid decarboxylase). On the contrary, MCGEER et al. (1969) reported no significant differences either in brain 5-HT concentrations between susceptible and nonsusceptible mice or in brain 5-HT levels and tryptophan hydroxylase activity between sensitive and nonsensitive rats. However, these results – at least in mice – should be interpreted with caution as the authors used mice of the susceptible strain (DBA/2J) at an age of 6 weeks when – according to SCHLESINGER et al. (1965) – their reactivity to audiogenic shock is very low.

Table 6. The effects of drugs affecting serotonergic activity in susceptibility to audiogenc seizures in mice (R)

Drug	Susceptibility to seizures	References
Drugs reducing serotonergic activity		
PCPA	Increase	SCHLESINGER et al. (1968a, 1970)
	No effect	LEHMANN (1968)
	Decrease	ALEXANDER et al. (1971), ALEXANDER and KOPELOFF (1976), KOSTOWSKI et al. (1978)
α-Propyldopacetamide	No effect	ALEXANDER and KOPELOFF (1976)
Methysergide	Decrease	ANLEZARK et al. (1976), KOSTOWSKI et al. (1978)
Cyproheptadine	Decrease	KOSTOWSKI et al. (1978)
Metergoline	Decrease	KOSTOWSKI et al. (1978)
Drugs enhancing serotonergic activity		
5-HTP[a]	Decrease	ALEXANDER and KOPELOFF (1976), BOGGAN et al. (1971), KELLOGG (1976), KOSTOWSKI et al. (1978), SCHLESINGER et al. (1968, 1970)
5-HT (intracranial)	Decrease	SCHLESINGER et al. (1969)
p-Chloro-*N*-methyl-amphetamine	Decrease	LEHMANN (1967)
LSD	Decrease	ANLEZARK et al. (1976, 1978)
Quipazine	Decrease	ANLEZARK et al. (1978)

[a] In some experiments mice pretreated with MAO inhibitors were used

Pharmacological intervention in the activity of the 5-HT system modifies susceptibility to audiogenic seizures in mice and rats; however, the results obtained do not permit any definite conclusion. The effects of such substances as reserpine, tetrabenazine, Ro 4-1284, and MAO inhibitors have already been discussed (Sect. B.III.1). The effects observed in mice under the influence of substances intervening in a more selective manner in the activity of the 5-HT system are shown in Table 6. They show that the activation of that system leads to a decrease in susceptibility to seizures since the anticonvulsant effect was found not only after the intracranial administration of 5-HT but also after administration of 5-HTP, the 5-HT receptor agonists quipazine and LSD, and the 5-HT-releasing agent *p*-chloro-*N*-methylamphetamine. Inasmuch, however, as the effect of 5-HTP was correlated with an enhancement of brain 5-HT level (ALEXANDER and KOPELOFF 1976; SCHLESINGER et al. 1970), the decrease in susceptibility to seizures after quipazine and LSD, observed after high doses of these drugs (50 and 9 mg/kg, respectively) questions the specificity of their effect. For example, DA receptor stimulation induced by LSD cannot be excluded as a mechanism responsible for the anticonvulsant effect of the drug (ANLEZARK et al. 1976, 1978).

Considerably more controversial results have been obtained when susceptibility to audiogenic seizures was influenced by substances reducing serotonergic transmission. Although SCHLESINGER et al. (1968a, 1970) – as could be expected – have shown that PCPA increases susceptibility to seizures in mice, other authors, however, have obtained different results. Thus, LEHMANN (1968) described the lack of effect of this inhibitor of 5-HT synthesis, and ALEXANDER et al. (1971), ALEXANDER and KOPELOFF (1976), and KOSTOWSKI et al. (1978) even observed its anticonvulsant activity in this species. Inasmuch, however, as ALEXANDER et al. (1971) and ALEXANDER and KOPELOFF (1976) found such an effect shortly (2–4 h) after PCPA administration – when the 5-HT level in the brain had not yet been lowered and the above pharmacological effect could have been associated with the activity of the amino acid itself – KOSTOWSKI et al. (1978) observed a decrease in susceptibility to seizures 24 and even 48 h after PCPA administration, with a concomitant profound reduction in brain 5-HT concentration. Moreover, ALEXANDER and KOPELOFF (1976) found no effect of α-propyldopacetamide (another inhibitor of 5-HT synthesis), and ANLEZARK et al. (1976) and KOSTOWSKI et al. (1978) reported the anticonvulsant effect of several 5-HT receptor antagonists (methysergide, cyproheptadine, metergoline). The effect of the least-mentioned drugs occurred, however, after relatively high doses and it is difficult to accept it as absolutely specific.

The role of 5-HT in audiogenic convulsions in rats is also not completely clear. JOBE et al. (1973a) found that Ro 4-1284 and PCPA increase susceptibility to seizures, whereas 5-HTP (in iproniazid-pretreated animals) decreases it. Moreover, the Ro 4-1284-induced effect was antagonized by iproniazid, and this action of the MAO inhibitor was completely prevented by PCPA. Interestingly, 5-HTP (plus MAO inhibitor) decreased susceptibility to seizures not only in normal rats, but also in animals with a severe depletion of brain catecholamines (α-MT and cold-induced stress). The increase in susceptibility to seizures in rats after administration of PCPA was confirmed by JERLICZ et al. (1978a), but they – on the other hand – could not demonstrate any effect for the lesion of the median or dorsal raphe nuclei. In the light of these results it is possible to suggest that depletion of whole brain 5-HT is more important for the increase in susceptibility to seizures in rats. Such an effect can be obtained under the influence of PCPA, in contrast to the raphe lesion which depletes 5-HT only in those areas of the brain which receive serotonergic input from the respective raphe nuclei.

There is also one report on the role of 5-HT in audiogenic seizures in rabbits (NELLHAUS 1968). The author found that rabbits of a genetic strain highly susceptible to the seizures had a lower brain 5-HT concentration than animals of a non-sensitive strain.

2. Photogenic Seizures

Several drugs increasing the activity of the central serotonergic system inhibit photically induced epileptic responses in baboons, *Papio papio*. Such an effect has been reported after administration of tryptophan (but only in animals pretreated with an MAO inhibitor – MELDRUM et al. 1972), 5-HTP (BALZANO and MELDRUM 1972; TRIMBLE et al. 1977), 5-HT receptor agonists LSD and *N,N*-dimethyltryptamine (MELDRUM and NAQUET 1970; WALTER et al. 1971), and the 5-HT-releasing drugs fenfluramine and norfenfluramine (KILLAM 1976). In addition, the serotonergic mechanism, besides the dopaminergic one, has been implicated in the anticonvulsant action of ergot alkaloids (ANLEZARK and MELDRUM 1978). On the other hand, when brain 5-HT is presumably depleted with PCPA, some enhancement of photosensitivity has been observed (BALZANO and MELDRUM 1972). All these results would indicate that central 5-HT serves an inhibitory function in the phenomenon of photically induced epilepsy.

There are, however, some other data which do not support such a hypothesis. First of all, 5-HT administered i.c.v. – in contrast to NA or adrenaline (Sect. B.III.2) – does not influence susceptibility to photogenic seizures (ALTSCHULER et al. 1976). Moreover, the 5-HT uptake inhibitor chlorimipramine lowered the seizure threshold (TRIMBLE et al. 1977), whereas 5-HT receptor antagonists (methysergide and metergoline) were shown to have anticonvulsant activity (MELDRUM and NAQUET 1970). However, the chlorimipramine-induced decreased in the seizure threshold was antagonized by 5-HTP, and the anticonvulsant action of the 5-HT receptor blockers was found after doses which produced sedation and loss of muscle tone. This suggests that the above effects of chlorimipramine and 5-HT antagonists may be unspecific.

D. Histamine

In contrast to the abundant literature on catecholamines and 5-HT, data on the role of histamine in susceptibility to seizures are rather sparse. KOHN and MILLICHAP (1958) have shown that the i.c.v. administration of histamine (200–500 μg) produced clonic convulsions in mice and guinea pigs. These convulsions were prevented not only by some anticonvulsants but also by antihistaminics (tripelennamine and diphenhydramine). However, the antagonistic effect of these antihistaminics was partial and was found only in guinea pigs, but not in mice. In contrast to these results GERALD and RICHTER (1976) observed no convulsions in mice after the i.c.v. administration of histamine, though lower doses of the amine (12.5–200 μg) were used in this study.

Some authors have also investigated the influence of various substances modifying the activity of the histaminergic system on the susceptibility of mice and rats to PTZ-induced seizures. In this respect ABBOZZO et al. (1951) have shown that the antihistaminic mepyramine antagonizes in low doses, but in higher doses potentiates this kind of convulsion in mice. DASHPUTRA et al. (1966) have investigated 11 antagonists of the H-1 receptor in rats. They have shown that these drugs fall into three different groups: those that prevent PTZ-induced convulsions (diphenhydramine, mepyramine, thonzylamine), those that potentiate them (antazoline, dimetindene), and those that have no effect (promethazine, pheniramine, chlorcyclizine, phenindamine, methapyrilene, thenalidine). A more precise investigation was carried out on mice by GERALD and RICHTER (1976). They showed that neither *l*-histidine nor i.c.v.-administered histamine affected the minimal (clonic) or maximal (tonic) seizures induced by PTZ. On the other hand, they found that brocresine (an inhibitor of histidine decarboxylase) enhanced the threshold for minimal seizures and decreased the threshold for maximal seizures. The same authors have also studied the influence of many H-1 receptor antagonists, and burimamide and metiamide (H-2 antagonists). Among the H-1 antagonists, cyclizine, diphenhydramine, mepyramine, and tripelennamine increased susceptibility to minimal seizures and reduced the incidence of maximal seizures. Chlorpheniramine and dexbrompheniramine increased susceptibility to minimal seizures, phenindamine antagonized maximal seizures, whereas chlorcyclizine and parathiazine were inactive. Burimamide and metiamide administered systemically did not affect the threshold for clonic convulsions, but metiamide increased susceptibility to maximal seizures. By contrast, after the i.c.v. administration of the latter drug an increase in risk to minimal seizures was observed. The above results show that whereas a reduction in histaminergic transmission modifies susceptibility to PTZ, an enhancement in the transmission is without effect. However, the fact that depletion of brain histamine (after brocresine) on the one hand and the blockade of H-1 or H-2 receptors on the other lead to rather opposite effects, shows that they are not specific.

E. Conclusions

The analysis of the data reviewed here indicates that the participation of central monoamines in convulsive phenomena is varied. The main role is undoubtedly played by NA, for which an inhibitory role was demonstrated in the vast majority of experimental seizure models. The inhibitory role of NA in susceptibility to seizures appears regardless of the convulsogenic factor (electric current, chemical substances, sound) and the type of seizures (clonic, tonic). All that is somewhat doubtful is the importance of NA in PTZ-induced seizures in mice (but not in rats), for photogenic seizures, and for the fully developed kindled seizures from the amygdala. The only clear exception is the low-frequency minimal electroshock seizure threshold; in this model the modification of activity of the NA system has no effect on susceptibility to seizures. Since this model reflects discharge of neurons responsible for a clonic seizure with little discharge spread and since, on the other hand, NA inhibits susceptibility to seizures in high-frequency minimal electroshock seizure threshold which reflects more intense discharge of neurons responsible for a clonic seizures and more discharge spread, this – taken all together – may indicate that NA does not participate in events directly initiating seizure activity, but may be important for the efficiency of the generation, spread, and propagation of the discharges from their initial site. A similar conclusion may be drawn from the results obtained in a different model – the development of kindling convulsions from the amygdala. A pharmacological manipulation of the NA system does not affect the afterdischarge threshold and the duration of the first afterdischarge, whereas it changes the number of stimulations necessary to produce behavioral seizures. This indicates that NA is not involved in the epileptogenicity of the amygdala, but participates in the spread of epileptiform activity from this stimulated structure.

There are relatively few studies on the role of NA in the various regions of the central nervous system. Thus, forebrain NA has been found to be involved in susceptibility to seizures in maximal electroshock seizures, in the development of kindling convulsions from the amygdala and in PTZ-induced tonic convulsions, but not in PTZ-induced clonic seizures. Brain stem NA seems to be important for PTZ-induced clonic convulsions, whereas cerebellar NA does not participate in this model. Spinal cord NA system has been shown to have an inhibitory function in maximal electroshock seizures but not in PTZ-induced clonic convulsions.

In contrast to NA, the cerebral DA seems to participate only in some types of convulsions. Many findings indicate its inhibitory role in the photogenic seizures in *Papio papio* baboons. Some, but not all, data also indicate its inhibitory role in some models of electrogenic seizures (high-frequency minimal electroshock seizure threshold, maximal electroshock seizures) and in audiogenic seizures in mice (but not in rats). In other models negative results concerning the involvement of DA predominate.

There is much controversy and doubt surrounding the role of 5-HT. This amine does not participate in low-frequency minimal electroshock seizure threshold, but possibly plays an inhibitory role in high-frequency minimal electroshock seizure threshold, in maximal electroshock seizures (in mice only), in PTZ-induced clonic and tonic convulsions (in rats only), in audiogenic convulsions (in rats only), and in photogenic seizures. However, even in these latter models results appear which contradict the assumption about the inhibitory role of 5-HT. The most controversial results were obtained in amygdaloid kindling convulsions (development of seizures and established seizures). In this model results were obtained which indicate either an inhibitory or a facilitatory role for 5-HT.

The participation of histamine has been the subject of only a few studies. Almost all the data pertain to PTZ-induced convulsions and suggest that histamine plays no significant role.

References

Abbozzo G, Genazzani E, Donatelli L (1951) L'action du neoantergan sur les convulsions au cardiazol et sur la narcose a l'avertine. Arch Int Pharmacodyn Ther 88:209–222

Alexander GJ, Kopeloff LM (1970) Metrazol seizures in rats: effect of *p*-chlorophenylalanine. Brain Res 22:231–235

Alexander GJ, Kopeloff LM (1976) Audiogenic seizures in mice: influence of agents affecting brain serotonin. Res Commun Chem Pathol Pharmacol 14:437–448
Alexander GJ, Kopeloff LM (1978) Effect of 6-hydroxydopamine. Delayed motor manifestations associated with high mortality in sound-induced seizures in mice. Neurochem Res 3:821–825
Alexander GJ, Kopeloff LM, Alexander RB (1971) Anticonvulsive effect of *p*-chlorophenylalanine in audiosensitive mice. Life Sci 10:877–882
Almatura AC, Bonati M, Brunello N, Giordano PL, Algeri S (1978) The activity of some neurotransmitter-synthesizing enzymes in experimental cobalt epilepsy. Neurosci Lett 7:83–87
Altshuler HL, Killam EK, Killam KF (1976) Biogenic amines and the photomyoclonic syndrome in the baboon, *Papio papio*. J Pharmacol Exp Ther 196:156–166
Anlezark GM, Meldrum BS (1975) Effects of apomorphine, ergocornine and piribedil on audiogenic seizures in DBA/2 mice. Br J Pharmacol 53:419–421
Anlezark GM, Horton RW, Meldrum BS (1978) Dopamine agonists and audiogenic seizures: the relationship between protection against seizures and changes in monoamine metabolism. Biochem Pharmacol 27:2821–2828
Anlezark G, Horton R, Meldrum B (1979) The anticonvulsant action of the (−)- and (+)-enantiomers of propranolol. J Pharm Pharmacol 31:482–483
Anlezark G, Meldrum B (1978) Blockade of photically induced epilepsy by "dopamine agonist" ergot alkaloids. Psychopharmacology (Berlin) 57:57–62
Anlezark G, Pycock C, Meldrum B (1976) Ergot alkaloids as dopamine agonists: comparison in two rodent models. Eur J Pharmacol 37:295–302
Arnold PS, Racine RJ, Wise RA (1973) Effects of atropine, reserpine, 6-hydroxydopamine and handling on seizure development in the rat. Exp Neurol 40:457–470
Ashton C, Anlezark G, Meldrum B (1976) Inhibition of reflex epilepsy by (±)-*N*-*n*-propylnorapomorphine. Eur J Pharmacol 39:399–401
Ashton D, Leysen JE, Wauquier A (1980) Neurotransmitters and receptor binding in amygdaloid kindled rats: serotonergic and noradrenergic modulatory effects. Life Sci 27:1547–1556
Ayhan IH (1976) Potentiation of morphine-induced seizure by 6-hydroxydopamine. Arch Int Pharmacodyn Ther 223:282–286
Azzaro AJ, Wenger GR, Craig CR, Stitzel RE (1972) Reserpine-induced alterations in brain amines and their relationship to changes in the incidence of minimal electroshock seizures in mice. J Pharmacol Exp Ther 180:558–568
Balzamo E, Meldrum BS (1972) Photic epilepsy in *Papio papio* and drugs modifying cerebral monoamine levels. Brain Res 42:543–544
Bhattacharya SK, Ghosh P, Bose R (1978) Pentylenetetrazol induced clonic convulsions in rat. Role of brain monoamines. Mater Med Pol 10:184–187
Billiet M, Bernard P, Delaunois A, De Schaepdryver A (1970) Induced changes in caudate nucleus dopamine and electroshock threshold. Arch Int Pharmacodyn Ther 188:396–400
Boggan WO (1973) Serotonin and convulsions. In: Barchas J, Usdin E (eds) Serotonin and behavior. Academic, New York, pp 167–172
Boggan WO, Seiden LS (1971) Dopa reversal of reserpine enhancement of audiogenic seizure susceptibility in mice. Physiol Behav 6:215–217
Boggan WO, Freedman DX, Lovell RA, Schlesinger K (1971) Studies in audiogenic seizure susceptibility. Psychopharmacologia (Berlin) 20:48–56
Bourn WM, Chin L, Picchioni AL (1972) Enhancement of audiogenic seizure by 6-hydroxydopamine. J Pharm Pharmacol 24:913–914
Bourn WM, Chin L, Picchioni AL (1977) Effect of neonatal 6-hydroxydopamine treatment on audiogenic seizures. Life Sci 21:701–705
Bourn WM, Chin L, Picchioni AL (1978) The role of dopamine in sound-induced convulsions. J Pharm Pharmacol 30:800–801
Browning RA, Maynert EW (1978a) Effects of intraventricularly administered monoamines on seizure susceptibility and body temperature in rats. Neuropharmacology 17:649–653

Browning RA, Maynert EW (1978b) Effect of intracisternal 6-hydroxydopamine on seizure susceptibility in rats. Eur J Pharmacol 50:97–101
Buterbaugh GG (1978) Effect of drugs modifying central serotonergic function on the response of extensor and nonextensor rats to maximal electroshock. Life Sci 23:2393–2404
Buterbaugh GG, London ED (1977) The relationship between magnitude of electroshock stimulation and the effects of digitoxigenin, pentylenetetrazol and brain monoamine reduction on electroshock convulsive thresholds. Neuropharmacology 16:617–623
Callaghan DA, Schwark WS (1979) Involvement of catecholamines in kindled amygdaloid convulsions in the rat. Neuropharmacology 18:541–545
Chen G, Bohner B (1956) A study of the neuropharmacologic properties of certain convulsants, anticonvulsants and reserpine. J Pharmacol Exp Ther 117:142–147
Chen G, Bohner B (1961) The anti-reserpine effects of certain centrally-acting agents. J Pharmacol Exp Ther 131:179–184
Chen G, Ensor CR, Bohner B (1954) A facilitation action of reserpine on the central nervous system. Proc Soc Exp Biol Med 86:507–510
Chen G, Ensor CR, Bohner B (1968a) Drug effects on the disposition of active biogenic amines in the CNS. Life Sci 7:1063–1074
Chen G, Ensor CR, Bohner B (1968b) Studies of drug effects on electrically induced extensor seizures and clinical implications. Arch Int Pharmacodyn Ther 172:183–218
Chimote KV, Moghe PJ (1977) Putative neurotransmitters in CNS and chemoconvulsions. Arch Int Pharmacodyn Ther 228:304–313
Chow MI, Hendley CD (1959) Effect of monoamine oxidase inhibitors on experimental convulsions. Fed Proc 18:376
Coleman DL, Schlesinger K (1965) Effects of pyridoxine deficiency on audiogenic seizure susceptibility in inbred mice. Proc Soc Exp Biol Med 119:264–266
Corcoran ME, Mason ST (1980) Role of forebrain catecholamines in amygdaloid kindling. Brain Res 190:473–484
Corcoran ME, Fibiger HC, McGeer EG, Wada JA (1973) Potentiation of leptazol seizures by 6-hydroxydopamine. J Pharm Pharmacol 25:497–499
Corcoran ME, Fibiger HC, McCaughran JA, Wada JA (1974) Potentiation of amygdaloid kindling and metrazol-induced seizures by 6-hydroxydopamine in rats. Exp Neurol 45:118–133
Cox B, Lomax P (1976) Brain amines and spontaneous epileptic seizures in the Mongolian gerbil. Pharmacol Biochem Behav 4:263–267
Crunelli V, Bernasconi S, Samanin R (1979) Evidence against serotonin involvement in the tonic component of electrically induced convulsions and in carbamazepine anticonvulsant activity. Psychopharmacology (Berlin) 66:79–85
Dashputra PG, Sharma ML, Jagtap MK, Khapre MD, Rajapurkar MV (1966) Modification of metrazol induced convulsions in rats by antihistaminics. Arch Int Pharmacodyn Ther 160:106–112
De la Torre JC, Mullan S (1970) A possible role for 5-hydroxytryptamine in drug-induced seizures. J Pharm Pharmacol 22:858–859
De la Torre JC, Kawanaga HM, Mullan S (1970) Seizure susceptibility after manipulation of brain serotonin. Arch Int Pharmacodyn Ther 188:298–304
De Schaepdryver AF, Piette Y, Delaunois AL (1962) Brain amines and electroshock threshold. Arch Int Pharmacodyn Ther 140:358–367
Dow RC, Hill AG, McQueen JK (1974) Effects of some dopamine receptor stimulants on cobalt-induced epilepsy in the rat. Br J Pharmacol 52:135P
Eichbaum FW, Yasaka WJ (1973) Inhibition of post-decapitation convulsions by reserpine. Experientia 29:816–817
Fariello RG, Hornykiewicz O (1979) Substantia nigra and pentylenetetrazol threshold in rats: correlation with striatal dopamine metabolism. Exp Neurol 65:202–208
Frey HH (1964) Note on the interactions of amphetamine with anticonvulsant drugs. Acta Pharmacol Toxicol (Copenh) 21:290–298

Fukuda T, Araki Y, Suenaga N (1975) Inhibitory effects of 6-hydroxydopamine on the clonic convulsions induced by electroshock and decapitation. Neuropharmacology 14:579–583
Gerald MC, Gupta TK (1977) Catecholaminergic involvement in the effects of amphetamine isomers on seizure susceptibility. Eur J Pharmacol 41:231–234
Gerald MC, Richter NA (1976) Studies on the effects of histaminergic agents on seizure susceptibility in mice. Psychopharmacologia (Berlin) 46:277–282
Gerald MC, Riffee WH (1973) Acute and chronic effects of *d*- and *l*-amphetamine on seizure susceptibility in mice. Eur J Pharmacol 21:323–330
Goldberg ME, Milmore JE, Haubrich MK, Haubrich DR (1975) Increased susceptibility to seizures and decreased catecholamine turnover in spontaneously hypertensive rats. Eur J Pharmacol 33:389–393
Gray WD, Rauh CE (1971) The relation between monoamines in brain and the anticonvulsant action of inhibitors of carbonic anhydrase. J Pharmacol Exp Ther 177:206–218
Gray WD, Rauh CE (1974) The anticonvulsant action of the carbonic anhydryse inhibitor methazolamide: possible involvement of a noradrenergic mechanism. Eur J Pharmacol 28:42–54
György L (1979) Role of dopaminergic and GABA-ergic interactions in seizure susceptibility. Arch Int Pharmacodyn Ther 241:280–286
Horton R, Anlezark G, Meldrum B (1980) Noradrenergic influences on sound-induced seizures. J Pharmacol Exp Ther 214:437–442
Jaeger V, Esplin B, Capek R (1979) The anticonvulsant effects of propranolol and β-adrenergic blockade. Experientia 35:80–81
Jenney EH (1954) Changes in convulsant thresholds after rauwolfia serpentina, reserpine and veriloid. Fed Proc 13:370
Jenney EH, Pfeiffer CC (1956) The predictable value of anticonvulsant indices. Ann NY Acad Sci 64:679–689
Jerlicz M, Kostowski W, Bidziński A, Hauptmann M (1978 a) Audiogenic seizure susceptibility in rats with lesioned raphe nuclei and treated with *p*-chlorophenylalanine. Pol J Pharmacol Pharm 30:63–68
Jerlicz M, Kostowski W, Bidziński A, Hauptmann M, Dymecki J (1978 b) Audiogenic seizures in rats: relation to noradrenergic neurons of the *locus coeruleus*. Acta Physiol Pol 29:409–412
Jobe PC, Picchioni AL, Chin L (1973 a) Role of brain 5-hydroxytryptamine in audiogenic seizure in the rat. Life Sci 13:1–13
Jobe PC, Picchioni AL, Chin L (1973 b) Effect of lithium carbonate and α-methyl-*p*-tyrosine on audiogenic seizure intensity. J Pharm Pharmacol 25:830–831
Jobe PC, Picchioni AL, Chin L (1973 c) Role of brain norepinephrine in audiogenic seizure in the rat. J Pharmacol Exp Ther 184:1–10
Jobe PC, Stull RE, Geiger PF (1974) The relative significance of norepinephrine, dopamine and 5-hydroxytryptamine in electroshock seizure in the rat. Neuropharmacology 13:961–968
Jones BJ, Roberts DJ (1968) The effects of intracerebroventricularly administered noradnamine and other sympathomimetic amines upon leptazol convulsions in mice. Br J Pharmacol 34:27–31
Kellogg C (1971) Serotonin metabolism in the brains of mice sensitive or resistant to audiogenic seizures. J Neurobiol 2:209–219
Kellogg C (1976) Audiogenic seizures: relation to age and mechanisms of monoamine neurotransmission. Brain Res 106:87–103
Kilian M, Frey HH (1973) Central monoamines and convulsive thresholds in mice and rats. Neuropharmacology 12:681–692
Killam EK (1976) Measurement of anticonvulsant activity in the *Papio papio* model of epilepsy. Fed Proc 35:2264–2269
Kleinrok Z, Przegaliński E, Czuczwar S (1977) Participation of 5-hydroxytryptamine in anticonvulsive action of benzodiazepines. Pol J Pharmacol Pharm 29:385–391
Kleinrok Z, Czuczwar S, Wójcik A, Przegaliński E (1978) Brain dopamine and seizure susceptibility in mice. Pol J Pharmacol Pharm 30:513–519

Kobayashi K, Shirakabe T, Kishikawa H, Mori A (1976) Catecholamine levels in penicillin-induced epileptic focus of the cat cerebral cortex. Acta Neurochir 23:93–100
Kobinger W (1958a) Reversibility of a facilitatory action of reserpine on the central nervous system, by methylamphetamine. Experientia 14:337–338
Kobinger W (1958b) Beeinflussung der Cardiazolkrampfschwelle durch veränderten 5-Hydroxytryptamingehalt des Zentralnervensystems. Naunyn Schmiedeberg's Arch Exp Pathol Pharmakol 233:559–566
Koe BK, Weissman A (1968) The pharmacology of *para*-chlorophenylalanine, a selective depletor of serotonin stores. In: Garattini S, Shore PA (eds) Advances in pharmacology, vol 6B. Academic, New York, pp 29–47
Kohn R, Millichap JG (1958) Properties of seizures induced by histamine. Proc Soc Exp Biol Med 99:623–628
Koslow SH, Roth LJ (1971) Reserpine and acetazolamide in maximum electroshock seizure in the rat. J Pharmacol Exp Ther 176:711–717
Kostowski W, Bidziński A, Hauptmann M, Malinowski JE, Jerlicz M, Dymecki J (1978) Brain serotonin and epileptic seizures in mice: a pharmacological and biochemical study. Pol J Pharmacol Pharm 30:41–47
Kovacs DA, Zoll JG (1974) Seizure inhibition by median raphe nucleus stimulation in rat. Brain Res 70:165–169
Lazarova MB, Roussinov KS (1978) On certain effects of dopaminergic agents in pentylenetetrazol convulsions. Acta Physiol Pharmacol Bulg 4:50–55
Lazarova M, Roussinov K, Kleinrok Z, Rajtar G (1980) On some relationship between GABA-ergic and 5-HT-ergic mechanisms in pentylenetetrazol convulsive-seizure reactions. Agressologie 21:253–257
Lazarova M, Roussinov K, Yanev S, Petkov V, Stach R, Kacz D (1981) Effect of chronic *para*-chlorophenylalanine treatment on convulsive-seizure reactions. Acta Biol Med Ger 40:309–316
Lehmann A (1967) Audiogenic seizure data in mice supporting new theories of biogenic amine mechanisms in the central nervous system. Life Sci 6:1423–1431
Lehmann A (1968) Modification de l'intensite de la crise audiogene par des substances actives sur le metabolisme des amines biogenes du cerveau de souris. C R Soc Biol (Paris) 162:24–27
Lehmann A (1977) Mechanisms underlying modifications in the severity of audiogenic convulsions. Life Sci 20:2047–2060
Lessin AW, Parkes MW (1959) The effects of reserpine and other agents upon leptazol convulsions in mice. Br J Pharmacol 14:108–111
Leszkovszky G, Tardos L (1965) Some effects of propranolol on the central nervous system. J Pharm Pharmacol 17:518–520
Little JM, Conrad EA (1960) Pentylenetetrazol seizure activity in mice as influenced by route of administration, acute adrenalectomy and reserpine. J Pharmacol Exp Ther 129:454–461
London ED, Buterbaugh GG (1978) Modification of electroshock convulsive responses and thresholds in neonatal rats after brain monoamine reduction. J Pharmacol Exp Ther 206:81–90
Lovell RA (1971) Some neurochemical aspects of convulsions. In: Lajtha A (ed) Handbook of neurochemistry, vol VI. Plenum, New York, pp 63–102
Madan BR, Barar FSK (1974) Anticonvulsant activity of some β-adrenoceptor blocking agents in mice. Eur J Pharmacol 29:1–4
Maj J, Vetulani J (1970) Some pharmacological properties of *N,N*-disubstituted dithiocarbamates and their effect on the brain catecholamine levels. Eur J Pharmacol 9:183–189
Mason ST, Corcoran ME (1978) Forebrain noradrenaline and metrazol-induced seizures. Life Sci 23:167–172
Mason ST, Corcoran ME (1979a) Seizure susceptibility after depletion of spinal or cerebellar noradrenaline with 6-OHDA. Brain Res 166:418–421
Mason ST, Corcoran ME (1979b) Catecholamines and convulsions. Brain Res 170:497–507
Maynert EW (1969) The role of biochemical and neurohumoral factors in the laboratory evaluation of antiepileptic drugs. Epilepsia 10:145–162

Maynert EW, Marczynski TJ, Browning RA (1975) The role of the neurotransmitters in the epilepsies. In: Friedlander WJ (ed) Advances in neurology, vol 13. Raven, New York, pp 79–147
McGeer EG, Ikeda H, Asakura T, Wada JA (1969) Lack of abnormality in brain aromatic amines in rats and mice susceptible to audiogenic seizure. J Neurochem 16:945–950
McIntyre DC, Saari M, Pappas BA (1979) Potentiation of amygdala kindling in adult or infant rats by injections of 6-hydroxydopamine. Exp Neurol 63:527–544
McKenzie GM, Soroko FE (1972) The effects of apomorphine, (+)-amphetamine and L-dopa on maximal electroshock convulsions – a comparative study in the rat and mouse. J Pharm Pharmacol 24:696–701
McKenzie GM, Soroko FE (1973) Inhibition of the anticonvulsant activity of L-dopa by FLA-63, a dopamine-β-hydroxylase inhibitor. J Pharm Pharmacol 25:76–77
Meldrum B, Anlezark G, Trimble M (1975) Drugs modifying dopaminergic activity and behaviour, the EEG and epilepsy in *Papio papio*. Eur J Pharmacol 32:203–213
Meldrum BS, Balzamo E (1971) Etude des effets de l'-α-methylparatyrosine chez le *Papio papio*. C R Soc Biol (Paris) 165:2379–2381
Meldrum BS, Naquet R (1970) Effects of psilocybin, dimethyltryptamine and various lysergic acid derivatives on photically-induced epilepsy in the baboon (*Papio papio*). Br J Pharmacol 40:144P–145P
Meldrum BS, Balzamo E, Wada JA, Vuillon-Cacciuttolo G (1972) Effects of L-tryptophan, L-3,4-dihydroxyphenylalanine and tranylcypromine on the electroencephalogram and on photically induced epilepsy in the baboon, *Papio papio*. Physiol Behav 9:615–621
Mennear JH, Rudzik AD (1968) The effect of pronethalol on the anticonvulsant action of acetazolamide. Life Sci 7:1265–1269
Mohr E, Corcoran ME (1981) Depletion of noradrenaline and amygdaloid kindling. Exp Neurol 72:507–511
Murmann W, Almirante L, Saccani-Guelfi M (1966) Central nervous system effects of four β-adrenergic receptor blocking agents. J Pharm Pharmacol 18:317–318
Nellhaus G (1968) Relationship of brain serotonin to convulsions. Neurology (Minneap) 18:298–299
Oishi R, Suenaga N, Fukuda T (1979a) Possible involvement of brainstem norepinephrine in pentylenetetrazol convulsions in rats. Pharmacol Biochem Behav 10:57–61
Oishi R, Suenaga N, Hidaka T, Fukuda T (1979b) The role of α-adrenoceptors in the regulation of pentylenetetrazol convulsions in mice. J Pharm Pharmacol 31:709–710
Osuide G, Wambebe C (1979) The influence of intraperitoneally injected 6-hydroxydopamine on electroshock seizure in chicks and rats. Clin Exp Pharmacol Physiol 6:367–372
P'an SY, Funderburk WH, Finger KF (1961) Anticonvulsant effect of nialamide and diphenylhydantoin. Proc Soc Exp Biol Med 108:680–683
Pfeifer AK, Galambos E (1965) Action of alpha-methyldopa on the pharmacological and biochemical effect of reserpine in rats and mice. Biochem Pharmacol 14:37–40
Pfeifer AK, Galambos E (1967a) The effect of reserpine, α-methyl-*m*-tyrosine, prenylamine, and guanethidine on metrazol-convulsions and the brain monoamine level in mice. Arch Int Pharmacodyn Ther 165:201–211
Pfeifer AK, Galambos E (1967b) The effect of (±)-*p*-chloroamphetamine on the susceptibility to seizures and on the monoamine level in brain and heart of mice and rats. J Pharm Pharmacol 19:400–402
Pfeifer AK, Vizi ES, Satory E (1964) Studies on the action of guanethidine on the central nervous system and on the norepinephrine content of brain in rats. In: Bradley PB, Flügel F, Hoch PH (eds) Neuro-psychopharmacology, vol 3. Elsevier, Amsterdam, pp 417–419
Picchioni AL, Chin L, Breitner C (1962) Relationship between brain levels of 5-hydroxytryptamine (5-HT) and norepinephrine (NE) and susceptibility to electrically-induced seizures. Fed Proc 21:416
Plotnikoff N (1960) Ataractics and strain differences in audiogenic seizures in mice. Psychopharmacologia (Berlin) 1:429–432
Prockop DJ, Shore PA, Brodie BB (1959) Anticonvulsant properties of monoamine oxidase inhibitors. Ann NY Acad Sci 80:643–651

Przegaliński E (1975) The role of 5-hydroxytryptamine in the mechanism of action of anticonvulsant drugs. Pol J Pharmacol Pharm 27 [Suppl]: 195–199

Przegaliński E (1976a) Convulsive thresholds and the activity of anticonvulsants in electroseizure test. The role of serotoninergic system. Pol J Pharmacol Pharm 28:143–155

Przegaliński E (1976b) The role of cerebral 5-hydroxytryptamine for convulsive threshold and anticonvulsant effect of acetazolamide in rats. Arch Immunol Ther Exp (Warsz) 24:821–827

Quattrone A, Samanin R (1977) Decreased anticonvulsant activity of carbamazepine in 6-hydroxydopamine-treated rats. Eur J Pharmacol 41:333–336

Quattrone A, Crunelli V, Samanin R (1978) Seizure susceptibility and anticonvulsant activity of carbamazepine, diphenylhydantoin and phenobarbital in rats with selective depletions of brain monoamines. Neuropharmacology 17:643–647

Racine R, Coscina DV (1979) Effects of midbrain raphe lesions or systemic *p*-chlorophenylalanine on the development of kindled seizures in rats. Brain Res Bull 4:1–7

Riffee WH, Gerald MC (1976) Effects of amphetamine isomers and CNS catecholaminergic blockers on seizures in mice. Neuropharmacology 15:677–682

Riffee WH, Gerald MC (1977) The effects of chronic administration of (+)-amphetamine on seizure threshold and endogenous catecholamine concentrations and their rates of biosynthesis in mice. Psychopharmacology (Berlin) 51:175–179

Roussinov KS, Lazarova MB (1978) On certain relationships between gamma-aminobutyric acid (GABA) and dopaminergic agents in pentylenetetrazol convulsions. Acta Physiol Pharmacol Bulg 4:43–49

Roussinov KS, Lazarova MB, Atanassova-Shopova S (1976) On certain relationships between gamma-aminobutyric acid (GABA) and adrenergic mechanisms in convulsive-seizure reactions. Acta Physiol Pharmacol Bulg 2:69–76

Rudzik AD, Johnson GA (1970) Effect of amphetamine and amphetamine analogs on convulsive thresholds. In: Costa E, Garattini S (eds) Amphetamines and related compounds. Raven, New York, pp 715–728

Safta L, Cuparencu B, Danau M, Comes L (1976) Some behavioural changes induced by amantadine (adamantine). Acta Biol Med Ger 35:229–233

Schlesinger K, Boggan W, Freedman DX (1965) Genetics of audiogenic seizures: I. Relation to brain serotonin and norepinephrine in mice. Life Sci 4:2345–2351

Schlesinger K, Boggan W, Freedman DX (1968a) Genetics of audiogenic seizures: II. Effects of pharmacological manipulation of brain serotonin, norepinephrine and gamma-aminobutyric acid. Life Sci 7:437–447

Schlesinger K, Boggan WO, Griek BJ (1968b) Pharmacogenetic correlates of pentylenetetrazol and electroconvulsive seizure threshold in mice. Psychopharmacologia (Berlin) 13:181–188

Schlesinger K, Stavnes KL, Boggan WO (1969) Modification of audiogenic and pentylenetetrazol seizures with gamma-aminobutyric acid, norepinephrine and serotonin. Psychopharmacologia (Berlin) 15:226–231

Schlesinger K, Boggan WO, Freedman DX (1970) Genetics of audiogenic seizures: III. Time response relationships between drug administration and seizure susceptibility. Life Sci 9:721–729

Schlesinger K, Harkins J, Deckard BS, Paden C (1975) Catechol-*O*-methyl transferase and monoamine oxidase activities in brains of mice susceptible and resistant to audiogenic seizures. J Neurobiol 6:587–596

Schonfeld AR, Glick SD (1980) Neuropharmacological analysis of handling-induced seizures in gerbils. Neuropharmacology 19:1009–1016

Scudder CL, Karczmar AG, Everett GM, Gibson JE, Rifkin M (1966) Brain catecholamines and serotonin levels in various strains and genera of mice and a possible interpretation for the correlations of amine levels with electroshock latency and behavior. Int J Neuropharmacol 5:343–351

Scuvee-Moreau J, Lepot M, Brotchi J, Gerebtzoff MA, Dresse A (1977) Action of phenytoin, ethosuximide and of the carbidopa-L-dopa association in semi-chronic cobalt-induced epilepsy in the rat. Arch Int Pharmacodyn Ther 230:92–99

Siegel J, Murphy GJ (1979) Serotonergic inhibition of amygdala-kindled seizures in cats. Brain Res 174:337–340
Simonton RL, Browning RA (1977) Increased sensitivity to maximal electroshock seizures following selective destruction of noradrenergic neurons with 6-hydroxydopamine. Neurosci Abst 3:145–148
Spencer PSJ, Turner TAR (1969) Blockade of biogenic amine synthesis: its effect on the responses to leptazol and dexamphetamine in rats. Br J Pharmacol 37:94–103
Spoerlein MT, Ellman AM (1961) Facilitation of metrazol-induced seizures by iproniazid and beta-phenylisopropylhydrazine in mice. Arch Int Pharmacodyn Ther 133:193–199
Stach R, Lazarova MB, Kacz D (1981) Serotonergic mechanism in seizures kindled from the rabbit amygdala. Naunyn Schmiedebergs Arch Pharmacol 316:56–58
Stull RE, Jobe PC, Geiger PF, Ferguson GG (1973) Effects of dopamine receptor stimulation and blockade on Ro 4-1284-induced enhancement of electroshock seizure. J Pharm Pharmacol 25:842–844
Stull RE, Jobe PC, Geiger PF (1977) Brain areas involved in the catecholamine mediated regulation of electroshock seizure intensity. J Pharm Pharmacol 29:8–11
Trimble M, Anlezark G, Meldrum B (1977) Seizure activity in photosensitive baboons following antidepressant drugs and the role of serotoninergic mechanisms. Psychopharmacology (Berlin) 51:159–164
Truitt EB Jr, Ebersberger EM (1962) Decarboxylase inhibitors affect convulsion thresholds to hexafluorodiethyl ether. Science 135:105–106
Walter S, Balzano E, Vuillon-Cacciuttolo G, Naquet R (1971) Effets comportementaux et electrographiques du diethylamide de l'acide *d*-lysergique (LSD 25) sur le *Papio papio* photo-sensible. Electroencephalogr Clin Neurophysiol 30:294–305
Wenger GR, Stitzel RE, Craig CR (1973) The role of biogenic amines in the reserpine-induced alteration of minimal electroshock seizure thresholds in the mouse. Neuropharmacology 12:693–703
Wolf HH, Stock GA Jr (1966) Utility of two convulsant techniques as indicators of CNS excitability. J Pharm Sci 55:1455–1457
Wolf HH, Rollins DE, Rowland CR, Reigle TG (1969) The importance of endogenous catecholamines in the activity of some CNS stimulants. Int J Neuropharmacol 8:319–328
Worms P, Lloyd KG (1979) The anticonvulsant effect of neuroleptics: dependence on intact noradrenergic transmission. In: Usdin E, Kopin IJ, Barchas J (eds) Catecholamines: basic and clinical frontiers. Pergamon, New York, pp 1643–1645
Yeoh PN, Wolf HH (1968) Effects of some adrenergic agents on low frequency electroshock seizures. J Pharm Sci 57:340–342

CHAPTER 6

Acetylcholine

C. Bianchi and L. Beani

A. Introduction

It is generally accepted that transmitters and modulators play a key role in epilepsy and that they are involved in attack initiation, spread, and termination. Thus, the altered synaptic availability of some excitatory and inhibitory messengers could represent an essential bridge between nerve cell physiology and pathology. To date, scientists dealing with epilepsy have focused their attention on the possible role played by the better known putative transmitters, like monoamines, gamma-aminobutyric acid (GABA), and acetylcholine (ACh) (Maynert et al. 1975; Karkzmar 1979). Following the development of new experimental models, such as kindling, the value of ACh in the field of epileptogenesis has recently increased dramatically (McNamara et al. 1980; Girgis 1981).

B. Effect of Cholinergic Drugs on Susceptibility to Seizures

The large body of contradictory results makes it difficult to draw definitive conclusions about susceptibility to seizures caused by drugs acting on the cholinergic system.

In view of their desynchronizing properties cholinomimetic compounds may counteract particular types of seizures, such as the repetitive discharges of cortical isolated slabs (Vasques and Kripp 1973) and cobalt-induced epilepsy (Hoover et al. 1977), although by themselves they are epileptogenic and lower the threshold of convulsant drugs and electric shock (Chen et al. 1968; Karczmar 1967).

Similarly atropine, perhaps as a consequence of its hypersynchronizing action, may facilitate other kinds of convulsions, such as the repetitive discharges of cortical isolated slabs (Vasques and Kripp 1973), although by itself it is capable of counteracting clonic seizures (Greer and Alpern 1977) or electrically induced extensor seizures (Chen et al. 1968). To make this picture even more complicated, both ACh agonists and antagonists cause seizures when they are locally applied to the cortex at high concentrations.

In order to propose an acceptable explanation for these contradictory findings, a distinction is needed between general and local drug treatment. When ACh antagonists or agonists are given systemically, they can change the safety factor in nicotine excitatory synapses and the extent and duration of muscarinic inhibitory and excitatory modulation. Assuming that both functional components (nicotinic and muscarinic) are involved in controlling brain excitability, it is not surprising that ACh-related drugs may reduce or increase susceptibility to seizures, depending on the dose and experimental conditions.

Recently, KRNJEVIC and ROPERT (1981) described the positive muscarinic control exerted by the cholinergic septohippocampal pathways on the firing rate of CA_1 pyramidal cells, normally inhibited by other noncholinergic cells. Since nicotinic receptors are also present in this area, their involvement in the regulation of the inhibitory input, as happens in the somesthetic cortex, caudate, and thalamus, cannot be excluded.

Consequently, depending on this particular circuit arrangement, the antimuscarinic or antinicotinic agents may counteract or favor the repetitive firing rate. Similar two-sided consideration can also be given to the ACh agonists. The generally recognized desynchronizing action of the ACh agonists may support the claims concerning the antiepileptic properties sometimes displayed by physostigmine (KARCZMAR 1979). On the other hand, the excessive, prolonged activation of the cholinoceptive cells is capable of promoting certain alterations in their membrane properties, similar to those found in the epileptic neurons. Therefore, the use of ACh agonists can resolve or worsen the convulsive state.

Examining now the topical application of ACh agonists and antagonists, our first criticism concerns the extremely high concentrations (1%–10%) generally used. In our opinion, cholinergic block is the most probable consequence of such procedures. In fact, agonists such as ACh at 1%–5% can be suspected to induce receptor desensitization, while antagonists such as atropine at 1% surely cause a full muscarinic blockade, together with other unspecific "local anesthetic" effects. In both circumstances, excluding cholinergic (and other) signals from the multitransmitter interplay could cause functional imbalance between inhibitory and excitatory inputs and induce hypersynchrony.

C. Effect of Experimental and Spontaneous Seizures on the Cholinergic System

I. Electroshock and Convulsant Drugs

In anesthetized animals, EEG seizures or motor convulsions caused by pentylenetetrazol, strychnine, picrotoxin, or bicuculline are associated with increased ACh efflux from the cerebral cortex (MITCHELL 1963; BELESLIN et al. 1965; HEMSWORTH and NEAL 1968; CELESIA and JASPER 1968; PEPEU 1974; GARDNER and WEBSTER 1977).

This suggests cholinergic activation during drug-induced imbalance between excitatory and inhibitory mechanisms controlling the cortex. The cholinergic pathways, related to both the primary sensory inflow through the thalamus and the diffuse "reticular" and "limbic" projections, could be simultaneously activated (COLLIER and MITCHELL 1966; DUDAR and SZERB 1969). The partial dissociation reported between ACh release and EEG activity may be due to cholinergic interspike activity inhibition (PHILLIS and YORK 1968; STONE 1972).

As a logical consequence of increased ACh release, not only compensatory increase in ACh synthesis (SIMON et al. 1976) but also a reduction in transmitter brain levels would be expected. However, the reports of different groups conflict.

According to RICHTER and CROSSLAND (1949) and KUROKAVA et al. (1963), a single electroshock lowers brain ACh levels, but after multiple electroshocks the transmitter content quickly returns to or exceeds the control levels. These observations have been refuted by HERKEN and NEUBERT (1953). Probably ACh released during seizures induces feedback inhibition in cholinergic cells (SAELENS and SCHUMAN 1974), and the procedures of killing affect the results.

As a rule, convulsant drugs lower the brain ACh content (ELLIOT et al. 1950; GIARMAN and PEPEU 1962; BEANI et al. 1969; KUROKAVA et al. 1963). However, in some species (e.g., mouse) the central stimulants have no appreciable effect on transmitter levels (CONSOLO et al. 1972), while in others (e.g., rat) bicuculline increases ACh in the frontal cortex, hippocampus, midbrain, and medulla pons, at variance with pentylenetetrazol, which causes reduction in the same areas. Interestingly, strychnine-induced convulsions are associated with decreased ACh levels in the hippocampus and caudate nucleus only (PEDATA et al. 1976). In conclusion, most of the above reports agree that brain ACh levels are reduced during experimental convulsions. Since, in some instances, increase or no change of ACh content has been found, the possible dissociation between convulsions and cholinergic-cell activity must be considered.

II. Spontaneous and Audiogenic Convulsions

The existence of genetically determined animal strains which are susceptible to sensory or postural convulsions is well known, but very little data concerning the cholinergic mechanism involvement in these particular models is available (MAYNERT et al. 1975). NARUSE et al. (1960) found that mice susceptible to seizures induced by physical stimuli exhibited high levels of brain ACh, the increase in susceptibility to seizures and in ACh levels being directly related to age. KUROKAVA et al. (1963) reported that during seizures certain strains of highly susceptible mice showed a marked reduction of "bound" ACh, which during interictal periods was twice as high as in normal animals.

Recently a comparison was made between acetylcholinesterase (AChE) and choline acetyltransferase (CAT) content in the brains of homozygous epileptic and heterozygous nonepileptic chicks (JOHNSON et al. 1979). The epileptic animals showed higher AChE activities in their cerebral hemispheres and lower CAT activities than the nonepileptic fowl.

In agreement with KUROKAVA et al. (1963) and JOHNSON et al. (1979), FUJIWARA (1980) found higher ACh levels and AChE activity in the brain (mostly in the diencephalon) of mice with inbred convulsive disposition to postural stimuli, i.e., E_1 and CBA mice. EBEL et al. (1975) reported abnormally high CAT activity in the cochlea of mice sensitized for audiogenic seizures, as well as in the cochlea of mice susceptible to audiogenic seizures. Therefore, at the level of the auditory input, some changes in the cholinergic system are demonstrable.

It remains to be elucidated whether the higher levels of ACh and CAT in the first acoustic relay represent an epileptogenic cofactor or are a consequence of excessive sensory input. CAT was also reported higher in the brains of mice susceptible to audiogenic seizures (SHENOY et al. 1981). This differs from JOHNSON's report and may depend on the various animal species and epilepsy models. When limiting analysis to audiogenic seizures, the above-summarized circumstantial evidence points to cholinergic activation during the seizures (as shown by increased ACh release) and intervention of compensatory mechanisms (as shown by increased CAT and AChE activities). Exclusion of the cholinergic system from the etiopathogenesis of these seizures, however, is strengthened by the fact that oxotremorine antagonizes attacks (ARONSTOM et al. 1979).

III. Focal Epilepsy

Focal epilepsies may be useful models for simultaneously studying different functional parameters and for assessing drug effects on them. In freely moving guinea pigs, provided with cortical electrodes and epidural cups (to collect the transmitters released from the cerebral cortex), acute focal epilepsy is easily produced, e.g., by warming the eserinized solution filling the cup to 40 °C. This experimental approach allowed BIANCHI et al. (1975) to investigate behavior, electrocorticogram (ECoG), and cortical ACh release and to establish how the antiepileptic drugs affected the investigated parameters.

Focal epileptogenesis is also induced or favored by many drugs and procedures, i.e., cobalt, alumina gel, penicillin, freezing, undercutting, periodic subliminal electrical stimulation, and "kindling" (WARD 1969; PURPURA et al. 1972; PENRY and PORTER 1979).

The experimentally induced foci are characterized by unspecific increased excitability of the involved neuronal population and derangement of the cell membrane electrical properties (KRNJEVIC et al. 1970). Indeed, certain similarities exist between the behavior of denervated skeletal muscle and epileptic neurons. Not only is the membrane potential reduced and unstable, while the electrical input resistance is almost doubled, but often a certain degree of ACh supersensitivity has been found. The lack of general agreement on this point could depend on the fact that loss of dendritic spines, characteristic of the epileptic neurons, could be accompanied by an increase in the number of dendritic, but not somatic, cholinergic receptors. Since the usual microionophoretic procedure considers only soma responses, dendritic activity cannot be detected (KRNJEVIC et al. 1970).

Apart from these considerations, the epileptic neurons show: (a) spontaneous interictal spikes, i.e., sharp waves detected in the EEG recording between seizures (AYALA et al. 1973), which are inhibited by cholinomimetic agents (PHILLIS and YORK 1968; STONE 1972) and/or, (b) interictal large paroxysmal depolarization with superimposed high-frequency spiking, followed by hyperpolarization (CRILL 1980). The possible ACh involvement in the epilepsy models is now briefly discussed:

1. Undercutting

After weeks or months, the isolated cortex shows spontaneous epileptic discharges. At the same time, increased ACh sensitivity has been reported (FERGUSON and JASPER 1971; ECHLIN 1975; FERGUSON and CORNBLATH 1975; CORNBLATH and FERGUSON 1976). However, SPEHLMAN (1971) and SPEHLMAN et al. (1971) found no selective ACh supersensitivity in the denervated occipital cortex and considered the increased ACh effectiveness in inducing seizures as an obvious consequence of the intrinsic focus abnormality. Furthermore, the spontaneous discharges were inhibited not by atropine but by GABA. Thus, SPEHLMAN concluded that the seizure activity in isolated slabs did not involve a cholinergic step and that ACh supersensitivity, if present, was not essential to neuron discharges.

2. Penicillin

Sodium benzyl penicillin is often used to induce quickly an acute epileptic focus in different parts of the brain, mostly in the cortex. The paroxysmal depolarization shift (PDS) is similar to that found in other models of focal epilepsy. Both indirect and direct evidence support the contention that PDS is a large excitatory postsynaptic potential (EPSP), but its exclusive synaptic origin remains to be settled (CRILL 1980).

Around the penicillin focus, neuronal hyperpolarization prevails, possibly representing a protective mechanism against the spread of seizure activity. Cholinergic involvement in this experimental model is uncertain. GUBERMAN and GLOOR (1974) found that cholinomimetic drugs sometimes have an anticonvulsant effect and concluded that no simple, unified role could be ascribed to ACh.

GOODMAN and LEBOVITZ (1982), however, reported that lesions of medial septal nucleus, i.e., removal of the tonic excitation cholinergic input to the hippocampus, decrease the excitability within the penicillin focus, while the interictal spikes can be accelerated by physostigmine or carbachol.

Recently, DINGLEDIN and GJERSTAD (1980) found that penicillin reduced the GABAergic inhibitory postsynaptic potentials (IPSP) evoked by subthreshold antidromic stimulation in CA_1 hippocampal pyramidal cells studied in vitro (see Chap. 7, this volume). Consequently, the mixed EPSP-IPSP induced by orthodromic stimulation was converted by penicillin into a pure EPSP, with a higher probability of causing cell discharges. Although additional observation suggested the existence of increased neuronal excitability, the prevailing penicillin mechanism could be due to disinhibition and not to an enhanced cholinergic excitatory signal.

3. Alumina and Cobalt

The chronic histological lesions produced by local alumina or cobalt application are associated with increased neuronal excitability, which is responsible for recurrent epileptic attacks. In guinea pigs with alumina-induced hippocampal epileptic foci, a generalized AChE increase in both cortical and subcortical structures was found. Increased enzyme activity was more pronounced in the hemisphere containing the secondary focus and was interpreted as compensating for increased synaptic ACh availability (GUERRERO-FIGUEROA et al. 1964). Similar observations were reported by BAXTER (1967) and GROSSMAN (1963).

BAKAY's (1981) report concerning the biochemical changes found in alumina-induced foci in the monkey cortex agrees with these conclusions (see also MCNAMARA 1978; ASHTON et al. 1980). The epileptic cortex showed a markedly reduced receptor binding to GABA (70%) and quinuclidyl-benzylate (QNB) (30%), together with a nonspecific cellular dropout, involving other neurotransmitter receptors.

In the primary focal area of "cobalt" rats, GOLDBERG et al. (1972) detected a significant reduction in cholinergic enzymes. A similar trend was observed in the controlateral cortex. Neuronal loss of transsynaptic influences could be responsible for the above changes, since histological examination showed terminal and fiber degeneration in ispilateral brain areas connected with the focus, as well as in homotropic contralateral areas (EMSON and JOSEPH 1975).

Reduction of many transmitter-related enzymes, such as glutamate decarboxylase, aromatic acid decarboxylase, AChE, and CAT, were simultaneously measured. Thus, it was impossible to establish the net effect (i.e., corrected for neuronal loss) of cobalt focus on the cholinergic system. On the other hand, the threshold for homocysteate excitation of cortical neurons and the proportion of acetylcholine-sensitive cells revealed no consistent changes in the motor cortex of cobalt rats (PUMAIN et al. 1977).

Moreover, 3 weeks after cobalt application on the rat frontal cortex (i.e., when the epileptiform activity was well established): (a) the ACh content in the tissue surrounding the necrotic area was normal; (b) physostigmine or diiosopropyl fluorophosphate (DFP) reduced both seizure activity and interictal spiking; and (c) hemicholinum-3 was less effective in depleting ACh levels in the cerebral cortex around cobalt lesions than in control rats. Therefore, cholinergic neurons adjacent to the cobalt implant were less active than normal cells, and anti-ChE agents antagonized the focal hypersynchrony, which is responsible for recurrent attacks. In summary, in neither alumina nor cobalt epilepsy do the cholinergic structures seem to play a direct role. Instead, the variations observed appear to depend on tissue damage or adaptive processes.

FARIELLO (1976) did not reach the same conclusions, experimenting with amygdaloid acute focus induced in the cat by locally injecting conjugated estrogens. While caudate nucleus stimulation inhibited interictal epileptic activity in the homolateral amygdala (probably by enhancing DA and GABA control), septal stimulation at a low frequency triggered amygdaloid spiking, and, at high frequencies, invariably evoked seizures. Consequently, FARIELLO (1976) postulated that septal stimulation caused a massive ACh release in the amygdala, thus facilitating seizures.

D. Kindling and the Cholinergic System

In general, the hippocampal formation shows a low seizure threshold. A possible cause of this is the presence of Schaffer collaterals, which originate from pyramidal cell axons and make excitatory synaptic connections with the apical dendrites of neighboring pyramidal cells and with the granule cells located in the dentate gyrus. Thus, strong excitation in one cellular population can be immediately transmitted to other parts of the whole structure. Since the hippocampal neurons are unusually tightly packed, increased concentration of extracellular K^+ (due to increased neuronal firing) could be an essential link in the chain of events initiating seizure (SMYTHIES and ADEY 1970; MAYNERT 1975).

Therefore, the particular cytoarchitecture of the limbic system determines its plasticity (RACINE et al. 1971; BLISS and LOME 1973) and its tendency to show the kindling phenomenon (McNamara et al. 1980). The hippocampus and the amygdala receive both interoceptive and exteroceptive inputs. Visceral information elaborated in the basal forebrain reaches the hippocampus via the cholinergic pathway from the septum (Dudar 1975) while most somatic information, processed in the thalamus and in the entorhinal cortex, is sent to the hippocampus via the perforant noncholinergic pathway (Smyties and Adey 1970). The ratio between these two inputs changes during waking and sleep and, in this context, it may be of interest to draw attention to certain forms of epilepsy which occur exclusively during sleep, i.e., when the septohippocampal input predominates.

Looking now at limbic kindling from the cholinergic point of view, some reports are in favor and some are against the cholinergic hypothesis.

Arnold et al. (1973) reported that atropine treatment delayed kindling in rats. Similarly, Vosu and Wiser (1975) showed that repeated carbamylcholine injections in the amygdala cause a gradual seizure development, antagonized by atropine.

Similar findings were presented by Wasterlain et al. (1978) and Albright et al. (1979). Girgis (1981) reported that few electrical stimuli potentiate physostigmine seizures. The hypersensitivity to anti-ChE agents paralleled kindling progression and scopolamine suppressed kindling-induced seizures.

Recently Kimura et al. (1981) proved that the presence of a cholinergic input favors development of kindling. In fact, lesions in substantia innominata significantly reduced amygdala kindling. Finally, Cain (1982) reported the bidirectional transfer between electrical kindling of the rat amygdala and intracerebrally administered carbachol. In summary, the presence or enhancement of the cholinergic signal in the limbic system seems to induce or favor kindling.

In agreement with a cholinergic link in limbic kindling, Burchfield et al. (1979) reported the parallel development of prolonged neuronal hypersensitivity to microionophoretically applied acetylcholine (with no change compared with GABA and glutamate) and the progression of kindled epileptic patterns. However, the increased responsiveness to muscarinic agents does not necessarily mean generalized worsening of the focal electroencephalographic signs. For instance, spontaneous interictal spiking (SIS) in the amygdala is activated by atropine and antagonized by physostignine (Fitz and McNamara 1979). Therefore, the stimulation of muscarinic receptors, per se capable of determining kindling and seizures, suppresses peculiar signs of electrical abnormality such as SIS. It has been suggested that SIS may reflect some protective inhibitory mechanisms, designed to reduce the likelihood of subsequent seizures; consequently, ACh could mediate a breakdown of this inhibition (Mucha and Pinel 1977; Fitz and McNamara 1979).

Enhanced ACh sensitivity and SIS development are associated with other relevant changes, such as reduction in the number of muscarinic receptors in the limbic system of kindled animals (McNamara 1978; Fitz and McNamara 1979; Byrne et al. 1980; Savage and McNamara 1981; Dasheiff et al. 1981; but see Noda et al. 1981).

On the other hand, the time course of receptor reduction has suggested a muscarinic step in the development (but not in the maintenance) of kindling and strenghthened the idea that the decrease in cholinergic neuronal communications was a consequence of/or a compensatory mechanism to seizures (DASHEIFF et al. 1981).

Such a mechanism is not localized to the stimulated areas but is well evident in other functionally interconnected regions. Thus, amygdala kindling is associated with cholinergic receptor decline not only in the amygdala, but also in both hippocampal formations (BYRNE et al. 1980), which could be considered the target structure of kindled amygdala. On the other hand, evidence exists that the down regulation of muscarinic receptors is independent of cholinergic input.

In fact, DASHEIFF and MCNAMARA (1980) reported that, during amygdala kindling, hippocampal muscarinic receptors continued to decline in rats previously submitted to medial septum lesions. Therefore, muscarinic receptor reduction can only represent one of the compensatory mechanisms to repeated neuronal depolarization (FISHMAN and NELSON 1981) and is independent of cholinergic pathway activation. To date, there is no information about possible changes in the number of nicotinic receptors which are surely present in the hippocampus (KRNJEVIC and ROPERT 1981).

The complexity of brain adjustments to kindling is confirmed by the contradictory reports about cholinergic enzyme changes. CAT activity increases according to NODA et al. (1981), but neither CAT nor AChE change in DASHEIFF's experiments (1981). Similarly, high-affinity choline uptake (HACU) is unchanged by amygdala kindling, while it is increased by pentylentetrazol (PTZ) convulsions (DASHEIFF et al. 1981).

There is doubt that increased ACh responsiveness, muscarinic receptor reduction, and other biochemical and functional changes involving other neuronal pools (KALICHMAN et al. 1980; ASHTON et al. 1980; GODDARD 1980; SHAVIT et al. 1981; TUFF et al. 1981) constitute a complex intertwining of causative and compensatory factors, simultaneously involved in the kindling process. This is morphologically demonstrated by the sprouting of fibers into the neuronal circuit, which is altered by repetitive stimulation (RACINE et al. 1971; MESSENHEIMER et al. 1979). On the other hand, the term "kindling" may represent a class of different pathological conditions with seizures as the end effect. Recently, KILBEY et al. (1979) showed that periodic systemic administration of subconvulsive doses of cocaine and other local anesthetics ultimately leads to generalized seizures. LAL et al. (1981) and CAIN (1981) reported that chronic PTZ treatment causes a progressive sensitization to the drug convulsant property and to electrically induced kindling, with no appreciable changes in benzodiazepine or QNB binding. Also penicillin injections in the neocortex cause kindling (COLLINS 1978). Therefore, systems other than the cholinergic are involved in drug-induced kindling.

E. Conclusions

At the end of this brief survey, a definitive answer concerning the pathophysiological role of ACh in epilepsy cannot be given. The few certainties are overshadowed by many negative and contradictory reports. Clearly, the cholinergic system, which originates in the basal nuclei, controls the whole neo- and archicortex, as well as other subcortical structures, where it mainly exerts excitatory influence through muscarinic (and also nicotinic) receptors.

No doubt, the increased cholinergic activity obtained with cholinomimetic drugs, however they are applied, causes generalized or localized convulsions, counteracted by proper antagonists. In addition, convulsant drugs or procedures simultaneously induce seizures and increased ACh release, whereas spontaneous epilepsies are associated with biochemical signs of cholinergic "hyperactivity."

On the other hand, the desynchronizing properties of the physiological ACh signal argue against the hypothesis of a cholinergic hypersynchrony, which is an essential prerequisite for inducing an epileptic focus. Since hypersynchrony is obtained only with very high, toxic doses of cholinomimetics, receptor desensitization or blockade is suspected.

The proved ACh involvement in certain types of local epilepsy does not necessarily mean that the increased ACh synaptic availability is a causative, essential step for epileptogenesis. In fact, the operative model of cholinergic transmission is characterized by a high degree of safety, and many synaptic mechanisms cooperate to reduce temporary excessive neurosecretion.

Considering now human pathology, increased AChE in epileptic focus has been definitively excluded (Tower and Elliot 1952; Pappius and Elliot 1958; Rapport et al. 1975).

To date, no additional reports on this point or on other possible traces of altered cholinergic activity in human epileptic foci have been published. In other words, a morphological or biochemical basis to support cholinergic involvement in human epilepsy is lacking.

These negative conclusions are strengthened by other arguments. The old observations that atropine was able to block spontaneous and hyperventilation-induced spike-and-wave discharges in patients with petit mal and, occasionally, in grand mal seizures (Williams 1941) have not been confirmed. A proper assessment of this antimuscarinic agent as an antiepileptic drug is precluded by its widespread peripheral and central actions, as pointed out by Wolff (1956) and Gardner and Webster (1977).

Furthermore, the presence of muscarinic excitatory and inhibitory receptors in the cortex (Stone 1972) makes drug end effects difficult to establish.

In contrast to the cholinergic hypothesis, Karczmar (1976) has reviewed the circumstances in which physostigmine, because of its desynchronizing effects, was capable of reducing or preventing petit mal seizures. The only field which remains to be investigated concerns the possible usefulness of scopolamine in preventing late, post-traumatic limbic epilepsy, which may be related in some way to experimental kindling (Girgis 1981). Indeed, this is not sufficient to support the hypothesis that the cholinergic system plays a key role in convulsive disorders.

References

Albright PS, Burnhan WM, Okazaki M (1979) Effect of atropine sulphate on amygdaloid kindling in the rat. Exp Neurol 66:409–412

Arnold PS, Racine RJ, Wise RA (1973) Effects of atropine, reserpine, 6-hydroxydopamine and handling on seizure development in the rat. Exp Neurol 40:457–470

Aronstom RS, Kellog C, Abood LG (1979) Development of muscarinic cholinergic receptors in inbred strains of mice: identification of receptor heterogeneity and relation of audiogenic seizure susceptibility. Brain Res 162:231–241

Ashton O, Leysen JE, Wanquier A (1980) Neurotransmitter and receptor binding in amygdaloid kindled rats: serotoninergic and noradrenergic modulatory effects. Life Sci 27:1547–1556

Ayala GF, Dichter M, Gumnit RJ, Matsumoto H, Spencer WA (1973) Genesis of epileptic interictal spikes, new knowledge of cortical feedback systems suggests a neurophysiological explanation of brief paroxysms. Brain Res 52:1–17

Bakay RAE (1981) Neurotransmitter, receptor and biochemical changes in monkey cortical epileptic foci. Brain Res 206:387–404

Baxter BL (1967) Comparison of the behavioral effects of electrical of chemical stimulation applied at the same brain loci. Exp Neurol 19:412–432

Beani L, Bianchi C, Megazzini P, Ballotti L, Bernardi G (1969) Drug-induced changes in free, labile and stabile acetylcholine of guinea-pig brain. Biochem Pharmacol 18:1315–1324

Beleslin D, Polak RL, Sproull DH (1965) The effect of leptazol and strychnine on the acetylcholine release fron the cat brain. J Physiol (Lond) 181:308–316

Bianchi C, Beani L, Bertelli A (1975) Effect of some antiepileptic drugs on brain acetylcholine. Neuropharmacology 14:327–332

Bliss TV, Lomo T (1973) Long-lasting potentiation of synaptic transmission in the dentate area of the anaesthetized rabbit following stimulation of the perforant path. J Physiol 232:331–356

Burchfield J, Dunchowny M, Duffly F (1979) Neuronal supersensitivity to acetylcholine induced by kindling in the rat hippocampus. Science 204:1096–1098

Byrne MC, Gottlieb R, McNamara JO (1980) Amygdala kindling induces muscarinic cholinergic receptors declines in a highly specific distribution within the limbic system. Exp Neurol 69:85–98

Cain DP (1981) Pentylenetetrazol sensitization facilitates subsequent amygdaloid kindling in the rat. Soc Neurosci 587 (abstract)

Cain DP (1982) Transfer between electrical kindling of the amygdala and intracerebral carbachol or pentylenetetrazol. Soc Neurosci 24.6 (abstract)

Celesia CG, Jasper HH (1966) Acetylcholine released from cerebral cortex in relation to state of activation. Neurobiology 16:1053–1067

Chen G, Ensor CR, Bohner B (1968) Studies of drug effects on electrically-induced extensor seizures and clinical implications. Arch Int Pharmacodyn Ther 172:183–218

Collier B, Mitchell JF (1967) The central release of acetylcholine during consciousness and after brain lesions. J Physiol (Lond) 188:83–98

Collins RC (1978) Kindling of neuroanatomic pathways during recurrent focal penicillin seizures. Brain Res 150:503–517

Cornblath DP, Ferguson JH (1976) Distribution of radioactivity from topically applied [^{3}H] acetylcholine in relation to seizure. Exp Neurol 50:495–504

Consolo S, Ladinsky H, Peri G, Garattini S (1972) Effect of central stimulants on mouse brain acetylcholine and choline levels. Eur J Pharmacol 18:251–255

Crill WE (1980) Neuronal mechanisms of seizures initiation. Adv Neurol 27:169–183

Dasheiff RM, McNamara JO (1980) Evidence for the agonist independent down regulation of hippocampal muscarinic receptors in kindling. Brain Res. 195:345–354

Dasheiff RM, Byrne MC, Patrone V, McNamara JO (1981) Biochemical evidence of decreased muscarinic cholinergic neuronal communication following amygdala-kindled seizures. Brain Res 206:233–238

Dingledine R, Gjerstad L (1980) Reduced inhibition during epileptiform activity in the in vitro hippocampal slice. J Physiol (Lond) 305:297–313

Dudar JD (1975) The effect of septal nuclei stimulation on the release of acetycholine from the rabbit hippocampus. Brain Res 83:123–134

Dudar JD, Szerb JC (1969) The effect of topically applied atropine on resting and evoked cortical acetylcholine release. J Physiol (Lond) 203:741–762

Ebel A, Ayad G, Simmer S, Stefanovic V, Collins R, Mandel P (1975) Activity of cholinergic system enzymes in the cochlea of mice sensitized for audiogenic seizure. Life Sci 17:641–644

Echlin FA (1975) Time course of development of supersensitivity to topical acetylcholine in partially isolated cortex. Electroencephalogr Clin Neurophysiol 38:225–233
Elliot KAC, Swank RL, Henderson N (1950) Effects of anaesthetics and convulsivant on acetylcholine content of brain. Am J Physiol 162:469–474
Emson PC, Joseph NH (1975) Neurochemical and morphological changes during the development of cobalt-induced epilepsy in the rat. Brain Res 93:91–110
Fariello R (1976) Forebrain influence on an amygdaloid acute focus in the cat. Exp Neurol 51:515–528
Ferguson JH, Cornblath DR (1975) Acetylcholine epilepsy: relationship of surface concentration, chronicity of denervation and focus size. Exp Neurol 46:302–314
Ferguson JH, Jasper HH (1971) Laminal DC studies of acetylcholine-activated epileptiform discharge in cerebral cortex. Electroencephalogr Clin Neurophysiol 30:377–390
Fishman MC, Nelson PG (1981) Depolarization-induced synaptic plasticity at cholinergic synapses in tissue culture. J Neuroscience 1:1043–1051
Fitz JG, McNamara JO (1979) Muscarinic cholinergic regulation of epileptic spiking in kindling. Brain Res 62:497–507
Fujiwara M (1980) Acetylcholine levels of mouse brain in preconvulsive states. Neuroscience 6:192–202
Gardner CR, Webster RA (1977) Convulsivant-anticonvulsivant interactions on seizure activity and cortical acetylcholine release. Eur J Pharmacol 42:247–256
Giarman NJ, Pepeu G (1962) Drug induced changes in brain acetylcholine. Br J Pharmacol 19:226–234
Girgis M (1981) Kindling as a model for limbic epilepsy. Neuroscience 6:1695–1706
Goddard GV (1980) Kindling model in limbic epilepsy. In: Girgis M, Kiloh (eds) Limbic epilepsy and the dyscontrol syndrome. Elsevier North Holland, Biomedical Press, Amsterdam, pp 108–116
Goldberg AM, Pollock JJ, Hartman ER, Craig CR (1972) Alterations in cholinergic enzymes during the development of cobalt induced epilepsy in the rat. Neuropharmacology 11:253–259
Goodman JH, Lebovitz RM (1982) Modulation of penicillin-induced interictal spikes by cholinergic agents and medial septal lesions. Soc Neurosci 24.4 (abstract)
Greer CA, Alpern HP (1977) Mediation of myoclonic seizures by acetylcholine and GABA. Life Sci 21:285–392
Grossman SP (1983) Chemically induced epileptiform seizures in the cat. Science 142:409–411
Guberman A, Gloor P (1974) Cholinergic drug studies of generalized penicillin epilepsy in the cat. Brain Res 78:203–222
Guerrero-Figueroa R, De Babbian Vester F, Barros A, Heat RG (1964) Cholinergic mechanisms in subcortical mirror focus and effects of gamma-aminobutyric acid and acetylcholine. Epilepsia 5:140–155
Hemsworth BA, Neal MJ (1968) The effect of central stimulant drugs on acetylcholine release from rat cerebral cortex. Br J Pharmacol 34:543–550
Herken H, Neubert D (1953) Der Acetylcholin Gehalt des Gehirns bei verschiedenen Funktionszuständen. Naunyn Schmiedeberg's Arch Exp Pharmacol 219:223–233
Hoover DB, Craig CR, Colasanti BK (1977) Cholinergic involvement in cobalt induced epilepsy in the rat. Exp Brain Res 29:501–513
Johnson DD, Davis HL, Crawford RD (1979) Pharmacological and biochemical studies in epileptic fowl. Fed Proc 38:2417–2423
Kalichman MW, McIntyre DC, Burnhan W (1980) Locomotor and convulsive responses to picrotoxin in amygdala-kindled rats. Exp Neurol 70:167–172
Karczmar AG (1967) Pharmacologic and therapeutic properties of anticholinesterases. In: Root WS, Hofman FG (eds) Physiological pharmacology. Academic, New York, pp 163–322
Karczmar AG (1976) Central actions of acetylcholine, cholinomimetics and related drugs. In: Goldberg AM, Hanin I (eds) Biology of cholinergic function. Raven, New York, pp 395–449

Karczmar AG (1979) Acetylcholine and animal electrophysiology. In: Davis KL, Berger PA (eds) Brain acetylcholine and neuropsychiatric disease. Plenum, New York, pp 265–310
Kilbey MM, Ellinwood EH, Easler ME (1979) The effect of chronic cocaine pretreatment on kindled seizures and behavioral stereotypes. Exp Neurol 64:306–314
Kimura H, Kambo Y, Wadi JA (1981) Catecholamine and cholinergic system and amygdaloid kindling. In: Wada (ed) Kindling, 2nd edn. Raven, New York, pp 265–284
Krnjevic K, Ropert N (1981) Cholinergic nature of septohippocampal modulation of pyramidal cell firing. Soc Neurosci 831 (abstract)
Krnjevic K, Reiffenstein RI, Silver A (1970) Chemical sensitivity of neurons in long-isolated slabs of cat cerebral cortex. Electroencephalogr Clin Neurophysiol 29:269–282
Kurokava M, Machiyama Y, Kato M (1963) Distribution of acetylcholine in the brain during various states of activity. J Neurochem 10:341–348
Lal H, Manu PA, Sherman GT, Lippa AS (1981) Effect of acute and chronic pentylenetetrazol treatment on benzodiazepine and cholinergic receptor binding in rat brain. Eur J Pharmacol 75:115–119
Maynert EW, Marczynsky TJ, Browing RA (1975) The role of the neurotransmitters in the epilepsies. Adv Neurol 13:79–147
McNamara JO (1978) Muscarinic cholinergic receptors participate in the kindling model of epilepsy. Brain Res 154:415–420
McNamara JO, Byrne MC, Dasheiff RM, Fitz JG (1980) The kindling model of epilepsy: a review. Progr Neurobiol 15:139–159
Messenheimer J, Harris E, Steward ON (1979) Sprouted fibers gain access to circuitry transsynaptically altered by kindling. Exp Neurol 64:469–481
Mitchell JF (1963) The spontaneous and evoked release of acetylcholine from the cerebral cortex. J Physiol (Lond) 165:98–116
Mucha RF, Pinel JPS (1977) Post-seizure inhibition of kindled seizures. Exp Neurol 54:266–282
Naruse H, Kato M, Kurokava M, Haba R, Yabe T (1960) Metabolic defects in a convulsive strain of mouse. J Neurochem 5:359–369
Noda Y, Vemura S, McGeer EG, Wada JA (1981) Lasting influence of amygdaloid kindling on cholinergic neurotransmission. Soc Neurosci 585 (abstract)
Pappius HM, Elliot KAC (1958) Acetylcholine metabolism in normal and epileptogenic brain tissue: failure to repeat previous findings. J Appl Physiol 12:319–323
Pedata F, Mulas A, Marconcini-Pepeu I, Pepeu G (1976) Changes in regional brain ACh levels during drug-induced convulsion. Eur J Pharmacol 40:329–335
Penry JK, Porter RJ (1979) Epilepsy – mechanisms and therapy. Med Clin North Am 63:802–812
Pepeu G (1974) The release of acetylcholine from the brain: an approach to the study of the central cholinergic mechanisms. Prog Neurobiol 2:257–288
Phillis JW, York DH (1968) Pharmacological studies on a cholinergic inhibition in the cerebral cortex. Brain Res 10:297–306
Pumain R, Louvel J, Chanvel P (1977) Chemical sensitivity of neurons in chronic epileptogenic foci. Electroencephalogr Clin Neurophysiol 44:E426
Purpura DP, Penry JK, Tower, D, Woodburg DM, Walter R (1972) Experimental models of epilepsy. Raven, New York
Racine R, Gartner J, Burnham W (1971) Epileptiform activity and neural plasticity in limbic structures. Brain Res 47:262–268
Rapport RL, Harris AB, Friel PN, Ojemann GA (1975) Human epileptic brain. Arch Neurol 32:549–554
Richter D, Crossland J (1949) Variations in acetylcholine content in the brain with the physiological state. Am J Physiol 159:247–255
Saelens JK, Schuman J (1974) Effect of multiple electroshock on acetylcholine (ACh) metabolism in mouse brain. Fed Proc 33:477
Savage DD, McNamara JO (1981) In vitro autoradiographic localization of muscarinic cholinergic binding sites in rat hippocampal formation: effects of amygdala kindling. Soc Neurosci 592 (abstract)

Shavit Y, Caldecott-Hazard S, Liebeskin JC (1981) Anticonvulsant effects of electroconvulsive shock (ECS) on subsequent kindled seizure in rats. Soc Neurosci 579 (abstract)
Shenoy AK (1981) Choline acetyltransferase and glutamic acid decarboxylase activities in audiogenic seizure susceptible (frings) mouse brain. Fed Proc 40:271
Simon JR, Atwch S, Kuhar MJ (1976) Sodium dependent high affinity choline uptake: a regulatory step in the synthesis of acetylcholine. J Neurochem 26:909–922
Smythies JR, Adey WK (1970) Brain mechanisms and behavior. Academic, New York
Spehlman R (1971) Acetylcholine and the epileptiform activity of chronically isolated cortex. II. Microelectrode studies. Arch Neurol 24:495–502
Spehlman R, Daniels JC, Chang CM (1971) Acetylcholine and the epileptiform activity of chronically isolated cortex. I. Macroelectrode studies. Arch Neurol 24:401–408
Stone TW (1972) Cholinergic mechanisms in the rat somatosensory cerebral cortex. J Physiol (Lond) 225:485–499
Tower DB, Elliot KAC (1952) Activity of acetylcholine system in human epileptogenic focus. J Appl Physiol 4:669–676
Tuff LP, Racine R, Mishra R (1981) Long-lasting alterations in inhibitory processes in kindled rats. Soc Neurosci 584 (abstract)
Vasquez AJ, Krip G (1973) Evidence for an inhibitory role for acetylcholine, catecholamines and serotonin on the cerebral cortex. In: Sabelli HC (ed) Chemical modulation of brain function. Raven, New York
Vosu H, Wiser RA (1975) Cholinergic seizure in the rat: comparison of caudate, amygdala and hippocampus. Behav Biol 13:491–495
Ward AA Jr (1969) The epileptic neuron: chronic foci in animals and man. In: Jasper HH, Ward AA (eds) Basic mechanisms of the epilepsies. Little Brown, Boston, pp 329–348
Wasterlain CG, Jonec V, Folm SJ (1978) Cholinergic receptors. Neurology 28:346
Williams D (1941) The effect of choline like substances on the cerebral electrical discharges in epilepsy. J Neurol Neurosurg Psychiatr 4:32–43
Wolff VH (1956) Die Behandlung zerebraler Anfälle mit Scopolamin: Ein Beitrag zur Klinik des „synkopalen“ Syndroms. Dtsch Med Wochenschr 81:1358–1360

CHAPTER 7

GABA and Other Amino Acids

B. S. MELDRUM

A. Introduction: Amino Acids as Neurotransmitters

Among the neutrotransmitter substances so far identified in the mammalian nervous system the amino acids are by far the most ubiquitous (in terms of the proportion of neurons containing them) and the most functionally consistent (in terms of their postsynaptic actions). Thus the neutral amino acids, glycine and GABA (gamma-aminobutyric acid), when tested iontophoretically are universally inhibitory, and the dicarbocylic amino acids, asfartate and glutamate are universally excitatory (CURTIS and WATKINS 1963; CURTIS and JOHNSTON 1974). Comparable generalisations are not possible in the case of noradrenaline (norepinephrine), dopamine, serotonin, or acetylcholine, which occur in a very restricted proportion of neurons and have actions that vary according to the site and other local circumstances.

Many convulsant and anticonvulsant drugs have potent effects on amino acid metabolism or on their synaptic function. Impairment of GABAergic or of glycinergic inhibition can explain the convulsant action of several different classes of convulsant drugs.

Enhancement of GABAergic inhibition probably plays an important part in the anticonvulsant actions of barbiturates and benzodiazepines and possibly other clinically useful antiepileptic agents such as valproate. However, a great deal remains to be elucidated in relation to amino acids and epilepsy. In particular, excitatory amino acids probably play a major role in the development and spread of seizure activity but their involvement in antiepileptic drug effects is poorly understood.

This chapter summarises biochemical, physiological and pharmacological data relating to inhibitory and excitatory amino acids in the brain. It indicates key elements linking them to pathophysiological mechanisms in epilepsy, and thus provides part of the basic science background to consideration of the mechanism of action of anticonvulsant drugs.

B. Amino Acids Producing Inhibition

I. Introduction

Table 1 lists amino acids that both occur naturally in the brain and inhibit neuronal firing when applied iontophoretically at the single-cell level. These amino acids are characterised by a zwitterionic state in neutral solution. They vary greatly in the concentration in which they occur and in their regional distribution within the brain.

Table 1. Inhibitory amino acids in mammalian brain

		pK (25 °C)		Concentration (µmol/g wet weight)		
				Rat brain	Human biopsy	
					A	B
Glycine	$CH_2(NH_2)COOH$	2.35	9.78	1.06	0.85	0.40
L-α-Alanine	$CH_3CH(NH_2)COOH$	2.35	9.81	0.42	0.49	0.25
L-Serine	$CH_2(OH)CH(NH_2)COOH$	2.21	9.15	0.84	0.49	0.44
β-Alanine	$NH_2CH_2CH_2COOH$	3.55	10.24	0.05–0.11 [a]		0.01
γ-Aminobutyric acid	$NH_2CH_2CH_2CH_2COOH$	4.03	10	1.79	0.93	0.42
δ-Amino-*N*-valeric acid	$NH_2CH_2CH_2CH_2CH_2COOH$	4.27	10.69			
Hypotaurine	$NH_2CH_2CH_2SOOH$	–	–	0.04		
Taurine	$NH_2CH_2CH_2SO_3H$	1.5	0.82	3.92	1.15	0.93
L-Cystathionine	$COOHCH(NH_2)CH_2{-}S{-}CH_2CH_2CH(NH_2)COOH$	–	–	0.08		2.02
Imidazoleacetic acid	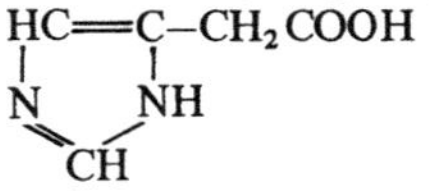	2.96	7.35			
Pipecolic acid	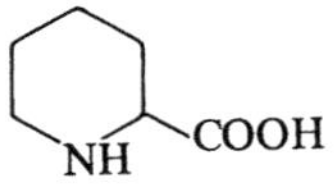	–	10.38			
L-Proline	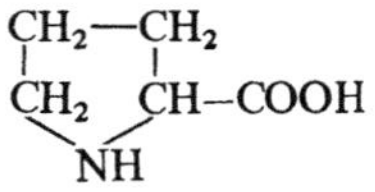	1.95	10.64	0.01	0.05	0.04

Dissociation constants (pK) at 25 °C from PERRIN (1965, 1972) and GREENSTEIN and WINITZ (1961)
Concentrations in rat brain from PERRY et al. (1981) and MARTIN DEL RIO et al. 1977 ([a])
Concentrations in human biopsies from PERRY et al. (1971) (B), 1981 (A)

Evidence of several kinds is required to establish that an amino acid acts as an inhibitory transmitter at a specific site in the brain. This includes evidence that the amino acid occurs in relatively high concentration in synaptosomes (or in synaptic vesicles), that the enzyme or enzymes responsible for its synthesis are similarly concentrated in synaptosomes (or are selectively localised in nerve terminals in histochemical or immunocytochemical studies), that the amino acid is released in a calcium-dependent fashion following electrical stimulation of the neuronal pathway, and that the action of the amino acid when applied exogenously is physiologically and pharmacologically comparable to the action of the endogenously released compound. A selective sodium-dependent reuptake system seems to be characteristic of amino acid transmitter systems. However, the presence of a sodium-dependent high- (or low-) affinity uptake system for an amino acid is only evidence of a secondary or supporting nature. Similarly the presence of a "receptor" for an amino acid, as demonstrated either by a physiological response or by binding of isotopically labelled ligand helps confirm the status of an already identified neurotransmitter, but is not itself persuasive evidence.

Of the neutral amino acids, GABA is undoubtedly an inhibitory transmitter at sites in the cortex, hippocampus, cerebellum, basal ganglia, etc. (see CURTIS 1979), and glycine is very probably a transmitter in the spinal cord and brain stem, and elsewhere (CURTIS and JOHNSTON 1974). β-Alanine has been proposed as a transmitter in the superior colliculus (SANDBERG and JACOBSON 1981). Taurine may be a transmitter in the cerebellum and in other brain regions, but the evidence is not yet decisive (MANDEL and PASANTES-MORALES 1978). All the inhibitory amino acids so far studied utilise the same ionic mechanism to induce inhibition, namely an increase in chloride conductance. Where there is a high external $[Cl^-]$ and a low internal $[Cl^-]$, as in the soma of most neurons, increasing the membrane chloride conductance hyperpolarises or stabilises the resting membrane potential and reduces the probability of an impulse being initiated at the initial segment of the axon. On hippocampal dendrites a depolarising action of GABA (associated with increased membrane conductance) provides a purely local shunting or inhibition of afferent excitatory inputs (ANDERSEN et al. 1980, 1982). Additional ionic conductance changes due to GABA, involving potassium and calcium, have been described, particularly in invertebrate preparations (YAROWSKY and CARPENTER 1978).

Differences between amino acid inhibitory mechanisms are not confined to the transmitter recognition sites. Associated membrane structures also differ, as demonstrated by the selective effects of benzodiazepines and barbiturates, or of picrotoxin, on GABAergic receptor systems as compared with glycinergic receptors. Furthermore the chloride ionophores themselves show distinctive properties according to the amino acid receptor activated. Thus in spinal neurons in tissue culture, analysis of the conductance change, and its duration, associated with activation of a single channel distinguishes between channels activated by GABA, glycine or β-alanine (BARKER et al. 1982). This suggests that there are at least three endogenous inhibitory amino acid transmitters. It does not prove which they are, as, for example, the endogenous amino acid for the "β-alanine receptor" could be taurine or some other compound (see OKAMOTO and SAKAI 1980).

Any amino acid may act on several different receptor sites. There may be more than one type of receptor that is selective for that neurotransmitter. This principle of "multiple receptors" is well established for monoamine neurotransmitters (SNYDER and GOODMAN 1980), covering subtypes not only of postsynaptic receptors but also of receptors on presynaptic terminals, including autoreceptors. There may also be receptor sites with multiple physiological agonists, i.e.responding to more than one amino acid, perhaps with variable selectivity according to ionic or other circumstances.

Selective antagonists that compete for the receptor recognition site provide a means of differentiating both receptors specific for particular amino acids and receptor subtypes for one amino acid. They also provide valuable evidence concerning the identity of exogenous and endogenous amino acid neurotransmitters. Strychnine has been widely used as an antagonist selective for postsynaptic glycine receptors and bicuculline and picrotoxin as antagonists for postsynaptic GABA receptors. However, it is now apparent that of these only bicuculline competes directly for the amino acid recognition site. Strychnine and picrotoxin act selectively on the glycine- and GABA-activated ionophores.

Amino acid analogues that are selective agonists also facilitate such differentiation both in pharmacological experiments and radioactive ligand studies. This approach has permitted the differentiation of "GABA A receptors", at which muscimol and THIP (4,5,6,7-tetrahydroisoxalo[5,4-C]pyridine-3-ol) are selective agonists, and "GABA B receptors", at which baclofen is a selective agonist (BOWERY et al. 1980).

The range of presynaptic receptors influencing neurotransmitter release is extremely wide (VIZI 1979) and includes various metabolites that probably cannot be considered as "neurotransmitters". GABA A type receptors are present on GABAergic and on glutamatergic neurons (LEVI et al. 1981; MITCHELL and MARTIN 1978; MITCHELL 1980). GABA B type receptors occur on monoaminergic terminals; GABA, or baclofen, acts to decrease the release of noradrenaline, dopamine and serotonin. L-Proline apparently acts on presynaptic receptors to inhibit glutamate release (KELLER et al. 1981).

II. GABA

GABA, 4-aminobutyric acid, is the major inhibitory transmitter in the mammalian brain. It provides intrinsic inhibition in the cortex, hippocampus, thalamus and cerebellum (see below) and because of this plays a critical role in several aspects of epileptogenesis. Any significant interference with GABA-mediated postsynaptic inhibition in the cortex or hippocampus leads to local or generalised seizure activity (MELDRUM 1975). Enhancement of GABA-mediated inhibition produces anticonvulsant effects in a wide range of animal models of epilepsy and at least two of the major classes of anticonvulsant drugs significantly enhance GABA-mediated inhibition.

1. Metabolism

GABA is synthesised within the nervous system from glutamic acid (see Fig. 1). Although the latter can be derived from dietary protein and is transported into

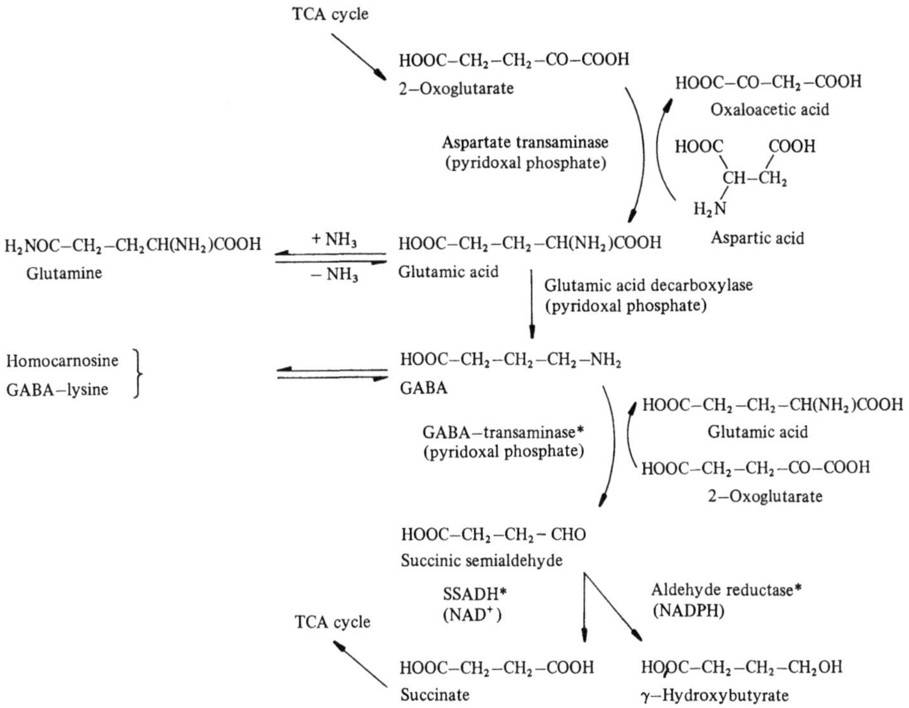

Fig. 1. Metabolic pathways of GABA. The route from 2-oxoglutarate to succinate is the "GABA shunt" on the tricarboxylic acid (TCA) cycle. Enzymes inhibited by anticonvulsant drugs (sodium valproate, phenobarbitone) in vitro are *asterisked*

the brain, most glutamate acting as a precursor for neurotransmitter GABA is derived from glucose by transamination from 2-oxoglutarate. Within the brain, glutamine also acts as a precursor of glutamate and GABA (Berl et al. 1961).

a) Synthesis

Glutamic acid decarboxylase (L-glutamate 1-carboxy-lyase: EC 4.1.1.15) is a cytosolic enzyme that requires pyridoxal phosphate as coenzyme. It is specifically localised in GABAergic neurons. It is highly concentrated in synaptosomal fractions of brain homogenates and is seen in perisomatic synaptic terminals in immunocytochemical studies employing specific antibodies of glutamic acid decarboxylase (Saito et al. 1974; Oertel et al. 1981 a; Ribak 1978).

Glutamic acid decarboxylase (GAD) activity can be inhibited by three types of compounds: (1) those interfering with the synthesis or coenzymic function of pyridoxal phosphate, (2) those competing with the substrate, and (3) compounds that are non-competitive inhibitors, including catalytic (K_{cat}) inhibitors (see Table 2). All these classes of GAD inhibitors can produce seizures in man and experimental animals – the latency to seizure onset and the pattern of seizures show distinct differences according to the type of inhibitor.

Competitive inhibitors such as 3-mercaptopropionic acid produce seizures with a very short latency (2 min in the baboon), indicating the very short half-life

Table 2. Compounds inhibiting the synthesis of GABA

	Convulsant dose in rats or mice (mmol/kg)	Seizure latency (min)
1. Pyridoxal phosphate antagonists		
Hydrazine	–	–
Methyldithiocarbazinate	0.12	30–45
Thiosemicarbazide	0.27	60–240
Isoniazid	1.2	7–40
4-Deoxypyridoxine	1.2	15–45
Methoxypyridoxine	–	–
2. Competitive antagonists		
D-Glutamate	–	–
2-Ketoglutarate	–	–
3-Mercaptopropionic acid	1.1	2–6
4-Mercaptobutyric acid	–	–
Thiomalic acid	–	–
3-Mercaptopyruvate	–	–
3. Non-competitive inhibition		
L-Allylglycine	1.0	60–120
D-Allylglycine	4.0	60–180
2-Keto-4-pentenoic acid	–	–

References: HORTON et al. (1978), TABERNER et al. (1977), REINGOLD and ORLOWSKI (1978), WU and ROBERTS (1974), and MELDRUM et al. (1975)

of neurotransmitter GABA. Pyridoxal phosphate antagonists produce partial seizures with secondary generalisation after a long latency (see MELDRUM 1979). The long latency of seizures induced by D,L-allylglycine is related to its initial conversion to 2-keto-4-pentenoic acid, which is an irreversible inhibitor of GAD. A different pattern of seizure activity is seen after D-allyglycine, compared with the L-isomer, because the D-isomer is activated by D-amino acid oxidase, which in mammals is found only in the hindbrain. Thus the fall in GABA content after D-allyglycine is restricted to the hindbrain, but is generalised after L-allyglycine (HORTON et al. 1978).

The 2-keto acids derived from cysteine and homocysteine by transamination or by L-amino acid oxidase (3-mercaptopyruvate and 2-keto-4-mercaptobutyrate) are very potent inhibitors of glutamic acid decarboxylase activity (REINGOLD and ORLOWSKI 1978). Formation of these compounds in the brain could explain the seizures observed in homocystinuria.

Infants suffering from dietary deficiency of pyridoxine show seizures which are almost certainly due to impaired synthesis of GABA and are rapidly terminated by parenteral administration of pyridoxine. There is also a rare inborn metabolic disorder, pyridoxine dependency, in which the requirement for pyridoxine is greatly increased (COURSIN 1954, 1964).

A fall in GAD activity can be produced by oestrogens, given either systemically or focally on, or in, the brain (WALLIS and LUTTGE 1980; MCGINNIS et al. 1980). The mechanism is not known but the phenomenon could contribute to changes in seizure threshold produced by oestrogens.

b) Further Metabolism

Two enzymes complete the further metabolism of GABA, within the GABA shunt, to succinic acid. These are GABA-transaminase (4-aminobutyrate: 2-oxo-glutarate aminotransferase, EC 2.6.1.19, GABA-T), which like GAD requires pyridoxal phosphate as cofactor, and succinic semialdehyde dehydrogenase (succinate-semialdehyde: NAD(P) oxidoreductase, EC 1.2.1.16, SSADH). GABA-T and SSADH are mitochondrial enzymes found in both neurons and the glia.

Succinic semialdehyde can alternatively be converted to 4-hydroxybutyrate, by an NAPDH-dependent aldehyde reductase (KAUFMAN et al. 1979). The reverse reaction is catalysed by the same enzyme (with $NADP^+$).

α) GABA-Transaminase Inhibition. Compounds inhibiting GABA-transaminase activity fall into two main categories: (1) carbonyl-trapping agents complexing with pyridoxal phosphate, which are therefore not specific, and commonly also inhibit GAD activity, and (2) compounds that are "catalytic" or irreversible inhibitors of GABA-T (METCALF 1979; PALFREYMAN et al. 1981; BEY et al. 1981). Anticonvulsant effects of amino-oxyacetic acid have been reported in many animal test systems but a dose slightly greater than the anticonvulsant dose precipitates seizures (MELDRUM et al. 1970).

However, the catalytic inhibitors of GABA-T have powerful anticonvulsant effects in baboons with photosensitive epilepsy (MELDRUM and HORTON 1978) and in a wide range of rodent models, including audiogenic seizures, electroshock and various chemically induced seizures (ANLEZARK et al. 1976; HORTON et al. 1977; PALFREYMAN et al. 1981). The action of γ-acetylenic GABA and γ-vinyl GABA against GABA-antagonist drugs shows some anomalies in terms of dose-response relations and time course of action (PALFREYMAN et al. 1981; KENDALL et al. 1981).

In rodents there is a massive increase in the cerebral GABA content (by four- to tenfold over 6–48 h) after administration of ethanolamine-*O*-sulphate and γ-vinyl GABA or γ-acetylenic GABA (SCHECHTER et al. 1977; HORTON et al. 1977; PALFREYMAN et al. 1981; CHAPMAN et al. 1982). There is evidence that there is a preferential increase in synaptosomal GABA concentration after γ-vinyl GABA administration in mice (SEILER and SARHAN 1980). Release of GABA into cortical superfusates is enhanced shortly after the intraperitoneal administration of γ-vinyl GABA or γ-acetylenic GABA in rats (ABDUL-GHANI et al. 1980). This test system does not differentiate enhanced synaptic release from impaired GABA reuptake. However, rat cortical synaptosomes show an enhanced release of preloaded GABA in the presence of γ-vinyl-GABA or γ-acetylenic GABA (ABDUL-GHANI et al. 1981). It is likely that the catalytic inhibitors of GABA-transaminase produce an anticonvulsant effect by increasing the quantity of GABA released physiologically at synapses, but some direct or indirect effect on GABA uptake cannot be excluded.

β) Succinic Semialdehyde Dehydrogenase. This enzyme has been purified from rat and human brain (as two isoenzymes in the latter case) (CASH et al. 1978). It is inhibited by 4-hydroxybenzaldehyde and various branched chain fatty acids including sodium valproate (MAÎTRE et al. 1976; ANLEZARK et al. 1976). The activity of SSADH is substantially greater than that of GABA-T (DE BOER and

BRUINVELS 1977), and the substrate, succinic semialdehyde, is found only in very low concentration in human or rat brain.

Inhibitors of SSADH have been reported not to increase brain GABA content (BAXTER and ROBERTS 1961; MAÎTRE et al. 1976); however the increase in brain GABA that follows ischaemia or hypoxia is thought to be due to cessation of SSADH activity in the absence of oxidised NAD. Indirect inhibition of GABA-transaminase activity through an increased succinic semialdehyde concentration has also been postulated as a mechanism of action of valproate (VAN DER LAAN et al. 1979).

γ) Aldehyde Reductases. Among the aldehyde reductases found in brain at least two can convert succinic semialdehyde to 4-hydroxybutyrate (linked to NADPH) or perform the reverse action (linked to NADP) (TABAKOFF and ERWIN 1970; KAUFMANN et al. 1979). The true metabolic or physiological function of these enzymes is not known. 4-Hydroxybutyrate is found in brain at a low concentration (DOHERTY et al. 1978). Given systemically 4-hydroxybutyrate has numerous effects on cerebral metabolism and function (SNEAD 1977) and induces EEG spike discharges and a trance-like state that has been compared to petit mal "absence" (WINTERS and SPOONER 1965; SNEAD 1978; GODSCHALK et al. 1877).

One isoenzyme of NADPH-dependent aldehyde reductase with a broad substrate specificity (RUMIGNY et al. 1980) (ARI, high-K_m form) is highly susceptible to inhibition by ionisable anticonvulsant drugs, including barbiturates, hydantoins, carbamezepine, succinimides, benzodiazepines, and valproic acid (ERWIN and DEITRICH 1973; RIS et al. 1975; JAVORS and ERWIN 1980; WHITTLE and TURNER 1981), but not non-ionisable forms (trimethadione, methsuximide). Rat brain 4-hydroxybutyrate concentration increases quickly after acute administration of ethosuximide, trimethadione and valproate but decreases after chronic phenobarbital, ethosuximide or trimethadione (SNEAD et al. 1980). The isoenzyme of aldehyde reductase with the higher specificity for succinic semialdehyde is not inhibited by anticonvulsant drugs (RUMIGNY et al. 1980). The isoenzyme inhibited by anticonvulsant drugs (ARI) is more potently inhibited by various flavonoids (quercetin, rutin and derivatives). These compounds appear not to posses anticonvulsant activity (WHITTLE and TURNER 1981).

2. GABAergic Pathways

Pathways releasing GABA were initially tentatively identified by a combination of neurophysiological, neuropharmacological and biochemical techniques (see ITO 1976; CURTIS 1979). However, the introduction of sensitive and specific immunocytochemical procedures for demonstrating glutamic acid decarboxylase in fixed or frozen sections (SAITO et al. 1974; OERTEL et al. 1981 a) has permitted the precise identification of cell types that synthesise GABA and the neuronal pathways that release it. These studies are now being supplemented by an immunocytochemical method for visualising GABA (STORM-MATHISEN et al. 1983).

Detailed GAD-immunocytochemical studies have been made in the cerebellum, basal ganglia, thalamus, hippocampus and neocortex (RIBAK et al. 1976, 1978; SAITO et al. 1974; OERTEL et al. 1981 b; HENDRICKSON et al. 1981; SOMOGYI et al. 1983). These have confirmed earlier neurophysiological and biochemical evidence for important intrinsic GABAergic inhibitory systems in the neocortex and hippocampus.

In the neocortex large aspinous stellate neurons form a horizontal GABAergic network (principally in lamina IV) that provides symmetrical endings on the somata of pyramidal cells. Activation of this inhibitory network leads to hyperpolarisation of pyramidal somata and reduced impulse generation at the initial segments of the axons (RIBAK 1978). The afferent and efferent connections of this system ensure that it provides feedforward and feedback collateral inhibition. The intrinsic GABAergic neurons in the hippocampus are similarly activated by feedback inhibition from pyramidal neurons. Thus in the two brain regions most significantly involved in partial or focal epileptic activity (i.e. the neocortex and hippocampus) the GABAergic inhibitory system is, in terms of structure and connectivity, ideally arranged to prevent or terminate the excessively synchronous or sustained firing of the neurons that constitute the output system, and thus to prevent or minimise epileptic activity.

3. Convulsant Drugs and GABA

Compounds that impair the functioning of the GABAergic system will, if given focally into the cortex or hippocampus, induce local seizure activity, and if they enter the brain following systemic administration will induce partial or generalised seizures (MELDRUM 1975, 1979).

The two major categories of convulsant compounds acting on GABAergic inhibition are those impairing the synthesis of GABA by inhibiting GAD activity and those preventing the postsynaptic action of GABA. Inhibition of GAD activity has been considered in Sect. A.II.1.a (see Table 2).

The postsynaptic inhibitory action of GABA can be blocked by drugs acting either at the GABA recognition site, such as bicuculline, or at a site closely related to the Cl^- ionophore, such as picrotoxinin, the cage convulsants (tetramethylenedisulphotetramine, *p*-chlorophenylsilatrane and various bicyclophosphate esters) and the convulsant barbiturates. The two sites can be differentiated in radioactive ligand studies using brain membrane preparations. Bicuculline competes with GABA or muscimol for binding (ENNA and SNYDER 1975; ENNA et al. 1977 a). Dihydropicrotoxinin competes with the cage convulsants, with barbiturates and with various other anticonvulsant drugs (OLSEN et al. 1979; OLSEN 1981a, b), Convulsants acting at the picrotoxinin binding site prevent the increase in chloride conductance induced by GABA acting at its recognition site.

4. Pathophysiology in Epilepsy

The evidence for a failure in GABAergic inhibition as the primary cause of any syndrome of epilepsy in man at the present moment is inconclusive, except for the syndromes of pyridoxine deficiency and dependence in infants (COURSIN 1964; SCHLESINGER and UPHOUSE 1972) and poisoning with drugs inhibiting glutamic acid decarboxylase.

However, three kinds of evidence support this concept.

a) GABA in Cerebrospinal Fluid

Pilot studies of CSF GABA content that compared patients with epilepsy and patients with other neurological disorders found no significant change (ENNA et al. 1977b; SCHMIDT and LÖSCHER 1981). However, when patients are compared with normal controls, a reduced mean GABA content is often, but not invariably, found. This apparently does not depend on seizure type (partial or generalised) nor on the kind of drug therapy. The significant reduction in GABA content in the CSF of children with febrile convulsions (LÖSCHER et al. 1981) must be interpreted cautiously, as the probands were febrile and directly postictal when sampled, and the control group was significantly older.

Caution is also required with regard to most published reports on CSF GABA content because of the possibility that both control and patient values are artefactually high, through hydrolysis of conjugated forms of GABA (such as homocarnosine, γ-aminobutyryl choline or unidentified peptides) which are present in CSF in concentrations 15–40 times higher than GABA itself (GROVE et al. 1981; PERRY et al. 1982).

b) GABAergic Systems in Experimental Focal Epilepsy

Measurements of GABA content in epileptogenic foci induced by cobalt in the cortex of rats and cats (KOYAMA 1972; VAN GELDER and COURTOIS 1972) show a reduction in GABA associated with severe convulsive activity.

Focal lesions induced by alumina in the monkey neocortex are associated with a reduction in the number of axon terminals (per unit volume) staining immunocytochemically for glutamic acid decarboxylase (RIBAK et al. 1979). This result has been confirmed at the fine structural level by evidence of a reduction in the relative number of symmetrical (inhibitory) synapses compared with asymmetrical (excitatory) synapses (RIBAK et al. 1981). Experiments in infant monkeys suggest that hypoxia, or focal ischaemia, in early life may cause a selective loss of GABAergic interneurons (SLOPER et al. 1980).

c) Human Epileptogenic Foci

Neurosurgical studies using appropriate control cortical material (PERRY et al. 1975b; PERRY and HANSEN 1981) have shown no reduction in GABA content in temporal or frontal foci. In contrast a significant elevation is found (0.63 ± 0.06 µmol GABA/g wet weight in 14 controls vs 0.82 ± 0.05 in 51 foci).

A preliminary study of GAD activity, GABA-T activity and GABA-binding sites in neurosurgically resected material (LLOYD et al. 1981) suggests that decreases occur in about one-third of patients and increases in another third. The significance of these observations is not yet clear.

5. Pharmacological Enhancement of GABA-Mediated Inhibition

GABAergic inhibition cannot normally be enhanced by the systemic administration of either GABA or of its precursor glutamic acid, primarily because of lack of access to the synaptic site.

However, there are many possible mechanisms for enhancing GABAergic inhibition pharmacologically. Seven of these are listed in Table 3 and discussed below.

Table 3. Mechanisms by which drugs enhance GABA-mediated inhibition

1. GABA agonist
   e.g. muscimol, THIP, imidazoleacetic acid
2. GABA prodrug
   e.g. cetyl-GABA, benzoyl-GABA, Progabide (?)
3. Facilitating GABA release
   e.g. baclofen (?), γ-acetylenic GABA (?)
4. Increasing presynaptic concentrations of GABA and/or GABA-transaminase inhibition
   e.g. valproate, γ-vinyl-GABA, ethanolamine-*O*-sulphate
5. Allosteric enhancement of affinity of GABA recognition site
   e.g. benzodiazepines, triazolopyridazines, barbiturates
6. Action on chloride ionophore
   e.g. barbiturates
7. Inhibition of GABA reuptake
   e.g. nipecotic acid: ethylnipecotate

a) GABA Agonists

A GABA agonist acts at the GABA recognition site to reproduce the physiological action of GABA (see BARKER and MATHERS 1981). There are two problems with this as a pharmacological approach to antiepileptic therapy.

Firstly there are structurally similar receptors on non-synaptic sites, including axons (BROWN and MARSH 1978; ALLAN et al. 1980) and presynaptic (autoreceptor) sites where GABA and other agonists act to reduce GABA release (MITCHELL and MARTIN 1978). There are also pharmacologically dissimilar GABA recognition sites, the GABA B receptors of BOWERY et al. (1980), which are sensitive to a different class of GABA agonists (e.g. baclofen) and which modify monoaminergic release.

Secondly agonists which are selective for the postsynaptic GABA recognition site and which produce bicuculline-sensitive inhibition when applied at the single-cell level [such as the fungal toxin muscimol and the synthetic bicyclic analogue of GABA, 4,5,6,7-tetrahydroisoxazolo[5,4-C]pyridine-3-ol (THIP)] appear to be anticonvulsant when tested in rodent models of epilepsy (ANLEZARK et al. 1978; LLOYD et al. 1979), but when evaluated in a primate model (photosensitive epilepsy in *Papio papio*) are not anticonvulsant, but facilitate spike-and-wave discharges and induce diffuse peripheral myoclonus (PEDLEY et al. 1979; MELDRUM and HORTON 1980; MELDRUM 1981). Muscimol given experimentally to patients with schizophrenia or movement disorders induces similar paroxysmal EEG appearances and diffuse myoclonus (TAMMINGA et al. 1978; SHOULSON et al. 1978). This proconvulsant action of specific and potent GABA agonists may be the result of an action at sites other than the postsynaptic GABA receptor (e.g. the autoreceptor). Alternatively action at GABA receptors that is not spatially and temporally integrated with ongoing physiological activity may be proconvulsant.

b) GABA Prodrugs

Lipid-soluble GABA derivatives that enter the brain and are subsequently hydrolysed to yield GABA have been tested as anticonvulsants in rodent models.

These include benzoyl GABA, pivaloyl GABA (GALZIGNA et al. 1978) and cetyl GABA (FREY and LÖSCHER 1980). High doses are required to block pentylenetetrazol seizures in rats or mice. It is not proven that an increase in synaptic GABA, due to hydrolysis of the prodrug, is responsible for the anticonvulsant effect. A cyclic prodrug, Δ'-pyrroline, is oxidised in the brain to 2-pyrrolidinone, which is hydrolysed to GABA (CALLERY et al. 1982).

c) Enhancing or Facilitating GABA Release

There is little definitive evidence for this as a direct action, but it may be one of the effects of γ-vinyl GABA and γ-acetylenic GABA (ABDUL-GHANI et al. 1980) and of benzodiazepines (CURTIS et al. 1976c).

d) Inhibition of GABA-transaminase

The anticonvulsant action of catalytic inhibitors of GABA-T has been discussed above. It is not clear to what extent the anticonvulsant effect depends on secondary effects such as enhanced synaptic GABA release and impaired glial uptake.

e) Allosteric Enhancement of the Affinity of the GABA Recognition Site

A mechanism of this type has been proposed (COSTA and GUIDOTTI 1979) to explain the enhancement by benzodazepines of the postsynaptic inhibition due to GABA (see HAEFELY et al. 1981; Sect. II.6, below). It was suggested that benzodiazepines compete with an endogenous peptide, "GABAmodulin", whose physiological function is to reduce the affinity of the GABA recognition site for GABA (COSTA and GUIDOTTI 1979; GUIDOTTI et al. 1979). This mechanism has yet to be confirmed although it is clear that many endogenous compounds (including GABA itself) reduce the binding of labelled GABA to brain membrane preparations. There is also evidence that β-carboline derivatives bind with high affinity at the benzodiazepine-binding site and have physiological actions comparable to, or opposing, those of benzodiazepines (BRAESTRUP et al. 1980; SKOLNICK et al. 1981; TENEN and HIRSCH 1980; OLSEN 1981; MELDRUM and BRAESTRUP 1983).

Radioactive ligand studies provide convincing evidence for interactions between (a) ligands which bind to the GABA recognition site, (b) ligands which compete with benzodiazepines for high-affinity binding and (c) ligands which compete with dihydropicrotoxinin for binding (OLSEN 1981).

The most precise studies (in terms of molecular structure for agonist action and in terms of kinetics) concern the potentiation of benzodiazepine binding by GABA agonists (KAROBATH and LIPPITSCH 1979; KAROBATH and SPERK 1979; BRAESTRUP et al. 1979; KAROBATH et al. 1979). Using thoroughly washed membrane preparations GABA enhances the affinity of the benzodiazepine-binding site in a concentration-dependent manner. This effect is reproduced by muscimol and blocked by bicuculline. However, 3-aminopropane sulphonic acid and isoguvacine are partial agonists (mixed agonists/antagonists) in this system and piperidine-4-sulphonic acid and THIP are competitive antagonists, i.e. they prevent the enhancement of benzodiazepine binding induced by GABA or muscimol (BRAESTRUP et al. 1979). These data can be interpreted in terms of multiple classes of GABA receptors with different coupling to benzodiazepine-binding site, or in terms of a conformational change in the receptor complex following the binding of GABA to the recognition site that modifies the properties of the benzodiazepine receptor. According to the latter concept certain GABA analogues are capable of binding to the recognition site but the complex is not then capable of the conformational change.

Neurophysiological studies of single-cell responses in vivo show an enhancement of inhibitory responses to GABA after focal or systemic benzodiazepines (see below). Studies of Cl^- ion channels in the membranes of cultured mouse spinal neurons demonstrate that benzodiazepines increase the frequency of channel activation by GABA rather than the properties of the open channel, as occurs during potentiation with pentobarbital (STUDY and BARKER 1981).

High-affinity GABA binding to crude synaptic membrane preparations is enhanced by pentobarbital (in concentrations similar to those occurring in the brain during surgical anaesthesia) (JOHNSTON and WILLOW 1981; WILLOW and JOHNSTON 1981). Barbiturate enhancement of GABA binding occurs only in chloride-containing media and depends on an interaction between the picrotoxinin-binding site and the GABA recognition site (OLSEN and LEEB-LUNDBERG 1981; OLSEN 1981 b; ASANO and OGASAWARA 1981).

f) Action on the Chloride Ionophore

Anaesthetic barbiturates can, by direct action, open Cl^- channels in the neuronal membrane and can additionally prolong the opening induced by GABA (NICOLL 1972; BARKER and RANSOM 1978; MACDONALD and Barker 1979; Study and Barker 1981). Anticonvulsant barbiturates (such as phenobarbital) do not directly activate Cl^- ion conductance. They do prolong the duration of GABA-activated channels (BARKER and MCBURNEY 1979), but this effect occurs only at concentrations ten times greater than those found in clinical use (MACDONALD 1983).

Both effects appear to be dependent on an action at the picrotoxinin-binding site, at which cage-convulsants and convulsant barbiturates compete for binding with dihydropicrotoxinin (OLSEN 1982).

g) Inhibition of GABA Reuptake

Local application of compounds that inhibit the reuptake of GABA into neurons or the glia enhances (a) the inhibitory effect of iontophoretically applied GABA (CURTIS et al. 1976a, b) physiologically evoked GABA-mediated postsynaptic inhibition (MATTHEWS et al. 1981). Some inhibitors of GABA uptake are also inhibitors of the enzymes of GABA metabolism or are active at the GABA recognition site. However, the structural features of the Na-dependent GABA carrier in membranes differ from the GABA recognition site, so that it has been possible to identify natural and synthetic compounds that are highly selective as GABA uptake inhibitors (JOHNSTON et al. 1976; KROGSGAARD-LARSEN 1980). There is also evidence for at least a partial selectivity for neuronal versus glial GABA uptake (IVERSEN and KELLY 1975; SCHOUSBOE et al. 1979; KROGSGAARD-LARSEN 1980; BRECKENRIDGE et al. 1981). Most of the selectively active compounds have a high

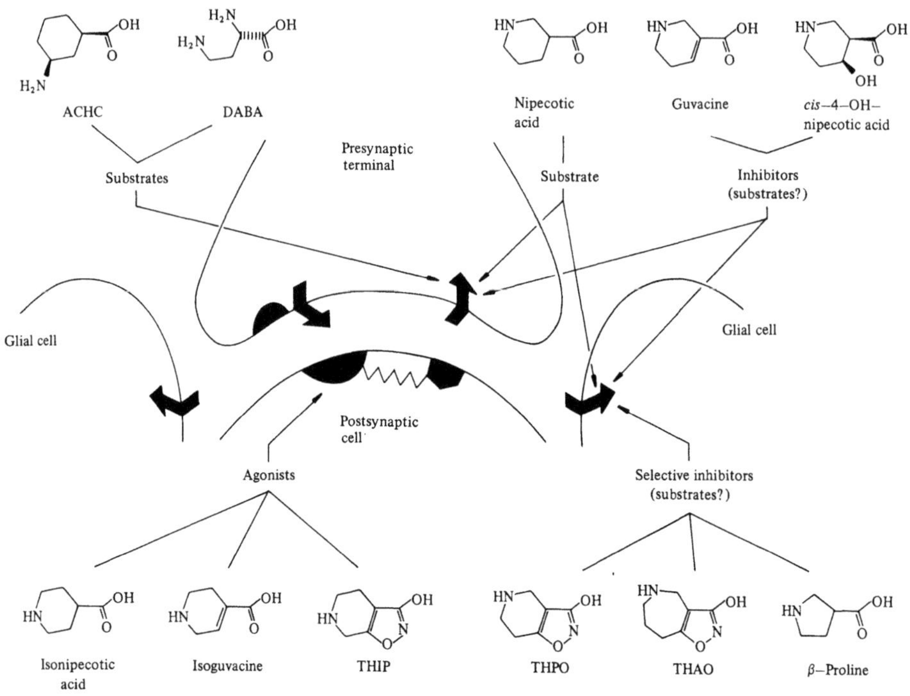

Fig. 2. Schematic diagram of GABAergic axosomatic synapse (KROGSGAARD-LARSEN 1980). *Thick arrows* indicate GABA release from, and reuptake into, a presynaptic terminal, and uptake into glial cells. *Black semicircles* indicate GABA autoreceptor (on presynaptic terminal) and GABA recognition site, connected to chloride ionophore, on the postsynaptic cell membrane

Molecular formulae of various analogues of GABA are grouped to indicate their preferential sites of action. *ACHC* (3-aminocyclohexanecarboxylic acid) and *DABA* (2,4-diaminobutyric acid) are substrates and competitive inhibitors of the neuronal GABA uptake system. *THPO* (4,5,6,7-tetrahydroisoxazolo [4,5-c] pyridin-3-ol) and *THAO* (5,6,7,8-tetrahydro-4*H*-isoxazolo [4,5-c] azepin-3-ol) are selective inhibitors of GABA uptake into glial cells

ionised/un-ionised ratio and enter the brain only to a very limited extent when given systemically (KROGSGAARD-LARSEN et al. 1981). Thus the comparative evaluation of GABA-uptake inhibitors as anticonvulsants requires intracerebroventricular injection. By this route several compounds are active against audiogenic seizures in mice [including nipecotic acid, *cis*-4-hydroxynipecotic acid and THPO (4,5,6,7,8-tetrahydro-4*H*-isoxazolo [4,5-c] azepin-3-ol)] (HORTON et al. 1979; MELDRUM et al. 1982). The two compounds that are selective inhibitors of neuronal versus glial GABA uptake, 2,4-diaminobutyric acid and *cis*-3-aminocyclohexanecarboxylic acid (NEAL and BOWERY 1977) (see also Fig. 2), both induce clonic jerks and seizures

Esters of nipecotic acid (e.g. ethyl or pivaloyloxymethyl) or of *cis*-4-*OH*-nipecotic acid (methyl) act as lipid-soluble prodrugs of the GABA uptake inhibitors and have anticonvulsant action in mouse models when given systemically (FREY et al. 1979; HORTON et al. 1979; KROGSGAARD-LARSEN et al. 1981; MELDRUM et al. 1982).

h) Enhanced GABA-Mediated Inhibition: Summary

The use of pharmacological tools of moderate or high selectivity has established that anticonvulsant effects are seen after any procedure that enhances the action of physiologically released GABA. At least four distinct mechanisms achieve this (a) enhanced release (following GABA-T inhibition), (b) increase in number of chloride channels opened by GABA (due to action on "benzodiazepine site"), (c) prolongation of opening of Cl^- channels (due to action at "barbiturate binding site"), and (d) impaired reuptake of GABA into neurons and the glia. A direct GABA agonist action that does not respect the critical spatial and temporal features of activity within the GABAergic nerve net is of doubtful value as an anticonvulsant procedure.

6. Anticonvulsant Drug Action and GABAergic Inhibition

Electrophysiological studies of single unit responses both in vivo and in vitro consistently show that barbiturates and benzodiazepines enhance the effect of exogenous GABA and of endogenously released GABA. The dual mechanism for enhancement of the chloride conductance increase produced by GABA, i.e. prolonging the open time of the Cl^- channels or increasing the frequency of their opening (STUDY and BARKER 1981), seems to be the electrophysiological counterpart of the differential effects of barbiturates and benzodiazepines observed in binding studies with washed membrane preparations.

There is less certain evidence for enhancement by valproate of the inhibition due to exogenous GABA in vivo and in vitro. Iontophoretic application of valproate enhances inhibition due to GABA in cultured spinal neurons (MACDONALD and BERGEY 1979), but this effect is not seen with bath-applied valproate, up to 1 m*M* (Barker, unpublished).

The studies utilising exogenous GABA in vitro and in vivo indicate a postsynaptic site of action of barbiturates and benzodiazepines on GABAergic inhibition. They do not exclude the possibility that there are also presynaptic actions of anticonvulsant drugs that may augment or oppose the postsynaptic action (e.g. AICKIN and DEISZ 1981; NESTOROS and NISTRI 1978; COLLINS 1981). Presynaptic actions involving GABA autoreceptors are possible, but the GABA receptor may well be different at this site (BRENNAN 1982). A general mechanism of anticonvulsant action shown potently by hydantoins and carbamazepine, but also by benzodiazepines, involves Ca^{++} calmodulin-activated protein phosphorylation in nerve terminals (DELORENZO 1980; DELORENZO et al. 1981) and is associated with a reduced release of both inhibitory and excitatory neurotransmitters (see Sect. B.I.4).

This mechanism will oppose any postsynaptic GABA-enhancing action of hydantoins, thus explaining the poor efficacy of hydantoins in some animal tests.

That enhancement of GABAergic postsynaptic inhibition is a common mechanism of action of anticonvulsant drugs is supported by biochemical evidence relating to GABA turnover. GABA turnover can be measured in vivo by two techniques, namely, (a) rate of incorporation of labelled precursor into GABA (FONNUM 1981; CHAPMAN et al. 1982) and (b) initial maximal rate of accumulation of GABA following inhibition of GABA-T by amino-oxyacetic acid, gabaculine or γ-vinyl GABA (BERNASCONI et al. 1982). Both methods show that after valproate, barbiturates and benzodiazepines the rate of GABA synthesis is significantly reduced (CHAPMAN et al. 1982; CHAPMAN 1984; BERNASCONI et al. 1984). This is consistent with a postsynaptic enhancement of GABA-mediated inhibition, leading to reduced physiological activity in the system by neuronal feedback.

III. Glycine

The highest concentrations of glycine are found in the brain stem and spinal cord (6.0 µmol/g in grey matter) (JOHNSTON 1968). There is conclusive physiological and pharmacological evidence that glycine is an inhibitory transmitter within the spinal cord, providing direct and reciprocal inhibition on motoneurons via interneurons in the anterior horn (CURTIS and JOHNSTON 1974). On motoneurons, inhibition invoked physiologically and that due to iontophoretically applied glycine can be blocked by strychnine and a variety of related alkaloids, including brucine and thebaine (CURTIS and JOHNSTON 1974). There is also physiological and biochemical evidence for glycine acting as an inhibitory transmitter in the cortex (LEVI et al. 1982).

Pathophysiology in Spasticity and Epilepsy

The concentration of glycine is reportedly elevated in cobalt-induced epileptogenic foci in the cat (KOYAMA 1972; KOYAMA and JASPER 1977), but not in similar foci in the rat (JOSEPH and EMSON 1976).

In neurosurgical patients with epilepsy, focal cortical glycine content was reported to be elevated relative to literature values (VAN GELDER et al. 1972). The mean glycine level was found to be normal in a limited controlled study (PERRY et al. 1975 b) but a more extensive study shows a significant elevation, with 7 out of 51 samples showing glycine levels more than 2 SD above control means (PERRY and HANSEN 1981). This elevation in glycine could be a consequence of hydantoin therapy.

Infants with hyperglycinaemia, an inherited disorder of amino acid metabolism, have markedly elevated plasma and CSF glycine concentration. The main clinical correlate, muscular hypotonia, is consistent with an action of glycine on spinal motoneuron receptors. However, generalised myoclonic jerks and spike wave discharges on the EEG and seizures are commonly observed in the nonketotic form of hyperglycinaemia (PERRY et al. 1975 c; MARKAND et al. 1982).

Seizures produced by strychnine (in animals and in man) and other alkaloids that selectively block glycinergic inhibition are almost certainly due to this action on inhibitory transmission. The seizures are primarily spinal; the cortical EEG activity (and consciousness) can remain unaltered. The systemic doses required to produce seizures are similar to those blocking glycine-induced inhibition in the spinal cord. However, no spontaneous syndromes of epilepsy in man or animals are comparable in seizure pattern to seizures induced by strychnine.

Effects of anticonvulsant drugs on glycine metabolism or on glycinergic mechanisms have frequently been reported, but no such mechanism can be definitively linked to anticonvulsant action. For example, pentobarbital inhibits D-amino acid oxidase in vitro (GOLDSTEIN 1966). Increases in plasma and urinary glycine concentration are sometimes seen in patients receiving sodium valproate, apparently through inhibition of the hepatic glycine cleavage system (JAEKEN et al. 1977; MORTENSEN et al. 1980). However, the effect appears unrelated to the anticonvulsant action of valproate. CSF glycine content is not elevated by valproate in patients, nor is brain glycine content elevated in experimental animals (GODIN et al. 1969; CHAPMAN et al. 1982).

The interpretation based on membrane-binding studies that benzodiazepines act on glycine receptors (YOUNG et al. 1974) is not supported by physiological studies (CURTIS et al. 1976b).

On spinal neurons, barbiturates prolong inhibition due to GABA but not that due to glycine (LODGE and CURTIS 1978; BARKER and RANSOM 1978).

IV. Taurine

In the mammalian brain the concentration of taurine is comparable to that of aspartate and glutamate, but with a different regional distribution. The highest concentration is found in the cerebellum and the lateral geniculate (PERRY et al. 1971; GUIDOTTI et al. 1972). The pituitary and pineal glands, the retina and the heart also contain taurine in high concentration.

Taurine is partially derived from the diet and partially by synthesis (from methionine or homocysteine and serine, or from cysteine). Dietary deficiency of taurine in the cat leads to retinal degeneration (HAYES et al. 1975) but is not known to produce cerebral pathology. Synthesis from methionine or cysteine can be demonstrated in the brain (GAITONDE 1970).

Release of taurine from brain cortex, slices or cubes or synaptosomes can be detected following physiological or electrical stimulation (JASPER and KOYAMA 1969; WHELER et al. 1979; COLLINS et al. 1981). The stimulated release of taurine is entirely or partially calcium dependent according to the preparation (non-calcium-dependent release may be from glial cells).

Iontophoretic experiments have shown that inhibition produced by taurine in the spinal cord can largely be blocked by strychnine (but not by bicuculline), whereas in the cortex and lateral geniculate both strychnine and bicuculline block the inhibition of neuronal firing produced by taurine (CURTIS and JOHNSTON 1974). This might suggest that taurine is acting on glycine and GABA receptors, with regional differences depending on receptor densities. However, in a careful comparison of the efficacy of different amino acids at various levels in the molecular layer of the guinea pig cerebellum (OKAMOTO and SAKAI 1980) it appeared that the inhibitory action of taurine at the Purkinje-cell soma was due to an action on GABA receptors (that is blocked by picrotoxin and bicuculline), whereas in the superficial layers the action is blocked by strychnine, but does not correspond precisely to the laminar pattern of glycine receptors (FREDERICKSON et al. 1978). Taurine has been proposed as the transmitter of stellate cells in the cerebellar molecular layer (MCBRIDE et al. 1976). However, release studies do not support this proposal (FLINT et al. 1981).

Taurine has effects on excitable membranes that are apparently separate from any postulated neurotransmitter function. In heart and skeletal muscle taurine modifies calcium and potassium fluxes, which probably explains its digitalis-like effect on the heart.

Pathophysiology in Epilepsy

In the past 10 years several hypotheses relating taurine to pathophysiological mechanisms have been developed, but none is adequately established.

Several studies of plasma or serum amino acid concentrations in patients with epilepsy and their relatives have indicated that there may be an abnormality in taurine metabolism or transport. Results on plasma concentration are divergent; most patients with epilepsy have plasma taurine levels within the normal range. An increased plasma taurine concentration in some patients has been found in three studies, and has been attributed to impaired renal excretion of taurine, probably as part of a genetic defect in amino acid transport (GOODMAN et al. 1980). A tendency to a lowered plasma taurine level has been reported in children with 3/s spike-and-wave discharge and their close relatives (VAN GELDER et al. 1980). This has also been tentatively attributed to a genetically determined general defect in amino acid transport.

Studies on the concentration of taurine in the cerebral cortex in the region of an epileptogenic focus, in man or in experimental animals, have yielded divergent results. In man the concentration of taurine was reported to be low in tissue from cortical foci (relative to literature taurine values) (VAN GELDER et al. 1972). Comparison of cortical epileptogenic foci with cortical biopsy samples (tumour patients without epilepsy) showed an elevation of taurine in the epileptogenic cortex in a small series (PERRY et al. 1975b) but no significant change in a larger series (PERRY and HANSEN 1981).

In focal epilepsy induced by cobalt, taurine concentration is elevated in the cat (KOYAMA 1972) and decreased in the mouse (VAN GELDER 1972) and rat (CRAIG and HARTMAN 1973; JOSEPH and EMSON 1976).

Therapeutic effects of taurine administration have been reported in certain animal models and in man. In animals, intraventricular administration has an acute protective effect against seizures induced by ouabain or pentylenetetrazol (IZUMI et al. 1973, 1974) or by sound in genetically susceptible rodents (LAIRD and HUXTABLE 1978).

Intraperitoneal or intravenous injection of taurine had acute protective effects against focal seizures induced by cobalt or alumina (VAN GELDER 1972; VAN GELDER et al. 1977), or penicillin or strychnine (MUTANI et al. 1974a, b). Photically induced myoclonus in baboons is also depressed by multiple injections of taurine (although these animals, like the focal models, had locally impaired blood-brain barrier due to multiple depth electrodes) (WADA et al. 1975).

An apparent reduction in seizure incidence has been described in patients (BARBEAU and DONALDSON 1974; BERGAMINI et al. 1974), although the effect appears transient at best (TAKAHASHI and NAKANE 1978).

The interpretation of the apparent antiepileptic effects of taurine remains speculative. Acute effects of intracerebroventricular injection could be due to direct actions on GABA, glycine, β-alanine or taurine membrane receptors. Effects of systemic drug administration could be due to changes in amino acid transport, storage or release, or to effects on excitable membranes relating to ionic fluxes.

Table 4. Excitatory amino acids in mammalian brain

		pK (25 °C)			Concentration (μmol/g wet weight)	
		pK_1	pK_2	pK_3	Rat brain	Human biopsy
Aspartic acid	$COOHCH(NH_2)CH_2COOH$	2.01	3.80	9.93	2.60	1.18
Glutamic acid	$COOHCH(NH_2)CH_2CH_2COOH$	2.13	4.31	9.76	11.29	10.16
Cysteine sulphinic acid	$COOHCH(NH_2)CH_2SOOH$	–	–	–	0.012[a]	
Cysteic acid	$COOHCH(NH_2)CH_2SO_3H$	1.89	8.70	12.70	0.01–0.10[a]	
Homocysteic acid	$COOHCH(NH_2)CH_2CH_2SO_3$	–	–	–		
Quinolinic acid	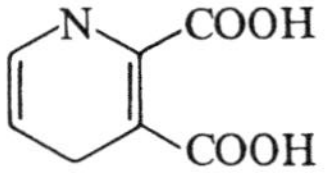	2.43	5.06	–		

Dissociation constants (*pK*) at 25 °C from Perrin (1965, 1972) and Merck index (1976)
Concentrations from Perry et al. (1981) and Rassin et al. (1981) ([a])

C. Amino Acids Producing Excitation

Table 4 lists various amino acids that occur in the mammalian brain and are excitatory when applied iontophoretically (CURTIS and JOHNSTON 1974; STONE and PERKINS 1981). There is substantial evidence that aspartic and glutamic acids are neurotransmitters in many brain regions. There is very little evidence concerning the sulphur-containing analogues or various cyclic analogues.

The intracortical or intracerebroventricular injection of any of these excitant amino acids, or other natural or synthetic analogues, produces focal or generalised seizure activity (HAYASHI 1954; CRAWFORD 1963). Kainic acid, a toxin derived from seaweed (SHINOZAKI and KONISHI 1970), is a very potent excitant and convulsant (OLNEY et al. 1974; OLNEY 1979).

Systemic administration of these excitant amino acids (in very high doses) also induces seizures (BRADFORD and DODD 1975; JOHNSTON 1973). Glutamate enters the brain from plasma by carrier (at 0.1–2 μmol/h per gram tissue) and is probably converted directly to glutamine in the glial compartment. However, entry into the periventricular organs is unrestricted (PRICE et al. 1981); seizure activity is presumably initiated at these points. Predominantly limbic seizures are seen after systemic kainic acid (JOHNSTON 1973; BRADFORD and DODD 1975; COLLINS et al. 1980).

Excitatory amino acid neurotransmitters probably play a role in the spread of focal and generalised seizure activity. An abnormality in excitatory transmission may contribute to the pathogenesis of focal seizures, e.g., supersensitivity of dicarboxylic amino acid receptors, enhanced release or impaired reuptake of excitatory compounds.

There is also evidence for diminished excitatory transmission as part of the mechanism of action of anticonvulsant drugs, particularly barbiturates (BARKER and RANSOM 1978).

I. Dicarboxylic Amino Acids

1. Physiological Role

The evidence concerning the neurotransmitter role of glutamic and aspartic acids in the brain is less complete than that for GABA and glycine. This is partly because highly specific antagonists are only now becoming available, partly because enzymic markers for the histochemical or immunocytochemical delineation of pathways have so far not been established (see NADLER et al. 1978) (but aspartate aminotransferase appears a possible marker for aspartergic neurons) and partly because the principal excitatory synapses are dendritic rather than somatic, making electrophysiological studies more difficult. The clearest evidence that glutamic acid is an excitatory transmitter in most brain regions, including the neocortex, thalamus, striatum hippocampus, brain stem and cerebellum, derives from biochemical data including that for Ca^{++}-dependent release following stimulation and from electrophysiological data.

Studies of high-affinity uptake systems (utilising labelled glutamic acid or L- or D-aspartic acid) do not distinguish between the two amino acids, but when compared with lesion studies have proved a useful tool (FONNUM et al. 1981).

Excitatory pathways which appear on these biochemical criteria to be glutamatergic and/or aspartergic include corticofugal pathways to the striatum, nucleus accumbens and thalamus (FONNUM et al. 1981); the perforant path from the entorhinal cortex to dentate granule cells (molecular layer) (NADLER and SMITH 1981); hippocampal output via the fornix to the lateral septum nucleus accumbens and mediobasal hypothalamus (ZACZEK et al. 1979; MALTHE-SØRENSEN et al. 1979, 1980); CA_3 pyramidal neurons via the Schaffer collaterals to CA_1 neurons (stratum radiatum) (STORM-MATHISEN 1981); and in the cerebellum excitation of Purkinje cells due to climbing fibres from the inferior olive or due to the parallel fibre endings (from granule cells) (FLINT et al. 1981).

By the same criteria several important excitatory pathways appear not to be glutamatergic/aspartergic, e.g. specific thalamocortical afferents to laminae III and IV.

In some of the pathways described it appears possible that both glutamate and aspartate may be involved as neurotransmitters (as they both show Ca^{++}-dependent release on stimulation and changes in concentration of both are found after focal lesions). These include optic nerve to tectum (CANZEK et al. 1981), visual cortex, layer 6, to lateral geniculate nucleus (BAUGHMAN and GILBERT 1980), cerebellar granule cell to Purkinje cell (FLINT et al. 1981) and auditory nerve to cochlear nucleus (WENTHOLD 1980). In the rat olfactory tract aspartate alone appears to be the transmitter (COLLINS and PROBETT 1981).

The principal action of glutamic and aspartic acids at postsynaptic receptors in the mammalian nervous system is to induce depolarisation by enhancing conductance to Na^+ (CURTIS and JOHNSTON 1974; SEGAL 1981). Glutamate is the excitatory transmitter at certain invertebrate neuromuscular junctions, where it acts to increase conductance to Na^+, K^+, and Ca^{++}. However, at some extrajunctional receptors it acts to hyperpolarise the membrane by opening Cl^- gates (USHERWOOD 1978). Hyperpolarising responses to glutamate have been reported in the mammalian cerebellum (YAMAMOTO et al. 1976).

Some amino acids not naturally occurring in the brain (including *N*-methyl-D-aspartate, ibotenic acid and D-homocysteate) can produce excitation, apparently by decreasing K^+ conductance (ENGBERG et al. 1979; LAMBERT et al. 1981).

2. Agonists and Antagonists

Testing non-endogenous analogues of the excitatory amino acids in the spinal cord has indicated that there are three pharmacologically distinct receptors for dicarboxylic amino acids (DAVIES and WATKINS 1979; DAVIES et al. 1980; WATKINS and EVANS 1981). These receptors are preferentially activated by *N*-methyl-D-aspartate, by quisqualate or by kainic acid, respectively.

Many compounds have been tested as antagonists of excitation due to iontophoretically applied glutamic or aspartic acid or their analogues. Among effective antagonists some have a highly selective action against excitation due to *N*-methyl-D-aspartate. These include D-amino adipic acid, 2-amino-5-phosphonovaleric acid and 2-amino-7-phosphonoheptanoic acid (EVANS et al. 1982). Glutamic acid diethylester is a relatively selective antagonist for excitation due to quisqualic acid. Excitation due to kainic acid can be blocked by γ-D-glutamyl glycine and by *cis*-2,3-piperidine dicarboxylic acid, but these are relatively non-selective antagonists, being active also against quisqualic acid and *N*-methyl-D-aspartic acid.

Several of these antagonists have been evaluated against synaptically evoked excitation. Glutamic acid diethyl ester blocks excitation in the striatum evoked by cortical stimulation (SPENCER 1976) or excitation of cortical interneurons induced by pyramidal tract stimulation (STONE 1973) or excitation of hippocampal neurons by perforant path stimulation (HICKS and MCLENNAN 1979; WHEAL and MILLER 1980). D-Amino adipic acid blocks excitation synaptically evoked in the spinal cord (EVANS et al. 1979), cochlea nucleus (MARTIN 1980; MARTIN and ADAMS 1979), cerebral cortex and striatum (STONE 1979).

3. Pathophysiology in Epilepsy

Apparent reductions in the concentration of glutamic and aspartic acids in human epileptogenic foci were described in a preliminary report (VAN GELDER et al. 1972). A larger controlled study shows a highly significant increase in glutamic acid concentration (+25%) and no change in aspartic acid in focal epileptogenic cortex (PERRY et al. 1975b; PERRY and HANSEN 1981).

Cortical foci induced experimentally by cobalt in the cat or rat consistently show a decrease in glutamic acid (up to −50%) and aspartic acid content (KOYAMA 1972; VAN GELDER and COURTOIS 1972; EMSON and JOSEPH 1975; KOYAMA and JASPER 1977). Release of glutamic acid into cortical superfusates is enhanced over a cobalt focus and correlates with the severity and time course of epileptic activity (DODD and BRADFORD 1976; DODD et al. 1980). An increased release into superfusates could arise from enhanced release of glutamic acid at excitatory synapses or from impaired reuptake of glutamic acid into neurons or the glia.

Plasma glutamic acid concentration is increased and aspartic acid concentration decreased in patients with 3/s spike-and-wave epilepsy and in their first-degree relatives (VAN GELDER et al. 1980). This may indicate an abnormality in amino acid transport, predisposing to one form of primary generalised epilepsy.

Many convulsant drugs interfere with glutamic acid metabolism. The majority of these inhibit glutamic acid decarboxylase, and the consequent impairment of GABA synthesis appears to be the critical factor (see above). Methionine sulphoximine inhibits glutamine synthetase (SELLINGER and WEILER 1963) and thus interrupts the glial glutamic acid-glutamine stage of the proposed recycling of glutamate. It is not clear whether excitatory amino acid neurotransmission is impaired or enhanced in this form of epilepsy.

A rare familial syndrome characterised by neonatal seizures (and early death) is associated with abnormally elevated CSF aspartic acid concentration (WEITZ et al. 1981).

4. Anticonvulsant Drugs

The specific antagonists of the excitatory action of dicarboxylic acids described above have not been extensively tested as potential antiepileptic agents. The relatively weak glutamate antagonist HA 966 (1-hydroxy-3-amino-pyrrolidone-2) protects against strychnine-induced seizures (DAVIES and WATKINS 1973; BONTA et al. 1971). In rats with cobalt-induced focal seizures, cortical superfusion with solutions of 2-amino-4-phosphonobutyric acid or 2-D-aminoadipic acid decreased EEG spikes or limb jerks (COUTINHO-NETTO et al. 1981).

In the only studies showing a quantitative relationship between antagonist action and anticonvulsant effect, blockade of sound-induced seizures in genetically susceptible mice correlates with antagonist action at *N*-methyl-D-aspartic acid preferring receptors (CROUCHER et al. 1982; MELDRUM et al. 1983 a). The most potent anticonvulsant of a series of glutamate/aspartate antagonists is 2-amino-7-phosphono heptanoic acid. This is effective in a wide range of animal models of epilepsy including photosensitive baboons (MELDRUM et al. 1983 b; MELDRUM and CHAPMAN 1983).

Established anticonvulsant drugs have effects both on the metabolism of dicarboxylic acids and on synaptically induced excitation. Phenobarbital produces an increase in cortical aspartic acid concentration (+33%) and a decrease in glutamic acid content (CHAPMAN et al. 1978). Diazepam also increases brain aspartic acid and slightly reduces glutamic acid (CARLSSON and CHAPMAN 1981). In contrast sodium valproate increases cortical glutamic acid concentration and markedly decreases aspartic acid content (SCHECHTER et al. 1978; KUKINO and DEGUCHI 1977; CHAPMAN et al. 1982).

Depression of excitatory transmission by barbiturates has been described in a wide variety of preparations, some of which involve excitatory amino acids. Both reduced release of transmitter and a reduced postsynaptic effect have been described. Thus the calcium-dependent stimulated release of glutamic and aspartic acids from midbrain slices is reduced by pentobarbital (WALLER and RICHTER 1980). A reduced entry of calcium into presynaptic terminals is thought to be responsible for this diminished release (GOLDRING and BLAUSTEIN 1980). Aspartate release from the lateral olfactory tract is reduced by chlordiazepoxide (COLLINS 1981).

Excitatory responses to iontophoretically administered glutamate are reduced by anaesthetic barbiturates (BARKER and GAINER 1973; BARKER and RANSOM 1978; LAMBERT and FLATMAN 1981).

II. Sulphinic and Sulphonic Acids

The sulphur-containing analogues of aspartic and glutamic acid (cysteine sulphinic acid, cysteic acid, homocysteine sulphinic acid and homocysteic acid) are found in the brain at much lower concentrations than aspartic acid and glutamic acid. However, they have no obvious metabolic function so the possibility that they are neurotransmitters requires consideration. They are formed in the brain by oxidation of cysteine or homocysteine.

Studies that delineate pathways using these amino acids as excitatory transmitters (involving release, lesions or immunohistochemistry) are not available.

Pathophysiology

Very little information is available concerning the possible involvement in epilepsy. Seizures are a common feature of homocystinuria and autosomal recessive inherited disorder due to deficiency of cystathionine synthase. Accumulation of homocysteine in the brain is thought to contribute to the induction of seizures.

Administration of homocysteine to animals induces generalised seizures (FOLBERGROVA 1974). This may be due to interference with the coenzymic function of pyridoxal phosphate or to oxidation to directly excitant amino acids (JOHNSTON 1973).

D. Concluding Remarks

I. Inherited Abnormalities of Amino Acid Metabolism and Epilepsy

The biochemical basis of the principal syndromes of epilepsy that are genetically determined (i.e. generalised seizures with 3/s spike-and-wave discharge; photosensitive epilepsy; febrile convulsions) is not known. These syndromes appear to be inherited in an autosomal dominant pattern with variable penetrance (METRAKOS and METRAKOS 1974; NEWMARK and PENRY 1979). Thus the biochemical defect probably lies in a structural protein or polypeptide rather than in an enzyme (HARRIS 1980). It has been proposed that the defect responsible for generalised seizures with 3/s spike-and-wave modifies the transport of amino acids, including taurine and glutamic acid (VAN GELDER et al. 1980). A relative deficiency in GABAergic inhibition could underly photosensitive epilepsy, as the syndrome can be induced or enhanced by compounds that impair GABA synthesis (MELDRUM 1975, 1979).

More precise biochemical information is available concerning the genetically determined abnormalities of amino acid metabolism, commonly referred to as "aminoacidurias". Seizures are seen either as an occasional feature or sometimes as a consistent and dominant sign in the aminoacidurias (CROME and STERN 1967; WELLNER and MEISTER 1981). Phenylketonuria is relatively common (1 in 15,000 infants) but hyperlysinaemia and hyperprolinaemia are rare disorders. Although the enzyme deficiencies are precisely known in many cases and the metabolites that accumulate in the brain are largely identified, the mechanisms favouring seizure induction remain uncertain. In several syndromes (hyperglycinaemia, hyperprolinaemia, histidinaemia) there is an excess of substances with an inhibitory action in the brain. This might favour seizures by inactivating physiological inhibitory processes. An excess of directly excitant amino acids (homocysteate, aspartate) could be significant in homocystinuria and in the syndrome of raised CSF aspartate content described in Sect. B.I.3. Accumulation of excess ammonia may be the neurotoxic factor in the disorders of the urea cycle.

A possible mechanism favouring seizures in homocystinuria and in phenylketonuria is inhibition of glutamic acid decarboxylase activity by excess of abnormal metabolites (e.g. 3-mercaptopyruvate and phenyllactic acid). The transport of amino acids into the brain and between cellular compartments is also secondarily deranged in many syndromes and this may modify amino acid neurotransmitter metabolism.

II. Amino Acids and Antiepileptic Drugs

The actions of antiepileptic drugs on neurotransmission mediated by amino acids fall into three principal types.

a) Enhancement of the Postsynaptic Inhibitory Action of GABA

The known function of the intrinsic inhibitory systems in the cortex and hippocampus suggests that this mechanism would be highly effective for preventing or arresting seizure activity.

The neurophysiological and biochemical evidence for this mechanism has been summarised in Sect. A.II. This is probably the most functionally significant mechanism of action for certain classes of anticonvulsant drugs. For benzodiazepines there is a good correlation between potency for enhancement of GABA-mediated inhibition and potency against pentylentetrazol seizures in rodents (see KRALL et al. 1978). In man this mechanism probably provides protection against myoclonic seizures and against primary, or secondary, generalised seizures.

b) Impairment of the Postsynaptic Excitatory Action of Dicarboxylic Acids and Their Sulphinic or Sulphonic Analogues

This mechanism is most prominently shown by barbiturates. It may relate more to anaesthetic actions than to anticonvulsant actions.

c) Impairment of the Synaptic Release of Excitatory and Inhibitory Amino Acids

This mechanism is apparently related to inhibition of a calcium-calmodulin activated protein phosphorylase in synaptic endings. Hydantoin, carbamazepine and benzodiazepines are active in this biochemical system and are also the most potent anticonvulsant drugs when tested against tonic extension induced by maximal electroshock. Because of its action on both inhibitory and excitatory transmission this mechanism appears of little value in most animal models of epilepsy. However, it is clinically effective against many forms of partial epilepsy – perhaps because of the role of excitatory amino acids in the spread of focal seizures.

This crude, tentative explanation in terms of three mechanisms will undoubtedly undergo modification in the light of further research. However, amino acid transmitters are likely to be central to future studies of anticonvulsant drug action, because of their dominant role in excitatory and inhibitory neurotransmission.

Acknowledgments. I thank Dr. A. G. Chapman and Dr. J. L. Barker for helpful comments on the manuscript; Mrs G. Muller and Mrs E. Williams for secretarial assistance; and the Medical Research Council, the Wellcome Trust and the British Epilepsy Association for financial support.

References

Abdul-Ghani AS, Coutinho-Netto J, Bradford HF (1980) The action of γ-vinyl-GABA and γ-acetylenic GABA on the resting and stimulated release of GABA in vivo. Brain Res 191:471–481

Abdul-Ghani AS, Norris PJ, Smith CCT, Bradford HF (1981) Effects of γ-acetylenic GABA and γ-vinyl GABA on synaptosomal release and uptake of GABA. Biochem Pharmacol 30:1203–1209

Aickin CC, Deisz RA (1981) Pentobarbitone interference with inhibitory synaptic transmission in crayfish stretch receptor neurons. J Physiol (Lond) 315:175–187

Allan RD, Evans RH, Jonston GAR (1980) γ-Aminobutyric acid agonists: an in vitro comparison between depression of spinal synaptic activity and depolarisation of spinal root fibres in the rat. Br J Pharmacol 79:609–615

Andersen P, Dingledine R, Gjerstad L, Langmoen IA, Mosfeldt-Laursen A (1980) Two different responses of hippocampal pyramidal cells to application of gamma-aminobutyric acid. J Physiol (Lond) 305:279–296

Andersen P, Bie B, Ganes T (1982) Distribution of GABA sensitive areas on hippocampal pyramidal cells. Exp Brain Res 45:357–363

Anlezark G, Horton RW, Meldrum BS, Sawaya MCB (1976) Anticonvulsant action of ethonalamine-*O*-sulphate and di-*n*-propylacetate and the metabolism of γ-aminobutyric acid (GABA) in mice with audiogenic seizures. Biochem Pharmacol 25:413–417

Anlezark G, Collins J, Meldrum B (1978) GABA agonists and audiogenic seizures. Neurosci Lett 7:337–340

Asano T, Ogasawara N (1981) Chloride-dependent stimulation of GABA and benzodiazepine receptor binding by pentobarbital. Brain Res 225:212–216

Barbeau A, Donaldson J (1974) Zinc, taurine and epilepsy. Arch Neurol 30:52–58

Barker JL, Gainer H (1973) Pentobarbital: selective depression of excitatory synaptic potentials. Science 182:720–722

Barker JL, Mathers DA (1981) GABA analogues activate channels of different duration on cultured mouse spinal neurons. Science 212:358–361

Barker JL, McBurney RN (1979) Phenobarbitone modulation of postsynaptic GABA receptor function on cultured mammalian neurons. Proc Roy Soc Lond B 206:319–328

Barker JL, Ransom BR (1978) Pentobarbitone pharmacology of mammalian central neurones grown in tissue culture. J Physiol (Lond) 280:355–372

Barker JL, McBurney RN, MacDonald JF (1982) Fluctuation analysis of neutral amino acid responses in cultured mouse spinal neurones. J Physiol (Lond) 322:365–387

Baughman RW, Gilbert CD (1980) Aspartate and glutamate as possible neurotransmitters of cells in layer 6 of the visual cortex. Nature 287:848–850

Baxter C, Roberts E (1961) Elevation of γ-amino-butyric acid in brain: selective inhibition of γ-amino-butyric α-ketoglutamic acid transaminase. J Biol Chem 12:3287–3294

Bergamini L, Mutani R, Delsedime M, Durelli L (1974) First clinical experience on the antiepileptic action of taurine. Eur Neurol 11:261–269

Berl S, Lajtha A, Waelsch H (1961) Amino acid and protein metabolism. VI. Cerebral compartments of glutamic acid metabolism. J Neurochem 7:186–197

Bernasconi R, Schmutz M, Martin P, Hauser K (1984) The GABA hypothesis of the mechanism of action of antiepileptic drugs: its usefulness and limitations. In: Fariello RG, Morselli P (eds) Neurotransmitters in epilepsy. Raven, New York

Bernasconi R, Maître L, Martin P, Raschdorf F (1982) The use of inhibitors of GABA-transaminase for the determination of GABA turnover in mouse brain regions: an evaluation of amino-oxyacetic acid and gabaculine. J Neurochem 38:57–66

Bey P, Jung MJ, Gerhart F, Schirlin D, Van Dorsselaer V, Casara P (1981) ω-Fluoromethyl analogues of ω-amino acids as irreversible inhibitors of 4-aminobutyrate: 2-oxoglutarate aminotransferase. J Neurochem 37:1341–1344

Bonta IL, De Vos CJ, Grijsen H, Hillen FC, Noach EL, Sim AEW (1971) 1-Hydroxy-3-aminopyrrolidone-2 (HA-966): new GABA-like compound, with potential use in extrapyramidal diseases. Br J Pharmacol 43:514–535

Bowery NG, Hill DR, Hudson AL, Doble A, Middlemiss DN, Shaw J, Turnbull M (1980) (−)Baclofen decreases neurotransmitter release in the mammalian CNS by an action at a novel GABA receptor. Nature 283:92–94

Bradford HF, Dodd PR (1975) Convulsions and activation of epileptic foci induced by monosodium glutamate and related compounds. Biochem Pharmacol 26:253–254

Braestrup C, Nielsen M, Krogsgaard-Larsen P, Falch E (1979) Partial agonists for brain GABA/benxodiazepine receptor complex. Nature 280:331–333

Braestrup C, Nielsen M, Olsen CE (1980) Urinary and brain β-carboline-3-carboxylates as potent inhibitors of brain benzodiazepine receptor. Proc Natl Acad Sci 77:2288–2292

Breckenridge RJ, Nicholson SH, Nicol AJ, Suckling CJ (1981) Inhibition of neuronal GABA uptake and glial β-alanine uptake by synthetic GABA analogues. Biochem Pharmacol 30:3045–3049

Brennan MJW (1982) GABA autoreceptors are not coupled to benzodiazepine receptors in rat cerebral cortex. J Neurochem 38:264–266

Brown DA, Marsh S (1978) Axonal GABA-receptors in mammalian peripheral nerve trunks. Brain Res 156:187–191

Callery PS, Geelhaar LA, Balachandran Nayar MS, Stogniew M, Gurudath Rao K (1982) Pyrrolines as prodrugs of γ-aminobutyric acid analogues. J Neurochem 38:1063–1067

Canzek V, Wolfensberger M, Amsler U, Cuenod M (1981) In vivo release of glutamate and aspartate following optic nerve stimulation. Nature 293:572–574

Carlsson C, Chapman AG (1981) The effect of diazepam on the cerebral metabolic state in rats and its interaction with nitrous oxide. Anaesthesiology 54:488–495

Cash CD, Maître M, Ossola L, Mandel P (1978) Purification and properties of two succinate semialdehyde dehydrogenases from human brain. Biochem Biophys Acta 524:26–36

Chapman AG (1984) The effect of anticonvulsant drugs on rat cerebral amino acid metabolism and cortical GABA turnover. In: Fariello RG, Morselli P (eds) Neurotransmitters in epilepsy. Raven, New York

Chapman AG, Nordström CH, Soesjö BK (1978) Influence of phenobarbital anaesthesia on carbohydrate and amino acid metabolism in rat brain. Anesthesiology 48:175–182

Chapman AG, Riley K, Evans MC, Meldrum BS (1982) Acute effects of sodium valproate and γ-vinyl GABA on regional amino acid metabolism in the rat brain. Neurochem Res 7:1089–1105

Collins GGS (1981) The effects of chlordiazepoxide on synaptic transmission and amino acid neurotransmitter release in slices of rat olfactory cortex. Brain Res 224:389–404

Collins GGS, Probett GA (1981) Aspartate and not glutamate is the likely transmitter of the rat lateral olfactory tract. Brain Res 209:231–234

Collins RC, McLean M, Olney J (1980) Cerebral metabolic response to systemic kainic acid: ^{14}C-deoxyglucose studies. Life Sci 27:855–862

Collins GGS, Anson J, Probett GA (1981) Patterns of endogenous amino acid release from slices of rat and guinea-pig olfactory cortex. Brain Res 204:103–120

Costa E, Guidotti A (1979) Molecular mechanisms in the receptor action of benzodiazepines. Ann Rev Pharmacol Toxicol 19:531–545

Coursin DB (1954) Convulsive seizures in infants with pyridoxine deficient diet. JAMA 154:406–408

Coursin DB (1964) Vitamin B_6 metabolism in infants and children. Vitam Horm 22:775–783

Coutinho-Netto J, Abdul-Ghani AS, Collins JF, Bradford HF (1981) Is glutamate a trigger factor in epileptic hyperactivity? Epilepsia 22:289–296

Craig CR, Hartman ER (1973) Concentration of amino acids in the brain of cobalt-epileptic rat. Epilepsia 14:409–414

Crawford JM (1963) The effect upon mice of intra-ventricular injection of excitant and depressant amino acids. Biochem Pharmacol 12:1443–1444

Crome LC, Stern J (1967) The pathology of mental retardation. Churchill, London, p 406

Croucher MJ, Collins JF, Meldrum BS (1982) Anticonvulsant action of antagonists of neuronal excitation due to dicarboxylic amino acids. Science 216, 899–901

Curtis DR (1979) GABAergic transmission in the mammalian central nervous system. In: Krogsgaard-Larsen P, Scheel-Krüger J, Kofod H (eds) GABA neurotransmitters. Munksgaard, Copenhagen, pp 17–27

Curtis DR, Johnston GAR (1974) Amino acid transmitters in the mammalian nervous system. In: Reviews of Physiology, Pharmacology and Biochemistry, vol 69. Springer, Berlin Heidelberg New York, pp 97–188

Curtis DR, Watkins JC (1963) Acidic amino acids with strong excitatory actions on mammalian neurones. J Physiol (Lond) 166:1–14

Curtis DR, Game CJA, Lodge D (1976a) The in vivo inactivation of GABA and other inhibitory amino acids in the cat nervous system. Exp Brain Res 25:413–428

Curtis DR, Game CJA, Lodge D (1976b) Benzodiazepines and central glycine receptors. Br J Pharmacol 56:307–311
Curtis DR, Lodge D, Johnston GAR, Brand SJ (1976c) Central actions of benzodiazepines. Brain Res 118:344–347
Davies J, Watkins JC (1973) Microelectrophoretic studies on the depressant action of HA-966 on chemical and synaptically excited neurones in the cat cerebral cortex and cuneate nucleus. Brain Res 59:311–322
Davies J, Watkins JC (1979) Selective antagonism of amino acid-induced and synaptic excitation in the cat spinal cord. J Physiol (Lond) 297:621–635
Davies J, Evans RH, Francis AA, Jones AW, Watkins JC (1980) Excitatory amino acid receptors in the vertebrate central nervous system. In Littauer UZ, Dudai Y, Silman I (eds) Neurotransmitters and their receptors. Wiley, Chichester, pp 333–347
De Boer Th, Bruinvels J (1977) Assay and properties of 4-amino-butyric-2-oxoglutaric acid transaminase and succinic semialdehyde dehydrogenase in rat brain tissue. J Neurochem 28:471–478
DeLorenzo RJ (1980) Phenytoin: calcium- and calmodulin-dependent protein phosphorylation and neurotransmitter release. In: Glaser GH, Penry JK, Woodbury DM (eds) Antiepileptic drugs: mechanisms of action. Raven, New York, pp 399–414
DeLorenzo RJ, Burdette S, Holderness J (1981) Benzodiazepine inhibition of the calcium-calmodulin protein kinase system in brain membrane. Science 213:546–549
Dodd PR, Bradford HF (1976) Release of amino acids from the maturing cobalt-induced epileptic focus. Brain Res 111:377–388
Dodd PR, Bradford HF, Abdul-Ghani AS, Cox DWG, Coutinho-Netto J (1980) Release of amino acids from chronic epileptic and sub-epileptic foci in vivo. Brain Res 193:505
Doherty JD, Hattox SE, Snead OC, Roth RH (1978) Positive identification of endogenous gamma-hydroxybutyrate in human, guinea pig, and rhesus monkey brain. J Pharmacol Exp Ther 207:130–139
Emson PC, Joseph MH (1975) Neurochemical and morphological changes during the development of cobalt-induced epilepsy in the rat. Brain Res 93:91–110
Engberg I, Flatman JA, Lambert JDC (1979) The actions of excitatory amino acids on motoneurones in the feline spinal cord. J Physiol(Lond) 288:227–261
Enna SJ, Snyder SH (1975) Properties of gamma-aminobutyric acid binding to receptor sites in central nervous system. Brain Res 100:81–97
Enna SJ, Collins JF, Snyder S (1977a) Stereospecificity and structure-activity required of GABA receptor binding in rat brain. Brain Res 124:185–190
Enna SJ, Wood JH, Snyder SH (1977b) γ-Aminobutyric acid (GABA) in human cerebrospinal fluid: radioreceptor assay. J Neurochem 28:1121–1124
Erwin VG, Deitrich RA (1973) Inhibition of bovine brain aldehyde reductase by anticonvulsant compounds in vitro. Biochem Pharmacol 22:2615–2624
Evans RH, Francis AA, Hunt K, Oakes DJ, Watkins JC (1979) Antagonism of excitatory amino acid-induced responses and of synaptic excitation in the isolated spinal cord of the frog. Br J Pharmacol 67:591–603
Evans RH, Francis AA, Jones AW, Smith DAS, Watkins JC (1982) The effects of a series of ω-phosphonic-α-carboxylic amino acids on electrically evoked and excitant amino acid-induced responses in isolated spinal cord preparations. Br J Pharmacol 75:65–75
Flint RS, Rea MA, McBride WJ (1981) In vitro release of endogenous amino acids from granule cell-, stellate cell-, and climbing fiber-deficient cerebella. J Neurochem 37:1425–1430
Folbergrova J (1974) Energy metabolism of mouse cerebral cortex during homocysteine convulsions. Brain Res 81:443–454
Fonnum F (1981) The turnover of transmitter amino acids, with special reference to GABA. In: Pycock CJ, Taberner PV (eds) Central neurotransmitter turnover. Croom Helm, London, pp 105–124
Fonnum F, Storm-Mathisen J, Divac I (1981) Biochemical evidence for glutamate as neurotransmitter in corticostriatal and corticothalamic fibres in rat brain. Neuroscience 6:863–973

Frederickson RCA, Neuss M, Morzorati SL, McBride WJ (1978) A comparison of the inhibitory effects of taurine and GABA on identified Purkinje cells and other neurons in the cerebellar cortex of the rat. Brain Res 145:117–126

Frey H-H, Löscher W (1980) Cetyl GABA: effect on convulsant thresholds in mice and acute toxicity. Neuropharmacology 19:217–220

Frey H-H, Popp C, Löscher W (1979) Influence of inhibitors of the high affinity GABA uptake on seizure thresholds in mice. Neuropharmacology 18:581–590

Gaitonde MK (1970) Sulfur amino acids. In: Lajtha A (ed) Handbook of neurochemistry, vol 3. Plenum, New York, pp 225–287

Galzigna L, Garbin L, Bianchi M, Marxotto A (1978) Properties of two derivatives of γ-aminobutyric acid (GABA) capable of abolishing cardiazol- and bicuculline-induced convulsions in the rat. Arch Int Pharmacodyn Therap 235:73–85

Godin Y, Heiner L, Mark J, Mandel P (1969) Effects of di-*n*-propylacetate, an anticonvulsive compound, on GABA metabolism. J Neurochem 16:869–873

Godschalk M, Dzoljic MR, Bonta IL (1977) Slow wave sleep and a state resembling absence epilepsy induced in the rat by γ-hydroxybutyrate. Eur J Pharmacol 44:105–111

Goldring JM, Blaustein MP (1980) Barbiturates: physiological effects II. In: Glaser GH, Penry JK, Woodbury DM (eds) Antiepileptic drugs: Mechanisms of action. Raven, New York, pp 523–531

Goldstein DB (1966) D-Amino acid oxidase in brain: distribution in several species and inhibition by pentobarbitone. J Neurochem 13:1011–1016

Goodman HO, Connolly BM, McLean W, Resnick M (1980) Taurine transport in epilepsy. Clin Chem 26:414–419

Greenstein JP, Winitz M (1961) Chemistry of the amino acids, vol I. Wiley, New York, London, p 487

Grove J, Schechter PJ, Tell G, Koch-Weser J, Sjoerdsma A, Warter JM, Marescauzx C, Rumbach L (1981) Increased GABA, homocarnosine and β-alanine in cerebrospinal fluid of patients treated with γ-vinyl-GABA (4-amino-hex-5-enoic acid). Life Sci 28:2431–2439

Guidotti A, Badiani G, Pepeu G (1972) Taurine distribution in cat brain. J Neurochem 19:431–435

Guidotti A, Toffano G, Baraldi M, Schwartz JP, Costa E (1979) A molecular mechanism for the facilitation of GABA receptor function by benzodiazepines. In: Krogsgaard-Larsen P, Scheel-Krüger J, Kofod H (eds) GABA-Neurotransmitters. Munksgaard, Copenhagen, pp 406–415

Haefely W, Pieri L, Polc P, Schaffner R (1981) General pharmacology and neuropharmacology of benzodiazepine derivatives. In: Hoffmeister F, Stille G (eds) Handbook of experimental pharmacology, 55/II. Springer, Berlin Heidelberg New York, pp 13–262

Harris H (1980) The principles of human genetics, 3rd edn. Elsevier/North Holland, Amsterdam, p 554

Hayashi T (1954) The effects of sodium glutamate on the nervous system. Keio J Med 3:183

Hayes KC, Casey RE, Schmidt SY (1975) Retinal degeneration associated with taurine deficiency in the cat. Science 188:949–951

Hendrickson AE, Hunt SP, Wu J-Y (1981) Immunocytochemical localization of glutamic acid decarboxylase in monkey striate cortex. Nature 292:605–607

Hicks TP, McLennan H (1979) Amino acids and the synaptic pharmacology of granule cells in the dentate gyrus of the rat. Can J Physiol Pharmacol 57:973–978

Horton RW, Anlezark GM, Sawaya MCB, Meldrum BS (1977) Monoamine and GABA metabolism and the anticonvulsant action of di-*n*-propylacetate and ethanolamine-*O*-sulphate. Eur J Pharmacol 41:387–397

Horton RW, Chapman AG, Meldrum BS (1978) Regional changes in cerebral GABA concentration and convulsions produced by D- and L-allylglycine. J Neurochem 30:1501–1504

Horton RW, Collins JF, Anlezark GM, Meldrum BS (1979) Convulsant and anticonvulsant actions in DBA/2 mice of compounds blocking the reuptake of GABA. Eur J Pharmacol 59:75–83

Ito M (1976) Roles of GABA neurons in integrated functions of the vertebrate CNS. In: Roberts E, Chase TN, Tower DB (eds) GABA in nervous system function. Raven, New York, pp 427–448

Iversen LL, Kelly J (1975) Uptake and metabolism of γ-amino-butyric acid by neurones and glial cells. Biochem Pharmacol 24:933–939

Izumi K, Donaldson J, Minnich JL, Barbeau A (1973) Ouabain induced seizures in rats: suppressive effects of taurine and γ-aminobutyric acid. Can J Physiol Pharmacol 51:885–889

Izumi K, Igisu H, Fukuda T (1974) Suppression of seizures by taurine – specific or non-specific?. Brain Res 76:171–173

Jaeken J, Corbeel L, Casaer P, Carchon H, Eggermont E, Eeckels R (1977) Dipropylacetate (valproate) and glycine metabolism. Lancet II:617

Jasper HH, Koyama I (1969) Rate of release of amino acids from the cerebral cortex in the cat as affected by brainstem and thalamic stimulation. Can J Physiol Pharmacol 47:889–905

Javors M, Erwin VG (1980) Effects of benzodiazepines and valproic acid on brain aldehyde reductase and a proposed mechanism of anticonvulsant action. Biochem Pharmacol 29:1703–1708

Johnston GAR (1968) The intraspinal distribution of some depressant amino acids. J Neurochem 15:1013–1017

Johnston GAR (1973) Convulsions induced in 10-day-old rats by intraperitoneal injection of monosodium glutamate and related excitant amino acids. Biochem Pharmacol 22:137

Johnston GAR, Stephanson AL, Twitchin B (1976) Inhibition of the uptake of GABA and related amino acids in rat brain slices by the optical isomers of nipecotic acid. J Neurochem 26:1029–1032

Johnston GAR, Willow M (1981) Barbiturates and GABA receptors. In: Costa E, Di Chiara G, Gessa GL (eds) GABA and benzodiazepine receptors. Raven, New York, pp 191–198

Joseph MH, Emson PC (1976) Taurine and cobalt induced epilepsy in the rat: a biochemical and electrographic study. J Neurochem 27:1495–1501

Karobath M, Lippitsch M (1979) THIP and isoguvacine are partial agonists of GABA-stimulated benzodiazepine receptor binding. Eur J Pharmacol 58:485–488

Karobath M, Sperk G (1979) Stimulation of benzodiazepine receptor binding by γ-aminobutyric acid. Proc Natl Acad Sci 76:1004–1006

Karobath M, Placheta P, Lippitsch M, Krogsgaard-Larsen P (1979) Is stimulation of benzodiazepine receptor binding mediated by a novel GABA receptor? Nature 278:748–749

Kaufman EE, Nelson T, Goochee C, Sokoloff L (1979) Purification and characterization of an $NADP^+$-linked alcohol oxido-reductase which catalyses the interconversion of γ-hydroxybutyrate and succinic semialdehyde. J Neurochem 32:699–712

Keller E, Davis JL, Tachiki KH, Cummins JT, Baxter CF (1981) LProline inhibition of glutamate release. J Neurochem 37:1335–1337

Kendall DA, Fox DA, Enna SJ (1981) Effect of γ-vinyl GABA on bicuculline-induced seizures. Neuropharmacology 20:351–355

Koyama I (1972) Amino acids in the cobalt-induced epileptogenic and non-epileptogenic cat's cortex. Can J Physiol Pharmacol 50:740–752

Koyama I, Jasper H (1977) Amino acid content of chronic undercut cortex of the cat in relation to electrical after discharge: comparison with cobalt epileptogenic lesions. Can J Physiol Pharmacol 55:523–535

Krall RL, Penry JK, White BG, Kupferberg HJ, Swinyard EA (1978) Antiepileptic drug development: II. Anticonvulsant drug screening. Epilepsia 19:409–428

Krogsgaard-Larsen P (1980) Inhibitors of the GABA uptake systems. Mol Cell Biochem 31:105–121

Krogsgaard-Larsen P, Labouta IM, Meldrum B, Croucher M, Schousboe A (1981) GABA uptake inhibitors as experimental tools and potential drugs in epilepsy research. In: Morselli PL, Lloyd KG, Löscher W, Meldrum B, Reynolds EH (eds) Neurotransmitters, seizures and epilepsy. Raven, New York, pp 23–35
Kukino K, Deguchi T (1977) Effects of sodium dipropylacetate on γ-aminobutyric acid and biogenic amines in rat brain. Chem Pharm Bull 25:2257–2262
Laird HE, Huxtable RJ (1978) Taurine and audiogenic epilepsy. In Barbeau A, Huxtable RJ (eds) Taurine and neurological disorders. Raven, New York, pp 339–357
Lambert JCD, Flatman JA, Engberg I (1981) Actions of excitatory amino acids on membrane conductance and potential in motoneurones. In: Di Chiara G, Gessa GL (eds) Glutamate as a neurotransmitter. Raven, New York, pp 205–216
Lambert JDC, Flatman JA (1981) The interaction between barbiturate anaesthetics and excitatory amino acid responses on cat spinal neurones. Neuropharmacology 20:227–240
Levi G, Gallo V, Raiteri M (1981) GABA potentiates the depolarization-induced release of glutamate from cerebellar nerve endings. In: Di Chiara G, Gessa GL (eds) Glutamate as a neurotransmitter. Raven, New York, p 127
Levi G, Bernardi G, Cherubini E, Gallo V, Grazia Marciani M, Stanzione P (1982) Evidence in favor of a neurotransmitter role of glycine in the rat cerebral cortex. Brain Res 236:121–131
Lloyd KG, Worms P, Deportere H, Bartholini G (1979) Pharmacological profile of SL 76002, a new GABA-mimetic drug. In: Krogsgaard-Larsen P, Scheel-Krüger J, Kofod H (eds) GABA-neurotransmitters. Munksgaard, Copenhagen, pp 308–325
Lloyd KG, Munari C, Bossi L, Bancaud J, Talairach J, Morselli PL (1981) Biochemical evidence for the alterations of GABA-mediated synaptic transmission in human epileptic foci. In: Morselli PL, Lloyd KG, Löscher W, Meldrum B, Reynolds EH (eds) Neurotransmitters, seizures and epilepsy. Raven, New York, pp 325–338
Lodge D, Curtis DR (1978) Time course of GABA and glycine actions on cat spinal neurones: effect of pentobarbitone. Neurosci Lett 8:125–129
Löscher W, Rating D, Siemes H (1981) GABA in cerebrospinal fluid of children with febrile convulsions. Epilepsia 22:697–702
MacDonald RL (1983) Mechanisms of anticonvulsant drug action. In: Pedley TA, Meldrum BS (eds) Recent advances in epilepsy I. Churchill Livingstone, Edinburgh, pp 1–23
MacDonald RL, Barker JL (1979) Enhancement of GABA-mediated postsynaptic inhibition in cultured mammalian spinal cord neurons: a common mode of anticonvulsant action. Brain Res 167:323–336
MacDonald RL, Bergey GK (1979) Valproic acid augments GABA-mediated postsynaptic inhibition in cultured mammalian neurons. Brain Res 170:558–562
Maître M, Ossola L, Mandel P (1976) In vitro studies into the effect of rat brain succinic semialdehyde dehydrogenase on GABA synthesis and degradation. FEBS Lett 72:53–57
Malthe-Sørenssen D, Skrede KK, Fonnum F (1979) Calcium-dependent release of D-^{3}H-aspartate evoked by selective electrical stimulation of excitatory afferent fibres to hippocampal pyramidal cells in vitro. Neuroscience 4:1255–1263
Malthe-Sørenssen D, Skrede KK, Fonnum F (1980) Release of D-^{3}H aspartate from the dorsolateral septum after electrical stimulation of the fimbria in vitro. Neuroscience 5:127–133
Mandel P, Pasantes-Morales H (1978) Taurine in the nervous system. In: Ehrenpreis S, Kopin I (eds) Reviews of neuroscience, vol 3. Raven, New York, pp 157–193
Markand ON, Garg BP, Brandt IK (1982) Nonketotic hyperglycinemia electroencephalographic and evoked potential abnormalities. Neurology 32:151–156
Martin MR (1980) The effects of ionotophoretically applied antagonists on auditory nerve and amino acid evoked excitation of anteroventral cochlear neurons. Neuropharmacology 19:519–528
Martin MR, Adams JC (1979) Effects of DL-α-aminodipate on synaptically and chemically evoked excitation of anteroventral cochlear nucleus neurons of the cat. Neuroscience 4:1097–1105

Martin del Rio R, Orensanz Munox LM, De Feudis FV (1977) Contents of β-alanine and γ-aminobutyric acid in regions of rat CNS. Exp Brain Res 28:225–227

Matthews WD, McCafferty GP, Setler PE (1981) An electrophysiological model of GABA-mediated neurotransmission. Neuropharmacology 20:561–565

McBride WJ, Nadi NS, Altman J, Aprison MH (1976) Effects of selective doses of X-irradiation on the levels of several amino acids in the cerebellum of the rat. Neurochem Res 1:141–152

Mc Ginnis MY, Gordon JH, Gorski RA (1980) Time course and localization of the effects of estrogen on glutamic acid decarboxylase activity. J Neurochem 34:786–792

Meldrum BS (1975) Epilepsy and GABA-mediated inhibition. Int Rev Neurobiol 17:1–36

Meldrum B (1979) Convulsant drugs, anticonvulsants and GABA-mediated neuronal inhibition. In: Krogsgaard-Larsen P, Scheel-Krüger J, Kofod H (eds) GABA-neurotransmitters. Munksgaard, Copenhagen, pp 395–405

Meldrum B (1981) GABA-agonists as anti-epileptic agents. In: Costa E, Di Chiara G, Gessa GL (eds) GABA and benzodiazepine receptors. Raven, New York, pp 207–217

Meldrum B, Braestrup C (1983) GABA and the anticonvulsant action of benzodiazepines and related drugs. In: Bowery N (ed) Actions and interactions of GABA and benzodiazepines. Raven, New York

Meldrum BS, Chapman AG (1983) Excitatory amino acids and anticonvulsant drug action. In: Hertz L, Kvamme E, McGeer EG, Schousboe A (eds) Glutamine, glutamate, and GABA in the central nervous system. AR Liss, New York, pp 625–642

Meldrum B, Horton R (1978) Blockade of epileptic responses in the photosensitive baboon, *Papio papio,* by two irreversible inhibitors of GABA-transaminase, γ-acetylenic GABA (4-amino-hex-5-ynoic acid) and γ-vinyl GABA (4-amino-hex-5-enoic acid). Psychopharmacology 59:47–50

Meldrum B, Horton R (1980) Effects of the bicyclic GABA agonist, THIP, on myoclonic and seizure responses in mice and baboons with reflex epilepsy. Eur J Pharmacol 61:231–237

Meldrum BS, Balzano E, Gadea M, Naquet R (1970) Photic and drug-induced epilepsy in the baboon (*Papio papio*): the effects of isoniazid, thiosemicarbazide, pyridoxine and amino-oxyacetic acid. Electroencephalogr Clin Neurophysiol 29:33–347

Meldrum BS, Horton RW, Sawaya MCCB (1975) The convulsant action of methyldithiocarbazinate: a comparison with other sulphur containing hydrazides. J Neurochem 24:1003–1010

Meldrum BS, Croucher MJ, Krogsgaard-Larsen P (1982) GABA-uptake inhibitors as anticonvulsant agents. In: Okada Y, Roberts E (eds) Problems in GABA research: from to bacteria. Excerpta Medica, Amsterdam, pp 182–191

Meldrum BS, Croucher MJ, Czuczwar SJ, Collins JF, Curry K, Joseph M, Stone TW (1983) A comparison of the anticonvulsant potency of (±) 2-amino-5-phosphonopentanoic acid and (±) 2-amino-7-phosphonoheptanoic acid. Neuroscience 9:925–930

Meldrum BS, Croucher MJ, Badman G, Collins JF (1983) Antiepileptic action of excitatory amino acid antagonists in the photosensitive baboon, *Papio papio*. Neurosci Lett 39:101–104

Merck Index (1976) Merck and Co., Rathway, New Jersey

Metcalf BW (1979) Inhibitors of GABA metabolism. Biochem Pharmacol 28:1705–1712

Metrakos K, Metrakos JD (1974) Genetics of Epilepsy. In: Magnus O, Lorentz de Haas (eds) Handbook of clinical neurology, vol 15. The epilepsies. Amsterdam North/Holland, pp 429–439

Mitchell PR, Martin IL (1978) Is GABA release modulated by presynaptic receptors? Nature 274:904–905

Mitchell R (1980) A novel GABA receptor modulates stimulus-induced glutamate release from cortico-striatal terminals. Eur J Pharmacol 67:119–122

Mortensen PB, Kølvraa S, Christensen E (1980) Inhibition of the glycine cleavage system: hyperglycinaemia and hyperglycinuria caused by valproic acid. Epilepsia 21:563–569

Mutani R, Bergamini L, Delsedime M, Durelli L (1974a) Effects of taurine in chronic experimental epilepsy. Brain Res 79:330–332

Mutani R, Bergamini L, Fariello R, Delsedime M (1974b) Effects of taurine on cortical acute epileptic foci. Brain Res 70:170–173
Nadler JV, Smith EM (1981) Perforant path lesion depletes glutamate content of fascia dentata synaptosomes. Neurosci Lett 25:275–280
Nadler JV, White WF, Vaca KW, Perry BW, Cotman CW (1978) Biochemical correlates of transmission mediated by glutamate and aspartate. J Neurochem 31:147–155
Neal MJ, Bowery NG (1977) *cis*-3-Aminocyclohexanecarboxylic acid: a substrate for the neuronal GABA transport system. Brain Res 138:169–174
Nestoros JN, Nistri A (1978) A presynaptic component of the action of iontophoretically applied flurazepam on feline cortical neurones. Can J Physiol Pharmacol 56:889–892
Newmark ME, Penry JK (1979) Genetics of epilepsy: a review. Raven, New York, p 130
Nicoll RA (1972) The effect of anaesthetics on synaptic excitation and inhibition in the olfactory bulb. J Physiol (Lond) 223:803–814
Oertel WH, Schmechel DE, Tappaz ML, Kopin IJ (1981a) Production of a specific antiserum to rat brain glutamic acid decarboxylase by injection of an antigen-antibody complex. Neuroscience 6:2689–2700
Oertel WH, Schmechel DE, Mugnaini E, Tappaz ML, Kopin IJ (1981b) Immunocytochemical localization of glutamate decarboxylase in rat cerebellum with a new antiserum. Neuroscience 6:2715–2735
Okamoto K, Sakai Y (1980) Localization of sensitive sites to taurine, γ-aminobutyric acid, glycine and β-alanine in the molecular layer of guinea-pig cerebellar slices. Br J Pharmacol 69:407–413
Olney JW (1979) Excitotoxic amino acids: research applications and safety implications. In: Filer LJ, Garattini S, Kare MR, Reynolds WA, Wurtman RJ (eds) Glutamic acid. Raven, New York, pp 287–319
Olney JW, Rhee V, Ho OL (1974) Kainic acid: a powerful neurotoxic analogue of glutamate. Brain Res 77:507–512
Olsen RW (1981) GABA-benzodiazepine-barbiturate receptor interactions. J Neurochem 37:1–17
Olsen RW (1982) Drug interactions at the GABA receptor ionophore complex. Ann Rev Pharmacol Toxicol 22:245–277
Olsen RW, Ticku MK, Greenlee D, Van Ness P (1979) GABA receptor and ionophore binding sites: interaction with various drugs. In: Krogsgaard-Larsen P, Scheel-Krüger J, Kofod H (eds) GABA-neurotransmitters. Munksgaard, Copenhagen, pp 165–178
Olsen RW, Leeb-Lundberg F (1981) Convulsant and anticonvulsant drug binding sites related to the GABA receptor/ionophore system. In: Morselli PL, Lloyd KG, Löscher W, Meldrum B, Reynolds EH (eds) Neurotransmitters, seizures and epilepsy. Raven, New York, pp 151–163
Palfreyman MG, Schechter PJ, Buckett WR, Tell GP, Koch-Weser J (1981) The pharmacology of GABA-transaminase inhibitors. Biochem Pharmacol 30:817–824
Pedley TA, Horton RW, Meldrum BS (1979) Electroencephalographic and behavioural effects of a GABA agonist (muscimol) on photosensitive epilepsy in the baboon, *Papio papio*. Epilepsia 20:409–416
Perrin DD (1965) Dissociation constants of organic bases in aqueous solutions. Butterworths, London
Perrin DD (1972) Dissociation constants of organic bases in aqueous solutions: Supplement 1972. Butterworths, London
Perry TL, Hansen S (1981) Amino acid abnormalities in epileptogenic foci. Neurology 31:872–876
Perry TL, Berry K, Hansen S, Diamond S, Mok C (1971) Regional distribution of amino acids in human brain at autopsy. J Neurochem 18:513–519
Perry TL, Hansen S, Kennedy J (1975a) CSF amino acids and plasma-CSF amino acid ratios in adults. J Neurochem 24:587–589
Perry TL, Hansen S, Kennedy J, Wada JA, Thompson GB (1975b) Amino acids in human epileptogenic foci. Arch Neurol 32:752–754

Perry TL, Urquhart N, MacLean J, Evans ME, Hansen S, Davidson GF, Applegarth DA, MacLeod PJ, Lock JE (1975c) Non-ketotic hyperglycinaemia. Glycine accumulation due to absence of glycine cleavage in brain. New Engl J Med 292:1269–1273
Perry TL, Hansen S, Gandham SS (1981) Postmortem changes of amino compounds in human and rat brain. J Neurochem 36:406–412
Perry TL, Hansen S, Wall RA, Gauthier SG (1982) Human CSF GABA concentrations: revised downward for controls, but not decreased in Huntington's chorea. J Neurochem 38:766–773
Price MT, Olney JW, Lowry OH, Buchsbaum S (1981) Uptake of exogenous glutamate and aspartate by circumventricular organs but not other regions of brain. J Neurochem 36:1774–1780
Rassin DK, Sturman JA, Gaull GE (1981) Sulfur amino acid metabolism in the developing rhesus monkey brain: subcellular studies of taurine, cysteinesulfinic acid decarboxylase, γ-aminobutyric acid and glutamic acid decarboxylase. J Neurochem 37:740–748
Reingold DF, Orlowski M (1978) Inhibition of human and mouse brain glutamate decarboxylase by the α-keto-analogs of cysteine and homocysteine. Biochem Pharmacol 27:2567–2570
Ribak CE (1978) Aspinous and sparsely-spinous stellate neurons in the visual cortex of rats contain glutamic acid decarboxylase. J Neurocytol 7:461–478
Ribak CE, Vaughn JE, Saito K, Barber R, Roberts E (1976) Immunocytochemical localization of glutamate decarboxylase in rat substantia nigra. Brain Res 116:287–298
Ribak CE, Vaughn JE, Saito K (1978) Immunocytochemical localization of glutamic acid decarboxylase in neuronal somata following colchicine inhibition of axonal transport. Brain Res 140:315–332
Ribak CE, Harris AB, Vaughn JE, Roberts E (1979) Inhibitory, GABAergic nerve terminals decrease at sites of focal epilepsy. Science 205:211–214
Ribak CE, Harris AB, Vaughn JE, Roberts E (1981) Immunocytochemical changes in cortical, GABA neurons in a monkey model of epilepsy. In: Morselli PL, Lloyd K, Löscher W, Meldrum B, Reynolds E (eds) Neurotransmitters, seizures and epilepsy. Raven, New York, pp 11–22
Ris MM, Deitrich RA, von Wartburg N-P (1975) Inhibition of aldehyde reductase isoenzymes in human and rat brain. Biochem Pharmacol 24:1865–1869
Rumigny JF, Maître M, Cash C, Mandel P (1980) Specific and non-specific succinic semialdehyde reductase from rat brain: isolation and properties. FEBS Lett 117:111–116
Saito K, Barber R, Wu J-Y, Matsuda T, Roberts E, Vaughn JE (1974) Immunohistochemical localization of glutamate decarboxylase in rat cerebellum. Proc Natl Acad Sci 71:269–273
Sandberg M, Jacobson I (1981) β-Alanine, a possible neurotransmitter in the visual system. J Neurochem 37:1353–1356
Schechter PJ, Tranier Y, Jung MJ, Böhlen P (1977) Audiogenic seizures protection by elevated GABA concentration in mice effects γ-acetylenic GABA and γ-vinyl GABA, two irreversible GABA-T inhibitors. Eur J Pharmacol 45:319–328
Schechter PJ, Tranier Y, Grove J (1978) Effect of dipropylacetate on amino acid concentrations in mouse brain: correlation with anticonvulsant activity. J Neurochem 31:1325–1327
Schlesinger K, Uphouse LL (1971) Pyridoxine dependency and central nervous system excitability. Adv Biochem Psychopharmacol 4:105–140
Schmidt D, Löscher W (1981) GABA concentrations in cerebrospinal fluid and plasma of patients with epileptic seizures. In: Morselli PL, Lloyd KG, Löscher W, Meldrum B, Reynolds EH (eds) Neurotransmitters, seizures and epilepsy. Raven, New York, pp 315–324
Schousboe A, Thorbek P, Hertz L, Krogsgaard-Larsen P (1979) Effects of GABA analogues of restricted conformation on GABA transport in astrocytes and brain cortex slices and on GABA receptor binding. J Neurochem 33:181–189
Segal M (1981) The actions of glutamic acid on neurons in the rat hippocampal slice. In: Di Chiara G, Gessa GL (eds) Glutamate as a neurotransmitter. Raven, New York, pp 217–225

Seiler N, Sarhan S (1980) Drugs affecting GABA. In: Neurochemistry and clinical neurology. Liss, New York, pp 425–439

Sellinger OZ, Weiler P (1963) The nature of the inhibition in vitro of cerebral glutamine synthetase by the convulsant, methionine sulfoximine. Biochem Pharmacol 12:989–1000

Shinozaki H, Konishi S (1970) Actions of several anthelmintics and insecticides on rat cortical neurones. Brain Res 24:368–371

Shoulson I, Goldblatt D, Charlton M, Joynt RJ (1978) Huntington's disease: treatment with muscimol, a GABA-mimetic drug. Ann Neurol 4:279–284

Skolnick P, Paul S, Crawley J, Rice K, Barker S, Weber R, Cain M, Cook J (1981) 3-Hydroxymethyl-β-carboline antagonizes some pharmacologic actions of diazepam. Eur J Pharmacol 69:525–527

Sloper JJ, Johnson P, Powell TPS (1980) Selective degeneration of interneurons in the motor cortex of infant monkeys follwing controlled hypoxia: a possible cause of epilepsy. Brain Res 198:204–209

Snead OC (1977) Gamma hydroxybutyrate. Life Sci 20:1935–1944

Snead OC (1978) Gamma-hydroxybutyrate in the monkey. I. Electroencephalographic behavioural and pharmacokinetic studies. Neurology 28:636–642

Snead OC, Bearden LJ, Pegram V (1980) Effect of acute and chronic anticonvulsant administration on endogenous γ-hydroxybutyrate in rat brain. Neuropharmacology 19:5–15

Snyder S, Goodman RR (1980) Multiple neurotransmitter receptors. J Neurochem 35:5–15

Somogyi P, Smith AD, Nunzi MG, Gorio A, Takagi H, Wu JY (1983) Glutamate decarboxylase immunoreactivity in the hippocampus of the cat: distribution of immunoreactive synaptic terminals with special reference to the axon initial segment of pyramidal neurons. J Neuroscience 3:1450–1468

Spencer HJ (1976) Antagonsim of cortical excitation of striatal neurons by glutamic acid as an excitatory transmitter in the rat striatum. Brain Res 102:91–102

Stone TW (1973) Cortical pyramidal tract interneurones and their sensitivity to L-glutamic acid. J Physiol (Lond) 233:211–225

Stone TW (1979) Amino acids as neurotransmitters of corticofugal neurons in the rat: a comparison of glutamate and aspartate. Br J Pharmacol 67:545–551

Stone TW, Perkins MN (1981) Quinolinic acid: a potent endogenous excitant at amino acid receptors. Eur J Pharmacol 72:411–412

Storm-Mathisen J (1981) Glutamate in hippocampal pathways. In: Di Chiara G, Gessa GL (eds) Glutamate as a neurotransmitter. Raven, New York, pp 43–55

Storm-Mathisen J, Leknes AK, Bore AT, Vaaland JL, Edminson P, Haug FS, Ottersen OP (1983) First visualisation of glutamate and GABA in neurons by immunocytochemistry. Nature 301:517–520

Study RE, Barker JL (1981) Diazepam and (–)pentobarbital: fluctuation analysis reveals different mechanisms for potentiation of GABA responses in cultured central neurons. Proc Natl Acad Sci 78:7180–7184

Tabakoff B, Erwin VG (1970) Purification and characterization of a reduced nicotinamide adenine dinucleotide phosphate-linked aldehyde reductase from brain. J Biol Chem 245:3263–3268

Takahashi R, Nakane Y (1978) Clinical trial of taurine in epilepsy. In: Barbeau A, Huxtable RJ (eds) Taurine and neurological disorders. Raven, New York, pp 375–385

Tamminga CA, Crayton JW, Chase TN (1978) Muscimol: GABA agonist therapy in schizophrenia. Am J Psychiatry 135:746–747

Tenen SS, Hirsch JD (1980) β-Carboline-3-carboxylic acid ethyl ester antagonizes diazepam activity. Nature 288:609–610

Usherwood PNR (1978) Amino acids as neurotransmitters. Adv Comp Physiol Biochem 7:227–309

Van Der Laan JW, De Boer Th, Bruinvels J (1979) Di-*n*-propylacetate and GABA degradation. Preferential inhibition of succinic semialdehyde dehydrogenase and indirect inhibition of GABA-transaminase. J Neurochem 32:1769–1780

Van Gelder NM (1972) Antagonism by taurine of cobalt-induced epilepsy in cat and mouse. Brain Res 47:157–165
Van Gelder NM, Courtois A (1972) Close correlation between changing content of specific amino acids in epileptogenic cortex of cats, and severity of epilepsy. Brain Res 43:477–484
Van Gelder NM, Sherwin AL, Rasmussen T (1972) Amino acid content of epileptogenic human brain: focal versus surrounding regions. Brain Res 40:385–393
Van Gelder NM, Koyama I, Jasper H (1977) Taurine treatment of spontaneous chronic epilepsy in a cat. Epilepsia 18:45–54
Van Gelder NM, Janjua NA, Metrakos K, MacGibbon B, Metrakos JD (1980) Plasma amino acids in 3/sec spike/wave epilepsy. Neurochem Res 5:659–670
Vizi ES (1979) Presynaptic modulation of neurochemical transmission. Prog Neurobiol 12:181–290
Wada JA, Osawa T, Wake A, Corcoran ME (1975) Effects of taurine on kindled amygdaloid seizures in rats, cats, and photosensitive baboons. Epilepsia 16:229–234
Waller MB, Richter JA (1980) Effects of pentobarbital and Ca^{+} on the resting and K^{+}-stimulated release of several endogenous neurotransmitters from rat midbrain slices. Biochem Pharmacol 29:2189–2198
Wallis CJ, Luttge WG (1980) Influence of estrogen and progesterone on glutamic acid decarboxylase activity in discrete regions of rat brain. J Neurochem 34:609–613
Watkins JC, Evans RH (1981) Excitatory amino acid transmitters. Ann Rev Pharmacol Toxicol 21:165–204
Weitz R, Merlob P, Amir J, Reisner SH (1981) A possible role for spartic acid in neonatal seizures. Arch Neurol 38:258–259
Wellner D, Meister A (1981) A survey of inborn errors of amino acid metabolism and transport in man. Ann Rev Biochem 50:911–968
Wenthold RJ (1980) Glutaminase and aspartate aminotransferase decrease in the cochlear nucleus after lesion of the auditory nerve. Brain Res 190:293–297
Wheal HV, Miller JJ (1980) Pharmacological identification of acetylcholine and glutamate excitatory systems in the dentate gyrus of the rat. Brain Res 182:145–155
Wheler GHT, Bradford HF, Davison AN, Thompson EJ (1979) Uptake and release of taurine from cerebral cortex slices and their subcellular compartments. J Neurochem 33:331–337
Whittle SR, Turner AJ (1981) Anticonvulsants and brain aldehyde metabolism. Biochem Pharmacol 30:1191–1196
Willow M, Johnston GAR (1981) Dual action of pentobarbitone on GABA binding: role of binding site integrity. J Neurochem 37:1291–1294
Winters WD, Spooner CE (1965) Various seizure activities following gamma-hydroxybutyrate. Int J Neuropharmacol 4:197–200
Yamamoto C, Yamashita H, Chujo T (1976) Inhibitory action of glutamic acid on cerebellar interneurones. Nature 262:786–787
Yarowsky PJ, Carpenter DO (1978) Receptors for gamma-aminobutyric acid (GABA) on aplysia neurons. Brain Res 144:75–94
Young AB, Zukin SR, Snyder SH (1974) Interaction of benzodiazepines with central nervous glycine receptors: possible mechanism of action. Proc Natl Acad Sci 71:2246–2250
Zaczek R, Hedreen JC, Coyle JT (1979) Evidence of a hippocampal-septal glutamatergic pathway in the rat. Exp Neurol 65:145–156

CHAPTER 8

Prostaglandins

K. Wiśniewski and H.-H. Frey

A. Introduction

Prostaglandin (PG) $F_{2\alpha}$ in ox brain was the first PG to be discovered (Samuelsson 1964). The occurrence of PGs in the brain of man and different animal species was confirmed in the following years by several groups (Bergström and Samuelsson 1965; Horton and Main 1967; Wolfe et al. 1967; Kataoka et al. 1967; Holmes and Norton 1968a, b; Wolfe et al. 1976c): PGE_1, PGE_2, $PGF_{1\alpha}$, $PGF_{2\alpha}$, and thromboxane B_2 were all identified.

Generally, the PG level in brain tissue is very low (Wolfe et al. 1976a) since PGs do not accumulate in the tissues, but are synthetized de novo upon stimulation (Hinman 1972). The PGs are distributed uniformly throughout the brain, but higher concentrations were found in the cerebrocortical gray matter (Wolfe et al. 1967; Kataoka et al. 1967; Holmes and Horton 1968a), suggesting that they are mainly associated with neurons and their function. More recent results have shown that the PG content is greater in the corpus striatum and middle brain than in the other parts of the brain (Hedqvist 1973; Kröner and Peskar 1976).

Biosynthesis of PGs in brain tissue takes place rapidly (van Dorp 1966; Kataoka et al. 1967; Wolfe et al. 1967; Pace-Asciak and Rangaraj 1976a, b). The enzyme system responsible for biosynthesis is located in the microsomal fraction. Biosynthesis can be stimulated by a variety of physiological and nonphysiological factors, e.g., destruction of cell membranes, ischemia, or incubation in vitro, as well as catecholamines (Wolfe et al. 1976a, b). Biosynthesis is also increased by electroconvulsive shock (Zatz and Roth 1975) and by convulsant and even subconvulsant doses of pentetrazole (Folco et al. 1977). Wolfe et al. (1976 b) found increased concentrations of $PGF_{2\alpha}$ in the cerebrospinal fluid of patients suffering from epilepsy, meningoencephalitis, and stroke.

A release of PGs has been shown in superfusates of cerebral cortex (Ramwell and Shaw 1966; Ramwell et al. 1966; Bradley et al. 1969; Galli et al. 1980), cerebellum (Coceani and Wolfe 1965) and spinal cord (Ramwell et al. 1966; Coceani et al. 1971). This release occurs spontaneously (Horton 1969) or, at a higher rate, following electrical stimulation or administration of drugs (Bradley et al. 1969), neurotransmitters (Wolfe et al. 1976b), and putative neurotransmitters (Ramwell and Shaw 1966; Holmes 1970).

The actions of PGs within the (CNS) have been reviewed by Horton (1972) and by Potts et al. (1974). In the following, only data regarding an effect of PGs on experimentally induced seizures, susceptibility to seizures, as well as relations between PGs and the metabolism of neurotransmitters within the CNS will be discussed.

B. Effects of Prostaglandins on Experimentally Induced Convulsions

Anticonvulsant and proconvulsant effects of PGs were first studied by HOLMES and HORTON (1968b). In mice, a dose of 0.5 mg/kg PGE_1 s.c. provided partial protection and a dose of 1 mg/kg total protection against seizures and death elicited by i.p. injection of 100 mg/kg pentetrazole 10 min later. In a later study, 10 mg/kg PGE_1 was found necessary for protection against pentetrazole seizures (HORTON 1972). In the original study of HOLMES and HORTON (1968b), and s.c. dose of 1 mg/kg PGE_1 showed slight protection against the convulsant and lethal effects of 1 mg/kg strychnine, but was without effect against seizures induced by 2 mg/kg strychnine or 10 mg/kg picrotoxin. $PGF_{2\alpha}$, on the other hand, had no anticonvulsant effect against pentetrazole, but, at doses of 1 and 2 mg/kg s.c., even enhanced the convulsant effect of a threshold dose of the convulsant (40 mg/kg). It resembled amphetamine in this respect. In the maximal electroshock test, 0.2 mg/kg PGE_1, injected 10 min before electroshock, protected completely against death, which occurred in 70% of the controls, but the incidence of tonic hindlimb extension was reduced to only 50% by a dose of 1 mg/kg.

In the experiments of DURU and TÜRKER (1969), i.p. doses of 20 and 30 μg/kg PGE_1 delayed the seizures induced by 2 mg/kg strychnine sulfate significantly, but increased their duration. Only the higher dose protected against the lethal effect of strychnine. The observed effect is most probably the consequence of an interference with the absorption of strychnine and thus no central nervous effect.

PODDUBIUK (1976) studied, in rats, the effect of PGA_1, PGE_1, PGE_2, $PGF_{1\alpha}$, and $PGF_{2\alpha}$ injected intraventricularly in doses of 0.02–4 μg against maximal electroconvulsions. The hindlimb extension was not suppressed, but its duration was reduced dose dependently. Threshold doses for a significant reduction were 0.2 μg for both PGEs and 2 μg for $PGF_{1\alpha}$, 4 μg for $PGF_{2\alpha}$, and PGA_1 was ineffective. The most active PG was PGE_1, which induced a 40% reduction in the duration of the tonic extension at a dose of 4 μg. In a parallel study, PODDUBIUK and KLEINROK (1976) described the effect of the PGs used on concentration and turnover of neurotransmitters in brain. The only parameters paralleling the "anticonvulsant" effect were an increase in noradrenaline turnover and an increase in the levels of free acetylcholine in brain after doses of 4 μg of the PGEs.

The group of ROSENKRANZ compared the anticonvulsant effect of PGE_1, PGE_2, and prostacyclin (PGI_2) in mice after intracerebroventricular injection (ROSENKRANZ 1978; ROSENKRANZ and KILLAM 1978, 1979, 1981). The results are summarized in Table 1. With the exception of strychnine convulsions, PGE_1 always proved to be more potent than PGE_2, which might be the consequence of the greater lipophility of PGE_1. The dose-effect curves for both PGEs were parallel, suggesting the same mechanism of action. All three PGs shortened the duration of the tonic hindlimb extension in the electroshock model. After i.p. administration in doses up to 2 (PGI_2) or 4 mg/kg (PGE_2), the tonic extension could

Table 1. ED_{50} of PGE_1 and PGE_2 after intracerebroventricular injection against experimentally induced convulsions in mice. The ED_{50} is given in micrograms per mouse with the 95% confidence limits (from ROSENKRANZ 1978; ROSENKRANZ and KILLAM 1978, 1979). PGE_1 and E_2 were given 5 min and PGI_2 2 min before induction of seizures

Seizure model	ED_{50}		
	PGE_1	PGE_2	PGI_2
Electroshock (11 mA) (maximal)	6.6 (4.3–12)	13.3 (8.9–22.4)	6.3 (2.5–11.1)
Electroshock (50 mA) (supramaximal)	$\gg 20$ [b]	$\gg 20$ [b]	$\gg 140$ [b]
Pentetrazole (100 mg/kg s.c.)	5.8 (2.9–13)	14 (6.9–29)	Not tested
Picrotoxin (12 mg/kg i.p.)	3.8 (2.1–6.4)	6.3 (3.6–10)	Not tested
Strychnine (2 mg/kg i.p.)	58 (41–80)	46 (31–67)	Not tested
Isoniazid [a] (200 mg/kg i.p.)	4.8 (2.9–7.4)	9.7 (5.5–17)	Not tested

[a] PGs were injected 35 min after isoniazid
[b] No effect with the dose indicated

not be suppressed, but its duration as well as the death rate were reduced. 6-Keto-$PGF_{1\alpha}$, a metabolite of PGI_2, was devoid of an anticonvulsant effect, but also reduced the duration of the extension and the death rate. $PGF_{2\alpha}$ proved to have a proconvulsant effect: When injected 5 min before a 7-mA electroshock which did not induce a tonic hindlimb extension in control mice, $PGF_{2\alpha}$ induced tonic seizures with an ED_{50} of 48 μg/mouse. PGE_2 increased the cerebral gamma-aminobutyric acid (GABA) levels in mice considerably and abolished the decrease of this transmitter induced by isoniazid (ROSENKRANZ and KILLAM 1981). The experiments of ROSENKRANZ have recently been repeated by CLIMAX and SEWELL (1981), who found similar ED_{50} values for PGE_1 against maximal electroconvulsions (11 mA) and penetrazole convulsions (11 and 4.8 μg/mouse, respectively). They confirmed the proconvulsant effect of $PGF_{2\alpha}$ in the threshold electroshock (7 mA) and report an ED_{50} of 14.5 μg/mouse for potentiation of pentetrazole seizures. Arachidonic acid increased the incidence of electrically induced seizures (ED_{50} 46 μg/mouse), but provided partial protection against pentetrazole seizures (ED_{50} 23 μg/mouse). On i.c.v. injection, lysine acetylsalicylate, an inhibitor of PG biosynthesis, potentiated both threshold electroshock and pentetrazole-induced convulsions in the dose range of 10–40 μg/mouse.

Convulsions elicited in baboons by photic stimulation could be completely suppressed by i.c.v. injection of 50–100 μg PGE_2; their duration was already reduced by 12.5 μg PGE_2 (ROSENKRANZ and KILLAM 1981).

PGE_2, 5 and 10 mg/kg i.p., strongly reduced the myoclonic activity induced by oral administration of 600 mg/kg chlorophenothane (dichloro-diphenyl-trichloroethane, DDT) in mice. This effect was antagonized by polyphloretin-phosphate, a PG antagonist, as well as by methysergide, 5 mg/kg, the latter finding pointing to an involvement of 5-HT in the mediation of the effect (van Woert and Hwang 1981). The authors assume that PGE_2 potentiates the 5-HT-induced production of cAMP in the inferior olive neurons, either by stimulation of adenylate cyclase or by enhancing the effect of the regulatory protein. Bhattacharya and Sanyal (1978) had previously pointed to a role of 5-HT in the mediation of the anticonvulsant effect of PGE_1 against pentetrazole in rats. This effect was antagonized by agents reducing the 5-HT activity in brain (*p*-chlorophenylalanine, methysergide, reserpine) but not by drugs influencing the metabolism of catecholamines.

C. Convulsant Effect of Prostaglandins

Contrary to the above findings in mice and rats, Wallenstein and Bito (1977) demonstrated a convulsant effect of PGE_1 and PGE_2 in rabbits. Superfusion of the visual cortex of conscious rabbits provoked seizure activity on the electrocortigram (ECoG) on photic stimulation when the rabbits had been pretreated with probenecid or bromcresol green, which are known to inhibit the transport of PGs. Pretreatment with inhibitors of PG synthesis, indometacin or paracetamol, also induced a convulsant effect of a superfusion with PGE_1, but not before 90 min after administration of the inhibitors. The effect is explained by a suppression of inhibitory postsynaptic potentials in the presence of high concentrations of PGEs (inhibitors of PG transport) or by development of supersensitivity (inhibitors of PG biosynthesis). Superfusion with $PGE_{2\alpha}$ had no comparable effect.

Five out of 320 women in whom high doses of $PGF_{2\alpha}$ were injected intraamniotically for abortion showed clinical seizures between 7 and 30 h after the first administration of the PG. Only two had a history of epilepsy. In five out of eight patients in whom the EEG was recorded during abortion with $PGF_{2\alpha}$, spike-and-wave activity was noticed (Lyneham et al. 1973). Wolfe et al. (1976b) reported increased CSF concentrations of $PGF_{2\alpha}$ in epileptic patients.

D. Release of Prostaglandins During Convulsions

In rats, cortical PGF concentrations were increased by a factor of 3–5 after corneal electroshock. This increase, but not the convulsions, could be inhibited by pretreatment with indometacin (Zatz and Roth 1975). The authors mention an increase of PGE and PGF concentrations on i.p. injection of 50 mg/kg pentetrazole. The reaction of PGE_2 and $PGF_{2\alpha}$, as well as of cGMP and cAMP, on convulsant and subconvulsant doses of pentetrazole was later studied by Folco et al. (1977) in rat brain. Ninety seconds after 100 mg/kg pentetrazole i.p., brain concentrations of $PGF_{2\alpha}$ had increased from 126 to 1,425 pg/mg protein and those of PGE_2 from 148 to 579 pg/mg. cGMP increased at the same time from 0.24 to 0.69 pmol/mg protein and cAMP from 7.9 to 18.2 pmol/mg. When, however, the subconvulsant dose of 50 mg/kg pentetrazole was used, only $PGF_{2\alpha}$ increased significantly to 396 pg/mg protein, PGE_2 not significantly to 203 pg/mg, but no changes of the cyclic nucleotides were observed. The authors conclude therefore that the change in PG concentrations is the primary event. Förster-

MANN et al. (1982) found increases of PGD_2, $PGE_{2\alpha}$, PGE_2, 6-keto-$PGF_{1\alpha}$, and TXB_2 in the brain of mice after electro- or pentetrazole-induced convulsions and gathered indirect evidence for an anticonvulsant effect of these endogenous PGs.

E. Conclusions

The evidence for a role of PGs in seizure activity is rather inconclusive at present. During clinical epilepsy as well as during seizure activity induced by electric stimulation or by pentetrazole, particularly the concentrations of $PGF_{2\alpha}$, and to a lesser degree those of PGE_2, seem to be considerably elevated, and an increase in the concentration of cyclic nucleotides seems to be secondary to the rise in PG concentrations (WOLFE et al. 1976b; ZATZ and ROTH 1975; FOLCO et al. 1977). Some results point to a mediation of the anticonvulsant effects of PGEs by 5-HT (BHATTACHARYA and SANYAL 1978) or GABA (ROSENKRANZ and KILLAM 1981), but an influence on cAMP as second messenger has been postulated by VAN WOERT and HWANG (1981). The experiments of PODDUBIUK and KLEINROK (1976), on the other hand, do not indicate a clear correlation between anticonvulsant PG effects and the metabolism of neurotransmitters. Interaction between the effect of PGs on susceptibility to seizures and the GABA system have so far not been studied.

After intracerebroventricular injection of PGE_1, PGE_2, and PGI_2, anticonvulsant effects against electroshock seizures – as long as the stimulation is not supramaximal – and chemoseizures have been reported rather univocally, whereas this effect was far less convincing after systemic administration. $PGF_{2\alpha}$ has mostly proved proconvulsant in these tests. The actions of PGs have been rather short lasting in all these experiments in spite of the fairly high doses necessary. Direct effects of the PGs on blood supply and distribution within the brain cannot be ruled out as causative factors (YAMAMOTO et al. 1972).

References

Bergström S, Samuelsson B (1965) Prostaglandins. Ann Rev Biochem 34:101–108

Bhattacharya SK, Sanyal AK (1978) Inhibition of pentylenetetrazole-induced convulsions in rats by prostaglandin E_1: role of brain monoamines. Psychopharmacology 56:235–237

Bradley PB, Samuels GMR, Shaw JE (1969) Correlation of prostaglandin release from the cerebral cortex of cats with electro-corticogram following stimulation of the reticular formation. Br J Pharmacol 37:151–157

Climax J, Sewell RDE (1981) Modification of convulsive behaviour and body temperature in mice by intracerebroventricular administration of prostaglandins, arachidonic acid and the soluble acetylsalicylic acid salt lysine acetylsalicylate. Arch Int Pharmacodyn Ther 250:254–265

Coceani F, Wolfe LS (1965) Prostaglandins in brain and the release of prostaglandin-like compounds from the cat cerebellar cortex. Can J Physiol Pharmacol 43:445–450

Coceani F, Puglisi L, Lavers B (1971) Prostaglandins and neuronal activity in spinal cord and cuneate nucleus. Ann NY Acad Sci 180:289–301

Duru S, Türker RK (1969) Effect of prostaglandin E_1 on the strychnine-induced convulsion in the mouse. Experientia 25:275–277

Förstermann V, Heldt R, Knappen E, Hertting G (1982) Potential anticonvulsive properties of endogenous prostaglandins formed in mouse brain. Brain Res 240:303–310

Folco GC, Longiave D, Bosisio E (1977) Relations between prostaglandin E_2, $F_{2\alpha}$ and cyclic nucleotides. Levels in rat brain and induction of convulsions. Prostaglandins 13:893–900

Galli C, Spagnuolo C, Petroni A (1980) Factors affecting brain prostaglandin formation. Adv Prostaglandin Thromboxane Res 8:1235–1239

Hedqvist P (1973) Autonomic neurotransmission. In: Ramwell PW (ed) The prostaglandins, vol 1. Plenum, New York, pp 101–131

Hinman JW (1972) Prostaglandins. Ann Rev Biochem 41:161–178

Holmes SW (1970) The spontaneous release of prostaglandins into the cerebral ventricles of the dog and the effect of external factors on this release. Br J Pharmacol 37:635–658

Holmes SW, Horton EW (1968a) The identification of four prostaglandins in dog brain and their regional distribution in the central nervous system. J Physiol (Lond) 195:731–741

Holmes SW, Horton EW (1968b) Prostaglandins and the central nervous system. In: Ramwell PW, Shaw JE (eds) Worcester symposium on prostaglandins. Wiley, New York, pp 21–36

Horton EW (1969) Hypothesis on physiological roles of prostaglandins. Physiol Rev 49:152–161

Horton EW (1972) Prostaglandins. Monographs on endocrinology, vol 7. Springer, Berlin Heidelberg New York, pp 117–149

Horton EW, Main JHM (1967) Identification of prostaglandins in central nervous tissues of the cat and chicken. Br J Pharmacol 30:582–602

Kataoka K, Ramwell PW, Jessup S (1967) Prostaglandins: localization in subcellular particles or rat cerebral cortex. Science 157:1187–1189

Kröner EE, Peskar BA (1976) On the metabolism of prostaglandins by rat brain homogenate. Experientia 32:1114–1115

Lyneham RC, Low PA, McLeod JG, Shearman RP, Smith ID, Korda AR (1973) Convulsions and electroencephalogram abnormalities after intraamniotic prostaglandin $F_{2\alpha}$. Lancet II:1003–1005

Pace-Asciak CR, Rangaraj G (1976a) Prostaglandin biosynthesis and catabolism in the developing fetal sheep brain. J Biol Chem 251:3381–3385

Pace-Asciak CR, Rangaraj G (1976b) Distribution of prostaglandin biosynthetic pathways in organs and tissues of fetal lamb. Biochim Biophys Acta 528:512–514

Poddubiuk ZM (1976) A comparison of the central actions of prostaglandins A_1, E_1, E_2, $F_{1\alpha}$ and $F_{2\alpha}$ in the rat. I. Behavioral, antinociceptive and anticonvulsant actions of intraventricular prostaglandins in the rat. Psychopharmacology 50:89–94

Poddubiuk ZM, Kleinrok Z (1976) A comparison of the central actions of prostaglandins A_1, E_1, E_2, $F_{1\alpha}$ and $F_{2\alpha}$ in the rat. Psychopharmacology 50:95–102

Potts WJ, East PF, Mueller RA (1974) Behavioral effects. In: Ramwell P (ed) Prostaglandins, vol 2. Plenum, New York, pp 157–173

Ramwell PW, Shaw JE (1966) Spontaneous and evoked release of prostaglandins from cerebral cortex of anesthetized cats. Am J Physiol 211:125–134

Ramwell PW, Shaw JE, Jessup R (1966) Spontaneous and evoked release of prostaglandins from frog spinal cord. Am J Physiol 211:998–1104

Rosenkranz RP (1978) Effects of intracerebroventricular administration of PGE_1, E_2 and $F_{2\alpha}$ on electrically induced convulsions in mice. Prostaglandins 15:925–942

Rosenkranz RP, Killam KF (1978) Effects of prostacyclin and 6-keto $PGF_{1\alpha}$ on electrically induced convulsions in mice. Life Sci 23:2609–2616

Rosenkranz RP, Killam KF (1979) Effects of intracerebroventricular administration of prostaglandins E_1 and E_2 on chemically induced convulsions in mice. J Pharmacol Exp Ther 209:231–237

Rosenkranz RP, Killam KF (1981) Anticonvulsant effects of PGE_2 on electrical, chemical and photomyoclonic animal models in epilepsy. Progr Lipid Res 20:515–522

Samuelsson B (1964) Identification of a smooth muscle-stimulating factor in bovine brain. Biochim Biophys Acta 84:218–219

Van Dorp DA (1966) The biosynthesis of prostaglandins. Mem Soc Endocrinol 14:39–47

Van Woert MH, Hwang EC (1981) Role of brain serotonin in myoclonus. In: Morselli PL, Lloyd KG, Löscher W, Meldrum B, Reynolds EH (eds) Neurotransmitters, seizures, and epilepsy. Raven, New York, pp 239–247
Wallenstein MC, Biko LZ (1977) Prostaglandin E_1-induced alterations in visually-evoked response and production of epileptiform activity. Neuropharmacology 16:687–694
Wolfe LS, Coceani F, Pace-Asciak C (1967) Brain prostaglandins and studies of the action of prostaglandins on the isolated rat stomach. In: Bergström S, Samuelsson B (eds) Nobel Symposium 2 on Prostaglandins. Almqvist and Wiksell, Stockholm, pp 265–275
Wolfe LS, Rostworowski K, Pappius HM (1976a) The endogenous biosynthesis of prostaglandins by brain tissue in vitro. Can J Biochem 54:629–640
Wolfe LS, Pappius HM, Marion J (1976b) The biosynthesis of prostaglandins by brain tissue in vitro. Adv Prostaglandin Thromboxane Res 1:345–365
Wolfe LS, Rostworowski K, Marion J (1976c) Endogenous formation of prostaglandin endoperoxide metabolite thromboxane B_2 by brain tissue. Biochem Biophys Res Comm 70:907–913
Yamamoto YL, Feindel W, Wolfe LS, Katch H, Hedge GP (1972) Experimental vasoconstriction on cerebral arteries by prostaglandins. Neurosurgery 37:385–397
Zatz M, Roth RH (1975) Electroconvulsive shock raises prostaglandins F in rat cerebral cortex. Biochem Pharmacol 24:2101–2103

General Pharmacology of Antiepileptic Drugs

CHAPTER 9

Chemical Constitution and Pharmacological Effect

H. SCHÄFER

A. Introduction

It is generally approved that there is a further need for more selective and less toxic antiepileptic drugs (KRALL et al. 1978a, b). In the search for optimal designs for new drugs, medicinal chemists and pharmacologists would benefit from consideration of the rules which emerge from comparison of the structures of active and inactive compounds. It is therefore the aim of this chapter to give an impression of structure-activity relationships mainly of those classes of compounds which include well-known antiepileptic drugs. In general the specification of anticonvulsant activity will be restricted to data from electroshock and pentylenetetrazol-induced shock tests.

It would be beyond the scope of this chapter also to discuss problems of quantitative structure-activity relationships (QSAR) including cluster analysis of antiepileptic drugs; these are much better outlined elsewhere (KRALL 1980; DESMEDT et al. 1976; LIEN et al. 1979). That also applies to the stereochemistry of antiepileptic drugs. Numerous studies have been performed to correlate the activity of various antiepileptic drugs with their stereochemistry. Obviously there are certain relationships between the space-filling properties of some compounds, bearing in mind their so-called active centers and their biological activity. These relationships are well reviewed by CAMERMAN and CAMERMAN (1980). On the other hand, STERNBACH et al. (1974) demonstrated that conformational similarities may be only one criterion for biological activity. Diazepam and two other structurally very closely related 1,4-benzodiazepines were crystallographically compared. All three compounds showed practically superimposable structures. However, only diazepam has known biological activity, while the derivatives mentioned were found to be only minimally active.

Many of the statements made so far on structure-activity relationship in the field of CNS active substances require qualification. This is because the biological, and in particular anticonvulsant, effects have usually been related to the given dose instead of to the concentration of the effective drug at the active site, e.g., the brain. Future animal studies on structure-activity relationships in the field of antiepileptic drugs should include quantitative determinations of active substances in the brain – as has been demonstrated in some papers (e.g., CACCIA et al. 1980a–c; JONES et al. 1981; MARCUCCI et al. 1972).

Recently, comprehensive reviews on qualitative structure-activity relationships of antiepileptic drugs have been published (MERCIER 1973; VIDA 1977). These provide complete information on all substances found to exhibit anticonvulsant activity.

B. Five-Membered Heterocyclic Compounds

Some of the most important antiepileptic drugs, which were first developed in the 1940s, belong to this group of chemical compounds, being characterized by the common formula

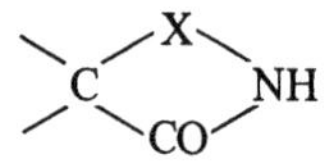

These are: 2,4-imidazolidine dione = hydantoin, X = NH–CO
2,4-oxazolidine dione, X = O–CO
2,4-pyrrolidine dione = succinimide X = CH_2–CO

I. Hydantoins

One of the most frequently used antiepileptic drugs is 5,5-diphenylhydantoin (phenytoin) (1). Other hydantoins such as 5-ethyl-3-methyl-5-phenylhydantoin (mephenytoin) (2) and 3-ethyl-5-phenylhydantoin (ethotoin) (3) have been accepted for limited use in the treatment of epilepsy or have been evaluated during extensive clinical trials, i.e., 3-allyl-5-isobutyl-2-thiohydantoin (albutoin) (4).

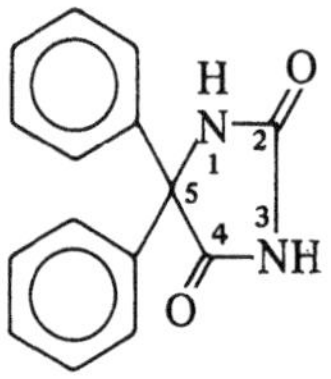

(1)

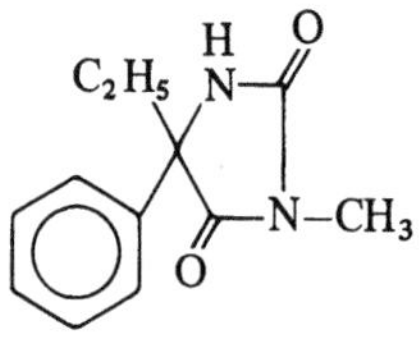

(2)

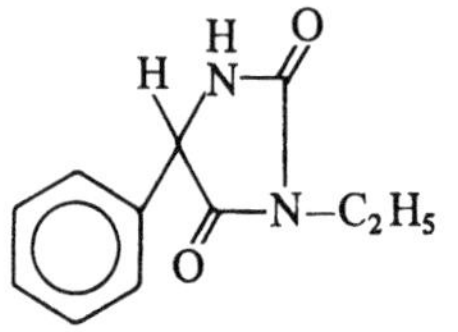

(3)

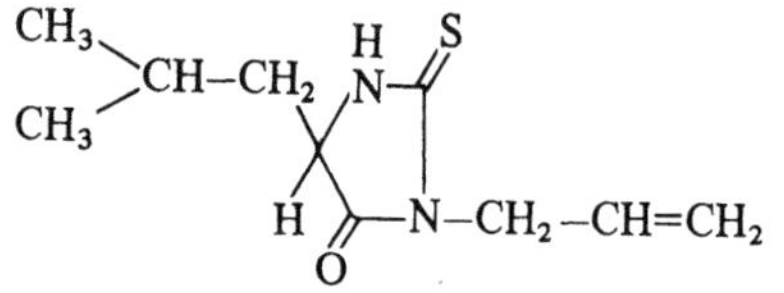

(4)

The discovery of the anticonvulsant activity of phenytoin by MERRITT and PUTNAM in 1938 and its introduction as an antiepileptic drug was a milestone in the development of antiepileptic therapy, insofar as their studies demonstrated for the first time that it was possible by an experimental method using animal models to develop clinically reliable antiepileptic drugs. By 1945 nearly 700 substances from various classes of chemical compounds had been tested for their anticonvulsant activity [maximal electroshock seizures (MES)] in cats (MERRITT and PUTNAM 1945).

More than 200 of the evaluated substances were hydantoins. These and further studies have elucidated many structure-activity relationships in the hydantoin series, the following of which are the most important:

1. The hydantoin ring must be provided with at least one phenyl or another aromatic hydrocarbon group at carbon-5 to show significant MES activity.

2. If two phenyl groups are attached to carbon-5, the resulting 5,5-diphenylhydantoin (phenytoin) will achieve maximal MES activity.
3. Replacement of one phenyl group of phenytoin by lower alkyl groups imparts moderate Metrazol(pentylenetetrazol)-induced seizure (Met) activity with a slight decrease in MES activity.
4. Replacement of both phenyl groups in phenytoin
   a) by isobutyl groups decreases MES activity.
   b) by other alkyl groups abolishes MES activity but elevates Met activity; two short alkyl groups favor Met activity.
   c) by benzyl groups abolishes MES activity.
5. Met activity is increased by substitution by lower alkyl groups, preferably methyl groups, on N3 and possibly on N1 and N3 of the hydantoin ring.
6. Any substitution on the phenyl groups in phenytoin suppresses MES activity.
7. MES activity of phenytoin is also decreased by substitution of H_2 for O in 5,5-diphenylimidazoline-4-one = doxenitoine (5) (GOODMAN et al. 1954), by substitution of S for O at carbon-2 in 5,5-diphenyl-2-thiohydantoin (6) (KNOEFEL and LEHMANN 1942; SOHN et al. 1970), or by hydrolytic cleavage of the hydantoin ring to 2-amino-2,2-diphenylacetamide (7) (BILLMAN and HIDY 1943; NAKAMURA et al. 1966).

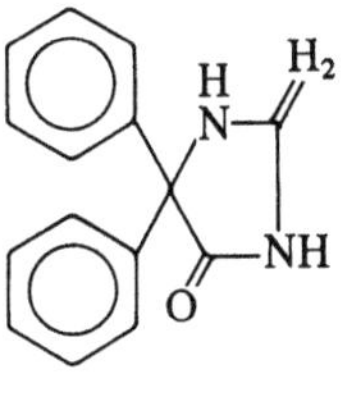

(5)

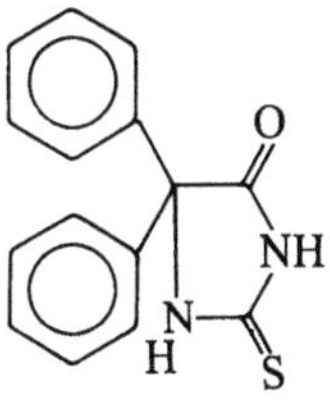

(6)

8. MES activity is almost or completely abolished in the products of phenytoin hydrolysis, 2,2-diphenyl-2-ureidoacetic acid (8) and 2-amino-2,2-diphenylacetic acid (9) (NAKAMURA et al. 1966), and in the phenytoin main metabolite 5-*p*-hydroxyphenyl-5-phenylhydantoin (10) (HPPH) (NAKAMURA et al. 1966).

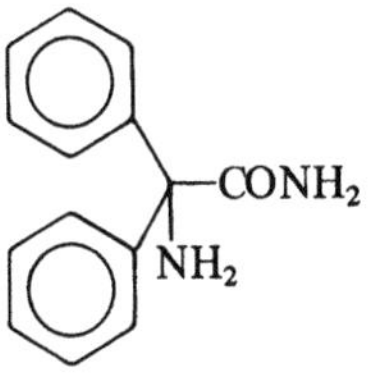

(7)

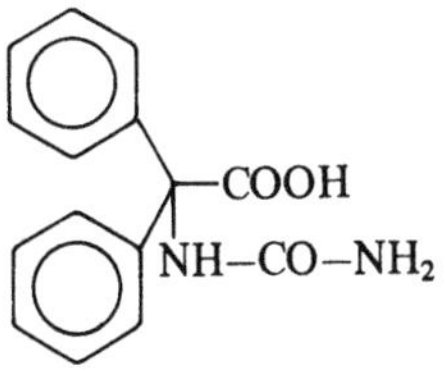

(8)

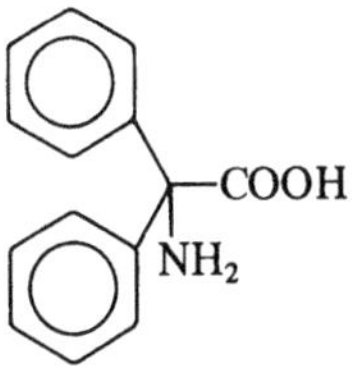

(9)

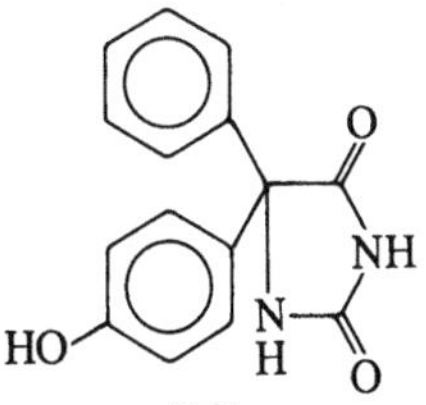

(10)

Additional alterations in the chemical structure of the clinically very important phenytoin have been attempted in order to extend its anticonvulsant activity profile as well as to reduce or even abolish its unfavorable side effects.

*N*3-Hydroxyphenytoin (CALL 1970) has not shown any anticonvulsant activity in animal models. SCHLÖGL et al. (1961), WINSTEAD et al. (1965), WINSTEAD

Table 1. Anticonvulsant activity of hydantoins cited in the text compared with phenobarbital and trimethadione in mice (m) and rats (r). MES and/or Met methods used; according to SWINYARD et al. (1952) (A); according to TOMAN et al. (1946) (B); or no details available (C)

	Route	MES ED_{50} (mg/kg)	Met ED_{50} (mg/kg)	NTD_{50} [a] (mg/kg)	Ref.
Phenytoin	p.o.	18.9 rB	167 rA		NAKAMURA et al. (1966)
	p.o.	12 mA	– mA	165	GESLER et al. (1961)
		9 mC	– mC	92	MILLICHAP (1972)
Mephenytoin		37 mC	53 mC	97	MILLICHAP (1972)
Ethotoin		350 mC	350 mC	400	MILLICHAP (1972)
Albutoin	p.o.	211 mA	40 mA	170	GESLER et al. (1961)
Phenobarbital	p.o.	24 mA	15 mA	113	GESLER et al. (1961)
Trimethadione	p.o.	>400 mA	225 mA	1240	GESLER et al. (1961)
3-Methylphenytoin		< 6.3 mA	>200 mA		VIDA et al. (1975)
1,3-Dimethylphenytoin		~ 50 mA	~ 25 mA		Vida et al. (1975)
2-Thiophenytoin	i.p.	25 rA	(–) rA		SOHN et al. (1970)
Doxenitoine	p.o.	32 mA	172 mA	320	GOODMAN et al. (1966)
2-Amino-2,2-diphenylacetamide	p.o.	45 rB	51 rA		NAKAMURA et al. (1966)
2-Amino-2,2-diphenylacetic acid	p.o.	>114 rB	>114 rA		NAKAMURA et al. (1966)
2,2-Diphenylhydantoic acid	p.o.	<135 rB	>135 rA		NAKAMURA et al. (1966)
HPPH	p.o.	>134 rB	>134 rA		NAKAMURA et al. (1966)

(–), weakly active; –, inactive
[a] Neurotoxin dose

Table 2. Anticonvulsant activity of hydantoins of the general formula 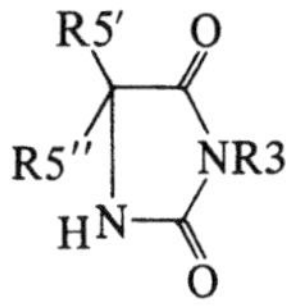 (SCHLÖGL et al. 1961). MES according to SWINYARD et al. (1952) in mice p.o.

Formula No.	R5′	R5″	R3	MES ED_{50} (mg/kg)	LD_{50} (mg/kg)	Peak time of activity (h)	Thera-peutic index
2	C_2H_5	C_6H_5	CH_3	30	1,460	0.5	48.7
11	C_2H_5	C_6H_5	CH_2OH	7	405	2	57.9
12	C_2H_5	C_6H_5	$CH_2 \cdot CH_2 \cdot OH$	68	>2,000	1	>30
	C_2H_5	p-C_6H_4–F	$CH_2 \cdot CH_2 \cdot OH$	180	3,000	2	16.7
	C_2H_5	p-C_6H_4–Br	$CH_2 \cdot CH_2 \cdot OH$	59	1,300	0.5	22
	C_6H_5	C_6H_5	$CH_2 \cdot CH_2 \cdot OH$	48	530	1	11
	C_6H_5	C_6H_5	$CH_2 \cdot CH_2 \cdot N\ (C_2H_5)_2$	113		0.5	
	C_6H_5	C_6H_5	$CH_2 \cdot CO \cdot NH\ (CH_2)_2OH$	>600			

and HAMEL (1965), and SHAFFER et al. (1968) demonstrated that both N3-substituted active and inactive derivatives of phenytoin and of 5-phenyl-5-alkyl-hydantoins could be prepared; activity is strongly dependent on the type of substituent: Anticonvulsant activity is decreased when $-CH_2-COOR$ or $-CH_2-NH_2$ is introduced in N3 of the above-mentioned hydantoins. Other polar groups such as $-CH_2-CH_2-COOH$, $-CH_2-CH_2-CONH_2$, or $-CH_2-CH_2-CN$ connected with N3 completely abolish the activity of the basic hydantoins in the MES or the Met tests. On the other hand, some of these hydantoins with *N*3-alkyl-*N*< and *N*3-alkyl-OH groups showed remarkable anticonvulsant activity (Table 2).

The most active compound of this series was the N3-CH_2OH derivative of the 5-ethyl-5-phenylhydantoin (11). It is noteworthy that the anticonvulsant effectivity of β-hydroxyethyl hydantoin (12), as measured by the therapeutic index (LD_{50}/ED_{50}), is also nearly in the same range as that of mephenytoin, although β-hydroxyethyl hydantoin (12) is much more soluble in water and possibly has a different partition coefficient.

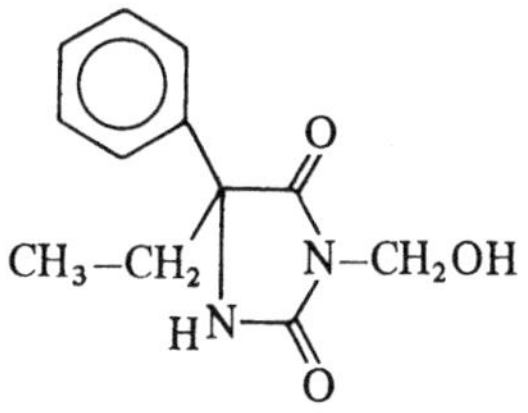

(11)

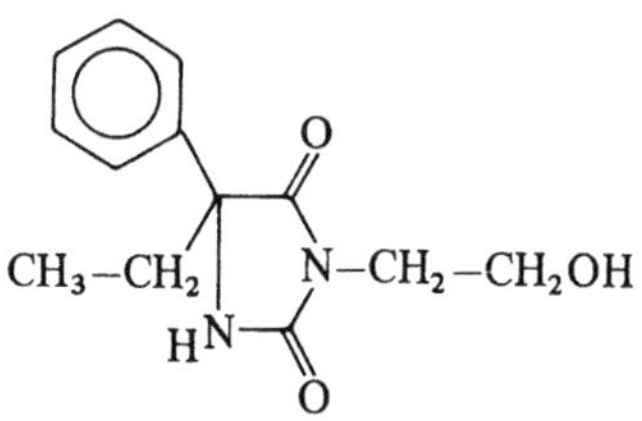

(12)

SAMOUR et al. (1971) have found that *N*3-alkoxymethyl derivatives of phenytoin are active anticonvulsants. The most effective derivative in the MES test is substituted at N3 with a methoxy methyl group (13), whereas phenytoin-*N*3-$CH_2-O-CH_2-C_6H_5$ exhibits remarkable activity in the Met test. Additional *N*3-

Table 3. Anticonvulsant activity of phenytoin derivatives with substituents on nitrogen-1 and nitrogen-3. MES and Met according to SWINYARD et al. (1952) in mice p.o.

R1	R3	MES ED_{50} (mg/kg)	Met ED_{50} (mg/kg)	Peak time of activity	Ref.
H	$CH_2 \cdot O \cdot CH_3$	~ 6	(−)	3	SAMOUR et al. (1971)
H	$CH_2 \cdot O \cdot CH_2 \cdot C_6H_5$	>25	< 50	1	SAMOUR et al. (1971)
$CH_2 \cdot O \cdot CH_3$	$CH_2 \cdot O \cdot CH_3$	~25	~600	0.5	VIDA et al. (1975)
H	CH_3	3.1–6.2	>200	2	VIDA et al. (1975)
CH_3	CH_3	~50	~ 25	3	VIDA et al. (1975)
H	$CH_2 \cdot O \cdot CO \cdot CH_3$	<12.5	–	1	VIDA et al. (1971)
Phenytoin		~ 7.5	–	3	VIDA et al. (1975)
Mephenytoin		~10	~ 30	1	VIDA et al. (1975)

(−), weakly active; –, inactive, no hypnotic activity except at lethal doses

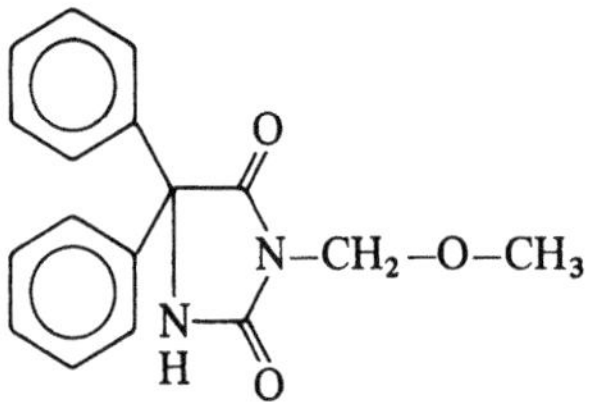

(13)

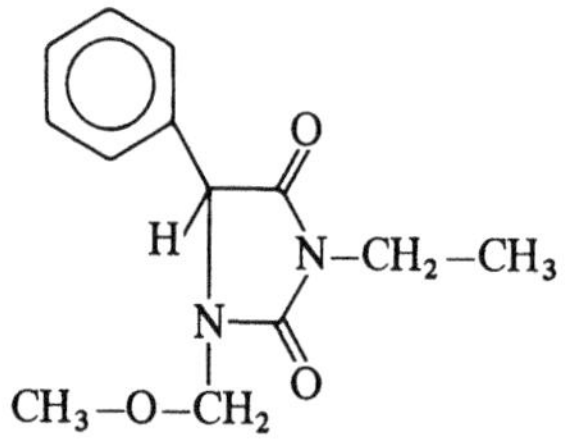

(14)

and/or N1-alkoxymethyl or -acyloxymethyl derivatives have been evaluated by SAMOUR et al. (1971) and VIDA et al. (1971, 1975). Examples of these series are shown in Table 3. An only weakly active N1-methoxymethyl derivative of ethotoin (14), MES $ED_{50} \sim 300$ mg/kg, Met $ED_{50} \sim 100$, neurotoxic $dose_{50}$ $(NTD)_{50} \sim 300$ mg/kg mouse, was screened in the Antiepileptic Drug Development Program (ADDP) (GAL 1979).

–COOR groups as substituents at N3 of phenytoin markedly increase its anticonvulsant activity (NAKAMURA et al. 1965, 1966; SCHÄFER 1969). It is safe to assume that the principal share of the biological activity of these N3-carbalkoxy derivatives is due to phenytoin resulting from chemical or enzymatic hydrolysis of the drug after being absorbed and distributed in tissues and cells. Nevertheless, it is readily understandable that these N3-carbalkoxy phenytoins display increased anticonvulsant activity, since unlike phenytoin some of the N3-COOR derivatives penetrate the blood-brain barrier better and show better retention in

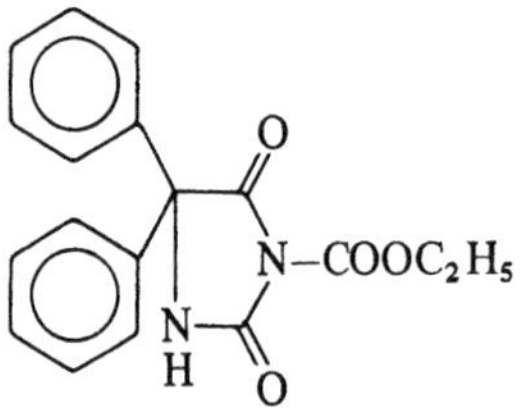

(15)

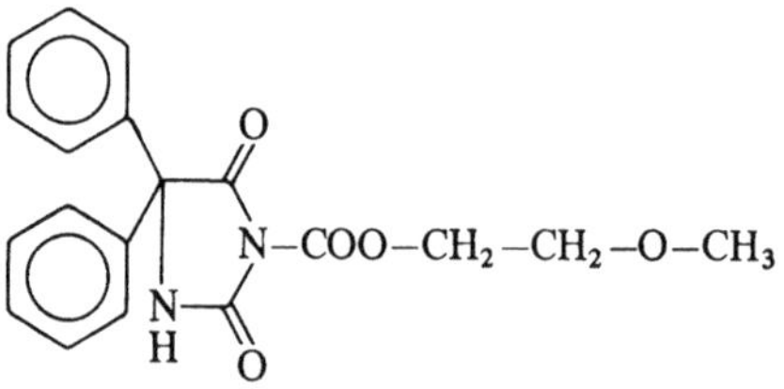

(16)

Table 4. Results with the minimal electroshock seizure threshold (MET) method (BROWN et al. 1953) and duration of action (DA_{50}) show that 50% of the animals were protected from tonic hindlimb extensor seizure after being treated with the respective dose of the test substance of the general formula (SCHÄFER 1969; SCHÄFER and LEUSCHNER unpublished data)

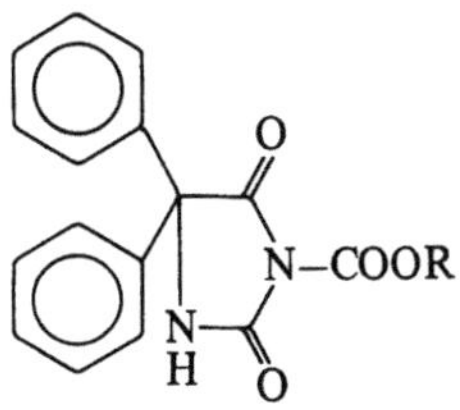

R	MET dose administered (mmol/kg)		DA_{50}	
	Mice	Rats	Mice (h)	Rats (h)
Phenytoin	0.048	0.044	10	8
$-CH_3$	0.026	0.048	26	
$-C_2H_5$	0.023	0.046	8	10
$-CH_2\cdot CH_2\cdot O\cdot CH_3$	0.040	0.014	20	10
$-CH_2\cdot CH_2\cdot O\cdot C_2H_5$	0.049	0.033	26	
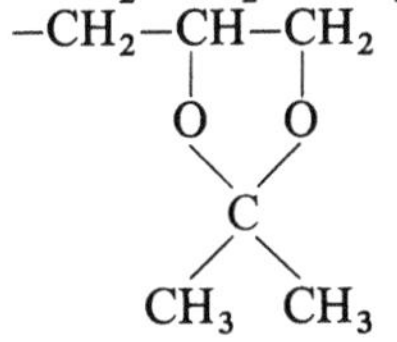	0.027	0.029	14	

brain, as has been demonstrated with *N*3-ethoxycarbonyl phenytoin (15) in dogs and cats (NAKAMURA et al. 1966). The better retention of these compounds and particularly that of *N*3-*β*-methoxyethoxycarbonyl phenytoin (16) in brain also shows itself in their increased duration of action (Table 4).

Efforts have been made to optimize the activity of phenytoin by connecting the two phenyl rings directly or via a C_x-bridge (17). FABING et al. (1947) has presented the results of clinical trials of diphenylenhydantoin (17, single bond instead of X), which is reported to have a therapeutic index similar to phenytoin. Spirohydantoins (17 with X = $-CH_2-CH_2-$, $-CH=CH-$, and $-CH_2-CH_2-CH_2-$) have been evaluated by DAVIS et al. (1964 b). None of these derivatives shows any advantage over phenytoin. The spirohydantoin with X = $-CH_2-CH_2-CH_2-$ is even a highly toxic convulsant. A series of cycloalkanspiro-5′-hydantoins have been tested by OLDFIELD and CASHIN (1965) for their biological activity. Only the cycloheptanespiro-5′-hydantoins (18) have been found to have some anticonvulsant

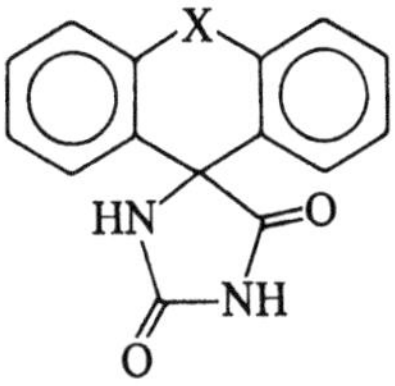

(17)

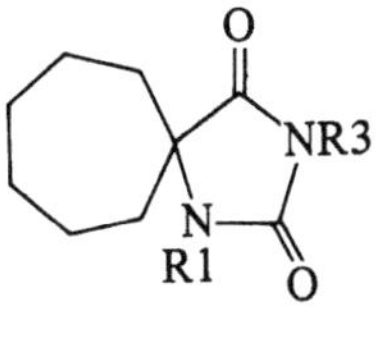

(18)

activity against electroshock, pentylenetetrazol, and strychnine; whereas cyclopentanespiro-5'-hydantoins have shown low sedative activity; certain cyclohexanespiro-5'-hydantoins have shown analgesic and anti-inflammatory properties; and the few cyclooctanespiro-5'-hydantoins have possessed weak hypnotic activities.

The anticonvulsant activity of phenytoin is decreased by the introduction of a 3-CF_3 group on the phenyl ring. However, if the phenyl ring in 5-benzyl hydantoin is substituted with a 3-CF_3 (19), a compound will result with anti-MES activity in rats comparable to that of phenytoin but with increased neurotoxicity and acute lethality in mice (MEHTA et al. 1981) (Table 5).

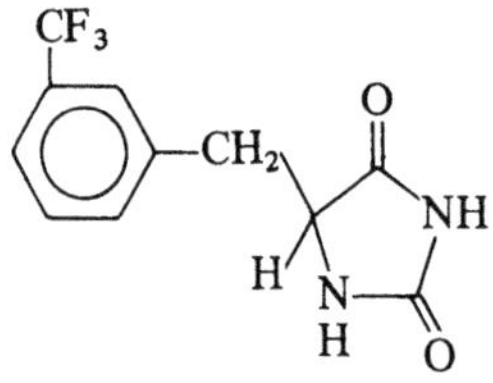

(19)

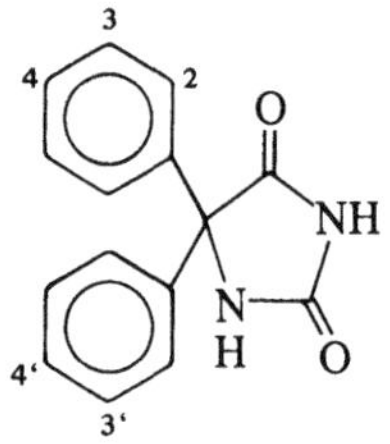

(20)

Phenytoin is mainly metabolized and renally excreted by enzymatic phenyl-C4 hydroxylation, with subsequent glucuronidation. Therefore, it might be possible to develop a phenytoin-like drug with a delayed metabolic rate and with a different spectrum of activity by blocking the phenyl-C4 position with substituents as small as possible. Thus, the addition of fluorine atoms especially in C4 is likely to be the smallest possible change to the phenytoin molecule with regard to its steric properties. NELSON et al. (1979) has prepared six fluorinated phenytoin analogues (20) with a = 4-F, b = 3-F, c = 2-F, d = 4-F, 4'-F, e = 3-F, 3'-F, and f = 4-F, 3'-F. Only three of these compounds (a, c, f) exhibit measurable anticonvulsant

Table 5. Anticonvulsant activity and neurotoxicity of hydantoins with fluorinated substituents on carbon-5. MES and Met according to the ADDP in mice i.p. for the first four compounds, and MES according to WOODBURY and DAVENPORT and Met according to SWINYARD et al. (1952) in mice and (rats) i.p. for the last three compounds

R5'	R5"	MES ED_{50} (mg/kg)	Met ED_{50} (mg/kg)	NTD_{50} (mg/kg mouse)	Ref.
C_6H_5	C_6H_5	9.5	–	65	NELSON et al. (1979)
4-F–C_6H_5	C_6H_5	61	–	1,190	NELSON et al. (1979)
2-F–C_6H_5	C_6H_5	23	–	158	NELSON et al. (1979)
4-F–C_6H_5	3'-FC_6H_4	270	–	>2,000	NELSON et al. (1979)
C_6H_5	C_6H_5	8.5 (9.6)	50 (–)	135	MEHTA et al. (1981)
C_6H_5	m-CF_3–C_6H_4	(>50)	(>200)		MEHTA et al. (1981)
H	m-CF_3–C_6H_4–CH_2	70 (23)	17.5 (~100)	65	MEHTA et al. (1981)

(–), inactive (in rats)

activity (Table 5). The most potent substance of this series is 5-(2-fluorophenyl)-5-phenylhydantoin, which is not only slightly less than half as active but also less than half as neurotoxic as phenytoin on a molar basis. The low activity of the 4-fluorinated phenytoins is difficult to explain satisfactorily. However, it is obvious that fluorine, the strongest electronegative element, being a substituent will change the polar properties of the molecule and in the same way its biological activities markedly and more than often assumed.

3-Allyl-5-isobutyl-2-thiohydantoin (albutoin), (4) was found to be the most potent compound in a series of 16 3,5-disubstituted-2-thiohydantoins (21) (GESLER et al. 1961).

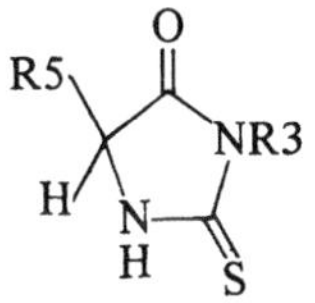

(21)

In animal models albutoin (4) exhibits anti-Metrazol activity more evident than that measured in the MES test (Table 1).

Therefore, albutoin has been assumed to be an effective drug in controlling absences. In contrast to this assumption and in clinical practice albutoin has been found to be more or even especially active in the treatment of grand mal attacks (DAVIES and SCHWADE 1959; MILLICHAP and ORTIZ 1967).

Though some authors have maintained the contrary (DAVIS et al. 1964b; MEHTA et al. 1981), phenytoin is generally considered to have no anti-Met activity. On the other hand, *N*1,*N*3-dimethyl phenytoin exhibits increased activity in the Met test (Table 1). CHIU et al. (1979) proposed the preparation of a phenytoin derivative showing anti-Met activity by substituting the hydantoin ring-N3 with a tertiary butyl group. The authors discovered that inactive hydantoins may be changed into active compounds by introducing a tertiary butyl group on N3. Thus, 5-methyl hydantoin (22) is inactive whereas the tertiary butyl compound 23

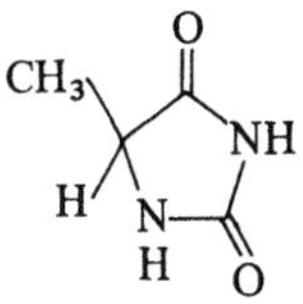

(22)

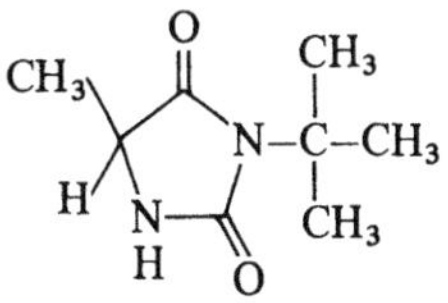

(23)

is active in the Met test in mice, with an ED_{50} of 130 mg/kg and an NTD_{50} of 343 mg/kg. However, it is uncertain whether or not the above-mentioned working hypothesis may be realized, because the N3-tertiary butyl-5-phenylhydantoin was proved to have "merely" an MES ED_{50} of 80 mg/kg but to have no Met activity at all.

Recently, the MES effectiveness and the acute toxicity of *N*-aminophenytoin (24) (probably the *N*3-amino compound) were shown to be similar to those of phenytoin (RUMP et al. 1981).

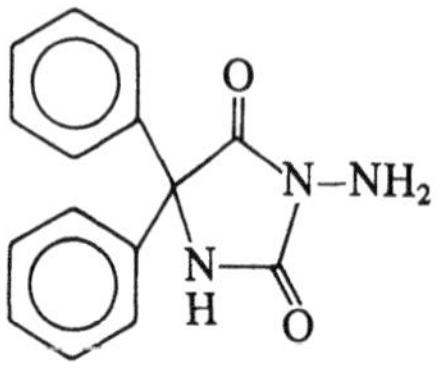

(24)

II. Oxazolidinediones

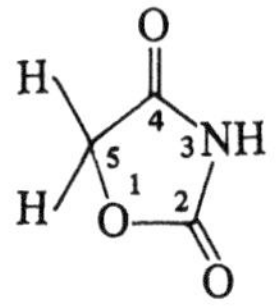

(25)

Recently the 2,4-oxazolidinediones (25) have been largely superseded by less toxic and more effective drugs (ethosuximide, valproic acid, and benzodiazepines). Nevertheless, they are mentioned in this chapter for several reasons. Firstly, trimethadione as the most important compound of this series is still in use as a well-known standard substance in animal studies and is therefore included in some of the tables. Secondly, these compounds are of considerable historical interest because they opened a new era in the drug therapy for epilepsy. GOODMAN et al. (1946) confirmed earlier findings that trimethadione [3,5,5-trimethyloxazolidine-2,4-dione (26)] is an effective anticonvulsant and is able to raise the threshold for both chemically and electrically induced seizures. Moreover, it was very important when GOODMAN et al. (1946) and above all PERLSTEIN and ANDELMAN (1946) found that for the first time absence seizures could be selectively controlled by trimethadione.

Later on other 2,4-oxazolidinedione derivatives were proposed for the treatment of absence seizures: 3-ethyl-5,5-dimethyloxazolidine-2,4-dione [ethadione (27)] and 3,5-dimethyl-5-ethyloxazolidine-2,4-dione [paramethadione (28)]. In

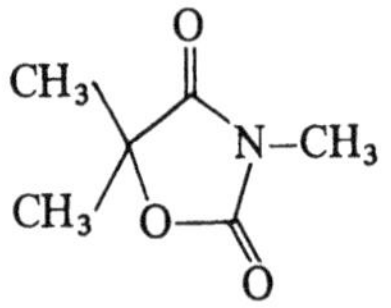

(26)

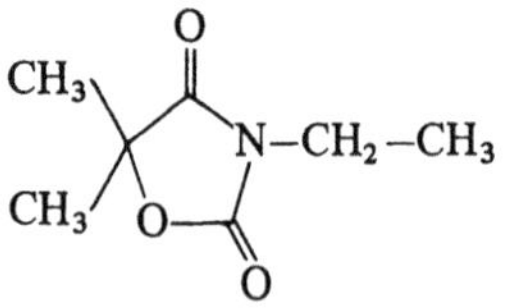

(27)

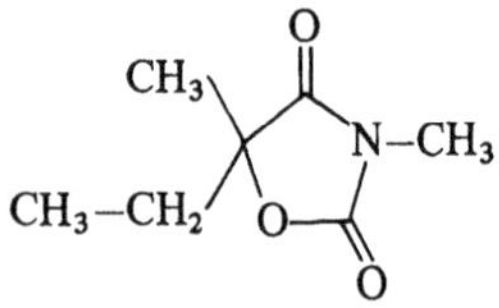

(28)

animal models the oxazolidinediones exhibit similar structure-activity relationships, as will be shown in Sect. B.-III on the succinimide series (VIDA and GERRY 1977). These are very briefly:

1. Substitution on carbon-5 by small alkyl groups results in substances with increased anti-Met activity
2. Phenyl groups on carbon-5 yield substances with more potent anti-MES activity
3. Substitution on NH by small alkyl groups for H increases anticonvulsant activity mainly in the Met test.

With respect to the *N*-lower alkyl oxazolidine-2,4-diones an important problem is the contribution of the unmetabolized drugs to anticonvulsant activity. BUTLER et al. (1952) showed that trimethadione is metabolically demethylated to 5,5-dimethyloxazolidine-2,4-dione [dimethadione (29)]. On a molar basis the un-

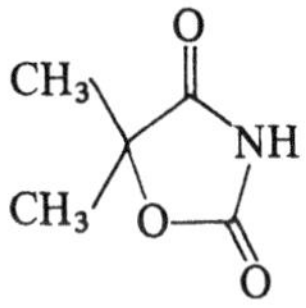

(29)

metabolized trimethadione has 1.25 times the anticonvulsant potency of dimethadione, as determined by the Met test (FREY 1969). FREY and SCHULZ (1970) have shown the half-life of demethylation to be about 45 min in mice, whereas the half-life of dimethadione excretion was found to be about 30 h. Similar differences have been found in dogs (8 h and 50–80 h, respectively). 5,5-Dimethyl-3-ethyloxazolidine-2,4-dione (27) is deethylated to dimethadione at nearly the same metabolic rate (BUTLER and WADDELL 1957). Thus data collected on animal models using single doses are not representative of real conditions during chronic treatment. The above-mentioned findings are early and useful examples for the indispensability of taking into consideration the potential metabolism of a potent drug leading to other active substances not only during pharmacological screening but in particular also during all discussions on structure-activity relationships.

III. Succinimides

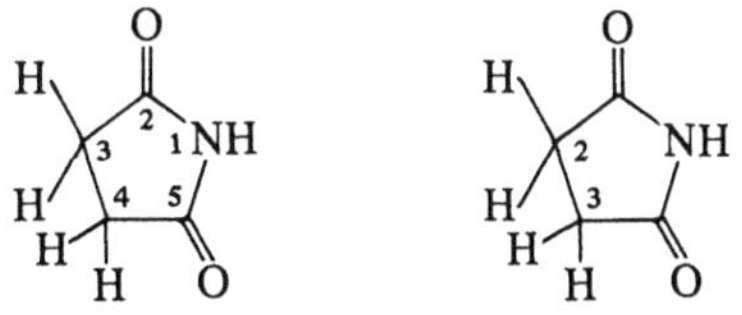

2,5 – Pyrrolidine dione Succinimide

(30)

Substituted 2,5-pyrrolidinediones = succinimides, containing a basic structure similar to those of the hydantoins and oxazolidinediones are clinically well-established antiepileptic drugs. Stimulated by the discovery of antipentylenetetrazol activity and the therapeutic usefulness of trimethadione, CHEN et al. (1951), MILLER and LONG (1951, 1953 a, b), and MILLER et al. (1951) evaluated a great many succinimides alkyl, and/or aryl substituted at C2, C2/N, C2/C3, and C2/C3/N which were shown to be active in MES and Met tests. Important drugs useful in the treatment of absence seizures such as *N*,2-dimethyl-2-phenylsuccinimide [methsuximide (31)], *N*-methyl-2-phenylsuccinimide [phensuximide (32)], and 2-ethyl-2-methylsuccinimide [ethosuximide (33)] (ZIMMERMANN and BURGEMEISTER 1958; CHEN et al. 1963) resulted from these studies. Preliminary but well-substantiated rules on structure-activity relationships were constructed from all these findings. To extend the above-mentioned investigations and to obtain more de-

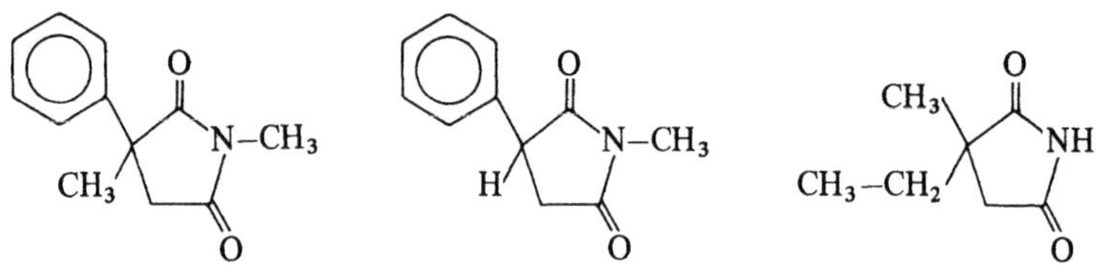

(31) (32) (33)

tailed information about their minimal electroshock seizure threshold (MET) and Met activity in the early 1960s we performed a comprehensive and comparative study on 2,2-di and 2,2,3-trisubstituted but *N*-unsubstituted succinimides, determining their ED_{50} values (Schäfer and Leuschner, unpublished). The compounds to be tested were of very different molecular size. Therefore the comparison of the ED_{50} data on a molecular basis in millimoles per kilogram mouse was preferred in this study (Fig. 1).

In accordance with the other authors mentioned we briefly stated the following relationships between the activity and structure of *N*-unsubstituted succinimides.

1. Unsubstituted phenyl groups on carbon-2 ensure activity in the electroshock test as well as in the pentylenetetrazol test; 2,2-diphenylsuccinimide, similar to 5,5-diphenylhydantoin, is devoid of antipentylenetetrazol activity
2. If there is one straight chained alkyl group out of two alkyl groups of at least three C-atoms on carbon-2 the activity in both convulsant tests will increase markedly
3. Two lower alkyl groups CH_3 and/or C_2H_5 on carbon-2 resulted only in weak activity in the animal models mentioned. Activity is evidently increased by an additional alkyl or phenyl group on carbon-3
4. In the 2′-spirocycloalkyl succinimide series the optimum is about a C_8 ring. It is noteworthy that the spirocyclohexyl succinimide, being rather inactive in the electroshock and Met tests, has the maximum toxicity of the tested spiro compounds.

While the unsubstituted succinimide seems to be inactive, tetra-substituted derivatives such as 2,3-diethyl-2,3-dimethyl- and 2,2,3,3-tetraethylsuccinimide were reported to be quite toxic, the main symptoms being muscular incoordination and convulsions with no evidence of sedative action (DOX 1925).

JUCKER and SÜESS (1961) tested a great many spiro-2′-*N*-methylpiperidyl-succinimides similar to compounds of Fig. 1. None of these compounds showed any anticonvulsant activity. However, some of these predominantly tertiary amines were found to have significant parasympathomimetic properties.

Succinimides with spirodibenzocycloalkadiene and -triene groups in 2′ were evaluated by DAVIS et al. (1964b). The tests were performed similarly to those of

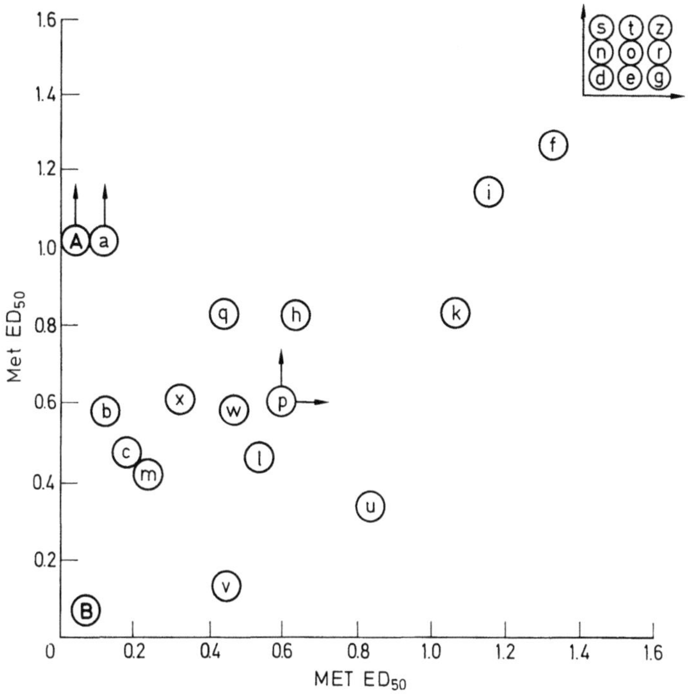

Fig. 1. Anticonvulsant activity of di- or trisubstituted succinimides given orally to NMRI mice. Minimal electroshock seizure threshold (MET) (10 mA, 0.6 s) according to BROWN et al. (1953), Met (100 mg/kg pentylenetetrazol s.c.); drugs were usually administered 1 h before the respective test. Key: substituents are specified as 2,2|| or 2,2||3. →, more than. *a*, C_6H_5, C_6H_5||; *b*, CH_3, C_6H_5||; *c*, C_2H_5, C_6H_5||; *d*, CH_3, CH_3||; *e*, CH_3, C_2H_5||; *f*, CH_3, n-C_3H_7||; *g*, CH_3, i-C_3H_7||; *h*, CH_3, n-C_4H_9||; *i*, C_2H_5, C_2H_5||; *k*, C_2H_5, n-C_3H_7||; *l*, C_2H_5, n-C_4H_9||; *m*, n-C_3H_7, n-C_3H_7||; *n*, i-C_4H_9, i-C_4H_9||; *o*, spirocyclo C_5||; *p*, spirocyclo C_6||; *q*, spirocyclo C_8||; *r*, spirocyclo C_{12}||; *s*, CH_3–N 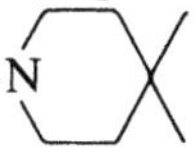 ||; *t*, CH_3, H||C_2H_5; *u*, CH_3, C_2H_5||C_2H_5; *v*, CH_3, C_2H_5||C_6H_5; *w*, spirocyclo C_5||C_6H_5; *x*, spirocyclo C_6||C_6H_5; *z*, CH_3–N 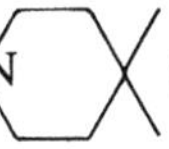 ||C_6H_5; *A*, phenytoin; *B*, phenobarbital

SWINYARD et al. (1952). Thus, compound 34 exhibited an MES ED_{50} of 38 mg/kg, an Met ED_{50} of 33 mg/kg, and a rotorod NTD_{50} of 430 mg/kg after oral administration to mice. A desoxy analogue of 34, the pyrrolidinone 35, showed simi-

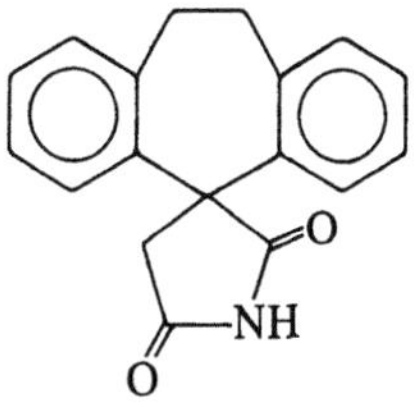

(34)

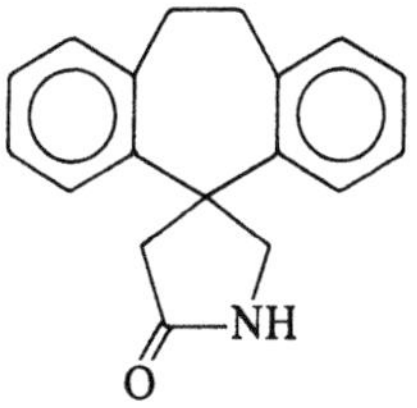

(35)

lar anticonvulsant activity in the mentioned tests but showed increased neurotoxicity with an NTD_{50} of 112 mg/kg.

Succinimides dialkylamino substituted exclusively on carbon-2 seem to be inactive as mentioned above; those containing an additional phenyl group on carbon-2 have been shown to have some anticonvulsant activity (CLEMSON et al. 1968). A series of phensuximide derivatives with additional tertiary amino groups (36, 37) were also evaluated at the dose level of 200 mg/kg i.p. in mice. All of the

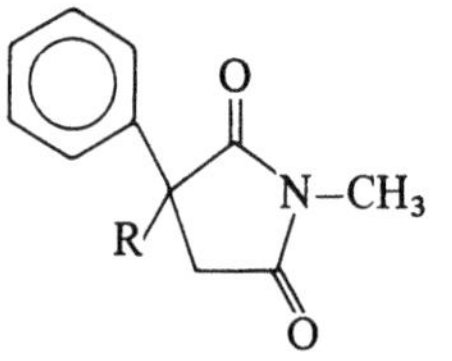

(36) R = $-CH_2-N<$

(37) R = $-CH_2-CH_2-N<$

test compounds were found to be ineffective against pentylenetetrazol-induced convulsions. However, in the MES test some of the compounds exhibited increased activity compared with the parent substance phensuximide, which was found to protect 20% of the test animals against electroshock (Table 6).

It is noteworthy that only small alterations in the amino group provoke a dramatic variation in MES activity: As shown in Table 7 the piperidyl derivative 38 protected 90% of the test animals against electroshock, while at the same dose level there is no protection when a pyrrolidyl group as in 39 is introduced instead of piperidyl.

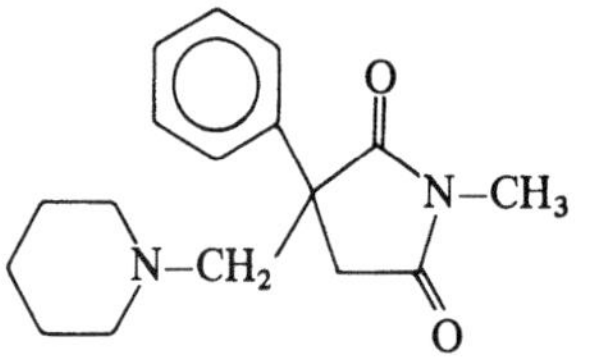

(38)

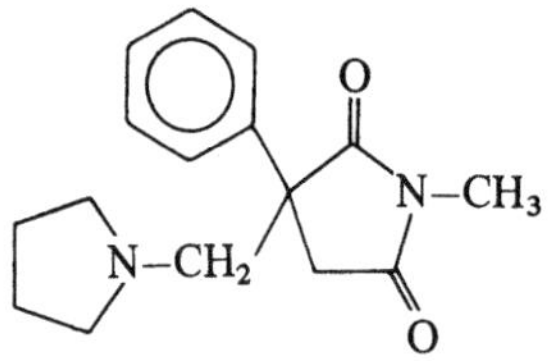

(39)

Some Mannich base derivatives of 2-phenylsuccinimide compared well with the anticonvulsant efficacy of the standard substance phensuximide. Particularly the *N*-substituted mono-Mannich bases (40) were generally more active than the corresponding *N*2 disubstituted analogues (41) in preventing the tonic extensor phase of the seizure pattern during the pentylenetetrazol test (MAGARIAN et al. 1973). In the above-mentioned alkylamino alkyl compounds structural elements of phensuximide or methsuximide have been included. If the phenyl group, supposed to be essential to MES activity, is attached to the nitrogen ring directly or

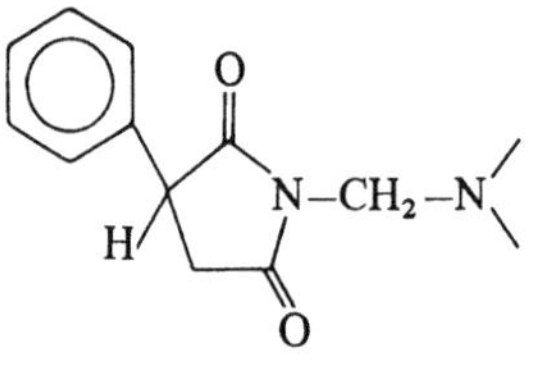

(40)

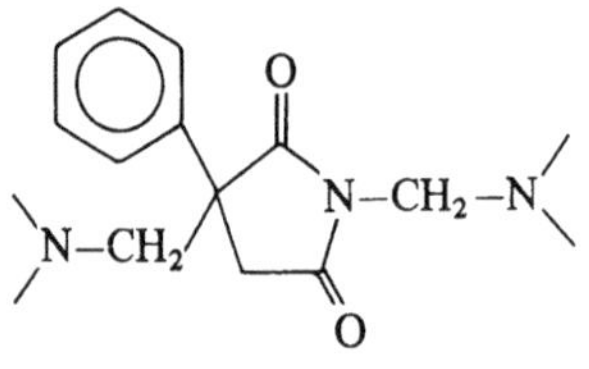

(41)

Table 6. Protection of mice in the electroshock test according to TOMAN et al. (1946) by alkylaminoalkyl-substituted succinimides of the general formula (CLEMSON et al. 1968).

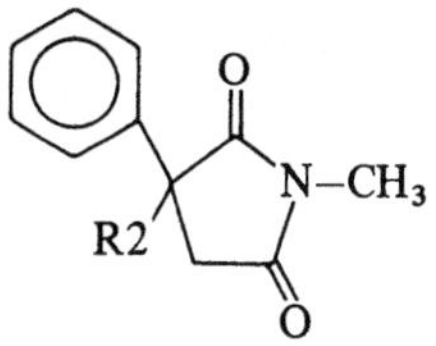

MES activity expressed in % protection of mice after i.p. administration of 200 mg/kg

R2 (HCl salts)	MES (% protection)
$-CH_2\cdot N(CH_3)_2$	60
$-CH_2\cdot N(C_2H_5)_2$	30
$-CH_2\cdot CH_2-N(CH_3)_2$	20
$-CH_2\cdot CH_2-N(C_2H_5)_2$	50
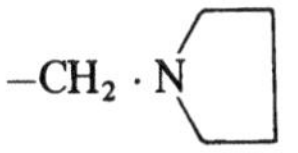	0
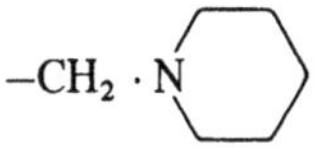	90
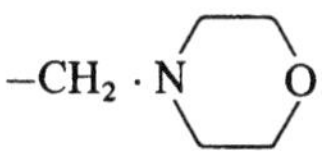	0
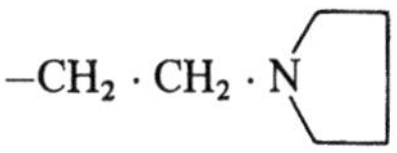	70
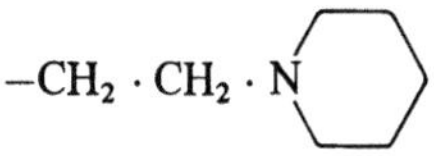	44 (at 100 mg/kg)
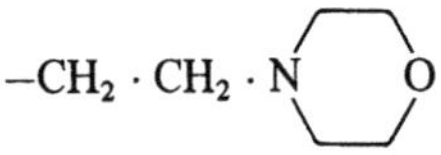	44
Phensuximide	20

via a CH_2-bridge, another type of amino-substituted succinimide will result (42) (WITIAK et al. 1977). These compounds exhibit moderate activity mainly in the electroshock test. With relation to its protective index (NTD_{50}/ED_{50}MES of 4, the index of phenytoin was found to be 10) the *N*-benzyl-substituted succinimide 43 was shown to be the most potent compound of this series.

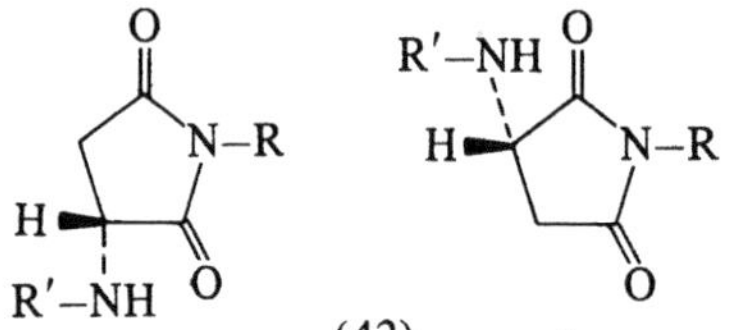

a (42) b

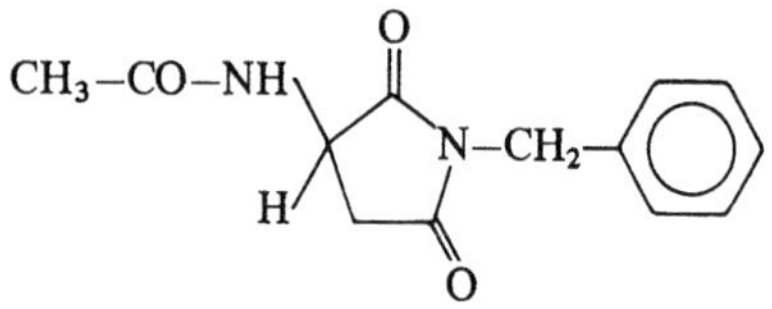

(43)

The authors (WITIAK et al. 1977) also separated the enantiomeres (42a, b) of these compounds. No significant differences in anticonvulsant potency between the activities of the members of the same enantiomeric pairs were observed while more striking differences between the activities of some enantiomeric pairs were noted for instance with regard to their influence on amphetamine-induced stereotyped behavior and in antagonizing oxotremorine-induced tremor.

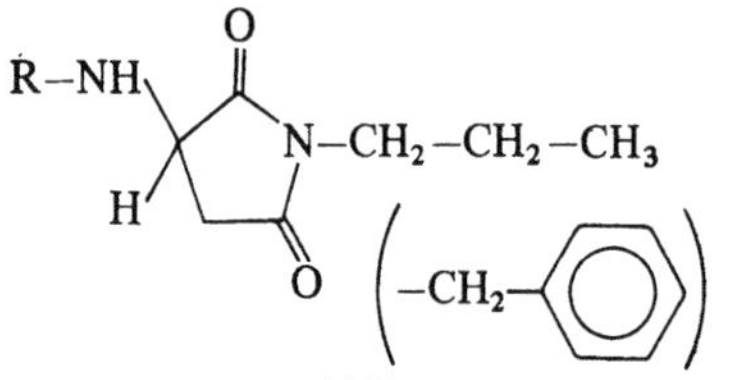

(44)

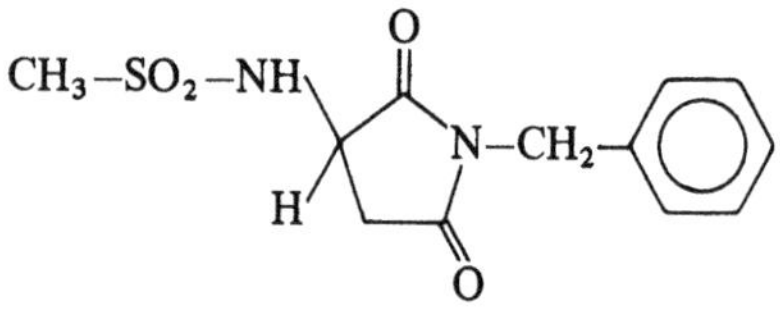

(45)

Table 7. Anticonvulsant activity of succinimide derivatives of the general formula

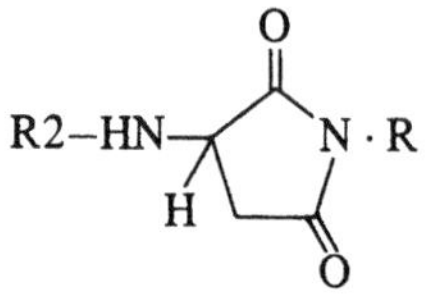

(CRIDER et al. 1981) tested in mice i.p. (ADDP method)

R2	R	MES at 0.5 h[a]	s.c. Met at 0.5 h[a]	NTD_{50}
H	$-CH_2C_6H_5$	++ (4/4)	++ (4/4)	4/4 at 600 mg/kg
$CH_3 \cdot NH \cdot CO-$	$-C_3H_7$	−	−	0/4
$CH_3 \cdot NH \cdot CO-$	$-CH_2 \cdot C_6H_5$	−	−	0/4
$C_4H_9NH \cdot CO-$	$-C_3H_7$	+	+ (2/4)	3/4 at 600 mg/kg
$C_4H_9 \cdot NH \cdot CO-$	$-CH_2 \cdot C_6H_5$	−	++ (1/4)	0/4
CH_3-CO-	$-C_3H_7$	−	+ (1/4)	0/4
CH_3-CO-	$-CH_2 \cdot C_6H_5$	+	++ (2/4)	0/4
CH_3-SO_2-	$-CH_2 \cdot C_6H_5$	288	120	422
Phensuximide		112	50	232

[a] ED_{50} (mg/kg), ++, +, or −, denoting activity at 300 and 600 mg/kg or no activity at 600 mg/kg. Numbers in parentheses indicate the number of protected animals or those exhibiting neurotoxicity as determined by the rotorod test

N-*n*-Propyl and *N*-benzyl succinimides of the general formula 44 have been evaluated (CRIDER et al. 1981); R represents H, $-COCH_3$, $-CONHR'$, and $-SO_2CH_3$. The most potent compound of this series was shown to be the racemic (R,S)*N*-benzyl-2-(methansulfamido)succinimide (45), which is active against both electroshock- and pentylenetetrazol-induced seizures (Table 7).

Attempts have been made to prepare potential long-acting anticonvulsants by attaching alkylating groups to either the carbon-2 of the phensuximide molecule or to the para position of the 2-phenyl substituent (KORNET et al. 1977a, b). $-CO-CH_2$-halogen, $-NH-CO-CH_2$-halogen, $-\overline{N-CO-CH=CH-CO}$ (maleimido), and $-NH-CO-CH=CH-COOH$ (maleamyl-) were the most-used alkylating

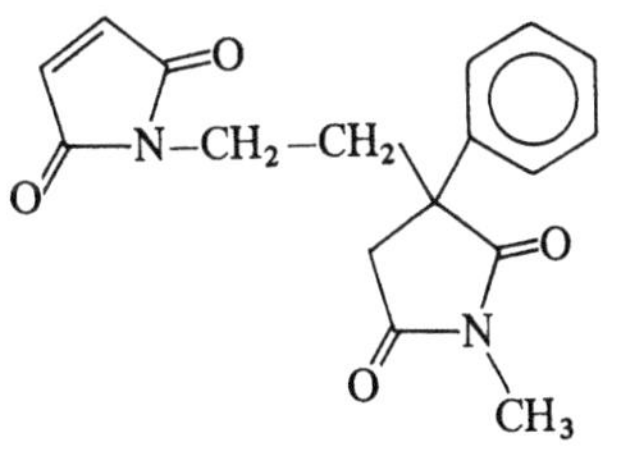

(46)

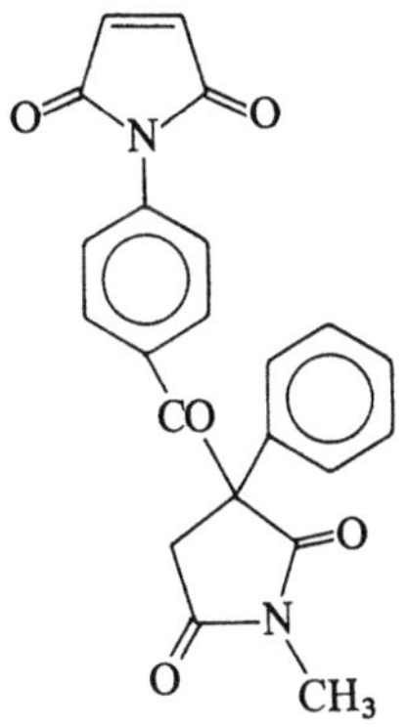

(47)

groups. An active compound of this series is 46, which exhibits a duration of action of at least 3.5 h, while 47 is an example of an inactive substance. Thus most bulky compounds were completely devoid of activity. The inactivity may be caused by a steric effect due to the inability in the complexing of these compounds to any active site.

The investigations of MILLER and LONG (1953b) confirmed that the anticonvulsant activity of succinimides in both electroshock and pentylenetetrazol tests did not improve by attaching halogen atoms as substituents to a phenyl ring on carbon-2. Nevertheless, studies were conducted to find succinimides that might exhibit a particular spectrum of anticonvulsant activity.

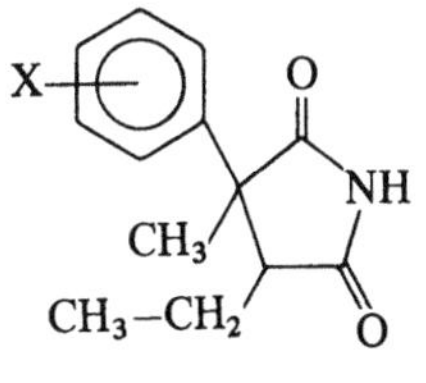

(48)

After 2-methyl-2-phenyl-3-ethylsuccinimide (48, $X=H$) was found to show tranquillizing or even hypnotic properties (CHEN and BASS 1964), a series of derivatives of 48 with $X=$ *o*-, *m*-, or *p*-halogen; *o*-, *m*-, or *p*-CH_3; *o*-, *m*-, or *p*-OCH_3;

p-NO_2; *p*-NH_2; or *m*-CF_3 were prepared and examined for their anticonvulsant activities. In derivatives of 48 containing *o*- and *p*-halogen, and *o*- and *p*-CH_3, the anti-MES and anti-Met activities of the parent compound were almost maintained. Other derivatives were less active or even inactive (HAUCK et al. 1967).

SCOULAR et al. (1976) investigated the influence of *p*-NO_2 and *p*-NH_2 substitution on the phenyl ring of methsuximide and phensuximide on the anticonvulsant activity of the parent compound; it had been anticipated that *p*-amino substitution would increase the anticonvulsant potency while decreasing the sedative action, by analogy with *p*-aminoglutethimide. However, there are no general rules for the structure-activity relationships of these *p*-substituted phenyl succinimides: *p*-Aminophensuximide (49) showed slightly increased anti-Met potency and nearly the same degree of sedative effect as phensuximide, whereas *p*-aminomethsuximide (50) exhibited decreased anti-Met activity compared with methsuximide. However, the largest changes of activity were observed when methsuximide or phensuximide were para-substituted by a nitro group. When phensuximide was *p*-NO_2-substituted (51) a compound with strongly increased anti-

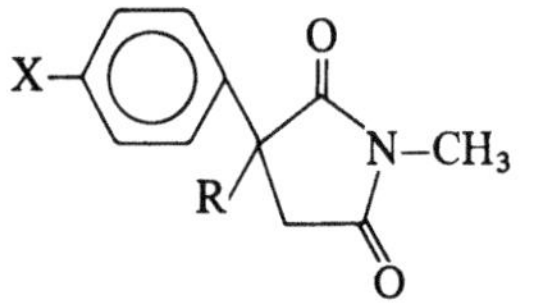

	X	R
(49) =	NH_2	H
(50) =	NH_2	CH_3
(51) =	NO_2	H
(52) =	NO_2	CH_3

Met potency resulted. On the other hand, the *p*-NO_2 compound 52 was virtually inactive in the Met test. Finally, LANGE et al. (1977a, b, 1979) prepared a series of new 2-phenylsuccinimides of the general formula 53, the phenyl groups of which are preferably meta-substituted by -halogen, -NO_2, and -CF_3. R mostly represents -H, -lower alkyl, -NH_2, and -dialkylaminoalkyl (Mannich bases). *N*-Morpholinomethyl-2-(3′-bromophenyl)succinimide (54) was considered to be an

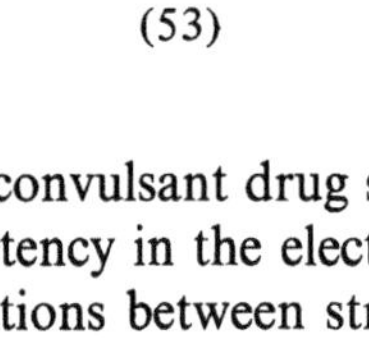

(53)

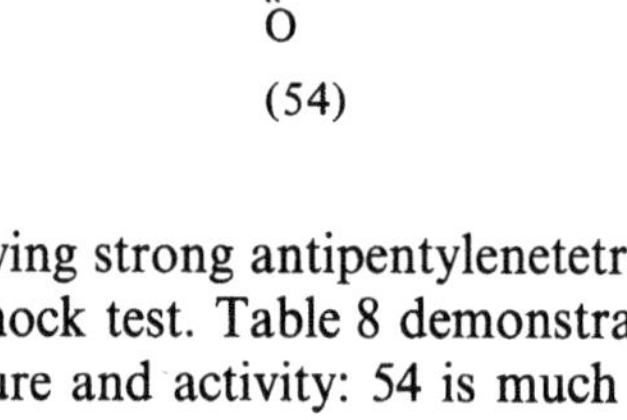

(54)

interesting anticonvulsant drug showing strong antipentylenetetrazol activity as well as high potency in the electroshock test. Table 8 demonstrates some more striking correlations between structure and activity: 54 is much more active in both tests than its 3′-fluoro analogue. When the morpholino group in 54 is exchanged for a piperidino moiety the resulting compound proves to be much more toxic and less potent in the anticonvulsant test (cf. Table 6).

Table 8. Anticonvulsant activity and acute toxicity of succinimides of the general formula

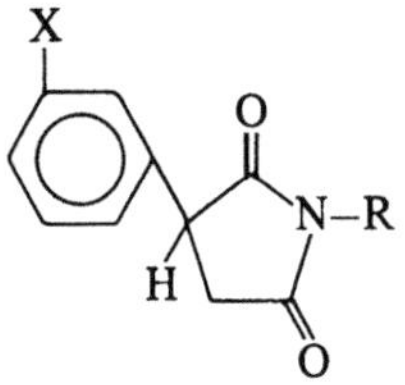

(LANGE et al. 1977a, b, 1979) tested in mice i.p. Drugs dissolved in dimethylsulfoxide/H_2O, 2:3. MES according to SWINYARD et al. (1952), Met, ED_{50} (after s.c. pentylenetetrazol, 119 mg/kg) or as factor of efficacy [ratio of convulsant $dose_{50}$ (CD_{50}) for treated animals to that of untreated animals]

X	R	MES ED_{50} (mg/kg)	Met		LD_{50} 24 h mg/kg	LD_{50}/ED_{50} (MES)
			ED_{50} (mg/kg)	Factor of efficacy		
H	CH_3 (phensuximide)	78.1	42	3.0	485	6.2
H	$-C_2H_5$	160.3	210		690	4.3
H	$-NH_2$	108.0		3.0	767	7.1
Br	H	48.4		2.0	310	6.4
Br	NH_2	37.3		1.6	387	10.4
F	NH_2	−(1/4 LD_{50})	261		555	–
Br	CH_2 · 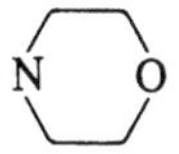	54.5		2.6	443	8.1
Br	CH_2 · 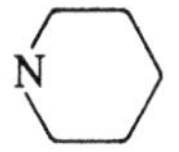	>1/4 LD_{50}		1.6	145	–
F	CH_2 · 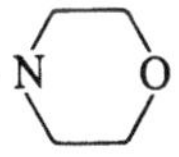	147.6		1.4	456	3.1
CF_3	H	42.1		2.6	252	6.0

C. Six-Membered Heterocyclic Compounds

I. Barbiturates and Other Compounds

As late as the 1960s a common structure such as –CO–NH–C(=X)– with X=O or H_2 was believed to be a prerequisite for a compound to be effective as a central-acting, e.g., antiepileptic, drug. Thus it happened that not only was phenobarbital introduced as an antiepileptic drug in 1912 by HAUPTMANN, but also other barbiturates and other six-membered heterocyclic compounds containing the above-mentioned structure moiety were screened for their anticonvulsant activity. Within the scope of a complete list of all the chemical compounds they had tested, MERRITT and PUTNAM (1945) published data on the anticonvulsant activity of 32 barbiturates administered to cats by different routes. Only the following substances were found to elevate the convulsive threshold to at least 50 mA at a dose of up to approximately 50 mg/kg in the electroshock test: 5-ethyl-5-phenyl barbituric acid [phenobarbital (55)], 5-butyl-5-phenyl barbituric acid, 5,5-diallyl barbituric acid, 5-ethyl-5-isoamyl barbituric acid, 5-ethyl-5-propyl-*N*-phenyl barbituric acid, and 5-allyl-5-cyclopentenyl barbituric acid. However, all of these compounds except phenobarbital were of no use as anticonvulsants on account of their predominantly hypnotic or even toxic properties at the dosage which sufficiently elevated the convulsive threshold.

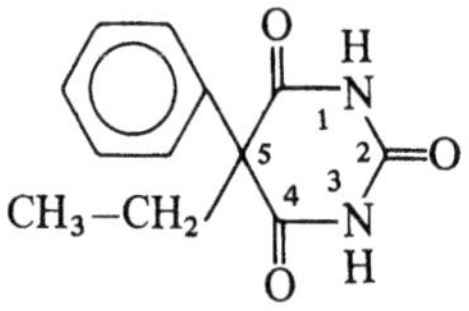

(55)

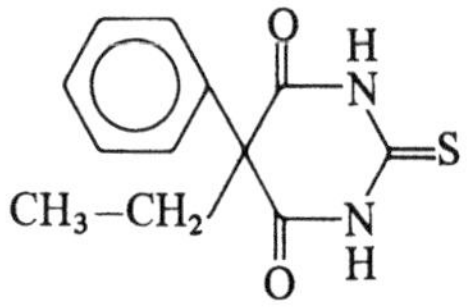

(56)

2-Thiophenobarbital (56) and 5-methyl-5-phenyl barbituric acid failed to elevate the anticonvulsive seizure threshold in the electroshock test up to 210 and 100 mg/kg, respectively.

Since 5,5-diphenylhydantoin is the most effective derivative in the hydantoin series it was assumed that 5,5-diphenyl barbituric acid (57) might also be a

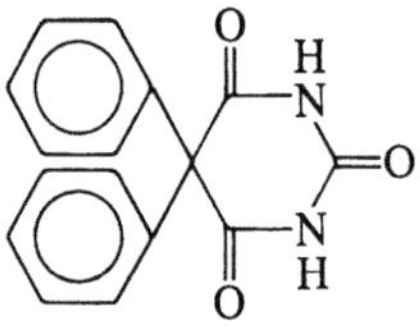

(57)

strongly active anticonvulsant. This expectation seemed to be disproved when 5,5-diphenylbarbituric acid was given to mice and was found to be less active than phenobarbital in the MES test (RAINES et al. 1973). In 1975, RAINES et al. repeated these investigations in rats. By this time 5,5-diphenylbarbituric acid appeared equipotent with phenobarbital on account of its improved absorption in this species. This conclusion was confirmed by the determination of the brain levels of 5,5-diphenylbarbituric acid and phenobarbital in rats being treated with MES protective doses of both these substances. The concentrations in brain associated with substantial protection were found to be: 2–6 µg/g for 5,5-diphenylbarbituric acid and 3.5–9 µg/g for phenobarbital (RAINES et al. 1975). 5,5-Diphenylbarbituric acid exhibits little or no hypnotic activity and might therefore be a favorable antiepileptic drug if, among other things, it were more readily available than hitherto by means of improved synthesis. The high efficiency of compound 57 was recently confirmed compared with the activity and neurotoxicity of several other barbiturates (RAINES et al. 1979).

This study and other above-mentioned examples show that in the barbiturate series small variations of the structure result in more extensive alterations of activity than in the previously discussed classes of compounds.

Thus a convulsant and some anesthetic and anticonvulsant barbiturates are distinguished by only minor structural changes in their side chains (ANDREWS et

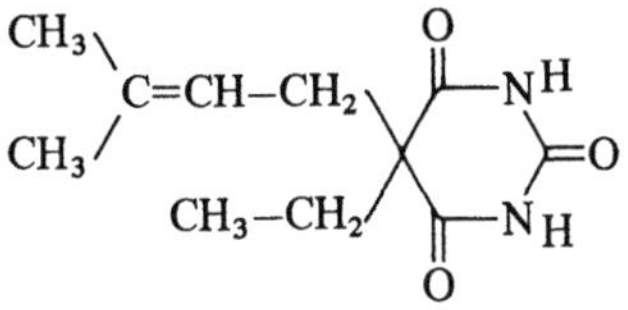

(58)

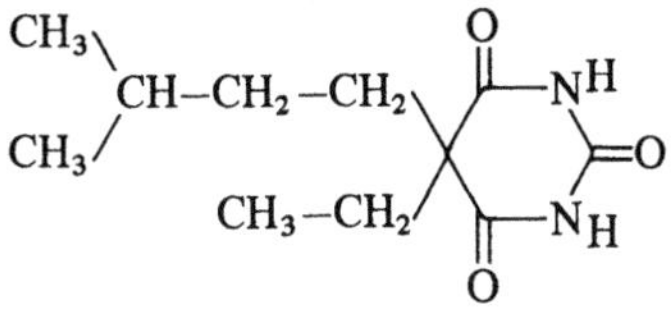

(59)

al. 1979). The convulsant 5-ethyl-5-(3′-methyl-but-2′-enyl) barbituric acid (58) and amobarbital (59), a useful anesthetic with a Met activity of 15 mg/kg only differ in the saturation of the side chain. Probably these differences in activity are primarily dependent on molecular conformation. This may be influenced not only by the shape and orientation of the C_5 side chain on carbon-5 but also by the accessibility of alternative conformations of the C5-ethyl group, and by slight deviations from planarity in the barbiturate ring (ANDREWS and JONES 1981; ANDREWS et al. 1981, 1982).

Hypnotic activity of a barbiturate might be changed to anticonvulsant activity by the introduction of a phenyl group on N_1 (60) (CZARNECKI and SOBANSKI 1980). However, it seems that the observed activity of compound 60 is mainly due to its biotransformation to compound 61 by lactonization.

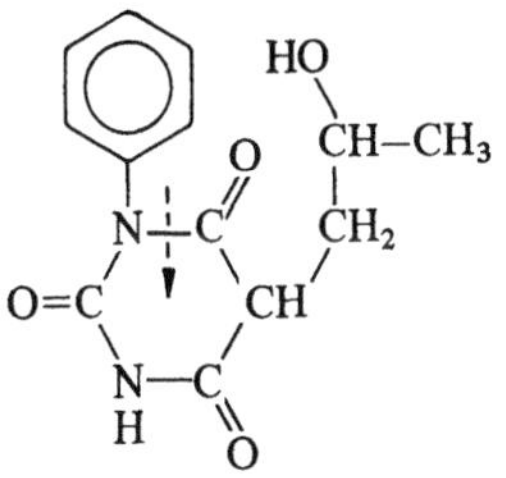

(60)

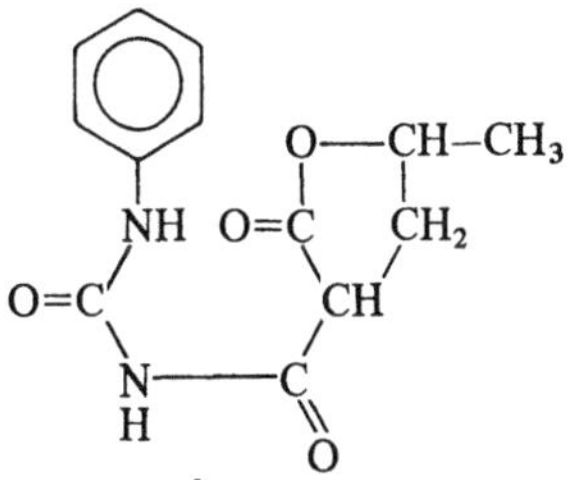

(61)

In an outline study we compared the MET activity of five- and six-membered heterocyclics of the general formula 62 (Schäfer and Leuschner unpublished

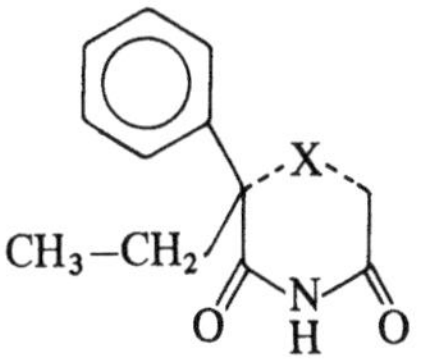

(62)

data). As shown in Table 9, none of the compounds has anti-MET activity corresponding to that of phenobarbital. On the other hand, the sedative-hypnotic glutethimide (63) is fairly similar to phenobarbital in its anti-MET behavior.

Table 9. Anti-MET activity (10 mA, 0.6 s, drugs administered orally, mice) of some five- and six-membered *N*-heterocyclics containing the common formula moiety

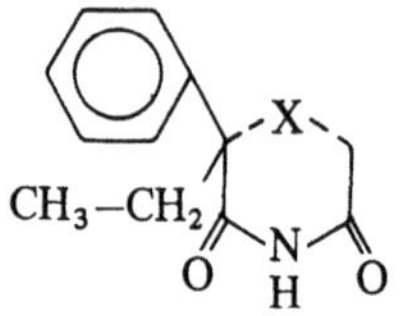

(SCHÄFER and LEUSCHNER, unpublished)

X	ED_{50} (mg/kg)
$-CH_2-$	70
$-NH-$	35
$-CH_2-CH_2-$	45
$-CH_2-NH-$	>500
$-NH-CH_2-$	60
$-C(=O)-NH-$	7

p-Aminoglutethimide (64) has even been used clinically as an antiepileptic drug, but it has been withdrawn because of its serious side effects. A series of glutethimide derivatives (65) was evaluated by ABOUL-ENEIN et al. (1975). It is remarkable that the introduction of an OH– or NH_2– group as a substituent on the heterocyclic ring does not change MES activity fundamentally. A similar observation will be discussed in the benzodiazepine series.

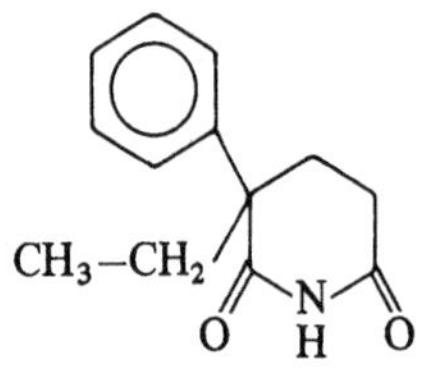

(63)

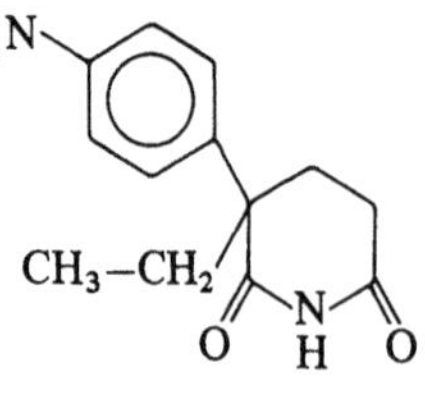

(64)

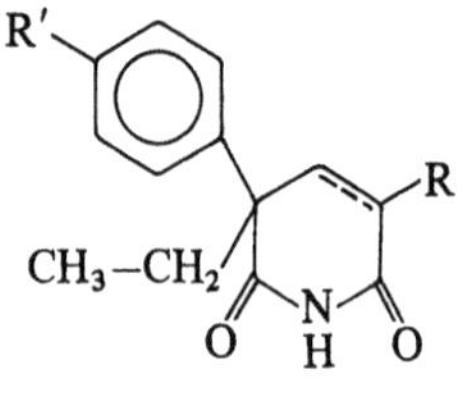

(65)

II. Phenobarbital and Primidone

Since the majority of barbiturates are clinically suitable only as hypnotics or even anesthetics, the 5-ethyl-5-phenyl moiety of phenobarbital is clearly the first essential for potent antiepileptic activity in doses with only marginal hypnotic action. Thus, only variations in nonessential parts of the phenobarbital molecule caused promising alterations in the mode of its action.

N-Methylphenobarbital (mephobarbital) (66) was proved to be an antiepileptic drug as early as 1932 by WEESE. Though its anticonvulsant activity in animal models was about the same, its hypnotic effectiveness was found to be lower. 1,3-Dimethylphenobarbital exhibits strong anti-MES and anti-Met activity. The most favorable *N*-substituted phenobarbital derivatives have been evaluated by SAMOUR et al. (1971) and VIDA et al. (1971, 1973a, b).

As is shown in Table 10 some of these *N*-substituted phenobarbitals exhibit strong anticonvulsant activity in both the MES and Met tests and have only weak or no hypnotic efficacy. All the *N*-substitutes mentioned in Table 10, unlike $-CH_3$ or $-C_2H_5$, are characterized by the sequence $-CH_2-X-$ (67), where X is –O–, $-N<$, -halogen, or –CS–. However, only those phenobarbital derivatives that are

Table 10. Anticonvulsant activity of some N1 and/or N3 substituted phenobarbitals of the general formula

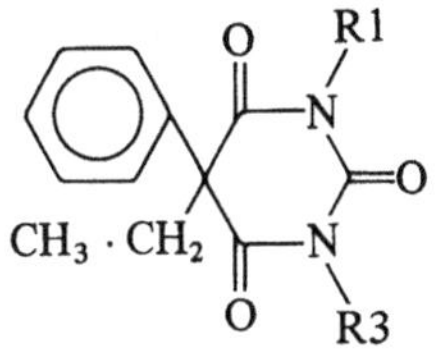

MES (60 mA) and Met (pentylenetetrazol, 106 mg/kg) according to SWINYARD et al. (1952)

R1	R3	MES ED_{50} (mg/kg)	Met ED_{50} (mg/kg)	HD_{50} (mg/kg)	Ref.
H (Phenobarbital)	H	20	10	100	VIDA et al. (1973a)
H	$-CH_3$	16	24	180	VIDA et al. (1973a)
$-CH_3$	$-CH_3$	~ 21	~ 15	~ 190	VIDA et al. (1973b)
H	$-CH_2 \cdot O \cdot CH_3$	22.5	4	> 100	VIDA et al. (1973b)
$-CH_3$	$-CH_2 \cdot O \cdot CH_3$	~ 50	16	> 500 < 1,000	VIDA et al. (1973a)
$-CH_3$	$-CH_2 \cdot O \cdot C_4H_9$	~125	32	> 1,000	VIDA et al. (1973b)
$-CH_2 \cdot O \cdot CH_3$	$-CH_2 \cdot O \cdot CH_3$	13.5	47.0	None (470)	VIDA et al. (1973a)
$-CH_2Br$	$-CH_2Br$	Inact.	~ 27	None (> 1,000)	VIDA et al. (1973a)
$-CH_2 \cdot O \cdot CO \cdot CH_3$	$-CH_2 \cdot O \cdot CO \cdot CH_3$	28	104		VIDA et al. (1971)
H	$-CH_2-N<$	< 12.5	~3	> 250 < 500	VIDA et al. (1973a)
$-CH_2 \cdot S \cdot C(=NH) \cdot NH_2$	$-CH_2 \cdot S \cdot C(=NH) \cdot NH_2$	In-active	In-active	> 1,000	VIDA et al. (1971)

HD_{50}, hypnotic $dose_{50}$; none, sleep did not appear except at lethal doses (in parentheses)

connected via N1 and/or N3 with moieties such as $-CH_2-O-$ or $-CH_2-N<$ show strong anticonvulsant activity in mice.

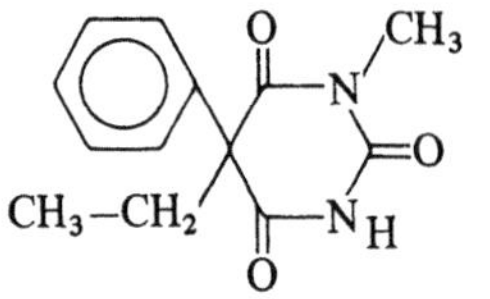

(66)

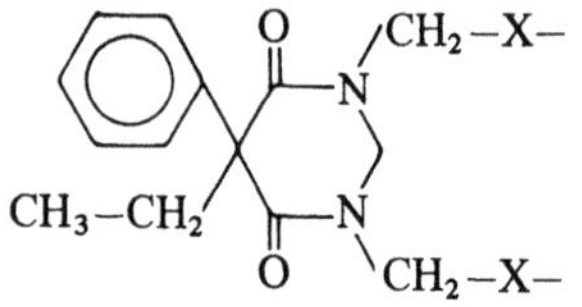

(67)

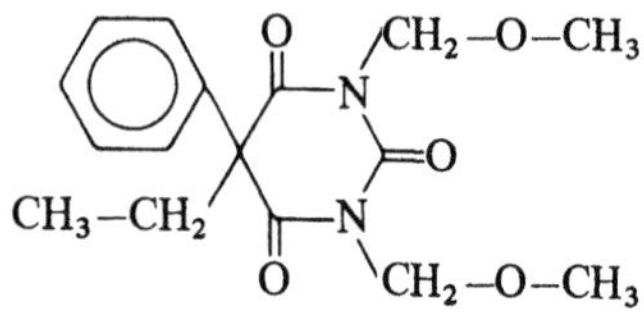

(68)

From these data it is likely that a new antiepileptic drug could be developed which displays activity similar to that of phenobarbital but without the latter's strongly sedative or even hypnotic effect. 1,3-Dimethoxymethyl-phenobarbital [eterobarb, DMMP (68)] was believed to be such an ideal barbiturate (GALLAGHER et al. 1975). However, these expectations have not been fulfilled during chronic treatment with this drug, and it must be assumed that, ultimately, phenobarbital itself, formed by progressive biotransformation, gradually becomes the biologically active agent (GOLDBERG et al. 1979).

When the 2-CO group of phenobarbital is replaced by $-CH_2$, a highly active anticonvulsant results (BOGUE and CARRINGTON 1953; GOODMAN et al. 1953). 5-Ethyl-5-phenyl-hexahydropyrimidine-2,4-dione [primidone (69)] is a very weak acid, which actually does not belong to the barbiturate class. Data on its anticonvulsant activity are compared in Table 12. The contribution of primidone itself to its antiepileptic activity is still under discussion. During chronic administration in man its efficiency is partly due to its metabolites phenobarbital and 2-ethyl-2-

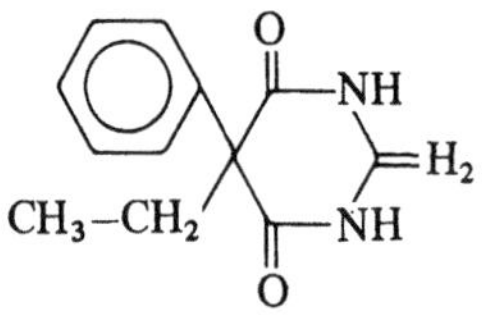

(69)

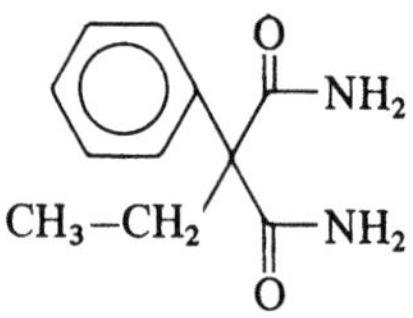

(70)

phenylmalonamide (PEMA) (70), the activity of which is under investigation. On the other hand, pretreatment of epileptic domestic fowl with SKF 525 A to inhibit the metabolism of primidone to phenobarbital has demonstrated primidone itself to exhibit strongly anticonvulsant efficiency (JOHNSTON et al. 1978). The preparation and testing of a primidone derivative substituted by a lower alkyl group on carbon-2 would yield much useful information on structure-activity relationships: such a compound would have to be prevented from being metabolized to phenobarbital.

D. Acyl Ureas

SPIELMAN et al. (1948) investigated more than 50 noncyclic acyl ureas structurally resembling the anticonvulsant barbiturates and the hydantoins. Barbiturates are malonyl ureas; however, like the hydantoins they also contain an acetyl urea moiety (71) as part of a heterocyclic ring system. Two of the straight-chained acyl ureas, phenylacetyl urea (phenacemide) (72) and 2-phenylbutyryl urea (pheneturide) (73) were really found to exhibit good anticonvulsant properties in animals and were mainly introduced in the therapy of psychomotor attacks.

EVERETT and RICHARDS (1952) gave more details on the pharmacological profile of phenacemide and summarized some structure-activity relationships in the series of substituted phenylacetyl ureas (74).

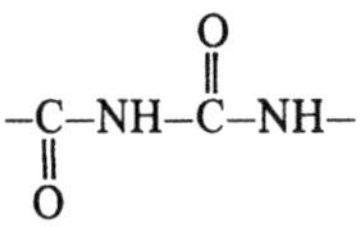

(71)

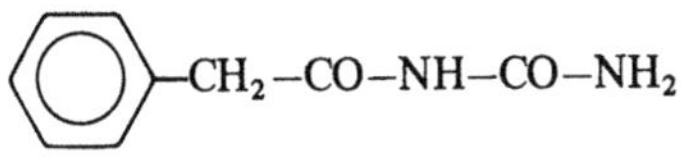

(72)

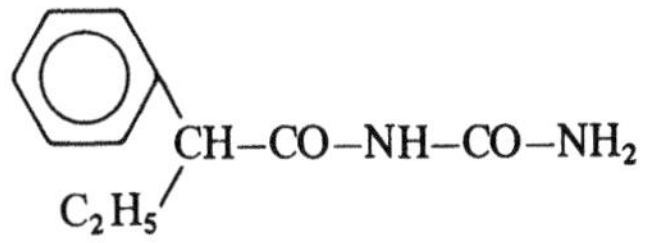

(73)

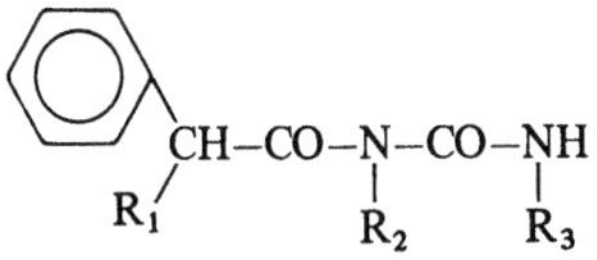

(74)

The unsubstituted phenyl group in (74) seems to be essential for adequate anticonvulsant activity. It is noteworthy that in mice antipentylenetetrazol activity is abolished when R_1 is C_2H_5 (with R_2 and R_3=H) in pheneturide, while excellent activity is found in the Met test when R_1 is H in phenacemide. When R_1 is phenyl (with R_2 and R_3=H) the resulting compound is most similar to phenytoin. However, unlike hydantoin with its high effectivity, the open-chained diphenylacetylurea was first found to be nearly inactive in animal tests (SWINYARD and TOMAN 1950), possibly due to its extremely low solubility in water. Though its anticonvulsant activity in mice may be enhanced by i.p. administration of sonicated suspensions (AMATO and JONES 1982), the relative potency of diphenylacetylurea (in terms of blood and brain concentrations) is nevertheless low compared with phenytoin and phenobarbital.

Phenacemide and pheneturide possess a number of side effects. Looking for a less toxic and more effective acyl ureide, NAKAMURA et al. (1968) proposed *N*-α-ethyl phenylacetyl-*N'*-acetyl urea ($R_1=C_2H_5$, R_2=H, $R_3=CO \cdot CH_3$, acetylpheneturide) (74). In mice, acetylpheneturide compared with phenacemide and pheneturide was found to have the strongest preventive effect against tonic extensor reflexes in MES and Met tests.

E. Tricyclic Compounds: Carbamazepine

5-Carbamoyl-5*H*-dibenz-*b,f*-azepine [carbamazepine (75)] was the first tricyclic compound to be clinically useful in the treatment of complex partial seizures and also beneficial in the management of generalized tonic-clonic convulsions. Developed in the 1950s and introduced in Europe in 1962 its anticonvulsant properties were described by THEOBALD and KUNZ (1963). Compared with other antiepi-

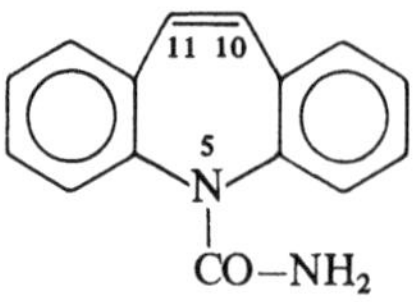

(75)

leptic drugs such as phenobarbital, phenytoin, valproic acid, diazepam, and clonazepam, carbamazepine was shown to exhibit remarkable anticonvulsant effects in a number of animal "epilepsy models" (KOELLA et al. 1976) and to be effective against electroshock-, pentylenetetrazol-, strychnine-, and picrotoxin-induced seizures. Furthermore, the "afterdischarge" in response to electrical stimulation of the hippocampus in unanesthetized cats was more effectively controlled than with phenytoin. Modifications of the substituents of the –10,11-double bond significantly alter the anti-MES activity of carbamazepine (GAGNEUX 1976; Table 11).

Table 11. Effect of minor molecular modifications on anti-electroshock activity (mice, 16 mA, 0.2 s) of carbamazepine (a) and some 10,11-derivatives (b–g) according to GAGNEUX (1976)

			MES ED_{50} (mg/kg)
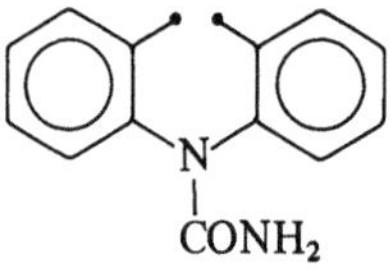	a	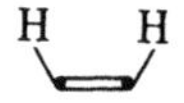	10
	b	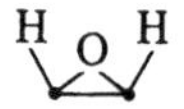	15
	c	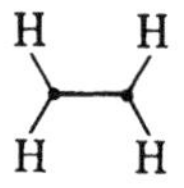	30
	d	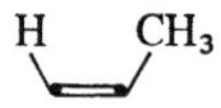	60
	e	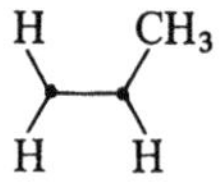	> 200
	f	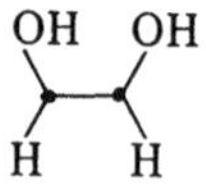	> 200
	g	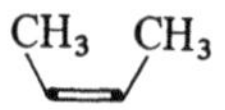	> 200

While *a* (Table 11) (carbamazepine) and *b* (carbamazepine-10,11-epoxide, the main metabolite of carbamazepine in serum) behave rather similarly in the MES test, *c* and *d* show decreased MES activity. The substituents in *e,f* (10,11-dihydro-diol-carbamazepine, another renally excreted metabolite of carbamazepine) and *g* abolish the protective action against the electroshock.

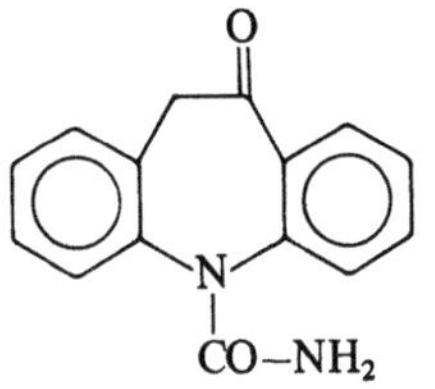

(76)

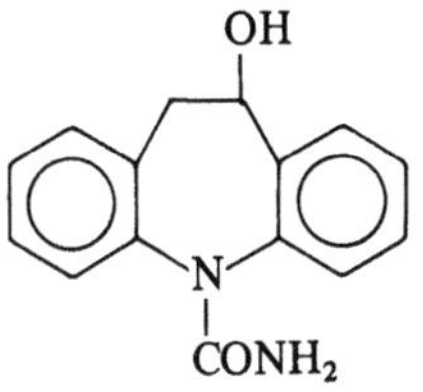

(77)

In some tests like electroshock and administration of pentylenetetrazol, strychnine, and picrotoxin, 5-carbamoyl-10,11-dihydro-10-oxo-5*H*-dibenz-*b,f*-azepine (76) and its main metabolite, the 10-hydroxy derivative (77), show favorable anticonvulsive activity in rats and mice (Baltzer and Schmutz 1977). However, compounds 76 and 77 are somewhat less potent than carbamazepine.

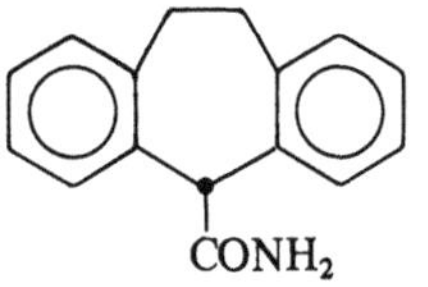

(78)

Dibenzo-*a,d*-cycloheptadiene-5-carboxamide (cyheptamide) (78), a compound similar to carbamazepine, was prepared by Davies et al. (1964a) and was also found to possess a high order of anticonvulsant activity. The anticonvulsant properties of cyheptamide and its open-ring analogue diphenylacetamide (79) were compared in a comprehensive study with the activities of other tricyclic carboxamides (80), including carbamazepine (75), its 10,11-dihydro-congener, and the analogue phenothiazine-*N*-carboxamide (77) (Table 12).

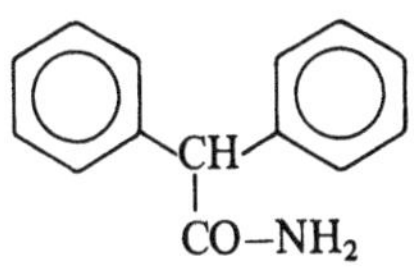

(79)

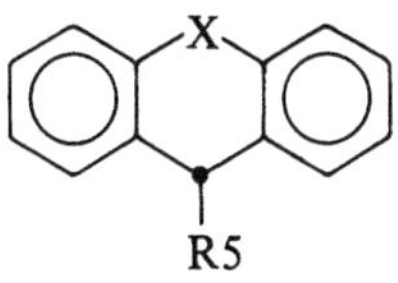

(80)

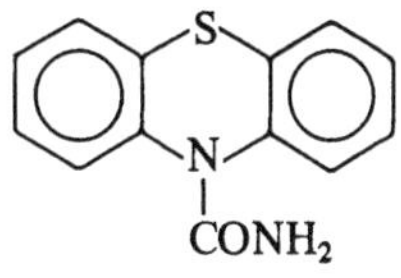

(81)

Some structure-activity relationships in the carbamazepine and congener series result from Table 12 and further data published by Davis et al. (1964a): Though there are significant differences in ED_{50} values, in general MES activity seems to be rather insensitive to the type and size of X provided that X is S or a lower nonbranched C-bridge and that position-5 (C or N) is substituted by a

Table 12. Anticonvulsant activity of tricyclic compounds (*80*) in mice p.o. selected from DAVIS et al. (1964a). MES (30 mA, 0.2 s) and Met (i.p. 100 mg/kg) according to SWINYARD et al. (1952), NTD_{50} values were determined by the rotorod test

X	R5	Ring-substituent	MES ED_{50} (mg/kg)	Met ED_{50} (mg/kg)	NTD_{50} (mg/kg)	NTD/Met
$-CH_2-CH_2-$	$-CO \cdot NH_2$		33	14.5	400	27.6
$-CH_2-CH_2-$	$-CO \cdot NH_2$	3-Cl	69	49	465	9.5
$-CH=CH-$	$-CO \cdot NH_2$		22.5	13	165	12.7
$-CH=CH-$	$-CO \cdot NH_2$	3-Cl	35	8	310	38.8
$-CH_2-$	$-CO \cdot NH_2$		42	15	175	11.7
$-CH_2-CH_2-CH_2-$	$-CO \cdot NH_2$		68	29	205	7.1
$-S-$	$-CO \cdot NH_2$		66			
[a]	$-CO \cdot NH_2$		62	22.5	~500	22.2
$-CH_2-CH_2-$	$-NH \cdot CO \cdot NH_2$		>400	53	>400	> 7.5
(*79*)			56	30.5	470	15.4
(*81*)			34.5	20	>300	> 15
(10,11-Dihydro-75)			20.5	21.5	176	8.2
Carbamazepine			18.5	11.5	66	5.7
Phenobarbital			17.8	3.6	76	20.8
Phenytoin			8.9	7[b]	84	12
Primidone			16	2[b]	>250	>125

[a] Single bond between two rings
[b] These data seem doubtful; see Chaps. 14 and 16

$CONH_2$. The C-bridge may be replaced by a single bond between the two phenyl rings or there may be no connection between the phenyl groups as in compound 79. If carbon-5 is substituted by other groups such as –NHR, MES activity will rise or toxicity will increase substantially. There are further differences in Met activity also with regard to the protective indices, which are dependent on the substituents of the tricyclic compounds. It is remarkable that the most active anti-Met substance is a ring-halogen derivative, 3-chlorodibenzo-*a,e*-cycloheptatriene-5-carboxamide (82), which has an NTD/Met index of 38.8. Cyheptamide

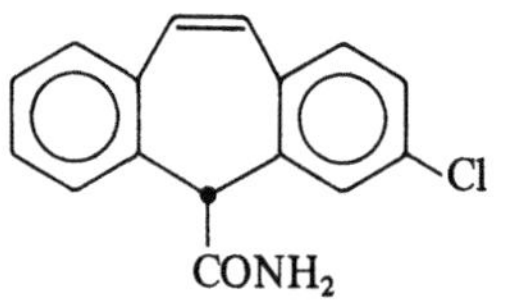

(82)

(78) was further investigated by FUNCKE et al. (1970). Though their investigation resulted in much lower Met activity than that found by DAVIS et al. (1964a) (Met ED_{50} 235 mg/kg and 14.5 mg/kg, respectively), the authors claimed cyheptamide to be a promising anticonvulsant. In view of its very low neurotoxicity and lethality, *N,N*-dimethyl dibenzo-*a,d*-cycloheptadienyl oxyacetamide (83) is worth mentioning (FUNCKE and ZANDBERG 1970). Out of a series of N-substituted 10,11-dihydrodibenz-*b,f*-1,4-oxazepines, none of which were active against

pentylenetetrazol-induced convulsions, the compound 84 was found to be active in the MES test (COYNE and CUSIC 1968; MES, 50 mA, 0.2 s; ED_{50} of 42 mg/kg, duration of effect of 2.5 h) and showed the relatively high ratio of neurotoxic to anticonvulsant effect of 10:1.

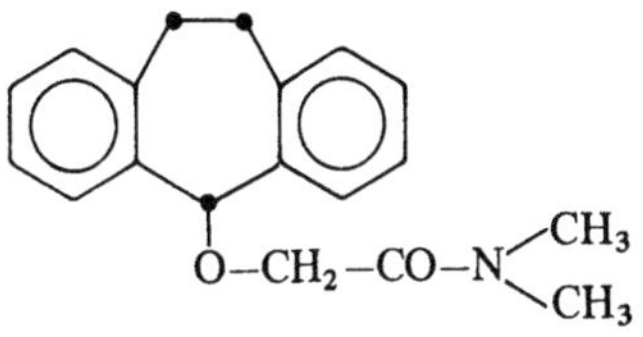

(83)

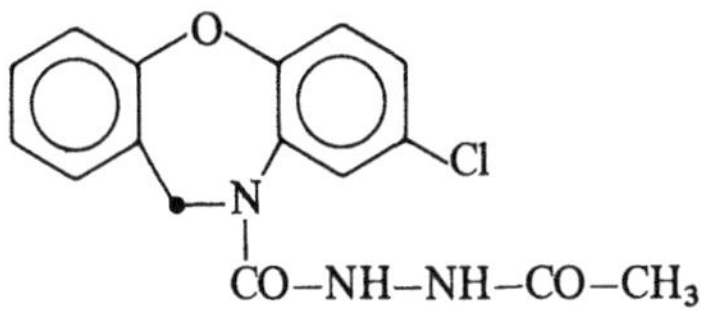

(84)

F. Benzodiazepines

The discovery of the central acting 1,4-benzodiazepines initiated a fascinating and successful chapter in the development of a new class of compounds, which have since superseded a previous generation of sedative drugs (STERNBACH 1973, 1980; STERNBACH et al. 1968; SWINYARD and CASTELLION 1966).

Since 1957, more than 3,000 of these and similar compounds have been prepared and pharmacologically screened. About 30 benzodiazepines have been clinically introduced as sedatives, tranquillizers, antianxiety agents, and last but not least antiepileptic drugs. Diazepam (85), nitrazepam (86), and clonazepam (87) are of current clinical interest and have proved to be very effective in the treatment of different types of epilepsy. On the other hand, there are some problems with side effects as well as with tolerance during chronic treatment. These problems will be discussed elsewhere. Further research activities to discover new antiepileptic drugs in this series are therefore indispensable.

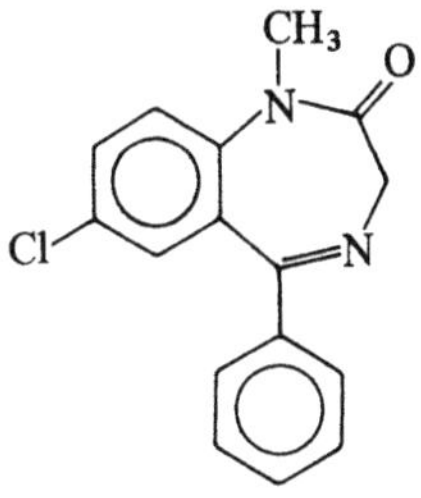

(85)

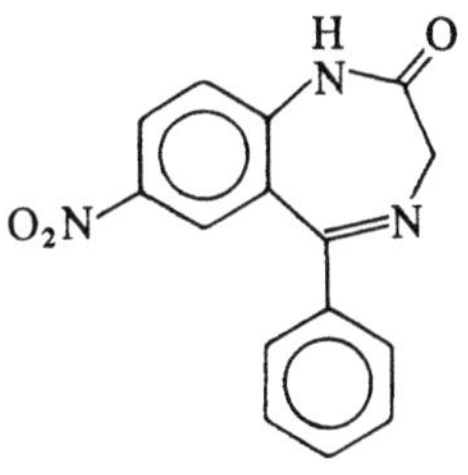

(86)

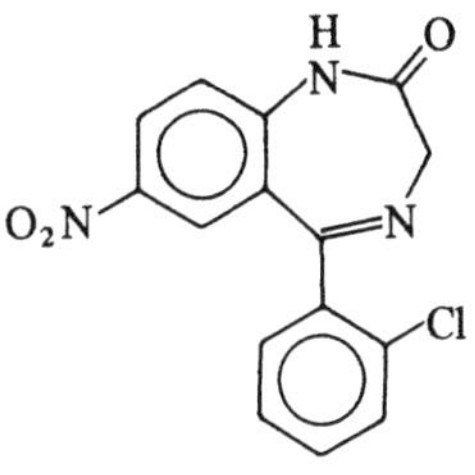

(87)

The high efficiency of diazepam and other 1,4-benzodiazepines as CNS-active drugs has initiated an intensive search for other active benzodiazepines, different in the positions of the two nitrogens in the seven-membered ring. Thus the *N*-desmethyldiazepam analogues of 1,3- (88, THOMAS, cited in CAMERMAN and CAMERMAN 1980) and 2,4-benzodiazepine (89, GOLIK 1975) have been synthesized and pharmacologically screened. While compound 89 seems to have a similar activity to diazepam, the 1,3-analogue (88) was reported to be rather inactive as an anticonvulsant. A differently substituted 5*H*-2,3-benzodiazepine (tofizopam) (90) was synthesized in Hungary (KÖRÖSI and LÁNG 1975).

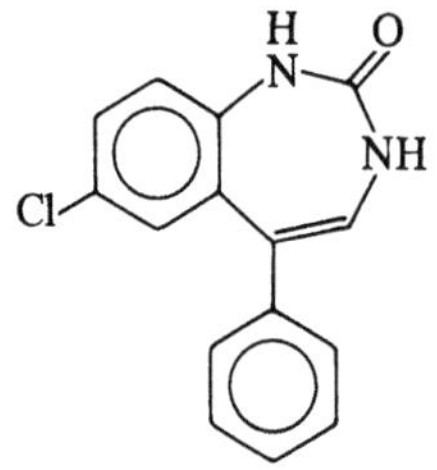
(88)

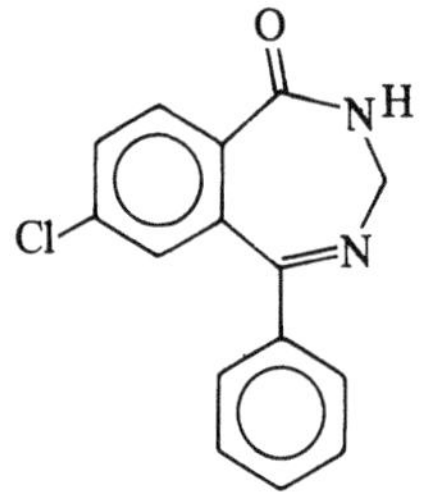
(89)

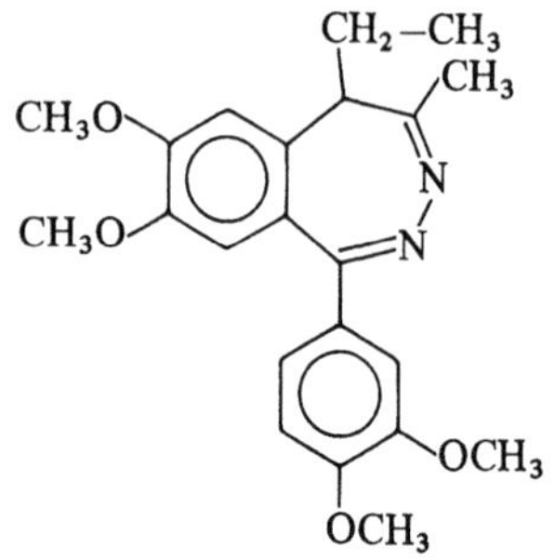
(90)

This compound was classified as a tranquillizer but was found to be inactive in antiseizure tests (PETÖCZ and KOSOCZKY 1975). Besides the original 1,4-benzodiazepines, some compounds in the 1,5 series with a structure following general rules similar to those valid in the 1,4 series are useful CNS-active drugs and will be discussed subsequently.

The basic structure of the biologically important 2,3-dihydro-1*H*-1,4-benzodiazepine-2-ones bearing a phenyl group in the 5-position of the heterocyclic ring is illustrated by the common formula 91, which also contains a schedule of substituents of some 1,4-benzodiazepines.

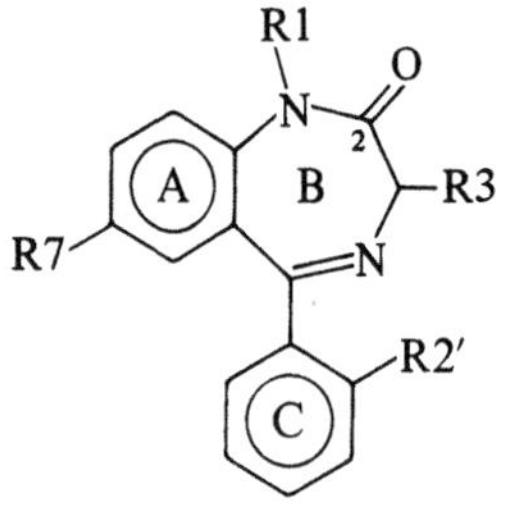
(91)

	R1	R3	R7	R2′	
Nitrazepam	H	H	NO_2	H	
Diazepam	CH_3	H	Cl	H	
Prazepam	$CH_2-\triangleleft$	H	Cl	H	
Flurazepam	$CH_2CH_2N(C_2H_5)_2$	H	Cl	H	
Oxazepam	H	OH	Cl	H	
Temazepam	CH_3	OH	Cl	H	
Clonazepam	H	H	NO_2	Cl	
Flunitrazepam	CH_3	H	NO_2	F	
Lorazepam	H	OH	Cl	Cl	
Camazepam	CH_3	$O-CON(CH_3)_2$	Cl	H	
Chlorazepate	H	COOK	Cl	H	2<(OK)(OH)
Medazepam	CH_3	H	Cl	H	(2)>CH_2

Ring A: A substituent in the 7-position is essential. The character of this substituent is also of great importance. Electron-withdrawing substituents, e.g., $-Cl$, $-Br$, $-NO_2$, and $-CF_3$, generally ensure high activity, whereas electron-releasing groups like $-CH_3$ or $-OCH_3$ lower the activity considerably. Substituents in any other position than 7 decrease the activity.

Ring B: Nitrogen-1 may be substituted preferably by a methyl group, by a lower alkyl group, or by a dialkylaminoalkyl group as in flurazepam. Carbon-3 may also be substituted by a $-COOH$ group as in chlorazepate. Free or esterified OH groups in position-3 do not significantly alter the activity of the compounds, e.g., in oxazepam and camazepam, respectively.

If the 2-C=O group is replaced by $-CH_2$ the anticonvulsant activity of the resulting medazepam mainly in the MES test is markedly decreased (RANDALL et al. 1968).

Table 13. Anticonvulsant activity of some benzodiazepines and their metabolites in mice p.o. (RANDALL and KAPPELL 1973). MES (30 mA) and Met (125 mg/kg) according to the methods of SWINYARD et al. (1952) and EVERETT and RICHARDS (1944), respectively. NTD_{50} values were determined by the rotorod test

	MES ED_{50} (mg/kg)	Met ED_{50} (mg/kg)	NTD_{50} (mg/kg)	LD_{50} (mg/kg)
Chlordiazepoxide	37	8	31	530
Diazepam	22	2	6	970
1-Desmethyldiazepam	19	1	4	2,950
3-Hydroxydiazepam	12	0.7	4	2,600
1-Desmethyl-4′-hydroxydiazepam	>200	>800	>200	> 800
Oxazepam	28	0.7	7	>4,000
Medazepam	36	7	4	820
Flunitrazepam	12	0.1	0.1	1,380
Nitrazepam	31	0.7	0.8	2,300
7-Aminometabolite of nitrazepam	600	>800	27	> 800
Clonazepam	400	0.2	0.2	>4,000
Phenobarbital	22	26	31	242

Ring C: Increasing activity is observed when halogens such as –F or –Cl are positioned in 2′ (=ortho). Any substituent in 3′ or 4′ decreases or abolishes the activity.

A strong correlation was demonstrated between the kinetics of a chemical reaction, namely the reduction of these benzodiazepines by sodium borohydride, and their ED_{50}s against pentylenetetrazol-induced seizures in mice, depending on the character of electron-withdrawing or -releasing groups especially in position-7 (SADAGOPA RAMANUJAM and TREFF 1978). It may be that the transition state between the benzodiazepinones and the postulated biological receptor (MÜLLER 1981) is similar to the transition state occurring in the sodium borohydride reduction of these compounds. Data in Table 13 compare the activity of the clinically used antiepileptic benzodiazepines, their main metabolites, and some important congeners. Furthermore, it may be mentioned that lorazepam is more active than oxazepam in the electroshock test and about ten times more effective in the pentylenetetrazol test than oxazepam (GLUCKMAN 1971). One of its metabolic precursors 2′-chlor-desmethyldiazepam is also very active in the Met test (TRAVERSA et al. 1977).

Ring A may be exchanged for other heterocyclic rings. Some of the resulting diazepines, which should preferably be similar to diazepam in rings B and C, were also found to be as active as diazepam in the pentylenetetrazol test: -pyrazolo[3,4-*e*][1,4]diazepine-7[1*H*]ones (92) (DEWALD et al. 1977); -1*H*-thieno[2,3-*e*][1,4]diazepines-2-ones (93) (TINNEY et al. 1974); and -pyrrolo[3,4-*e*][1,4]diazepine-2[1*H*]ones (94) (FONTANELLA et al. 1976). Benzodiazepines containing a C–N–N-bridge between nitrogen-1 and carbon-2 of ring B are the 6-phenyl-4*H*-*s*-triazolo[4,3-*a*][1,4]benzodiazepines. They have also been proved to be substances with strong CNS depressant activity. Estazolam, alprazolam, and triazolam (95)

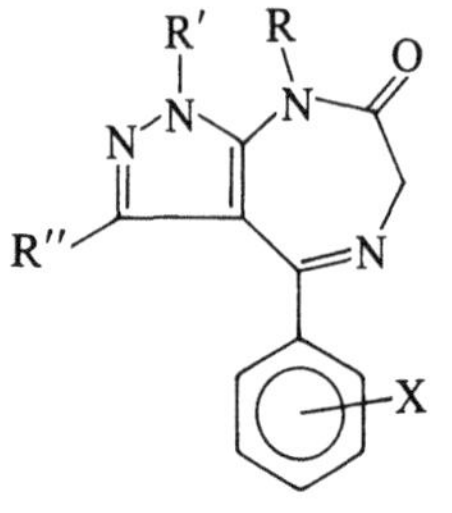

(92)

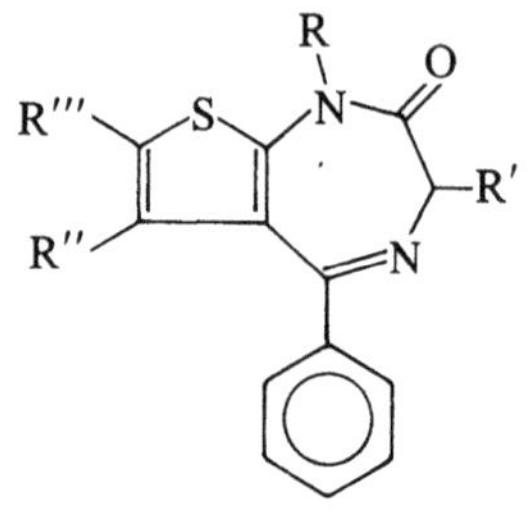

(93)

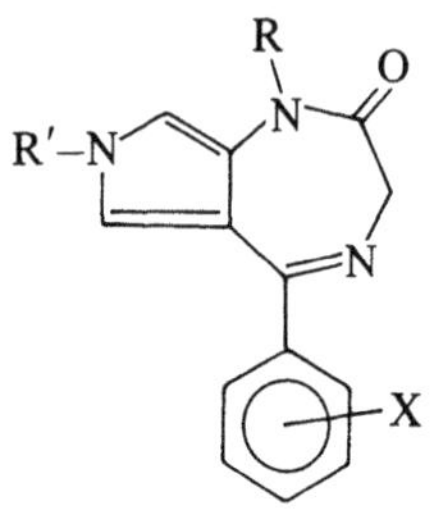

(94)

(HESTER et al. 1971) show efficiency against electroshock similar to that of diazepam. Some derivatives of compound 95 with an -alk(-en,-in)yl-N< group on carbon-1 strongly protect mice against bicuculline (tonic-extensor) and pentylenetetrazol (clonic) convulsions (HESTER et al. 1980 a). When the 6-phenyl group in alprazolam is replaced by piperidyl the pharmacological profile is hardly changed (HESTER et al. 1980 b).

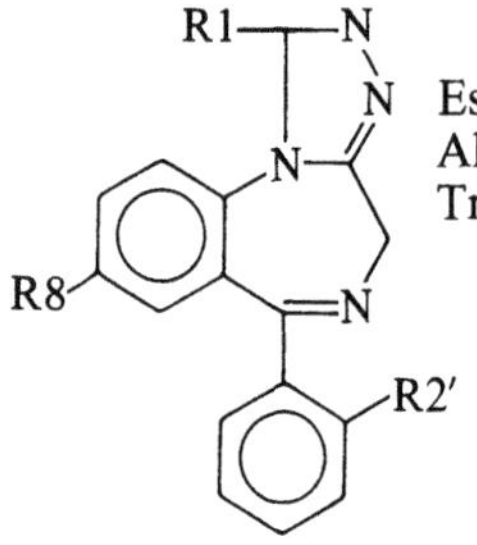

	R1	R8	R2'
Estazolam	H	Cl	H
Alprazolam	CH_3	Cl	H
Triazolam	CH_3	Cl	Cl

(95)

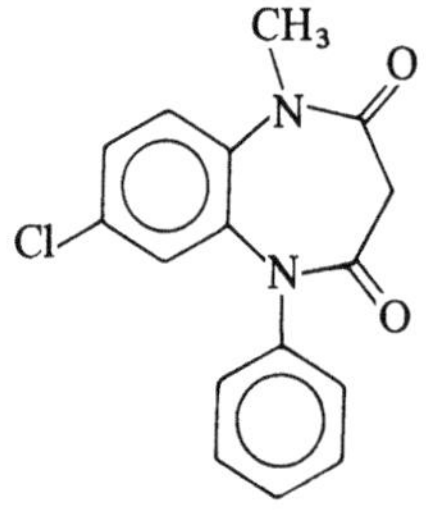

(96)

1,5-Benzodiazepines were synthesized by ROSSI et al. (1969). One of the most interesting compounds of this series, clobazam (7-chloro-1-methyl-5-phenyl-1*H*-1,5-benzodiazepine-2,4-3*H*,5*H*-dione) (96), was pharmacologically evaluated by BARZAGHI et al. (1973). Clobazam is active in mice against the tonic phase of seizures induced by pentylenetetrazol (oral $ED_{50} = 1.6$ mg/kg) or by maximal electroshock (oral $ED_{50} = 23$ mg/kg). In a comparative study clobazam and diazepam were found to be equipotent in the Met test in mice whereas clobazam was slightly more active than diazepam against the tonic extensor phase of the electroshock response (FIELDING and HOFFMANN 1979). On the other hand, the protection from pentylenetetrazol convulsions given by clobazam is weaker and shorter lasting in the rat than in the mouse (CACCIA et al. 1980 a). It may be that this difference in anti-Met activity is brought about by a difference in the brain levels of clobazam and its main metabolite *N*-desmethylclobazam, which contributes significantly to the high and long-lasting activity of the parent compound in mice (CACCIA et al. 1980 b).

From a chemical point of view the pharmacological similarity between clobazam and diazepam or even their equipotency is surprising. In ring B both molecules differ markedly with respect to their basicity (acid methylene protons on C3 of clobazam in contrast to the weakly basic imine group on N4 of diazepam), lipophilicity, and electronic charge distribution (KUCH 1979).

This structure-activity relationship between clobazam and diazepam demonstrates again that relatively large alterations in ring B influence the overall efficiency of the benzodiazepines to a lesser degree than small alterations caused mainly by substituents in ring A or C.

In clinical trials clobazam has been found to be active against all varieties of epilepsy. However, like or even more than other benzodiazepines its antiepileptic effectiveness diminishes after only a few weeks in one-third of all cases (Gastaut and Low 1979).

G. Valproic Acid

Though short-chain fatty acids with optimal activity at about C_8 had been known to cause CNS depression (Samson et al. 1956), it was very surprising when Meunier et al. (1963) found by chance that a simple C_8 fatty acid, 2-*n*-propyl pentanoic acid [valproic acid (97)], shows pronounced anticonvulsant activity, which was further studied in several seizure models (Frey and Löscher 1976). Valproic acid has since proved to be an efficient antiepileptic drug especially active against generalized seizures of the absence type.

$$\left.\begin{matrix} CH_3-CH_2-CH_2 \\ CH_3-CH_2-CH_2 \end{matrix}\right\rangle CH-CO-R \qquad \begin{matrix} (97)\ R = OH \\ (98)\ R = NH_2 \end{matrix}$$

Many esters and amides of valproic acid have been prepared and tested against pentylenetetrazol-induced seizures. The esters have proved barely active or inactive. Only dipropyl acetamide (98), which is therapeutically used in some countries, valproyl ureide, and a valproyl hydantoin derivative have been found to be active in the same range as valproic acid (Benoit-Guyod et al. 1968). The activity of valproic acid derivatives seems to be closely connected with the free acid or with a derivative which is quickly metabolized to the free acid. Thus the *N*-methylamide of valproic acid is barely active in single-dose Met tests. Valproyl anilide shows no anticonvulsant activity (Benoit-Guyod et al. 1969).

Concerning its antipentylenetetrazol activity valproic acid is only one active branched chained fatty acid among others similarly structured. Carraz (1967) demonstrated that the mortality of mice intoxicated with 80 mg/kg pentylenetetrazol depends on the size and structure of the fatty acid molecule used for pretreatment. The dosages of the compounds tested i.p. (Table 14) were equimolar to 200 mg valproic acid/kg mouse. Some α-ketocarbonic acids (C_4–C_6) were inactive in this experiment. On the other hand, the activity of the fatty acids rose with increase in molecular size and with increase in branching of the CH-chain, though it is incomprehensible that there is a sudden halt in the increase in activity: it remains to be confirmed that dibutyl acetic acid is indeed inactive.

Taillander et al. (1975) investigated a series of branched chained fatty acids and found that those containing 9–11 C-atoms were more active than valproic acid at a 0.9 mmol dose in the Met test. Thus dipropyl butanoic acid ($n=2$) (99) and dipropyl pentanoic acid ($n=3$) (99) demonstrated not only higher activity than valproic acid but also a longer duration of action. This may be due to consecutive metabolic degradation to valproic acid. C_8- and C_9-branched chain eth-

Table 14. Protection of mice intoxicated with 80 mg/kg pentylenetetrazol, by means of i.p. 200 mg/kg valproic acid (2-propylpentanoic acid) or of equimolar amounts of the C_4–C_{10} fatty acids shown (CARRAZ 1967)

	Number of C-atoms	Percentage of surviving mice
$CH_3 \cdot CH_2 \cdot CH_2$╲ $CH \cdot COOH$ $CH_3 \cdot CH_2 \cdot CH_2$╱	8	100
CH_3╲ $CH \cdot COOH$ CH_3╱	4	20
CH_3╲ $CH{-}CH_2{-}COOH$ CH_3╱	5	0
CH_3╲ $CH_3{-}C{-}COOH$ CH_3╱	5	80
$CH_3 \cdot CH_2$╲ $CH{-}COOH$ $CH_3 \cdot CH_2$╱	6	80
CH_3╲ $C{-}CH_2{-}COOH$ CH_3╱ | ╱CH╲ CH_3 CH_3	8	100
$CH_3 \cdot CH_2 \cdot CH_2 \cdot CH_2$╲ $CH \cdot COOH$ $CH_3 \cdot CH_2 \cdot CH_2 \cdot CH_2$╱	10	0

ylenic acids and amides have been investigated by TAILLANDER et al. (1977). The authors demonstrated that 2,3-unsaturated acids, i.e., 2-propyl-2-pentenoic acid, a metabolite of valproic acid, are somewhat less active than the corresponding saturated acids. 3-Propyl-2-hexenamide (100) was described to be a mildly hypnotic drug in mice.

$$(CH_3{-}CH_2{-}CH_2)_2CH(CH_2)_n{-}COOH$$

(99)

$$(CH_3{-}CH_2{-}CH_2)_2C{=}CH{-}CONH_2$$

(100)

It would be of great pharmacological and clinical interest to know whether or not active metabolites of valproic acid may contribute to its antiepileptic activity. Some metabolites have been prepared (SCHÄFER and LÜHRS 1978; SCHÄFER et al. 1980) and exact data on their effects on electro- and chemoconvulsive thresholds

Table 15. Anticonvulsant efficiency of metabolites of valproic acid on the threshold for electroshock and pentylenetetrazol convulsions in mice. The potency relative to valproic acid (=1) was calculated on a molar basis. (LÖSCHER 1981)

Metabolite (prop = $CH_3 \cdot CH_2 \cdot CH_2-$)	Potency relative to valproic acid		
	Electro shock threshold	Pentylenetetrazol seizure threshold	
		Clonic	Tonic
$CH_3-CH_2-CH=C(prop)-COOH$	0.49	Not tested	Not tested
$CH_3-CH=CH-CH(prop)-COOH$	0.36	Not tested	Not tested
$CH_2=CH-CH_2-CH(prop)-COOH$	0.87	0.59	0.57
$CH_3-CH_2-CH(OH)-CH(prop)-COOH$	0.13	0.45	0.34
$CH_3-CH_2-CO-CH(prop)-COOH$	0.17	Inactive	0.28
$CH_3-CH(OH)-CH_2-CH(prop)-COOH$	0.26	0.48	0.33
$CH_2(OH)-CH_2-CH_2-CH(prop)-COOH$	Inactive	0.21	0.29

in mice have been collected (LÖSCHER 1981). Table 15 shows the potency of the tested compounds relative to valproic acid in both threshold tests.

BENOIT-GUYOD et al. (1972, 1973) tested the anticonvulsant activity of compounds which resulted from replacing the biologically active dipropylacetyl moiety in 101 A by the amino compound of the general formula 101 B. Only the acetamide of 1-methyl-2-propylpentylamine (102) exhibited some anticonvulsant and tranquilizing activity.

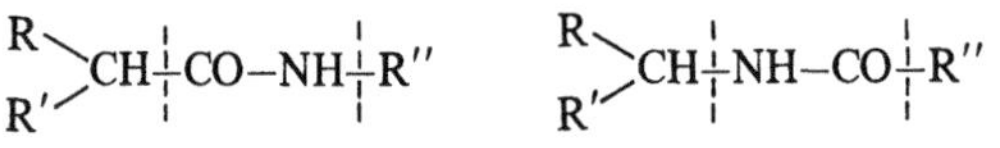

A (101) *B*

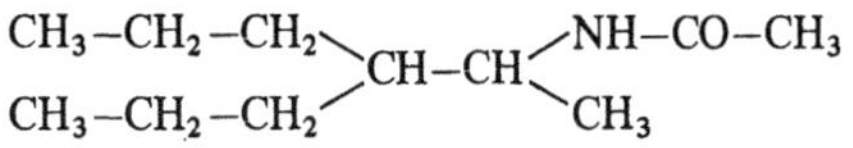

(102)

H. Miscellaneous Compounds

In the final section of this chapter on chemical constitution and anticonvulsant activity we will briefly summarize some recent developments in the field of new anticonvulsant drugs. Our aim has been to demonstrate the widest possible selection from the different structures of compounds which have been found to show promising anticonvulsant activity and which are therefore undergoing clinical trial.

Sulfonamides are known to exhibit anticonvulsant activity. Benzene-sulfonamides (103) *p*-substituted by electron-withdrawing substituents are highly active in protecting mice against maximal electroshock seizures. Due to their simple chemical structure these aromatic sulfonamides are favored objects of QSAR studies (HAGEN et al. 1980).

The sulfonamides sulthiame (104) and acetazolamide (105) have been used sporadically for the treatment of psychomotor and other types of seizures. Both drugs are powerful inhibitors of carbonic anhydrase; this inhibition seems to be partly responsible for their antiepileptic action. The usefulness of acetazolamide is limited because of the rapid development of tolerance to its anticonvulsant effect. Sulfanilamide itself (106) shows moderate activity against electrically in-

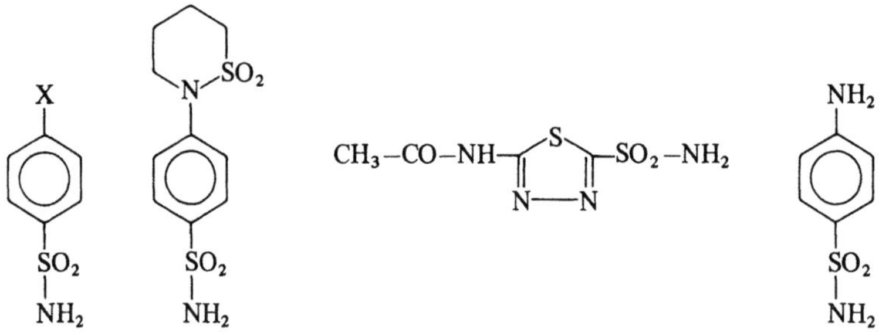

(103) (104) (105) (106)

duced seizures, which could be enhanced by substitution of the phenyl ring with a halogen atom (GANZ et al. 1978). In this series the relationship between anticonvulsant activity and inhibition of the renal and cerebral carbonic anhydrase has been discussed but not clarified.

WASER et al. (1977a–c; 1978) tested a great many derivatives of sulfanilamide, the *p*-amino group of which was part of a heterocyclic ring such as succinimide, hydantoin, pyrrolidone, or imidazolidone. Out of this class of sulfonamide compounds, 3-chloro-4-(2-phenylsuccinimido)-benzenesulfonamide (107) with a MET (5 mA, 0.35 s) ED_{50} of 7.8 mg/kg and a Met (100 mg/kg pentylenetetrazol) ED_{50} of 64 mg/kg in mice was selected for clinical trials (TCHICALOFF and MITROI 1975).

While (107) still contains structural components of previously known antiepileptic drugs, the following examples demonstrate novel types of compounds.

In Japan an aliphatic sulfonamide, 3-sulfamoylmethyl-1,2-benzisoxazole (108) was found to be more active and less neurotoxic than many of the known antiepileptic drugs (UNO et al. 1979; MASUDA et al. 1980). From its pharmacological profile this drug can be classified as an effective agent for treatment of grand

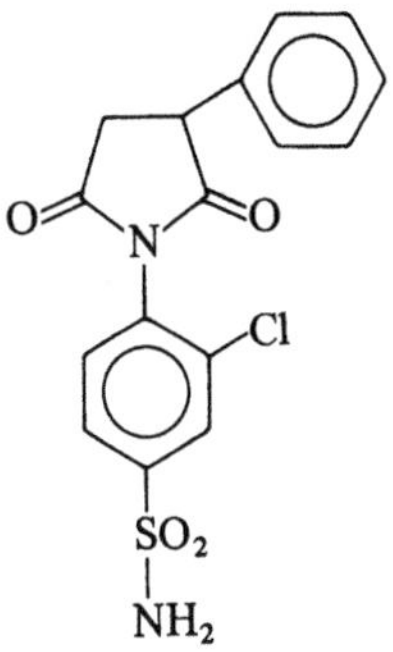

(107)

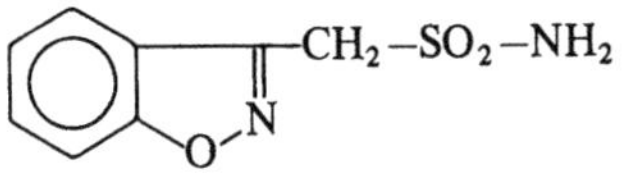

(108)

mal epilepsy. No tolerance develops to its anticonvulsant activity against MES and obviously it does not exert its anticonvulsant efficiency through inhibition of carbonic anhydrase. Thus the mechanism of action of this aliphatic sulfonamide is different from that of the above-mentioned aromatics.

In Italy 1-[4-(phenylethyl)phenyl]-2-(*N*-imidazolyl)ethanol (109), with an ED_{50} of 5.3 mg/kg in the electroshock test after i.p. treatment in mice, has been selected for further studies (NARDI et al. 1981). In the United States a similar compound 1-(2-naphthoylmethyl)imidazole-HCl (110) was developed and designed for testing in humans (WALKER et al. 1981).

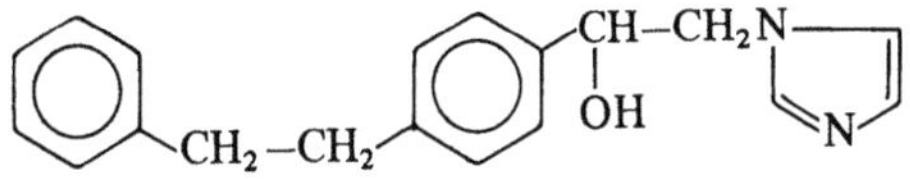

(109)

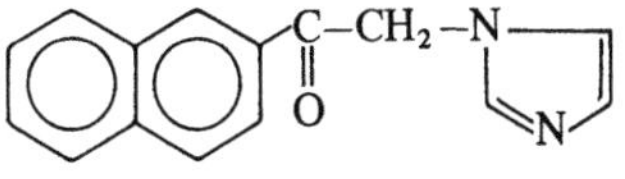

(110)

After selection from a great number of α-ethylene alcohols exhibiting CNS activity (ASTOIN et al. 1978), 4,4-dimethyl-1(3′,4′-methylenedioxy phenyl)-pentene-1-ol-3 [stiripentol (111)] has been suggested for clinical trials.

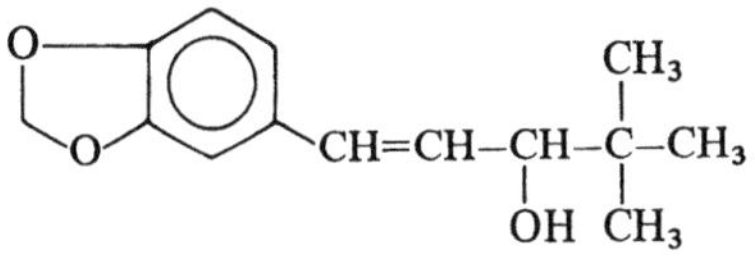

(111)

BALSAMO et al. (1975, 1977, 1981) investigated a series of cinnamamides which were predominantly α,β-dimethyl substituted with different R groups (Cl, CF_3, OCH_3) in the *m*- or *p*-position (112) and showed that some of them prevented maximal extensor seizures induced by pentylenetetrazol in mice. Another compound from this class, more simple in structure, 3-bromo-*N*-ethylcinnamamide [cinromide (113)], seems to be favorable not only in its pharmacological profile,

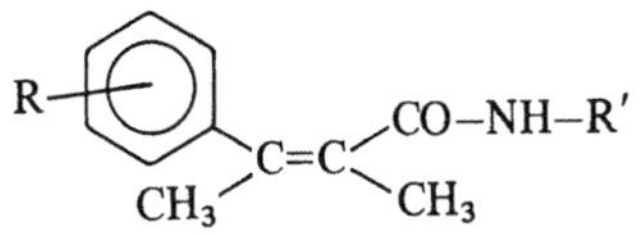

(112)

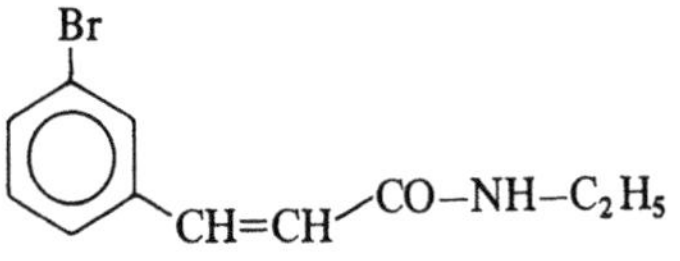

(113)

which shows a broad spectrum of anticonvulsant activity (SOROKO et al. 1981), but also as a useful antiepileptic drug in current clinical trials.

Schiff bases of γ-aminobutyric acid (GABA) or its amide represent another type of compound with potential anticonvulsant activity. They serve as a carrier for GABA, which by itself cannot easily cross the blood-brain barrier. 4-[[(4-Chlorophenyl)(5-fluoro-2-hydroxyphenyl)-methylene]amino]butanamide [progabide (114)] or the corresponding acid (OH instead of NH_2) was considered as a GABA agonist, releasing the γ-aminobutyric acid moiety of the molecule after distribution into brain. This mechanism of action is obvious from the displacement of [^{3}H]-GABA from its membrane-binding sites by progabide (KAPLAN et al. 1980).

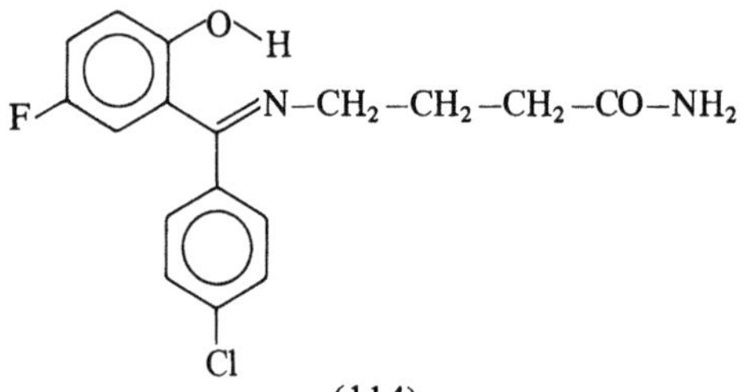

(114)

References

Aboul-Enein HY, Schauberger ChW, Hansen AR, Fischer LJ (1975) Synthesis of an active hydroxylated glutethimide metabolite and some related analogs with sedative-hypnotic and anticonvulsant properties. J Med Chem 18:736–741

Amato RJ, Jones GL (1982) Reassessment of the anticonvulsant activity of diphenylacetyl urea. Drug Dev Res 2:47–53

Andrews PR, Jones GP (1981) Convulsant and anticonvulsant barbiturates. 2. Molecular orbital calculations. Eur J Med Chem 16:139–143

Andrews PR, Jones GP, Lodge D (1979) Convulsant, anticonvulsant and anaesthetic barbiturates. 5-Ethyl-5-(3′-methyl-but-2′-enyl)-barbituric acid and related compounds. Eur J Pharmacol 55:115–120

Andrews PR, Jones AJ, Jones GP, Marker A, Owen EA (1981) Convulsant and anticonvulsant barbiturates. 3. Conformational analysis by ^{1}H and ^{13}C NMR. Eur J Med Chem 16:145–150

Andrews PR, Jones GP, Poulton DB (1982) Convulsant, anticonvulsant and anaesthetic barbiturates. In vivo activities of oxo- and thiobarbiturates related to pentobarbitone. Eur J Pharmacol 79:61–65

Astoin J, Marivain A, Riveron A, Crucifix M, Lapotre M, Torrens Y (1978) Action de nouveaux alcools – éthyléniques sur le système nerveux central. Eur J Med Chem 13:41–47

Balsamo A, Barili PL, Crotti P, Macchia B, Macchia F, Pecchia A, Cuttica A, Passerini N (1975) Structure-activity relationships in cinnamamides. 1. Synthesis and pharmacological evaluation of some (E)- and (Z)-*N*-alkyl-α,β-dimethylcinnamamides. J Med Chem 18:842–846

Balsamo A, Barili PL, Crotti P, Macchia B, Macchia F, Cuttica A, Passerini N (1977) Structure-activity relationships in cinnamamides. 2. Synthesis and pharmacological evaluation of some (E)- and (Z)-*N*-alkyl-α,β-dimethylcinnamamides substituted on the phenyl group. J Med Chem 20:48–53

Balsamo A, Crotti P, Lapucci A, Macchia B, Macchia F, Cuttica A, Passerini N (1981) Structure-activity relationship in cinnamamides. 3. Synthesis and anticonvulsant activity evaluation of some derivatives of (E)- and (Z)-*m*-(trifluoromethyl)cinnamamide. J Med Chem 24:525–532

Baltzer V, Schmutz M (1977) Experimental anticonvulsive properties of GP 47680 and of GP 47779, its main human metabolite; compounds related to carbamazepine. In: Meinardi H, Rowan AJ (eds) Advances in epileptology. Proceedings of the 13th congress of the international league against epilepsy and 9th symposium of the international bureau for epilepsy. Swets and Zeitlinger, Amsterdam, p 295

Barzaghi F, Fournex R, Mantegazza P (1973) Pharmacological and toxicological properties of clobazam (1-phenyl-5-methyl-8-chloro-1,2,4,5-tetrahydro-2,4-diketo-3*H*-1,5-benzodiazepine), a new psychotherapeutic agent. Arzneimittelforsch 23:683–686

Benoit-Guyod JL, Boucherle A, Benoit-Guyod M, Dardas A, Rupp R, Eymard P, Carraz G, Boitard M, Lebreton S, Beriel H, Meunier H (1968) Dérivés de l'acide dipropylacétique. III. Nouveaux amides et esters. Chim Ther 5:336–342

Benoit-Guyod JL, Benoit-Guyod M, Boucherle A, Eymard P, Carraz G, Meunier H (1969) Dérivés de l'acide dipropylacétique. IV. Etude des relations entre la structure et l'activité antalgique de quelques dipropylacétanilides substitués. Chim Ther 1:17–20

Benoit-Guyod M, Benoit-Guyod JL, Boucherle A, Broll M, Eymard P (1972) Recherches dans la série dipropylacétique. VII. Structures homologues: amides et urées substituées provenant de la propyl-1 butylamine. Eur J Med Chem 5:388–392

Benoit-Guyod M, Benoit-Guyod JL, Boucherle A, Broll M, Eymard P (1973) Recherches dans la série dipropylacétique. IX. Structures homologues: methyl-1 propyl-2 pentylamine, amides et urées substituées. Eur J Med Chem 4:412–418

Billman JH, Hidy PhH (1943) *N,N'*-Substituted α-aminodiphenylacetamides. J Am Chem Soc 65:760–761

Bogue JY, Carrington HC (1953) The evaluation of "Mysoline" – a new anticonvulsant drug. Br J Pharmacol 8:230–236

Brown WC, Schiffman DO, Swinyard EA, Goodman LS (1953) Comparative assay of antiepileptic drugs by "psychomotor" seizure test and minimal electroshock threshold test. J Pharmacol Exp Ther 107:273–283

Butler TC (1953) Quantitative studies of the demethylation of trimethadione (TRIDIONE®). J Pharmacol Exp Ther 108:11–17

Butler TC, Waddell WJ (1957) Metabolic deethylation of 5,5-dimethyl-3-ethyl-2,4-oxazolidinedione (dimedion). Arch Int Pharmacodyn 111:308–313

Caccia S, Carli M, Garattini S, Poggesi E, Rech R, Samanin R (1980a) Pharmacological activities of clobazam and diazepam in the rat: relation to drug brain levels. Arch Int Pharmacodyn Ther 243:275–283

Caccia S, Guiso G, Garattini S (1980b) Brain concentrations of clobazam and *N*-desmethylclobazam and antileptazol activity. J Pharm Pharmacol 32:295–296

Caccia S, Ballabio M, Garattini S (1980c) Relationship between camazepam, *N*-methyloxazepam and oxazepam brain concentrations and antileptazol effect in the rat. J Pharm Pharmacol 33:185–187

Call L (1970) 5,5-Diphenyl-3-hydroxy-hydantoin. Monatsschr Chem 101:228–239

Camerman A, Camerman N (1980) Structure-activity relationships. Stereochemical similarities in chemically different antiepileptic drugs. In: Glaser GH, Penry JK, Woodbury DM (eds) Antiepileptic drugs: mechanism of action. Raven, New York, p 223

Carraz G (1967) Approches pour une théorie sur l'activité de la structure die -*n*-propylacétique. Agressologie 8:13–20

Chen G, Bass P (1964) Certain pharmacological properties of 3-ethyl-2-methyl-2-phenylsuccinimide. Arch Int Pharmacodyn Ther 152:115–120

Chen G, Portman R, Ensor ChR, Bratton AC (1951) The anticonvulsant activity of α-phenyl succinimides. J Pharmacol Exp Ther 103:54–61

Chen G, Weston JK, Bratton AC (1963) Anticonvulsant activity and toxicity of phensuximide, methsuximide and ethosuximide. Epilepsia 4:66–76

Chiu S, Keifer L, Timberlake JW (1979) Synthesis of imidazolidinediones and oxazolidinediones from cyclization of propargylureas and propargyl carbamates. J Med Chem 22:746–748

Clemson HC, Magarian EO, Fuller GC, Langner RO (1968) Synthesis of derivatives of *N*-methyl-2-phenylsuccinimide involving a lithium salt condensation and a novel application of the Mannich reaction. J Pharm Sci 57:384–389

Coyne WE, Cusic JW (1968) Anticonvulsant semicarbazides. J Med Chem 11:1158–1160
Crider AM, Kolcynski ThM, Miskell DL (1981) Synthesis and anticonvulsant activity of racemic 2-amino-*N*-substituted succinimide derivatives. J Pharm Sci 70:192–195
Czarnecki R, Sobanski H (1980) Anticonvulsant properties of 5-allyl-(β-hydroxy)propyl-*N*-phenylbarbituric acid and the corresponding lactone. Farmaco [Sci] 31:945–950
Davis JP, Schwade ED (1959) Anticonvulsant effects of 3-allyl-5-isobutyl-2-thiohydantoin (BAX 422Z). Fed Proc 18:380
Davis MA, Winthrop StO, Thomas RA, Herr F, Charest MP, Gaudry R (1964a) Anticonvulsants. I. Dibenzo[*a,d*]cycloheptadiene-5-carboxamide and related compounds. J Med Chem 7:88–94
Davis MA, Winthrop StO, Thomas RA, Herr F, Charest MP, Gaudry R (1964b) Anticonvulsants. II. Spiro compounds. Dibenzo[*a,d*]cycloheptadiene-5,5′-hydantoins, -5,5′-oxazolidinediones, and -5,2′-succinimides. J Med Chem 7:439–445
Desmedt IKC, Niemegeers CJE, Lewi PJ, Janssen PAJ (1976) Antagonism of maximal Metrazol seizures in rats and its relevance to an experimental classification of antiepileptic drugs. Arzneimittelforsch 26:1592–1603
De Wald HA, Lobbestael S, Butler DE (1977) Pyrazolodiazepines. 2. 4-aryl-1,3-dialkyl-6,8-dihydropyrazolo[3,4-*e*][1,4]diazepine-7-(1*H*)-ones as antianxiety and anticonvulsant agents. J Med Chem 20:1562–1569
Dox AW (1925) Tetra-alkyl-succinimides and their pharmacological action. J Am Chem Soc 47:1471–1477
Everett GM, Richards RK (1952) Pharmacological studies of phenylacetylurea (Phenurone) an anticonvulsant drug. J Pharmacol Exp Ther 106:303–313
Fabing HD, Gayle RF, Hawkins JR (1947) The treatment of epilepsy with sodium diphenylene hydantoin. Assoc Res Publ Nerv Ment Dis 26:398–403
Fielding St, Hoffmann I (1979) Pharmacology of anti-anxiety drugs with special reference to clobazam. Br J Clin Pharmacol 7:7S–15S
Fontanella L, Mariani L, Tarzia G, Corsico N (1976) 3,7-Dihydro-5-phenylpyrrolo[3,4-*e*][1,4]-diazepine-2(1*H*)-ones. Synthesis and pharmacological properties. Eur J Med Chem 11:217–220
Frey HH (1969) Determination of the anticonvulsant potency of unmetabolized trimethadione. Acta Pharmacol Toxicol 27:295–300
Frey HH, Löscher W (1976) Di-*n*-propylacetic acid – profile of anticonvulsant activity in mice. Arzneimittelforsch 26:299–301
Frey HH, Schulz R (1970) Time course of the demethylation of trimethadione. Acta Pharmacol Toxicol 28:477–483
Funcke ABH, Zandberg P (1970) The anticonvulsive activity in mice of a number of derivatives of 5*H*-dibenzo[*a,d*]cycloheptene and its 1- and 3-aza analogues, in comparison with some therapeutically used anticonvulsants. Arzneimittelforsch 20:1896–1900
Funcke ABH, van Beek MC, van Hell G, Lavy UI, Timmermann H, Zandberg P (1970) Cyheptamide. A pharmacological evaluation. Arch Int Pharmacodyn Ther 187:174–191
Gagneux AR (1976) The chemistry of carbamazepine. In: Birkmayer W (ed) Epileptic seizures-behaviour-pain. Huber, Bern, p 120
Gal J (1979) Convenient synthesis of *N*-alkoxymethylbarbituric acids and *N*-alkoxymethylhydantoins. J Pharm Sci 68:1562–1564
Gallagher BB, Baumel IP, Woodbury SG, Dimicco JA (1975) Clinical evaluation of eterobarb, a new anticonvulsant drug. Neurology 25:399–404
Ganz AJ, Waser PG, Pfirrmann RW (1978) Die Entwicklung neuer Antiepileptika. V. Pharmakologische Wirkungen einiger Sulfanilamidderivate. Arzneimittelforsch 28:1331–1334
Gastaut H, Low MD (1979) Antiepileptic properties of clobazam, a 1,5-benzodiazepine, in man. Epilepsia 20:437–446
Gesler RM, Lints CE, Swinyard EA (1961) Pharmacology of some substituted 2-thiohydantoins with particular reference to anticonvulsant properties. Toxicol Appl Pharmacol 3:107–121

Gluckmann MI (1971) Pharmacology of 7-chloro-5-(*o*-chlorophenyl)-1,3-dihydro-3-hydroxy-2*H*-1,4-benzodiazepine-2-one (lorazepam; WY 4036). Arzneimittelforsch 21:1049–1055

Goldberg MA, Gal J, Cho AK, Jenden DJ (1979) Metabolism of dimethoxymethyl phenobarbital (eterobarb) in patients with epilepsy. Ann Neurol 5:121–126

Golik U (1975) The synthesis of some 2,4-benzodiazepine-1-ones, potent CNS agents. J Heterocyclic Chem 12:903–908

Goodman LS, Toman JEP, Swinyard EA (1946) The anticonvulsant properties of tridione. Am J Med 1:213–228

Goodman LS, Swinyard EA, Brown WC, Schiffman DO, Grewal MS, Bliss EL (1953) Anticonvulsant properties of 5-phenyl-5-ethyl-hexahydropyrimidine-4,6-dione (Mysoline), a new antiepileptic. J Pharmacol Exp Ther 108:428–436

Goodman LS, Swinyard EA, Brown WC, Schiffman DO (1954) Anticonvulsant properties of 5,5-diphenyl-tetrahydroglyoxaline-4-one. (SKF NO. 2599) J Pharmacol Exp Ther 110:403–410

Hagen V, Morgenstern E, Göres E, Franke R, Sauer W, Heine G (1980) Quantitative Struktur-Wirkungs-Beziehungen bei antikonvulsiv wirksamen Benzensulfonamiden. Pharmazie 35:183–185

Hauck FP, Demick J, Fan J (1967) Preparation and anticonvulsant activity of some aryldialkylsuccinimides. J Med Chem 10:611–614

Hauptmann A (1912) Luminal bei Epilepsie. MMW 59:1907–1909

Hester JB, Rudzik AD, Kamdar BV (1971) 6-Phenyl-4*H*-*s*-triazolo[4,3-*a*][1,4]benzodiazepines which have central nervous system depressant activity. J Med Chem 14:1078–1081

Hester JB, Rudzik AD, von Voigtlander PHF (1980a) 1-(Aminoalkyl)-6-aryl-4*H*-*s*-triazolo[4,3-*a*][1,4]benzodiazepines with antianxiety and antidepressant activity. J Med Chem 23:392–402

Hester JB, von Voigtlander Ph, Evenson GN (1980b) 6-(Substituted-amino)-4*H*-*s*-triazolo[4,3-*a*][1,4]benzodiazepines and 4-(substituted-amino)-6*H*-*s*-triazolo[4,3-*a*][1,4]benzodiazepines with potential antianxiety activity. J Med Chem 23:873–877

Johnson DD, Davis HL, Crawford RD (1978) Epileptiform seizures in domestic fowl. VIII. Anticonvulsant activity of primidone and its metabolites, phenobarbital and phenylethylmalonamide. Can J Physiol Pharmacol 56:630–633

Jones GL, Amato RJ, Wimbish GH, Peyton GA (1981) Comparison of anticonvulsant potencies of cyheptamide, carbamazepine, and phenytoin. J Pharm Sci 70:618–620

Jucker E, Süeß R (1961) Über neuartige Spiro-succinimide. Arch Pharm 4:210–220

Kaplan JP, Raizon BM, Desarmenien M, Feltz P, Headley PM, Worms P, Lloyd KG, Bartholini G (1980) New anticonvulsants: Schiff bases of γ-aminobutyric acid and γ-aminobutyramide. J Med Chem 23:702–704

Knoefel PK, Lehmann G (1942) The anticonvulsant action of diphenylhydantoin and some related compounds. J Pharmacol Exp Ther 76:194–201

Koella WP, Levin P, Baltzer V (1976) The pharmacology of carbamazepine and some other anti-epileptic drugs. In: Birkmayer W (ed) Epileptic seizures-behaviour-pain. Huber, Bern, p 32

Körösi J, Láng T (1975) Forschungsarbeit auf dem Gebiet der 5*H*-2,3-benzodiazepine. Ther Hung 23:141–142

Kornet MJ, Crider AM, Magarian EO (1977a) Potential long-acting anticonvulsants. 1. Synthesis and activity of succinimides containing an alkylating group at the 2 position. J Med Chem 20:405–409

Kornet MJ, Crider AM, Magarian EO (1977b) Potential long-acting anticonvulsants. 2. Synthesis and activity of succinimides containing an alkylating group on nitrogen or at the 3 position. J Med Chem 20:1210–1213

Krall RL (1980) Structure-activity relationships. Quantitative structure-activity relationship studies of anticonvulsant drugs. In: Glaser GH, Penry JK, Woodbury DM (eds) Antiepileptic drugs: mechanisms of action. Raven, New York, p 233

Krall RL, Penry JK, Kupferberg HJ, Swinyard EA (1978a) Antiepileptic drug development. I. History and a program for progress. Epilepsia 19:393–408

Krall RL, Penry JK, White BG, Kupferberg HJ, Swinyard EA (1978 b) Antiepileptic drug development. II. Anticonvulsant drug screening. Epilepsia 19:409–428
Kuch H (1979) Clobazam: chemical aspects of the 1,4- and 1,5-benzodiazepines. Br J Clin Pharmacol 7:17S–21S
Lange J, Rump S, Galecka E, Ilczuk I, Lechowska-Postek M, Rabsztyn T, Szymańska T, Walczyna K (1977 a) Synthesis and properties of new cyclic derivatives of succinic acid with anticonvulsant activity. Pharmazie 32:82–84
Lange J, Rump S, Ilczuk I, Lapszewicz J, Rabsztyn T, Walczyna K (1977 b) Synthesis and properties of cyclic derivatives of succinic acid with anticonvulsant activity. Pharmazie 32:579–581
Lange J, Rump S, Ilczuk I, Lapszewicz J, Rabsztyn T, Walczyna K (1979) Synthesis and properties of cyclic derivatives of succinic acid with anticonvulsant activity. Pharmazie 34:794–795
Lien EJ, Liao RCH, Shinouda HG (1979) Quantitative structure-activity relationships and dipole moments of anticonvulsants and CNS depressants. J Pharm Sci 68:463–465
Löscher W (1981) Anticonvulsant activity of metabolites of valproic acid. Arch Int Pharmacodyn Ther 249:158–163
Magarian EO, Becker GW, Diamond L (1973) Anticonvulsant properties of Mannich base derivatives of 2-phenylsuccinimide III. J Pharm Sci 62:325–327
Marcucci F, Mussini E, Airoldi L, Guaitani A, Garattini S (1972) Brain concentrations of lorazepam and oxazepam at equal degree of anticonvulsant activity. J Pharm Pharmacol 24:63–64
Masuda Y, Karasawa T, Shiraishi Y, Hori M, Yoshida K, Shimizu M (1980) 3-Sulfamoylmethyl-1,2-benzisoxazole, a new type of anticonvulsant drug. Arzneimittelforsch 30:477–483
Mehta NB, Risinger Diuguid ChA, Soroko FE (1981) Potential anticonvulsants. 1,5-benzylhydantoins. J Med Chem 24:465–468
Mercier J (1973) Chemical compounds possessing anticonvulsant activity. Structure-activity relationships of the antiepileptics. In: Radouco-Thomas C (ed) International encyclopedia of pharmacology and therapeutics, section 19. Anticonvulsant drugs 1. Pergamon, Oxford, p 203
Merritt HH, Putnam TJ (1945) Experimental determination of anticonvulsive activity of chemical compounds. Epilepsia 3:51–75 (sec series, Banta, Menasha, Wisconsin)
Meunier H, Carraz G, Meunier Y, Eymard P, Aimard M (1963) Propriétés pharmacodynamiques de l'acide *n*-dipropylacétique. Therapie 18:435–438
Miller CA, Long LM (1951) Anticonvulsants. I. An investigation of N-R-α-R_1-α-phenylsuccinimides. J Am Chem Soc 73:4895–4898
Miller CA, Lono LM (1953a) Anticonvulsants. III. A study of N,α,β-alkylsuccinimides. J Am Chem Soc 75:373–375
Miller CA, Long LM (1953 b) Anticonvulsants. IV. An investigation of α-(substituted phenyl)-succinimides. J Am Chem Soc 75:6256–6258
Miller CA, Scholl HI, Long LM (1951) Anticonvulsants. II. A study of N-R-α,β-substituted succinimides. J Am Chem Soc 73:5608–5610
Millichap JG, Ortiz WR (1967) Albutoin, a new thiohydantoin derivative for grand mal epilepsies. Comparison with diphenylhydantoin in a double-blind, controlled study. Neurology 17:162–165
Millichap JG (1972) Mephenytoin, Ethotoin, and albutoin. In: Penry JK, Schmidt RP, Woodbury DM (eds) Antiepileptic drug. Raven, New York, p 275
Müller WE (1981) The benzodiazepine receptor. Pharmacology 22:153–161
Nakamura K, O'Hashi K, Nakatsuji K, Hiroka T, Fujimoto K, Ose S (1965) The anticonvulsant activity of 3-ethoxycarbonyl-5,5-diphenylhydantoin (P-6127) in animals. Arch Int Pharmacodyn Ther 156:261–270
Nakamura K, Masuda Y, Nakatsuji K, Hiroka T (1966) Comparative studies on the distribution and metabolic fate of diphenylhydantoin and 3-ethoxycarbonyldiphenylhydantoin (P-6127) after chronic administrations to dogs and cats. Arch Exp Pathol Pharmacol 254:406–417
Nakamura K, Murai K, Nakatsuji K, Kobayashi M, Masuda Y, Kadokawa T, Soji Y, Nakamura H, Hiroka T, Senda H (1968) Neuropharmacological and toxicological stu-

dies on a new anti-epileptic, *N*-α-ethyl-phenylacetyl-*N'*-acetyl urea in experimental animals. Arzneimittelforsch 5:524–529
Nardi D, Tajana A, Leonardi A, Penini R, Portioli F, Magistretti MJ, Subissi A (1981) Synthesis and anticonvulsant activity of *N*-(benzoylalkyl)imidazoles and *N*-(ω-phenyl-ω-hydroxyalkyl)imidazoles. J Med Chem 24:727–731
Nelson WL, Kwon YG, Marshall GL, Hoover JL, Pfeffer GT (1979) Fluorinated phenytoin anticonvulsant analogs. J Pharm Sci 68:115–117
Oldfield W, Cashin CH (1965) The chemistry and pharmacology of a series of cycloalkanespiro-5'-hydantoins. J Med Chem 8:239–249
Perlstein MA, Andelman MB (1946) Tridione, its use in convulsive and related disorders. J Pediatr 29:20–40
Petöcz L, Kosóczky I (1975) Die wichtigeren pharmakologischen Parameter von Grandaxin (Tofizopam; egyt-341) Ther Hung 23:143–147
Raines A, Niner JM, Pace DG (1973) A comparison of the anticonvulsant, neurotoxic and lethal effects of diphenylbarbituric acid, phenobarbital and diphenylhydantoin in the mouse. J Pharmacol Exp Ther 186:315–322
Raines A, Baumel I, Gallagher BB, Niner JM (1975) The effects of 5,5-diphenylbarbituric acid on experimental seizures in rats: correlation between plasma and brain concentrations and anticonvulsant activity. Epilepsia 16:575–581
Raines A, Blake GJ, Richardson B, Gilbert MB (1979) Differential selectivity of several barbiturates on experimental seizures and neurotoxicity in the mouse. Epilepsia 20:105–113
Randall LO, Schallek W, Scheckel C, Banziger R, Moe RA (1968) Zur Pharmakologie des neuen Psychopharmakons 7-chlor-2,3-dihydro-1-methyl-5-phenyl-1*H*-1,4-benzodiazepin (Ro 5-4556). Arzneimittelforsch 18:1542–1545
Randall LO, Kappell B (1973) Pharmacological activity of some benzodiazepines and their metabolites. In: Garattini S, Mussini E, Randall LO (eds) The benzodiazepines. Raven, New York, p 27
Rossi S, Pirola O, Maggi R (1969) Sintesi di 1,2,4,5-tetraidro-2,4-dicheto-3*H*-1,5-benzodiazepine. Chim Ind (Milan) 51:479–483
Rump S, Ilczuk I, Rabsztyn T, Walczyna K (1981) Pharmacological properties of *N*-aminodiphenylhydantoin, a new hydantoin derivative with anticonvulsant activity. Pharmazie 36:780–781
Sadagopa Ramanujam VM, Trieff NM (1978) Structure activity relation for some 1,4-benzodiazepinones: correlation between rate constants for reduction by sodium borohydride and antileptazol ED_{50}. J Pharm Pharmacol 30:542–546
Samour CM, Reinhard JF, Vida JA (1971) Anticonvulsants. 1. Alkoxamethyl derivatives of barbiturates and diphenylhydantoin. J Med Chem 14:187–189
Samson FE, Dahl N, Dahl DR (1956) A study on the narcotic action of the short chain fatty acids. J Clin Invest 35:1291–1298
Schäfer H (1969) 5,5-Diphenylhydantoin-*N*3-carbonsäureester. German Patent 1966802 (Desitin-Werk Carl Kinke GmbH)
Schäfer H, Lührs R (1978) Metabolite pattern of valproic acid. Part I: gas chromatographic determination of the valproic acid metabolite artifacts, heptanone-3, 4- and 5-hydroxyvalproic acid lactone. Arzneimittelforsch 28:657–662
Schäfer H, Lührs R, Reith H (1980) Chemistry, pharmacokinetics, and biological activity of some metabolites of valproic acid. In: Johannessen SI, Morselli PL, Pippenger CR, Richens A, Schmidt D, Meinardi H (eds) Antiepileptic therapy: advances in drug monitoring. Raven, New York, p 103
Schlögl K, Wessely F, Kraupp O, Stormann H (1961) Synthese und Pharmakologie einiger 3,5-di- und trisubstituierter Hydantoine. J Med Pharm Chem 4:231–258
Scoular IT, Nicholls PJ, Smith HJ (1976) Anticonvulsant properties of some new 3-phenyl-2,5-pyrrolidinediones. Eur J Med Chem 11:91–93
Shaffer JW, Steinberg E, Krimsley V, Winstead MB (1968) Substitution in the hydantoin ring. VII. *N*-3-propionic acid and its ethyl ester and *N*-3-(2-cyanoethyl) derivatives. J Med Chem 11:462–466
Sohn YJ, Levitt B, Raines A (1970) Anticonvulsant properties of diphenylthiohydantoin. Arch Int Pharmacodyn Ther 188:284–289

Soroko FE, Grivsky E, Maxwell RA (1981) Cinromide (3-bromo-*N*-ethylcinnanamide), a novel anticonvulsant agent. J Pharm Pharmacol 33:741–743

Spielman MA, Geiszler AO, Close WJ (1948) Anticonvulsant drugs. II. Some acylureas. J Am Chem Soc 70:4189–4191

Sternbach LH (1973) Chemistry of 1,4-benzodiazepines and some aspects of the structure-activity relationship. In: Garattini S, Mussini E, Randall LO (eds) The benzodiazepines. Raven, New York, p 1

Sternbach LH (1980) The benzodiazepine story. In: Priest RG, Vianna Filho U, Amrein R, Skreta M (eds) Benzodiazepines today and tomorrow. MTP, Falcon House, England, p 5

Sternbach LH, Randall LO, Banziger R, Lehr H (1968) Structure-activity relationships in the 1,4-benzodiazepine series. In: Burger A (ed) Drugs affecting the central nervous system. Dekker, New York, p 237

Sternbach LH, Sancilio FD, Blount JF (1974) Quinazolines and 1,4-benzodiazepines. 64. Comparison of the stereochemistry of diazepam with that of close analogs with marginal biological activity. J Med Chem 17:374–377

Swinyard EA, Castellion AW (1966) Anticonvulsant properties of some benzodiazepines. J Pharmacol Exp Ther 151:369–375

Swinyard EA, Toman JEP (1950) A comparison of the anticonvulsant actions of some phenylhydantoins and their corresponding phenylacetylureas. J Pharmacol Exp Ther 100:151–157

Swinyard EA, Brown WC, Goodman LS (1952) Comparative assays of antiepileptic drugs in mice and rats. J Pharmacol Exp Ther 106:319–330

Taillandier G, Benoit-Guyod JL, Boucherle A, Broll M, Eymard P (1975) Recherches dans la série dipropylacétique. XII. Acides et alcools aliphatiques ramifiés anticonvulsivants. Eur J Med Chem 10:453–462

Taillandier G, Benoit-Guyod JL, Laruelle C, Boucherle A (1977) Investigation in the dipropylacetic acid series, C_8 and C_9 branched chain ethylenic acids and amides. Arch Pharm 310:394–403

Tchicaloff M, Mitroi G (1975) Prüfung des neuen Antiepileptikums G 385. Z EEG EMG 6:133–136

Theobald W, Kunz HA (1963) Zur Pharmakologie des Antiepileptikums 5-carbamyl-5*H*-dibenzo[*b,f*]azepin. Arzneimittelforsch 13:122–125

Tinney FJ, Sanchez JP, Nogas JA (1974) Synthesis and pharmacological evaluation of 2,3-dihydro-1*H*-thieno[2,3-*e*][1,4]diazepines. J Med Chem 17:624–630

Toman JEP, Swinyard EA, Goodman LS (1946) Properties of maximal seizures, and their alteration by anticonvulsant drugs and other agents. J Neurophysiol 9:231–239

Traversa U, De Angelis L, Vertua R (1977) On the hypnogenic and anticonvulsant activities of demethyldiazepam and chlordemethyldiazepam: time-effect relations. J Pharm Pharmacol 29:504–506

Uno H, Kurokawa M, Masuda Y, Nishimura H (1979) Studies on 3-substituted 1,2-benzisoxazole derivatives. 6. Syntheses of 3-(sulfamoylmethyl)-1,2-benzisoxazole derivatives and their anticonvulsant activities. J Med Chem 22:180–183

Vida JA (1977) Anticonvulsants. Academic, New York

Vida JA, Gerry EH (1977) Cyclic ureides. In: Vida JA (ed) Anticonvulsants. Academic, New York, p 151

Vida JA, Wilber WR, Reinhard JF (1971) Anticonvulsants. 2. Acyloxymethyl and halomethyl derivatives of barbituric acid and diphenylhydantoin. J Med Chem 14:190–193

Vida JA, Hooker ML, Reinhard JF (1973 a) Anticonvulsants. 3. Phenobarbital and mephobarbital derivatives. J Med Chem 16:602–605

Vida JA, Hooker ML, Samour CM (1973 b) Anticonvulsants. 4. Metharbital and phenobarbital derivatives. J Med Chem 16:1378–1381

Vida JA, O'Dea MH, Samour CM, Reinhard JF (1975) Anticonvulsants. 5. Derivatives of 5-ethyl-5-phenylhydantoin and 5,5-diphenylhydantoin. J Med Chem 18:383–385

Walker KAM, Wallach MB, Hirschfeld DR (1981) 1-(Naphthylalkyl)-1*H*-imidazole derivatives, a new class of anticonvulsant agents. J Med Chem 24:67–74

Waser PG, Ganz AJ, Pfirrmann RW (1977a) Die Entwicklung neuer Antiepileptika. I. Antikonvulsive Wirkung von *N*-(*p*-Sulfamoylphenyl)-succinimid-Derivaten. Arzneimittelforsch 27:1942–1953

Waser PG, Ganz AJ, Pfirrmann RW (1977b) Die Entwicklung neuer Antiepileptika. II. Antikonvulsive Wirkung einiger Hydantoin-Derivate. Arzneimittelforsch 27:2125–2128

Waser PG, Ganz AJ, Pfirrmann RW (1977c) Die Entwicklung neuer Antiepileptika. III. Antikonvulsive Wirkung einiger 1-(*p*-Sulfamoylphenyl)-imidazolidinon-5-Derivate. Arzneimittelforsch 27:2336–2341

Waser PG, Ganz AJ, Pfirrmann RW (1978) Die Entwicklung neuer Antiepileptika. IV. Antikonvulsive Wirkung einiger 1-(*p*-Sulfamoyl-phenyl)-pyrrolidin-2-on-Derivate. Arzneimittelforsch 28:952–956

Weese H (1932) Pharmakologie des Prominal. Dtsch Med Wochenschr 58:696

Winstead MB, Hamel CR (1965) Substitution in the hydantoin ring. II. *N*-3-acetic acid derivatives. J Med Chem 8:120–123

Winstead MB, Barr DE, Hamel CR, Renn DJ, Parker HI, Neumann RM (1965) Substitution in the hydantoin ring. I. *N*-3-aminomethyl derivatives. J Med Chem 8:117–120

Witiak DT, Vishnuvajjala BR, Cook WL, Minatelli JA, Gupta TK, Gerald MC (1977) 3,4-Methylenedioxyphenyl-, isopropylidenedioxyphenyl-, and benzyl-substituted chiral 2-aminosuccinimides and 3-aminopyrrolidines. Stereoselective investigations of potential anti-parkinsonian, antipsychotic, and anticonvulsant activities. J Med Chem 20:801–805

Zimmermann FT, Burgemeister BB (1958) A new drug for petit mal epilepsy. Neurology 8:769–775

CHAPTER 10

Biochemistry

G. L. JONES and D. M. WOODBURY

A. Introduction

Although the mechanisms of anticonvulsant action remain uncertain, numerous physiological and biochemical correlates of such action have been documented, and it is possible that one or more of such correlates bears a causal (i.e., mechanistic) relationship with action. The physiological correlates of anticonvulsant action are discussed in Chap. 23; the present chapter will focus on biochemical correlates, with an analysis of the possible mechanistic significance of each.

Correlates most often cited in discussions of anticonvulsant action include effects on membrane function, particularly ionic conductances, and effects on neurotransmitter metabolism and/or disposition. Collectively, anticonvulsants have been shown to affect membrane permeability to sodium, calcium, potassium, and chloride, although selectivity for each effect varies with the particular compound. Anticonvulsants may also affect the synthesis, degradation, utilization, or dynamics of gamma-aminobutyric acid (GABA), glycine, aspartic acid, glutamic acid, acetylcholine, norepinephrine, and other neurotransmitter substances. Again, however, selectivity for each effect varies with the particular compound. While each of these effects might be expressions of an anticonvulsant action, lack of consistency among drugs known to be effective in a particular seizure type has prevented the unambiguous interpretation of mechanism.

B. Ionic Permeability

I. Effects on Sodium Conductance

Much of the early evidence that changes in sodium conductance were involved in anticonvulsant action was acquired for phenytoin. Two of the more popular theories of phenytoin action are each based upon a decrease of intracellular sodium, but differ with respect to the mechanism of such decrease. WOODBURY (1955) suggested that phenytoin might facilitate active sodium transport by stimulating Na^+-K^+-ATPase, an effect later observed by others in selected systems (FESTOFF and APPEL 1968; LEWIN and BLECK 1977). However, a more recent theory suggests that phenytoin acts in a tetrodotoxin-like manner to limit passive sodium influx (AYALA et al. 1977; LIPICKY et al. 1972). Each of these theories will be discussed in some detail.

1. Active Sodium Transport

Phenytoin has been reported to increase Na^+-K^+-ATPase activity in brain both in vivo (LEVIN and BLECK 1977; LEZNICKI and DYMECKI 1974) and in vitro (FES-

TOFF and APPEL 1968; SIEGLE and GOODWIN 1972; WILENSKY and LOWDEN 1972). A similar effect was seen in skeletal muscle (KOOTSTRA and WOODHOUSE 1974) and in cardiac muscle (GOLDSTEIN et al. 1973). However, other studies have reported negative results, both in brain (DEUPREE 1977; SCHWARTZ et al. 1975) and cardiac muscle (SPAIN and CHIDSEY 1971); and in some cases, phenytoin actually decreased Na^+-K^+-ATPase activity (GILBERT and WYLLIE 1976; GOLDSTEIN et al. 1973).

Much of the above controversy might be rationalized on the basis of the number of variables that seem to affect Na^+-K^+-ATPase activity. For example, it has been suggested that phenytoin stimulates the enzyme only under conditions where intracellular sodium concentration is elevated and potassium concentration is decreased, or alternatively, when the total concentration of sodium and potassium is low (DELGADO-ESCUETA and HORAN 1980). Indeed, epileptogenic foci may be characterized by high intracellular Na^+/K^+ ratios (ESCUETA et al. 1974). At lower Na^+/K^+ ratios there might be no effect, or even inhibition. WOODBURY (1980) has discussed still other variables that might affect Na^+-K^+-ATPase activity.

There is much experimental support for the hypothesis that phenytoin acts in part by stimulating Na^+-K^+-ATPase. FERTZIGER et al. (1971) demonstrated that phenytoin increased potassium influx in lobster nerve, which is consistent with a stimulatory effect on the ATPase. [However, proof of the active nature of the influx has been questioned; see DEWEER (1980).] Others (WATSON and WOODBURY 1973; BASKIN et al. 1973) have reported that phenytoin may antagonize the effects of ouabain on cardiac muscle by decreasing sodium and increasing potassium concentrations. Results consistent with the above findings have also been recorded for nonexcitable tissue. For example, it was reported that phenytoin stimulates the sodium pump in frog skin and toad bladder (WATSON and WOODBURY 1972; DESOUSA and GROSSO 1973), an effect that probably occurs in other epithelial cells as well, including choroid plexus, glial cells, and secretory cells.

In epithelial cells, in contrast to excitable tissue, phenytoin increases permeability of the mucosal membrane to sodium, possibly by an effect on membrane calcium binding (WOODBURY 1980). The effect is different from that of vasopressin, because at concentrations of phenytoin producing a maximal response vasopressin produces an additional response, and vice versa. Therefore, some of the observed increase in Na^+-K^+-ATPase activity is likely due to an increased sodium concentration (since the sodium pump is sensitive to the intracellular sodium concentration). However, the concentration of sodium in these cells is eventually decreased (below control) after the initial increase due to enhanced sodium permeability, and the intracellular potassium concentration is increased as sodium is decreased. Thus, the sodium pump is stimulated to a greater extent than that which is accountable for by increased sodium concentration. This apparent direct effect on Na^+-K^+-ATPase may be due either to an activation of the enzyme or to an increase in its synthesis. Such an effect in the choroid plexus and/or glial cells would result in an increase in CSF sodium and a decrease in potassium. The decrease in extracellular potassium might thereby limit the increase normally observed secondary to excessive neuronal activity, as occurs in seizures (see below).

Other studies (WOODBURY 1978) have shown that phenytoin is transported by toad bladder epithelium in the same direction as potassium. When placed on the mucosal side of the cell, phenytoin does not accumulate on the serosal side; however, accumulation does occur on the mucosal side if placed initially on the serosal side. Thus, it was postulated that phenytoin might be transported across the cell membrane by attachment to the potassium arm of the Na^+-K^+ pump. If this is the case, phenytoin and ouabain might compete for transport, because it is known that ouabain transport into cells is blocked by high potassium concentrations (BRONSTED and WOODBURY 1973). To investigate this possibility further WATSON and WOODBURY (1973) administered phenytoin either simultaneously or 15 min prior to ouabain injection, and observed the relative effect of phenytoin on the usual ouabain-induced changes in sodium and potassium concentrations in cardiac cells. When given prior to ouabain, phenytoin prevented the ouabain-induced increase in intracellular sodium. Also, BASKIN et al. (1973) reported that phenytoin blocks ouabain uptake in cardiac cells. The possible transport of phenytoin by the potassium arm of the Na^+-K^+ pump is significant because, as discussed above, the concentration of potassium and the Na^+/K^+ ratio appear to determine the response of Na^+-K^+-ATPase to phenytoin. Thus, the failure in certain cases to demonstrate a stimulatory effect of phenytoin on the sodium pump might be explained by competition by potassium for the active transport of phenytoin into the cell.

The actions of phenytoin on epithelial as well as excitable cells pose interesting possibilities with respect to mechanism. For example, it has been suggested that increased activity of glial-cell Na^+-K^+-ATPase might increase the clearance of potassium from interstitial fluid. Since potassium concentration appears to be higher in epileptogenic tissue, this effect might be particularly relevant to an anticonvulsant action. Experiments by HEINEMANN and LUX (1973) have shown that phenytoin does indeed enhance potassium removal from brain extracellular fluid. Additional evidence that phenytoin acts on glial cells was provided by WOODBURY (1980). The intriguing observation was made that phenytoin lacks anticonvulsant properties in neonatal animals; in fact, it is excitatory. Furthermore, phenytoin does not decrease intracellular sodium concentration in neonatal animals, as it does in the adult animal.

However, after 10 days of age phenytoin begins to exert its anticonvulsant properties. This corresponds precisely with the onset of development of the glial-cell population in brain. The properties of phenytoin as a function of postnatal maturation might also be explained using the concept that phenytoin's actions are primarily excitatory. Since inhibitory neurons develop slowly during postnatal maturation, the delayed appearance of phenytoin's anticonvulsant properties, presumed in this case to be due to an excitatory action on inhibitory neurons, might thus be rationalized. However, the present experimental evidence weighs in favor of an action on epithelial Na^+-K^+-ATPase.

As already mentioned, much of the evidence that anticonvulsants affect sodium conductance has been acquired for phenytoin. This is especially true when considering drug effects on active sodium transport. Although phenobarbital reduced sodium uptake in lobster nerves (PINCUS et al. 1970), the mechanism of such decrease may not be attributable to an effect on Na^+-K^+-ATPase, and its potency for this effect was much less than that for phenytoin. Likewise, there is little if any evidence that other anticonvulsants act by stimulating active sodium transport.

2. Passive Sodium Influx

A more recent theory is that phenytoin interacts with the neuronal membrane in a tetrodotoxin-like manner to block sodium channels (although different sites in the sodium channel might be involved), and thereby decreases sodium influx (LIPICKY et al. 1972). Unlike the activation of Na^+-K^+-ATPase, the reduction of passive sodium influx has been observed with several anticonvulsants in addition to phenytoin. For example, carbamazepine is capable of blocking sodium permeability in *Myxicola* giant axons (SCHANT et al. 1974). However, much of the evidence for this action is from neurophysiological studies, and is discussed in more detail in Chap. 23, and in Chap. 13, which covers the specific pharmacology of hydantoin derivatives. Whether or not such an effect is an expression of a "membrane-stabilizing" action cannot be ascertained with certainty, but it is of interest that phenytoin normalized the increased membrane fluidity observed in erythrocytes from patients with myotonic dystrophy, while exerting no effect on fluidity of membranes derived from normal donors (ROSES et al. 1975). However, such a correlation would imply that phenytoin exerts a selective action on neuronal membranes that are "abnormal" with respect to fluidity; yet, there is no evidence to support this contention. In fact, most evidence supports the idea of an action on normal neurons to prevent their detonation by rapidly firing neurons located at an epileptogenic focus.

Although most studies of anticonvulsant effects on passive sodium influx were conducted using neurophysiological models, indirect evidence of such effects has been obtained using synaptosomes isolated from rat cerebral cortex (SOHN and FERRENDELLI 1973, 1976; FERENDELLI and DANIELS-MCQUEEN 1982). Because of the coupling between sodium and calcium permeability, these studies will be discussed in the next section (Sect. B.II), which deals with anticonvulsant effects on calcium conductance.

II. Effects on Calcium Conductance

Phenytoin, carbamazepine, diazepam, phenobarbital, and several other drugs have been shown to decrease calcium influx across synaptosomal membranes (SOHN and FERRENDELLI 1973, 1976; FERRENDELLI and DANIELS-MCQUEEN 1982), and this effect has also been reported for phenytoin in lobster walking nerves (HASBANI et al. 1974). In addition, phenytoin inhibits intracellular uptake of calcium by subcellular fractions (YAARI et al. 1977). However, the precise mechanism of these effects is not yet known.

The inhibition of influx across cellular and subcellular membranes might be due either to a direct effect to block calcium channels or to an indirect effect secondary to a decrease in passive sodium influx. For example, phenytoin inhibits active calcium uptake in mitochondria by a process that is independent of sodium influx. This effect, which is seen with higher doses of phenytoin, may actually increase intracellular free calcium and might be responsible for the excitatory effects sometimes seen in phenytoin toxicity. Thus, decreased calcium flux might be due to a primary action of phenytoin to block calcium channels directly. However, it is also apparent that a decrease in sodium influx across synaptosomal membranes can significantly reduce presynaptic calcium concentration. The decreased calcium might be due in part to a direct block of calcium channels, and in part to a blockade of sodium channels, through which calcium also enters (BAKER et al. 1971), but the most significant factor is probably the steepened sodium electrochemical gradient caused by blockade of passive sodium influx. Not only does the resulting hyperpolarization close the "late" calcium channels (BAKER et al. 1971), but the steepened sodium electrochemical gradient will also increase the calcium electrochemical gradient (i.e., lower intracellular calcium) by virtue of the sodium-calcium countertransport mechanism (BAKER et al. 1969).

FERRENDELLI and DANIELS-MCQUEEN (1982) have addressed some of these questions in their biochemical studies. In isolated synaptosomes, calcium uptake was increased by both potassium and veratridine in a concentration-dependent manner. Tetrodotoxin (a specific blocker of sodium channels) was shown to block the action of veratridine by as much as 90%, but it had no effect on the action of potassium. In contrast, manganese ion inhibited calcium uptake whether it was stimulated by potassium or by veratridine. Thus, potassium and veratridine stimulate calcium uptake by different mechanisms. Increased intracellular potassium will reduce the large intra- to extracellular potassium concentration gradient and thereby cause membrane depolarization. Veratridine is an alkaloid that prevents inactivation of sodium channels, leading to an accumulation of intracellular sodium and thereby depolarization. Depolarization by either mechanism augments calcium influx. Because the effect of veratridine is sodium dependent, it is inhibited by tetrodotoxin. In contrast, the action of potassium is not sodium dependent, and is unaffected by tetrodotoxin. Manganese ion, which acts primarily by blocking calcium channels (NACHSHEN and BLAUSTEIN 1980), has the same effect on both potassium- and veratridine-induced calcium uptake.

Phenytoin inhibits the action of both veratridine and potassium to activate calcium uptake, but (like tetrodotoxin) it is much more effective against veratridine (FERRENDELLI and DANIELS-MCQUEEN 1982). Thus, phenytoin appears to have both tetrodotoxin-like and manganese-like properties. Potassium-induced uptake was inhibited only 20% by 0.1 mM phenytoin, and this inhibition was unaffected by tetrodotoxin. In contrast, 0.1 mM phenytoin inhibited veratridine-induced uptake by 80%, an effect that was sensitive to tetrodotoxin. Thus, phenytoin inhibits veratridine- and potassium-induced calcium uptake by different mechanisms, suggesting that phenytoin can inhibit both sodium and calcium conductance by separate and independent processes. In one case, phenytoin might act at sites on or near sodium channels to block sodium conductance (and, secondarily, calcium conductance), while in the other case it might act directly to block calcium channels. However, because much lower concentrations of phenytoin (and carbamazepine and lidocaine; see below) are needed to inhibit veratridine-induced uptake than are required to inhibit potassium-induced uptake, it is felt that their antiepileptic effects are most likely due to blockade of sodium uptake rather than a direct action on calcium conductance.

FERRENDELLI and DANIELS-MCQUEEN (1982) reported that carbamazepine, phenobarbital, lidocaine, and diazepam also inhibit stimulated calcium uptake in synaptosomes, while ethosuximide and valproic acid exert no significant effect. Similar to phenytoin, carbamazepine and lidocaine blocked veratridine-induced uptake better than potassium-induced uptake. In contrast, phenobarbital and diazepam have little or no selective effect on the two depolarizing agents. In comparing the inhibitory effects of the above drugs with clinically effective blood levels, these authors concluded that inhibition of sodium and/or calcium uptake could be a mechanism of action underlying the clinical effects only for phenytoin, carbamazepine, and lidocaine, but not for the remaining drugs studied.

GOLDBERG and TODOROFF (GOLDBERG 1980) made several observations possibly relevant to calcium transport mechanisms. They reported that: (a) phospholipids show variable degrees of phenytoin binding; (b) phenytoin binding to brain tissue is enhanced by removal of tissue lipids, suggesting that phenytoin binds to protein sites normally occupied by charged lipids; and (c) phenytoin increases the binding of calcium by certain phospholipids. CHWEN and LESLIE (1981) reported that phenytoin enhanced the binding of $^{45}Ca^{++}$ to phosphatidic acid and phosphatidylserine, and suggested that enhanced binding to acidic lipids might be involved in an alteration of sodium or potassium transport. Indeed, it is thought that phosphatidic acid may act as an ionophore selective for both mono- and divalent cations. It is also conceivable that phenytoin binding to protein sites normally occupied by acidic phospholipids might selectively increase calcium binding to these lipids by increasing the availability of anionic sites. Thus, these lipids might serve as ion-exchange sites for sodium and potassium; calcium might be removed from these sites during depolarization, allowing the site to bind and transport sodium. Enhancement of calcium binding could result in inhibition of sodium influx by an inhibition of binding to its carrier. The enhanced binding of calcium might also allow less calcium to penetrate the membrane and thereby decrease calcium influx.

Collectively, these data imply that the so-called "boundary lipid" may be of profound significance with respect to anticonvulsant mechanisms of action. ("Boundary lipid" is usually thought of as a monomolecular layer of phospholipid surrounding an integral membrane protein, determining to some degree the structural and functional properties of that protein.) For example, it is thought that "boundary lipid" might in many cases consist of acidic (as opposed to neutral) phospholipids. If anticonvulsants interact with the interface of this lipid with functional protein, not only might enzyme activities (e.g., Na^+-K^+-ATPase) be directly altered, but ion channel size and shape might also be affected. Such a selective action might account for the lack of effect of anticonvulsants on normal membrane systems studied by spectroscopic and other physical methods; a subtle perturbation at a functional lipid-protein interface, such as might occur at the sodium channel, would likely go undetected by even the most sensitive spectroscopic methods.

The pharmacological consequences of decreased intracellular calcium are manifold. Because calcium is known to enhance a variety of secretory processes, the phenytoin-induced decrease in intracellular calcium might generally compromise all such processes. This is supported by the observations that phenytoin can inhibit the release of insulin from pancreatic islet cells (COHEN et al. 1973), vasopressin (FICHMAN et al. 1970) and oxytocin (MITTLER and GLICK 1972) from the neurohypophysis, thyrotropin from the adenohypophysis (WOODBURY 1969), glucagon from pancreas (GERICH et al. 1972), catecholamines from adrenal medulla (GUTMAN and BOONYAVIROG 1977), and yet other hormones. Since intracellular calcium affects neurotransmitter release, phenytoin also exerts effects on synaptic transmission. YAARI et al. (1977) reported that phenytoin markedly decreased synaptic efficacy in the frog neuromuscular synapse by reducing evoked neurotransmitter release, an effect presumably due to an inhibition of calcium influx. However, when synaptic transmission was depressed by lowering the calcium concentration of the medium, phenytoin augmented neurally evoked transmitter release. This was thought to be due to the inhibition by phenytoin of the intracellular uptake of calcium by subcellular particles. Assuming that such an effect predominates (over synaptic uptake) in low calcium solutions, or low phenytoin concentrations, the increased transmitter release could be due to higher intracellular calcium concentration. A similar dependence on phenytoin concentration was seen in its effect on thyrotropin release (WOODBURY 1969); low doses of phenytoin stimulated rather than decreased release, perhaps because of a selective action on calcium uptake by subcellular organelles.

Another calcium-dependent event altered by phenytoin is the production of cyclic nucleotides (FERRENDELLI and KINSCHERF 1977). The accumulation of cyclic GMP and cyclic AMP, which normally occurs in response to depolarization, is inhibited by phenytoin, presumably secondary to its effects on passive sodium.influx. It is believed that increased intracellular calcium resulting from depolarization leads to increased cyclic GMP levels; and that depolarization-induced release of neurotransmitter substances elevate cyclic AMP, through their actions on adenylate cyclase. Thus, the actions of phenytoin might be both direct and indirect, as discussed already.

Although depolarization-induced increases in these cyclic nucleotides may be inhibited by phenytoin, basal levels are decreased only for cyclic GMP and only in the cerebellum. Other drugs that selectively depress basal cyclic GMP levels in the cerebellum include phenobarbital, ethosuximide, valproic acid, bromide, and diazepam. However, nonanticonvulsant drugs may also produce this effect, as seen with phenothiazines, ethanol, reserpine, general anesthetics, and other drugs. Thus, it is not presently clear whether the effect of anticonvulsants on basal cyclic GMP levels in the cerebellum is relevant to antiepileptic mechanisms, or simply reflects a sedative-depressant action of these drugs. Although increased levels of cyclic nucleotides may have excitatory effects which might be prevented by phenytoin, the role of such an effect in the antiepileptic action of phenytoin is questionable.

III. Effects on Potassium Conductance

Apart from changes in potassium conductance due to effects on Na^+-K^+-ATPase activity, certain anticonvulsants are thought selectively to alter potassium permeability in epithelial cells. For example, the convulsant pentylenetetrazol (PTZ) is known to increase the short-circuit current (SCC) across isolated toad bladders by enhancing the potassium permeability of the serosal membrane (GROSS and WOODBURY 1972). The antiabsence drugs trimethadione, dimethadione, ethosuximide, and diazepam competitively inhibit the increase in SCC induced by PTZ. Because these drugs inhibit the SCC increase in proportion to their relative potencies against PTZ-induced seizures in mice and absence seizures in humans, it was proposed that their antiepileptic action is due to a decrease in potassium permeability (WOODBURY 1974). It is intriguing that absence seizures are characterized by spikes and large, slow waves, the latter of which are the EEG manifestation of inhibitory discharges. By increasing potassium permeability of the serosal membrane, PTZ might hyperpolarize the membrane and, if this effect occurs in the neuronal membrane, produce an inhibitory wave characteristic of absence seizures. Thus, the massive inhibitory stimulus characteristic of the spike-wave discharges seen in both absence and PTZ-induced seizures can be blocked by reducing the inhibitory drive (i.e., decreasing potassium permeability), and this might represent the action of the antiabsence class of drugs.

Because drugs such as phenytoin increase SCC by increasing mucosal permeability to sodium (see Sect. B.II), but are ineffective in the PTZ-stimulated system, it is believed that the toad bladder might be a useful in vitro model to distinguish between drugs effective against absence seizures and those effective against tonic-clonic seizures. As further support for the premise that antiabsence action results from decreased potassium permeability, it might be noted that ethosuximide does not inhibit passive calcium conductance, nor does it affect stimulated calcium flux in systems depolarized with veratridine or high potassium concentrations; and it does not block sodium influx into nervous tissue (SOHN and FERRENDELLI 1976).

Also, there is substantial electrophysiological data that support the role of decreased potassium permeability in the action of valproic acid (SLATER and JOHNSTON 1978; NOSEK 1981).

IV. Effects on Chloride Conductance

Several chemical classes of anticonvulsants, including valproic acid and the benzodiazepines, have been postulated to act by the activation of chloride channels. These effects will be discussed in the section (C.III) below that deals with drug effects on the dynamics of neurotransmitter-receptor interactions.

C. Neurotransmitter Metabolism, Disposition, and Dynamics

I. Effects on Intracellular Processes Related to Transmitter Release

Like many of the other effects of phenytoin already discussed, its effects on various aspects of neurotransmitter metabolism and disposition are complex. KATZ and MILEDI (1970) showed that depolarization of the presynaptic nerve ending causes increased calcium permeability in the nerve terminal membrane. The subsequent entry of calcium into the terminal has been shown to release neurotransmitter (MILEDI 1973). The actual role of calcium in transmitter release appears to be indirect, through an action of calcium on the phosphorylation of specific brain proteins; calcium ions stimulate the endogenous level of phosphorylation of these proteins (DELORENZO 1977). It was reasoned that if calcium-dependent protein phosphorylation mediates calcium-dependent neurotransmitter release, phenytoin would be expected to inhibit this process, since phenytoin inhibits the effects of calcium on neurotransmitter release. That this does indeed occur was shown by DELORENZO and co-workers (DELORENZO 1980) for two particular brain proteins, which they designated DPH-L and DPH-M. Phenytoin caused a substantial decrease in the calcium-dependent incorporation of labeled phosphate (from ATP) into these proteins. Furthermore, this effect was demonstrated in a highly enriched synaptic vesicle preparation, and was shown to be dependent upon an endogenous calmodulin-like protein present in association with the vesicles. Phenytoin supposedly, inhibits the effects of the calcium-calmodulin complex, and not the binding of calcium to calmodulin.

Therapeutic concentrations of phenytoin reduced the effectiveness of calmodulin by about 10%–20%, and similar results were found for carbamezepine. Phenobarbibtal, ethosuximide, and trimethadione had no significant effects on either protein phosphorylation or neurotransmitter release. These data suggest that drugs lacking significant effect on post-tetanic potentiation (PTP) (phenobarbital, ethosuximide, and trimethadione) also fail to affect calcium- and calmodulin-dependent protein phosphorylation, while those that do modify PTP (phenytoin and carbamazepine) also inhibit phosphorylation. Thus, the ability of phenytoin to inhibit PTP might be related to its inhibition of calcium- and calmodulin-stimulated protein phosphorylation (presumably by inhibiting an associated protein kinase), and the consequent decrease in neurotransmitter release.

The neurotransmitter studied by DELORENZO (1980) was norepinephrine, and this presents several problems of interpretation. Because norepinephrine is an inhibitory transmitter in the brain, the role that decreasing its calcium-dependent release might play in the antiepileptic action of phenytoin is uncertain, unless it involved an effect on presynaptic inhibition of inhibitory neurons. While the role of norepinephrine as an inhibitory transmitter involved in presynaptic inhibition of inhibitory neurons is conceptually possible, it has not been documented experimentally. Also, WEINBERGER et al. (1976) reported that phenytoin failed to affect norepinephrine release. However, the stimulus for release in their study was potassium rather than calcium. Yet another problem of interpretation arises because phenytoin is a noncompetitive inhibitor of norepinephrine uptake in synaptosomes (WEINBERGER et al. 1976), and as such would tend to increase inhibitory tone in the central nervous system by allowing norepinephrine to accumulate at the synapses. (Apparently the sodium electrochemical gradient, which is heightened by phenytoin, does not effectively "drive" the reuptake of norepinephrine in the presence of noncompetitive inhibition.) This would counteract the inhibitory effect of phenytoin on norepinephrine release. However, it is clear that the above principles can be applied not just to norepinephrine, but to most other transmitters as well, with a net anticonvulsant effect a conceptual possibility.

II. Effects on Neurotransmitter Metabolism and Disposition

VERNADAKIS and WOODBURY (1960) reported that phenytoin decreased glutamic acid and slightly increased gamma-aminobutyric acid (GABA) levels in rat cerebral cortex. SAAD et al. (1972) also showed that brain GABA levels were increased by phenytoin. Because glutamic acid and GABA are excitatory and inhibitory transmitters, respectively, such changes might conceivably result in an anticonvulsant effect. However, PATSALOS and LASCELLES (1981) reported that phenytoin reduced both cerebellar and hypothalamic GABA, and the excitatory neurotransmitter aspartic acid was also decreased. Phenobarbital (SAAD et al. 1972), ethosuximide (SAWAYA et al. 1975), and diazepam (OSTRAVSKAYA et al. 1975) have also been shown to increase brain GABA levels. However, the mechanisms for such changes are apparently complex. For example, the increase in GABA levels caused by phenytoin is thought to result from increased synthesis (SAWAYA et al. 1975), because therapeutic concentrations of this drug do not inhibit GABA transaminase (GABA-T) or succinate semialdehyde dehydrogenase (SSD), two enzymes responsible for GABA degradation. Similarly, phenobarbital inhibits GABA-T only at supratherapeutic concentrations (SAWAYA et al. 1975). However, ethosuximide (SAWAYA et al. 1975) in therapeutic concentrations inhibits both GABA-T and SSD; and diazepam inhibits GABA-T (OSTRAVSKAYA et al. 1975).

Valproic acid (VPA) is a relatively "broad spectrum" anticonvulsant that has been postulated to act by increasing brain GABA concentrations (although direct postsynaptic mechanisms also appear to be involved; see below). Reports indicate that the activity of L-glutamic acid decarboxylase (GAD), the enzyme that catalyzes the biosynthesis of GABA, is increased, perhaps by the action of the only significant metabolite of VPA, 2-propyl-2-pentenoic acid (NAU and LÖSCHER 1982). These authors showed that VPA in mice increased the activity of GAD and elevated GABA concentrations, and that these effects paralleled the duration of anticonvulsant activity and the timecourse of the principal metabolite. GODIN et al. (1969) found that VPA increased brain GABA levels and inhibited the activitiy of GABA-T. However, NAU and LÖSCHER (1982) reported that VPA had no effect on GABA-T activity in their studies. FOWLER et al. (1975) studied the inhibition of GABA-T by VPA and several other monocarboxylic acids, and found VPA to be a relatively weak inhibitor. Although with clinical dosages inhibition of GABA-T by a few percent is possible, inhibition by at least 50% is required to produce any functional change in experimental animals (ANLEZARK et al. (1976).

HARVEY et al. (1975) found that VPA inhibited not only GABA-T, but also SSD; and that inhibition of SSD was greater than that of GABA-T. However, MAITRE et al. (1976) showed that the total inhibition of SSD by *p*-hydroxybenzaldehyde had no effect on brain GABA levels. Furthermore, it seems unlikely that normal doses of VPA as used clinically would produce brain concentrations sufficient to inhibit GABA-T significantly (HAMMOND et al. 1981). Another enzyme involved in GABA degradation, aldehyde reductase, is reportedly more sensitive to inhibition by VPA than either GABA-T or SSD (WHITTLE and TURNER 1978), which suggests that it might be a key site in the action of VPA.

Nonuniform data have also been reported for GABA disposition. WEINBERGER et al. (1976) reported that both phenytoin and phenobarbital stimulate the high-affinity uptake of glutamic acid and GABA into rat brain synaptosomes; on the other hand, diazepam inhibits GABA uptake into mouse brain synaptosomes

(OLSEN et al. 1977). The ability of phenytoin to stimulate uptake of glutamic acid and GABA contrasts with its inhibition of norepinephrine uptake already discussed. These different effects of phenytoin might be rationalized on the basis of the observation that GABA is degraded outside the synapse (e.g., in glia), while norepinephrine is metabolized largely within the synapse. Thus, increasing GABA uptake would minimize the extent of degradation, and make more of the transmitter available for release. The increased uptake of glutamate might afford the same result, since glutamic acid is converted to GABA. The mechanism for the increased uptake of these amino acids is probably the heightened sodium electrochemical gradient, which would provide a driving force for membrane penetration.

Acetylcholine metabolism and disposition might also be affected by certain anticonvulsants. MCLENNAN and ELLIOT (1951) reported that production of acetylcholine by brain slices is increased by low concentrations of phenytoin and decreased by high concentrations. These effects might be due to the ability of low concentrations of phenytoin to block calcium uptake by subcellular particles, thus increasing cytosolic calcium and consequently neurotransmitter release; and the ability of high phenytoin concentrations to block calcium flux across the synaptic membrane, thus decreasing cytosolic calcium and transmitter release. Because acetylcholine causes depolarization by opening sodium channels, an effect of phenytoin to block sodium channels (as already discussed) would be expected to prevent such depolarization, and could account for an anticonvulsant effect. The effect of low doses of phenytoin to stimulate acetylcholine release might explain the excitatory effects sometimes encountered with this drug. Others have also demonstrated the inhibitory effects of phenytoin on acetylcholine release (YAARI et al. 1977), and phenytoin has also been shown to decrease total brain acetylcholine concentrations (AGARWAL and BHARGAVA 1964). However, BIANCHI et al. (1975) report that phenytoin has no effect on acetylcholine concentration or release in normal guinea pig cortex.

III. Effects on Receptor-Ionophore Dynamics

Effects on GABAergic transmission may occur by interactions at the postsynaptic receptor-ionophore as well as by actions on GABA metabolism and disposition. The activity of GABAergic synapses is potentiated by anticonvulsant drugs such as benzodiazepines, barbiturates, phenytoin, valproic acid, and others; and evidence is accruing that many of these drugs act on discrete receptors that are related to the action of GABA on chloride channels. The action of GABA involves rapid and reversible binding to a specific receptor site in the postsynaptic membrane. Binding to this site regulates the opening and closing of membrane chloride ion channels. However, the GABA receptor-ionophore appears in reality to be a receptor complex that includes sites for three chemical classes of ligand: the GABA (and GABA-mimetic) receptor site; the benzodiazepine receptor site; and the picrotoxinin/barbiturate receptor site. Ligand interactions at these sites could modulate activation of chloride channels; positive modulation might result in potentiation of chloride conductance, while negative modulation might block chloride conductance. Thus, drugs might mimic or inhibit the actions of natural substances at each site in the complex. Furthermore, interactions might occur among the three subunits. In each case, an anticonvulsant effect might be rationalized on the basis of a net physiological response to activate chloride conductance and thus hyperpolarize the neuronal membrane, while a convulsant effect might be rationalized in the reciprocal manner.

All compounds which inhibit the binding of GABA to its subunit have been found either to mimic or to inhibit the action of GABA at synapses (OLSEN et al. 1978). In particular, agonists such as muscimol, isoguvacine, 3-aminopropane sulfonic acid, and piperidine-4-sulfonic acid (GREENLEE et al. 1978), and antagonists such as bicuculline, each inhibit the binding of GABA. Thus, the synaptic activity of a large series of GABA analogues correlates very well with binding to the GABA subunit (KROGSGAARD-LARSEN et al. 1979). However, GABA receptor binding is not inhibited by GABA analogues such as nipecotic acid, which specifically inhibit GABA uptake but have no postsynaptic agonist or antagonist activity (JOHNSTON 1978).

Drugs which appear to act directly (and competitively) at the GABA subunit are for the most part physiological agonists. However, the potential use of such agents as anticonvulsants is restricted by their inability to penetrate the blood-brain barrier, a property they share with GABA itself. Although inhibition of GABA-T might allow higher concentrations of GABA-mimetics to enter the brain (ENNA et al. 1980), GABA therapy for epilepsy has generally proved unsuccessful (MELDRUM et al. 1980). However, some promise as anticonvulsants can be seen for the hydrophobic analogues of GABA such as 4,5,6,7-tetra hydroisoxazolo [5,4-C]pyridine-3-ol (THIP) (MELDRUM and HORTON 1980), which enter the brain more readily, or for drugs such as cetyl-GABA (FREY and LÖSCHER 1980), which are metabolized to GABA.

As noted above, GABA binding might also be inhibited by specific GABA antagonists. The convulsant bicuculline, which is the best known of such antagonists (JOHNSTON 1978), appears to block GABA binding directly (GREENLEE et al. 1978), while many other GABA antagonists appear to act at sites distinct from the GABA subunit. These include the convulsants picrotoxin (NICOLL and WOJTOWIEZ 1980), PTZ (MACDONALD and BARKER 1978), convulsant barbiturates (DOWNES and WILLIAMS 1969), and a convulsant benzodiazepine (SCHLOSSER and FRANCO 1979).

It is also known that certain GABA-mimetic drugs can affect GABA-mediated inhibition by interaction at sites distinct from the GABA receptor subunit. For example, radiolabeled diazepam or flunitrazepam binding is potently inhibited by pharmacologically active benzodiazepines, but by very few other drugs. Phenytoin and the convulsant PTZ are weak inhibitors. The binding affinities are in the nanomolar range, and correlation analysis of relative inhibitory potencies suggest that the binding sites are related to anxiolytic, anticonvulsant (anti-PTZ), sedative, and muscle relaxant actions. Furthermore, the receptor sites appear to be physically coupled to GABA receptor sites, and both appear to be coupled to the chloride ion channel. Evidence for such coupling comes from interaction studies with various ligands and from anion effects on such interactions. Thus, GABA binding in vitro was enhanced by benzodiazepines, and benzodiazepine binding was enhanced by GABA (GUIDOTTI et al. 1979), and both interactions are strictly dependent on the presence of anions that can penetrate the chloride ion channel.

Yet another site at which GABA-mimetic drugs might interact is the so-called picrotoxinin/barbiturate site. Interaction of picrotoxinin with the GABA receptor complex blocks GABAergic transmission without blocking GABA binding to its subunit. Dihydropicrotoxinin (DHP), a biologically active analogue of picrotoxinin, has been used to assay picrotoxinin-binding sites (OLSEN et al. 1979). It was found that radiolabeled DHP binding was inhibited by many convulsant drugs known to inhibit GABA synapses, including convulsant barbiturates (TICKU and OLSEN 1978) and a convulsant benzodiazepine (OLSEN et al. 1980). Also, anticonvulsant barbiturates (TICKU and OLSEN 1978), carbamazepine (LEEB-LUNDBERG et al. 1981), and phenytoin (TICKU et al. 1978) were reported to inhibit DHP binding at therapeutically relevant concentrations. Binding potency correlates well with the activity of barbiturates in enhancing the postsynaptic chloride conductance activated by GABA (MACDONALD and BARKER 1979) and with the reversal by barbiturates of GABAergic antagonism caused by bicuculline and picrotoxin (OLSEN 1981).

As with the benzodiazepine site, the picrotoxinin/barbiturate site appears to be physically coupled to the GABA site; and coupling also occurs with the benzodiazepine site. In vitro, depressant barbiturates enhance benzodiazepine binding, and the relative potency for this effect correlates well with their potency in reversing the actions of GABA antagonists (DRAY and BOWERY 1979). Picrotoxinin competitively inhibits the enhancement of benzodiazepine binding by such drugs. OLSEN (1981) has also shown that depressant barbiturates enhance GABA receptor binding, which is to be expected on the basis of the established coupling between benzodiazepine and GABA receptors. However, phenytoin, carbamazepine, valproic acid, and the anticonvulsant barbiturates do not enhance benzodiazepine binding (although they do inhibit DHP binding). Thus, anticonvulsants appear to interact with the barbiturate receptor in a qualitatively different manner than do the anesthetic/hypnotic barbiturates. Finally, barbiturate enhancement of both benzodiazepine and GABA binding was found to be dependent on the presence of chloride, which suggests that the same picrotoxinin/barbiturate receptor is involved in both interactions, and the receptor is coupled to the GABA receptor (OLSEN 1981).

A matter worthy of discussion is that the high-affinity (nanomolar) benzodiazepine-binding sites do not account for the activity of these drugs in the treatment of generalized tonic-clonic (GTC) convulsions. While their nanomolar affinity constants correlate very well with potencies in the PTZ threshold test (used to predict drugs useful in absence seizures), and account for their very high potency in this test, the correlation of such constants with activity against maximal electroshock seizures (as a predictor of activity against GTC seizures) is very poor. This, and the finding that micromolar concentrations of benzodiazepine in brain are associated with pharmacological activity (BOWLING and DELORENZO 1982), led to the search for selective benzodiazepine receptors with binding affinities in the micromolar range. Such receptors were recently reported by BOWLING and DELORENZO (1982), who demonstrated that the binding was both saturable and stereospecific. For a series of benzodiazepines, the correlation of micromolar binding with potency against maximal electroshock seizures in mice was very good ($r = 0.953$, $P < 0.001$). Furthermore, phenytoin in therapeutic concentrations displaced specifically bound diazepam from the micromolar receptors with a K_i of 155 μM, suggesting that the micromolar receptor is also a phenytoin receptor. Unlike the nanomolar sites, the binding affinity of the micromolar receptors was not significantly enhanced by GABA or muscimol, a GABA agonist. This is consistent with the failure of phenytoin, carbamazepine, and other anticonvulsants effective against GTC seizures to enhance GABA binding (see above). Thus, it appears that the micromolar binding sites are more closely related (functionally) to the picrotoxinin/barbiturate site than to the high-affinity benzodiazepine sites.

The demonstration of micromolar benzodiazepine sites is particularly gratifying because of the Camermans (CAMERMAN and CAMERMAN 1970) demonstration that marked structural similarities exist between diazepam and phenytoin. If we are to infer from such similarities in structure that a common mechanism exists, it would be useful to demonstrate an experimental model in which both drugs are active. However, until now this was lacking, because phenytoin is notably inactive in the PTZ threshold test for which the nanomolar affinities correlate so well with potency. New developments in this area will be anxiously awaited.

D. Perspective

It is important to recognize that the effects of phenytoin on any one biochemical or physiological parameter cannot necessarily be interpreted as a separate mechanism of action. The bewildering complexity of the central nervous system and the large variety of seizure types known to occur certainly provide ample justification for the hypothesis of multiple antiepileptic mechanisms. Such a hypothesis receives further support from the selectivity of the drugs used to treat such seizures. However, it is possible that several of the above effects are related as different effects in a common effector system, or as components of different effector systems arising from a common action. For example, the inhibition of passive sodium influx might be correlated with inhibition of PTP, as pointed out by PINCUS (1972). Yet, because of the coupling between sodium and calcium conductance, it is possible that the primary action of phenytoin is to antagonize calcium transport. Furthermore, presynaptic calcium concentration might affect PTP independently of changes in sodium flux; thus, the action of phenytoin to antagonize calcium movements might directly determine its affect on PTP. Yet another possibility is that inhibition of PTP might be due to inhibition of calcium- and calmodulin-dependent phosphorylation of specific proteins associated with synaptic vessels.

In conclusion, phenytoin affects numerous indices of neurophysiological function. The changes induced are almost always compatible with an anticonvulsant action. Stimulation of the sodium pump, inhibition of passive sodium influx, inhibition of calcium influx or the effect of the calcium-calmodulin complex on protein phosphorylation, increasing GABA concentrations, and many other observable correlates of phenytoin action might all provide logical explanations for the ability of this drug to stabilize the hyperexcitable brain.

References

Agarwal SL, Bhargava V (1964) Effect of drugs on brain acetylcholine level in rats. Indian J Med Res 52:1179–1182

Anlezark G, Horton RW, Meldrum BS, Sawaya MCB (1976) Anticonvulsant action of ethanolamine-*o*-sulfate and di-*n*-propylacetate and the metabolism of γ-aminobutyric acid (GABA) in mice with audiogenic seizures. Biochem Pharmacol 25:413–417

Ayala GF, Lin G, Johnston D (1977) The mechanism of action of diphenylhydantoin on invertebrate neurons: I. Effects on basic membrane properties. Brain Res 121:245–258

Baker PF, Blaustein MP, Manil J, Steinhardt RA (1969) The influence of calcium on sodium efflux in squid axons. J Physiol (Lond) 200:431–458

Baker PF, Hodgkin AC, Ridgway EF (1971) Depolarization and calcium entry in squid giant axons. J Physiol (Lond) 218:709–755

Baskin SI, Dutta S, Marks BH (1973) The effects of diphenylhydantoin and potassium on the biological activity of ouabain in the guinea pig heart. Br J Pharmacol 47:85–96

Bianchi C, Beani L, Bertelli A (1975) Effects of some anti-epileptic drugs on brain acetylcholine. Neuropharmacology 14:327–332

Bowling AC, DeLorenzo RJ (1982) Micromolar affinity benzodiazepine receptors: identification and characterization in central nervous system. Science 216:1247–1250

Bronsted HE, Woodbury DM (1973) Uptake and distribution of ^{3}H-ouabain in brain and other tissues of developing rats. In: Boreus L (ed) Fetal pharmacology. Raven, New York, pp 89–92

Camerman A, Camerman N (1970) Diphenylhydantoin and diazepam: molecular structure similarities and steric basis of anticonvulsant activity. Science 168:1457–1458

Chwen AY, Leslie SW (1981) Enhancement of $^{45}Ca^{++}$ binding to acidic lipids by barbiturates, diphenylhydantoin, and ethanol. J Neurochem 36:1865–1867

Cohen MS, Bower RH, Fidler SM, Hohnsonbaugh RE, Sode J (1973) Inhibition of insulin release by diphenylhydantoin and diazoxide in a patient with benign insulinoma. Lancet 1:40–41

Delgado-Escueta AV, Horan MP (1980) Antiepileptic drugs. Phenytoin: biochemical membrane studies. In: Glaser GH, Penry JK, Woodbury DM (eds) Antiepileptic drugs: mechanisms of action. Raven, New York, pp 337–396

DeLorenzo RJ (1977) Antagonistic action of diphenylhydantoin and calcium on the level of phosphorylation of particular rat and human brain proteins. Brain Res 134:125–138

DeLorenzo RJ (1980) Antiepileptic drugs. Phenytoin: calcium- and calmodulin-dependent protein phosphorylation and neurotransmitter release. In: Glaser GH, Penry JK, Woodbury DM (eds) Antiepileptic drugs: mechanism of action. Raven, New York, pp 399–414

DeSousa RC, Grosso A (1973) Effects of diphenylhydantoin on transport processes in frog skin (*Rana ridibunda*). Experientia 29:1097–1098

Deupree JD (1977) The role or non-role of ATPase activation by phenytoin in the stabilization of excitable membranes. Epilepsia 18:309–315

DeWeer P (1980) Antiepileptic drugs. Phenytoin: blockage of resting sodium channels. In: Glaser GH, Penry JK, Woodbury DM (eds) Antiepileptic drugs: mechanisms of action. Raven, New York, pp 353–361

Downes H, Williams JK (1969) Effects of a convulsant barbiturate on the spinal monosynaptic pathway. J Pharmacol Exp Ther 168:283–289

Dray A, Bowery NH (1979) GABA convulsants and their interactions with central depressant agents. In: Krogsgaard-Larsen P, Scheel-Krüger J, Kofod H (eds) GABA-neurotransmitters. Munksgaard, Copenhagen, pp 376–389

Enna SJ, Maggi A, Worms P, Lloyd KG (1980) Muscimol: brain penetration and anticonvulsant potency following GABA-T inhibition. Brain Res Bull 5 (Suppl 2):461–464

Escueta AV, Davidson O, Hartwig G, Reilly E (1974) The freezing lesion. III. The effects of diphenylhydantoin on potassium transport within the nerve terminals from the primary foci. Brain Res 86:85–96

Ferrendelli JA, Daniels-McQueen S (1982) Comparative actions of phenytoin and other anticonvulsant drugs on potassium- and veratridine-stimulated calcium uptake in synaptosomes. J Pharmacol Exp Ther 220–29–34
Ferrendelli JA, Kinscherf DA (1977) Phenytoin: effects on calcium flux and cyclic nucleotides. Epilepsia 18:331–336
Fertziger AP, Liuzzi SE, Dunham PB (1971) Diphenylhydantoin (Dilantin): stimulator of potassium influx in lobster axons. Brain Res 33:592–596
Festoff BW, Appel SH (1968) Effect of diphenylhydantoin on synaptosome sodium-potassium-ATPase. J Clin Invest 47:2752–2758
Fichman MP, Kleeman CR, Bethune JE (1970) Inhibition of antidiuretic hormone secretion by diphenylhydantoin. Arch Neurol 22:45–53
Fowler LJ, Beckford J, John RA (1975) An analysis of the kinetics of the inhibition of rabbit brain γ-aminobutyrate aminotransferase by sodium *n*-dipropylacetate and some other simple carboxylic acids. Biochem Pharmacol 24:1267–1270
Frey HH, Löscher W (1980) Cetyl GABA: effect on convulsant thresholds in mice and acute toxicity. Neuropharmocology 19:217–220
Gerich JE, Charles MA, Levin SR, Forsham PH, Grodsky GM (1972) In vitro inhibition of pancreatic glucagon secretion by diphenylhydantoin. J Clin Endocrin Metab 35:823–824
Gilbert JC, Wyllie MG (1976) Effects of anticonvulsant and convulsant drugs on the ATPase activities of synaptosomes and their components. Br J Pharmacol 56:49–57
Godin Y, Heiner L, Mark J, Mandel P (1969) Effects of di-*n*-propylacetate, an anticonvulsive compound, on GABA metabolism. J Neurochem 16:869–873
Goldberg MA (1980) Antiepileptic drugs. Phenytoin: binding. In: Glaser GH, Penry JK, Woodbury DM (eds) Antiepileptic drugs: mechanisms of action. Raven, New York, pp 323–337
Goldstein RE, Penzotti C, Kuehl KS, Prindle HK Jr, Hall CA, Titus EO (1973) Correlation of antiarrhythmic effects of diphenylhydantoin with digoxin-induced changes in myocardial contractility, sodium-potassium adenosine triphosphatase activity, and potassium efflux. Circ Res 33:823–824
Greenlee DV, Van Ness PC, Olsen RW (1978) Gamma-aminobutyric acid binding in mammalian brain: receptor-like specificity of sodium independent sites. J Neurochem 31:933–938
Gross GJ, Woodbury DM (1972) Effects of pentylenetetrazole on ion transport in the isolated toad bladder. J Pharmacol Exp Ther 181:257–272
Guidotti A, Toffano G, Baraldi M, Schwartz JP, Costa E (1979) Molecular mechanism for the facilitation of GABA receptor function by benzodiazepines. In: Krogsgaard-Larsen P, Scheel-Krüger J, Kofod H (eds) GABA-neurotransmitters. Munksgaard, Copenhagen, pp 406–415
Gutman Y, Boonyaviroj P (1977) Mechanism of inhibition of catecholamine release from adrenal medulla by diphenylhydantoin and by low concentrations of ouabain (10^{-10} *M*). Naunyn Schmiedebergs Arch Pharmacol 296:293–296
Hammond EJ, Wilder BJ, Villarreal HJ, Perchalski RJ (1981) Central nervous system penetration of valproic acid. Epilepsia 22:227
Harvey PKP, Bradford HF, Davison AN (1975) The inhibitory effect of sodium *n*-dipropyl acetate on the degradative enzymes of the GABA shunt. FEBS Lett 52:251–254
Hasbani M, Pincus J, Lee SH (1974) Diphenylhydantoin and calcium movement in lobster nerves. Arch Neurol 31:250–254
Heinemann LI, Lux HD (1973) Effects of diphenylhydantoin on extracellular [K^+] in cat cortex. Electroencephalogr Clin Neurophysiol 34:735
Johnston GAR (1978) Neuropharmacology of amino acid inhibitory transmitters. Ann Rev Pharmacol Toxicol 18:269–289
Katz B, Miledi R (1970) Further study of the role of calcium in synaptic transmission. J Physiol (Lond) 207:789–801
Kootstra A, Woodhouse SP (1974) The effect of diphenylhydantoin on the Na^+-K^+-stimulated ouabain inhibited ATPase. Proc Univ Otago Med Sch 52:6–7

Krogsgaard-Larsen P, Hjeds H, Curtis DR, Lodge D, Johnston GAR (1979) Dihydromuscimol, thiomuscimol and related heterocyclic compounds as GABA analogues. J Neurochem 32:1717–1724

Leeb-Lundberg F, Snowman A, Olsen RW (1981) Some anticonvulsants interact with the GABA receptor-ionophore complex at barbiturate/picrotoxin receptor sites. Fed Proc 40:309

Lewin E, Bleck V (1977) The effect of diphenylhydantoin administration on sodium-potassium-activated ATPase in cortex. Neurology 21:647–651

Leznicki AL, Dymecki J (1974) The effect of certain anticonvulsants in vitro and in vivo on enzyme activities in rat brain. Neurol Neurochir Pol 24:413–419

Lipicky RJ, Gilbert DK, Stillman IM (1972) Diphenylhydantoin inhibition of sodium conductance in squid giant axon. Proc Natl Acad Sci NY 69:1758–1760

Maitre M, Ossola L, Mandel P (1976) In vitro studies into the effect of inhibition of rat brain succinic semialdehyde dehydrogenase on GABA synthesis and degradation. FEBS Lett 72:53–57

McDonald RL, Barker JL (1978) Specific antagonism of GABA-mediated postsynaptic inhibition in cultured mammalian spinal cord neurons: a common mode of convulsant action. Neurology (Minneap) 28:325–330

McDonald RL, Barker JL (1979) Enhancement of GABA-mediated postsynaptic inhibition in cultured mammalian spinal cord neurons: a common mode of anticonvulsant action. Brain Res 167:323–336

McLennan H, Elliot KAC (1951) Effects of convulsant and narcotic drugs on acetylcholine synthesis. J Pharmacol Exp Ther 103:35–43

Meldrum B, Hortin R (1980) Effects of the bicyclic GABA agonist, THIP, on myoclonic and seizure responses in mice and baboons with reflex epilepsy. Eur J Pharmacol 61:231–237

Meldrum B, Pedley T, Horton R, Anlezark G, Franks A (1980) Epileptogenic and anticonvulsant effects of GABA agonists and GABA uptake inhibitors. Brain Res Bull 5 (Suppl 2):685–690

Miledi R (1973) Transmitter release induced by injection of calcium ions into nerve terminals. Proc R Soc Lond (Biol) 183:421–425

Mittler JC, Glick SM (1972) Radioimmunoassayable oxytocin release from isolated neural lobes; responses to ions and drugs. IV International congress of endocrinology, Washington, 1972. Excerpta Medica Abstracts of Communications No. 177, p 46

Nachshen DA, Blaustein MP (1980) Some properties of potassium-stimulated calcium influx in presynaptic nerve endings. J Gen Physiol 76:709–728

Nau H, Löscher W (1982) Valproic acid: brain and plasma levels of the drug and its metabolites, anticonvulsant effects and γ-aminobutyric acid (GABA) metabolism in the mouse. J Pharmacol Exp Ther 220:654–659

Nicoll RA, Wojtowicz JM (1980) The effects of pentobarbital and related compounds on frog motoneurons. Brain Res 191:225–237

Nosek TM (1981) How valproate and phenytoin affect the ionic conductance and active transport characteristics of the crayfish giant axon. Epilepsia 22:651–665

Olsen RW (1981) The GABA postsynaptic membrane receptor-ionophore complex. Site of action of convulsant and anticonvulsant drugs. Mol Cell Biochem 39:261–279

Olsen RW, Lamar EE, Bayless JD (1977) Calcium-induced release of γ-aminobutyric acid from synaptosomes: effects of tranquilliser drugs. J Neurochem 28:299–305

Olsen RW, Greenlee D, Van Ness P, Ticku MK (1978) In: Fonnum F (ed) Amino acids as chemical transmitters. Plenum, New York, pp 467–486

Olsen RW, Ticku MK, Greenlee D, Van Ness P (1979) GABA receptor and ionophore binding sites – interaction with various drugs. In: Krogsgaard-Larsen P, Scheel-Krüger J, Kofod H (eds) GABA-neurotransmitters. Munksgaard, Copenhagen, pp 165–178

Olsen RW, Leeb-Lundberg F, Napias C (1980) Picrotoxin and convulsant binding sites in mammalian brain. Brain Res Bull 5 (Suppl 2):217–221

Ostravskaya RU, Molodavkin GM, Porfireva RP, Zubovskaya AM (1975) Mechanism of the anticonvulsant action of diazepam. Bull Exp Biol Med 79:270–273

Patsalos PN, Lascelles PT (1981) Changes in regional brain levels of amino acid putative neurotransmitters after prolonged treatment with the anticonvulsant drugs diphenylhydantoin, phenobarbitone, sodium valproate, ethosuximide, and sulthiame in the rat. J Neurochem 36:688–695

Pincus JH (1972) Diphenylhydantoin and ion flux in lobster nerve. Arch Neurol 26:4–10

Pincus JH, Grove I, Marino BB, Glaser GB (1970) Studies on the mechanism of action of diphenylhydantoin. Arch Neurol 22:566–571

Roses AD, Butterfield A, Appel SH, Chestnut DR (1975) Phenytoin and membrane fluidity in myotonic dystrophy. Arch Neurol 33:535–538

Saad SF, El-Masry AM, Scott PM (1972) Influence of certain anticonvulsants on the concentration of gamma-aminobutyric acid in the cerebral hemisphere of mice. Eur J. Pharmacol 17:386–392

Sawaya MCB, Horton RW, Meldrum BS (1975) Effects of anticonvulsant drugs on the cerebral enzymes metabolizing GABA. Epilepsia 16:649–655

Schant CL, Davis FA, Marder V (1974) Effects of carbamazepine on the ionic conductance of *Myxicola* giant axons. J Pharmacol Exp Ther 189–538–543

Schlosser W, Franco S (1979) Reduction of γ-aminobutyric acid (GABA)-mediated transmission by a convulsant benzodiazepine. J Pharmacol Exp Ther 211:290–295

Schwartz A, Lindenmayer GE, Allen JC (1975) The sodium-potassium adenosine triphosphatase: pharmacological and biochemical aspects. Pharmacol Rev 27:3–134

Siegle GJ, Goodwin BB (1972) Sodium-potassium-activated adenosine triphosphatase of brain microsomes: modification of sodium inhibition by diphenylhydantoin. J Clin Invest 51:1164–1169

Slater GE, Johnston D (1978) Sodium valproate increases potassium conductance in *Aplysia* neurons. Epilepsia 19:379–384

Sohn RS, Ferrendelli JA (1973) Inhibition of Ca^{++} transport into rat brain synaptosomes by diphenylhydantoin (DPH). J Pharmacol Exp Ther 185:272–275

Sohn RS, Ferrendelli JA (1976) Anticonvulsant drug mechanisms. Phenytoin, phenobarbital, and ethosuximide and calcium flux in isolated presynaptic endings. Arch Neurol 33:626–629

Spain RC, Chidsey CA (1971) Myocardial Na/K adenosine triphosphatase activity during reversal of ouabain toxicity with diphenylhydantoin. J Pharmacol Exp Ther 179:594–598

Ticku MK, Olsen RW (1978) Interaction of barbiturates with dihydropicrotoxinin binding sites related to the GABA receptor-ionophore system. Life Sci 22:1643–1651

Ticku MK, Ban M, Olsen RW (1978) Binding of [^{3}H]-dihydropicrotoxinin, a γ-aminobutyric acid synaptic antagonist, to rat brain membranes. Mol Pharmacol 14:391–402

Vernadakis A, Woodbury DM (1960) Effects of diphenylhydantoin and adrenocortical steroids on free glutamic acid, glutamine and gamma-aminobutyric acid concentrations of rat cerebral cortex. In: Roberts E (ed) Inhibition in the nervous system and gamma-aminobutyric acid, Pergamon, Oxford, pp 242–248

Watson EL, Woodbury DM (1972) Effects of diphenylhydantoin on active sodium transport in frog skin. J Pharmacol Exp Ther 180:767–776

Watson EL, Woodbury DM (1973) The effect of diphenylhydantoin and ouabain, alone and in combination, on the electrocardiogram and on cellular electrolytes of guinea pig heart and skeletal muscle. Arch Int Pharmacodyn 20:389–399

Weinberger J, Nichlas WJ, Berl S (1976) Mechanism of action of anticonvulsants. Neurology (Minneap) 26:162–166

Whittle SR, Turner AJ (1978) Effects of the anticonvulsant sodium valproate on γ-aminobutyrate and aldehyde metabolism in ox brain. J Neurochem 31:1453–1459

Wilensky AJ, Lowden JA (1972) The inhibitor effect of diphenylhydantoin on microsomal ATPase. Life Sci 11:319–327

Woodbury DM (1955) Effects of diphenylhydantoin on electrolytes and radiosodium turnover in brain and other tissues of normal, hyponatremic and postictal rats. J Pharmacol Exp Ther 115:74–95

Woodbury DM (1969) Role of pharmacological factors in the evaluation of anticonvulsant drugs. Epilepsia 10:121–143

Woodbury DM (1974) Antiepileptic drugs: pharmacology and mechanisms of action. In: Harris P, Mawdsley C (eds) Epilepsy. Proceedings of the Hans Berger centenary symposium, Churchill Livingstone, Edinburgh, pp 78–95

Woodbury DM (1978) Metabolites and the mechanisms of action of antiepileptic drugs. In: Meinardi H, Rowan AJ (eds) Advances in epileptology, 1977: Psychology, pharmacotherapy, and new diagnostic approaches. Proceedings of the thirteenth congress of the International League Against Epilepsy and ninth symposium of the International Bureau for Epilepsy, Amsterdam, September 1977, Swets and Zeitlinger, Amsterdam, pp 134–150

Woodbury DM (1980) Antiepileptic drugs. Phenytoin: proposed mechanisms of anticonvulsant action. In: Glaser GH, Penry JK, Woodbury DM (eds) Antiepileptic drugs: mechanisms of action. Raven, New York, pp 447–471

Yaari Y, Pincus JH, Argov Z (1977) Depression of synaptic transmission by diphenylhydantoin. Ann Neurol 1:334–338

CHAPTER 11

Tolerance and Dependence

H.-H. FREY

A. Introduction

The existence of tolerance to or dependence on antiepileptic drugs remains a controversial issue. While there is considerable and convincing experimental evidence for both phenomena, clinical experience and opinion are equivocal. Observations that can only be interpreted as tolerance or dependence are often merely described in the clinical literature, and the authors avoid drawing conclusions from their observations.

The following review will be confined to tolerance and dependence in connection with the anticonvulsant effect or the clinical use of antiepileptic drugs. A general review of the phenomena of tolerance to and dependence on nonopiate drugs appeared some years ago in the *Handbook of Experimental Pharmacology* (SMITH 1977). This provided general information on both phenomena, and the reader should consult this review for all aspects outside the scope of antiepileptic drugs.

Similarly, the field of "metabolic tolerance" or the induction of microsomal liver enzymes responsible for the metabolic inactivation and termination of pharmacological effect have been reviewed (CONNEY 1967). It is obvious that metabolic tolerance developing to the sedative effect of an antiepileptic drug will have the same significance for its very antiepileptic effect. Therefore the topic of metabolic tolerance to antiepileptic drugs will be dealt with fairly briefly, and this chapter will consider in extenso the experimental and clinical findings which are of importance for the treatment of epileptic patients.

It is often hardly possible to decide whether metabolic or functional tolerance is the factor responsible for the observations reported, especially in the earlier clinical literature. This is in fact valid for all clinical reports in which drug concentrations in plasma have not been determined. Since the clinical significance of the phenomenon of tolerance is independent of its exact mechanisms of action, such reports have been included and are tentatively dealt with under "Functional Tolerance" (Sect. B.II).

B. Tolerance

The term "tolerance" means, generally speaking, that higher doses of a drug become necessary during treatment in order to maintain the initial therapeutic effect. This merely descriptive term can experimentally be subdivided into

I. *Metabolic tolerance,* i.e., enhanced metabolic inactivation that makes an increase in dose necessary in order to maintain the original therapeutic drug concentrations and therapeutic efficacy

II. *Functional tolerance* characterized by adaptive processes in the neurons requiring higher drug concentrations in order to maintain the therapeutic effect

There are other factors in patients which may induce or mimic a phenomenon of decreasing drug efficacy during antiepileptic treatment. Besides metabolic and functional tolerance, the following have been put forward (BROWNE 1976): (1) variability of seizure incidence, (2) noncompliance, i.e., the patient does not take the drug as prescribed, (3) growth of the patient that will reduce the relative dosage, and (4) metabolites that might interfere with the effect of the parent drug. Strictly speaking, factors (1)–(3) have nothing to do with tolerance, but they may mimic tolerance when the treatment is not closely monitored by determination of plasma concentrations and – especially in children – increases in body weight are not compensated for by an adjustment of dose.

I. Metabolic Tolerance

As outlined in the "Introduction", only reports which have given special attention to antiepileptic drug action will be reviewed in this section. Drug interactions with an influence on the rate of elimation of antiepileptic drugs will be covered by the respective drug chapters and the section on "Clinical Pharmacology" in this volume.

1. Experimental Evidence

CUCINELL et al. (1963) reported a remarkable shortening of the elimination half-life of *phenytoin* in dogs when these animals were treated with high doses of phenobarbital. Initial half-lives were in the range of 5.5–12.5 h; they declined to 1.5–2.5 h after phenobarbital treatment. In the light of more recent results in dogs it remains dubious whether this observation really represented the result of enzyme induction by phenobarbital as postulated by the authors. FREY and LÖSCHER (1980b) found phenytoin to be an excellent inducer of its own metabolic inactivation in dogs. When the animals were treated with doses of 20 mg/kg t.i.d., there was some accumulation resulting in therapeutic drug concentrations in plasma on days 2 and 3 of treatment, but subsequently plasma concentrations rapidly declined so that only a few micrograms per millimeter of phenytoin could be detected after 1 week of treatment. The elimination half-life had fallen from an average value of 4.4 h before to 1–2 h after 1 week of treatment. In the rat, a decline in plasma concentrations of phenytoin was also found, and the tolerance observed to the anticonvulsant effect was therefore interpreted as a metabolic phenomenon (MASUDA et al. 1979). In parallel experiments with *phenobarbital* the protective effect waned in spite of constant plasma concentrations. In mice receiving phenobarbital with drinking water for 1–14 days, the resulting tolerance was analyzed by FREY and KAMPMANN (1965) as follows: The relative increases in the daily dose necessary for 50% protection and in the serum concentration at this level of protection were compared. When the relative increase in the daily dose exceeded that in serum concentrations, tolerance was considered to be metabolic, whereas in the case of a parallel rise in both parameters functional tolerance was assumed. Functional tolerance prevailed from day 1 to day 4, but subsequently the daily drug intake für 50% protection against electroconvulsions had to be increased more than the rise in serum concentrations necessary for this level of protection, so that metabolic tolerance was predominant from day 4 to day 14.

There is general agreement about the significance of the development of metabolic tolerance to *carbamazepine*. During treatment with this drug a strong enzyme induction with corresponding declines in plasma concentrations has been seen in dogs (FAIGLE et al. 1976; FREY and LÖSCHER 1980 a) and monkeys (PATEL et al. 1978; LOCKARD et al. 1979). In experiments with dogs (FREY and LÖSCHER 1980 a), unchanged carbamazepine or its active metabolite carbamazepine-10,11-epoxide could hardly be detected in plasma after only 5 days of treatment in spite of daily oral doses of 90 mg/kg! In the rat a functional tolerance seems to exist besides the metabolic one: In one study plasma concentrations declined, but at a given concentration fewer rats proved to be protected against electroconvulsions than in nontolerant animals (MASUDA et al. 1979).

Enzyme induction has been shown for moderate doses of *succinimides* in rats (ORTON and NICHOLLS 1972). For *benzodiazpines* metabolic tolerance seems not to play a major role with the usually small doses employed in the treatment of epilepsies. In the case of diazepam, the metabolite desmethyldiazepam even inhibits further demethylation (KLOTZ et al. 1976). However, nitrazepam metabolism can be accelerated in dogs by treatment with phenobarbital (ELIANDER and PEKKARINEN 1980). In mice treated twice daily with 75 mg/kg *methaqualone*, the protective effect against electroconvulsions fell from 70% to 23% within 1 week (BOGGAN et al. 1977). Since plasma concentrations of the drug were lower on day 4 than after the first administration, the authors regarded the tolerance as "metabolic".

2. Clinical Evidence

The existence of metabolic tolerance against the antiepileptic drug effect in man is best documented for *carbamazepine* (FAIGLE et al. 1976). In single-dose experiments, carbamazepine has an elimination half-life in the range of 30–55 h, which, during treatment of 2–4 weeks' duration, is reduced to about one-half of the initial value (MORSELLI et al. 1975; EICHELBAUM et al. 1975). The total body clearance was also increased in children, rising from 28 to 56 ml/kg per hour after 17–32 days of treatment (BERTILSSON et al. 1980). During combined antiepileptic treatment a plasma half-life of only 5–14 h was found by EICHELBAUM et al. (1979), who used [^{15}N]carbamazepine for the repeated determination of pharmacokinetics. The relative degree of metabolite tolerance to carbamazepine is thus the same as in the dog experiments of FREY and LÖSCHER (1980 a), but since the initial half-life of the drug is fairly long in man, the drug retains its therapeutic usefulness.

The enzyme induction by carbamazepine also accelerates the metabolic inactivation of other antiepileptic drugs: The elimination half-life of clonazepam fell from 32 to 22.5 h and that of ethosuximide from 54 to 45 h during concomitant carbamazepine therapy (LAI et al. 1978; WARREN et al. 1980). The elimination of valproate can also be accelerated by concomitant therapy with other antiepileptic drugs, as, e.g., carbamazepine or phenytoin, resulting in plasma concentrations lower than expected from previous single-dose studies (MIHALY et al. 1979).

The question of the existence of metabolic tolerance to *diazepam* remains controversial. Tolerance should not usually occur with the relatively low doses used in the therapy of epileptic disorders (KLOTZ et al. 1976; GREENBLATT and SHADER 1978), but SELLMAN et al. (1975) have reported an accelerated decline of diazepam plasma concentrations in patients treated with daily doses of 10–30 mg for 0.4–5 years. These patients had considerably higher plasma concentrations of desmethyldiazepam than in single-dose studies. KANTO et al. (1974) advocated the existence of enzyme induction during chronic misuse of the drug, but did not exclude a parallel development of functional tolerance.

II. Functional Tolerance

1. Experimental Evidence

The first drug which was studied experimentally for the development of tolerance to its anticonvulsant effect was *acetazoleamide*. This drug had an ED_{50} in the maximal electroshock test in mice of 75 mg/kg, but, when the animals received this dose twice daily for 6 days, the anticonvulsant ED_{50} had risen to 480 mg/kg (MILLICHAP et al. 1955). These results were confirmed by KOCH and WOODBURY (1958) in rats. The ED_{50} against maximal electroconvulsions was 2 mg/kg orally after the first exposure, but, when redetermined with intervals of 2 days, it rapidly rose to about 10 mg/kg, and then remained in this range. A similar increase was found in the anticonvulsant concentration of carbon dioxide: its median effective concentration EC_{50} rose from 2% to 5.2%. There is cross-tolerance between acetazoleamide and carbon dioxide (WOODBURY 1980). The tolerance to acetazoleamide was explained by an induction of carbonic anhydrase in glial cells or by a numerical increase of these cells with normal enzyme activity.

The development of tolerance to the anticonvulsant effect of *phenytoin* against maximal electroconvulsions in mice has been studied by FREY and KAMPMANN (1965). The animals received phenytoin with the drinking water, and the drug concentration in drinking water, the drug concentration in plasma, as well as the daily drug intake necessary for 50% protection were determined after 1, 2, 4, 7, and 14 days of treatment. The phenytoin concentration in drinking water providing 50% protection was about 0.21–0.22 mg/ml after 1 and 2 days of treatment, and then rose to 0.27 mg/ml after 4 days, 0.42 mg/ml after 7 days, and 1.4 mg/ml after 14 days. Since the mice reduced their water consumption when concentrations in the drinking water exceeded 0.3 mg/ml, the daily drug intake increased from 21–22 mg/kg on the first 2 days to only 59 mg/kg after 14 days. The serum concentration at 50% protection was 11 µg/ml after 1 day, and had significantly risen to 18 µg/ml after 4 days, to 24 µg/ml after 1 week, and to 47 µg/ml after 2 weeks. The relative increase of serum drug concentrations necessary for 50% protection exceeded that of drug intake. This unusual observation was explained as central adaptation to an accumulating drug. In the mice used phenytoin had an elimination half-life of 33 h. However, a contribution of metabolic tolerance to the phenomenon observed could not be excluded. That the latter in fact plays a certain role has since been stated by MASUDA et al. (1979) in rats. In mice daily treated i.p. with 7 mg/kg phenytoin, the protective effect declined from 70% on day 1 to only 5% on day 4 (KARLER et al. 1974). This tolerance was paralleled by an only moderate decrease in hexobarbital sleeping times, and the authors therefore regard central adaption to the drug effect as the most likely explanation for the tolerance observed. In later experiments, KARLER and TURKANIS (1980) did not see tolerance to the anticonvulsant effect of phenytoin in mice. However, these animals received injections of 9 mg/kg i.p. for only 4 days, and this time may have been too short for the manifestation of tolerance.

Tolerance to the anticonvulsant effect of *phenobarbital* was demonstrated in mice by the same experimental design as that described for phenytoin (FREY and KAMPMANN 1965). In order to achieve 50% protection against maximal electroconvulsions the drug concentration in drinking water had to be increased from 0.19 mg/ml for the 1st day of treatment to 1.1 mg/ml after 14 days of administration. The daily drug intake had to be increased from 30 to 100 mg/kg over this period. Serum concentrations at 50% protection increased rapidly from 12 to 22 μg/ml during the first 4 days, and then more slowly to 30 μg/ml after 14 days. For the first 4 days the relative increases in drug intake and serum phenobarbital concentrations required for 50% protection were identical and that was interpreted as tolerance by cerebral adaption. During the last 10 days of the study, drug intake for 50% protection had to be increased more than the rise in serum concentrations at this level of protection, so that, in this period, metabolic tolerance must be assumed to have played a role too. In a later study the results were reproduced in another strain of mice, and were also extended to the effect of phenobarbital on pentylenetetrazol-induced seizures (KILIAN and FREY 1973). In this test the daily drug intake in drinking water necessary for 50% protection rose from 110 mg/kg after 4 days to 160 mg/kg after 14 days. Brain concentrations of phenobarbital at 50% protection against electroconvulsions likewise rose from 20 to about 30 μg/g during the 2nd week of treatment. In the study by KARLER et al. (1974) mice were injected i.p. with 12 mg/kg phenobarbital for 4 days and the protective effect of this dose fell from 75% on day 1 to less than 20% on day 4. Hexobarbital sleeping time was not altered by this treatment, and the tolerance was thus regarded as functional. SCHMIDT et al. (1978, 1980) treated mice with daily i.p. injections of 25 mg/kg phenobarbital, and saw a decline in the anticonvulsant effect against maximal electroconvulsions from 95% on day 1 to 45% on day 5. Brain and plasma concentrations of phenobarbital, determined 2 h after the daily injection, remained constant throughout the study. No tolerance was seen in the minimal electroshock seizure threshold test, but treatment lasted only 3 days. The pentylentetrazol threshold for the first clonic jerk of the forelimbs was also not altered when determined 2 h after the daily injection of phenobarbital for 8 days. These latter results are in conflict with the study of KILIAN and FREY (1973) and the difference is difficult to explain. However, one possible reason might be the difference in drug administration: in the drinking water in one study and by single-drug injections in the other. MASUDA et al. (1979) have also observed tolerance to the anticonvulsant effect of phenobarbital in mice. In their study the protective effect against maximal electroconvulsions declined though plasma concentrations remained at the initial level, thus pointing to functional tolerance. When treated for 4 days with daily i.p. injections of 12 mg/kg phenobarbital, the convulsive threshold for the 6/s and 60/s electroshock, but not for the maximal electroshock, were lower than after a single i.p. dose of the drug (KARLER and TURKANIS 1980).

When rats were treated daily with phenacemide the effect of the drug against pentylenetetrazol-induced seizures was clearly reduced after 1 week of treatment: The initial ED_{95} protected only 50% of the animals, and the initial ED_{50} had no effect at all (DESALVA 1956). When the electroshock threshold of rats treated daily with oral doses of 200 mg/kg phenacemide or 500 mg/kg *trimethadione* was determined, it was increased for the first 2 weeks, then remained constant for 1 week, and fell rapidly during the next week (DESALVA 1956). Tolerance to the anticonvulsant effect of trimethadione was also shown by FREY and KRETSCHMER (1971). The mice were given the drug in the drinking water, and a 0.5% solution provided 20% protection against pentylenetetrazol-induced convulsions from day 1 to day 4, but only 10% protection after 7 days of treatment. Plasma concentrations of unmetabolized trimethadione remained between 18 and 27 µg/ml during the study, but the concentrations of the active metabolite dimethadione had risen from 670 µg/ml after 24 h to 1 800 µg/ml after 7 days. Experimental results of LOCKARD et al. (1977) in a monkey model might be interpreted as evidence for tolerance to *valproic acid*, but the experimental design seems too complex to permit valid conclusions.

The development of tolerance to the anticonvulsant effect of *benzodiazepines* has been studied by several authors. KILLAM et al. (1973), working with photically induced epilepsy in baboons, reported an escape from the anticonvulsant effect of diazepam and clonazepam. In order to keep the seizures under control the daily doses of diazepam had to be increased from 0.025 mg/kg to 0.2–0.4 mg/kg, and those of clonazepam from 0.005 mg/kg to 0.02 mg/kg in the course of the study, which lasted for 8–16 weeks. FUXE et al. (1975) reported that mice injected daily with 10 mg/kg diazepam i.p. developed tolerance from day 5, when 30%–40% of the animals were no longer protected against pentylenetetrazol-induced seizures. The acute ED_{50} for diazepam had been determined as 0.63 mg/kg! These authors assume a relation between dopamine turnover in the limbic forebrain and the anticonvulsant effect of the drug. FILE (1983) confirmed the development of tolerance to the anti-pentylenetetrazol effects of diazepam in mice. Contrary to the results of these authors, JUHASZ and DAIRMAN (1977) saw no tolerance to the anticonvulsant effect in mice treated orally with 2 mg/kg diazepam for 4 days when pentylenetetrazol was used as convulsant. But the same dose regimen clearly produced tolerance to the anticonvulsant effect of diazepam against bicuculline. By day 6 of a regimen using two daily oral doses of 1 mg/kg diazepam in mice, the drug had lost its anticonvulsant effect against seizures induced by 3-mercaptopropionic acid (TURNBALL et al. 1981). No tolerance to the anticonvulsant effect of triazolam developed, although the drug was administered for 25 days (PAKES et al. 1981). A rapid onset of tolerance to the anti-pentylenetetrazol effect of the 1,5-benzodiazepine clobazam was described by GENT and HAIGH (1983).

The biochemical background of tolerance to the actions of benzodiazepines has attracted considerable interest. At least the main approaches of research will be mentioned here, though only the study of SHER (1983) has been specially designed to study tolerance to the anticonvulsant effect. The close relationship between benzodiazepine receptors and the receptors for the inhibitory transmitter gamma-aminobutyric acid (GABA) in the CNS has focused great interest on alterations of binding to the benzodiazepine receptor during prolonged treatment. When rats were treated with extremely high doses of flurazepam for 4–8 weeks, the maximum binding capacity (B_{max}) for benzodiazepines was reduced by 15% –20%, but only for less than 24 h after termination of treatment. The dissociation constant was not changed (CHIU and ROSENBERG 1978; ROSENBERG and CHIU 1981). Similar results have been reported for clonazepam (CRAWLEY et al. 1982). These authors feel that the reduction in binding capacity might be related to the development of tolerance. MÖHLER et al. (1978), treating rats with more reasonable doses of 3 mg/kg diazepam daily, could not find a decrease in benzodiazepine-binding sites and considered this to be in "agreement with the general absence of tolerance during benzodiazepine therapy"! A decrease of GABA-binding sites in the striatum found by these authors remained unclear in its significance. BRAESTRUP et al. (1979) were not able to reproduce the results of ROSENBERG and CHIU. Recently, SHER (1983) has shown a significant dose-dependent reduction of benzodiazepine receptor binding in cell cultures from fetal mouse cerebral cortex which were exposed to diazepam concentrations of 0.45–3.6 μg/ml for 10 days. JENNER et al. (1975) found brain concentrations of 5-hydroxytryptamine (5-HT) and 5-hydroxyindoleacetic acid (5-HIAA) significantly increased when mice had been treated once with doses of 0.5–0.8 mg/kg clonazepam, but this increase had disappeared after 8 days of treatment. Since 5-HIAA concentrations in cerebrospinal fluid of patients treated with clonazepam for myoclonic fits were also higher as long as the clinical effect lasted, 5-HT metabolism might be of relevance for the development of tolerance. Especially in the case of diazepam, an interference with the main metabolite desmethyldiazepam at the receptor site might be implicated with respect to tolerance. GALLAGER et al. (1984) found a subsensitivity of the dorsal raphé nucleus to iontophoretically applied GABA after 3 weeks' treatment of rats with reasonable doses of diazepam. This finding might provide an explanation for the development of tolerance. If desmethyldiazepam occupies a greater part of benzodiazepine receptors by a higher affinity or simply by mass action, the sedative – and possibly also the anticonvulsant – effect of the parent drug might be attenuated (ELSASS et al. 1980).

As early as 1949, ALLAN and SWINYARD reported the development of tolerance to the anticonvulsant effect of *ethanol*. Rats were given ethanol daily in doses of 1–4 mg/kg orally, which, at the start, protected between 20% and 100% of the animals against electroshock seizures. The increase in electroconvulsive threshold vanished after 3 weeks and then even increases in the dose of ethanol produced only minor increases in the convulsive threshold. Similar results were later presented both for electro- and chemoconvulsions in mice treated with *phenaglycodol* or *meprobamate* (CHIN and SWINYARD 1958, 1959).

2. Clinical Evidence

Although HAUPTMANN (1912) in his classical paper on the use of phenobarbital in epilepsy has already pointed to the development of tolerance (*Gewöhnung*) during prolonged use of the drug, genuine clinical evidence for functional tolerance is still rare. Mostly, a more or less pronounced escape from the beneficial effects of antiepileptic drugs is merely stated, but, since adequate determinations of drug concentrations or elimination rates before and during tolerance have not been performed, the question of the nature of tolerance must remain open.

a) Proven Functional Tolerance

One of the few studies documenting genuine functional tolerance to the clinical effect of phenobarbital was published by BUCHTHAL et al. (1968). In most of 15 hospitalized patients in whom drug concentrations were monitored, seizures and paroxysmal EEG discharges were controlled by phenobarbital serum concentrations of 8–15 μg/ml in some patients even by 3–4 μg/ml. In three patients suffering from grand mal, whose seizures were initially controlled by serum concentrations of between 8 and 12 μg/ml, phenobarbital was withdrawn for 1–3 weeks. On renewed medication the paroxysmal discharges could only be controlled when phenobarbital concentrations of 18–25 μg/ml, i.e., twice the original concentration, were reached. This observation was interpreted as "tolerance" by the authors, but, some years later, the same observation was regarded as "most likely to be a withdrawal effect than evidence of tolerance" (BUCHTHAL and LENNOX-BUCHTHAL 1972). BOOKER (1972) cited the patients of BUCHTHAL et al. as evidence for genuine tolerance, and mentioned examples of "clinical breakthrough," i.e., fits, at serum concentrations of trimethadione, dimethadione, diazepam, and primidone which were higher than at the time of the initial "dramatic response" to these drugs. Unfortunately, no details were given.

b) Clinical Evidence of Tolerance Without Proof of Its Functional Nature

The author is unaware of any clinical studies reporting the development of tolerance to phenytoin.

The existence of tolerance to the antiepileptic effect of *phenobarbital* is mentioned especially in the earlier literature (HAUPTMANN 1912; FOX 1927; GRINKER 1929). Only the paper of FOX gives some quantitative data: Tolerance developed in 51 out of 167 patients (31%) who were followed for periods of 6 months to 8 years. During the first 6 months the incidence of fits increased from 2.8 to 4.8/month, and for the longer observation periods from an average of 3.47 or 3.25 fits/month during the first 6 months to 5.33 or 4.6 fits/month during the last 6 months' period of 2 or 8 years of observation.

A decline in the therapeutic effect of *valproic acid* after 4–6 months of treatment has been repeatedly mentioned but seems not to be too pronounced. In only some of the cases could the effect be reinstituted by increasing the dose (RITZ and JACOBI 1973; SCHÄFER and KETTNER 1974; FRÖSCHER et al. 1978).

LOMBROSO and FORXYTHE (1959) note that the therapeutic effect of *trimethadione* in patients with petit mal fell from 41% with complete or near-complete protection during the 1st month to 18% after 1 year and only 7% after 2 years of treatment.

Tolerance to the antiepileptic effect of *benzodiazepines* seems fairly common and has often been described. In reviewing the role of benzodiazepines in the treatment of epilepsy, BROWNE and PENRY (1973) mentioned 222 cases of tolerance to diazepam, nitrazepam, or clonazepam from 20 publications. These drugs were used for treatment of petit mal, infantile, and other myoclonic fits. Tolerance developed within a few days or after up to 18 months of treatment in 8%–52% (median 26%) of patients. The question of "metabolic" or "functional" nature of tolerance remains open though general experience with small doses of these drugs should speak for the latter type.

Tolerance to *diazepam* may appear within several weeks (GASTAUT et al. 1967) or 6–10 months (TROLLE 1965) in up to 40% of patients. By small increases of the doses which were well tolerated, it was possible to keep the disease under control so that tolerance did not pose an outstanding problem in the opinion of GELLER and CHRISTOFF (1971). Tolerance to the antiepileptic effect of *nitrazepam* developed in some cases after a few days, in others after months of treatment (JONG 1964; GIBBS and ANDERSON 1965; HAGBERG 1968; HAMBERT and PETERSEN 1970). MILLICHAP and ORITZ (1966) found it necessary to increase the dose in 29 out of 36 patients with myoclonus epilepsy from the initial dose of 0.1–0.7 mg/kg to final doses of 0.3–4.0 mg/kg. Tolerance appeared after an average time of 12 weeks in this study. Sometimes the doses necessary finally provoked signs of general depression, and thus the usefulness of the drug was limited (HAMBERT and PETERSEN 1970). In a review on *clonazepam* BROWNE (1976) reports that tolerance to the antiepileptic effect against many different forms of epilepsy develops in 11%–100% (median 33%) of patients. In approximately two-thirds of the patients who had become tolerant, considerable beneficial effects could be maintained by the initial or a greater dose of the drug, whereas the rest could no longer be controlled even with large doses. Tolerance became evident after 1–6 months of administration. Similar experiences have been published by other authors (BERGAMINI et al. 1970; DUMERMUTH and KOVACS 1974, KICK and DREYER 1973; MASLAND 1975). KRUSE and BLANKENHORN (1973) described the progressive loss of antiepileptic effect: In patients with minor fits, clonazepam had a positive effect (complete freedom of fits or reduction by at least 50%) in 62% during the 1st month; this effect declined to 45% after 3 months, to 34% after 6 months, to 25% after 1 year, to 18% after 2 years, and finally to 14% after 2½ years. In myoclonic-astatic fits a similar course was observed, whereas grand mal and/or tonic seizures were ameliorated to a lesser degree by clonazepam. The initial rate of effect in these patients was 41%, but after 6–12 months the antiepileptic effect had in fact been lost and could not even be reinstituted by increases in dose. Also ROSSI et al. (1973) note a rapid loss of the effect against seizures and EEG manifestations in patients with generalized epilepsies. The loss of these effects began as soon as the 1st week of treatment and was complete after 1 month. On the other hand, in the opinion of HANSON and MENKES (1972), tolerance in children with minor motor seizures is less pronounced with clonazepam than with other benzodiazepines. Regarding the development of tolerance, there seems to be no difference between the classical 1,4-benzodiazepines and the 1,5-analogue clobazam (GASTAUT and LOW 1979).

Acetazoleamide became known relatively early to induce tolerance to its anticonvulsant effect. Tolerance developed within weeks to some months; the effect could be maintained for some time by increases in dose, but finally patients became resistent even to doses of 20 mg/kg (ANSELL and CLARKE 1956; MILLICHAP 1956). In the study of LOMBROSO and FORXYTHE (1959) seizures in 42% of 91 patients with petit mal were controlled after the first 3 weeks; this dropped to 25% after the 1st year, to 14% after the 2nd year, and to 10% after the 3rd year.

HAMBERT and PETERSEN (1970) have reported tolerance to the antiepileptic effect of *clomethiazol* in patients with myoclonus epilepsy.

III. Acute Tolerance

Acute tolerance is usually defined as a subsensitivity developing during the time of action of a single drug dose, i.e., the drug effect ceases at higher drug concentrations than it started with. The terms is, however, sometimes used in a way that covers "tachyphylaxis," which is defined as a loss of drug effect on rapidly repeated injections. For the phenomenon described especially for diazepam, tachyphylaxis seems in fact more adequate than acute tolerance.

PARSONAGE and NORRIS (1967) described this phenomenon in patients with severe status epilepticus treated with diazepam. Tolerance developed during continued i.v. infusion of total doses of 300–500 mg over periods of 2–3 days and usually became apparent within the first 24 h. The drug lost its efficacy against the seizures and this could not even be restored by intermittent injections of diazepam.

Acute tolerance to diazepam has been studied experimentally in cats in which focal seizures were elicited by application of penicillin on the motor cortex (SHARER and KUTT 1971). This provoked peripheral motor jerking which could be abolished by infusion of 0.5 mg/kg diazepam over 2 min for periods of 3–90 min. When the jerking recurred, an average dose of 1.8 mg/kg was necessary in order to suppress it again. The authors believe that a rapid metabolic detoxification cannot be the explanation since diazepam is slowly metabolized and its metabolites retain pharmacological activity. A similar observation was reported by BARNETT and FIORE (1971, 1973), who studied the effect of diazepam on the linguomandibular reflex in cats. Tolerance appeared when increasing doses of the drug were injected with intervals greater than 15 min. Tolerance was more pronounced after intraduodenal than after i.v. administration. However, no tolerance developed to the metabolite desmethyldiazepam, which had only one-fifth of the potency of diazepam. Desmethyldiazepam, given before diazepam, also attenuated the effect of the parent drug. Similar results were obtained when the effects of diazepam on the flexor reflex in spinal cats or the depression of the EEG amplitudes were studied. The development of acute tolerance is explained by the accumulation of the metabolite desmethyldiazepam which occupies the benzodiazepine receptors and thus prevents the access of the more potent parent drug to the receptor site. The same explanation may be valid also for the mechanisms of acute tolerance to the anticonvulsant action of diazepam, which seems to be a clinical problem in the treatment of status epilepticus.

For phenobarbital a phenomenon quite opposite to acute tolerance has been reported by FREY and MAGNUSSEN (1971). When the ED_{50} in the maximal electroshock test was determined in mice at intervals ranging from 2 to 24 h after oral administration, protection was afforded by progressively lower drug concentrations in serum and brain. After administration of the ED_{50} for 2 h, the time of the maximum effect of phenobarbital, a brain concentration of 21 μg/g was determined, whereas, after 24 h, only 9 μg/g was found in the brain after administration of the respective ED_{50}. An imbalance in the turnover of noradrenaline and 5-HT may explain this phenomenon. At shorter time intervals the turnover of noradrenaline was depressed and that of 5-HT unaltered, but at 20–24 h after administration of phenobarbital, noradrenaline turnover had normalized while that of 5-HT was significantly depressed.

IV. Conclusions

Tolerance to the anticonvulsant effect of antiepileptic drugs has been well documented in animal experiments, and has also been described for the clinical effect of many antiepileptic drugs such as the benzodiazepines, valproic acid, and carbamazepine. However, for two of the most widely used drugs, namely phenytoin and phenobarbital, no clinical tolerance has been reported or the evidence is at least equivocal.

Though there is general agreement as to the existence of tolerance to the sedative and hypnotic effect of phenobarbital, tolerance to its antiepileptic effect has only been reported occasionally and is even denied by many authors. The problem was discussed by BUTLER et al. (1954) at a time when tolerance to antiepileptic effects had hardly been studied. The authors described the development of tolerance to the behavioral effects of phenobarbital in man and dog, and expressed the opinion that the existence of tolerance to the antiepileptic effect would be difficult to prove since tolerance to the sedative-hypnotic effect appears within a few days, i.e., long before a steady state is attained. This argument seems quite convincing especially in view of the fact that up to 3 weeks elapse before a steady state with phenobarbital is reached in man.

The half-life of phenytoin is considerably shorter than that of phenobarbital, but, if tolerance should also develop rapidly, a similar mechanism might be considered. If no clinical control of seizures is achieved within the 1st week of treatment, the physician will increase the dose without thinking of the possibility of tolerance. The usual range of therapeutic concentrations of the antiepileptic drugs might thus very well represent the tolerant state of the patient. Such an interpretation would be in agreement with the clinical experience that tolerance does not present major problems for therapy with these classical antiepileptic drugs.

There is a dual problem with benzodiazepines: the acute tolerance and the tolerance developing after weeks or even months of therapy. The former is of importance for the treatment of status epilepticus when diazepam has to be given repeatedly or by infusion, and might be explained by interference of a metabolite at the receptor site. On the other hand, the slowly developing tolerance to diazepam, nitrazepam, and clonazepam has often been described, but so far its nature has not been elucidated.

C. Physical Dependence

The possibility of development of physical dependence to sedative and hypnotic drugs, mostly after longer times of abuse, is well known and documented (for review see SMITH 1977). As far as drugs with sedative or hypnotic potencies are concerned that are used in the treatment of epileptic disorders the appearance of signs of physical dependence on withdrawal will not be surprising, though the doses used in the antiepileptic indication are usually smaller than in drug abuse cases.

I. Experimental Evidence

Using the electro- or chemoconvulsive threshold in mice, withdrawal hyperexcitability has been shown relatively early for meprobamate, ethanol, and phenaglycodol (SWINYARD et al. 1957; MCQUARRIE and FINGL 1958; CHIN and SWINYARD 1958, 1959). When mice were treated orally with fairly high doses of these drugs for 2–3 weeks, the convulsive thresholds increased, but when treatment was terminated, the threshold values fell below the values for untreated controls. The duration of this hyperexcitability varied somewhat: After administration of meprobamate the control threshold was reached 28 h after withdrawal, with phenaglycodol after more then 32 h for the electroconvulsive threshold and after 60 h for the pentylenetetrazol seizure threshold, and with ethanol withdrawal symptoms reached their maximum after 2 days and recurrence to the control threshold for minimal electroconvulsions was seen only after 10 days.

RÜMKE (1967) saw a lowered convulsive threshold in mice for bemegride 48 and 72 h after one single dose of 100 mg/kg phenobarbital s.c., as well as 48 h after 100 mg/kg primidone orally or 60 mg/kg methoin orally, and 96 h after 50 mg/kg phenytoin s.c. Similar results were obtained when pentylenetetrazol or dioxone were used as convulsants. Neither after single doses nor following a 6-day regimen with phenobarbital, primidone, trimethadione, or phenytoin was the incidence of electroconvulsions increased. In these experiments the current was adjusted so that 50% of untreated mice displayed the extensor component of the maximal electroshock seizure. The fall in the chemoconvulsant threshold could be prevented when 250 mg/kg ethionine was injected 30 min before the anticonvulsants. In rats no decrease in threshold values was observed.

A significantly lowered electroconvulsive threshold was determined 24 h after withdrawal in mice that had been given phenobarbital in the drinking water for 4, 7, or 14 days. Whereas the electroconvulsive threshold had returned to control values 48 h after withdrawal, the pentylenetetrazol threshold remained lowered for 48 h after 7 or 14 days of drug administration. During the 3 days following withdrawal of phenobarbital, an average weight loss of 1–2 g/mouse was observed (KILIAN and FREY 1973). KARLER and TURKANIS (1980) treated mice for 4 days with daily i.p. injections of 12 mg/kg phenobarbital and noted a decrease in the electroconvulsive threshold 24 h after the last dose. No corresponding changes were seen when the animals were treated with phenytoin. Rats that were treated with phenytoin doses of up to 200 mg/kg for 20 days were more sensitive to audiogenically or electrically induced seizures 48 and 72 h after withdrawal (DELIMA and PALERMO-NETO 1981).

In rhesus monkeys made epileptic by injection of aluminum hydroxide gel into the pre- and postcentral gyrus, the number of seizures increased from an average of 13/2 weeks during primidone treatment to 55/2 weeks after withdrawal of the drug. The incidence of withdrawal seizures was thus more pronounced than after treatment with phenytoin or phenobarbital (LOCKARD et al. 1975).

In the experiments of TURNBULL et al. (1981) mice received two daily oral doses of 1 mg/kg diazepam for 28 days; 24 h after the last dose the convulsive threshold for 3-mercaptopropionic acid had dropped from a control value of 34 mg/kg to 26 mg/kg, and the halothane sleeping time (after 5 min exposure to 3% halothane) was shortened from 84 to 38 s.

The withdrawal hyperexcitability (lowered pentylenetetrazol seizure threshold) after treatment with phenobarbital was not abolished by pretreatment with 6-hydroxydopamine (TABAKOFF et al. 1978), and BRAESTRUP et al. (1979) found no relation between abstinence to diazepam and the number of benzodiazepine-binding sites or the drug's affinity to these.

For valproic acid a "quasi morphine abstinence behavior" has been described in rats by DEBOER et al. (1977). It appears during the first 15 min after i.p. injection of the drug in doses of 200–400 mg/kg, and is similar to the syndrome seen on withdrawal of morphine: escape digging, body and foreleg shaking, and yawning. This syndrome is, however, too closely related to the injection of the drug as to allow an interpretation as physical dependence but must be regarded as an acute pharmacodynamic effect of valproic acid.

II. Clinical Evidence

Withdrawal symptoms on termination of antiepileptic drug therapy with phenobarbital are relatively common observations. Early reports agree on the occurrence of frequent seizures, sometimes even status epilepticus, after withdrawal of the drug. The incidence of seizures then returns slowly to the level before initiation of treatment (FOX 1927; GRINKER 1929; SCHMIDT 1938; VIUKARI and TAMMISTO 1969). Withdrawal symptoms were not so severe in all cases; SCHMIDT (1938) describes some patients in whom only headache and vertigo, cardiovascular depression, or absences were seen. In patients with a previous history of convulsions, severe withdrawal reactions were more common than in patients without former convulsions (WULFF 1959). This author noted paroxysms in the EEG at phenobarbital plasma concentrations of 13 and 21 μg/ml, whereas similar EEG changes were only seen when phenobarbital plasma levels had fallen to about 3 μg/ml. However, changes may also be the consequence of tolerance in patients treated with the drug for a longer time. Withdrawal symptoms in newborn infants from epileptic mothers treated with phenobarbital have been reported: tremor, hyperexcitability, hypotonia, vomiting, and diarrhea (MARTINEZ and SNYDER 1973; ERITH 1965; DOOSE 1980). No corresponding observations exist for phenytoin or carbamazepine (DOOSE 1980).

Signs of physical dependence on benzodiapines have been seen mostly in psychiatric patients after withdrawal from high doses or in abusers. Dependence on the rather low doses used in the treatment of epilepsy has rarely been reported. MILLICHAP and ORTIZ (1966) mention 9 out of 36 children treated with nitrazepam for myoclonic epilepsies who showed an increase in fits after withdrawal, and KRUSE and BLANKENHORN (1973) state that some patients treated with clonazepam showed a temporary deterioration when the drug was stopped. This was even the case when the drug no longer had a clinical effect on account of tolerance. The observation was interpreted as withdrawal syndrome. DOOSE (1980), however, states clearly that abrupt termination of clonazepam therapy in epileptic children can lead to considerable signs of withdrawal, with an increased incidence of seizures. In newborn infants from epileptic mothers treated with diazepam, signs of physical dependence similar to those seen after treatment with phenobarbital developed within hours or even some days (REMENTERIA and BHATT 1977; DOOSE 1980).

Cases of acute psychosis on withdrawal of antiepileptic treatment consisting of three different drugs have been described; the symptoms disappeared as soon as the patients were put back on the original anticonvulsant medication (DEMERS-DESROSIERS et al. 1978).

III. Conclusions

Physical dependence may well develop after prolonged administration of antiepileptic drugs in doses necessary for the control of seizures. Dependence has, however, only been observed with drugs having a sedative or hypnotic potency, i.e., barbiturates,, primidone, benzodiazepines, ethanol, and meprobamate. On the other hand, dependence to phenytoin has only rarely been noted in experimental models but not in patients. No experimental or clinical evidence exists for the occurrence of withdrawal reactions after termination of treatment with carbamazepine, oxazolidinediones, succinimides, or valproic acid.

CARRANZA (1980) has recently denied the existence of withdrawal reactions after termination of benzodiazepine administration and expressed the opinion that the seizures seen after withdrawal are simply the result of the lack of antiepileptic protection by the drug. Clinical observations reporting only temporary increases in seizure frequency and general deterioration of patients are evidence against this interpretation. Generally, speaking, physical dependence seems not to be a great problem in antiepileptic drug therapy as long as drugs are withdrawn slowly. Slow withdrawal seems necessary even when an objective clinical effect of the drug can no longer be verified on account of the development of tolerance (KRUSE and BLANKENHORN 1973).

References

Allan FD, Swinyard CA (1949) Evaluation of tissue tolerance to ethyl alcohol by alterations in electroshock seizure threshold in rats. Anat Rec 103:419

Ansell B, Clarke E (1956) Acetazolamide in treatment of epilepsy. Br Med J I:650–654

Barnett A, Fiore JW (1971) Acute tolerance to diazepam in cats and its possible relationship to diazepam metabolism. Eur J Pharmacol 13:239–243

Barnett A, Fiore JW (1973) Acute tolerance to diazepam in cats. In: Garattini S, Mussini E, Randall LO (eds) The benzodiazepines. Raven, New York, pp 545–557

Bergamini L, Utani R, Fariello R, Liboni W (1970) Elektroenzephalographische und klinische Bewertung des neuen Benzodiazepin Ro 5/4023. EEG/EMG 1:182–188

Bertilsson L, Höjer B, Tybring G, Osterloh J, Rane A (1980) Autoinduction of carbamazepine metabolism in children examined by a stable isotope technique. Clin Pharmacol Ther 27:83–88

Boggan WO, Meyer JS, Steinberg RM, Worthington C (1977) The effects of methaqualone on the seizure susceptibility of mice. Psychopharmacology 54:45–49

Booker HE (1972) Phenobarbital, mephobarbital, and metharbital. Relation of plasma level to clinical control. In: Woodbury DM, Penry JK, Schmidt RP (eds) Antiepileptic drugs. Raven, New York, pp 329–334

Braestrup C, Nielsen M, Squires RF (1979) No changes in rat benzodiazepine receptors after withdrawal from continuous treatment with lorazepam and diazepam. Life Sci 24:347–350

Browne TR (1976) Clonazepam. A review of a new anticonvulsant drug. Arch Neurol 33:326–332
Browne TR, Penry JK (1973) Benzodiazepines in the treatment of epilepsy. A review. Epilepsia 14:277–310
Buchthal F, Lennox-Buchthal MA (1972) Phenobarbital. Relation of serum concentration to control of seizures. In: Woodbury DM, Penry JK, Schmidt RP (eds) Antiepileptic drugs. Raven, New York, pp 335–343
Buchthal F, Svensmark O, Simonsen H (1968) Relation of EEG and seizures to phenobarbital in serum. Arch Neurol 19:567–572
Butler TC, Mahaffee C, Waddell WJ (1954) Phenobarbital: studies on elimination, accumulation, tolerance, and dosage schedules. J Pharmacol Exp Ther 111:425–435
Carranza J (1980) Long term use and abuse of benzodiazepines. Pharmakopsychiatrie Neuropsychopharmakol 13:254–258
Chin L, Swinyard EA (1958) Tolerance and withdrawal hyperexcitability induced in mice by chronic administration of phenaglycodol. Proc Soc Exp Biol Med 97:251–254
Chin L, Swinyard EA (1959) Pentylenetetrazol seizure threshold in meprobamate- and phenaglycodol-treated mice. J Am Pharm Assoc Sci Ed 48:6–8
Chiu TH, Rosenberg HC (1978) Reduced diazepam binding following chronic benzodiazepine treatment. Life Sci 23:1153–1158
Conney AH (1967) Pharmacological implications of microsomal enzyme induction. Pharmacol Rev 19:317–366
Crawley JN, Marangos PJ, Stivers J, Goodwin FK (1982) Chronic clonazepam administration induces benzodiazepine receptor subsensitivity. Neuropharmacology 21:85–89
Cucinell SA, Koster R, Conney AH, Burns JJ (1963) Stimulatory effect of phenobarbital on the metabolism of diphenylhydantoin. J Pharmacol Exp Ther 141:157–160
De Boer T, Metselaar HJ, Bruinvels J (1977) Suppression of GABA-induced abstinence behaviour in naive rats by morphine and bicuculline. Life Sci 20:933–942
DeLima TCM, Palermo-Neto J (1981) Effects of withdrawal from longterm diphenylhydantoin treatment on audiogenic and maximal electroshock-induced seizures in rats. Acta Neurol Scand 63:189–196
Demers-Desrosiers LA, Nestoros JN, Vaillancourt P (1978) Acute psychosis precipitated by withdrawal of anticonvulsant medication. Am J Psychiatr 135:981–982
DeSalva SJ (1956) Tolerance development to anticonvulsive drugs. J Pharmacol Exp Ther 116:15–16
Doose H (1980) Zerebrale Anfälle im Kindesalter, 6th edn. Desitin-Werk Carl Klinke, Hamburg
Dumermuth G, Kovacs E (1974) Die Wirkung von Clonazepam in der peroralen Langzeittherapie schwerer Epilepsieformen des Kindesalters. Schweiz Med Wochenschr 104:608–617
Eichelbaum M, Ekbom K, Bertilsson L, Rane A (1975) Plasma kinetics of carbamazepine and its epoxide metabolite in man after single and multiple doses. Eur J Clin Pharmacol 8:337–341
Eichelbaum M, Köthe KW, Hoffmann F, v. Unruh GE (1979) Kinetics and metabolism of carbamazepine during combined antiepileptic therapy. Clin Pharmacol Ther 26:366–371
Eliander H, Pekkarinen A (1980) Enzyme inducing effects of phenobarbital on nitrazepam metabolism in dogs. Acta pharmacol Toxicol (Copenh) 47:171–174
Elsass P, Hendel J, Hvidberg EF, Hansen T, Gymoese E, Rathje J (1980) Kinetics and neuropsychologic effects of iv. diazepam in the presence and absence of its active *N*-desmethyl metabolite in humans. Psychopharmacology 70:307–312
Erith MJ (1975) Withdrawal symptoms in newborn infants of epileptic mothers. Br Med J III:40
Faigle JW, Brechbühler S, Felmann KF, Richter WJ (1976) The biotransformation of carbamazepine. In: Birkmayer W (ed) Epileptic seizures – behavior – pain. Huber, Bern, pp 127–140
File SE (1983) Tolerance to the anti-pentylenetetrazole effects of diazepam in the mouse. Psychopharmacology 79:284–286

Fox JT (1927) Luminal-sodium in the treatment of epilepsy. Lancet 589–592
Frey H-H, Kampmann E (1965) Tolerance to anticonvulsant drugs. Acta Pharmacol Toxicol (Copenh) 22:159–171
Frey H-H, Kretschmer B-H (1971) Anticonvulsant effect of trimethadione in mice during continued treatment via the drinking water. Arch Int Pharmacodyn Ther 193:181–190
Frey H-H, Löscher W (1980a) Pharmacokinetics of carbamazepine in the dog. Arch Int Pharmacodyn Ther 243:180–191
Frey H-H, Löscher W (1980b) Clinical pharmacokinetics of phenytoin in the dog: a reevaluation. Am J Vet Res 41:1635–1638
Frey H-H, Magnussen MP (1971) A hitherto undescribed feature in the anticonvulsant effect of phenobarbital. Pharmacology 5:1–8
Fröscher W, Schulz H-U, Gugler R (1978) Valproinsäure in der Behandlung der Epilepsien unter besonderer Berücksichtigung des Serumspiegels. Fortschr Neurol Psychiatr 46:327–341
Fuxe K, Agnati LF, Bolme P, Hökfelt T, Lidbrink P, Ljungdahl A, Perez de la Mora M, Ögren S-O (1975) The possible involvement of GABA mechanisms in the action of benzodiazepines on central catecholamine neurons. Adv Biochem Pharmacol 14:45–61
Gallager DW, Lakoski JM, Gonsalves SF, Rauch SL (1984) Chronic benzodiazepine treatment decreases postsynaptic GABA sensitivity. Nature (Lond.) 308:74–77
Gastaut H, Low MD (1979) Antiepileptic properties of clobazam, a 1–5 benzodiazepine, in man. Epilepsia 20:437–446
Gastaut H, Roger J, Lob H (1967) Le diazepam dans les épilepsies chroniques. Sem Hop Paris 43:462–467
Geller M, Christoff N (1971) Diazepam in the treatment of childhood epilepsy. J Am Med Assoc 215:2087–2090
Gent JP, Haigh JRM (1983) Development of tolerance to the anticonvulsant effects of clobazam. Europ J Pharmacol 94:155–158
Gibbs FA, Anderson EM (1965) Treatment of hypsarrhythmia and infantile spasms with a Librium analogue. Neurology 15:1173–1176
Greenblatt DJ, Shader RI (1978) Dependence, tolerance and addiction to benzodiazepines: clinical and pharmacokinetic considerations. Drug Metab Rev 8:13–28
Grinker RR (1929) The proper use of phenobarbital in the treatment of the epilepsies. J Am Med Assoc 93:1218–1219
Hagberg B (1968) The chlordiazepoxide HCl (Librium) analogue nitrazepam (Mogadon) in the treatment of epilepsy in children. Dev Med Child Neurol 10:302–308
Hambert O, Petersen I (1970) Clinical, electroencephalographical and neuropharmacological studies in syndromes of progressive myoclonus epilepsy. Acta Neurol Scand 46:149–186
Hanson FA, Menkes JH (1972) A new anticonvulsant in the management of minor motor seizures. Dev Med Child Neurol 14:3–14
Hauptmann A (1912) Luminal bei Epilepsie. MMW 59:1907–1909
Jenner P, Chadwick D, Reynolds EH, Marsden CD (1975) Clonazepam-induced changes in 5-hydroxytryptamine (5-HT) metabolism in animals and man. J Pharm Pharmacol 27:38 P
Jong TH (1964) Klinische Erfahrungen mit dem Benzodiazepinderivat Ro 4–5360 bei der Behandlung der Epilepsie. Schweiz Med Wochenschr 94:730–733
Juhasz L, Dairman W (1977) Effect of subacute diazepam administration in mice on the subsequent ability of diazepam to protect against metrazol and bicuculline induced convulsions. Fed Proc 36:377
Kanto J, Ilsalo E, Lehtinen V, Salminen J (1974) The concentration of diazepam and its metabolites in the plasma after an acute and chronic administration. Psychopharmacologia (Berlin) 36:123–131
Karler R, Turkanis SA (1980) Subacute cannabinoid treatment: anticonvulsant activity and withdrawal excitability in mice. Br J Pharmacol 68:479–484
Karler F, Cely W, Turkanis SA (1974) A study of the development of tolerance to an anticonvulsant effect of Δ^9-tetrahydrocannabinol and cannabidiol. Res Commun Chem Pathol Pharmacol 9:23–39

Kick H, Dreyer R (1973) Klinische Erfahrungen mit Clonazepam unter besonderer Berücksichtigung psychomotorischer Anfälle. Acta Neurol Scand 49:[Suppl 53] 54–59
Kilian M, Frey H-H (1973) Thresholds for electro- and chemoconvulsions in mice after treatment with phenobarbital. Pharmacology 10:169–177
Killam EK, Matsuzaki M, Killam KF (1973) Effects of chronic administration of benzodiazepines on epileptic seizures and brain electrical acitivity in *Papio papio*. In: Garattini S, Mussini E, Randall LO (eds) The benzodiazepines. Raven, New York, pp 443–460
Klotz U, Antonin KH, Bieck PR (1976) Comparison of the pharmacokinetics of diazepam after single and subchronic doses. Eur J Clin Pharmacol 10:121–126
Koch A, Woodbury DM (1958) Effects of carbonic anhydrase inhibition on brain excitability. J Pharmacol Exp Ther 122:335–342
Kruse R, Blankenhorn V (1973) Zusammenfassender Erfahrungsbericht über die klinische Anwendung und Wirksamkeit von Ro 5-4023 (Clonazepam) auf verschiedene Formen epileptischer Anfälle. Acta Neurol Scand 49:[Suppl 53] 60–71
Lai AA, Levy RH, Cutler RE (1978) Time-course of interaction between carbamazepine and clonazepam in normal man. Clin Pharmacol Ther 24:316–323
Lockard JS, Uhler V, DuCharme LL, Farquhar JA, Huntsman BJ (1975) Efficacy of standard anticonvulsants in monkey model with spontaneous motor seizures. Epilepsia 16:301–317
Lockard JS, Levy RH, Congdon WC, DuCharme RL, Patel IH (1977) Efficacy testing of valproic acid compared to ethosuximide in monkey model: II. Seizures, EEG, and diurnal variations. Epilepsia 18:205–224
Lockard JS, Levy RH, DuCharme, LL, Congdon WC, Patel IH (1979) Carbamazepine revisited in a monkey model. Epilepsia 20:169–173
Lombroso CT, Forxythe I (1959) A long-term follow-up of acetazolamide (Diamox) in the treatment of epilepsy. Epilepsia 1:493–500
Martinez G, Snyder RD (1973) Transplacental passage of primidone. Neurology 23:381–383
Masland RL (1975) A controlled trial of clonazepam in temporal lobe epilepsy. Acta Neurol Scand [Suppl] 60:49–54
Masuda Y, Utsui Y, Shiraishi Y, Karasawa T, Yoshida K, Shimizu M (1979) Pharmacokinetic and pharmacodynamic tolerance of a new anticonvulsant agent (3-sulfamoylmethyl-1,2-benzisoxasole) compared to phenobarbital diphenylhydantoin and carbamazepine in rats. Arch Int Pharmacodyn Ther 240:79–89
McQuarrie DG, Fingl E (1958) Effects of single doses and chronic administration of ethanol on experimental seizures in mice. J Pharmacol Exp Ther 124:264–271
Mihaly GW, Vauda FJ, Miles JL, Louis WJ (1979) Single and chronic dose pharmacokinetic studies of sodium valproate in epileptic patients. Eur J Clin Pharmacol 16:23–29
Millichap JG (1956) Anticonvulsant action of Diamox in children. Neurology 6:552–559
Millichap JG, Ortiz WR (1966) Nitrazepam in myoclonic epilepsies. Am J Dis Child 112:242–248
Millichap JG, Thatcher LD, Williams PM (1955) Anticonvulsant action of acetazolamide, alone and in combination with ammonium chloride. Fed Proc 14:370–371
Möhler H, Okada T, Enna SJ (1978) Benzodiazepine and neurotransmitter receptor binding in rat brain after chronic administration of diazepam or phenobarbital. Brain Res 156:391–395
Morselli PL, Gerna M, de Maio D, Zanda G, Viani F, Garattini S (1975) Pharmacokinetic studies on carbamazepine in volunteers and in epileptic patients. In: Schneider H, Janz D, Gardner-Thorpe C, Meinardi H, Sherwin AL (eds) Clinical pharmacology of antiepileptic-drugs. Springer, Berlin Heidelberg New York, pp 166–179
Orton TC, Nicholls PJ (1972) Effect in rats of subacute administration of ethosuximide, methsuximide and phensuximide on hepatic microsomal enzymes and porphyrin turnover. Biochem Pharmacol 21:2253–2261
Pakes GF, Brogden RN, Heel RC, Speight TM, Avery GS (1981) Triazolam: a review of its pharmacological properties and therapeutic efficacy in patients with insomnia. Drugs 22:81–110

Parsonage MJ, Norris J (1967) Use of diazepam in treatment of severe convulsive status epilepticus Br Med J III:85–88
Patel IH, Levy RH, Trager WF (1978) Pharmacokinetics of carbamazepine-10,11-epoxide before and after autoinduction in rhesus monkeys. J Pharmacol Exp Ther 206:607–613
Rementeria JL, Bhatt K (1977) Withdrawal symptoms in neonates from intrauterine exposure to diazepam. J Pediatr 90:123–126
Ritz A, Jacobi G (1973) Zur Behandlung kindlicher Epilepsien mit Dipropylessigsäure (DPA). Fortschr Med 91:590–596
Rosenberg HC, Chiu TH (1981) Tolerance during chronic benzodiazepine treatment associated with decreased receptor binding. Eur J Pharmacol 70:453–460
Rossi GF, diRocco C, Maira G, Megilo M (1973) Experimental and clinical studies of the anticonvulsant properties of a benzodiazepine derivative, clonazepam (RO 5-4023). In: Garattini S, Mussini E, Randall LO (eds) The benzodiazepines. Raven, New York, pp 461–488
Rümke CL (1967) Increased susceptibility of mice to seizures after some anticonvulsant drugs. Eur J Pharmacol 1:369–377
Schäfer J, Kettner I (1974) Erfahrungen mit Dipropylacetat in der Behandlung therapieresistenter erwachsener Anfallskranker. Med Welt 25:561–563
Schmidt D, Kupferberg HJ, Yonekawa W, Penry JK (1978) Toleranzentwicklung bei mehrtägiger Phenobarbitalgabe. Arzneimittelforsch 28:1515–1516
Schmidt D, Kupferberg HJ, Yonekawa W, Penry JK (1980) The development of tolerance to the anticonvulsant effect of phenobarbital in mice. Epilepsia 21:141–147
Schmidt G (1938) Erscheinungen bei Luminalentzug. MMW 85:1944–1946
Sellman R, Kanto J, Raijola E, Pekkarinen A (1975) Induction effect of diazepam on its own metabolism. Acta Pharmacol Toxicol (Copenh) 37:345–351
Sharer L, Kutt H (1971) Intravenous administration of diazepam. Effects on penicillin-induced focal seizures in the cat. Arch Neurol 24:169–175
Sher PK (1983) Reduced benzodiazepine receptor binding in cerebral cortical cultures chronically exposed to diazepam. Epilepsia 24:313–320
Smith CM (1977) The pharmacology of sedative/hypnotics, alcohol, and anesthetics: sites and mechanism of action. In: Martin WR (ed) Handbook of experimental pharmacology, vol 45/1. Springer, Berlin Heidelberg New York, pp 496–587
Swinyard EA, Chin L, Fingl E (1957) Withdrawal hyperexcitability following chronic administration of meprobamate to mice. Science 125:739–741
Tabakoff B, Yanai J, Ritzmann RF (1978) Brain noradrenergic systems as a prerequisite for developing tolerance to barbiturates. Science 200:449–451
Trolle E (1965) Diazepam (Valium) in the treatment of epilepsy. A report of fifty cases. Acta Neurol Scand 41:[Suppl 13] 535–539
Turnbull MJ, Watkins JW, Wheeler H (1981) Demonstration of withdrawal hyperexcitability following administration of benzodiazepines to rats and mice. Br J Pharmacol 72:495 P
Viukari NMA, Tammisto P (1969) Central effects of diphenylhydantoin (Dilantin®) in epileptic oligophrenics during phenobarbital-primidone withdrawal, sodium bicarbonate, and ammnoium chloride administration. Behav Neuropsychiatr 1:13–16
Warren JW, Benmaman JD, Wannamaker BB, Levy RH (1980) Kinetics of carbamazepine-ethosuximide interaction. Clin Pharmacol Ther 28:646–651
Woodbury DM (1980) Carbonic anhydrase inhibitors. In: Glaser GH, Penry JK, Woodbury DM (eds) Antiepileptic drugs. Mechanisms of action. Raven, New York, pp 617–633
Wulff MH (1959) The barbiturate withdrawal syndrome. A clinical and electroencephalographic study. Electroenceph Clin Neurophysiol [Suppl] 14:73

CHAPTER 12

Animal Experimental Methods in the Study of Antiepileptic Drugs

W. P. KOELLA

A. Introduction

Animal experiments with antiepileptic drugs serve a variety of purposes. First, they are used for *screening* newly synthesized chemical compounds before these are investigated in patients; i.e., animals are used at an early stage to provide information which is more or less reliable, on whether a new agent is able to combat, with adequate efficacy, potency, and duration of action, the most important symptom of epilepsy, the seizure. In a more advanced phase of the screening procedure, animal experiments, usually of a more complex nature, are used to test the possible specific efficacies of new compounds against *distinct forms of seizures*.

Second, animal experiments of a more detailed nature serve to detect and clarify the (putative) mode, locus, and *mechanism of action* of a chemical agent in its effect on seizures.

Third, animal experiments are employed for the discovery and characterization of a variety of *side effects*. Early knowledge of such additional actions enables a new drug to be eliminated from further development if its side effects are strong and "undesirable"; on the other hand, if they are of a "desirable" nature, it permits the prediction of advantageous additional actions in the treatment of epilepsy. Early detection of side effects may also open pathways for the development of a new drug in the direction of other, additional, indications, not necessarily related to epilepsy.

Fourth, many animals of a variety of species are used for the determination of *toxic, cancerogenic, mutagenic*, and *teratogenic* effects; studies indispensable in the development of new compounds.

Fifth, studies are needed on the absorption, internal transport across various barriers, storage, binding, local concentrations, metabolism, and excretion of the compounds under investigation; information about these *kinetic* aspects forms the background for such studies in man at a later stage, in both volunteers and patients.

Sixth, investigations with antiepileptic drugs in what are usually quite complex animal experimental procedures offer an excellent opportunity for learning more – by "feedback" – about the *pathoneurophysiology of seizures* or, more globally, the pathogenesis or basic mechanisms of the different types of epilepsy.

The mechanisms of action of antiepileptic drugs are dealt with in other chapters of this volume; so too are the basic mechanisms of epilepsy. The techniques for, and the concepts involved in, studies concerning side and toxic effects – including cancerogenic, mutagenic, and teratogenic effects – are not specific for antiepileptic compounds. Neither are the methods used in investigation of the kinetics of drugs. This chapter will not therefore deal with these topics at any length, but will be mainly devoted to a discussion of *screening procedures,* both primary and advanced, i.e., a description of those animal models that are used for the characterization of a chemical compound *as an antiepileptic drug* and its possible further characterization as an agent effective *against special forms of convulsions,* or epilepsies.

Yet, before these themes can be dealt with in more detail, there are several concepts pertaining mainly to the nature of screening and of therapeutic action in general which require discussion and clarification. This should not only facilitate the readers' understanding of what such screening models are capable of revealing, or not revealing, but should also help the reader to grasp the not always easy problems occurring with considerations of phenomena borderline between "applied" research (viz., screening) and "basic" research (viz., studies on the mechanisms of action of antiepileptic drugs).

In discussing these various "models," in addition to the *gross symptomatology,* signs of function or malfunction at the network and neuronal level are also mentioned. This will not only expand the spectrum of "symptoms" of these screening models, but will also furnish additional information to be used as a cross-reference for a better conceptual understanding of the facts and theories presented in the chapters on "mechanisms." Screening is performed preferably in *"symptomatic models,"* i.e., in animals which in response to a variety of inducing – "etiological" – factors reveal behavioral, neurological, and/or electrographic signs of seizures and, in subchronic and chronic preparations, signs of interictal phenomena. These models exhibit epileptiform symptoms of a considerable variety of form, distribution, duration, development, and time course. The main aim in screening is to record attenuation or complete block of the gross symptoms through application – at a proper dose and by a proper route of application – of the drug under investigation. The mechanisms of action by which these drugs combat epileptiform symptoms in these models are largely unknown; hence the effect must be interpreted as being *symptomatic* and not causal *in nature,* and thus is not much different from the largely anticonvulsive treatment effected by so-called antiepileptic remedies in cases of epilepsy in man. Our insight into the mechanisms of action could be somewhat improved if more often we were to use (symptomatic) models with probes penetrating into the more detailed neurophysiological malfunctions which (may) underlie overt convulsions and which, by their very reaction to the drug, may signal *a* mechanism of action.

Such more detailed investigations may, however, reveal that our treatment of experimental epilepsy is still symptomatic in nature for the following reasons: anticonvulsants may in fact act not by affecting and improving the behavior of malfunctioning "epileptic" neurons in an "epileptic" network, but rather by *compensation* through the modulation of activity in an antagonistic, yet basically normal, pathway. If we assume, for the sake of argument, that a convulsing focus is solely the manifestation of an exaggerated excitatory input to a pool of neurons, then checking and reducing this input with our drug would constitute a case of causal treatment. However, if the drug in question enhances activity in the – basically normal – inhibitory pathways also impinging on this pool, then treatment would be symptomatic in nature. The late DON ESPLIN, in his excellent review of "synaptic system models" (ESPLIN 1972), quite evidently favored this "indirect" or symptomatic mechanism of action when he asked: "do those agents exert their basic antiepileptic action on the abnormal neuron [the epileptogenic neuron] or do they prevent the manifestations of epilepsy by actions primarily upon normal neurons?" In fact, ESPLIN takes "the easier course and assume(s) that most antiepileptic drugs exert their beneficial actions on normal neurons." We prefer a still easier course, and admit that we do not know as yet.

For similar reasons, even detailed neurophysiological studies in *nonsymptomatic models* – experiments in basically normal, nonepileptic animals – do not always permit us to decide unequivocally between a symptomatic and a causal effect. An alteration of any functional activity as induced by a drug may signal an effect exerted either on a potentially (in an epileptic focus) disturbed ("epileptic") or on a potentially normal neuron. But even if we can localize a drug effect to a neuron which in the actual experiment is still "normal" (but may be one that is typically affected in epilepsy), it cannot be transposed to the latter's abnormal state: sensitivity and *Ausgangslage* happen to differ in health and disease.

There is one exception, however, to these general statements about "uncertainty." It is well established – also through experiments discussed in this chapter (Sect. B. V) – that an initially well-confined discharging focus can spread the propensity to produce epileptiform discharge – possibly by a mechanism akin to posttetanic potentiation – to neighboring and/or remote, initially healthy areas. This "contamination" is clearly *the etiological factor* for epileptogenesis in the secondary sites. A drug that typically stems such a spread would unequivocally exert a *causal therapeutic effect* on the developing secondary focus while still (possibly) acting as a *symptomatic remedy* with respect to the primary focus.

Following such conceptual considerations the chapter then addresses the main topic: the description of animal experimental methods for the study of antiepileptic drugs. As already briefly indicated, this will be mainly a presentation of animal models showing a variety of epilepsies or – better – *convulsive and/or interictal phenomena*. These will be introduced with "etiology" as an independent variable. Where appropriate, a description of more detailed biophysical and biochemical pathoneurophysiology will be included. Although used mainly in investigations pertaining to "mechanism of action" a few remarks about *nonsymptomatic models* will be added. For the presentation of both the "symptomatic" and "nonsymptomatic models," either the procedure is introduced with a brief description – whenever the model is well established – or as well as a description the "classical" experiment is outlined and more recent developments in the particular field are added. In the last section an attempt is made to assign a "function" to some – but not all – of these models in the sense where in our primary and advanced screening procedures such models should, if not must, be used.

B. Models of Epileptiform Phenomena in Animals

A variety of methods – physical, physicochemical, chemical, pharmacological – are available to induce epileptiform seizures in animals. According to the nature and power of the inducing means, its temporal characteristics, the site and spatial distribution of its application, and also the particular animal species employed and its momentary level of "sensitivity," focal, spreading or initially generalized, grand or petit mal-type, acute, subchronically repeated, or chronically recurring seizures can be produced. Among the physical methods, electrical current of various shapes and intensities, and in various modes of application always was, and still is, one of the most used "epileptogenic" agents. Also, focal freezing and, to a lesser extent, local pressure or other types of mechanical irritation and changes in the blood supply, and induction of alterations in local O_2 and CO_2 levels have been used to produce ictal phenomena. The "chemical" methods include metals of various kinds, hormones, antibiotics, a variety of neurotransmitters, some psychotropic drugs (antidepressants, neuroleptics), local anesthetics, ammonia, receptor-blocking agents, and, of course, the "classical epileptogenic" drugs (strychnine, pentylenetetrazol, picrotoxin).

Of the many types of ictogenic factors and the many types of epileptiform phenomena produced by them, only a limited number can be discussed here. The reader interested in considerably more detail and a considerably larger variety of "models" is referred to the not so recent, but still excellent, compilation in *Experimental Models of Epilepsy,* edited by PURPURA et al. (1972). STUMPF's article in the *Handbuch für experimentelle Pharmakologie* (1962) also still has a great deal to offer as to pertinent information about animal models of epilepsy, especially in small rodents.

I. Electrically Induced Seizures

1. "Simple" Models of Generalized or Partial Seizures in Rodents

SWINYARD (1972) characterized in detail the electroshock (ES)-induced seizure in the rat and mouse. In the same article, he offered directions as to particular procedures to be followed in the use of this technique for research, and he described the history and development of this "classical" model in epileptology. Using either mice or rats (although other species such as frogs, hamsters, rabbits, cats, sloths, and monkeys have served as test animals) and (preferably) corneal electrodes, either a sine-wave alternating current (60 Hz) for 0.2 s or a asymmetrical pulsating direct current usually at a low rate (6 pps, pulse width about 0.2 ms, for 3 s) is applied. Depending on intensity, wave form, and pulse rate or frequency, two extreme types of attacks occur; the *threshold* or *minimal* seizure, on the one hand, and the *maximal* seizure, on the other. The *threshold seizure* in mice or rats is precipitated by low-rate pulse trains or by 60-Hz alternating current and, in mice only, by high-rate pulse trains adjusted in strength (or voltage) to induce a limited discharge only, manifested – in order of increasing stimulus intensity – by a *stun reaction* [designated by SWINYARD (1972) as catatonia] and *localized clonic movements* of the vibrissae, face, pinnae, and forelimbs. The *maximal seizure* is usually induced by supramaximally intense 60-Hz trains. It is characterized by tonic flexion, followed by tonic extension including the hindlegs (i.e., increased tonus in the "antigravity" muscles) and by terminal clonus of all four legs and the trunk. While mice invariably react to a (supramaximal) stimulus with this characteristics sequence, about 10% of all rats fail to do so.

The various levels of *minimal seizures* are obtained by proper adjustment of stimulus intensity. According to SWINYARD, a (60-Hz current-induced) minimal seizure consists of about 7–12 s of clonic activity in the "focal" areas mentioned earlier but without loss of posture. The *maximal seizure* (usually produced with 60-Hz AC, 50 mA in mice, 150 mA in rats) consists, after a short latency, of a tonic flexion of about 1.5 s duration, followed by tonic extension of about 13 s duration and an approximately 7 ½ s period of clonus.

2. Electrically Induced Localized Cortical Afterdischarges

The first detailed study on electrically induced localized cortical afterdischarges was carried out by ROSENBLUETH und CANNON (1941/1942), who did their work mainly in rhesus monkeys and occasionally in dogs and cats. The monkeys and dogs were under chloralose and the cats were under sodium pentobarbital anesthesia. The authors recorded muscular activity (mainly gracilis, semimembranosus, quadriceps, or flexor digitorum) by tension myograph, and the cortical electrographic phenomena, using surface or transcortical silver electrodes, by inkwriter via capacity-coupled amplifiers. Stimulation of the cortex was done by "Harvard coil" or by a condenser-discharge apparatus, through silver ball electrodes applied directly to the area under investigation in acutely craniotomized animals.

Dependent on locus, intensity, frequency, and duration of stimulation, a variety of motor responses were obtained. Typically the involved muscles (contralateral to the stimulation) contracted first in direct response to the stimulus; this was followed by an initial phase of high tension (the tonic phase), then by a phase of relative inactivity developing into a phase of often irregular clonic activity. The attack then slowed down and eventually ceased abruptly. Such localized fits were produced most readily in contralateral muscles from points in area 4; but also in ipsilateral muscle from areas 4 and 6, as well as from areas 8, 9, 1, 2, 5, and 7.

Electrical recordings from points near to the stimulation site revealed a characteristic "afterdischarge" phenomenon (referred to by these authors also as "tonic-clonic"). After a brief period of "silence," a series of "fine, rapid (18–30/s)" regular oscillations of quickly increasing amplitude developed which, after a few seconds, converted into even larger oscillations with a frequency of 6–15/s. This was then followed by more irregular, although still rhythmic, activity in which some fast ("spikes") and slow components were present. The end of the electrographic response was again sudden and the resting electrogram reappeared. During the period of clonic activity of the muscle the rhythmic pattern of the cortical response correlated in rate and amplitude with the (clonic) muscular contractions. The slow decline of clonic muscular activity paralleled the decline of cortical "clonical" activity.

A decade later, FRENCH et al. (1956) reinvestigated in immobilized, awake, and acutely prepared monkeys regional differences in susceptibility to neocortical seizures. Using a modern EEG and a square-wave stimulator, they monitored the response to local stimuli in craniotomized animals (50 pps, 5-ms pulse duration, 5, 10, or 15-V amplitude). *No-response, locally-confined* response (including the thalamic area "belonging" to that cortical site), and *expansion* of the discharge over widespread cortical areas, including propagation to a variety of "subcortical" (including limbic) structures, were the three levels, which, in addition to duration of discharge, subserved quantification of the activities observed. In this important piece of research it was noted that the most susceptible "epileptogenic" neocortical areas were located in the motor and premotor cortex, the posterior cingulate region, the superior temporal gyrus, and the parietal area. Other surface areas displayed little or no propensity to develop spreading afterdischarge. Subcortical structures, most commonly involved together with the cortically evoked seizures, were the reticular formation, septal region, amygdala and, as already mentioned, "cortical areas" of the thalamus.

WALKER et al. (1956) studied the (downstream) spread of electrically induced cortical afterdischarges in monkeys. They observed that afterdischarges from frontal, central, temporal, and occipital cortices spread to different subcortical nuclei. Discharge originating in the frontal cortex propagated to the caudate nucleus, to the contralateral frontal cortex, and, subsequently, to other subcortical structures. Discharge from the central cortex spread to the putamen and to contralateral homotopic areas; discharge from the temporal cortex spread toward the amygdala and hippocampus, then to the septum, hypothalamus, and medial thalamus.

PINSKY and BURNS (1962) investigated the quantitative aspects of afterdischarge production in cats. Experimenting on isolated "unanesthetized" cortical slabs (for this technique see BURNS 1951) they varied such parameters as site, surface area of the stimulated cortex, stimulus strength, pulse duration, pulse number, and stimulation frequency. A number of highly interesting findings resulted from this work: (1) Varying just *pulse amplitude* (bipolar electrodes at a distance of 2.5 mm, 20 pps for 4 s) revealed an all-or-none kind of pattern; once the threshold for the elicitation of an afterdischarge was reached, a further increase in pulse voltage did not prolong the afterdischarge beyond the initial (threshold) duration. (2) A similar pattern evolved with respect to *pulse duration;* for a given stimulus voltage and rate, pulse durations below 0.3 ms proved to be subthreshold; increases up to 9 ms did not prolong the afterdischarge beyond the "threshold value." *Current density* for threshold effects was shown to be independent of the surface area of the stimulating electrode. (4) Varying *pulse number* again revealed an all-or-none pattern; increasing the pulse number past the threshold value (usually 40–80, occasionally as low as 20) did not prolong the duration of the afterdischarge. (5) However, *frequency* (with number of pulses, pulse duration, and voltage kept constant) proved to have a decisive – though not linear – influence on the duration of the afterdischarge. The afterdischarge increased in duration with increasing rates up to between 32 and 63/s and decreased with still higher rates. The authors concluded from these findings that "the establishment in the cortex of a focus for paroxysmal afterdischarge is dependent in an all-or-nothing manner upon the excitation of a *critical minimum number of neurons.*" They also stated that the "critical number of neurons will act as a focus for afterdischarge only if a *minimum density of neurons* per unit area of cortex is excited by the stimulus." Furthermore, "the afterdischarge results from recovery of neurons from an exhausted state; it breaks out only during recovery and *not during a period of driven activity.*"

In their work in immobilized cats, LECLERCQ and SEGAL (1965) and SEGAL and LECLERCQ (1965) investigated the thresholds of electrically (and mechanically) elicited afterdischarge in different areas of the cortex as well as of some deeper structures of the brain. They found "highly electrically sensitive centers" in the cortex, amygdala and hippocampus. Due to their large number of stimulation points they were able to map out "isoliminal" regions. These maps clearly demonstrated gradients in threshold surrounding the spots of highest sensitivity. Highly epileptogenic "spots" were found to be situated mainly "at the limit of the gray and white matter in the walls of the sulci." Furthermore, the authors noted a relationship between highly responsive areas (in the cortex) and the presence of large nucleated cells.

HUGHES (1959a, b) investigated motor and electrical signs of electrically induced, local or spreading afterdischarges in the mesial cortex of freely moving *cats,* chronically implanted with stimulating and recording electrodes. For stimulation 5-s trains of bidirectional pulses of variable rate and amplitude were used. Through careful gauging of voltage and frequency of stimulation, the author was able to separate, over the various areas of the mesial cortex, thresholds for movements only and – with stronger stimuli – for electrographic afterdischarges. The latter were carefully analyzed with regard to duration, amplitude, frequency, and waveform. In areas in close proximity to the stimulating electrodes (in most of the areas of the mesial cortex) the characteristic afterdischarge began with a phase of waxing and waning regular waves with a frequency of 16–18/s; after a few seconds these gave place to bi- or multiphasic waves at "subharmonic" frequencies of 8–9/s. This pattern was seen especially in the anterior mesial cortex. Full-blown clinical and electrographic seizures of this limbic area, lasting from 1 to 2 min usually began with similar rhythmical activity, which after 10–20 s gave way to high-amplitude 2–3/s spike-and-wave complexes.

HUGHES and MAZUROWSKI (1962, 1964) performed similar work in the awake *rhesus monkey,* chronically prepared with 50(!) stimulating and recording electrodes mounted over extensive regions of the supracallosal mesial surface of the hemispheres. Stimulation parameters were similar to those used in the investigations on cats. As in the cat, low-level stimuli tended to elicit movements coinciding with stimulation and involving different areas of the body, depending on the exact site stimulated.

With repetitive and stronger stimuli a number of electrographic signs, in particular *K*-complexes and typical afterdischarges, were elicited. The afterdischarges consisted of rhythmical sharp spikes or of "quasi-sinusoidal" waves. Toward the end of longer-lasting discharges, the regular frequency either just slowed down or turned into spike-and-wave complexes or a series of double or triple spikes.

In an excellent review, AJMONE-MARSAN (1972) summarized the pertinent points of (mainly) cortical epileptiform afterdischarge as they had been worked out by previous workers. This review includes, besides a fine description of afterdischarges (mostly from human epileptics), a set of valuable methodological recommendations for the use and performance of this model.

3. Electrically Induced Afterdischarges in the Hippocampus of Cats

This model relates directly to the experimental afterdischarge phenomena discussed in the preceding section. However as it presents a special case with its phenomenology and, in particular, with its behavioral concomitants, it is described separately. GIBBS and GIBBS (1936), RENSHAW et al. (1940), and KAADA (1951), among many others,, have noted that the hippocampus is characterized by a rather low threshold in reacting to electrical stimulation with an afterdischarge. LIBERSON and his collaborators (LIBERSON and AKERT 1953, 1955; LIBERSON and CADILHAC 1953 a, b) and ANDY and AKERT (1953) were among the first to describe these afterdischarges and their electroencephalographic and behavioral manifestations in detail. Since the present author has acquired a good deal of experience with this model during the past 10 years or so, he can take the liberty to refer to his own procedure for a description of the "classical" experiment.

This experiment is usually carried out in the *chronically prepared, unrestrained,* i.e., freely moving, cat; this enables the electroencephalographic phenomena *and* the behavior during and after the discharge proper to be observed. The gallamine-immobilized, artificially ventilated cat, in which only the electrographic manifestations of the discharge are considered, has also sometimes been used (see KOELLA 1980 a). For the "chronic" preparation, which also makes repeated use of the same animal possible, e.g., in drug studies or investigations pertaining to kindling, stimulating electrodes – preferably of the concentric or double-barred bipolar type – are implanted, usually unilaterally, into the dorsal or ventral hippocampus. For recording purposes the same electrodes may be used for monitoring hippocampal electrographic parameters. For the observation of possible spread to other limbic structures and – rather rarely, if stimulation intensity does not exceed critical values – to neocortical and brain stem areas, additional recording electrodes must be implanted in a variety of neocortical and deep structures.

Using an adequate, preferably "constant", current – pulsating DC-stimulus source that enables pulse rate, width, and height (measured in volts or milliamperes) to be adjusted independently, the experiment is usually started with the application of a pulse rate of 50 pps, a pulse duration of 1–2 ms and trains of usually 5 s duration, and a slowly increasing voltage (or amperage), until the animal reacts with an afterdischarge of the desired duration (0 up to 50 or 60 s). Two different threshold voltages can be determined with pulse rate and duration at constant values: (1) the (usually low, i.e., 0.8- to 1.5-V) threshold for the induction of a (minimal) afterdischarge and (2) the (usually considerably higher, i.e., about 5- to 8-V, depending on the size and shape of the electrodes) threshold for inducing generalization, i.e., spread to extralimbic areas.

The discharge usually starts, and rapidly builds up to high amplitude and frequency values, immediately after cessation of stimulation. The discharge is of the "spiky" type, with average spike rates of 25–35/s and some slowing toward the end of the discharge. In the cat, the discharge usually stops abruptly and leads into a postictal subnormal activity phase which may last from 30 to 180 s. Duration of discharge quite clearly depends – aside from such factors as level of vigilance, previous discharge history, influence of drugs, and electrode position – upon stimulus intensity. Usually the discharge readily spreads to the other areas

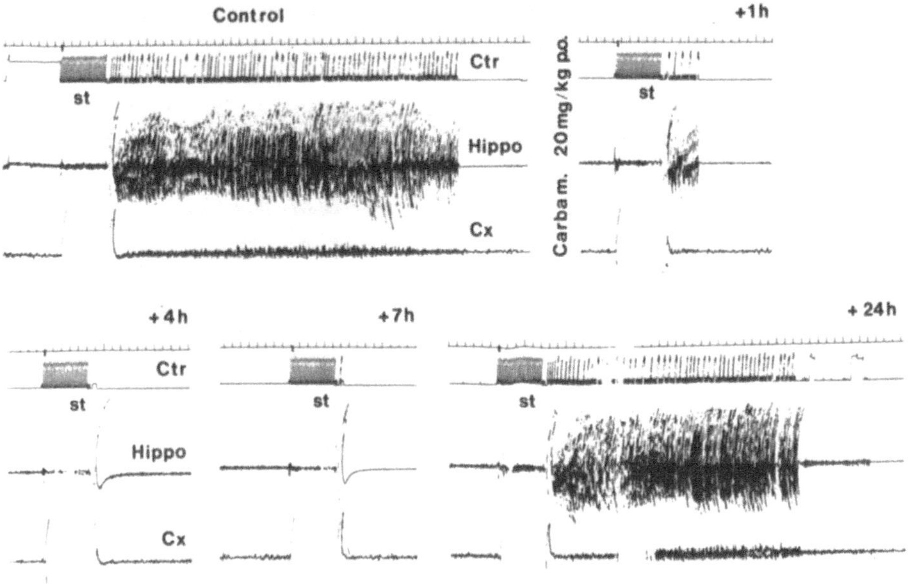

Fig. 1. Hippocampal afterdischarge in response to (local) hippocampal stimulation of the freely moving, "chronic" cat. Note in the *Control* part that the discharge is confined to the hippocampus, lasts 42 s, and does not "contaminate" the cortex (*Cx*). *Ctr,* automatic record for spike-counting. *St,* 5-s stimulation period. Influence of carbamazepine (20 mg/kg p.o.) on these convulsions 1, 4, 7, and 24 h after administration (KOELLA 1980a)

of the limbic system, viz., the contralateral hippocampus and the ipsilateral – more rarely the contralateral – amygdala. Figure 1 depicts a typical hippocampal discharge pattern elicited in the "chronic" cat.

Of importance – and, in view of the "diagnosis" of a particular type of epilepsy, of considerable significance – is the observation of the *behavior* of the animals during and after the (electrographic) afterdischarge. In our own experiments in the cat (KOELLA 1980a, b; KOELLA and SCHMUTZ 1981; SCHMUTZ et al. 1981) we usually saw, with the beginning of the stimulation train, a sudden arrest of ongoing activity; the animals would carry over their actual posture and position from the immediate prestimulus period; they would "freeze" in place (what may be refered to as an "arrest reaction") and they would stay in this posture usually up to the end of the seizure. The animals always stared in an "absence-like" manner at some ("absolutely uninteresting") point in the cage or the laboratory and did not deviate from this, even when there was a good deal of activity in the laboratory (light flashes, moving and "staring" visitors). The pupils were usually extremely wide. Often, and, in particular, with repeated stimulations there was salivation and licking. Very rarely though were there signs of myoclonus-like activity in the (fore-)legs.

With cessation of the afterdischarge the animals would quite suddenly begin to move, would change their posture, or would start walking around the cage. Usually there was mewing, and occasionally some abortive or real grooming.

These postictal activities usually disappeared (if not resumed again spontaneously) within 1 min, and the pupils would move back to their natural medium or small size.

According to MACLEAN (1954) the animals appear to be poorly in contact with the surrounding space during such afterdischarges; they do not avoid light flashes and they "do not cringe when one pretends to strike their face." However, when there was actual contact with some (potentially) noxious stimulus, e.g., a burning cigarette or pinching the tail, the animals would react with unduly strong aversive behavior; they would hiss, spit, and strike out. Prolonged or repeated noxious stimulation may lead to states of wild excitement, with poorly directed attack behavior, which then may terminate, while the afterdischarge still proceeds, in a "catatonic"-like stance. MACLEAN (1954) referred to such behavior as "schizophrenic."

4. Electrically Induced Afterdischarges in the Amygdala

KREINDLER and STERIADE (1963) described an experiment utilizing electrically induced afterdischarges in the amygdala as a model for limbic seizures. From their observations the authors drew conclusions not only about some special aspects of amygdalar "partial" epilepsy but also, on the basis of the particular propagating patterns within and without the amygdala (viz. toward the hippocampus), about "functional links" between the various amygdalar substructures per se and between the amygdala and the Ammonshorn.

The experiments were performed in cats, which, after spinal transsection at C1/C2 under ether anesthesia (*encéphale isolé* preparation), were supplied with gallamine, artificially ventilated, and given local anesthesia around the wound margins. Stimulating and recording electrodes were implanted into various substructures of the amygdaloid complex, hippocampus, pyriform cortex, various nuclei of the thalamus, and mesencephalic reticular formation. Recording electrodes were also placed on various areas of the neocortex. Stimulation (via closely set bipolar leads) was carried out by a square-wave "constant-current" generator so that trains (usually of 5-s duration) with pulse rates varying from 16 to 200/s could be applied. Iterative stimulation of the ventral amygdaloid structures (the parvocellular basal amygdalar nucleus and the ventral parts of the lateral and anterior amygdalar nuclei) induced paroxysmal discharge during current application, followed by an afterdischarge. Stimulation of the more dorsal amygdalar areas (lateral central nucleus and dorsal aspects of the lateral and anterior nuclei) induced an afterdischarge only following an initial arousal reaction occurring during stimulation. Optimal stimulation rates were found to vary, from area to area, from 50 to 100 pps. Lower critical stimulation rates were found to be about 30–35 pps in the lateral central nucleus and as low as 20 pps in the basal parvocellular nucleus. Minimal stimulation *intensities* necessary to induce an afterdischarge were found to be lower in the basal compared with the more dorsal levels.

5. Spike-Wave Pattern Induced in the Cat by Electric Stimulation of the Thalamus

This is the "classical" arrest-reaction model of HUNTER and JASPER (1949). This experiment is performed preferably in the chronically prepared, freely moving animal, lest behavioral symptoms be masked. Stimulating electrodes, preferably of the double-barred, or concentric, bipolar type, are introduced so that their exposed tip rests in the intralaminar nuclei of the thalamus. EEG-recording electrodes are placed over a variety of cortical structures, and additional electrodes may be implanted for recording of the EEG from a variety of "deep structures."

Typically, according to HUNTER and JASPER, stimulation in the intralaminar nuclei (usually 10–30 pps, 10- to 12-m pulse duration up to 12 V, produced behavioral and electrographic signs of a seizure, which the authors referred to as a *petit-mal attack*. Behaviorally, this seizure was characterized by the *arrest reaction*. Starting with the beginning of the stimulation period, the animal would stop walking (as though "frozen"), remain in a fixed or crouched stance, and "stare" with a rather stunned facial expression. It would stop eating and cease pursuing a mouse. Usually, the animal would resume the (prestimulation) activities with cessation of stimulation. Occasionally though the attack could outlast the stimulation period by a "few seconds or longer." There was no loss in muscle tone, nor any change in pupillary size (this in contrast to the hippocampal afterdischarge!). Reactions to sensory stimuli were slowed down or completely stopped, except withdrawal to noxious stimuli. These latter, again in contrast to the hippocampal seizure, did *not elicit undue general defense* reactions. As a rule strong motor activities did not accompany this arrest reaction. According to HUNTER and JASPER, and the present author can confirm this from his own experience, there are, however, occasional slight (myoclonic?) twitches in the face.

When the arrest reaction outlasted the stimulation train, and if the seizure did not develop into a grand-mal attack (which occurred when higher stimulation intensities were used), typical spike-and-wave patterns appeared in the cortical and thalamic leads at a rate of 3/s. They showed full amplitude immediately at the end of the stimulation period and ended as abruptly with the cessation of the arrest reaction and transition to normal behavior. The rhythmical pattern was found to show an astonishing degree of synchrony and phase coincidence between homologous areas of the two opposite hemispheres and synchrony between the cortices and thalamic record. Occasionally, particularly if the "petit-mal" seizure led over into a (generalized) grand-mal attack, the EEG showed, instead of a "slow" spike-and-wave pattern, an approximately 10/s rhythm of intermediate amplitude.

6. A Combined "Staring Look" – Myoclonus – Spike Wave-Pattern, Elicited by Bilateral Infraneocortical Stimulation in the Cat

Together with our collegues (SCHMUTZ et al. 1980) we searched for a better site of electrical stimulation for more reliable induction in the animal of a "typical" *petit-mal seizure,* i.e., a low-frequency spike-wave pattern, signs of a loss of consciousness or at least "awareness," and occasional signs of myoclonic activity. After trying out a variety of stimulation parameters through practically the whole of the cat CNS, we noted that bilateral iterative stimulation of the white matter, situated roughly between the sensory motor cortex (cruciate gyrus) and the upper-lateral limit of the thalamus-hippocampal complex, could produce, as an after effect, a seizure pattern that would fulfill the above-mentioned criteria of a petit-mal attack in man.

For repeated application in the course of drug research, as well as for possible insight into patterns of tolerance and kindling, the model was developed a priori as a "chronic" one. Adult cats of both sexes were supplied with (bipolar) stimulating electrodes (stainless steel, 0.25 mm diameter, 0.5 mm free tip) aimed bilaterally at the white matter under the sensorimotor area (coordinates: frontal, +10.0 and 12.0; lateral 5.5; vertical +21). Recording electrodes were placed through burr holes to rest on the sensorimotor area and the suprasylvian gyrus on both sides and, occasionally, on additional cortical areas or in deep structures. The electrode leads were connected to a lucite socket fastened to the skull. Con-

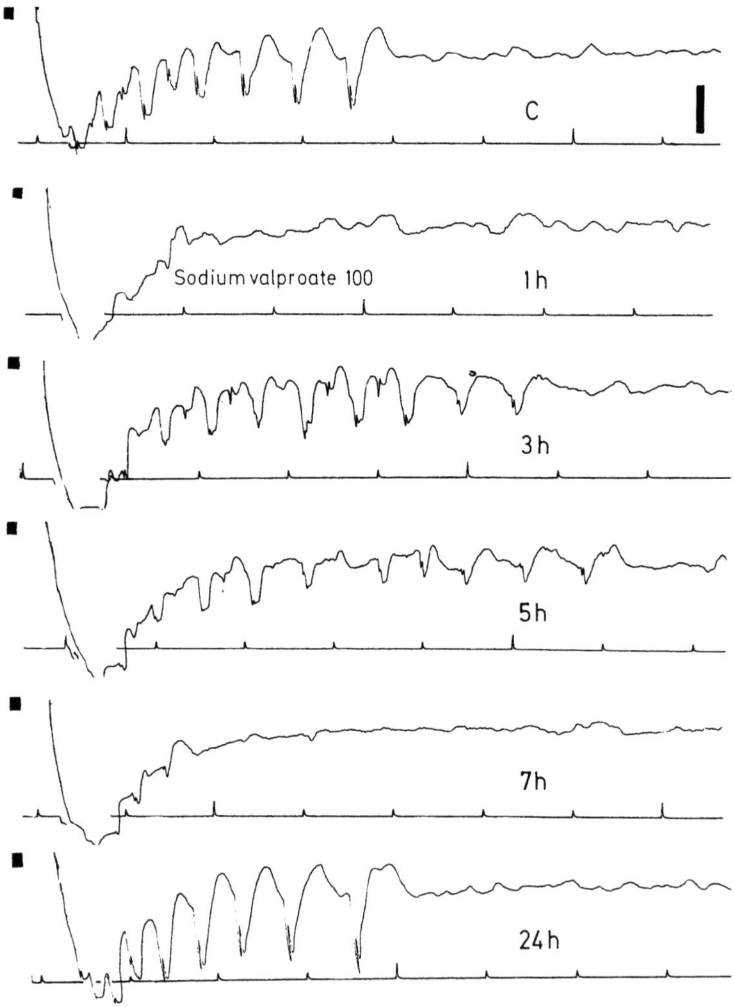

Fig. 2. Spike-wave discharges produced in the chronically prepared freely moving cat by electrical stimulation in "infra-sensorimotor" cortical white matter with 2.9-V 15-pps 1-ms pulses for 5 s. *Black mark on left-hand side* shows end of stimulation. Calibration, 1 and 5 s, and 100 μV. Also shown is the effect of sodium valproate (100 mg/kg p.o.) on this discharge 1, 3, 5, 7, and 24 h after administration. (Courtesy of CIBA-GEIGY Laboratories)

nection between the socket and swivel contact was made through a light, multilead cable. The stimulation parameters were 100 pps, 3-ms pulses for 3 s, and 1–3 V. Following such stimulation, a petit-mal seizure usually developed as an "afterdischarge," revealing a 1.5–3/s spike-wave pattern, often accompanied by myoclonic twitches of the face (rarely of the legs) and as often by a "staring" look. The attacks lasted, depending on stimulus strength and pattern of repetition, for 5–20 s (see Fig. 2). With stronger stimuli, high repetition rates, and placement of the stimulating electrodes below the level coinciding with the dorsal boundary of the thalamus, the "absence phase" often led into generalized seizures.

II. Chemically Induced Ictal and Interictal States (Exclusive of Metals)

A considerable number of chemicals can be used to produce epileptiform phenomena in experimental animals. Many of these compounds can be employed also to activate latent epileptogenic lesions. STONE (1972) and PRINCE (1972) published two excellent and detailed reviews on this topic. In some ways, the "chemical" models are – mutatis mutandis – of value equal to, if not higher than, that of the "electrical" models. As to advantages, the (systemic) application of a convulsant drug often proves to be an easier method – and thus apt to facilitate the procedures in large series – than is application of an electroshock. For determination of convulsant thresholds (and their elevation by anticonvulsants) the infusion at constant rates of convulsant drugs yields considerably more exact results than does, e.g., the use of a pulsed electrical stimulus, increasing steadily in a ramp-shaped fashion. The latter is bound to produce, at levels below convulsive threshold, a variety of alien effects (pain, excitement, withdrawal) that are bound to disturb the flow of the experiment. Such subthreshold effects are considerably less dramatic with chemical convulsants. As there is already some insight into the (mainly) biochemical or physicochemical mechanism of action of some of these convulsogenic agents, one may obtain information not only about the basic mechanism of epilepsy but also about some of the more intimate mechanisms of action of anticonvulsants. And, finally, "wet" convulsants applied systemically are an excellent means – as already mentioned – of activating, i.e., "seeking out," a latent or dormant lesion.

The convulsogenic chemicals, however also present some disadvantages. If given systemically, they make it difficult to determine the locus of action – unless a spatially well-defined lesion of latent epileptogenicity is present. Furthermore, while chemical convulsants may in some cases help in identifying the mechanism of action of antiepileptic drugs, they in turn may obscure the picture by inducing a variety of biochemical changes that are unrelated to their convulsogenic action and thus falsify the (biochemical) substrate upon which one wants to pinpoint the anticonvulsant's mechanism of action.

1. Pentylenetetrazol

Pentylenetetrazol (also pentamethylenetetrazol, Metrazol, Cardiazol) was synthesized by SCHMIDT (1924) and introduced as a convulsant by HILDEBRANDT

(1926). SWINYARD et al. (1952) and SWINYARD (1969) made the pentylenetetrazol convulsion in small rodents into a valuable, still very widely used, testing procedure by standardizing dose (systemic), route of application, observation technique, and species (mice). The methods and "clinical" semiology of the pentylenetetrazol convulsion test, according to SWINYARD'S account, can be described as follows: pentylenetetrazol (85 mg/kg, as 0.85% solution in 0.9% NaCl) is injected s.c. (or, in somewhat lower doses, i.p.) in mice (SWINYARD recommends the CF 1 strain, Charles River, but strain does not seem to play too much of a role). Within 60–210 s after injection, clonic convulsions appear that affect the whole body. One or several interruptions of the clonus are not rare. Occasionally a tonic extension phase, affecting all four extremities, follows the clonus. Animals exhibiting this tonic phase usually die, whereas mice not developing tonic extension most often survive the attack. A "*Straub* tail" often accompanies the clonic phase. In surviving animals the whole clonic phase may last up to 3 min. With the dose mentioned above, about 96%–98% of the animals (of the CF 1 strain) respond with convulsions. For different strains the proper ("supramaximal") dose should be carefully determined. A range of lower doses is indicated where manipulation of the "threshold" dose is one of the main aims of the experiment.

AJMONE-MARSAN and MAROSSERO (1950) investigated in chloralosed, curarized (Intocostrin), and artificially ventilated dogs and cats the effects of pentylenetetrazol (up to 130 mg/kg i.v.) on the electrogram of the cerebral cortex and of the spinal cord, in the ventral gray matter of the lumbar segment. In the cortical leads very fast sharp waves appeared within 10–15 s after injection that rapidly built up to amplitudes of easily 1,000 μV and also steadily increased in frequency. After about 30 s this pattern abruptly disappeared and gave way to virtual electrical silence. A second seizure would then start, exhibiting a pattern similar to the first one.

In the spinal electrogram changes took place under pentylenetetrazol that followed rather closely the various phases observed in the cortex; the "waves" though were simpler and also slower. Occasionally, the cortical ictal activity was not "faithfully" transmitted to the spinal cord in the sense that only the high-amplitude and high-frequency cortical spikes were followed by similar signs in the cord. In the non- or only slightly curarized animals, muscular jerks accompanied the cortical (and spinal) events.

Of interest in this piece of work is the observation that a transection of the brain stem at the mesencephalic level rendered the spinal cord unresponsive to pentylenetetrazol (in doses mentioned above). This clearly indicated that the forebrain – probably the cortex – was much more sensitive to the (convulsant) effect of this drug; the "grand mal" appearing in response to pentylenetetrazol was quite obviously of cortical origin (see also BIRCHER et al. 1962). Finally, it should be noted that in the records shown by these authors (e.g., their Fig. 2) some of the electrocortical potentials were easily recognized as *spike- (or polyspike-)wave* complexes. Such complexes were also noted by SWINYARD (1969) and WOODBURY (1972).

As already briefly mentioned, pentylenetetrazol (in appropriate dilution) can also be slowly infused, preferably in immobilized nonanesthetized animals supplied with recording electrodes in a variety of cortical and subcortical and limbic structures. This method is particularly suitable for obtaining information about changes in threshold dose (induced, e.g., by pretreatment with anticonvulsants).

2. Picrotoxin

This chemical convulsant has been investigated in comparison with bemegride and pentylenetetrazol in the mouse, rat, and rabbit by HAHN and OBERDORF (1962). Early experiments in dogs and monkeys were performed by STONE et al. (1960), BIRCHER et al. (1962), and CHUSID and KOPELOFF (1969).

Unless dose interactions or threshold-dose investigations are contemplated, the drug, diluted in water, is injected in mice in doses of 6.0–8.0 mg/kg. With i.v. or s.c. injections the maximal convulsive doses are somewhat lower or higher, respectively. As with pentylenetetrazol, but somewhat slower in onset, clonic convulsions of the whole body appear that may terminate in a tonic phase. If the latter occurs the animals usually die. According to HAHN and OBERDORF (1962) female mice are somewhat more sensitive than males; the average ED_{50} (with i.v. injections) is given by these authors as 2.44 (♀) and 2.90 (♂) mg/kg.

According to STONE et al. (1960) and STONE (1972) picrotoxin in dogs, supplied with EEG recording electrodes, induces a "slow build-up" of epileptiform activity in the cortex, when given in i.v. doses of 2 mg/kg. This abnormal activity consists mainly of spikes, slow waves, and spike-wave complexes. Similar observations (in dogs) were reported by BIRCHER et al. (1962).

3. Bicuculline

Bicuculline is a GABA-receptor blocking agent similar to, but probably more specific than, picrotoxin (see e.g. CURTIS et al. 1970a, b). If given in doses of 6 mg/kg i.p., this compound produces convulsions which in form, time course, and intensity differ little from those triggered by picrotoxin.

MELDRUM and HORTON (1971) investigated the convulsogenic activity of bicuculline, in addition to 4-deoxypyridoxine (a powerful and specific antagonist of pyridoxine and an inhibitor of glutamic acid decarboxylase), in the photomyoclonic baboon and rhesus monkey. Intravenous doses of 0.2–0.25 mg/kg induced, within 5–15 s, isolated jerks of the limbs and spike-wave complexes in the frontorolandic cortex, but which lasted only a few seconds. The effect of photic stimuli was enhanced in that on some occasions they could induce generalized myoclonus.

Doses of 0.2–0.6 mg/kg bicuculline were apt to induce convulsions within 2–11 s after injection. These started with a cry, followed by a few irregular generalized jerks and then by a tonic flexion spasm rapidly giving way to a generalized rhythmic myoclonus. The EEG indicated that the seizure usually began with a generalized spiky discharge. The myoclonic episodes were accompanied in the EEG by "asymmetrical, irregular" spike waves, whereas the tonic phases were accompanied by faster spiky rhythms.

In a later communication, MELDRUM'S group (BRIERLEY et al. 1972) reported on physiological changes accompanying bicuculline-induced (0.3–0.6 mg/kg i.v. up to three times) seizures in adolescent baboons. In this work they were also able to demonstrate the occurrence, within a few hours of the seizure, of brain damage "similar to that found in man after *status epilepticus*."

4. Strychnine

Strychnine is probably the "most classical" of chemical convulsants and a vast literature exists describing the various effects and mechanism(s) of action of this drug. For the epileptologist strychnine has served a role in the testing of potential antiepileptic drugs. Also, for many years, it has been a valuable instrument for producing, when locally applied, a spatially restricted *focus of excitation* leading to propagation of signals along "physiological" pathways.

An added advantage of strychnine must be seen in the fact that its mechanism of action – at least in part – is established: according to CURTIS et al. (1970a, b) and many others, this drug produces local excitation and the epileptiform motor activity by (antagonistic) interaction with glycine receptors; this is unlike, e.g. picrotoxin or bicuculline which both are gamma-aminobutyric acid antagonists. Yet, it was shown quite early (see, e.g., LONGO and CHIAVARELLI 1962) that strychnine, if given systemically, affects networks mainly in the spinal cord, brain stem, and cerebellum. This may be the reason, or one of the reasons, that strychnine-induced convulsions are not regarded as being truly epileptiform in nature (STONE 1972).

The strychnine experiment, in connection with testing for "antiepileptic" efficacy and/or potency of new drugs, is usually performed in *mice*. A dose of 2.5 mg/kg is given by the i.p. route. With a short delay, the animals develop *tonic* fore- and hindleg convulsions, including opisthotonus, but rarely clonic manifestations. Within 10 min they usually die. At the beginning of the attack, sensory stimulation, viz., handling or noise, can greatly enhance the intensity of the extensor cramp.

5. Enkephalin

In a recent paper URCA et al. (1977) presented evidence that enkephalin may well be used for the establishment of a new interesting "model" of epilepsy; interesting, as convulsive EEG activity is induced by application of a "natural product." Working in male Sprague-Dawley rats, these authors investigated changes in multiunit activity in the periaqueductal gray, and analgesia, in response to i.v.-administered (morphine and) methionine enkephalin. Enkephalin, while in the dosage given proved to be less efficient in inducing analgesia and in enhancing neuronal activity in the periaqueductal gray it changed, unlike morphine, the EEG activity (frontal and occipital leads) to a clearly convulsive pattern. Phases of "rapidly repetitive" spikes alternated with periods of high-amplitude sharp waves, with phases of almost flat EEGs and again with phases of repetitive spiking. There were also (2–3/s) spikes and spike-wave complexes. The "attack" usually petered out with a phase of spike- or polyspike-wave complexes at a rate of 1 in every 5–7 s. The animals were usually motionless during these attacks except for some periodic twitches and some "wet-dog-like shakes, coinciding with EEG spike, or spike-wave discharges. In a subsequent study, FRENK et al. (1978) showed that leucine enkephalin was even more potent than methionine enkephalin in inducing convulsions; the former induced epileptiform activity in (ventricular) doses as low as 10 μg.

6. Conjugated Estrogens (Premarin)

MARCUS and WATSON (1964, 1966, 1968) and MARCUS et al. (1968) showed that the bilateral application of conjugated estrogens (Premarin) to the cerebral cortex of cats and monkeys led to appearance of (bilaterally) synchronous discharges including 2–3/s spike-wave complexes associated with short "staring spells." In a more recent study in cats, JULIEN et al. (1975) used this "epileptogenic" technique for the establishment of a "model" to evaluate the potency of a variety of antiepileptic agents. Male or female cats were craniotomized under halothane anesthesia to expose bilaterally the sigmoid and coronal gyri. Screw electrodes were inserted through the (remaining) bone to rest over the frontal and parietal cortex and in the frontal sinus. After application of a local anesthetic to the wound margins and the external meatus, anesthesia was discontinued; the animals received *d*-tubocurarine and were artificially ventilated (end-tidal CO_2: 3.0%–3.2%).

Conjugated estrogens were dissolved in water. Pieces of filter paper were saturated with the solution (content ca. 0.4 mg) and applied bilaterally to the pial surface of the sensorimotor cortex. The pads were changed every hour. After a 10-min interval, such treatment invariably led to the appearance of bilaterally synchronous sharp waves. Within 30 min intermittent bursts or sustained discharges of 2–3/s spike-wave complexes dominated the picture and continued to do so for periods of up to 8 h. The authors emphasized the resemblance between these EEG patterns and the electrographic picture of human petit-mal attacks.

7. Tetanus Toxin

Early experimental studies with tetanus toxin-induced seizures were reported by CARREA and LANARI (1962) and BROOKS and ASANUMA (1962). MELLANBY et al. (1977) performed a very detailed investigation with this agent. Male Wistar rats (250–450 g body wt.), anesthetized with chloral hydrate and pentobarbital, were injected, using stereotactic techniques, with tetanus toxin bilaterally or unilaterally into the ventral hippocampus, parafascicular nucleus, or visual cortex. The actual dose was titrated against the LD_{50} for mice and rats. During the same session stainless steel screws were implanted to rest over the frontal and occipital areas and connected to a miniature socket. The animals were observed and recorded for several hours at a time over a period of up to 6 months. The (repeatedly occurring) seizures, developed within a day after injection of a few "mouse LD_{50}." Before a fit occurred, the rats would exhibit a "glazed expression" and stand motionless. After about 15 s the seizure began with clonic movements of one foreleg and, bilaterally, of the facial muscles. The mouth and eyes were opened, and the pinnae were held close to the head, which, in turn, "swung up and down." The animals would begin to rear whereupon the second forepaw also would start clonic movements. After occasional falls from the rearing posture the animals were able to right themselves immediately. Such ictal phases lasted (depending on dose) from a few up to 75 s. After a seizure the rats usually lay still for a few minutes. During such seizures, which often occurred at high rates (one or more per hour), the EEG was first characterized by frequent fast spikes, turning, with the onset of the myoclonus, into a high-amplitude slow-wave pattern which continued into the (postictal) "trance-like" state. In rats in which the toxin had been given together with a "neutralizing" dose of antitoxin, no fits were observed.

Within a few days after injection, the animals became quite aggressive and hyperreactive with intermittent "vicious behavior." This abnormal behavior as well as the frequency of the fits attenuated, depending on the dose given, after a few weeks or several months. Of interest in this model is the further observation that in none of the injected animals was there any grave histological change in the area injected or in other brain areas. The authors stressed the resemblance of the observed behavioral changes (and the abnormal EEG) to human temporal lobe epilepsy.

8. Acetylcholine and Cholinesterase Inhibitors

An involvement of acetylcholine (ACh), a natural central (and peripheral) nervous transmitter, in the forming of epileptic discharges has been well recognized for a number of years. POPE et al. (1947) observed an increase in ACh content in epileptic foci in man and animals. PHILLIS (1968) showed that convulsants such as pentylenetetrazol, strychnine, and bicuculline enhance ACh release from nerve terminals. In line with such observations was the discovery of RADOUCO-THOMAS et al. (1955) that an increase in cerebral ACh content enhanced sensitivity to convulsant agents and the discovery of STONE (1957) that a general – indirect – enhancement of synaptic cleft ACh concentrations through inhibition of ACh breakdown induced generalized convulsions.

ECHLIN (1954, 1959) used ACh to demonstrate *supersensitivity* of the *isolated* cerebral cortex of monkeys. He neuronally isolated (or partially isolated) slabs of frontal and parietal cortex by subpial section and "wide undercutting" (about 1 cm below the surface). Between 2 weeks and 2½ years later, the cortex was again exposed for (acute) recordings and applications of drugs. Such isolated cortices showed, even without treatment, an EEG record which was "unstable, abnormal in appearance, often paroxysmal and which bore little resemblance to that recorded from normal cerebral cortex." Applications of 0.2%–0.5% ACh over a wide area precipitated discharges of rhythmic spike-and-wave epileptiform electrical activity selectively from the isolated area. When applied to only partially isolated slabs, ACh produced a spread of epileptiform discharge from the undercut area to the motor cortex; it also induced clonic seizures and, less often, generalized electrical and clinical convulsions. In contrast, when applied to "normal" cortex, ACh (0.2%–0.5%) never caused epileptiform discharge.

FERGUSON and CORNBLATH (1974) performed a similar experiment in cats, in which the suprasylvian cortex was undercut. In such preparations (up to 82 days after surgery), ACh was applied through a nylon chamber placed over the cortex. Nonpolarizable gross electrodes and microelectrodes were used to record rhythmic as well as "steady" (i.e., DC) potentials. With ACh concentrations of 0.1%–2% in the chamber (including 100 μg/ml neostigmine bromide) epileptiform activity was observed which the authors described as "rhythmical oscillations (bursts) superimposed on a sudden DC shift, with periods of electrographic silence (suppression) in between."

The normal (i.e., not isolated) cortex was used by SZIRMAI et al. (1977) to study the local epileptiform activity induced by ACh, and to investigate its spread as well as the regional blood flow. The animals were immobilized and artificially ventilated. After placing a total of eight bipolar Ag-AgCl electrodes on the cortex, ACh was injected into the cortex in doses of 150–200 µg. Five different types of seizures were observed: (1) focal discharges that remained localized, (2) spreading discharges gradually involving neighboring cortical areas and the contralateral cortex (the most frequently observed type!); (3) spreading seizures that became generalized; (4) occasionally initially generalized seizures; and (5) spreading seizures that began in the noninjected cortex. In the generalized seizures, "synchronized" potentials in the frequency range of 4–5 and 8–9/s spikes (or waves) dominated the picture. Spreading was also observed to involve the mesencephalon. Typically, the seizures appeared "serially" with spontaneous reoccurrence of the fits and interictal periods of various duration. The velocity of spread was usually in the neighborhood of 10 mm/min.

The spread of seizures induced by intracortical injection of ACh in acutely prepared rabbits was also investigated by VOLLMER et al. (1979). By following the (spatial) development of the discharge over a row of linearly placed electrodes they concluded that the "walking" of such seizures was based on a "stepwise propagation of an active focus" and that the propagation was "strongly correlated with certain graphoelements and rhythms." Typically, in any one area the seizure would start as a high-frequency (up to 30 spikes/s) pattern that would slow down to a steady-state rate of about 9/s which was replaced, still later, by irregular seizure activity.

9. Penicillin

Penicillin by now is probably the most extensively used agent for the production of a chemical focus or series of foci. The discovery of the epileptogenic potency of penicillin goes back to WALKER et al. (1945). These authors noted that penicillin applied to the cerebral cortex of monkeys and man produces convulsive activity. In the meantime a good many investigators have made use of this antibiotic's "side effect" to induce, through topical application in a variety of places of the CNS, a focal or partial discharge, including "remote" consequences. Also, preferring the "generalized approach" of epileptogenesis, some investigators have used systemically given penicillin to induce widespread epileptiform discharge. The literature up to 1971 on the topic of penicillin epilepsy has been reviewed by AJMONE-MARSAN (1969) and PRINCE (1969, 1972).

MAREŠ (1973) applied the sodium salt of penicillin through trephine holes to the frontal, temporal, or occipital regions of immobilized (*d*-tubocurarine) male Wistar rats. Silver bead electrodes were used for recording the EEG. Some characteristic interictal discharges appeared within 3 min after application of penicillin, and were present for the whole of the 30-min recording period. Only 3 out of a total of 45 animals developed actual seizures.

Using a penetrating "multielectrode" with eight contacts PETSCHE et al. (1978) monitored the *intracortical spatiotemporal* behavior of seizures produced by local application of sodium penicillin G (1 *M*) to various areas of the (exposed) cerebral cortex of unanesthetized, immobilized rabbits. These and earlier studies led to the concept of "generator zones," i.e., "the volume of cortical tissue where a field potential of a distinct shape may be recorded." In an earlier study from the same laboratory (VOLLMER et al. 1974), in which a "surface multielectrode" (16 electrodes arranged in 4 rows to form a square of 3 × 3 mm) was used, the phase relations of the penicillin-induced wave were followed. It was noted that the potential fields typically performed *circling movements*.

REICHENTHAL and HOCHERMAN (1977) investigated the smallest critical size of penicillin focus in the rat brain, to yield seizures activity. Either by limiting the space covered by the penicillin solution (10% penicillin G) or by subpial undercut and thus isolating a given area of cortex, they found that an area of at least 0.5 mm^2 had to be exposed to penicillin in order to produce (local) discharge.

DICHTER and SPENCER (1969) investigated the epileptogenic effect of penicillin on the *hippocampus* of sodium thiopental-anesthetized cats. Application of sodium penicillin G crystals or of pieces of filter paper soaked with the penicillin solution on the exposed dorsal surface of the hippocampus (CA_1, CA_2, CA_3 regions) produced, after a delay of from 3 to 10 min, regularly spread spiky paroxysmal discharges of up to 1–2 mV amplitude. These would often continue "for hours," then occur less frequently, and finally stop altogether.

DICHTER et al. (1973) supplemented their earlier study by additional experiments on "isolated islands of the hippocampus." Through a variety of incisions in cats they separated pieces of the hippocampal formation from their connections via long extrahippocampal projections and afferents *and* the intrahippocampal loop of the "dentate gyrus-CA_3-CA_1 areas, subiculum-entorhinal area." Local application of penicillin to such "islands" was still found likely to produce epileptiform discharge. The authors concluded that "very local circuits in each region of the hippocampus can support epileptogenesis." Even the granule-cell layer (dentate gyrus) was not found "necessary for the development of interictal discharges or seizures."

Also in the cat, O'CONNOR and LEWIS (1974) noted that the rate of seizures produced by local application of penicillin to the hippocampus could be increased by an increase in K^+ concentration in the "bathing fluid."

The neuronal activities in epileptic foci induced by penicillin in the *immature cortex* were studied by PRINCE and GUTNICK (1972). Kittens (3–16 days of age) were operated on under general anesthesia to expose the cerebral cortex for recordings with gross and (intracellular) microelectrodes. The actual experiment was performed after discontinuation of anesthesia in the immobilized and artificially ventilated animals. An acute epileptiform focus was produced by application to the pial surface of the cortex of pieces of Gelfoam saturated with a solution of 100,000–500,000 U/ml sodium penicillin G. The authors noted that surface interictal discharges were associated with depolarizations in neurons. In comparison with such phenomena in mature animals (cats), the synaptic depolarizations and surface discharges were longer in duration and more variable in amplitude in the kittens. During depolarizations, most neurons generated bursts of one to five spikes at a frequency of 100/s or less in the kitten, whereas in mature cortices the units fired long bursts of high-frequency spikes accompanying each depolarization shift.

Also in connection with the focal lesions produced by topical application of penicillin, the study of GUTNICK et al. (1976) should be mentioned. These authors investigated the relative convulsant potencies of structural analogues of penicillin on the cortex of (pentobarbital-) anesthetized cats. The sodium salts of the various analogues were dissolved in saline and applied to the exposed cortex with a Gelfoam pledgette. They found that the most active compounds were benzylpenicillin and phenoxymethylpenicillin, whereas ampicillin and methicillin (and cephalothin) were weaker by a factor of 10–20.

In the experiments by GLOOR et al. (1977) pieces of filter paper soaked with weak penicillin G solutions (50–250 IU sodium penicillin/hemisphere) were applied *bilaterally* to the entire exposed surfaces of the cerebral cortices of immobilized, unanesthetized, and artificially ventilated (end-tidal CO_2: 4%) cats. Recording was carried out by a variable number of deep (thalamus, striatum, reticular formation, amygdala, hippocampus, corpus callosum, capsula interna) and surface electrodes (lateral, suprasylvian, ectosylvian gyri). Invariably such treatment resulted in bursts of bilaterally synchronous epileptiform discharges of the *spike-wave type*. These bursts, in contrast to experiments with systemic application of penicillin, were *not* attended by similar discharges in "subcortical structures." Single shock or repetitive stimulation of the intralaminar, or midline, nuclei of the thalamus (but of no other structures) were liable to precipitate such synchronous discharges. In turn, application of penicillin to these thalamic areas failed to elicit discharges in the (nontreated) cortex.

Using intracellular recording MATSUMOTO et al. (1969) and AYALA et al. (1970), after some preliminary observations by SAWA et al. (1963), discovered the *paroxysmal* depolarization shift (PDS) in neurons of penicillin-induced foci. The PDS is a graded potential which is frequently so large that it inactivates the spike-generating mechanism, although it is still often superimposed with "axon spikes." It is followed by a prominent hyperpolarization phase, attributable probably to recurrent inhibition. Moving away from a focus the depolarization phase becomes smaller while the inhibitory, hyperpolarizing part increases in size. AYALA et al. (1970) noted that with the transition from interictal to ictal patterns the decaying phase of the PDS gradually became longer and the depolarization state more sustained, "assuming the aspect of an afterdepolarization."

Gamma-aminobutyric acid (GABA) synthesis and uptake rates were studied (in cats) in penicillin C sodium or potassium penicillin (10^6 IU/ml)-induced foci in the cortex and its contralateral counterpart by GOTTESFELD and ELAZAR (1975). Glutamic acid decarboxylase (GAD) activity and GABA uptake rate were determined in tissue pieces from the focus and from the contralateral cortex. GAD activity was found to be significantly reduced in both the primary and secondary focus ($p < 0.002$ and < 0.01, respectively). This explained, in these authors' view, the reduced GABA content in discharging foci. GABA uptake was also found to be reduced in both the primary (penicillin-induced) and secondary focus ($p < 0.001$ and < 0.01, respectively). The authors tended to relate this latter finding to the increased interneuronal K^+ accumulation. Evidence for K^+ accumulation in the extracellular space in penicillin-induced epileptic neural tissue has been presented by MOODY et al. (1974).

III. Focal Epileptogenesis Through Local Application of Metals or Metal Salts

Local application of a variety of metals – either in "pure" form or as salts – has been shown to be a reliable means for the production of subacute and/or chronic foci of epileptiform discharge. CHUSID and KOPELOFF (1962), in an extended series of experiments performed under identical conditions, made a comparative study and found some metals to be more "epileptogenic" in nature than others. Some proved to be in fact quite ineffective, if applied "purely" to the motor cortex of the monkey. For the purpose of this chapter, we confine our discussion to just four such models: the alumina, the cobalt, the tungstic acid, and the iron focus.

1. Alumina Cream

This technique dates back to KOPELOFF et al. (1941/1942). They applied disks containing alumina cream (aluminum hydroxide) to the exposed motor cortex of monkeys in a "chronic" manner and then kept their animals for many months after proper surgical closure of the wound. They noted after an initial "silent" period (up to 60 days) the recurrent appearance of clinical seizures with a clear focal onset. The monkeys stayed "epileptic" for months, occasionally for years. Later, KOPELOFF et al. (1955) expanded the range of this model by applying the alumina cream also to subcortical sites.

WARD and his collaborators, seeing the obvious "similarities between chronically recurrent seizures in the monkey induced by this technique and the phenomenon of human epilepsy" (WARD 1969), began to use this method and developed it into a highly standardized model (WARD 1972).

In anesthetized monkeys (mainly *Macaca mulatta*) the sensorimotor cortex was exposed to the pial surface. The autoclaved alumina cream was injected at four points into the pre- and postcentral gyrus with a syringe and a 27-gauge needle in amounts to produce a barely visible hump at every injection site. Recording electrodes were mounted over the focus and in various other structures for (chronically) monitoring the electrographic manifestations of this epileptogenic lesion, both during seizures and the interictal intervals.

Monkeys, prepared and recorded in such a manner, exhibited signs of "spontaneous" clinical seizures after a delay of from 35 to 60 days. The frequency (and intensity) of attacks varied roughly in proportion to the size of cortical lesion produced; with a large number of local injections (i.e., >4, and possibly larger volumes per injection site) the seizures not only occurred with somewhat shorter delays but also increased in rate to give rise finally to status epileptici (which, for saving the animals, required adequate and speedy anticonvulsive treatment).

While "clinical" seizures (with foci in the senorimotor cortex) developed not before 5–9 weeks after surgery, some EEG signs – spikes, sharp waves – could be observed somewhat earlier. The overt appearance – the symptomatology – of the seizure depended of course upon the site of the (primary) lesion. With alumina deposits in the sensorimotor area (as usually in WARD's work) the seizures began, in a "focal" fashion, by synchronous twitching of the contralateral hand and face. These commonly progressed by Jacksonian spread to involve the musculature of the entire contralateral body and became generalized. With increasing frequency, the muscular contractions "fused" into tonic-type contractions, which could last from 30 s to several minutes and on which strong jerks were superimposed. After (usually abrupt) cessation of the seizure the animals were hypotonic and nonresponsive to external stimuli; often they hyperventilated. According to WARD (1972) "once the seizures were established, they recurred spontaneously, presumably for the life-span of the animal"; a relatively constant pattern of seizure frequency has been observed in such monkeys for at least 7 years.

MAYANAGY and WALKER (1974) produced epileptogenic lesions in a series of monkeys by applying alumina cream into either the second convolution of the temporal cortex or the "region of the amygdala." Recording electrodes were implanted again in a chronic fashion into the amygdala, hippocampus, thalamus, caudate nucleus, putamen, pallidum, septum, hypothalamus, subthalamus, and mesencephalic reticular formation. In addition, surface electrodes were placed (over the dura mater) to rest over the frontal, parietal, occipital, and temporal cortex. Of the nine animals that had alumina deposits of 0.2 or more milliliters of volume, one revealed only focal spikes; five animals developed clinical and electrographic seizures upon the (additional) administration of 20 mg pentylenetetrazol (i.v.); four monkeys, however exhibited "spontaneous clinical and electrographic seizures."

According to MAYANAGY and WALKER (1974), electrographic manifestations of the attack always preceded the appearance of clinical attacks, often by weeks. Any single one of the well-developed seizures started upon a background of slow waves or "slow spikes" in the focus; it began with fast spikes increasing in amplitude but decreasing in rate from about 12–14 to 6–7/s. Seizures originating in the *amygdala,* usually spread rapidly to adjacent structures, in particular to the hippocampus and the anterior temporal cortex. A few irregular movements of the limbs often initiated the "clinical" seizure. Thereafter the animals would become motionless in a kind of catatonic fashion. With the onset of the generalized seizures, this latter state led into ubiquitous clonic jerks.

DAVID and GREWAL (1978) further improved and simplified the technique of producing $Al(OH)_3$ (aqueous solution) lesions in rhesus monkeys. Confining their approach to cortical sites, they injected the epileptogenic agent through burr holes to cortical sites which previously had been shown to be responsive (with a motor activity) to electrical stimulations. Thus they were able to avoid craniotomy. With their method the authors were able (1) to reduce mortality and the occurrence of "premature" generalized reactions; (2) to increase reproducibility in latency (attacks appeared after a delay of 74 ± 4 days after introduction of the epileptogen) and extent and form of the seizures; and (3) to simplify the procedure. In this way they prepared a uniform and reliable population of epileptic animals "suitable for physiological and pharmacological studies."

There appear to exist species differences with respect to the occurrence of spontaneous seizures in response to the alumina deposit. According to WARD (1972), the occurrence of spontaneous convulsions "from a focus in the cerebral cortex appears unusual in any species below the primate" with "cortical foci induced by alumina." Somewhat in contradiction to WARD's claim, VELASCO et al. (1973, 1977) were able to induce focal electrographic and clinical seizures by injection of "critical amounts" of alumina cream into the *sensorimotor cortex* of the *cat*. They noted that "one type of cortical, paroxysmal EEG spikes, arising from the epileptic focus was consistently accompanied by clonic flexor contractions of the contralateral forelimb muscles and by contractions of the facial musculature."

Using extracellular tungsten microelectrodes, WYLER et al. (1973) investigated the spontaneous firing behavior of neurons in the *alumina-induced* epileptogenic lesion in the motor cortex of the awake *Macaca mulatta* monkey. They noted, in the quiescent animal, a characteristic pattern, in a number of "epileptic" cells, consisting of an *initial spike* followed first by a long interval and then by a high-frequency afterburst of variable duration. The latter tended to grow in length and total number of spikes, with shortening of the first interspike interval. In the view of WYLER et al. (1975) the *burst is the hallmark of an epileptic cell.* The same authors also established the term *"burst index"* (BI), this being the percentage ratio of interspike intervals (ISI) of less than 5 min duration to total ISIs per 15 s of epochs. Pyramidal tract neurons with a BI of less than 10 were considered to be "normal," whereas those with a BI of more than 10 were considered to be "epileptic." Furthermore, neurons with a BI variability of less than 10 were considered as being "strongly epileptic," whereas weakly epileptic neurons had a variability of more than 10. WYLER et al. (1975) also found that epileptic pyramidal tract neurons reacted to an antidromic pyramidal tract volley with a high-frequency burst whereas normal neurons responded with the usual single-action potential.

2. Cobalt

The technique of inducing epileptic foci by implantation of pure *metallic cobalt* also goes back to the fundamental studies of KOPELOFF (1960) and CHUSID and KOPELOFF (1962). While for KOPELOFF introduction of cobalt resulted in spontaneous seizures in the mouse, CHUSID and KOPELOFF did not succeed in inducing clinically visible attacks by implantation of metallic cobalt into the motor cortex of the monkey. However, DOW et al. (1962) were able "consistently" to produce a chronically discharging focus in the Sprague-Dawley *rat* through application of metallic cobalt powder to the cerebral cortex. Under thiopental anesthesia, about 30 mg metallic cobalt powder (200 mesh) was applied to an area measuring 10–15 mm^2 on the *right* motor cortex, representing the (contralateral) forelimb, head, and face musculature. In a number of animals the metal powder was applied to the temporal or parieto-occipital cortex. For recording of the electrocorticogram (ECoG), DOW and co-workers used plastic-mounted platinum wires, slipped between the skull and the dura mater, and connected to a female plug mounted on the skull. When prepared in this way, during the first few days after surgery the animals became restless, aggressive, and "hypersensitive", and often attempted to escape from the cage. By the 2nd week, clonic movements of the contralateral (i.e., left) "hemibody" developed in about half of the animals with implanted cobalt. These repetitive fits occurred over periods of a few days only; generalized seizures were seen only in a few animals.

The electrical recording within the first days after surgery revealed high-amplitude waves within the delta range. Actual epileptiform activity gradually developed within the 2nd (and 3rd) week and then slowly receded again in the course of the 4th to 6th week. At the height of the effect, high-amplitude spikes and polyspikes in and around the cobalt depot dominated the picture. Often the spikes appeared in isolation, as often they coincided with clonic movements in the contralateral musculature. In many rats the epileptic activity gradually spread to the contralateral cortex (mirror focus). Maximal activity was usually observed between the 10th and 20th days after surgery.

HENJYOJI and DOW (1965) used the cobalt method to induce focal epilepsy in the *cat*. From 50 to 100 mg of the metallic powder was applied to the right *anterior sigmoid gyrus* over an area of 30–50 mm^2. Six extradurally positioned electrodes were placed to rest over the frontal, medial, parietal, and occipital cortex on both sides. Within 30 h after the application of cobalt, seizure activity began to appear spontaneously or could be provoked (e.g., by shaking the contralateral foreleg). The spontaneous seizure were focal and clonic in nature. They involved the mouth area, eyelids, and occassionally the entire (contralateral) half of the face. Focal electrical seizures activity was preceded by high-voltage slow waves, later replaced by spiking arising near the cobalt area. Spiking then spread to adjacent electrodes in the ipsilateral cortex, occasionally also, but to smaller degree, to contralateral sites. Usually epileptiform activity decreased and disappeared 4–5 days after surgery.

FISCHER et al. (1967), again working on rats, rather than applying the metallic powder, constructed cobalt powder-gelatine sticks, which were inserted into the cortex. They found that this method improved reliability in eliciting epileptiform activity. MUTANI (1967) implanted cobalt into the hippocampus or the amygdala of cats. The foci became active within 2 days and remained active for 1–2 months. The attacks were typically "psychomotor" in nature: the animals became motionless, were "staring," and became unresponsive to external stimuli. As with electrically induced limbic afterdischarges, after cessation of the seizure the animals exhibited some emotional activity, meowed, and showed some ambulatory motor activity, or just changed their posture.

PAYAN and CONARD (1973) investigated the susceptibility of various strains of rats – as well as of guinea pigs, hamsters, and mongolian gerbils – in their epileptogenic response to application of a cobalt rod into the frontal lobes. On day 28 after surgery the animals were challenged with 3 × 15 mg/kg i.p. pentylenetetrazol (at 15-min intervals) and monitored for the development of generalized seizures. Of the seven strains of rats used, the inbred BNs were the most responsive and the Fischer 344 the least responsive, with the ACl, Lewis, Wistar, Sherman, and Sprague Dawley strains taking an intermediate position. The gerbils developed epilepsy to a degree comparable to the Fischer 344 variety, whereas hamsters and guinea pigs proved to be "resistent." In a later paper the same authors (PAYAN and CONARD 1974) claimed that there was an inverse relationship among the various rat strains between sensitivity to cobalt, on the one hand, and serum alkaline phosphatase, on the other.

In their investigations on the Wistar rat, ROLDAN et al. (1971 b) introduced a cobalt-gelatine rod unilaterally either in the dorsal hippocampus or the thalamus. Recording electrodes were placed onto the frontal cortex and into the dorsal hippocampus and the mesencephalic reticular formation. Within 1–2 days after implantation, over 80% of their animals developed spikes and spike-wave patterns that appeared, in waxing and waning trains of, on average, 7-s duration (range, 1–20 s). These discharges usually appeared not only in the structure bearing the cobalt but in both cortices, and also in the contralateral hippocampus and thalamus. While an absence-like posture sometimes appeared during the trains of (electrical) discharges, profound changes in behavior during or between these attacks were not observed.

In Sprague-Dawley rats, supplied with "chronic" recording electrodes over the cortex and temporal muscle, CALASANTI et al. (1974) produced epileptiform discharge by implantation of a 1- to 2-mm length of a 1-mm diameter cobalt wire into the (right) parietal cortex. They observed focal spiking to appear within a few days after the operation and – typically – at the end of sleep episodes. As of the 4th day, about half of all (implanted) rats had, in addition to focal spiking, incomplete secondary generalization. By the end of the 1st week all animals showed complete secondary generalization, with the seizures lasting about 1 min. By the 3rd week there were usually no more attacks.

MARCUS and his various collaborators [for a review of their work, see MARCUS (1972)] have also experimented extensively with cobalt. They found, in contrast to CHUSID and KOPELOFF (1962) that this agent is "useful for the production of unilateral foci in the motor cortex" of rhesus monkeys. In (acute) animals, kept under gallamine and artificial respiration, discharges were seen to start within 80–95 min after application of cobalt powder. In "chronic" animals, prepared under ketamine hydrochloride, focal spike discharge also appeared within less than 2 h after implantation of the convulsant and continued to recur for up to 72 h. Clinical focal seizures set in within 95–130 min.

Of particular interest in the work by MARCUS (MARCUS 1972) is the model with *bilateral cobalt foci* in male rhesus monkeys. Under pentobarbital anesthesia, an area of about 1 cm^2 on the right *and* the left premotor cortex was coated with cobalt powder (60 mg × 2) by means of a Gelfoam sheat. A total of ten screw electrodes were placed bilaterally to rest on the prefrontal, premotor, precentral, inferior, parietal, and occipital areas. Following recovery from anesthesia, usually about 5½ h after surgery and continuing for up to 96 h, absence-type seizures were recorded. They were characterized by 3/s spike-wave patterns over wide parts of the cortex together with myoclonic eyelid, eye, face, and arm movements.

In their "classical" study, VAN GELDER and COURTOIS (1972), using ion-exchange column chromatography in the cat, investigated the content of various amino acids in brain tissue pieces excised from the anterior motor cortex adjacent to a *cobalt focus,* or from the homotopic contralateral cortex of rats. They noted that brain tissue from the close vicinity of the lesion was deficient in GABA, glutamic acid (GA), and aspartic acid (AA), while levels of glutamine and glycine were above those found in controls. "A clear correlation was demonstrable between severity of epilepsy and the extent by which the concentration of all 5 amino acids deviated from normal." Low concentrations of GABA, GA, and AA were noted also in the contralateral (not primarily lesioned) motor cortex and the contralateral visual cortex.

WOODBURY and KEMP (1977) have shown that *carbonic anhydrase* activity followed *pari passu* the development and eventual drop in spiking activity in a focus produced by implantation of cobalt in the rat's frontal cortex. Such an increase in carbonic anhydrase activity was also seen in the (spiking) homotopical contralateral cortex, yet not in (nonspiking) heterotopical areas of the (ipsi- and) contralateral hemisphere.

3. Tungstic Acid

The first mention of this method dates back to the early sixties, when BLUM and LIBAN (1960) and BLUM et al. (1961) published their results obtained in *cats*. In the former paper the preparation of an adequate colloidal tungstic acid gel for injection and some first observations in cats were described. The second paper then gave a detailed account of the electrographic signs of epilepsy obtained in cats chronically supplied with surface and ventral hippocampal platinum-recording electrodes. The tungstic acid gel was injected, using stereotactic techniques, unilaterally into the ventral hippocampus. The first signs of epileptic abnormalities appeared within 1 day after surgery; spontaneous attacks usually occurred "at least every hour for a period of 2 to 3 or more days." Interictal anomalies were most conspicuous in the lesioned hippocampus, but readily traversed to the contralateral homotopic site, and also spread bilaterally to the suprasylvian gyrus and, ipsilaterally, to the temporal region. These interictal signs revealed themselves as single sharp waves, biphasic spikes, and polyspikes of rather high amplitude. Bursts of high-voltage spikes and sharp waves and (sporadic) spike-wave complexes in the hippocampus completed the picture.

The hippocampal seizures started out by the cat assuming a crouching posture and looking "apprehensive," followed by an ipsiversive turning movement, masticatory movements, clonus of the upper lip, hyperventilation, pupillary dilation, and further ipsiversive turning. In some cats, shortly before the seizure started, the (interictal) spikes increased in rate. The actual seizure would then begin in the "focal" lead and then spread, with a few seconds delay, to other leads. The seizure appeared as high-amplitude multiple spikes, often in the form of "doublettes." With a short period of reduced "organization" the seizures would then terminate. Such attacks lasted for, on average, about 40 s.

4. Iron

WILLMORE et al. (1978) supplied rats (Sprague-Dawley strain) or cats, with five epidurally placed recording (including one indifferent) electrodes. While still under pentobarbital anesthesia, the animals were injected subpially with either $FeCl_2$ or $FeCl_3$ (5 µl of a 100-nmol solution in the rat, 10 µl in the cat). Within 48 h after surgery the animals developed focal spiking with spread to the contralateral cortex. Frequent and sustained bursts of epileptic spikes (seizures) appeared within 10 days. During "generalized" seizures, the rats interrupted orienting activity; they revealed piloerection and twitching of the vibrissae and neck muscles. The cats (with left cruciate gyrus foci) displayed focal motor seizures in the limb muscles, followed occasionally by generalized attacks. Such seizure activity persisted, regardless of whether ferrous or ferric ions were injected in 94% of the (35 operated) rats and in all cats beyond the 12-week observation period. Four of the 14 control animals injected with similar volumes of saline "exhibited transient focal spike activity lasting less than 14 days."

IV. Local Freezing as Epileptogenic Factor

The technique of freezing a small area of an animal's cerebral cortex for the production of an epileptogenic lesion dates back to OPENCHOWSKI (1883), who used the method in rabbits and dogs. Speranski (cited by Lewin 1972) employed compressed carbon dioxide to freeze the cortex locally in dogs. Schneider and Epstein (1931) produced local lesions in the cerebral cortex of cats by application of dry ice. Nims et al. (1941) were the first to report electroencephalographic findings from such freezing-induced foci.

Smith and Purpura (1960) also worked in cats. After surgery under ether for vascular cannulation and exposure of the pial surface of various cortical structures, the animals were immobilized and artificially ventilated. The cortical lesion in the posterior sigmoid or the anterior suprasylvian gyrus was produced by gently touching the pial surface with the tip of a 2-mm diameter metal rod attached to a chamber containing dry ice. After the appearance of ice crystals adjacent to the cryoprobe, the cortex and rod were flushed with warm Ringer's solution to facilitate disengagement of the rod from the pia mater. Recording electrodes were placed in the form of an array over the lesion and on various other, nonlesioned areas.

According to Smith and Purpura (1960), such cortical lesions "became epileptogenic within an hour, but, in some instances, it was necessary to repeat the procedure in order to obtain a lesion with stable, low frequency discharge characteristics." In a few instances the lesion became progressively more epileptogenic. According to the authors, single spikes were almost always found to be initially surface negative. With "increasing" activity the spikes became diphasic, then multiphasic, and, finally, discharge terminated in a sustained focal seizure.

Stalmaster and Hanna (1972), also working on the cat, developed the cryoprobe further by consolidating the (aluminum) rod and chamber into one piece. The real innovation though was a "silver coating" of the rod which was connected to four "freezing contacts." This new arrangement made possible better control of the lesion. With dry ice-acetone or dry ice-alcohol mixtures in the chamber and application times of up to 100 s, the lesions produced were well confined to layers I and II of the cat's cortex. For electrographic recordings the authors used a "chronically" implanted electrode array on both (i.e., ipsilateral and contralateral) sensorimotor cortices. All surgical procedures including lesioning were carried out under barbiturate anesthesia. Hanna and Stalmaster (1973) described their observations as follows: after recovery from anesthesia the animals typically showed repetitive jerking movements involving the contralateral forelimb and, occasionally, the neck, trunk, face, and hindlimb. Generalized seizures were not seen, however, in this series of experiments. Within 2 h after left-sided freezing, the electrocorticogram showed multiple bilateral sites of epileptiform activity. Repetitive slow waves were prominent near the primary freeze lesion. They tended to be bisynchronous and were temporally associated with repetitive myoclonic jerking movements contralateral to the lesion. Such slow waves were always of maximum amplitude in the cortex immediately adjacent to the primary freeze lesion. Additionally, there were low-frequency spikes and sharp waves and paroxysmal bursts of high-frequency spiking. Both the paroxysmal bursts and low-frequency events appeared bilaterally; unlike the slow waves, they showed no particular tendency to be bisynchronous. They arose from multiple bilateral sites, neither necessarily adjacent nor contralateral to the primary lesion. Spiking sites tended to remain active throughout subsequent days of observation. Spontaneous epileptiform discharges were observed to persist as long as 20 days postoperatively. They occurred most often during the first few days of observation, diminishing gradually after the 1st week. During (electrically) quiet periods, spike-and-sharp wave discharges could be evoked on either side by repetitive, mild sensory stimulation of the contralateral forelimb.

Upon histological examination the lesions revealed gliosis, new vessel ingrowth, neuronal loss, and – more temporarily – edema and capillary dilatation. According to ESCUETA et al. (1974), *synaptosomes* derived from *freezing lesions* in the sigmoid cortex of cats revealed a reduced (by 59%) K^+ uptake in comparison with nonlesioned controls, if incubated in Tris medium.

To produce surface lesions (of the exposed cortex) of cats and rabbits, MORRELL (1959, 1960) and MORRELL and FLORENZ (1958) introduced the use of the ethyl chloride spray. Through a small burr hole in the cranium and an incision in the dura, a fine spray of the coolant was directed onto the pial surface (of a small predetermined cortical area) until the cortex whitened and swelled. The spraying was then discontinued and the opening closed. A number of recording electrodes were then implanted over the lesioned site – according to the particular questions being investigated – and over additional areas, e.g., homotopic points in the contralateral cortex. Local spiky discharge appeared within 1–3 h after freezing and remained with "fairly constant" intensity for up to 12 h. Thereafter the discharge became more variable but was evident for as long as 6 weeks and 3 months (in rabbits and cats, respectively). The discharge could be activated by systemic application of pentylenetetrazol. Of importance in MORRELL's studies was the development of secondary lesions; these will be discussed in the next section.

V. Models for Secondary and Progressive Epileptogenic Lesions

On a variety of occasions, the discussion of chronic or subacute convulsion models has offered an opportunity to point out cases where the epileptiform activity, in response to a strictly locally acting convulsant, not only invaded areas in the neighborhood of the (primary) focus, but also "jumping" to remote sites within the hemisphere bearing the focus and also to the contralateral hemisphere. This quite clearly indicated that *basically normal nervous* tissue can, and does, exhibit epileptiform activity once it is brought under the influence of an epileptiformly discharging "upstream" structure. Furthermore, such "sympathetic" epileptiform activity in an initially "virginal" tissue obviously seems able, if repeated and/or if lasting beyond a critical period, to induce *permanent functional* (or even structural) changes in that tissue that per se are convulsogenic in nature.

In fact, such considerations touch on the very heart of the problem as to what is the *nature of epilepsy* and what is the basic mechanism involved in the *development of epilepsy*. It is thus quite fortunate to have available two sets of animal experimental models that, due to their very nature and procedural characteristics, can be used to investigate exactly such problems. They can be employed also in connection with drug work, e.g., the influence of antiepileptic agents on such aspects of development.

1. Secondary Focus Models

MORRELL (1959, 1960, 1961, 1973) was the first to perform systematic investigations on "secondary epileptogenesis" (or development of secondary foci, homologous transfer, mirror focus, just to name a few of the terms applied to this phenomenon). He has recently reviewed his "classical" observations (MORRELL 1978).

For the production of the *primary lesion* in cats and rabbits, MORRELL used the freezing technique – *ethyl chloride* applied to the exposed cortex (see also p. 311 in this chapter). Electrodes of proper configuration and size were implanted to record the EEG from the site of the primary lesion, from the contralateral homotopic area, and from cortical areas adjacent (a few millimeters away), to these two loci. Recording electrodes may also be implanted into deep structures, in particular "downstream" from the cortical sites (i.e., the basal ganglia, brain stem, and limbic structures) for monitoring possible epileptogenesis in infracortical areas.

Within a few hours (to several days) – according to MORRELL – epileptiform spikes appeared in the site of the primary lesion and remained active in that area for days to weeks (in rabbits and cats). Yet, usually within a week spike discharges began in the homotopic area of the contralateral cortex, at first just a few in number and occurring in time to the spikes in the primary lesion with a delay of some 20–30 ms. These spikes in the secondary site were viewed as being *evoked potentials;* they were characteristic for the dependent *mirror focus*. Dependence could be demonstrated by *excision* (or undercutting) of the primary focus, which was followed immediately by cessation of epileptiform activity in the secondary site, i.e., the mirror focus disappeared. Injection of a depressant drug (e.g., sodium amobarbital) into the carotid artery ipsilateral to the primary focus yielded similar though not as reliable results.

If the primary lesion was left intact and in proper connection with the contralateral site, the focus in the latter, on its way to independence, went through an *intermediate state* (MORRELL 1978), which we prefer to refer to as *semi-independent*. Discharge in the secondary focus increased in rate and amplitude; spiking there also gradually became temporally independent of the spikes in the primary focus; the secondary focus would begin to discharge even more frequently and intensely than did the primary one; and it could develop into a source of discharge spreading to other areas including the primary focus. Yet, all these features still did not "make" the secondary focus an independent one. At this stage, excision of the primary focus in about 67% and 20% of the cases still led to a drop and eventually complete cessation of activity in the secondary focus, when excision was performed after 7 days and 4 weeks, respectively.

Only with delays of about 90 days for undercutting, or excision of, the primary focus, did the secondary focus persist (except for about 8%–20% of the animals) for at least 6 months (MORRELL's criterion of "true" independence). Yet, this particular time course in the development of the mirror focus seemed to be fairly specific for, and to depend on, the nature and developmental characteristics of the primary lesion. WYLER (1978) studied the behavior of identified pyramidal tract neurons in the "mirror focus" of *Macaca mulatta* monkeys after *at least 1 year* had elapsed following induction of the primary focus by *alumina cream*. The state of the neurons, i.e., "epileptic" or "normal", was determined using the criteria mentioned earlier (WYLER et al. 1975). None of the pyramidal tract neurons in the mirror focus could be diagnosed as "epileptic." They were rather "follower" neurons only that discharged in response to a transmitted spike.

So far we have centered on the description of the "classical" mirror focus, i.e., an epileptogenic lesion in a *homotopic point contralateral to an artificially induced primary focus*. One must be aware, though, that the mirror focus – regardless of whether it is of the dependent, semi-independent, or independent variety – is but one special case of a large variety of secondary foci. The common feature of all such secondary lesions is – quite probably – that they are situated "downstream," from, i.e., at a "projection site", of, the primary focus. The (epileptogenic) information is conveyed from the primary to the secondary lesion via "natural" mono- or oligosynaptic transmission channels (i.e., projecting axons).

Two examples of such "nonmirror type" cases of secondary epileptogenesis should illustrate this point. WADA and CORNELIUS (1960) produced (primary) lesions by local freezing or implantation of alumina gel in the pericruciate cortex of *cats*. They noted that independent discharging foci developed not only in the (homotopic area of the) contralateral cortex but also in cortical areas of the ipsilateral hemisphere, in the basal ganglia, and in the thalamus (both sites constituting "projection areas" of the sensorimotor cortex in this species!). The proof for "independence" was the persistence of these secondary foci after excision of the primary lesion.

WILDER and SCHMIDT (1965, see also WILDER 1972) investigated the development of secondary foci in *Macaca mulatta*. Their primary focus was produced by implantation of alumina gel into the sensorimotor cortex. They noted "preferential routes" of propagation toward the thalamus, basal ganglia, and reticular formation. All animals developed (secondary) focal motor and generalized seizures. Three of the animals, after an interval of 2–3 years, had "tonic fits" of up to 20 s in duration. When finally implanted with cortical and subcortical recording electrodes, the monkeys revealed epileptiform discharge not only in the area of the primary lesion, but in a variety of subcortical areas as well. Of interest is the authors' observation that propagation occurred from the primary focus to subcortical areas and from such subcortical to other deep areas but rarely back to the cortex (WILDER and SCHMIDT 1965; WILDER et al. 1969; WILDER 1972). In their work on rhesus monkeys NIE and ETTLINGER (1974) placed (primary) aluminum hydroxide lesions in the inferotemporal cortex. Through implanted recording electrodes they noted that, after ablation of the primary lesion, typical "class I events," i.e., "definite epileptiform abnormalities," occurred in neocortical areas, suggesting that they "genuinely" arose from an independent epileptic focus.

This section can be concluded by referring again to WILDER's paper (WILDER 1972), which offers, following a description of the (patho-)physiology, biochemistry, and histology of such projection and secondary epileptogenic phenomena, some excellent technical advice as to how to proceed in experiments dealing with secondary foci.

2. The Kindling Phenomenon

The kindling phenomenon is yet another manifestation of the fact that "epilepsy induces epilepsy." Evidently through a kind of a *positive feedback mechanism,* a local epileptiform discharge, confined initially to a small focus or network, will tend, if not "disturbed," to spread in *space* and in *severity*. DELGADO and SEVILLANO (1961) demonstrated experimental evidence for such "auto-amplifying" capabilities of epileptiform activity. They worked with *cats,* chronically implanted with electrodes in the hippocampus, septum, amygdala, cingulate gyrus, thalamus, and reticular formation. In response to electrical stimulation (5-s trains at 100 pps, 0.2-ms pulse duration) in the hippocampus, they observed not only electrographic afterdischarges in this structure, but also clinical manifestations such as "staring," movements of the vibrissae, of the face, of the eyelids, and of the head, and licking, salivation, postural disturbances, jumping and generalized convulsions. With repeated applications of the stimulus, these symptoms typically increased in severity.

STRAW and MITCHELL (1966) electrically stimulated the cerebral cortex of mongrel cats and recorded the ensuing electrographic afterdischarge through chronically implanted electrodes. In one group of animals, stimulation was carried out every 5 min for 5 h at either 25 or 50 pps. In the second group, the stimulation periods consisted of three trains given at 5-min intervals, and these periods were repeated eight times every 30 min (again rates of 25 or 50 pps were used). Quite typically, the duration of the afterdischarge increased with increasing number of stimulation periods. Furthermore, this increase was always more pronounced with the lower stimulus frequency (25 pps) than with the higher frequency.

GODDARD and his collaborators characterized, in detail, in a systematic manner, and with well-controlled technique, this phenomenon, which they came to refer to as *kindling*. In a first series of experiments GODDARD (1967) worked on Wistar rats, *Macaca mulatta*, and cats. They were chronically implanted with stimulation and recording electrodes in various areas of the limbic system and some other strategic structures. Stimulating electrodes were of the bipolar type, made of stainless steel, nichrome, or platinum, coated with Diamel or Teflon, and overcoated with Insl-X or Epoxylite. At least 1 week after surgery, stimulation of the amygdala was given once a day with the following parameters: biphasic pulses of 1-ms duration at a rate of 62.5 pps, trains of 1-s duration, and a peak-to-peak amplitude of 75 μA.

In the 1st-day trial there was neither an EEG response nor a behavioral response to stimulation. As of the 7th day there was, in response to stimulation, arrest, closing of the (ipsilateral) eyelid and some grooming movements. At this time the first afterdischarge occurred in the EEG. The first bilateral clonic convulsions were observed about 2 weeks after the beginning of stimulation; they set in 15 s after stimulation and lasted at first for only 7 s. The convulsions involved rearing back on the hindlimbs and tail, facial contractions, and forelimb clonus (contralateral before ipsilateral). Isolated spikes in the amygdala outlasted the clinical convulsions by 1–2 min. With ongoing trials the (clinical) convulsions occurred with progressively shorter latencies, and became longer in duration to level out, after another 10 days or so, at 5 and 20 s, respectively. Tonic convulsions were not seen. Additional experiments (in other animals) revealed that at this stage *clonic* convulsions could be triggered with an about 50% probability with stimulating currents as low as 5 μA. However, spontaneously occurring convulsions were not seen by this stage.

In an additional series of rats, GODDARD et al. (1969) investigated the *anatomical specificity* of kindling. In this series, a 60-Hz sine wave of 50 μA was applied once daily for 60 s to various structures. A variety of points in the "olfactory-limbic" system were found to be "positive," with the amygdala being the most responsive area. Yet, also from the striatum and, even more so, from the globus pallidus, kindling could be elicited.

Another part of this investigation dealt with questions of *permanence* of the kindling "trace." Again they worked in rats and used stimulation parameters identical to those in the previous series. They found that animals which had been "prekindled" and then had been given a 12-week rest required fewer trials of "rekindling" to reach the criterion than did animals that were not "prekindled". This clearly showed that "the changes which underlie the kindling process were relatively permanent changes which remained almost completely intact for at least 3 months without (re-)activation."

A third part of this work was devoted to the role of *stimulus parameters*. It was demonstrated that the optimal stimulation frequency for triggering convulsions in (pre-)kindled rats was 60 Hz; this was regardless of whether (pre-)kindling had been carried out with 25, 60, or 150 Hz. Also kindling was found to develop in an identical temporal pattern, irrespective of whether a 25-, 60-, or 150-Hz stimulus was used. Furthermore, it was shown that time to first clonic convulsions (stimulation in the amygdala for either 1 or 60 s) was from 10 to 15 days, regardless of stimulus intensity, which ranged from 0.05 to 10 mA. Finally, and possibly rather surprisingly, the probability of finally precipitating convulsions increased with interstimulus interval to reach a plateau with rates of one trial per 24 h.

By using two separete electrodes to stimulate two different brain areas (again in rats) the authors were able to demonstrate that the "kindled" state would "transfer" from one site to the other. The septal region required about one-third of the trials normally necessary to reach the "criterion," following (pre-)kindling in the amygdala.

GODDARD and co-workers also performed some experiments to demonstrate kindling proneness in different strains of rats and in the cat and the monkey. For these experiments the amygdala was stimulated. They showed that the reaction of the Royal Victoria hooded rat was quite similar to that of the Wistar rat, but that the Holtzman strain war more seizure prone. Also, kindling could be shown to occur in cats. Finally, using somewhat different stimulating electrodes (in the amygdala) and different stimulus parameters, evidence was obtained that also in the monkey, "as in the rat, stimulation led to development of clonic convulsions; the duration of clonus progressively increased with repetition, and stimulus threshold decreased."

MORRELL (1973) followed up GODDARD's work and performed an experimental series aimed at the demonstration of kindling in cats. Unilateral electrical stimulation (2-s trains, biphasic rectangular pulses, 2 × 1-ms duration, 62.5 pps, 100 μA per pulse) was given once a day between 10.00 and 11.00 hour through Nicrome electrodes with their tip in the lateral nucleus of the amygdala or in the adjacent pyriform cortex. Some animals were "pretreated" with a nonconvulsive "control current." All (18) cats developed behavioral and electrographic signs of seizures upon repeated stimulation, after a latency of 30–55 days (or 70 days for those that had received a particular control stimulation). In the 16 animals which "finished" the study, seizure activity was progressive and developed into full-blown fits, which lasted up to 100 s. Typically, the seizures began with arrest of ongoing activity, then exhibited some rhythmic twitching of the mouth, tongue, and ipsilateral eyelid. The contractions became more intense, including other facial muscles, and turned into head bobbing. Finally, the (contralateral) legs began to twitch and the seizure turned into a (bilateral) tonic-clonic fit. Earlier in every kindling series, i.e., during stages with no or few clinical signs, there were electrographic afterdischarges which typically lengthened with the increasing number of trials. They affected not only areas in proximity of, but also remote from, and opposite to ("mirror focus"!), the stimulated point.

According to MORRELL, a 50- to 100-pps current was optimal for production of kindling. He also emphasized the importance of intervals of several hours (up to several days) between trains of iterative stimulation, as a prerequisite for the development of kindling. He further stressed the permanence of the "trace," induced during development of kindling, and remaining unaltered even if the stimulation was interrupted for as long as several weeks. He finally pointed out the similarities between the kindling phenomenon and the *mirror focus,* another "model epilepsy" developed and experimentally clarified by himself.

RACINE et al. (1973) studied in the rat the influence of *interstimulus interval* on the rate of development of kindling generated by electrical stimulation of the amygdala. In this series they used 1-ms diphasic pulses (400 μA peak-to-peak) at a rate of 60 pps applied in trains of 1-s duration. Of interest – and in contrast to GODDARD's findings – is the observation that "there were no significant differences between 24-h, 2-h, or 1-h interstimulation intervals with respect to number of stimulations required to develop seizures." When stimulated at intervals of less than 1 h, the animals required more trials to reach the "criterion." Nevertheless, with the 0.5-h interval seizures developed within 13–46 trials, i.e., in less than a day! With the 1-h interval it took from 5 to about 43 h, and with the 24-h interval the "criterion" was reached in 8–28 days.

In experiments by PINEL and co-workers (PINEL et al. 1975), rats, continuing to be kindled past the criterion, i.e., past the time when motor seizures appeared in response to stimulation, developed the ability to produce spontaneous motor convulsions. Such seizures displayed a wide variety of symptomatology, ranging from mild running fits to severe myoclonic convulsions. According to PINEL (1981), kindled rats kept for 6–7 months continued to show such spontaneous seizures, even when not further stimulated.

WADA and SATO (1974), WADA and OSAWA (1976), and WADA et al. (1975) demonstrated the proneness toward kindling in cats, rhesus monkey, and baboon. WADA and SATO (1975) showed that kindling is producible in split-brain cats.

GILBERT and CAIN (1982) stimulated the amygdala in neonate (10 days of age), infant (14 days), weanling (21 days), juvenile (39 days), and adult (>200 days) hooded rats. While they found no difference in the rate of development of kindling between the weanlings, juveniles, and adults, they noted that neonate and infant rats kindled only partially and "unreliably." The authors attributed this to the "immaturity of various mechanisms of neural transmission."

Of interest, in terms of comparative physiology, is the study by MORRELL and TSURU (1976). They stimulated the hippocampus of partially immobilized *bullfrogs*, once per hour with 2-s trains of 62.5/s bipolar pulses of 1-ms duration and pulse amplitudes of 200 μA. Recording electrodes were placed bilaterally in the hippocampi. Initially, such trains induced a short afterdischarge which – with repeated stimulation – became progressively longer. After four to six such stimuli, there appeared isolated, still infrequent high-voltage discharges in the primary (stimulated) site. Somewhat later in the procedure, these discharges were transmitted to secondary sites, and after a few more stimuli they appeared there spontaneously and independently of the first focus. Shortening the stimulation intervals to as little as 5 min neither quantitatively nor qualitatively affected the afterdischarges in their dynamic development.

POST et al. (1976) chronically administered *cocaine* (10–17 mg/kg i.p. twice daily) to rhesus monkeys. Besides behavioral disturbances (stereotypies, catalepsy, and dyskinesias), in 7 out of 13 animals they also observed convulsions of increasing severity with increasing number of injections. On average, the first convulsions were seen after eight cocaine injections and developed into generalized tonic-clonic fits of short duration, reoccurring though at short intervals for periods of up to 15 min and more (in fact such longer-lasting status epileptici had to be blocked with diazepam or pentobarbital to save the animals!). Cocaine levels in the cerebrospinal fluid were not found to differ between animals tested after the first and after the tenth drug administration. POST and co-workers also noted that cocaine administration, regardless of whether performed acutely or chronically, led to an elevation of homovanillic acid (HVA) in the cerebrospinal fluid, paralleled by an increase (though not significant) in 5-hydroxyindoleacetic acid (5-HIAA).

Because of the similarity between the time course of the development of cocaine-induced convulsions and that of the convulsions induced by initially subthreshold, repetitive electrical stimulation of the amygdala, the authors concluded that with their repeated cocaine administration they "engaged a kindling-like mechanism."

In another investigation in Sprague-Dawley rats, POST (1981) used *lidocaine* (60–65 mg/kg i.p.) to induce kindling. After a number of daily ("subthreshold") applications, seizures started to occur that increased in intensity with increasing duration of "treatment." The seizures were characterized by recurrent episodes of clonic movements of the head, trunk, and forepaws, with the animals sitting on their haunches and "balanced" by a *Straub*-tail phenomenon. Seizures increased in intensity (i.e., number of repeated fits following each injection), but also displayed a rhythm-like pattern with 2–4 days periodicity that evolved with repeated injections of the drug. Rats that had been kindled by electrostimulation of the amygdala were more responsive to lidocaine 18 days after cessation of electrokindling; 88% of electrokindled rats showed convulsions to (one-time) lidocaine, in contrast to only 24% of a "sham-kindled" group. Finally, POST showed that rats which successfully kindled in response to repeated lidocaine, i.e., which developed seizures, reacted with increased aggressiveness. This was not so for rats that received saline and for rats that, though receiving lidocaine, did not kindle.

Also with rats, CAIN (1981) demonstrated kindling with pentylenetetrazol (20 mg/kg i.p.). In the course of 50 daily administrations, all animals showed an increasing frequency of facial twitching and myoclonic jerks; yet, only one rat had a generalized convulsion. CAIN also found, as did POST (1981), the phenomenon of "cross-kindling," but here in reverse. After having been "prekindled" by pentylenetetrazol, the rats needed on average only 7.6 electrically induced afterdischarges (amygdala) to produce a pronounced kindling effect, whereas controls (i.e., not "chemically" kindled animals) required 13.2 afterdischarges to reach the criterion.

VI. Animals with "Inborn" Epilepsy: Genetic Models

In the preceding sections we have described and discussed a number of "epilepsy models" in which the symptom "seizure" was induced, acutely or repetitive-chronically, by a physical or chemical agent in initially and basically healthy – nonepileptic – animals. Yet, this review has also shown that these agents are not similarly effective in all species tested (including submammals). In fact, in monkeys it is easier to produce (chronic) epilepsy by implantation of alumina than it is, e.g., in rats. In turn, frogs seem to kindle faster and with more ease than, say, cats or primates. This indicates that different species have a priori a different – possibly chemically determined – sensitivity to the various epileptogenic agents. Or to take the reverse view, the various species enjoy in their central nervous system a different degree of protection against epileptiform discharge.

In fact, it is by now well established that there are some species and strains that typically and repeatedly exhibit spontaneous seizures, or, at least, are characterized by an extremely low threshold to a number of "epileptogenic" (or better convulsogenic) agents such as stress and sensory stimulation. It is clear that animals that show seizures spontaneously or that show seizures in response to a low stimulus, i.e., animals that are "natural epileptics," may turn out to be better "models" than those in which the convulsions are induced by some possibly "alien" agents. Holliday's chapter in this volume (Chap. 3) describes a number of cases of such "spontaneous" epilepsies in a variety of species, and we can restrict our own treatment of this topic to "semispontaneous" epilepsy as revealed by audiogenic seizures in mice and rates.

According to KRUSHINSKY et al. (1970), audiogenic seizures in mice were first mentioned by STUDENTSOV in 1924. Later, DICE (1935) described "waltzing and epilepsy" in the genus *Peromyscus*, and MIRSKY et al. (1943) wrote about "sonogenic convulsions" in rats and mice. HALL (1947) noted a striking difference in susceptibility to noise (and the consequent behavior) between the C57 and DBA strains of mice.

In his chapter in *Experimental Models of Epilepsy* COLLINS (1972) gave an excellent description of audiogenic seizures in mice and rats, including some remarks on ontogenetic aspects and genetics. He added two valuable appendices on sources of adequate animal material and of information about such animals. As on earlier occasions, we follow COLLINS' presentation for the description of the "classical experiment." Of a variety of sound sources – jingling keys, jangling metal tubes, high-pressure air blasts, white noise, and high-pitch pure (sine wave) tones and sirens – the electric bell is probably the most widely used instrument. Sine wave frequencies below 8–10 kHz are ineffective (as being below the hearing range of mice). Sound intensities between 90 and 120 dB above 0.0002 dynes/cm^2 are necessary for the elicitation of seizures. The test should be performed in a quasi-soundproof chamber to protect the surroundings from repeated intense acoustic traumatization.

The whole response to such stimuli in mice usually consists of three phases: a *pretonic*, a *tonic*, and a *posttonic* one. Mice and rats, immediately after the onset of the sound, react first with an initial stun and/or startle response. After an intervening latent period, the animals follow with a burst of rapid running movements, interrupted by leaping. Then they fall over, and show a variety of clonic movements. The second phase begins with a tonic flexion of the hindlegs, followed by extension, which can be maintained for up to 20 s. Respiratory failure – which often proves to be fatal unless the animals are given artifical respiration – is signaled by relaxation of the pinnae. The posttonic phase consists of an initial period of clonic movements, followed by a stuporous state. According to COLLINS, some of the animals may go through a free interval after the running phase, followed by a second period of running which then leads into the actual convulsive phase. When one ear is occluded the motor patterns develop in a rather asymmetrical way. COLLINS, on the basis of temporal comparisons, suggested that audiogenic seizures can be regarded as generalized convulsions not much different from those induced by electroshock or pentylenetetrazol.

As to the proper (i.e., adequately sensitive) strain, COLLINS recommended DBA/2J mice; in his own experiments nearly 100% of this strain, tested at the age of 3–4 weeks, succumbed to (often fatal) seizures. SCHLESINGER et al. (1965, 1968, 1970) also offered some important information about "the genetics of sound-induced seizures in inbred mice." In two recent papers SEYFRIED (1979) and NOEBELS (1979) dwelled on the genetic factors controlling the susceptibility of various strains to sound stimulation. The former also discussed the role of age in the development of susceptibility to audiogenic seizures; in DBA/2J mice, susceptibility begins over a relatively short period of 12–17 days after birth. Also, according to SEYFRIED, susceptibility to sound can be induced in initially resistant animals by prior acoustic exposure.

Rats, not unlike mice, react to (intense) sound stimulation also with an initial startling response, followed, after a short quiescent phase, by violent running leading into a (generalized) tonic-clonic seizures; a postictal depression phase terminates the attack (CONSROE et al. 1979). According to the same authors, the "genetic profile of audiogenic (AG) rats has not been fully defined." Studies involving brain ablations, stimulations, and recordings suggested that audiogenic rats are deficient in neuronal inhibition at the cochlear and vestibular nuclei, as well as in the inferior colliculi and reticular formation.

VII. Circadian Aspects

In many of the experiments with the various "chronic symptomatic models" discussed in the preceding sections the investigators noted that the propensity toward epileptic discharge or overt seizures varied in the course of the 24-h day and/or with changes in behavioral activity. LOCKARD and BARENSTEN (1967) observed that the alumina-induced seizures of monkeys were concentrated in the night hours. According to MAYANAGY and WALKER (1974), spiking frequency (in an alumina focus in the monkey's cortex) varied with the "state of somnolence." Seven of their eight animals showed an increase in spiking rate during light and deep slow-wave sleep. The eighth monkey, however, developed spiking to waking levels when shifting from light to deep sleep. Two of the animals increased discharge rate when entering paradoxical (REM) sleep. VELASCO and co-workers (VELASCO et al. 1973, 1977) found that cats with cortical alumina cream lesions lost their peripheral manifestations of convulsions (twitches) during sleep while maintaining the electrocortical discharges. In fact, spiking in the cortex increased when shifting from waking to slow-wave sleep to decrease again in rate when entering paradoxical sleep. WYLER (1974) recorded with tungsten microelectrodes the activity of 40 normal and 17 "abnormal" neurons from alumina-induced neocortical epileptic foci in *Macaca mulatta* during waking and sleeping. During sleep, normal neurons were not found to change their firing pattern "from what would be expected from previous reports." The abnormal ("epileptic") neurons though produced, with the transition from waking to sleep, an increased number of spikes per burst or (if initially only slightly "epileptic") changed the firing pattern so drastically as to become indistinguishable from initially highly "epileptic" neurons.

ROLDAN et al. (1970) noted a striking correlation in Wistar rats between the incidence of (cobalt-induced) spike and spike-wave trains, on the one hand, and the state of vigilance, on the other. Typically, these trains occurred mostly and mainly during relaxed wakefulness whereas they were almost missing during deep (slow-wave) and paradoxical sleep. The same group (ROLDAN et al. 1971 a) found that rats, exhibiting spike and spike-wave discharges, had shortened slow-wave sleep time. COLASANTI et al. (1974) found that spiking in response to a cobalt insertion into the parietal cortex of rats appeared mainly at the end of sleep episodes.

Circadian and/or vigilance level-dependent variations in epileptogenic output also appear in "inborn"-type epilepsies in animals. As early as 1955, HALBERG had observed a clear circadian rhythm in the susceptibility of mice to audiogenic convulsions (HALBERG 1955). The photomyoclonic Senegal baboon shows, according to KILLAM (1979), the greatest seizure responsiveness at 0800 h and the least 12 h later, i.e., at 2000 h.

These findings in epileptic animals come as no surprise, if one knows that man's epilepsy is a time (of the day)-dependent variable. Among many others, JANZ (1962, 1975) has shown that particular types of epilepsies have their favorite "phase position(s)" in the circadian cycle. According to PASSOUANT (1977), slow-wave sleep favors focal (partial) epilepsies, including the tendency toward generalization. In turn, REM sleep rather inhibits generalized (grand mal) attacks but favors the appearance of petit-mal and temporal lobe seizures. Other examples of such time- and/or vigilance-dependent variations are cited in other chapters of this volume. For a quite detailed review the reader is referred to DALY's article (DALY 1973).

Such circadian and/or vigilance-dependent variations are of interest not only for the epileptologist involved in basic research (one may ask the question as to what factors control these variations); they are also of practical importance as well for the proper evaluation of efficacy and potency of potential anticonvulsant drugs in the various screening procedures. We have established an experimental paradigm that should be adequate for the physiologist and pharmacologist to investigate a variety of variables dependent on the time of day (KOELLA 1980a). This procedure is "statistical" in nature as it is based on the probability that n animals out of n_0 subjects per group respond with (maximal) convulsions in response to an electroshock of given intensity at any particular time of the (24-h) day. For this procedure it is of outmost importance that the animals (rats) are adjusted for at least 2 weeks to a constant light-dark schedule (in our experiments 1830–0630 dark). Electroshock (0.65-s train, 100 V, 50-Hz alternating current) is applied by corneal electrodes to groups of 20–30 animals at different time points regularly distributed over the 24-h day. Figure 3 shows that in three experimental settings (run in the course of a 4-month period) the percentage of convulsing animals varied quite distinctly, although with a similar pattern, over the 24-h day. Two *maxima* of responsiveness occur – one at the beginning, one toward the end – during the night ("dark") activity period; a first minimum occurs in the middle of the dark period and a second one toward the end of the rest (i.e., the "light") period. It is obvious that such experiments can be performed also with chemical convulsants, e.g., picrotoxin, bicuculline, pentylenetetrazol, and, possibly, strychnine. On the other hand, convulsants with longer delays until onset of action and lon-

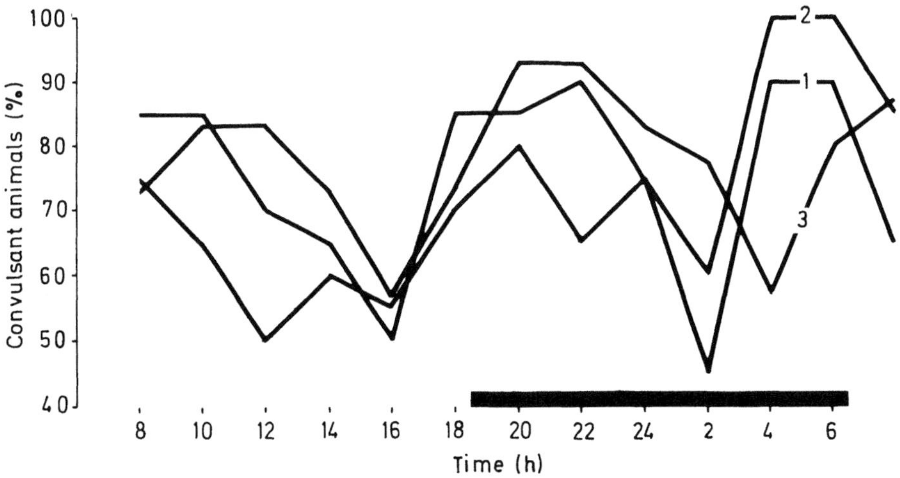

Fig. 3. Change over a full day in susceptibility to electroshock of three different groups of rats (*1, 2, 3*). Note the high seizure incidence at the beginning and toward the end of the dark ("active") period (*black bar*) with troughs at 1600 and 0200 h (KOELLA 1980a)

ger-lasting convulsive behavior would probably be less well suited for this kind of investigation.

C. Some Nonsymptomatic Models

Epileptologists quite often, and in particular in connection with questions concerning the *intimate mechanism of action of antiepileptic drugs,* use nonsymptomatic models; they administer their drugs to animals which exhibit no epileptiform symptomatology: animals which for all practical purposes have a "normal" brain except that they have been subjected to some nonspecific interventions such as anesthesia, decerebration, spinalization, or other "isolation" procedures; epileptologists investigate the effect of drugs on *normal* biophysical and biochemical, neural and/or neuronal processes. They do that for two reasons. Firstly, there is the strong possibility that, as outlined earlier, antiepileptic drugs act indirectly, in a sense *symptomatically,* and combat seizures, or seizure proneness, by an action on "normal" (e.g., inhibitory) neurons to counterbalance excessive excitation in "epileptic" (excitatory) units. Here, experiments in "normal" animals are likely to yield pertinent information. Yet, the investigator may also be inclined to interpret the drug effects obtained in normal tissues to have a similar significance for abnormal (e.g., "epileptic") neurons or networks. Here, though one must be aware that the reaction to a chemical in an "abnormal" substrate is often entirely different from that in a normal one, data obtained in normal tissue cannot a priori be assumed to be relevant for abnormal tissue. Secondly, as preliminary information, data obtained in such nonsymptomatic models are highly valuable if an effort is made to expand, where possible, the experiments to the *same "function"* in symptomatic models, viz., in a convulsing focus. A few of the more often used biophysical experimental paradigms together with some general remarks about biochemical studies are presented in the following sections.

I. Biophysical Approach

1. Spinal Synaptic Assemblies

The mono- and polysynaptic *spinal reflex* has always been a popular model for investigations with "antiepileptic" drugs. Such experiments are usually performed in spinalized, unanesthetized, or intact chloralose-anesthetized animals, preferably cats. For reliable and constant results adequate monitoring and control of body temperature and blood pressure is of the utmost importance. Electrical stimulation of the dorsal roots (preferably L7 or S1), or of a muscle nerve containing IA and II fibers, activates mononeurons, whose excitation can be recorded from the ventral roots. Recording from the ventral roots enables, together with those from dorsal roots, the *output/input relations* to be monitored. Intracellular recordings from motoneurons yield information about (possibly) subthreshold excitatory postsynaptic potentials (EPSPs) and their reaction to manipulations of synaptic "conductance." Drugs can be administered using either the i.v. or the (close) i.a. route.

Reducing stimulation intensity at the dorsal roots enables monosynaptic reflex activity to be "isolated" (through IA afferents), whereas higher intensities activate thinner (II, III and IV), as well as heavier, afferent fibers, thus producing a monosynaptic action potential followed by the *polysynaptic reflex*. Such differentiation is possible, to some extent too, by stimulation of either an afferent fiber from a muscle or one from the skin.

Through stimulation of afferents from antagonistic muscles, in addition to the monosynaptic reflex test procedure, the effect of polysynaptic or *direct inhibition* and its reaction to drugs can be investigated. Similarly, the inhibitory influence of cutaneous afferents on the motoneuron and its susceptibility to the effect of (antiepileptic) drugs can be studied. Through antidromic stimulation of the ventral root (motoneuron) fibers, one can activate the *Renshaw cells* and study the effect of drugs upon this inhibitory feedback system.

An often employed method, using principally the same procedure of reflex testing, is the *posttetanic potentiation paradigm (PTP)*. First introduced by LLOYD (1949), this method involves long-lasting (up to 60 s) high-frequency (50–500 pps) stimulation of the dorsal roots (or a muscle nerve) which results, after cessation of tetanization, in a remarkable increase of the ventral root response. ESPLIN (1972) has shown the time course of the increase of the ventral root potentials and the clear dependence of the effect upon tetanization frequency.

2. Supraspinal Models

FROMM and KILLIAN (1967) investigated synaptic transmission onto, and excitability of, postsynaptic cells in the oral part of the spinal trigeminal nucleus under the influence of a variety of anticonvulsants. In either pentobarbital- or chloralose-anesthetized cats, they introduced glass microelectrodes to monitor unit activity. Typically (orthodromic) single-pulse stimulation of the maxillary nerve elicited, with a latency of approximately 2 ms, a series of two to four postsynaptic potentials. In turn, (antidromic) lemniscal stimulation evoked only one response with a latency of only 1 ms, yet with good "following" of the stimulation rates up to 200 pps. In more recent work, FROMM et al. (1980, 1981) again recorded the response of units in the oral part of the spinal trigeminal nucleus to maxillary nerve stimulation, following an inhibitory conditioning stimulus to the contralateral hypothalamic periventricular gray matter. This conditioning stimulus typically increased the latency and decreased the number of the postsynaptic potentials recorded from trigeminal nucleus units.

ANDERSEN et al. (1977) and ANDERSEN (1978) investigated in isolated slices, cut perpendicularly from the hippocampus of guinea pigs, the "long-lasting facilitation of synaptic transmission." After tetanization of a variety of hippocampal afferent pathways (10–50 Hz for 5–15 s), they noted, through microelectrode recordings, an increased (postsynaptic) response in, e.g., CA_1 pyramidal cells, a typical PTP! This facilitation outlasted the period of tetanization by easily 25–75 min. The increased postsynaptic response was interpreted to be, in all probability, the consequence of enhanced release of synaptic transmitter – a mechanism also proposed to be responsible for (spinal) PTP. It seems that this model, if "epileptic" hippocampal tissue were also used, would be well suited to investigate the difference in the effects of anticonvulsants in normal and abnormal networks.

3. Invertebrate Models

The relatively simple nervous systems of invertebrate organisms, e.g., insects, mollusks, crustacea, cephalopods, offer welcome access to the study of a variety of neurophysiological processes and mechanisms of both the dry and wet type. Physiological properties of neuronal membranes, their reactivity to a variety of natural and "exogenous" inputs, conduction of impulses along elongated processes of the nerve cells, interactive patterns in the neuropil, and a host of other problems can be investigated in such "primitive" neuronal networks (see KANDEL 1976).

Of the numerous possible experimental approaches in a great variety of species, we mention a few to demonstrate the ready applicability of such models in epilepsy research.

Aplysia californica, the "sea hare," has in its abdominal ganglion a number of spontaneously "bursting" nerve cells – L_2, L_3, L_4, L_5, L_6, and R_{15}. The majority of the other cells are "silent" when investigated in the isolated ganglion. A short stretch of the typically "ever-lasting" bursting behavior of R_{15}, with the repeated trains of spikes and the intervening membrane hyperpolarization, as revealed by an intracellular microelectrode, is shown in Fig. 4. A certain similarity between the ("normal") behavior of this cell with the "symptomatic" seizure discharges in "epileptic" cells is obvious; this "epileptiform" behavior is reinforced by convulsants. FRAZIER et al. (1967), then WILSON and WACHTEL (1974, 1978), BARKER and SMITH (1978), and ADAMS et al. (1980) among many others have worked out some of the basic ionic and electrical mechanisms underlying this seizure-like discharge and the parallel shifts in the membrane polarization.

KLEE et al. (1973) showed that pentylenetetrazol (PTZ), applied to isolated abdominal ganglia of *Aplysia*, can induce "doublet" discharges "associated, in voltage clamp, with a decrease in the threshold for the inward current and a reduction and delayed onset of the outwart current." PTZ was also shown to produce oscillations and bursting behavior in normally silent cells.

SPECKMANN and CASPERS (1973) used isolated single cells for their work excised from the parietal and visceral ganglia of *Helix pomatia*. Intracellular recording was carried out with single or multiple KCl– or K-citrate-filled microcapil-

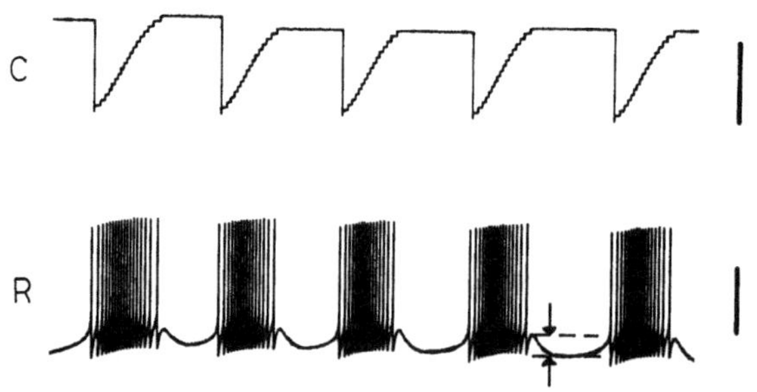

Fig. 4. Bursting activity and interburst hyperpolarization recorded intracellularly from the R_{15} cell of the (isolated) abdominal ganglion of *Aplysia californica*. *R*, original record; *C*, spike counter. Calibration, 50 mV; total length of record, 1 min, 40 s. (From author's laboratory)

laries. With proper injection of current they were able to measure membrane input resistance. Using PTZ added to the bath to yield 10–100 m*M* concentrations they either increased the spontaneous discharge rate of such cells, or even produced discharge in initially silent cells. The drug also induced changes reminiscent of paroxysmal depolarization in mammalian "epileptic" cells. Finally, PTZ was found to decrease the amplitude and to increase the duration of the action potentials and to reduce the extent of the afterhyperpolarization. Also with the help of PTZ, FAUGIER and WILLOWS (1973) and PARTRIDGE (1975) turned single bursting cells of Tritonia into – "symptomatic" – models to be used for measurements of a variety of membrane properties.

II. Biochemical Approach

The basic aim of such "biochemical" nonsymptomatic models is – as it was, mutatis mutandis, with the "biophysical" models – the establishment of "standards" pertaining to a vast variety of biochemical parameters for the investigation of the influence of antiepileptic drugs. With nonsymptomatic (as with the "symptomatic") models, a great variety of approaches are at hand. WOODBURY and KEMP (1977) have presented a list – together with valuable comments – of "biochemical changes in epileptic foci of animals and man". It seems that work pertaining to the behavior of the many different *neurotransmitter mechanisms* (aminergic, aminoacidergic, and polypeptidergic ones) should assume priority. Such investigations should be directed at one or more of the three phases of humoral transmission: release, inactivation, and receptor-bound transduction to obtain evidence at what point (or points) in the "wet" transmission mechanism a drug attacks. Here it is of interest – as it was with respect to biophysical studies – to spread the experimental probes to a variety of structures (not least those that are plagued by a notoriously high epileptogenic sensitivity) to obtain evidence about possible structure-specific influence of the antiepileptic drugs to be tested.

Studies on the levels *and* kinetics of the various *relevant ions* are probably as important with regard to the clarification of the modes and mechanisms of antiepileptic action. Here too, a structure-dependent approach is indicated. Finally, studies on a variety of *enzymes* (e.g., carboanhydrase) and on the various structured constituents of the neuronal and glia membranes – including proteins and lipids – should be used to broaden the spectrum of approaches and, thus, to increase the probability of finally pinpointing *the* important (yet "normal") substrate(s) for the action of antiepileptic drugs. For details the reader is referred to the chapter on "Pathophysiology of Epilepsy."

D. Discussion

In the two preceding sections we have described and discussed a variety of experimental procedures which, based on their very nature, lend themselves as *models* for the discovery and characterization of potential antiepileptic drugs. The bulk of these models are *symptomatic* in nature; they exhibit *convulsive activity* and/or *interictal phenomena* induced, in the majority of cases, artificially, by a variety of "epileptogenic" agents. In a few of these symptomatic models, though, the epileptiform symptoms appear "spontaneously", due evidently to genetic priming. Some of the experimental procedures described are basically *nonsymptomatic* in nature. Still, due to the particular neurophysiological system under scrutiny, these nonepileptic models are valuable instruments in the further characterization of antiepileptic agents.

In this concluding section, we shall now make an attempt to assign an experimental *function* to some of these models. We must decide – or at least suggest – what model(s) should preferably be used in realizing the *experimental aims* as outlined and defined in the introduction to this chapter: (1) qualitative and quantitative characterization of "unknown" chemicals as antiepileptic drugs in general, or *screening;* (2) determination of efficacy of such compounds in special forms of convulsive disease, or *testing for special indications.*

I. Models for Screening

Two important conditions must be imposed on any screening procedure: it must be *"fast and snappy"* and it must be (reasonably) *reliable.* On average it should be possible to test *two to three new substances,* together with standards, per day, and still have time available to run additional more time-consuming tests, e.g., time course studies or establishment of proper dose-response relations. As to *reliability,* the tests should be able to predict, with adequate probability, clinical efficacy – or inefficacy. These screening procedures should produce no, or only a minimal number of, *false positives.* Enough (potential) "true positives" must be discarded for a number of other reasons: too many and/or too severe side effects, toxicity, etc. So whatever passes the tests of further development should turn out to be a potent and efficient anticonvulsant drug. Also, and even more important, the screening procedures must not yield *false negatives,* lest potential clinically effective anticonvulsants are rejected at an early state of development. Inappropriate dose range, i.e., failure to test high doses when low doses proved to be ineffective, is one of the important causes for the production of such false negatives.

Most laboratories involved in the development of anticonvulsants (or antiepileptics) use two or more of the "simple" testing procedures for screening purposes: the *maximal electroshock procedure* and one or more of the "simple" chemically induced acute convulsion models. *Maximal electroshock (MES) testing in mice* ($n = 10$/dose) comes first. Doses of 3, 30, and 300 mg/kg p.o. give an initial indication of (possible) anticonvulsant efficacy. Depending on the results obtained in the first test, a second series is run with the same doses *and* doses intermediate to those in the *effective dose range.* Then, again in mice, the *pentylenetetrazol* MET or PTZ), *picrotoxin* (PIC) and, possibly, *strychnine* (STR) tests are performed, with doses within and around the range found effective in the MES. ED_{50}s are calculated for all these tests. Finally, and only with substances found effective in the preceding procedures, a MES test may be performed in *rats,* again with a range of doses the ED_{50}s found in mice. Some laboratories also use, in addition to (or replacing some of) the procedures just mentioned, the *audiogenic mice* test.

The *Epilepsy Branch* of the US National Institute of Neurological and Communicative Disorders and Stroke, *National Institute of Health,* has initiated an intramural program to screen – for "outsiders" – potential anticonvulsant drugs (KRALL et al. 1978).

To evaluate the time course of effectiveness of the drugs the NIH group recommends – as first approximation – testing for anticonvulsive activity 30 and 240 min after administration of the drug. We prefer a somewhat more detailed procedure and test – using MES in mice and rats – 0.5, 1, 2, 4, 8, 16, and 24 h after *oral* administration of the compound in question. Here, it is of importance to allow, through proper experimental design, for circadian influences on sensitivity to the drug *and* to the epileptogenic agent.

II. Testing for "Special Indications"

The description of the various models in Sect. B of this chapter has revealed that *convulsions,* precipitated acutely or chronically by a wide variety of physical or chemical factors, or occurring "spontaneously in genetically primed animals, as well as the many interictal phenomena, differ considerably in severity and form. Often the convulsions impress as being generalized attacks with a tonic-clonic sequence. Often the fits may have all the earmarks of a partial seizure which, though, may generalize. Behavioral indicators may indicate that we deal, in one or the other model, with a complex partial attack of limbic origin. Electrophysiological recordings enable us to differentiate at least two forms of discharge: a fast, spiky one that has all the characteristics of a focal or a "grand-mal" attack; or then the 2–4/s spike- (or polyspike-) wave patterns reminiscent of an absence seizure.

Quite evidently, the animal (at least down to amphibia, if not further) is apt to produce (or release) epileptiform activity which, in electrographic and behavioral appearance, is not far removed from such activity observed in man; this, in the first place, is *independent* of etiology! Thus, this gives us the idea of using such *special forms* of animal convulsions as models for testing putative antiepileptic drugs on special efficacy in the *various forms* of (human) convulsions. In recent years, a variety of compounds of known efficacy in special forms of seizures in man were tested in such special animal models. The results are encouraging; it seems possible to predict to some extent in what types of seizure a particular (putative) antiepileptic drug would be most efficacious – at what price and with how many "false positives" and "negatives" cannot be foreseen as yet. Still, some discussion of such procedures, making use of some of the models described earlier, is in place.

1. Testing Efficacy in Petit-Mal Epilepsy

According to WOODBURY (1972) and many others, a (relatively) high potency of a particular compound in the *pentylenetetrazol* test (in comparison with the maximal electroshock test) is characteristic for compounds with high efficacy in petit-mal epilepsy. WOODBURY (1972) also claimed that a strong (inhibitory) reaction of post-tetanic potentiation (PTP) to a drug is a good predictor of its high efficacy in petit-mal epilepsy. Furthermore, the *arrest reaction* (HUNTER and JASPER 1949, see Sect. B.I.5) has been suggested as a model for this purpose. Yet, in this experiment the electrically induced electrographic and behavioral reactions appear with considerable variability; as often as not the arrest reaction develops into an overt grand-mal seizure. This makes interpretation of results obtained with the drug somewhat difficult.

The research efforts of recent years have yielded a number of new "petit-mal" models that may be better suited and more reliable for prediction of anti-petit-mal efficacy. The "acute" model of MARCUS (1972) (see Sect. B. III.2) with *bilateral cobalt* application should be mentioned as one possibility. Not much work has been done with this experimental procedure for the testing of drugs (involving "old standards"), so that its suitability for discovering specific anti-petit-mal remedies cannot be judged. Also the use of a "high-standing" primate in an acute fashion would make one hesitate to utilize this model for routine exploration. "Acuteness," i.e., the necessity of using one animal for each experiment, and loss of behavioral manifestations due to immobilization are again the important drawbacks of the cat *Premarin model* (MARCUS et al. 1968; JULIEN et al. 1975; see Sect. B. II.6). Still, JULIEN and his co-workers obtained some relevant results with this procedure. It could be shown that acetazolamide, ethosuximide, and trimethadione strongly inhibited, whereas diphenylhydantoin intensified, the estrogen-induced spike-wave pattern.

GLOOR and TESTA (1974) and GLOOR et al. (1977) administered *penicillin* i.m. and (bilaterally) directly to the cortex, respectively, in "acute" immobilized cats and noted, in response to such treatment, a spike-wave pattern (see Sect. B. II.9). Little pharmacological work has been performed with this model, so its use as a "predictor" for anti-petit-mal efficacy cannot be jugded. As these models also rely on immobilization of the animals, the masking of behavioral manifestations and of their reaction to test drugs is certainly a drawback. This though is not the case with the experiment carried out by FISHER and PRINCE (1977), who worked in freely moving cats under i.m. or i.v.-administered *penicillin*. Again, no systematic work with a variety of antiepileptic agents has been done with this model, so its suitability for prediction purposes is far from being settled.

We described a model (Sect. B. I.6) in which cortical spike-wave (after-)discharges, accompanied by a "staring gaze" and myoclonic twitches of the face and occasionally of the legs, was elicited by bilateral electrical stimulation of the white matter (below the sensorimotor cortex) of chronically prepared freely moving cats. This model impressed by its reliability in revealing these "symptoms" over and over again during numerous repeated (at hourly, as well as at weekly intervals) sessions. The petit-mal features reacted well to typically antiabsence drugs, whereas substances such as phenobarbital, carbamazepine, but also methsuximide and trimethadione were effective in (relatively) high doses only (Table 1). Figure 2 illustrates the effect of sodium valproate on the spike-wave afterdischarge elicited by electrical stimulation of the cat's white matter. Also, the photomyoclonic baboon (see KILLAM 1979; also Chap. 3, this volume) may lend itself as a petit-mal model, as suggested by WOODBURY (1972). These animals, in reaction to an intermittent photic stimulus, revealed not only localized myocloniform movements but also spike-wave patterns in the EEG. However, the picture is often obscured by a generalized clonus and, in the EEG, by frequent spikes and polyspikes, so that the otherwise characteristic phenomenology of a petit-mal attack becomes ambiguous.

Table 1. Potency of a variety of antiepileptic drugs in the cat "petit-mal" model (PMM) (SCHMUTZ et al. 1980) compared with that in the electroshock test in mice (ESM). Potency in the former is expressed by the dose revealing "threshold" effects, in the latter by ED_{50}. R designates "relative potency" and is the quotient obtained by division of the ED_{50} (ESM) by threshold dose in PMM

Drug	PMM Threshold dose	ESM ED_{50}	R
Ethosuximide	30 mg/kg p.o.	1000 (40%)	> 30
Methsuximide	30 mg/kg p.o.	41	1.3
Trimethadione	300 mg/kg p.o.	430	1.4
Valproate sodium	30 mg/kg p.o.	210–530	~ 10
Clonazepam	0.3 mg/kg p.o.	1	3
Phenobarbital	10 mg/kg p.o.	13	1.3
Carbamazepine	3 mg/kg p.o.	10	3
Phenytoin	3 mg/kg p.o.	7–20	~ 5

2. Testing Efficacy in Grand-Mal Epilepsy

WOODBURY (1972) offered a choice of eight "symptomatic" models which, with their special reactivity to selected and/or "new" anticonvulsive drugs, should enable the effectiveness "in generalized seizures of the grand-mal type" to be predicted. He suggested maximal electroshock seizures (mouse), maximal pentylenetetrazol seizure (mouse), maximal audiogenic seizures (mouse), flurothyl-induced tonic-clonic seizures, chronic alumina lesions, freezing lesions, topical penicillin (or other convulsants), and focal (cortical) electrical stimulation (with afterdischarge). In first approximation, this choice can be supported. Still, for detailed drug work, it is important to distinguish between primarily and secondarily generalized seizures.

There is a good chance that antiepileptic drugs are able to differentiate in their effectiveness between spread arising from a focus and leading to (secondary) generalization, on the one hand, and a primarily generalized seizure, on the other. To obtain experimental evidence for such differential efficacy, *it is necessary* to test drugs in models of both kinds. For testing efficacy in primarily generalized attacks, the "old-fashioned" maximal electroshock paradigm still seems to be the model of choice. For testing efficacy against spread (and secondary generalization) a (preferably "chronic") model with a sustained large focus in one of the highly susceptible areas of the neocortex, including detailed and widespread electrographic pick-up for recording of the spread and generalization, should be used. Still, the question of spread will be dealt with in somewhat more detail in Sect. D.II.4.

3. Testing Efficacy Against Temporal Lobe Seizures

In principle any animal experiment in which seizures are induced by an epileptigenic focus, or lesion, placed into the temporal lobe area should lend itself as a model for *temporal lobe epilepsy*. The electrically induced hippocampal afterdischarge described in Sect. B. I.3, using cats either acutely or chronically prepared with stimulating and recording electrodes (KOELLA 1980 a, b), seems to serve this purpose adequately. Figure 1 shows the effect of carbamazepine, a drug said to be specially effective in temporal lobe epilepsy, on hippocampal afterdischarges in "chronic" preparation. In addition to this model with an electrically induced limbic afterdischarge, experiments with placements of chemicals or metals as epileptogenic agents in the hippocampus may be used here. The experiment carried out by MELLANBY et al. (1977) with tetanus toxin deposits, the method of ROLDAN et al. (1971 a) with cobalt application, and the experiment of BLUM et al. (1961) with tungstic acid (all described in Sects. B. II, B. III) deserve to be tried with established and putative antiepileptic drugs.

4. Testing Efficacy in Focal and Spreading Seizures and on Development of Epilepsy

Seizures arising in foci, in particular in those of the cerebral cortex, tend to spread and to lead, eventually, to (secondarily) generalized attacks. The therapeutic approach can be looked at as being twophased. Treatment may either confine itself merely to stem back the spread, or then, and preferably, may combat the seizure *in the focus* itself. Models used to characterize drugs as to their special application should allow differentiation between these two modes of action. Evidently, they must present a discharging epileptogenic focus and they must exhibit – possibly at a later state of the developing epilepsy – spread, either around the initial focus, or by "jumping" toward remote structures, e.g., the contralateral homotopic area. The primary focus produced in cats by local freezing (see MORRELL's work described in Sect. B. IV), together with the temporally well-defined development first of a dependent, and then of an independent, secondary focus probably satisfies these criteria best. Applications of drugs in identical doses, at various time points over the development of the primary *and* secondary focus, should enable the two targets of action to be differentiated.

It stands to reason that foci engendered by other agents, e. g., metals such as cobalt, tungstic acid, ferri- or ferrochloride, can serve the same purpose. In turn, foci produced acutely by electrical stimulation or by application of such chemical agents as penicillin may be apt to act as models for "purely" focal seizures and for the monitoring of the effect of antiepileptic drugs thereupon.

With the discussion of spread of the epileptiform discharge, we also have closed in on another – easily the most important – problem of epilepsy per se, namely its development. From an analysis of clinical cases, it has become quite clear that at least one mode of development involves "contamination": an initially well-confined discharging focus spreads – possibly by a mechanism akin to post-tetanic potentiation – the propensity to produce epileptiform discharge to neighboring and/or remote ("downstream"); initially healthy areas. It is easy to understand that the end point of such spread is *generalization,* possibly even *"primary" generalization,* if large areas of the brain have lowered – through such contamination – their threshold to any convulsogenic factor.

This is not the place to dwell too long on these and other mechanisms of development of epilepsy, but it seems that the *secondary focus paradigm* and, possibly even more so, the *kindling paradigm* can easily stand in as models of such development. If they do, they should be used to a greater extent as instruments for the testing of drugs that are potentially able specifically to slow down, or even stop, the development of epilepsy.

Thus, for testing drug efficacy in the development of epilepsy, the "nonsymptomatic" post-tetanic potentiation model should also be put to use. And finally, one or the other of the "genetic models" – in particular during their early stages of development – may lend themselves as valuable additional instruments for the discovery of truly *antiepileptogenic remedies,* i.e., drugs that not only combat "secondary" establishment – spread, "contamination" – but also primary development, the making of the very local epileptogenic lesion.

If the work on established and new anticonvulsant drugs in the many different animal models is to yield still better drugs – possibly true antiepileptic remedies – and improve our understanding of the very nature of epilepsy, then the use of such models in epileptology is well justified and the search for still superior experimental techniques must continue.

References

Adams WB, Parnas I, Levitan IB (1980) Mechanism of long-lasting synaptic inhibition in *Aplysia* neurons R 15. J Neurophysiol 44:1148–1160

Ajmone-Marsan C (1969) Acute effects of topical epileptogenic agents. in: Jasper HH, Ward AA, Pope A (eds) Basic mechanisms of epilepsies. Little Brown, Boston, pp 299–319

Ajmone-Marsan C (1972) Focal electrical stimulation. In: Purpura DP, Penry JK, Woodbury DM, Tower DB, Walter RD (eds) Experimental models of epilepsy – a manual for the laboratory worker. Raven, New York, pp 147–172

Ajmone-Marsan C, Marossero F (1950) Electrocorticographic and electrochordographic study of the convulsions induced by cardiazol: some observations on the combined action of CNS excitants. Electroencephalogr Clin Neurophysiol 2:133–142

Andersen P (1978) Long-lasting facilitation of synaptic transmission. In: Function of the septo-hippocampal system. CIBA-Foundation Symposium 58, Elsevier, Amsterdam, pp 87–102

Andersen P, Sundberg SH, Sveen O, Wigström H (1977) Specific long-lasting potentation of synaptic transmission in hippocampal slices. Nature 266:736–737

Andy OJ, Akert K (1953) Electrographic and behavioral changes during seizures induced by stimulation of ammonsformation in the cat and monkey. Electroencephalogr Clin Neurophysiol [Suppl] III:48

Ayala GF, Matsumoto H, Gumnit RJ (1970) Excitability changes and inhibitory mechanisms in neocortical neurons during seizures. J Neurophysiol 33:73–85

Barker JL, Smith TG (1978) Electrophysiological studies of molluscan neurons generating pacemaker potential activity. In: Chalozonitis N, Boisson M (eds) Abnormal neuronal discharges. Raven, New York, pp 359–387

Bircher RP, Kanai T, Wang SC (1962) Intravenous, cortical and intraventricular dose-effect relationship of pentylenetetrazol, picrotoxin and deslanoside in dogs. Electroencephalogr Clin Neurophysiol 14:256–267

Blum B, Liban E (1960) Experimental basotemporal epilepsy in the cat: discrete epileptogenic lesions produced in the hippocampus or amygdaloid by tungstic acid. Neurology 10:546–554

Blum B, Magnes J, Bental E, Liban E (1961) Electroencephalographic studies in cats with experimentally produced hippocampal epilepsy. Electroencephalogr Clin Neurophysiol 13:340–353

Brierley JB, Horton RW, Meldrum BS (1972) Physiological observations during prolonged epileptic seizures in primates and their relation to subsequent brain damage. J Physiol (Cambridge) 222:69P–70P

Brooks VB Asanuma H (1962) Action of tetanus toxin in the cerebral cortex. Science 137:674–676
Burns BD (1951) Some properties of isolated cerebral cortex in the unanaesthetized cat. J Physiol (Lond) 112:156–175
Cain DP (1981) Kindling: recent studies and new directions. In: Wada JA (ed) Kindling 2. Raven, New York, pp 49–62
Carrea R, Lanari A (1962) Chronic effect of tetanus toxin applied locally to the cerebral cortex of the dog. Science 137:342–343
Chusid JG, Kopeloff LM (1962) Epileptogenic effects of pure metals implanted in motor cortex of monkeys. J Appl Physiol 17:696–700
Chusid JG, Kopeloff LM (1969) Use of chronic irritative foci in laboratory evaluation of anti-epileptic drugs. Epilepsia 10:239–262
Colasanti BK, Hartman ER, Craig CR (1974) Electrocorticogram and behavioral correlates during the development of chronic cobalt experimental epilepsy in the rat. Epilepsia 15:361–373
Collins RL (1972) Audiogenic seizures. In: Purpura DP, Penry JK, Woodbury DM, Tower DB, Walter RD (eds) Experimental models of epilepsy – a manual for the laboratory worker. Raven, New York, pp 347–372
Consroe P, Picchioni A, Chin L (1979) Audiogenic seizure susceptible rats. Fed Proc 38:2411–2416
Curtis DR, Duggan AW, Felix D, Johnston GAR (1970 a) GABA, bicuculline, and central inhibition. Nature 226:1222–1224
Curtis DR, Duggan AW, Felix D, Johnston GAR (1970 b) Bicuculline and central GABA receptors. Nature 228:676–677
Daly DD (1973) Circadian cycles and seizures. In: Brazier (ed) Epilepsy, its phenomena in man. Academic, New York, pp 215–233
David J, Grewal RS (1978) A simplified technique for producing aluminium hydroxide-induced chronic focal seizures in monkeys. Indian J Exp Biol 16:96–99
Delgado JMR, Sevillano M (1961) Evolution of repeated hippocampal seizures in the cat. Electroencephalogr Clin Neurophysiol 13:722–733
Dice LR (1935) Inheritance of waltzing and of epilepsy in mice of the genus *Peromyscus*. J Mammol 16–25–35
Dichter M, Spencer WA (1969) Penicillin-induced interictal discharges from the cat hippocampus. II. Mechanisms underlying origin and restriction. J Neurophysiol 32:663–687
Dichter M, Herman C, Selzer M (1973) Penicillin epilepsy in isolated islands of hippocampus. Electroencephalogr Clin Neurophysiol 34:631–638
Dow RS, Fernández-Guardiola A, Manni E (1962) The production of cobalt experimental epilepsy in the rat. Electroencephalogr Clin Neurophysiol 14:399–407
Echlin FA (1954) Acetylcholine, supersensitivity and focal cortical seizures in chronically neuronally isolated and partially isolated cerebral cortex. Electroencephalogr Clin Neurophysiol 6:690
Echlin FA (1959) The supersensitivity of chronically "isolated" cerebral cortex as a mechanism in focal epilepsy. Electroencephalogr Clin Neurophysiol 11:697–722
Escueta AV, Davidson D, Hartwig G, Reilly E (1974) The freezing lesion. II. Potassium transport within nerve terminals isolated from epileptogenic foci. Brain Res 78:223–237
Esplin DW (1972) Synaptic system models. In: Purpura DP, Penry JK, Woodbury DM, Tower DB, Walter RD (eds) Experimental models of epilepsy – a manual for the laboratory worker. Raven, New York, pp 223–248
Faugier S, Willows AOD (1973) Behavioral and nerve cell membrane effects of an epileptic agent (Metrazol) in a mollusk. Brain Res 52:243–260
Ferguson JH, Cornblath DR (1974) Acetylcholine epilepsy: modification of DC shift in chronically undercut cat cortex. Electroencephalogr Clin Neurophysiol 36:113–122
Fischer J, Holubar J, Malik V (1967) A new method of producing chronic epileptogenic cortical foci in rats. Physiologia Bohemoslovaca 16:272–277
Fisher RS, Prince DA (1977) Spike-wave rhythms in cat cortex induced by parenteral penicillin. I. Electroencephalographic features. Electroencephalogr Clin Neurophysiol 42:608–624

Frazier WT, Kandel ER, Kupfermann I, Waziri R, Coggeshall RE (1967) Morphological and functional properties of identified neurons in the abdominal ganglion of *Aplysia californica*. J Neurophysiol 30:1288–1351
French JD, Gernandt BE, Livingston RB (1956) Regional differences in seizure susceptibility in monkey cortex. Arch Neurol Psychiat 75:260–274
Frenk H, Urca G, Liebeskind JC (1978) Epileptic properties of leucine- and methionine-enkephalin: comparison with morphine and reversibility by naloxone. Brain Res 147:327–337
Fromm GH, Killian JM (1967) Effect of some anticonvulsant drugs on the spinal trigeminal nucleus. Neurology 17:275–280
Fromm GH, Glass JD, Chattha AS, Martinez AJ, Silverman M (1980) Antiabsence drugs and inhibitory pathways. Neurology 30:126–131
Fromm GH, Glass JD, Chattha AS, Martinez AJ (1981) Effect of anticonvulsant drugs on inhibitory and excitatory pathways. Epilepsia 22:65–73
Gibbs FA, Gibbs EL (1936) The convulsive threshold of various parts of the cat's brain. Arch Neurol Psychiatr 35:109–116
Gilbert ME, Cain DP (1982) A developmental study of kindling in the rat. Dev Brain Res 2:321–328
Gloor P, Testa G (1974) Generalized penicillin epilepsy in the cat: effects of intracarotid and intravertebral pentylenetrazol and amobarbital injections. Electroencephalogr Clin Neurophysiol 36:499–515
Gloor P, Quesney LF, Zumstein H (1977) Pathophysiology of generalized penicillin epilepsy in the cat: the role of cortical and subcortical structures. II. Topical application of penicillin to the cerebral cortex and to subcortical structures. Electroencephalogr Clin Neurophysiol 43:79–94
Goddard GV (1967) Development of epileptic seizures through brain stimulation at low intensity. Nature 214:1020–1021
Goddard GV, McIntyre DC, Leech CK (1969) A permanent change in brain function resulting from daily electrical stimulation. Exp Neurol 25:295–330
Gottesfeld Z, Elazar Z (1975) GABA synthesis and uptake in penicillin focus. Brain Res 84:346–350
Gutnick MJ, Duijn H van, Citri N (1976) Relative convulsant potencies of structural analogues of penicillin. Brain Res 114:139–143
Hahn F, Oberdorf A (1962) Vergleichende Untersuchungen über die Krampfwirkung von Bemegrid, Pentetrazol und Pikrotoxin. Arch Int Pharmacodyn Ther 135:9–30
Halberg F (1955) Twenty-four-hour periodic susceptibility to audiogenic convulsions in several stocks of mice. Fed Proc 14:67–88
Hall CS (1947) Genetic differences in fatal audiogenic seizures. J Hered 38:2–6
Hanna GR, Stalmaster RM (1973) Cortical epileptic lesions produced by freezing. Neurology 23:918–925
Henjyoji EY, Dow RS (1965) Cobalt-induced seizures in the cat. Electroencephalogr Clin Neurophysiol 19:152–161
Hildebrandt F (1926) Pentamethylenetetrazol (Cardiazol®). Arch Exp Pathol Pharmakol 116:100–109
Hughes JR (1959a) Studies on the supracallosal mesial cortex of unanesthetized, conscious mammals. I. Cat. A. Movements elicited by electrical stimulation. Electroencephalogr Clin Neurophysiol 11:447–458
Hughes JR (1959b) Studies on the supracallosal mesial cortex of unanesthetized, conscious mammals. I. Cat. B. Electrical activity. Electroencephalogr Clin Neurophysiol 11:459–469
Hughes JR, Mazurowski JA (1962) Studies on the supracallosal mesial cortex of unanesthetized, conscious mammals. II. Monkey. A. Movements elicited by electrical stimulation. Electroencephalogr Clin Neurophysiol 14:477–485
Hughes JR, Mazurowski JA (1964) Studies on the supracallosal mesial cortex of unanesthetized, conscious mammals. II. Monkey. D. Vertex sharp waves and epileptiform activity. Electroencephalogr Clin Neurophysiol 16:561–574

Hunter J, Jasper HH (1949) Effects of thalamic stimulation in unanesthetized animals. Electroencephalogr Clin Neurophysiol 1:305–324
Janz D (1962) The grand mal epilepsies and the sleeping-waking cylce. Epilepsia 3:69–109
Janz D (1975) Types of epilepsy and types of sleepers. In: Hara T, Wada T (eds) Circadian rhythm and epilepsy. The Japanese branch of ILAE, pp 5–12. Available from: Natl. Musashi Res. Inst. for Mental and Nervous Diseases, 2620 Ogawa-higashi, Kodaira, Tokyo
Julien RM, Fowler GW, Danielson MG (1975) The effects of antiepileptic drugs on estrogen-induced electrographic spike-wave discharge. J Pharmacol Exp Ther 193:647–656
Kaada BR (1951) Somato-motor, autonomic and electrocorticographic responses to electrical stimulation of "rhinencephalic" and other structures in primates, cat and dog. Acta Physiol Scand 231:[Suppl] 83:1–285
Kandel ER (1976) Cellular basis of behavior. An introduction to behavioral neurobiology. Freeman, San Francisco
Killam EK (1979) Photomyoclonic seizures in the baboon *Papio papio*. Fed Proc 38:2429–2433
Klee MR, Faber DS, Heiss W-D (1973) Strychnine- and pentylenetetrazol-induced changes of excitability in *Aplysia* neurons. Science 179:1133–1136
Koella WP (1980a) Laboratory approaches to new antiepileptic drugs. In: Robb P (ed) Epilepsy updated: causes and treatment. Symposia Specialists, Miami, pp 71–84
Koella WP (1980b) Preclinical development of antiepileptic drugs. In: Wada, JA, Penry JK (eds) Advances in epileptology. The Xth Epilepsy International Symposium. Raven, New York, pp 289–294
Koella WP, Schmutz M (1981) Preclinical development of new antiepileptic drugs – the present and the future. In: Dam M, Gram L, Penry JK (eds) Advances in epileptology. XIIth Epilepsy International Symposium. Raven, New York, pp 7–12
Kopeloff LM (1960) Experimental epilepsy in the mouse. Proc Soc Exp Biol Med 104:500–504
Kopeloff LM, Barrera SE, Kopeloff N (1941/1942) Recurrent convulsive seizures in animals produced by immunologic and chemical means. Am J Psychiatry 98:881–902
Kopeloff LM, Chusid JG, Kopeloff N (1955) Epilepsy in *Macaca mulatta* after cortical or intracerebral alumina. Arch Neurol Psychiatr 74:523–526
Krall RL, Penry JK, White BG, Kupferberg H-J, Swinyard EA (1978) Antiepileptic drug development: II. Anticonvulsant drug screening. Epilepsia 19:409–428
Kreindler A, Steriade M (1963) Functional differentiation within the amygdaloid complex inferred from peculiarities of epileptic afterdischarges. Electroencephalogr Clin Neurophysiol 15:811–826
Krushinsky LV, Molodkina LN, Fless DA, Dobrokhotova LP, Steshenko AP, Semiokhina AF, Zorina ZA, Romanova LB (1970) The functional state of the brain during sonic stimulation. In: Welch BL, Welch AS (eds) Physiological effects of noise. Plenum, New York, pp 159–183
Leclercq B, Segal M (1965) An investigation of centers susceptible to mechanically and electrically induced afterdischarge in the cat brain. Can J Physiol Pharmacol 43:491–507
Lewin E (1972) The production of epileptogenic cortical foci in experimental animals by freezing. In: Purpura DP, Penry JK, Woodbury DM, Tower DB, Walter RD (eds) Experimental models of epilepsy – a manual for the laboratory worker. Raven, New York, pp 37–49
Liberson WT, Akert K (1953) Observations on electrical activity of the hippocampus, thalamus, striatum, and cortex under resting conditions and during experimental seizure states in guinea pigs. Electroencephalogr Clin Neurophysiol 5:320
Liberson WT, Akert K (1955) Hippocampal seizure states in guinea pig. Electroencephalogr Clin Neurophysiol 7:211–222
Liberson WT, Cadilhac JG (1953a) Further observation on DC potentials during electrically induced seizure discharge activity in guinea pig. Electroencephalogr Clin Neurophysiol 5:320

Liberson WT, Cadilhac JG (1953b) Further studies of hippocampal seizure states. Electroencephalogr Clin Neurophysiol. [Suppl] III:42
Lloyd DPC (1949) Post-tetanic potentiation of response in mono-synaptic reflex pathways of the spinal cord. J Gen Physiol 33:147–190
Lockard JS, Barensten RI (1967) Behavioral experimental epilepsy in monkeys. I. Clinical seizure recording apparatus and initial data. Electroencephalogr Clin Neurophysiol 22:482–486
Longo VG, Chiavarelli S (1962) Neuropharmacological analysis of strychnine-like drugs. In: Paton WDM (ed). Pharmacological analysis of central nervous action. Proceedings of the first international pharmacological meeting. Pergamon, Oxford, pp 189–198
MacLean PD (1954) The limbic system and its hippocampal formation. Studies in animals and their possible application to man. J Neurosurg 11:29–44
Marcus EM (1972) Experimental models of petit mal epilepsy. In: Purpura DP, Penry JK, Woodbury DM, Tower DB, Walter RD (eds) Experimental models of epilepsy – a manual for the laboratory worker. Raven, New York, pp 113–146
Marcus EM, Watson CW (1964) Bilateral "epileptogenic" foci in cat cerebral cortex: mechanisms of interaction in the intact, the bilateral cortical callosal and a diencephalic preparation. Electroencephalogr Clin Neurophysiol 17:454
Marcus EM, Watson CW (1966) Bilateral synchronous spike wave electrographic patterns in the cat. Arch Neurol 14:601–610
Marcus EM, Watson CW (1968) Symmetrical epileptogenic foci in monkey cerebral cortex. Arch Neurol 19:99–116
Marcus EM, Watson CW, Simon SA (1968) An experimental model of some varieties of petit mal epilepsy: electrical-behavioral correlations of acute bilateral epileptogenic foci in cerebral cortex. Epilepsia 9:233–248
Mareš P (1973) Bioelectrical activity of an epileptogenic focus in rat neocortex. Brain Res 56:203–213
Matsumoto H, Ayala GF, Gumnit RJ (1969) Neuronal behavior and triggering mechanism in cortical epileptic focus. J Neurophysiol 32:688–703
Mayanagi Y, Walker AE (1974) Experimental temporal lobe epilepsy. Brain 97:423–446
Meldrum BS, Horton RW (1971) Convulsive effects of 4-deoxypyridoxine and of bicuculline in photosensitive baboons (*Papio papio*) and in rhesus monkeys (*Macaca mulatta*). Brain Res 35:419–436
Mellanby J, George G, Robinson A, Thompson P (1977) Epileptiform syndrome in rats produced by injecting tetanus toxin into the hippocampus. J Neurol Neurosurg Psychiatry 40:404–414
Mirsky IA, Elgart S, Aring CD (1943) Sonogenic convulsions in rats and mice: I. control studies. J Comp Psychol 35:249–253
Moody WJ, Futamachi KJ, Prince DA (1974) Extracellular potassium activity during epileptogenesis. Exp Neurol 42:248–263
Morrell F (1959) Experimental focal epilepsy in animals. Arch Neurol 1:141–147
Morrell F (1960) Secondary epileptogenic lesions. Epilepsia 1:538–560
Morrell F (1961) Microelectrode studies in chronic epileptic foci. Epilepsia 2:81–88
Morrell F (1973) Goddard's kindling phenomenon: a new model of the "mirror focus". In: Sabelli HC (ed) Chemical modulation of the brain function. Raven, New York, pp 207–223
Morrell F (1978) Aspects of experimental epilepsy. In: Wada JA (ed) Modern perspectives in epilepsy. Eden, Montreal, pp 24–75
Morrell F, Florenz A (1958) Modification of the freezing technique for producing experimental epileptogenic lesions. Electroencephalogr Clin Neurophysiol 10:187
Morrell F, Tsuru N (1976) Kindling in the frog: development of spontaneous epileptiform activity. Electroencephalogr Clin Neurophysiol 40:1–11
Mutani R (1967) Cobalt experimental hippocampal epilepsy. Epilepsia 8:223–240
Nie V, Ettlinger G (1974) Ablation of the primary inferotemporal epileptogenic focus in rhesus monkeys with independent secondary spike discharges. Brain Res 69:149–152
Nims LF, Marshall C, Nielsen A (1941) Effect of local freezing on the electrical activity of the cerebral cortex. Yale J Biol Med 13:477–484

Noebels JL (1979) Analysis of inherited epilepsy using single locus mutations in mice. Fed Proc 38:2405–2410
O'Connor MJ, Lewis DV (1974) Recurrent seizures induced by potassium in the penicillin treated hippocampus. Electroencephalogr Clin Neurophysiol 36:337–345
Openchowski P (1883) Sur l'action localisée du froid appliqué à la surface de la région corticale du cerveau. C R Soc Biol (Paris) 35:38–43
Partridge LD (1975) Pentylenetetrazol-induced bursting activity in the absence of a negative conductance characteristic. Brain Res 94:161–166
Passouant P (1977) Influence des états de vigilance sur les épilepsies. In: Koella WP, Levin P (eds) Sleep 1976. Proceedings of 3rd European Congress on sleep research. Karger, Basel, pp 57–65
Payan HM, Conard JR (1973) Cobalt experimental epilepsy in various strains of rat. Epilepsia 14:415–421
Payan HM, Conard JR (1974) Cobalt-induced epilepsy in rats. A study in biochemical substances. Arch Pathol 97:170–172
Petsche H, Müller-Paschinger IB, Pockberger H, Prohaska O, Rappelsberger P, Vollmer R (1978) Depth profiles of electrocortical activities and cortical architectonis. In: Brazier MAB, Petsche H (eds) Architectonics of the cerebral cortex. Raven, New York, pp 257–280
Phillis JW (1968) Acetylcholine release from the cerebral cortex. Its role in cortical arousal. Brain Res 7:378–389
Pinel JPJ (1981) Spontaneous kindled motor seizures in rats. In: Wada JA (ed) Kindling 2. Raven, New York, pp 179–181
Pinel JPJ, Mucha RF, Phillips AG (1975) Spontaneous seizures generated in rats by kindling: a preliminary report. Physiol Psychology 3:127–129
Pinsky C, Burns BD (1962) Production of epileptiform afterdischarges in cat's cerebral cortex. J Neurophysiol 25:359–379
Pope A, Morris AA, Jasper HH, Elliot KAC, Penfield W (1947) Histochemical and action potential studies on epileptogenic areas of cerebral cortex in man and the monkey. Res Publ Assoc Res Nerv Ment Dis 26:218–227
Post RM (1981) Lidocaine-kindled limbic seizures: behavioral implications. In: Wada JA (ed) Kindling 2. Raven, New York, pp 149–157
Post RM, Kopanda RT, Black KE (1976) Progressive effects of cocaine on behavior and central amine metabolism in rhesus monkeys: relationship to kindling and psychosis. Biol Psychiatry 11:403–419
Prince DA (1969) Microelectrode studies of penicillin foci. In: Jasper HH, Ward AA, Pope A (eds) Basic mechanism of epilepsies. Little Brown, Boston, pp 320–328
Prince DA (1972) Topical convulsant drugs and metabolic antagonists. In: Purpura DP, Penry JK, Woodbury DM, Tower DB, Walter RD (eds) Experimental models of epilepsy – a manual for the laboratory worker. Raven, New York, pp 51–83
Prince DA, Gutnick MJ (1972) Neuronal activities in epileptogenic foci of immature cortex. Brain Res 45:455–468
Purpura DP, Penry JK, Woodbury DM, Tower DB, Walter RD (1972) Experimental models of epilepsy – a manual for the laboratory worker. Raven, New York
Racine RJ, Burnham WM, Gartner JG, Levitan D (1973) Rates of motor seizure development in rats subjected to electrical brain stimulation: strain and interstimulation interval effects. Electroencephalogr Clin Neurophysiol 35:553–556
Radouco-Thomas C, Frommel E, Radouco-Thomas S (1955) Médication antiépileptique et activité cholinestérasique. Helv Physiol Pharmacol Acta 13:1–13
Reichenthal E, Hocherman S (1977) The critical cortical area for development of penicillin-induced epilepsy. Electroencephalogr Clin Neurophysiol 42:248–251
Renshaw B, Forbes A, Morison BR (1940) Activity of isocortex and hippocampus. Electrical studies with micro-electrodes. J Neurophysiol 3:74–105
Roldań E, Radil-Weiss T, Chocholová L (1970) Paroxysmal activity of hippocampal and thalamic epileptogenic foci and induced or spontaneous changes of vigilance. Exp Neurol 29:121–130

Roldań E, Radil-Weiss T, Chocholová L (1971 a) Sleep cycle in rats with paroxysmal foci. Int J Neurosci 2:179–182
Roldań E, Radil-Weiss T, Chocholová L (1971 b) Epileptic electroencephalographic activity induced by cobalt foci in the dorsal hippocampus and/or thalamus. Int J Neurosci 2:293–300
Rosenblueth A, Cannon WB (1941/1942) Cortical responses to electric stimulation. Am J Physiol 135:690–741
Sawa M, Marnyama N, Kaji S (1963) Intracellular potential during electrically induced seizures. Electroencephalogr Clin Neurophysiol 15:209–220
Schlesinger K, Boggan W, Freedman DX (1965) Genetics of audiogenic seizures: I. Relation to brain serotonin and norepinephrine in mice. Life Sci 4:2345–2351
Schlesinger K, Boggan W, Freedman DX (1968) Genetics of audiogenic seizures: II. Effects of pharmacological manipulation of brain serotonin, norepinephrine and gamma-aminobutyric acid. Life Sci 7:437–447
Schlesinger K, Boggan W, Freedman DX (1970) Genetics of audiogenic seizures: III. Time response relationships between drug administration and seizure susceptibility. Life Sci 9:721–729
Schmidt KF (1924) Über den Imin-Rest. Ber Dtsch Chem Ges 57:704–706
Schmutz M, Klebs K, Koella WP (1980) A chronic petit mal model. In: Wada JA, Penry JK (eds) Advances in epileptology: the Xth epilepsy international symposium. Raven, New York, pp 311–314
Schmutz M, Bürki H, Koella WP (1981) Electrically induced hippocampal afterdischarge in the freely moving cat: an animal model of focal (possibly temporal lobe) epilepsy. In: Dam M, Gram L, Penry JK (eds) Advances in epileptology: XIIth epilepsy international symposium. Raven, New York, pp 59–65
Schneider A, Epstein B (1931) The effects of local freezing of the central nervous system of the cat. Arch Neurol Psychiatr 25:1264–1270
Segal M, Leclercq B (1965) Threshold studies and isolimital mapping of electrically elicited afterdischarge in the cat brain. Can J Physiol Pharmacol 43:685–697
Seyfried TN (1979) Audiogenic seizures in mice. Fed Proc 38:2399–2404
Smith TG Jr, Purpura DP (1960) Electrophysiological studies on epileptogenic lesion of cat cortex. Electroencephalogr Clin Neurophysiol 12:59–82
Speckmann E-J, Caspers H (1973) Paroxysmal depolarization and changes in action potentials induced by pentylenetetrazol in isolated neurons of *Helix pomatia*. Epilepsia 14:397–408
Stalmaster RM, Hanna GR (1972) Epileptic phenomena of cortical freezing in the cat: persistent multifocal effects of discrete superficial lesions. Epilepsia 13:313–324
Stone WE (1957) The role of acetylcholine in brain metabolism and function. Am J Phys Med 36:222–255
Stone WE (1972) Systemic chemical convulsants and metabolic derangements. In: Purpura DP, Penry JK, Woodbury DM, Tower DB, Walter RD (eds) Experimental models of epilepsy – a manual for the laboratory worker. Raven, New York, pp 407–432
Stone WE, Tews JK, Mitchell EN (1960) Chemical concomitants of convulsive activity in the cerebrum. Neurology 10:241–248
Straw RN, Mitchell CL (1966) A study on the duration of cortical afterdischarge in the cat. Electroencephalogr Clin Neurophysiol 21:54–58
Stumpf C (1962) Pharmakologische Methoden. In: Stumpf C, Petsche H (eds) Handbuch der experimentellen Pharmakologie. Vol XVI/7. Springer, Berlin p 1–105
Swinyard EA (1969) Laboratory evaluation of antiepileptic drugs. Epilepsia 10:107–119
Swinyard EA (1972) Electrically induced convulsions. In: Purpura DP, Penry JK, Woodbury DM, Tower DB, Walter RD (eds) Experimental models of epilepsy – a manual for the laboratory worker. Raven, New York, pp 433–458
Swinyard EA, Brown WC, Goodman LS (1952) Comparative assays of antiepileptic drugs in mice and rats. J Pharmacol Exp Ther 106:319–330
Szirmai I, Molnar M, Czopf J, Borsics K (1977) Spreading epileptiform discharges and cortical regional blood flow in rabbits. Electroencephalogr Clin Neurophysiol 42:238–247

Urca G, Frenk H, Liebeskind JC, Taylor AN (1977) Morphine and enkephalin: analgesic and epileptic properties. Science 197:83–86
Van Gelder NM, Courtois A (1972) Close correlation between changing content of specific amino acids in epileptogenic cortex of cats, and severity of epilepsy. Brain Res 43:477–484
Velasco M, Velasco F, Estrada-Villanueva F, Olivera A (1973) Alumina cream-induced focal motor epilepsy in cats. Part I. Lesion size and temporal course. Epilepsia 14:3–14
Velasco M, Velasco F, Cepeda C, Almanza X, Estrada-Villanueva F (1977) Alumina cream induced focal motor epilepsy in cats. I. Wakefulness-sleep modulation of cortical paroxysmal EEG spikes. Electroencephalogr Clin Neurophysiol 43:59–66
Vollmer R, Petsche H, Prohaska O, Rappelsberger P, Kaiser A (1974) Kreisende kortikale Potentialfelder beim epileptischen Anfall. Experientia 30:156–157
Vollmer R, Szirmai IG, Rappelsberger P (1979) Zur Ausbreitung von Azetylcholin-induzierten Anfällen. EEG/EMG 10:123–131
Wada J, Cornelius L (1960) Functional alterations of deep structures in cats and chronic initiative lesions. Arch Neurol 3:425–447
Wada JA, Osawa T (1976) Spontaneous recurrent seizure state induced by daily electric amygdaloid stimulation in Senegalese baboons (*Papio papio*). Neurology 26:273–286
Wada JA, Sato M (1974) Generalized convulsive seizure induced by daily electrical stimulation of the amygdala in cats: correlative electrographic and behavioral features. Neurology 24:565–574
Wada JA, Sato M (1975) The generalized convulsive seizure state induced by daily electrical stimulation of the amygdala in split brain cats. Epilepsia 16:417–430
Wada JA, Sato M, McCaughran JA Jr (1975) Cortical electrographic correlates of convulsive seizure development induced by daily electrical stimulation of the amygdala in rats and cats. Folia Psychiatr Neurol Jpn 29:329–339
Walker AE, Johnson HC, Kollros JJ (1945) Penicillin convulsions. The convulsive effects of penicillin applied to the cortex of monkey and man. Surg Gynecol Obstet 81:692–701
Walker AE, Poggio GF, Andy OJ (1956) Structural spread of cortically-induced epileptic discharges. Neurology 6:616–626
Ward AA (1969) The epileptic neuron: chronic foci in animals and man. In: Jasper HH, Ward AA, Pope A (eds) Basic mechanisms of the epilepsies. Little Brown, Boston, pp 263–288
Ward AA (1972) Topical convulsant metals. In: Purpura DP, Penry JK, Woodbury DM, Tower DB, Walter RD (eds) Experimental models of epilepsy – a manual for the laboratory worker. Raven, New York, pp 13–35
Wilder BJ (1972) Projection phenomena and secondary epileptogenesis – mirror foci. In: Purpura DP, Penry JK, Woodbury DM, Tower DB, Walter RD (eds) Experimental models of epilepsy – a manual for the laboratory worker. Raven, New York, pp 85–111
Wilder BJ, Schmidt RP (1965) Propagation of epileptic discharge from chronic neocortical foci in monkeys. Epilepsia 6:297–309
Wilder BJ, King RL, Schmidt RP (1969) Cortical and subcortical secondary epileptogenesis. Neurology 19:643–652
Willmore LJ, Sypert GW, Munson JB, Hurd RW (1978) Chronic focal epileptiform discharges induced by injection of iron into rat and cat cortex. Science 200:1501–1503
Wilson WA, Wachtel H (1974) Negative resistance characteristic essential for the maintainance of slow oscillation in bursting neurons. Science 186:932–934
Wilson WA, Wachtel H (1978) Prolonged inhibition in burst firing neurons; synaptic inactivation of the slow regenerative inward current. Science 202:772–775
Woodbury DM (1972) Applications to drug evaluations. In: Purpura DP, Penry JK, Woodbury DM, Tower DB, Walter RD (eds) Experimental models of epilepsy – a manual for the laboratory worker. Raven, New York, pp 557–583
Woodbury DM, Kemp JW (1977) Basic mechanisms of seizures: neurophysiological and biochemical etiology. In: Shagass C, Gershon S, Friedkoff AJ (eds) Psychopathology and brain dysfunction. Raven, New York, pp 149–182
Wyler AR (1974) Epileptic neurons during sleep and wakefulness. Exp Neurol 42:593–608

Wyler AR (1978) Single unit analysis of "mirror foci" in chronic epileptic monkeys. Brain Res 150:201–204
Wyler AR, Fetz EE, Ward AA (1973) Spontaneous firing patterns of epileptic neurons in the monkey motor cortex. Exp Neurol 40:567–585
Wyler AR, Fetz EE, Ward AA Jr (1975) Firing patterns of epileptic and normal neurons in the chronic alumina focus in undrugged monkeys during different behavioral states. Brain Res 98:1–20

APPENDIX TO CHAPTER 12

Antiepileptic Drug Development Program

G. D. GLADDING, H. J. KUPFERBERG, and E. A. SWINYARD

A. Antiepileptic Drug Development Program

The Antiepileptic Drug Development (ADD) Program of the National Institute of Neurological and Communicative Disorders and Stroke (NINCDS) is searching for more effective and less toxic drugs than those now available. This pursuit entails the integration of several activities: (a) synthesis of compounds; (b) evaluation of the anticonvulsant and toxicity profiles of compounds in mice and rats by use of several seizure models and various routes of administration; (c) study of the compounds' toxicity in rats and dogs after oral administration for 90 days; (d) determination of the compounds' pharmacokinetic parameters in the primate seizure model, healthy volunteers, and epileptic patients; and (e) appraisal of antiepileptic efficacy in controlled clinical trials.

In its first efforts to develop new antiepileptic drugs, the NINCDS sponsored clinical trials of drugs with antiepileptic potential marketed for other diseases or disorders or antiepileptic drugs under investigation in other countries. It soon became apparent, however, that too few promising drugs were available for clinical study and that the continued flow of new antiepileptic agents would require the involvement of the NINCDS in preclinical development of anticonvulsant drugs. Initially, emphasis was placed on the evaluation of available compounds. Thus, the Anticonvulsant Screening Project, the first preclinical segment of the ADD Program, was begun in 1975.

B. Anticonvulsant Screening Project

The Anticonvulsant Screening Project evaluates several aspects of drug action: (a) the existence, specificity, and profile of anticonvulsant activity; (b) the profile of toxicity, particularly in the central nervous system; (c) the therapeutic and protective indices; (d) the time course of activity; (e) the comparative activity following intraperitoneal and oral administration; and (f) the presence or absence of tolerance after repeated administration of the drug.

Compounds are submitted from suppliers throughout the world, including pharmaceutical firms, academic institutions, government organizations, and any other parties interested in antiepileptic drug research. Any substance of known matter or composition is accepted. The only substances not accepted are mixtures, such as extracts of natural products. The purity of the compounds must be assured by the suppliers. Suppliers retain all commercial rights to their compounds. The results of the screen are returned to the supplier quickly to expedite decisions about further development of the compound.

Water-soluble compounds are administered in 0.9% sodium chloride; water-insoluble subtances are either dissolved or suspended in 30% polyethylene glycol 400 (PEG 400) in water. PEG 400 was chosen as a solvent for water-insoluble compounds because it was found to have the least effect on anticonvulsant activity, time of peak effect, duration of action, slope of the probit regression line, and median effective dose.

The screening project is divided into seven phases, each serving as a decision point for further evaluation. The battery of screening tests is standardized, allowing comparison of anticonvulsant activity and neurotoxicity of the test compounds with a large number of prototype antiepileptic drugs. Table 1 shows the results from five phases of the screening project for most the currently marketed antiepileptic drugs in the United States.

I. Phase I

Phase I identifies the anticonvulsant activity and neurotoxicity of the compounds in mice. The maximal electroshock seizure (MES) test (SWINYARD et al. 1952) evaluates the ability of a substance to prevent seizure spread through neural tissue, and the subcutaneous pentylenetetrazol (scMet) test (SWINYARD 1972) estimates the ability to raise seizure threshold for excitation of neural tissue. The rotorod ataxia test assesses central nervous system toxicity. Neurological deficit is indicated by the inability of a mouse to remain on a 25.4-mm knurled plastic rod rotating at 6 rpm for 1 min (DUNHAM and MIYA 1957).

A dose of 30, 100, 300, or 600 mg/kg is administered intraperitoneally; four mice are tested at each dose level (16 animals). All mice are subjected to the rotorod test 30 min after drug administration. At the same time, and then 4 h later, two animals from each group are tested, one by the MES test and one by the scMet test. The results of these tests indicate the potency of the compound and allow an estimate of the protective index. Testing for anticonvulsant activity at both 30 min and 4 h after drug administration yields elementary pharmacokinetic information and minimizes the likelihood of failure to identify slowly absorbed compounds or compounds with anticonvulsant activity attributable to metabolites.

Compounds are divided into four categories on the basis of the data from phase I testing: (1) anticonvulsant activity at 100 mg/kg or less, (2) anticonvulsant activity at 300 mg/kg, (3) no anticonvulsant activity at all or activity only at 600 mg/kg, and (4) anticonvulsant activity and neurotoxicity at 30 mg/kg. Compounds in category 1 are usually advanced to phase II testing immediately, and compounds in category 4 are generally retested at doses of less than 30 mg/kg. Category 2 compounds may or may not undergo further evaluation, and compounds in category 3 are dropped from further consideration.

II. Phase II

Phase II quantitates the anticonvulsant activity and neurotoxicity of the compounds in mice, and determines the time of peak anticonvulsant and toxic effect. An estimated median effective dose (ED_{50}) or median toxic dose (TD_{50}) is administered intraperitoneally to four groups of four mice each, and the animals are tested by the MES or scMet test and the rotorod test at 30 min, and 1, 2, and 4 h, or until peak activity or toxicity has obviously passed. All further tests are then performed at the time of peak effect. The TD_{50} and ED_{50} are determined by establishing at least four dose levels between 0% and 100% minimal neurotoxicity or anticonvulsant effectiveness. Probit analysis of the data provides the 95% confidence intervals of the ED_{50} and TD_{50} and the slopes of regression lines (with standard errors). Data from phase II are essential to a critical evaluation of structure-activity relationships, as well as anticonvulsant activity and neurotoxicity.

III. Phase III

Phase III, the toxicity profile in mice, is established by a modification of the procedure of IRWIN (1968) and a determination of the median hypnotic dose (HD_{50}) and the median lethal dose (LD_{50}). The toxicity profile is determined by the intraperitoneal administration of the TD_{50}, twice the TD_{50}, and four times the TD_{50} to two mice at each dose level. The mice are then observed and tested at 10, 20, and 30 min and 1, 2, 4, 6, 8, and 24 h after drug administration for the onset, intensity, and nature of overt toxicity. The assessment considers approximately 40 signs and symptoms, including alterations in motor activity, overt central nervous system effects, respiratory changes, and various peripheral manifestations. These observations provide preliminary but essential pharmacological information about the effects of the test compounds on the central and autonomic nervous systems.

IV. Phase IV

Phase IV, quantitation of anticonvulsant activity in mice, provides the same kind of information as phase II, except that the compounds are administered orally. Data from this phase are important because they help define the absorption and metabolic characteristics of the agents. In some cases, anticonvulsant activity is greater after oral administration than after intraperitoneal injection, whereas in other cases activity is decreased or lost after oral administration. Moreover, if metabolic considerations are important (for example, first-pass metabolism), then structure modifications that change metabolic profile can be considered. If absorption factors are important, water-soluble pro-drugs can be made.

V. Phase V

Phase V delineates the antiepileptic potential of the compounds in mice. Selective chemical convulsants are administered subcutaneously to help elucidate differences in the mechanisms of action of the compounds. Strychnine, picrotoxin, and bicuculline are used, in addition to pentylenetetrazol, because they each induce seizures by different mechanisms (WOODBURY 1980). Strychnine (scStr) induces generalized tonic-clonic seizures by blocking postsynaptic inhibition mediated by the inhibitory transmitter glycine in the spinal cord. Picrotoxin (scPic) produces seizures by blocking gamma-aminobutyric acid (GABA) at a presynaptic inhibitory site. Bicuculline (scBic) blocks GABA receptors at the postsynaptic inhibitory terminals. The mechanism of pentylenetetrazol-induced threshold seizures (scMet) is still unkown, but it is believed to stimulate neuronal membranes directly.

Table 1. Anticonvulsant screening project: quantitation of anticonvulsant activity and neurotoxicity of most antiepileptic drugs marketed in the United States

Drug	Mice, i.p.								Mice, p.o.			Rats, p.o.		
	Phase III		Phase V			Phase II			Phase IV			Phase VI		
	Right-ing reflex	Le-thality test	scBic	scPic	scStr	MES	scMet	Tox	MES	scMet	Tox	MES	scMet	Tox
Phenytoin	178.3 (12)	229.6 (24)	NE (2)	NE (2)	Max. prot. 50% at 55–110 mg/kg (2)	9.5 (2)	NE	65.5 (2)	9.0 (2)	NE	86.7 (2)	29.8 (4)	NE	>3,000 (0.5)
Mephenytoin	406.0 (1)	568.0 (24)	124.1 (0.5)	101.0 (0.5)	Max. prot. 50% at 70–150 mg/kg (0.5)	60.5 (0.5)	30.5 (0.5)	153.8 (0.25)	65.9 (2)	36.3 (0.5)	353.9 (4)	18.1 (2)	21.7 (4)	85.7 (4)
Phenobarbital	135.5 (1)	264.7 (24)	37.7 (0.75)	27.5 (0.75)	95.3 (0.75)	21.8 (1)	13.2 (1)	69.0 (0.5)	20.1 (2)	12.6 (2)	96.8 (2)	9.1 (5)	11.6 (5)	61.1 (0.5)
Primidone	720.7 (48)	734.9 (48)	148.1 (3)	341.7 (3)	NE (3)	11.4 (3)	58.6 (3)	679.7 (24)	26.9 (6)	28.2 (6)	484.6 (24)	6.2 (6)	15.4 (6)	233.9 (6)
Trimethadione	1,689.2 (1)	2,511.8 (24)	532.1 (0.75)	408.1 (0.75)	Max. prot. 37% at 500–1,500 mg/kg (0.75)	627.5 (1)	300.5 (1)	819.1 (0.5)	1,012.5 (1)	233.7 (0.5)	1,326.9 (1)	1,278.4 (2)	108.9 (2)	390.5 (0.5)
Ethosuximide	850.6 (0.5)	1,752.2 (24)	459.0 (0.5)	242.7 (0.5)	Max. prot. 62% at 250–1,000 mg/kg (0.5)	>1,000 (0.5)	130.4 (0.5)	440.8 (0.5)	>2,000 (0.5)	192.2 (0.5)	879.2 (1)	>1,200 (2)	54.0 (2)	1,012.3 (2)
Methsuximide	376.8 (0.5)	789.6 (24)	127.4 (0.5)	210.8 (0.5)	Max. prot. 62.5% at 250 mg/kg (0.5)	76.3 (0.5)	68.3 (0.5)	187.6 (0.5)	163.4 (2)	130.2 (2)	511.2 (1)	45.7 (4)	25.3 (4)	59.8 (4)

Diazepam (adjunct only)	206.7 (0.5)	882.0 (24)	1.2 (0.5)	1.2 (0.5)	13.0 (0.5)	19.1 (0.5)	0.17 (0.5)	7.3 (0.25)	51.3 (0.5)	0.31 (0.5)	24.3 (0.5)	214.8 (1)	1.3 (1)	14.8 (1)
Clonazepam	> 6,000 (0.5)	> 6,000 (24)	0.009 (0.5)	0.04 (0.5)	NE (0.5)	86.6 (0.5)	0.02 (0.5)	0.18 (0.5)	78.4 (0.5)	0.06 (0.5)	3.4 (0.5)	186.0 (1)	0.06 (1)	71.6 (0.5)
Carbamazepine	172.2 (0.25)	628.7 (24)	Max. prot. 50% at 100 mg/kg(0.25)	37.2 (0.25)	78.8 (0.25)	8.8 (0.25)	NE (0.25)	71.6 (0.25)	15.4 (0.5)	48.1 (0.5)	217.2 (0.5)	8.5 (1)	NE	813.1 (2)
Valproic acid	885.5 (0.25)	1,104.6 (24)	360.0 (0.25)	387.2 (0.25)	293.0 (0.25)	271.7 (0.25)	148.6 (0.25)	425.8 (0.25)	664.8 (1)	388.3 (1)	1,264.4 (2)	489.5 (0.5)	179.6 (0.5)	280.3 (1)

i.p., intraperitoneal; p.o., oral; NE, not effective.
Values for righting reflex test are expressed as HD_{50} in mg/kg, those for lethality test as LD_{50} in mg/kg, those for tests of anticonvulsant activity (scBic, scPic, scStr, MES, scMet) as ED_{50} in mg/kg, and those for tests of neurotoxicity (Tox) as TD_{50} in mg/kg.
Numbers in parentheses give the time between drug administration and observation in hours

VI. Phase VI

Phase VI, quantitation of anticonvulsant activity in rats, verifies the anticonvulsant activity and neurotoxicity in another rodent species. More importantly, it provides essential information for determining whether the accumulated experimental data justify costly pharmacokinetic and long-term toxicity studies of the compounds. After oral administration, anticonvulsant activity is determined again by the MES and scMet tests. Instead of the rotorod test, however, the positional sense, gait, stance, and muscle tone tests are used to determine neurotoxicity. Generally, compounds found active in mice are active in rats, and differ only in the therapeutic or protective indices. Information obtained in this phase and in phase VII is important in choosing the oral doses for the 90-day toxicity studies in rats.

VII. Phase VII

Phase VII determines the minimal lethal dose (LD_3) and the effect of repeated administration on anticonvulsant activity of the compounds. The LD_3 is determined by orally administering the compound (estimated LD_3) to two groups of rats (one male group and one female group) for 5 days, and recording the body weight and number of deaths daily for 5 days thereafter. Tolerance to the anticonvulsant effect is determined by administering the compound (ED_{50}) to one group of male rats for 5 consecutive days; a second group of male rats receives only the requisite volume of solvent for the 5 days, and a third group receives only the requisite volume of solvent for 4 days and then a single dose of the compound (ED_{50}) on day 5.

C. Toxicity/Selected Pharmacology Project

For compounds that show outstanding activity in all seven phases of the Anticonvulsant Screening Project, pharmaceutical firms are urged to make a commitment to toxicological and pharmacological tests in collaboration with the Toxicity/Selected Pharmacology Project of the ADD Program, and academic suppliers are assisted in finding sponsors from the pharmaceutical industry. This project identifies potential sites of toxicity prior to clinical trials of the compounds. It includes 14- to 28-day studies to determine dose range and 90-day studies of toxicity after oral administration to rats and dogs. If the data from these studies warrant use of the drug in humans, the sponsor may file a Claimed Notice of Investigational Exemption for a New Drug (IND) with the Food and Drug Administration.

D. Primate Model of Epilepsy

Another important segment of the ADD Program is evaluation of the compounds in the primate model of epilepsy. This model of partial seizures in *Macaca mulatta* provides an advanced, specialized means of determining the efficacy and dose-related toxic side effects of investigational anticonvulsant drugs (LOCKARD 1980). This model has been standardized and developed with the integration of pharmacokinetic data so that important metabolic questions may also be answered.

E. Controlled Clinical Trials

Compounds judged in the foregoing antiepileptic drug development process to have potential clinical application will be considered for controlled clinical trials sponsored by the Epilepsy Branch. This group has been central in developing methodology and designs for controlled clinical trials, in identifying appropriate patient populations, and in monitoring and analyzing data accumulated during these trials. Controlled clinical trials, the ultimate segment of the ADD Program, continue to be the keystone to the evaluation and approval of new antiepileptic drugs in the United States.

References

Dunham NW, Miya TS (1957) A note on a simple apparatus for detecting neurological deficit in rats and mice. J Am Pharm Assoc 46:208–209

Irwin S (1968) Comprehensive observational assessment: a systematic, quantitative procedure for assessing the behavioral and physiological state of the mouse. Psychopharmacology (Berlin) 13:222–257

Lockard JS (1980) A primate model of clinical epilepsy: mechanism of action through quantification of the therapeutic effects. In: Lockard JS, Ward AA (eds) Epilepsy: a window to brain mechanisms. Raven, New York, pp 11–49

Swinyard EA (1972) Assay of antiepileptic drug activity in experimental animals: standard tests. In: Mercier J (ed) Anticonvulsant drugs. International encyclopedia of pharmacology and therapeutics. Pergamon, Oxford, pp 47–65

Swinyard EA, Brown WC, Goodman LS (1952) Comparative assays of antiepileptic drugs in mice and rats. J Pharmacol Exp Ther 106:319–330

Woodbury DM (1980) Convulsant drugs: mechanisms of action. In: Glaser GH, Penry JK, Woodbury DM (eds) Antiepileptic drugs: mechanisms of action. Raven, New York, pp 249–303

Specific Pharmacology of Antiepileptic Drugs

CHAPTER 13

Hydantoins

G. L. JONES and G. H. WIMBISH

A. Introduction

Selective antiepileptic therapy with organic compounds began in 1912 when Hauptmann (1912) reported on the clinical efficacy of phenobarbital. Prior to this the only effective drug therapy for epilepsy involved the bromide ion, introduced clinically in 1857 (LOCOCK 1857). Although modestly successful in the treatment of generalized tonic-clonic (GTC, grand mal) seizures, the bromide ion proved to be highly toxic at therapeutic concentrations. Phenobarbital, on the other hand, afforded a relatively low-risk modality of treatment, and proved to be effective against GTC seizures, as well as some of the partial (focal) seizures (e.g., Jacksonian). However, further significant advances were not realized until a quarter century later when MERRITT and PUTNAM (1938a, b) reported on the efficacy of phenytoin (5,5,-diphenylhydantoin) in GTC seizures.

Phenytoin was first synthesized in 1908 (BILTZ 1908), but pharmacological studies with the compound were not reported until 3 decades later. Preliminary screening for hypnotic action was conducted by Parke-Davis Laboratories (GRUHZIT 1939), and MERRITT and PUTNAM (1938a) subsequently tested its efficacy against electroshock-induced convulsions in cats. In the same year, MERRITT and PUTNAM (1938b) reported on its anticonvulsant efficacy in man. Because it proved to be highly effective in humans and lacked sedative properties in normal doses, phenytoin received immediate acceptance in therapeutics.

The introduction of phenytoin was of value for several reasons unrelated to its immediate therapeutic application. It provided the first evidence of the selective nature of antiepileptic therapy. Phenytoin was somewhat effective in the treatment of complex partial seizures (e.g., psychomotor epilepsy) as well as elementary partial and GTC seizures; phenobarbital was notably ineffective against the former. Furthermore, because it is not a sedative, phenytoin was also responsible for the recognition that sedation is not a requisite for anticonvulsant action. Thus, the hydantoins represent the second chemical class of organic compounds to find applicability in the treatment of epilepsy. Phenobarbital and phenytoin continue to this day as the two most useful antiepileptic agents.

Although there is much interest today in the study of novel antiepileptic compounds, the bulk of our present knowledge of antiepileptic mechanisms has derived from research with phenytoin and other hydantoins. A review of the literature through 1958 showed that there were 504 hydantoin derivatives synthesized and tested in various experimental models of epilepsy, compared with only 131 barbituric acid derivatives, 163 succinimides, and 80 substituted oxazolidinediones (CLOSE and SPIELMAN 1961). A similar review covering the period between 1958 and 1976 showed that 316 new hydantoins were tested, compared with 122 barbiturates, 145 oxazolidinediones, and 334 succinimides (VIDA and Gerry 1977). Thus, over 800 hydantoin derivatives were synthesized and tested as of 1976, compared with 497 succinimide derivatives, 253 barbiturates, and 225 oxazolidinediones.

Despite the very large number of hydantoin derivatives evaluated for anticonvulsant potency in laboratory animals, only three are in common use throughout the world today. These include phenytoin, mephenytoin (3-methyl-5-ethyl-5-phenylhydantoin), and ethotoin (3-ethyl-5-phenylhydantoin). Mephenytoin, introduced as an antiepileptic in 1945 (CLEIN 1945; LOSCALZO 1945), has a spectrum of activity similar to that of phenytoin. Although it might prove dramatically superior to phenytoin in selected cases of refractory epilepsy, serious toxicity is much more common than with phenytoin. The N-demethylated product of mephenytoin metabolism, Nirvanol, was employed clinically in the 1920s, but was abandoned because of a high incidence of serious toxicity. Ethotoin was introduced as an antiepileptic by SCHWADE et al. (1956). However, the apparent low efficacy and pharmacokinetic limitations of this drug have relegated its role to that of adjunctive status in the treatment of GTC seizures. A very limited number of additional hydantoins, or hydantoin-like derivatives, have found restricted use in a few countries. However, phenytoin is without question the most important of the hydantoin derivatives, both in terms of its therapeutic value und its heuristic value in the study of antiepileptic mechanisms. Therefore, emphasis will be given in this chapter to the experimental pharmacology of phenytoin; the other hydantoins will be discused where their properties differ significantly from those of phenytoin and where such properties are useful to an understanding of antiepileptic mechanisms.

B. Chemistry

I. Physicochemical Properties

Phenytoin is a weak organic acid (molecular weight 252.26; melting point 295°–298 °C). Its pK_a is not known with certainty, as estimates have varied between 8.06 (SCHWARTZ et al. 1977) and 9.2 (DILL et al. 1956). However, the most reliable estimate is probably that given by AGARWAL and BLAKE (1968), who reported an apparent pK_a of 8.31 based upon spectrophotometric titration in alcohol-water solution. This apparent pK_a value is for the dissociable hydrogen at the imide (N3) position of the hydantoin ring (Fig. 1 b). The hydrogen at the amide (N1) position is much less acidic. Because of alkyl substitution, mephenytoin and ethotoin lack a dissociably hydrogen at the N3 position in their structures. The molecular weights of mephenytoin and ethotoin are 218.25 and 204.22, respectively.

Phenytoin as the free acid is very poorly soluble in water, but it will dissolve readily in alkali and many organic solvents. Salt formation occurs by lactam-lactim tautomerism involving the imidic hydrogen at the N3 position. Although the amide (N1) hydrogen is much less acidic than the imidic hydrogen, it might also undergo lactam-lactim tautomerism under certain conditions (VIDA and GERRY 1977). The aqueous solubility of phenytoin at pH 7.5 is 21.9 μg/ml (at 25 °C), which just exceeds the usual therapeutic plasma concentrations. However, the apparent solubility in plasma is much greater (75 μg/ml at 37 °C), due to significant binding to plasma protein (GLAZKO 1972b).

The poor aqueous solubility of phenytoin is due largely to the hydrophobicity of the diphenyl moiety at the hydantoin C5 position. Hydrophobicity (or lipophilicity) estimates for phenytoin have been reported as the log of the partition coefficient (log P) measured in various two-phase systems. The log P value for the free acid in a standard octanol-water system has been reported as 2.47 (HANSCH and LEO 1979). A similar value (2.40) was reported for octanol equilibrated with aqueous buffer at pH 6.0 (LEPETIT 1977). At pH 10.49 the value in the octanol-buffer system was 0.14 (LEPETIT 1977). Lower values of log P were reported when mineral oils were used as the nonaqueous phase: 0.96 for an oil: water system (VEREBELY et al. 1970) and 0.83 for an oil: buffer system, pH 7.5 (OLDENDORF 1974). The partition of phenytoin between synaptosomal membranes and pH-10.49 buffer has been reported as 1.75 (SEEMAN et al. 1972). Experimental log P values have not been reported for mephenytoin or ethotoin. However, if the experimental log P value for hydantoin (−1.69; octanol: water system) is added to the lipophilicity constants (π) for the respective substituents, it is possible to estimate a relative order of lipophilicity for ethotoin, mephenytoin, and phenytoin (HANSCH and LEO 1979). Using π constants 2.13, 1.02, and 0.56 for phenyl, ethyl, and methyl substituents, respectively, the order of increasing lipophilicity is ethotoin ($\log P_{calc}=1.46$), mephenytoin ($\log P_{calc}=2.02$), and phenytoin ($\log P_{calc}=2.57$). The calculated log P of phenytoin is very close to the experimental value (2.47).

Little is known about the electronic structure of phenytoin and related hydantoins. One author (G. JONES) has performed iterative extended Huckel calculations (REIN et al. 1966) on phenytoin and ethotoin, and several non-hydantoin derivatives (unpublished data). The net atomic charges at each of the heavy atoms in phenytoin and ethotoin are depicted in Fig. 2. The relationships among the atoms in each molecule approximate what one would expect from chemical intuition, the more electronegative atoms carrying a greater negative charge. The influence of inductive effects can also be rationalized in terms of the depicted net charges.

II. Structure-Activity Relationships

An understanding of the qualitative structure-activity relationships (SARs) of anticonvulsants began to emerge several decades ago (GOODMAN et al. 1949; PUTNAM and MERRITT 1941). These relationships have been documented more recently in monographs by CLOSE and SPIELMAN (1961) and VIDA and GERRY (1977). One of the most serious limitations of these SAR data is that they were not obtained by application of uniform experimental models of epilepsy. Furthermore, the data were often reported simply as "active" or "inactive"; quantitative data amenable to parametric statistical analysis were often lacking. However, in recent reports KRALL et al. (1978a, b) have described a uniform approach to antiepilep-

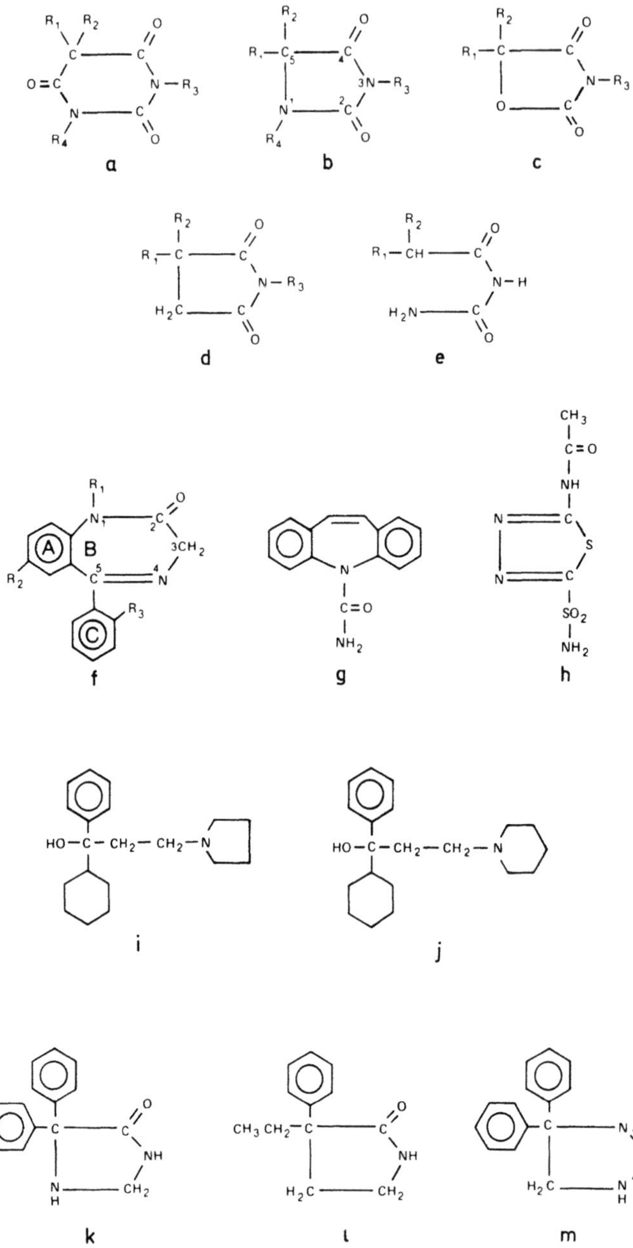

Fig. 1. Structures (*a–h*) are variety of substituted compounds found at one time to be clinically useful. (*a*), barbituric acid derivatives such as phenobarbital (R_1 = phenyl, R_2 = ethyl, R_3 = R_4 = hydrogen); (*b*), hydantoins such as phenytoin (R_1 = R_2 = phenyl, R_3 = R_4 = hydrogen); (*c*), oxazolidinediones such as trimethadione (R_1 = R_2 = R_3 = methyl); (*d*), succinimides such as ethosuximide (R_1 = ethyl, R_2 = methyl, R_3 = hydrogen); (*e*), acetylureas such as phenacemide (R_1 = phenyl, R_2 = hydrogen); (*f*), benzodiazepines such as diazepam (R_1 = methyl, R_2 = chlorine, R_3 = hydrogen); (*g*), tricyclic carboxamides such as carbamazepine; (*h*), sulfonamides such as acetazolamide. Structures (*f–h*) bear a less obvious

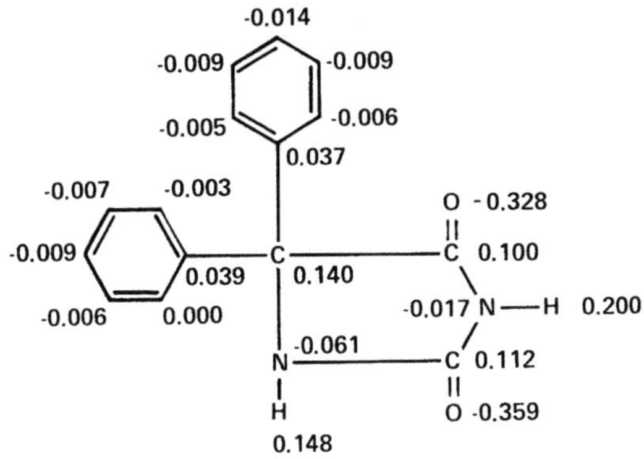

Phenytoin

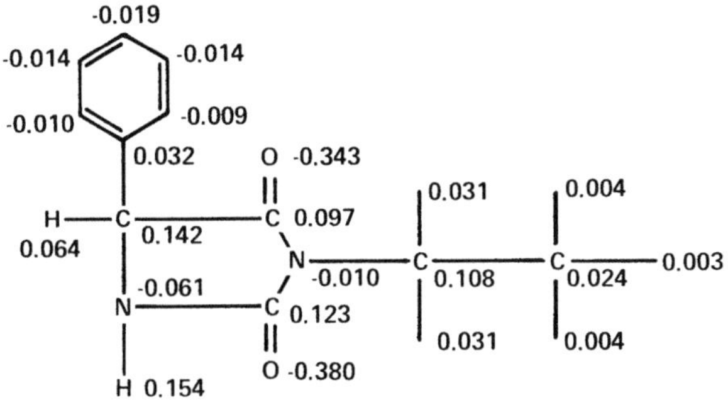

Ethotoin

Fig. 2. Net atomic charges at heavy atoms, calculated for phenytoin and ethotoin using iterative extended Huckel theory

tic drug development which will likely make future SAR data more amenable to study.

For the purposes of illustrating SARs, anticonvulsant activity will be defined only with respect to the maximal electroshock (MES) model of GTC seizures (Toman et al. 1946; Swinyard 1972) and the subcutaneous Metrazol (pentylenetetrazol) model of absence seizures (Swinyard et al. 1952; Woodbury 1972). The MES test represents the most thoroughly documented experimental model of GTC epilepsy, while drugs that are effective in the subcutaneous Metrazol (scMet) test are very often effective against the absence seizure in man (Woodbury 1972). Experimental models selective for partial seizures have not been ad-

structural similarity among themselves than do structures (*a–e*), and substituent effects on selectivity are different. Structures (*i–m*) have not been found clinically useful, but are active in various experimental models of epilepsy. Procyclidine (*i*) and trihexyphenidyl (*j*) lack obvious structural similarities to structures (*a–h*). Structures (*k–m*) possess greater structural similarity to structures (*a–e*), but the composition of the heterocyclic ring differs. See the text for discussion equately documented (Sect. C.I.2), nor do reliable in vitro models of epilepsy exist.

With reference to hydantoin derivatives (Fig. 1 b), at least one phenyl or similar aromatic group is required at R_1 or R_2 for optimal activity against MES-induced seizures. Alternatively, alkyl substitution (at R_1 or R_2) imparts efficacy against scMet-induced seizures. Alkyl substitution elsewhere on the molecule can attenuate to some degree the selective influence of aromatic or alkyl groups at R_1 or R_2. (The foregoing discussion pertains specifically to hydantoin derivatives, but most of the stated relationships also apply to other so-called "traditional" anticonvulsant structures, i.e., the oxazolidinediones, succinimides, barbiturates, and acetylureas. See Fig. 1 a–e.)

Maximal MES activity is achieved when there are two phenyl groups at the tetrahedryl (C5) carbon (phenytoin), although significant activity is retained with just one phenyl group at this position (5-phenylhydantoin). Replacement of one phenyl group in phenytoin with a methyl, ethyl, or thienyl group results in a variable decrease in MES activity, and in some cases an increase in scMet activity. Replacement of both phenyl groups in phenytoin by benzyl groups destroys both MES and scMet activity. Complete loss of MES activity also occurs when both phenyl groups are replaced by alkyl groups; an exception is that replacement by two isobutyl groups will decrease, but not abolish MES activity. Any substitution on the phenyl groups will also decrease activity. Alkyl groups at the C5 position impart scMet activity.

Introduction of a third phenyl group at the N3 nitrogen of phenytoin abolished activity. On the other hand, methylation at this position simply reduces MES activity. The introduction of *n*-butoxymethyl or benzyloxymethyl groups at N3 will decrease the MES activity slightly while increasing scMet activity.

Replacement of a phenyl group of phenytoin by an ethyl group, with the introduction of a methyl group at the N3 nitrogen (mephenytoin), confers significant scMet activity without decreasing MES activity. The introduction of a second methyl group at the N1 nitrogen of mephenytoin does not affect scMet activity, but decreases MES activity.

A more comprehensive appreciation of anticonvulsant SAR began to unfold as a result of the Camerman's X-ray crystallography studies, which have revealed conformational and other similarities among phenytoin (CAMERMAN and CAMERMAN 1971 a), diazepam (CAMERMAN and CAMERMAN 1972 a), procyclidine (CAMERMAN and CAMERMAN 1971 b), trihexyphenidyl (CAMERMAN and CAMERMAN 1972 b), and phenacemide and ethyphenacemide (CAMERMAN and CAMERMAN 1977). They found that all of these drugs possess hydrophobic regions and electron-donor groups with similar stereochemical features. For example, the two phenyl rings of phenytoin share a similar mutual orientation in space with the phenyl and chlorophenyl rings in diazepam, and with the phenyl-cyclohexyl moiety in procyclidine and trihexyphenidyl. When these hydrophobic groups were approximately superimposed, it was found that two electron-donor functions (either oxygen or nitrogen) also occupy similar positions and orientations in space. This was true even for the open-chained acetylureas (phenacemide and ethylphenacemide) because the acetylurea moiety folds back on itself to form a six-atom "ring" stabilized by hydrogen bonding. Such relationships can be clarified by reference to Fig. 1 a–j.

These observations led the Camermans to propose that stereochemical properties form the basis of selective anticonvulsant action, and that anticonvulsant potential in new compounds might be predictable from this knowledge (CAMERMAN and CAMERMAN 1980). A quantitative measure of the stereochemical similarities among these drugs was provided as the interatomic distance between electron donor atoms, and the distance between these atoms and the hydrophobic groups. For example, the two electronegative atoms in phenytoin thought best to approximate the optimal configuration for anticonvulsant action are the two carbonyl oxygens. The distance between these atoms is 4.56 Å. The respective atoms in diazepam (those that best approximate the carbonyl oxygens in phenytoin when the phenyl groups of the two molecules are superimposed) are the carbonyl oxygen and the trigonal nitrogen at the 4-position of the azepine ring. Their interatomic distance is 3.35 Å. Based upon a comparision of these distances with the respective interatomic distances for a variety of benzodiazepine (CAMERMAN and CAMERMAN 1980) and sulfonamide compounds (CAMERMAN and CAMERMAN 1975), the Camermans proposed that a critical lower limit (approximately 2.4 Å) must be exceeded before a particular compound will possess significant anticonvulsant activity (CAMERMAN and CAMERMAN 1980).

However, a simple quantitative relationship between interatomic distance and activity cannot be demonstrated. For example, drugs which are totally ineffective against scMet seizures have interatomic distances that include the extremes (i.e., trihexyphenidyl, 2.76 Å; procyclidine, 3.55 Å; phenytoin, 4.56 Å). Also, an 8.8-fold difference in scMet potency (comparing phenacemide and phenobarbital) can be compared with only a very modest difference in interatomic distance (4.13 Å vs 4.51 Å). The interatomic distances also fail to correlate with MES potency. The correlation coefficients (r) are only 0.29 in either comparison (scMet or MES).

These findings are not remarkable considering the diversity of potent anticonvulsants that clearly do not conform to the structural prescription discussed above. Doxenitoin, for example, is a phenytoin-like structure, the only difference being reduction of the carbonyl at the 2-position to a methylene group (Fig. 1 k). Yet this drug retains significant anticonvulsant potency when evaluated by the MES test (GOODMAN et al. 1954). It is possible that the nitrogen in the 1-position suffices as the second electron donor in the absence of the carbonyl oxygen; the distance between N1 and the remaining carbonyl oxygen is 3.5 Å (an estimate taken from Drieding stereomodels) compared with 4.56 Å between the two oxygens in phenytoin. The distance between the N3 nitrogen and the single oxygen in doxenitoin (approximately 2.3 Å, estimated) would not satisfy the critical distance defined in the above formulation. However, a reasonably potent 2-pyrrolidinone has been described which is in essence a hydantoin with the N1 nitrogen and the C2 carbonyl replaced by methylene groups (MARSHALL 1958) (Fig. 1 l). This compound, 3-ethyl-3-phenyl-2-pyrrolidinone, has two relatively electronegative atoms, but their separation is estimated to be only about 2.3 Å. Furthermore, an imidazole derivative, 4,4,-diphenylimidazolidine, is an effective anticonvulsant even though it is totally without oxygen (GOODMAN 1956) (Fig. 1 m).

Thus, the possibility exists that two nitrogens (approximately 2.2 Å apart) suffice as the requisite electron donors even though they are separated by less than the critical distance already discussed. These observations support a less rigorous hypothesis of anti-GTC activity: simply two electron donors are required in some proximity to a bulky hydrophobic group. For activity in the scMet model two electron donors would again be required, but in proximity to a smaller, less hydrophobic moiety. Although it is possible to cite exceptions even to the "two electron-donor" requirement (BRODIE et al. 1958), it is not clear that these exceptions represent drugs with "selective" anticonvulsant action (as opposed to general CNS depression).

III. Analytical Methods

Recent advances in microprocessor-based instrumentation, combined with the fundamental principles of analytical chemistry, have provided accurate and precise methods for the determination of hydantoins in biological specimens. The analytical methods currently available for the analysis of hydantoins are briefly described below.

1. Thin-Layer Chromatography

Although the primary use of thin-layer chromatography (TLC) has been for qualitative analysis (screening), recent advances in high-performance TLC (HPTLC) have permitted the quantitative analysis of several anticonvulsants, including phenytoin (DAVIS and FENIMORE 1981; FENIMORE and DAVIS 1978). These procedures require about 50 μl plasma. The drug is extracted into ethyl acetate, and the residue spotted (with standards) on an HPTLC plate. The developing solvent includes chloroform, isopropanol, and ammonium hydroxide (80:20:1). The use of HPTLC is a relatively new approach to quantitative analysis, and is not presently in wide use. HPTLC has some advantages in its ability to provide rapid analysis of multiple samples for direct comparison. However, the instrumentation required to adapt the procedure for quantitation approaches that of some of the methods described below, and the simplicity of the procedure is thereby lost. The scanning step alone approaches the elution time of other chromatographic methods; thus the time gained by the simultaneous development of many samples is lost.

2. Gas-Liquid Chromatography

A thorough treatment of the application of gas-liquid chromatography (GLC) to antiepileptic drug assay is provided in a book edited by PIPPENGER et al. (1978). GLC permits analysis not only of the parent compound, but also of major metabolites, which allows one to look at the metabolic profile of an individual by determining the ratio of parent compound to metabolites. The ability to select specialized columns and specific detectors to enhance sensitivity makes GLC one of the most powerful techniques available for drug and metabolite analysis. Sensitivity is normally in the microgram to picogram range.

In order for a drug to be analyzed by GLC it must be heat stable (50–300 °C), have a significant vapor pressure at these temperatures, and be extractable from the biological specimen. As with other chromatographic procedures, hydantoins are first extracted from their biological matrix with an organic solvent such as chloroform or toluene. The solvent is then evaporated and the residue analyzed by injection onto an appropriate column. Columns frequently used for hydantoins include 3% OV-17 on Gas Chrome Q; 3% SP2250 on Gas Chrome Q, or a special deactivated column of 2% SP2210 plus 1% SP2520DA on 100/120 mesh Supelcoport (Supelco, Inc.). The latter column allows the hydantoin to be analyzed without derivatization. However, the chromatographic properties of phenytoin are greatly improved by derivatization to an *N*-alkyl analogue (GREELEY 1974). Detection is most commonly by flame ionization, which has adequate sensitivity for the assay of hydantoins. If a more specifc or sensitive detector is required, the nitrogen-phosphorus detector (NPD) and the electron capture (EC) detector have particular advantages. The NPD detector allows selective detection of nitrogen atoms in the hydantoin molecule and is relatively insensitive to coextracted hydrocarbons. EC detection greatly increases the sensitivity and reduces the amount of sample required, but derivatization of the hydantoin to a corresponding halogenated analogue is required.

3. High-Pressure Liquid Chromatography

HPLC is an excellent alternative to GLC for compounds that lack volatility or thermal stability. In addition, both mobile and stationary phases usually affect separation, whereas in GLC only the stationary phase contributes to the separation. HPLC requires only that the analyte be soluble in the mobile phase, and detectable. Advances in bonded phases and detector systems (including ultraviolet, fluorescent, and electrochemical detection) have expedited the application of HPLC in therapeutic drug monitoring. A thorough discussion of the analysis of phenytoin and other antiepileptics was provided by HAWK and FRANCONI (1978). Although sample extraction is required, HPLC is similar to GLC in that it allows for the use of an internal standard. Columns frequently used for hydantoins include modified silica gel C-8 or C-18, for reverse-phase chromatography. The mobile phase usually consists of acetonitrile, methanol, and phosphate buffer ($1.5 \times 10^{-4} M$) in the volume ratio 210:120:670.

4. Immunoassay

The immunochemical techniques developed for anticonvulsant analysis include radioimmunoassay, homogenous enzyme immunoassay, nephelometric analysis, and fluorescence polarization immunoassay. Generally, these techniques are based on competitive binding between an unlabeled drug (analyte) and a labeled drug (tracer) for antibody raised against the analyte. In the presence of analyte (from specimen or standard), competition for antibody-binding sites results in an increase in free (unbound) tracer in proportion to the concentration of analyte. The procedures differ, however, in the method of relating drug concentration to that of the unbound tracer.

In the radioimmunoassay (RIA) the analyte is made radioactive (usually ^{125}I), so that it is only necessary to measure the radioactivity of either the free or the bound tracer. However, since both free and bond tracer are radioactive, it becomes very important to employ methods that achieve complete separation of these two entities. The double antibody method employed a second antibody that precipitates the soluble radioligand-antibody complex formed initially. Separation has also been achieved by the precipitation of antibody complex with salts or organic solvents, by solid-phase techniques, and by methods designed to absorb the free ligand to various substances. The application of RIA to the assay of phenytoin has been described in several recent publications (COOK et al. 1976, 1973; SPIEHLER et al. 1976).

The homogenous enzyme assay systems include the enzyme multiplied immunoassay technique (EMIT^R) and the substrate-labeled fluorescent immunoassay (SLFIA). Neither of these methods requires extraction or separation of the drugs from its plasma matrix. EMIT^R measures the rate of an enzyme reaction which is proportional to the concentration of drug in the specimen. The tracer is a complex formed between the analyte and the enzyme glucose-6-phosphate dehydrogenase, which is active only when it is not bound by antibody against the analyte. In the unbound state, the tracer catalyzes the oxidation of glucose-6-phosphate to 6-phosphoglucose-γ-lactone, with the accompanying reduction of NAD^+ to NADH. The rate of increase of NADH is measured spectrophotometrically at 340 nm. Thorough discussions of the application of EMIT^R to phenytoin and other antiepileptics have been provided by SCHOTTELIUS (1978) and others (PIPPENGER et al. 1975).

Substrate-labeled fluorescent immunoassay (Miles Laboratories) also employs the principle of competitive protein binding, but the competition in this case is between the drug (from specimen or standard) and an enzyme substrate-labeled drug for binding sites on a specific antibody. The substrate-drug complex formed with umbelliferyl-β-D-galactoside, is referred to as GUD. While GUD itself is nonfluorescent, reaction of unbound GUD with the enzyme β-galactosidase produces a fluorescent complex. In the absence of unlabeled drug (in specimen or standard), GUD binds to the drug-specific antibody and cannot be hydrolyzed by the enzyme to a fluorescent product. In the assay, unlabeled drug is allowed to compete with GUD for antibody-binding sites. The fluorescence produced is proportional to the amount of drug in the specimen (or standard). At present, this procedure is based on equilibrium rather than kinetic measurements, thus simplifying instrumentation.

The nephelometric inhibition immunoassay (NIIA) is designed to measure the change in light scattering due to a change in particle size during an antigen-antibody reaction. Both equilibrium (GAULDIE and BIENENSTOCK 1978) and rate (ANDERSON and STERNBERG 1978) NIIAs have been described. The analyte of interest is first linked to a carrier protein, and the resulting conjugate is used to raise an antibody. The analyte is then linked to an unrelated carrier protein, and the new conjugate allowed to react with a limited amount of antibody. The soluble immune complexes that form will scatter light, and the inhibition of light scattering by unbound analyte serves as a basis for its quantitation by NIIA. Specific assays for phenytoin have been developed for both equilibrium (NISHIKAWA et al. 1979) and rate (BECKMAN INSTRUMENTS, FULLERTON, CA) NIIAs. The sensitivity of the rate NIIA for phenytoin is about 2 µg/ml. Rate NIIA has the advantage of rapid analysis, but greater control over assay variables (especially the ratio of developer antigen to antibody) is often required. Other advantages include those common to all homogeneous immunoassays, and relate to the lack of an extraction requirement.

The most recent example of microcomputer-based methodology is the fluorescence polarization immunoassay (FPIA). FPIA is similar in principle to the immunoassay techniques already described, except that the tracer in this case is analyte labeled with a fluorescent probe (POPELKA et al. 1981). When the tracer is bound to antibody, the fluorophore is constrained from rotating during the interval of time that light is absorbed and emitted. Therefore, when plane-polarized light is used to excite the tracer, the fluorophore is still highly polarized upon emission. However, when the tracer is free (unbound), the rotational motion of the fluorophore is much greater and the emitted light is depolarized. The greater the concentration of analyte (in specimen or standard), the larger the fraction of unbound tracer; and the concentration of analyte can be estimated from a standard curve. The advantages of FPIA include the specificity, speed, and convenience characteristic of all homogenous immunoassays (see above).

C. Anticonvulsant Activity

I. Anticonvulsant Potency in Laboratory Animals

1. Standard Experimental Models in Small Rodents

The hydantoins as a class have been extensively investigated using both the MES and scMet models of GTC and absence seizures, respectively. The methodology and interpretation of these experimental models has been reviewed previously (SWINYARD 1972; WOODBURY 1972). Anticonvulsant activities based upon these models have been evaluated in both rats and mice, and for various routes of administration. A summary of selected data is presented in Table 1 for phenytoin, mephenytoin, and ethotoin. No attempt was made to provide comprehensive documentation of the multiplicity of reported values (for phenytoin in particular). Instead, an effort was made to select data which were obtained by reasonably uniform methods. In assessing the variability among estimates, however, it is important to recognize that factors other than "model," "species," and "route of administration" might influence potency. For example, differences in the administration vehicle might produce significant variations in bioavailability. While suspensions in gum acacia or tragacanth were often employed in early studies, aqueous solvents composed of methylcellulose, polyethylene glycol, and other alcohols, or detergents have been used more recently. Another possible source of variability might be the use of different strains of mice (or rats) or the use of different sexes. Although the standardized procedure for the MES test (SWINYARD 1972) employs male CF # 1 albino mice, some of the reported studies used other strains and mixed sex groups.

The failure of some studies to adhere rigidly to standardized models might also contribute to variability. For example, ACHARI and SINHA (1967) administered 240-mA current (0.4-s duration) to rats, compared with the standard 150 mA (0.2-s duration). Thus, it is difficult to determine whether their relatively low es-

Table 1. Anticonvulsant activity of hydantoin derivatives: a comparison using standard experimental models in small rodents

Derivative	Model	ED_{50} (mg/kg)	Species	Route of administration	Refs.
Phenytoin	MES	9.6	Mouse	i.p.	SLATER et al. (1950)
	MES	8.1	Mouse (young)	i.p.	PETTY and KARLER (1965)
	MES	14	Mouse (old)	i.p.	PETTY and KARLER (1965)
	MES	8.3	Mouse	i.p.	WITIAK et al. (1972)
	MES	9.5	Mouse	i.p.	Krall et al. (1978b)
	MES	7.1	Mouse	i.p.	JONES et al. (1981)
	MES	ca. 10	Mouse	s.c.	SWINYARD et al. (1952)
	MES	9.1	Mouse	s.c.	GOODMAN et al. (1953)
	MES	11.4	Mouse	p.o.	CHEN and ENSOR (1950)
	MES	12	Mouse	p.o.	GESLER et al. (1961)
	MES	16	Mouse	p.o.	WOLF et al. (1962)
	MES	17	Mouse	p.o.	NAKAMURA et al. (1965)
	MES	12.8	Mouse	p.o.	RAINES et al. (1973)
	MES	ca. 7.5	Mouse	p.o.	VIDA et al. (1975)
	MES	23	Rat	i.p.	HARNED et al. (1953)
	MES	11.3	Rat	i.p.	SWINYARD et al. (1950)
	MES	5.0	Rat (young)	i.p.	PETTY and KARLER (1965)
	MES	5.1	Rat (old)	i.p.	PETTY and KARLER (1965)
	MES	ca. 10	Rat	s.c.	SWINYARD et al. (1952)
	MES	42	Rat	s.c.	STILLE and BRUNCKOW (1954)
	MES	24	Rat	p.o.	CHEN and ENSOR (1950)
	MES	30.0	Rat	p.o.	SWINYARD and TOMAN (1950)
	MES	18.9	Rat	p.o.	NAKAMURA et al. (1965)
	scMET	NA	Mouse	i.p.	KRALL et al. (1978b)
	scMET	NA	Mouse	p.o.	VIDA et al. (1975)
	scMET	NA	Rat	p.o.	CHEN and ENSOR (1950)
Mephenytoin	MES	60.5	Mouse	i.p.	KRALL et al. (1978b)
	MES	45	Mouse	p.o.	CHEN and ENSOR (1950)
	MES	ca. 35	Mouse	p.o.	SWINYARD et al. (1952)
	MES	37.1	Mouse	p.o.	GOODMAN et al. (1953)
	MES	30	Mouse	p.o.	SCHLOGL et al. (1961)
	MES	46	Mouse	p.o.	WOLF et al. (1962)
	MES	80	Mouse	p.o.	NAKAMURA et al. (1965)
	MES	4.5	Rat	i.p.	SWINYARD (1949)
	MES	81.0	Rat	s.c.	ACHARI and SINHA (1967)
	MES	7.1	Rat	p.o.	CHEN and ENSOR (1950)
	MES	ca. 10	Rat	p.o.	SWINYARD et al. (1952)
	MES	5.0	Rat	p.o.	NAKAMURA et al. (1965)
	scMET	30.5	Mouse	i.p.	KRALL et al. (1978b)
	scMET	ca. 55	Mouse	p.o.	SWINYARD et al. (1952)
	scMET	40	Mouse	p.o.	WOLF et al. (1962)
	scMET	54.9	Rat	i.p.	SWINYARD (1949)
	scMET	97	Rat	s.c.	ACHARI and SINHA (1967)
	scMET	ca. 105	Rat	p.o.	SWINYARD et al. (1952)
Ethotoin	MES	85.5	Mouse	i.p.	KRALL et al. (1978b)
	MES	350	Mouse	p.o.	MILLICHAP (1972)
	scMET	48	Mouse	i.p.	KRALL et al. (1978b)
	scMET	350	Mouse	p.o.	MILLICHAP (1952)

NA, not active

timate of potency (81 mg/kg) for mephenytoin in rats is due to the use of higher current, or is caused by the subcutaneous administration of this drug (Table 1). Therefore, a knowledgeable assessment of the variability among the depicted data will require the reader to consult the original reports.

In the MES test, phenytoin appears to be slightly more potent in mice than in rats (Table 1). The opposite is found with mephenytoin, which is clearly more potent in rats than in mice. Phenytoin is more potent than mephenytoin in mice, but there appears to be little overall difference in their activity in rats. However, ethotoin is clearly less potent than either phenytoin or mephenytoin, an observation that is corroborated by clinical experience in humans. There does not appear to be a substantial difference in anti-MES potency when phenytoin is administered by the intraperitoneal or subcutaneous routes, but activity is expectedly somewhat lower by the oral route. There does not appear to be a significant age-related difference in the potency of phenytoin in rats, but the situation is less clear in mice.

In sharp contrast to its activity against MES seizures, phenytoin is essentially inactive in the scMet test. Single doses of phenytoin as large as 500 mg/kg failed to prevent clonic seizures in rats administered pentylenetetrazol (93 mg/kg, s.c.) (Chen and Ensor 1950), and a similar lack of activity was noted in mice (Vida et al. 1975). Although an anti-scMet effect was noted when phenytoin was administered per os twice daily (20–30 mg/kg) to mice (or rats) for 4–7 days (Reinhard and Reinhard 1977), the ED_{50} for single doses in rats was reported to exceed 3,200 mg/kg (Swinyard and Toman 1950). Unlike phenytoin, both mephenytoin and ethotoin are active in the scMet test. This effect is undoubtedly due partly to the replacement of a phenyl group at the hydantoin C5 position (in phenytoin) with smaller, nonaromatic groups, and the presence of substitution at the hydantoin N3 position (see Sect. B.II). However, neither mephenytoin nor ethotoin are effective in absence seizures, as their anti-scMet activity alone might suggest.

2. Special Experimental Models in Small Rodents

Many experimental models of epilepsy are not yet as thoroughly documented as the MES and scMet tests. These models include the 6-Hz minimal electroshock threshold (PsM) test, the 60-Hz minimal electroshock threshold (MET) test, the hyponatremic electroshock threshold (HET) test, the maximal Metrazol seizure (MMS) model, the audiogenic seizure model, and numerous others. Several experimental models have been reported which are primarily conducted with nonrodents, and these will be discussed in Sect. C.I.3.

a) 6-Hz Minimal Electroshock Threshold

Descriptions of the 6-Hz minimal electroshock threshold (PsM) method have been reported previously (Toman 1951; Brown et al. 1953). Available evidence indicates that the PsM test correlates well with minimal neuronal discharge and with minimal spread to adjacent areas of the brain. Thus, this test was originally thought to have value in the testing of drugs potentially effective against partial (focal, including psychomotor) seizures. However, its use as a specific "psychomotor" model is invalid, as pointed out by Brown et al. (1953). These authors

Table 2. Anticonvulsant activity of hydantoin derivatives: a comparison using special experimental models in small rodents

Derivative	Model	ED_{50} (mg/kg)	Species	Route of admin-istration	Refs.
Phenytoin	PsM	NA	Mouse	p.o.	BROWN et al. (1953)
	PsM	61	Mouse	p.o.	WOLF et al. (1962)
	MET	NA	Mouse	i.p.	CARRAZ and EMIN (1967)
	MET	NA	Mouse	p.o.	BROWN et al. (1953)
	MET	NA	Rat	s.c.	SWINYARD (1949)
	HET	ca. 40	Mouse	s.c.	SWINYARD et al. (1952)
	HET	94.5	Rat	s.c.	SWINYARD (1949)
	HET	ca. 187	Rat	s.c.	SWINYARD et al. (1952)
	MMS	42.9	Mouse	s.c.	GOODMAN et al. (1953)
	MMS	23	Mouse	i.p.	NAKAMURA et al. (1965)
	Audio	5	Mouse	p.o.	FINK and SWINYARD (1959)
	Audio	35	Mouse	p.o.	FINK and SWINYARD (1959)
	Audio	13.9	Mouse	i.p.	COLLINS and HORLINGTON (1969)
Mephenytoin	PsM	ca. 265	Mouse	p.o.	BROWN et al. (1953)
	PsM	65	Mouse	p.o.	WOLF et al. (1962)
	MET	ca. 40	Mouse	p.o.	BROWN et al. (1953)
	MET	72.5	Rat	i.p.	SWINYARD (1949)
	HET	ca. 43	Mouse	p.o.	SWINYARD et al. (1952)
	HET	35.2	Rat	i.p.	SWINYARD (1949)
	HET	ca. 107	Rat	p.o.	SWINYARD et al. (1952)
	MMS	74	Mouse	p.o.	GOODMAN et al. (1953)

found no correlation between relative potency in the PsM test and a drug's clinical value in psychomotor seizures. Drugs ineffective in psychomotor epilepsy (e.g., phenobarbital) ranked higher than did phenacemide, a drug recognized to be superior to most in the treatment of this disorder.

Furthermore, phenytoin was inactive in the PsM test (Table 2), even though it is known to be of value in the treatment of psychomotor seizures in humans. In fact, phenytoin exacerbated PsM seizures (BROWN et al. 1953). However, WOLF et al. (1962) reported that phenytoin was indeed effective in the PsM test; its ED_{50} was estimated at 61 mg/kg for oral administration (Table 2). The explanation for the conflicting reports is not clear, except that BROWN et al. (1953) used a test current four times the threshold value, while WOLF et al. (1962) employed a current only twice the threshold value.

This explanation is supported by comparison of the ED_{50} values reported for mephenytoin in the two studies: 265 mg/kg (BROWN et al. 1953), and 65 mg/kg (WOLF et al. 1962). The oral route was employed in both studies (Table 2).

According to WOLF et al. (1962), the potency of phenytoin and mephenytoin were about equal (ED_{50} values 61 and 65 mg/kg, respectively). Yet, mephenytoin is recognized as the more effective of the two drugs for clinical psychomotor seizures. Thus, the use of less current (i.e., twice threshold) probably offers little if any advantage to the PsM test as a model for selective anti-psychomotor drugs. The activity of ethotoin apparently has not been evaluated in this model.

b) 60-Hz Minimal Electroshock Threshold

Descriptions of the 60-Hz minimal electroshock threshold (MET) method have been reported previously (SWINYARD 1949; BROWN et al. 1953). Although technically different, it is thought that this model provides essentially the same ranking of relative potencies as provided by the PsM test (BROWN et al. 1953). However, in comparison with the PsM (6-Hz) model, MET (60-Hz) seizures result from a more intense discharge of neurons, and are associated with greater (but still limited) spread of the discharge to other brain areas (SWINYARD 1972). Thus, the MET and PsM models are interchangeable to a degree, although one might expect the two models to yield subtle differences in relative potencies, based on different degrees of seizure spread induced by each model.

Phenytoin was reported to be inactive in the MET test in at least three different studies (BROWN et al. 1953; CARRAZ and EMIN 1967; SWINYARD 1949), involving both mice and rats (Table 2). Phenytoin actually exacerbated MET seizures, as was observed in the PsM model; see above. Because phenytoin's inactivity contrasts with its documented effectiveness in certain partial seizures, the MET seizure appears to suffer the same limitations as a model of partial epilepsy, as does the PsM model in the representation of psychomotor seizures. Although the rank order of potencies based upon the two models differs somewhat, the correlation with clinical potency is equally poor for either model. In fact, BROWN et al. (1953) suggest that the MET and PsM tests measure similar or identical anticonvulsant properties.

In contrast with phenytoin, mephenytoin was reported active in both mice and rats; the ED_{50} values were about 40 mg/kg for mice (BROWN et al. 1953) and 72.5 mg/kg for rats (SWINYARD 1949) (Table 2). Mephenytoin usually provides some benefit in the treatment of partial seizures in man, and may be tried in place of phenacemide for psychomotor epilepsy refractory to safer drugs such as phenytoin or carbamazepine. The activity of ethotoin apparently has not been evaluated in this model.

The failure of phenytoin to elevate the threshold for 60-Hz stimulation in the adult rat has been attributed to a stimulatory effect on subcortical excitatory systems. For example, excitation of the hypothalamohypophyseal system would cause the release of adrenocortical steroids, which might antagonize any effect phenytoin might have to elevate electroshock threshold (VERNADAKIS and WOODBURY 1969). To test this hypothesis, VERNADAKIS and WOODBURY (1965) studied the effect of phenytoin on MET seizures as a function of age in both rats and mice. It is known that the hypothalamohypophyseal system does not function completely until about 2 weeks after birth (JAILER 1951). Accordingly, if their hypothesis is correct, phenytoin should elevate minimal electroshock threshold during the first 2 weeks of life, but not in older animals. The results supported their hypothesis.

c) Hyponatremic Electroshock Threshold

The hyponatremic electroshock threshold test (HET) is a threshold test similar to those described above, except that it employs animals rendered sensitive to seizures by acute hyponatremia. Descriptions of the method have appeared elsewhere (SWINYARD et al. 1952). In contrast to its failure to elevate threshold in the

MET test (and certain applications of the PsM model; see above), phenytoin does elevate the hyponatremic electroshock threshold (SWINYARD 1949). Mephenytoin is also active in this test; data for ethotoin are not available. The ED_{50} values are depicted in Table 2. The evidence suggests that mephenytoin is more potent than phenytoin in both rats and mice. However, several factors render this conclusion uncertain. For example, the large variability in ED_{50} values for phenytoin in rats (i.e., 187 mg/kg vs 94.5 mg/kg) cannot be explained by any documented variance in experimental procedure (SWINYARD 1949; SWINYARD et al. 1952), and one does not know which is the more accurate figure. Furthermore, phenytoin was administered to rats by the subcutaneous route, but mephenytoin was administered by either the oral or intraperitoneal routes. Although the ED_{50} values in mice are similar for the two drugs, phenytoin was administered subcutaneously and mephenytoin orally.

Despite the variability among the electroshock threshold models (PsM, MET, and HET) with respect to the activity of phenytoin, it is probable that all three models are measuring similar, if not identical, anticonvulsant properties. A comparison of relative potencies of drugs evaluated by these tests (SWINYARD et al. 1952; BROWN et al. 1953) will show that the correlation is quite good. The fact that phenytoin is inactive in certain tests might simply imply a special mechanism not shared by the other drugs.

d) Maximal Metrazol Seizure

In contrast to the scMet test, which employs subcutaneous dosage sufficient to elicit clonic (threshold) seizures in mice, the maximal Metrazol seizure (MMS) test is designed to produce a maximal (tonic) seizure reminiscent of that produced by MES. Accordingly, the MMS test requires either larger sucutaneous dosage or rapid intravenous administration of Metrazol. The MMS model has been described previously (WOODBURY 1972).

Phenytoin is highly effective in the MMS test, even though single doses fail to prevent the clonic seizures of the scMet test. Mephenytoin is also active in the MMS test, but is less potent than phenytoin (Table 2). This order of potencies is the same as that observed for the MES test in mice (Table 1). However, the MMS model of epilepsy is not nearly as well documented as are many other models, and a selective advantage over the MES test is seriously doubted. Data are not available for the anti-MMS potency of ethotoin.

e) Audiogenic Seizures

Audiogenic seizures are convulsions triggered by sound stimuli of adequate intensity within a delimited bandwidth. The audiogenic seizure in mice begins with an initial startle response shortly after the onset of sound, and is followed by a period of running and leaping, which gives way to clonic spasms as the animal loses postural tone. This is the so-called pretonic phase. The tonic phase begins with hindlimb flexion, which is followed by a more persistent hindlimb extension. If the animal survives the tonic extension, the post-tonic phase consists of clonus and postictal depression. Thorough descriptions of audiogenic seizures and test protocols have been reported previously (COLLINS 1972).

FINK and SWINYARD (1959) employed two end points for their study of drug effects on audiogenic seizures in mice: one based on abolition of the tonic extensor component and the other on the running response. Phenytoin was active in both tests; the ED_{50} values were 5 mg/kg and 35 mg/kg, respectively (Table 2). COLLINS and HORLINGTON (1969) used a different strain of mice and reported an ED_{50} value of 13.9 mg/kg (p.o.) for phenytoin (Table 2). However, their study has been criticized for their failure to make allowance for variance in peak time (REINHARD and REINHARD 1977). The activities of mephenytoin and ethotoin in this model have not been reported.

It is commonly held that audiogenic convulsions represent generalized seizures analogous to those provoked by other means (COLLINS 1972) and that compounds capable of inhibiting maximal audiogenic seizures have therapeutic potential in grand mal epilepsy (WOODBURY 1972). Although it has been difficult, due to technical limitations, to corroborate an analogous relationship between audiogenic and other "generalized" seizures, some pharmacological relationships support such a concept. A comparison of the rank order of potencies of several drugs tested in either the MES model (KRALL et al. 1978b) or the audiogenic model (SWINYARD et al. 1963) show remarkable correlation. For example, the ratio of ED_{50} values for trimethadione and the more potent phenytoin in the MES test is 66; the same ratio in the audiogenic model is almost identical at 75.

f) Other Models

Numerous other experimental models of epilepsy have been developed for use in small rodents. However, only a relatively few of these models have received much experimental documentation. A procedure designed to induce local epileptogenic activity involves the topical application of penicillin to the cerebral cortex; but tonic-clonic as well as purely clonic seizures may develop, and the selectivity of drug action on either type of seizure might give clues relevant to its clinical potential. Phenytoin has very low activity against the clonic seizures elicited by topical penicillin, but is highly active against the tonic-clonic variety in rats and other species. This would be expected on the basis of the ability of phenytoin to prevent seizure spread, but relative inability to elevate the threshold for focal discharge (WOODBURY 1972).

Elevated carbon dioxide concentrations, and sudden withdrawal from hypercarbia, can induce clonic seizures in both rats and mice (WITHROW 1972). The seizures produced by hypercarbia might be due to an effect of CO_2 to activate subcortical brain centers sufficiently to overcome CO_2-mediated cortical depression (WOODBURY and KARLER 1960), while the CO_2 withdrawal seizures have been explained on the basis of changes in intracellular pH affecting cellular permeability to sodium (WITHROW 1972). Phenytoin fails to protect against either seizure type; in fact, both types are exacerbated by phenytoin (WOODBURY et al. 1958). In contrast, many drugs that are effective as anti-petit mal (absence) agents also protect against CO_2 seizures. Thus, CO_2 seizures appear to have potential value in the experimental study of absence seizures, but not GTC (grand mal) epilepsy.

Bemegride is a systemic convulsant whose site of action in the brain (cortex) is thought to be the same as that of pentylenetetrazol (HAHN 1960); and was, therefore, thought to have predictive value for potential anti-petit mal drugs.

Both phenytoin and mephenytoin have been reported active against bemegride-induced seizures (RÜMKE 1967), but interpretation of these data are complicated. RÜMKE (1967) demonstrated that phenytoin (100 mg/kg, s.c.) and mephenytoin (60 mg/kg, p.o.) produced a significant elevation of the median convulsive dose (CD_{50}) of bemegride in mice. However, bemegride may cause both clonic and tonic convulsions, and it is not clear from the data whether these drugs had a selective effect on one or the other seizure type. Also, phenytoin had no effect on the CD_{50} when given 1½ h before the convulsant, a time which approximates that peak time in many experiments. However, an anticonvulsant effect of phenytoin was noted 24 h after its administration, and a proconvulsant effect (i.e., lower CD_{50}) after 96 h. Although the anticonvulsant action of mephenytoin occurred after 1½ h, it too had a proconvulsant effect, in this case after 48 h. Because the time course of phenytoin's action does not correspond to peak plasma levels, it appears to have a unique mechanism of action against bemegride seizures. Although an explanation for the proconvulsant effect was not offered, it was suggested to account for the withdrawal supersensitivity seen in epileptics who suddenly terminate their medication.

Other systemic convulsants against which phenytoin has been tested include picrotoxin and strychnine. Strychnine appears to act by competing with the inhibitory transmitter glycine at spinal motorneurons; picrotoxin may compete with the inhibitory transmitter gamma-aminobutyric acid involved in presynaptic inhibition. Phenytoin does not affect either seizure process in rats (VERNADAKIS and WOODBURY 1969).

3. Other Animal Species

Many of the experimental models already discussed have also been applied to nonrodent species. For example, the ED_{50} for phenytoin in the MES model is about 60 mg/kg (s.c.) in rabbits and 10 mg/kg (i.p.) in cats (TOMAN et al. 1946). Phenytoin is also active in both cats and monkeys against tonic convulsions induced by penicillin, but is only minimally effective against the clonic seizures induced in this model (WOODBURY 1972); it is active against tonic seizures induced in rabbits and monkeys by large doses of pentylenetetrazol (MMS model), but is inactive (in rabbits) against the threshold seizure (scMet); it is inactive against CO_2-withdrawal seizures in dogs (WYKE 1963); and is ineffective in the prevention of barbiturate-withdrawal convulsions in dogs. Data are not available for ethotoin and mephenytoin in other animal species.

In addition to those already discussed, several experimental models have been developed which employ nonrodent species almost exclusively. A notable example is the photomyoclonic model developed by KILLAM et al. (1967) using the baboon (*Papio papio*). It was found that intermittent light stimulation (25/s) produces a myoclonic seizure in baboons that closely resembles that seen in man, and electrographic evidence corroborates its epileptic-like status. The seizure consists of eyelid clonus, followed by clonus of facial muscles and jaws, and terminating in violent jerking movements involving the entire body. The activity occurs during the period of photic stimulation, and may persist as self-sustained discharges after the stimulus is terminated. Phenytoin is not very effective in this model, although chronic administration will produce some protection. In a related model,

BARNES (1954) reported that large doses of phenytoin failed to suppress the electrographic response to photic stimulation in the rabbit. Data are not available in either animal model for ethotoin or mephenytoin.

Another experimental model that employs nonrodent species involves topical application of alumina cream to the sensorimotor cortex of monkeys. The chronic, recurrent, and spontaneous seizures that result frequently resemble Jacksonian seizures in humans, and may become generalized with propagation to involve major motor convulsions. Phenytoin is only modestly effective in preventing the clonic seizures reminiscent of human Jacksonian epilepsy, and this is only after chronic dosage; acutely, there is no protection (WOODBURY 1972). Although phenytoin would presumably be much more effective against the tonic component, tonic-clonic seizures are not generally reproducible in chronic animals. Phenobarbital is much more effective in this model than is phenytoin, but mephenytoin and ethotoin have not been tested.

Cortical lesions induced by local freezing is another model of focal epilepsy in which phenytoin has been tested. Although phenytoin was effective in reducing discharge frequency and spread from secondary foci, it did not prevent focal spiking activity in cat (MUSGRAVE and PURPURA 1963).

II. Anticonvulsant Potency in Man

The relative clinical potencies of phenytoin, mephenytoin, and ethotoin were reviewed by MILLICHAP (1972), who compared their clinical potencies with anti-MES potencies in mice. The effective daily dose reported for man was 10 mg/kg each for phenytoin and mephenytoin, and 50 mg/kg for ethotoin; the anti-MES potencies (ED_{50}) in mice were 9, 37, and 350 mg/kg, respectively. Thus, the potency of mephenytoin and phenytoin are about equal in man, even though phenytoin is more potent in laboratory assays. However, the actual dosages reported by MILLICHAP (1972) for phenytoin and mephenytoin may be excessive. For example, the 10-mg/kg dose would require 700 mg daily for an average 70-kg adult. For seizures responsive to phenytoin, the usual adult dosage is 300–400 mg (or about 5–6 mg/kg) daily. Dosage may be increased to 600 mg/day if necessary, but care must be taken because of a disproportionate increase in serum concentration with increased dosage (see Sect. F.III). The initial pediatric dose is about 5 mg/kg per day, with increases to a maximum 300 mg/day if necessary. The daily maintenance dosage in children is usually in the 5–11 mg/kg range.

The usual adult dosage of mephenytoin is 200–600 mg daily; pediatric dosage varies from 100 to 400 mg/day (or 3–10 mg/kg per day), depending on the nature of seizures and age. The normal therapeutic serum concentration, based on the metabolite *N*-desmethylmephenytoin (Nirvanol), is 15–40 µg/ml. The usual maintenance dose of ethotoin is 2–3 g/day for adults, which is five to six times that for phenytoin or mephenytoin. Pediatric maintenance dosage is about 0.5–1 g daily, although higher doses may be required in some cases. The therapeutic range for serum concentrations is 15–50 µg/ml (LARSEN and NAESTOFT 1974).

The therapeutic serum concentration for phenytoin is about 10–20 µg/ml (some sources quote 15–25 µg/ml). However, efficacy may be encountered at lower concentrations, or some patients require much higher concentrations. With concentrations below 15 μg/ml, toxicity is usually not a problem. Above 15 μg/ml, toxicity increases in both frequency and severity; above 30 μg/ml, almost all patients will experience some manifestation of toxicity. In adults, the ratio of dose (mg/kg) to serum concentration (μg/ml) is about 3.5 to 10. That is, a 3.5-mg/kg dose will produce an approximate 10 μg/ml serum concentration. In the pediatric population serum phenytoin concentrations tend to be significantly lower than those in the adult population for equivalent (mg/kg) dosages; and children often must receive higher maintenance dosages to achieve optimal antiepileptic concentrations (Pippenger 1978). Thus, in children the ratio needs to be increased, so that 10 mg/kg may in some cases be required to produce a 10 μg/ml serum concentration (Buchthal and Lennox-Buchthal 1972). However, individual variations are substantial, and the above ratios for phenytoin should be used only as approximations. As noted above, the usual approach in children is to start with 5 mg/kg dosage, and make adjustments as required. Although a more accurate approach would involve the application of pharmacokinetic principles to individual patients, clinical surveillance and therapeutic drug monitoring will provide adequate results in most cases.

III. Mechanism of Anticonvulsant Action

1. Neuropharmacology and Biochemistry

The neuropharmacology and biochemical effects of hydantoin derivatives, phenytoin in particular, are legion. For example, phenytoin in various systems has been reported to: (1) produce a tetrodotoxin-like decrease in passive sodium conductance, both during the action potential and during the resting state (Neuman and Frank 1977; Selzer 1978; Perry et al. 1978); (2) produce a decrease in neuronal excitability due to an increase in chloride and/or potassium conductance (Ayala et al. 1977a); (3) produce a reduction in synaptic calcium uptake (Hasbani et al. 1974; Pincus and Lee 1973; Sohn and Ferrendelli 1976); (4) inhibit post-tetanic potentiation (PTP) (Esplin 1957; Raines and Standaert 1967); (5) inhibit axonal propagation of action potentials during high-frequency stimulation (Esplin 1957; Yaari et al. 1977); (6) produce changes in the amplitude of synaptic potentials, with excitation being reduced and inhibition increased (Ayala et al. 1977b; Selzer 1978); (7) elevate membrane potential (Perry et al. 1978; Schwarz and Vogel 1977); (8) raise threshold (Morell et al. 1958; Schwarz and Vogel 1977); (9) reduce conduction velocity and spike amplitude (Morell et al. 1958; Schwarz and Vogel 1977); (10) reduce repetitive firing (Ayala et al. 1977a); (11) suppress bursting activity of certain pacemaker cells (Johnston and Ayala 1975); (12) inhibit calcium- and calmodulin-dependent protein phosphorylation and neurotransmitter release (DeLorenzo 1980); (13) inhibit elevation of brain cyclic nucleotides (cyclic GMP and cyclic AMP) produced by electroshock, and decrease basal levels of cyclic GMP in cerebellum (Ferrendelli 1980); and (14) increase Purkinje-cell activity and decrease deep cerebellar nuclei activity (Laxer et al. 1980). Those acquainted with the antiepileptic field will recognize that the preceding is only a partial accounting of the myriad of effects documented for phenytoin and selected other hydantoins.

The efficacy of phenytoin in the treatment of various seizure disorders is well established, as is its value in certain cardiac arrhythmias. In addition, phenytoin has been reported to be of value in the control of insulin hypersecretion (COHEN et al. 1973) and antidiuretic hormone hypersecretion (FICHMAN et al. 1970; LANDOLT 1974), and in the treatment of a syndrome characterized by continuous muscle fiber activity (neuromyotonia) (MERTENS and ZSCHOCKE 1965). Although the clinical uses of phenytoin might conceivably be explained on the basis of one or more of the effects listed above, such an attribution has never been proven. However, several theories have been developed in an attempt to unify the neuropharmacological and biochemical effects on the one hand, and the clinical observations on the other. The two most popular theories are each based upon a decrease of intracellular sodium; but differ with respect to the mechanism of such decrease. The earlier theory argues that phenytoin might facilitate active sodium transport by stimulating Na^+-K^+-ATPase (WOODBURY 1955; FESTOFF and APPEL 1968; LEWIN and BLECK 1977); the more recent theory suggests that phenytoin acts to limit the inward current due to sodium (AYALA et al. 1977a; LIPICKY et al. 1972). Other theories have implicated effects on calcium fluxes (FERRENDELLI and KINSCHERF 1977; SOHN and FERRENDELLI 1973) or alterations of neurotransmitter disposition and metabolism (AYALA et al. 1977b; DELORENZO 1980; SAAD et al. 1972). These theories are discussed in more detail below.

2. Effects on Active Sodium Transport

The hypothesis that phenytoin acts by stimulating active sodium-potassium transport (WOODBURY 1955) is controversial. Phenytoin has been reported to increase Na^+-K^+-ATPase activity in brain both in vivo (LEWIN and BLECK 1977; LEZNICKI and DYMECKI 1974) and in vitro (FESTOFF and APPEL 1968; SIEGLE and GOODWIN 1972; WILENSKY and LOWDEN 1972a). Phenytoin was also reported to increase Na^+-K^+-ATPase activity in skeletal muscle (KOOTSTRA and WOODHOUSE 1974) and cardiac muscle (GOLDSTEIN et al. 1973). However, other studies have failed to demonstrate such an effect, either in brain (DEUPREE 1977; SCHWARZ et al. 1975) or cardiac muscle (SPAIN and CHIDSEY 1971). In some cases, phenytoin actually decreased Na^+-K^+-ATPase activity (GILBERT and WYLLIE 1976; GOLDSTEIN et al. 1973). See Chap. 10 this volume, for further discussion of anticonvulsant effects on active sodium transport.

3. Effects on Passive Sodium Influx

Although stimulation of the active sodium-potassium pump might explain many of the physiological and therapeutic effects of phenytoin, so might its effect to decrease passive sodium influx. For example, one result of a decrease in resting sodium permeability is membrane hyperpolarization. Hyperpolarization may elevate threshold, reduce firing, and generally "stabilize" membranes (an effect which might also apply to membranes of secretory cells). The first demonstration that phenytoin blocks sodium channels was provided by LIPICKY et al. (1972), using voltage-clamped squid giant axons. They reported that phenytoin altered only maximal sodium conductance, and did not affect the kinetic parameters or voltage dependence of the sodium channel. Thus, it appeared that phenytoin blocked the channel in a manner similar to tetrodotoxin. Additional research has indicated that phenytoin might also affect the kinetics and voltage dependence of the sodium channel (SCHWARZ and VOGEL 1977; NEUMAN and FRANK 1977). SCHWARZ and VOGEL (1977) observed that the reduction of sodium current by phenytoin was pH dependent and potential dependent, and postulated that phenytoin binds to sites in the sodium channel that are different from those of tetrodotoxin. They also observed that phenytoin hyperpolarized the membrane, an effect that could be due to inhibition of resting sodium conductance. But they did not conduct experiments which might validate this possibility, even though LIPICKY et al. (1972) stated that phenytoin did not affect resting membrane properties.

However, DEWEER (1980) was able to confirm the hyperpolarizing effect of phenytoin in squid giant axon, and he also demonstrated that this effect does indeed result from blockade of resting sodium channels. He specifically eliminated the possibility that an increase in potassium permeability or stimulation of an electrogenic sodium pump might be responsible for the hyperpolarization. DEWEER (1980) also demonstrated that phenytoin reverses a veratridine-induced depolarization in squid giant axon, alone or in combination with tetrodotoxin; and the effects of phenytoin and tetrodotoxin were nonadditive, suggesting a common action to interfere with the sodium channel gating mechanism. (Veratridine is an alkaloid that "holds open" the sodium channels of excitable cells by interfering with their inactivation mechanism.) He concluded that phenytoin, like tetrodotoxin, blocks sodium channels be they resting, excitable, or held open by veratridine.

Thus, is seems clearly established that phenytoin exerts a significant action on excitable membranes to decrease passive sodium influx, perhaps by blocking sodium channels in a manner similar to that of tetrodotoxin. Indeed, the experimental validation of such an effect has caused several investigators to call into question the validity of the earlier theory, which is confirmed only under a very specific set of conditions (e.g., high Na^+/K^+ ratios). DEWEER (1980) has shown that phenytoin had no detectable effect on active sodium efflux in the squid giant axon, and others have reported similar findings in different systems. JOHNSTON and AYALA (1975) reported that phenytoin decreased the bursting pacemaker activity in *Aplysia* neurons, an effect attributable to inhibition of passive sodium influx. However, it is still premature to award a decision on the relative merit of either theory as it applies to mechanism, because precisely those conditions which appear to be required to demonstrate a stimulatory effect on Na^+-K^+-ATPase seem to exist in epileptogenic tissue (see Chap. 10, this volume). Therefore, much further experimentation will be required to delineate the relevance of either action to the antiepileptic effects.

4. Effects on Calcium

Phenytoin has been demonstrated to decrease calcium influx across synaptosomal membranes prepared from cerebral cortex (SOHN and FERRENDELLI 1976), and it might also inhibit the intracellular uptake of calcium by subcellular fractions (YAARI et al. 1977). However, the mechanism of the decrease is not known with certainty. It might be due to a primary action of phenytoin to block calcium channels directly, but this has not been proven. On the other hand, phenytoin-induced hyperpolarization is known to close the "late" calcium channels (BAKER et al. 1971). Decreased calcium influx might also be due to blockade of sodium channels, through which calcium may also enter (BAKER et al. 1971). Yet another mechanism might involve the steepened sodium gradient across the plasma membrane, which results from the inhibition of passive sodium influx. Because of the sodium-calcium countertransport mechanism involved in removal of calcium ions from cells, an inhibition of passive sodium influx will heighten the electrochemical gradient of calcium as well as sodium; and this is thought by some to be the major regulator of intracellular calcium concentration. See Chap. 10, this volume, for further discussion of anticonvulsant effects on calcium metabolism.

5. Effects on Neurotransmitters

Phenytoin (and presumably other hydantoins) exert multiple effects on neurotansmitter metabolism, disposition, and dynamics. For example, phenytoin inhibits the release (DELORENZO 1980) and uptake (WEINBERGER et al. 1976) of norepinephrine, and possibly its metabolism by monoamine oxidase (AZZARO and GUTRECHT 1973). The inhibition of norepinephrine release is calcium dependent, and is discussed separately (below), while the inhibition of its reuptake is thought to be related to decreased sodium and/or calcium influx.

DELORENZO and co-workers (DELORENZO 1980) demonstrated that phenytoin inhibits the calcium-dependent protein phosphorylation that mediates calcium-dependent neurotransmitter release. Phenytoin caused a substantial decrease in the calcium-dependent incorporation of labeled phosphate (from ATP) into two particular brain proteins labeled DPH-L and DPH-M. Furthermore, this effect was demonstrated in a highly enriched synaptic vesicle preparation, and was shown to be dependent upon an endogenous calmodulin-like protein present in association with the vesicles. Phenytoin supposedly inhibits the effects of the calcium-calmodulin complex, and not the binding of calcium to calmodulin.

In contrast to norepinephrine, the uptake of both GABA and glutamate by synaptosomes is increased by phenytoin (WEINBERGER et al. 1976). Since the sodium gradient is the energy source for cellular uptake of many organic molecules, including neurotransmitters, the steepened sodium gradient produced by phenytoin is probably responsible for the enhanced uptake of GABA and glutamate. This appears to be a uniform effect for amino acid neurotransmitters. The failure of norepinephrine reuptake to be similarly effected is not clearly understood, except that phenytoin has been described as a pure blocker of norepinephrine uptake because of its noncompetitive characteristics (WEINBERGER et al. 1976).

VERNADAKIS and WOODBURY (1960) demonstrated that phenytoin decreased glutamic acid and slightly increased gamma-aminobutyric acid (GABA) levels in rat cerebral cortex. SAAD et al. (1972) reported similar findings for GABA. Because phenytoin stimulates the uptake of GABA (see above), its metabolism (which occurs outside the synapse, probably in glia) is probably reduced; and this might account for the slight increase in cerebral GABA levels. Furthermore, the increased uptake of glutamate might contribute to the slight increase in GABA levels, and also account for the lower brain glutamate concentrations, because glutamate is converted to GABA in the nerve terminal. Because glutamate and GABA are excitatory and inhibitory neurotransmitters, respectively, it is possible that such changes could account for an anticonvulsant effect. Although norepinephrine, like GABA, is an inhibitory transmitter in the central nervous system, its metabolism occurs largely within the synapse. Thus, the opposite effects of phenytoin on the uptake of norepinephrine and GABA probably both contribute to an anticonvulsant effect.

The involvement of GABA and other neurotransmitters in the antiepileptic effects of phenytoin might depend upon receptor phenomena as well as changes in transmitter metabolism/disposition. For example, phenytoin markedly increases the duration of the inhibitory postsynaptic potential (IPSP) in the crayfish stretch receptor neuron (SRN), presumably by prolonging and increasing the conductance change of the postsynaptic membrane to chloride (AYALA et al. 1977 b). Phenytoin also prolonged the GABA-induced hyperpolarization which results when GABA is applied iontophoretically to dendrites of the SRN (AYALA et al. 1977b; DEISZ and LUX 1977). DEISZ and LUX (1977) have shown that phenytoin protects the GABA receptor against the convulsant picrotoxin, which suggests competition between phenytoin and picrotoxin for a common site related to GABA-dependent chloride conductance changes. Indeed, phenytoin inhibits binding of dihydropicrotoxinin (DHP; a derivative of the active component of picrotoxin) to rat brain membranes (TICKU et al. 1978). Because the seizure activity induced by picrotoxin is thought to result from blockade of GABA-mediated presynaptic inhibition, one would expect the effect of such competition with phenytoin to be antagonism of the convulsive effects of picrotoxin. However, in mammals, phenytoin enhances the seizure activity induced by picrotoxin, an effect which cannot presently be explained. Furthermore, phenytoin fails to modify the chloride-dependent GABA response when studied in various other systems (AYALA und JOHNSTON 1980).

Phenytoin apparently exerts little effect on the acetylcholine-mediated chloride-dependent ("short") IPSP in *Aplysia* (AYALA et al. 1977b), which suggests that phenytoin might not act on the chloride channel of the GABA complex, but rather at the GABA receptor. However, phenytoin does enhance the acetylcholine-mediated potassium-dependent ("long") IPSP in *Aplysia* (AYALA and JOHNSTON 1980). This "long" IPSP is thought to be due to inactivation of the slow inward current responsible for bursting pacemaker activity (WILSON and WACHTEL 1978). The inward current is due primarily to calcium, but sodium might also be involved; the hyperpolarizing phase is due to slow potassium conductance activated by calcium influx (JONSTON 1976). Phenytoin in therapeutic concentrations significantly reduced bursting activity in *Aplysia* neurons, an effect attributable to a reduction in slow inward current (due to calcium and/or sodium) and slow outward potassium current (JOHNSTON and AYALA 1975). Phenytoin also suppressed bursting activity induced in these cells by application of the convulsant pentylenetetrazol, which is thought to act by blocking GABA-mediated presynaptic inhibition (possibly by binding to the DHP site of the GABA complex; LAL et al. 1981). However, in this case, phenytoin appeared to act by reducing the slow inward current, which is the basis of the "long" IPSP as discussed above. Phenytoin also decreased the amplitude of excitatory postsynaptic potentials

(EPSPs) in the frog neuromuscular junction (YAARI et al. 1977) and various other systems. See Chap. 10, this volume, for further discussion of anticonvulsant effects on neurotransmitter metabolism/disposition.

In summary, phenytoin affects numerous indices of neurophysiological function. The changes induced are almost always compatible with an anticonvulsant action. Stimulation of the sodium pump, inhibition of passive sodium influx, prolonging IPSPs, decreasing EPSP amplitude, inhibiting calcium influx or the effect of the calcium-calmodulin complex on protein phosphorylation, increasing GABA concentrations, and many other observable correlates of phenytoin action might all provide logical explanations for the ability of this drug to stabilize the hyperexcitable brain.

D. Other Central Nervous System Effects

Unlike many other antiepileptics, phenytoin is a remarkably selective drug. It lacks sedative properties in usual dosage and may, in fact, elicit "convulsions" if very large doses are administered (see below). In contrast to phenytoin, mephenytoin and ethotoin display significant sedative properties (although less than for phenobarbital) in animals and man, an effect attributed to the presence of alkyl substitution at positions 3 and 5 of the hydantoin ring. All three drugs may produce signs of cerebellar-vestibular toxicity as measured by the rotorod test of gross neurological deficit in rodents (see Sect. H). Signs and symptoms referable to the cerebellar-vestibular system in humans include ataxia, nystagmus, diplopia, and vertigo. Phenytoin is more likely to produce these effects in humans than are either mephenytoin or ethotoin. Other central nervous system effects may include blurred vision, mydriasis, hyperactivity, confusion, hallucinations, and behavioral changes (see Sect. H).

Although physical dependence is not a significant problem with the hydantoin derivatives, their sudden cessation, as for any antiepileptic medication, can result in "rebound" hyperexcitability, leading to status epilepticus in some patients. To investigate this phenomenon, RÜMKE (1967) evaluated the effect of phenytoin and mephenytoin on seizure threshold (in mice) to the convulsants pentylenetetrazol and bemegride. Phenytoin had no effect on the convulsive potency (CD_{50}) of either agent when evaluated 1½ h after phenytoin pretreatment. The CD_{50} was increased for both convulsants 1–2 days after a single dose of phenytoin, but significantly lower CD_{50} values (a proconvulsant effect) were recorded after a 96-h interval. In contrast, mephenytoin had an anticonvulsant effect (increased CD_{50}) if given 1½ h prior to convulsant administration, but a proconvulsant effect when the interval was increased to 48 h. Similar experiments using maximal electroshock rather than systemic convulsants demonstrated that neither phenytoin nor mephenytoin increased the incidence of seizures when evaluated 96 h and 48 h, respectively, after drug administration. These findings suggested to RÜMKE (1967) that a central origin of the increased sensitivity to bemegride and pentylenetetrazol was unlikely.

An often quoted toxicity of phenytoin is its ability in large dosage to produce "convulsions" (GRUBER et al. 1940). However, the characterization of these "convulsions" as actual seizures has been disputed by BAZEMORE and ZUCKERMANN

(1974). These authors reported that the seizure-like episodes that occur in mice following the intraperitoneal injection of 85 mg/kg phenytoin are not accompanied by electroencephalographic evidence of seizure activity. Furthermore, there was no postictal change in behavior, the eyes remained open, and the animal did not defecate or bleed from the mouth. The seizure-like activity was invariably related to the attempts of the animals to move about the cage, and frequently occurred as the animal lost its balance. No episodes occurred when the mice were immobilized by securing the limbs with tape on a platform. Similar findings were reported by these authors for rats, rabbits, and cats, none of which displayed clinical seizures with large doses of phenytoin. These observations suggested to the authors that the seizure-like episodes encountered with very large doses of phenytoin might actually be due to a central disturbance of vestibular integration. There was also speculation that phenytoin-induced cerebellar degeneration might play a role, since it is thought by some that phenytoin might cause the loss of cerebellar Purkinje cells (HABERLAND 1962).

E. Actions Outside the CNS

I. Cardiac Muscle

Phenytoin exerts significant effects on excitable tissues outside the CNS. For example, in isolated cardiac cells in tissue culture, phenytoin decreases the number of cells beating (automaticity) and antagonizes the digitalis-induced increase in automaticity (MERCER et al. 1967). Phenytoin also antagonizes the positive inotropic effect of ouabain (HELFANT et al. 1967). The antiarrhythmic effect has been demonstrated for acute arrhythmias occurring after myocardial infarction in experimental animals (ZEFT et al. 1968) and in man (BASHOUR et al. 1965); it has also been demonstrated for various other cardiac arrhythmias (BERNSTEIN et al. 1965; SCHERF et al. 1960) and for digitalis-induced arrhythmias in man and animals (WOODBURY 1969 a). The antiarrhythmic effects of phenytoin appear to be due to inhibition of spread of excessive activity from a focus, analogous to its presumed action in the brain to inhibit generalized tonic-clonic seizures (see Sect. C.III). WATSON and WOODBURY (1973) and BASKIN et al. (1973) observed that phenytoin antagonized the effect of ouabain to increase sodium and decrease potassium concentration in heart muscle cells. Thus, these drugs are possibly selective antagonists of the Na^+-K^+ pump. An action of phenytoin to "stimulate" the pump might underlie its antiarrhythmic action, as has been postulated for its antispread activity in the CNS. The greatest clinical value of phenytoin as an antiarrhythmic drug is in the treatment of ventricular ectopic rhythms, whether or not these are the result of digitalis toxicity.

II. Smooth Muscle

In addition to its activity in cardiac muscle, phenytoin exerts significant effects on both smooth and skeletal (see below) muscle. DRUCKMAN and MOORE (1955) studied the effect of phenytoin on isolated rabbit intestinal smooth muscle, and found that the amplitude of contractions was decreased. CHOU et al. (1972) reported that phenytoin reduced the contractile state in situ of canine ascending colon and terminal ileum segments, and attenuated both spontaneous and stimulated phasic motor activities of the colon. VANASIN et al. (1973) studied the effect of phenytoin on isolated strips of colon smooth muscle from canine and human sources. Phenytoin increased significantly the relaxation time and decreased contraction time when the strips were stimulated either electrically or by acetylcholine, and the authors conclude that phenytoin has a direct action on smooth muscle as well as on the neuromuscular junction. Each of the above authors have suggested that the observed effects might represent the basis for the therapeutic use of phenytoin in the treatment of intestinal hypermotility and the spastic colon syndrome.

In isolated rat ileum, low concentrations of phenytoin (0.1 μg/ml) caused an initial contraction, which was sensitive to blockade by atropine and potentiation by physostigmine (WOODBURY 1969a). Thus, it is possible that phenytoin causes the release of acetylcholine from parasympathetic nerve endings (VAN REES et al. 1969). Using brain slices, MCLENNAN and ELLIOT (1951) reported that low concentrations of phenytoin stimulate acetylcholine synthesis. These observations might explain some of the findings that phenytoin has excitatory effects in the brain. It has been postulated that low concentrations of phenytoin block calcium uptake by subcellular particles. This would lead to increased cytosolic calcium concentration and increased transmitter release. However, higher concentrations (1 μg/ml or higher) of phenytoin progressively inhibit the contraction produced by acetylcholine (GAYET-HALLION 1944), and the mechanism appears to be noncompetitive (WOODBURY and KEMP 1971). It is known that higher concentrations of phenytoin not only reduce calcium uptake by subcellular particles, but also reduce calcium influx across the synaptic membrane. Such an effect might result in a net decrease in transmitter release by lowering intracellular calcium. Also, WATSON (1978) showed that phenytoin inhibited the effects of the calcium ionophore A23187 to cause contractions of dog coronary artery and rabbit aortic strips. Thus, it is apparent that phenytoin might exert at least some of its effects on smooth muscle by an action to block calcium movements, either at the level of the excitation-contraction coupling system or at the synaptic level.

BIANCHI et al. (1975) reported that phenytoin had no effect on the level of acetylcholine or its release from the cerebral cortex in normal guinea pigs. But in epileptic guinea pigs, phenytoin suppressed convulsions and reduced the abnormally high cortical acetylcholine outflow. These findings suggest that phenytoin alters acetylcholine disposition only indirectly, by restraining paroxysmal neuronal activity, and does not affect its presynaptic release. Because acetylcholine depolarizes the postsynaptic membrane by opening sodium channels, an action of phenytoin to decrease sodium influx, by whatever mechanism (see Sect. C.III), would have the effect of blocking acetylcholine-stimulated excitatory receptors. This effect, which might be noncompetitive, could account for phenytoin's action (at higher concentration) on both smooth muscle and the CNS. Also, since the sodium gradient is a major regulator of intracellular calcium levels, such a primary action on sodium influx could explain its effects on calcium movements. However, other data (VAN REES et al. 1969; WOODBURY and KEMP 1971; YAARI et al. 1977) are clearly consistent with an effect either to increase or decrease acetylcholine release. Thus, the effects of phenytoin on acetylcholine metabolism and smooth muscle function remain ambiguous.

III. Skeletal Muscle

Phenytoin was reported by ISAACS (1961) to be of value in the treatment of a syndrome characterized by continuous muscle fiber activity. Later, MERTENS and ZSCHOCKE (1965) described three patients having in common a continuous spastic contraction of the entire skeletal musculature, which was not alleviated by sleep or anesthesia. Again, phenytoin provided significant relief. Numerous other reports have been made, each proclaiming the therapeutic value of phenytoin in the treatment of continous muscle fiber activity. In most cases, withdrawal of phenytoin resulted in recurrence of the syndrome.

The mechanism of the palliative action of phenytoin in this curious disorder is unknown. While normal skeletal muscle is electrically silent between contractions, the clinical problem in myotonia becomes apparent during relaxation, when a myotonic afterdischarge occurs (ISAACS 1967). Phenytoin presumably stabilizes the myotonic afterdischarge, as it reportedly stabilizes against post-tetanic potentiation and post-tetanic afterdischarge (processes thought to be involved in epileptogenesis). ISAACS (1964) postulated that the problem in continuous muscle fiber activity might involve the acetylcholine release mechanism. As noted in the above section on smooth muscle, it is conceivable that phenytoin primarily antagonizes calcium entry into the presynaptic terminal and thus reduces transmitter release. If this occurred at the neuromuscular synapse, phenytoin should reduce evoked neurosecretion.

YAARI et al. (1977) reported that under normal physiological conditions, phenytoin significantly depressed the evoked release of acetylcholine at the frog neuromuscular synapse. They also demonstrated that phenytoin increased the frequency of miniature end-plate potentials. Both of these effects were explained by a logic similar to that used to account for the effects of phenytoin on acetylcholine disposition in smooth muscle, i.e., blockade of calcium uptake at the axonal membrane and blockade of intracellular sequestration-extrusion of calcium, respectively. Phenytoin has long been known to reduce post-tetanic potentiation (PTP), a phenomenon that involves a prolonged increase in acetylcholine release following repetitive presynaptic stimulation. Calcium is required for PTP to occur, and when external calcium is decreased, PTP decays more rapidly. Assuming that the myotonic afterdischarge characteristic of continuous muscle fiber activity is likewise dependent on calcium, the inhibition of presynaptic calcium influx by phenytoin might provide the basis for its action in this disorder.

IV. Other Actions

Phenytoin has been reported to inhibit insulin release from isolated perfused rat pancreas (LEVIN et al. 1970) and isolated islets of Langerhans (KIZER et al. 1970). In the study by KIZER et al. (1970), the inhibitory action of phenytoin was found to be reversible by potassium and ouabain. Phenytoin was later shown to be effective in the treatment of patients with benign insulinoma (COHEN et al. 1973) and functional islet-cell tumors (BRODOWS and CAMPBELL 1974), and in other cases of functional hypoglycemia unresponsive to dietary management (STAMBAUGH and TUCKER 1974). However, the effectiveness of phenytoin in the treatment of insulinomas has been questioned by HOFELDT et al. (1974).

In a related study, GERICH et al. (1972) reported that low concentrations (25 μg/ml) of phenytoin markedly diminished glucagon release from the isolated perfused rat pancreas but did not inhibit insulin release. They note that the effects on insulin release reported by LEVIN et al. (1970) required higher phenytoin concentrations. GERICH et al. (1972) concluded that the pancreatic alpha cells are more sensitive to phenytoin than are the beta cells, and suggested that the potential action of phenytoin on both glucagon and insulin release might account for its reported ability to stabilize poorly controlled diabetes mellitus in humans (FABRYKANT and PACELLA 1948).

Phenytoin has also been reported to inhibit antidiuretic hormone (ADH) release from the neurohypophysis (FICHMAN et al. 1970; GUZEK et al. 1974), an effect shown to be of value in the treatment of the inappropriate ADH syndrome (LANDOLT 1974; LEE et al. 1961). LANDOLT (1974) noted that phenytoin corrected the abnormal condition, but did not affect normal water metabolism. In a related study, MITTLER and GLICK (1972) demonstrated that phenytoin inhibits potassium-stimulated oxytocin release from isolated rat pituitary gland.

An action of particular interest is the inhibition of thyrotropin release from the adenohypophysis (WOODBURY 1969b). Low doses (20 mg/kg) of phenytoin stimulated the uptake of iodide by the thyroid gland in rats, but larger doses (40–80 mg/kg) inhibited uptake. The inhibitory effect of phenytoin was absent in hypophysectomized rats, suggesting that uptake was mediated through the pituitary; and the inference was made that low doses of phenytoin stimulate and high doses inhibit the release of thyroid-stimulating hormone (TSH). Because strophanthin antagonized the inhibition of iodide uptake by phenytoin, it was reasoned that the action of phenytoin might involve the stimulation of sodium-potassium transport.

PENTO (1976) has demonstrated that phenytoin inhibits calcitonin secretion in the pig (see also PENTO et al. 1973). Normal basal levels of calcitonin secretion apparently were not significantly affected by phenytoin. However, when calcitonin secretion was stimulated by glucagon or calcium administration, phenytoin produced a measurable reduction. PENTO et al. (1973) have noted that these findings are in accord with other reports that phenytoin does not alter normal basal function, but that when unusual stimuli are present phenytoin exerts a regulatory influence.

Phenytoin also inhibits the release of adrenocorticotrophin from the adenohypophysis (RINNE 1966), the secretion of norepinephrine by the adrenal medulla (GUTMAN and BOONYAVIROJ 1977), salivary secretion (WATSON and SIEGEL 1976), and synaptic neurotransmitter release (see Sect. C.III). Thus, phenytoin appears to exert a general inhibitory effect on all secretory cells. Since calcium is known to increase secretion in the processes listed above, it is possible that phenytoin acts by blocking cellular calcium uptake (see Sect. C.III). However, as exemplified by its effects on thyrotropin release, small concentrations of phenytoin might stimulate release, an effect that might be explained by the inhibition of calcium uptake by subcellular particles.

Phenytoin exerts an effect on thyroid metabolism which is probably unrelated to secretory mechanisms. Serum protein-bound iodine may be reduced during phenytoin administration to levels as low as 2.5–3.8 μg/100 ml. The mechanism possibly involves the displacement of thyroxine from thyroxine-binding globulin (OPPENHEIMER and TAVERNETTI 1962), but this concept is controversial (see Sect. H.V). The free thyroxine presumably is eliminated more rapidly, resulting in a lower total serum thyroxine concentration. However, the free thyroxine *concentration* is not significantly altered (even though the free fraction is increased), and there are no signs or symptoms of hypothyroidism. The clinical significance of this phenytoin-thyroxine interaction is the diagnostic confusion it might cause.

F. Pharmacokinetics

Representative pharmacokinetic data for phenytoin are depicted in Table 3. Pharmacokinetic data for mephenytoin and ethotoin are extremely limited, but will be cited where appropriate in the following discussion.

I. Absorption and Bioavailability

As already noted, phenytoin is a weak acid with an approximate pK_a of 8.3 (AGARWAL and BLAKE 1968). As such, it should be predominantly nonionized at physiological pH (approximately 89% at pH 7.4). Furthermore, the drug is very lipid soluble as judged from estimates of its partition coefficient in various solvent systems (see Sect. B.I). Thus, phenytoin should have little difficulty penetrating membranes by nonionic diffusion. While this is in fact the case, the absorption of phenytoin is nevertheless slow and subject to substantial variability. Its absorption rate constant and half-life in man were reported as 0.569 h^{-1} and 1.62 h, respectively (GUGLER et al. 1976).

1. Oral Administration

The slow and variable absorption of phenytoin relates to several factors. Foremost is the fact that the nonionized (free acid) from is practically insoluble in water. Although the sodium salt has a much greater aqueous solubility than the free acid, oral administration of phenytoin in this form results in rapid conversion to the nonionized form in the acid contents (pH ~ 2) of the stomach. Thus, equivalent oral dosage of either chemical form might result in equivalent amounts of virtually insoluble drug in the stomach. Nevertheless, early observations suggested that greater bioavailability was attainable with the sodium salt (DILL et al. 1956). For example, LUND (1974) compared two formulations containing phenytoin sodium in capsules with a single formulation of phenytoin acid tablets. Much better bioavailability was reported for phenytoin sodium when the two forms were given as a single dose (300 mg or 400 mg) to healthy volunteers. In another report, patients who changed from phenytoin acid tablets to capsules containing phenytoin sodium experienced a two- to fourfold increase in serum phenytoin

Table 3. Pharmacokinetic data for phenytoin in various species

Parameter	Value	Notes	Refs.
Plasma protein binding (%)	77.5	Dog, i.v.	LÖSCHER (1979)
	76	Cat, 15 mg/kg, i.v.	FIREMARK et al. (1963)
	80	Rat, 33 mg/kg, i.p.	DILL et al. (1956)
	89 (69–96)	Man, 4.4 mg/kg, p.o.	WOODBURY and SWINYARD (1972)
	93	Man	BARTH et al. (1976)
V_d (liters/kg)	1.0	Dog, 10 mg/kg, i.v.	FREY and LÖSCHER (1980)
	2.22	Dog, 20 mg/kg, i.v.	DAYTON et al. (1967)
	6.3	Cat, 15 mg/kg, i.v.	FIREMARK et al. (1963)
	6.5	Rat, 33 mg/kg, i.p.	DILL et al. (1956)
	1.57	Man, 6.5 mg/kg, p.o.	WOODBURY and SWINYARD (1972)
	2.54	Man, 2 mg/kg, i.v.	SUZUKI et al. (1970)
	0.78	Man	CRANFORD et al. (1977)
K_m (μmol/liter)	5.9–23.0	Man	MAWER et al. (1974)
	4.8–96.0	Man	RAMBECK et al. (1979)
V_{max} (mg/day)	275–585	Man	MAWER et al. (1974)
	155–818	Man	RAMBECK et al. (1979)
Cl_{tot} (liters/kg/h)	0.168	Dog, 10 mg/kg, i.v.	FREY and LÖSCHER (1980)
	0.016	Man	CRANFORD et al. (1977)
	0.022	Man	GUGLER et al. (1976)
k_{elim} (h^{-1})	0.161	Dog, 10 mg/kg, i.v.	FREY and LÖSCHER (1980)
	0.199	Dog, 10 mg/kg, p.o.	FREY and LÖSCHER (1980)
	0.32	Gerbil, 20 mg/kg, i.p.	FREY et al. (1981)
Half-life (h)	3.4	Rat, 33 mg/kg, i.p.	DILL et al. (1956)
	5	Rat, 100 mg/kg, p.o.	DILL et al. (1956)
	72	Cat, 15 mg/kg, i.v.	FIREMARK et al. (1963)
	2.2	Dog, 20 mg/kg, i.v.	DAYTON et al. (1967)
	6.4	Dog, 50 mg/kg, i.v.	DAYTON et al. (1967)
	4.4	Dog, 10 mg/kg, i.v.	FREY and LÖSCHER (1980)
	2.1	Gerbil, 20 mg/kg, i.p.	FREY et al. (1981)
	10.5	Monkey, 10 mg/kg, i.v.	GABLER and HUBBARD (1973)
	15	Monkey, 30 mg/kg, i.v.	GABLER and HUBBARD (1973)
	22	Man, 4.4 mg/kg, p.o.	WOODBURY and SWINYARD (1972)
	59	Man, 13 mg/kg, p.o.	WOODBURY and SWINYARD (1972)
	9.5	Man, 2 mg/kg, i.v.	SUZUKI et al. (1970)
	10.2	Man, 4.4 mg/kg, i.v.	SUZUKI et al. (1970)

V_d, apparent volume of distribution [all data except those of FREY and LÖSCHER (1980) and CRANFORD et al. (1977) are based on plasma free drug concentrations]; K_m, Michaelis constant; V_{max}, maximum metabolic rate; Cl_{tot}, total body clearance; k_{elim}, elimination rate constant.

[a] Although half-life values have been reported for phenytoin, it is now established that the elimination of this drug is better described by Michaelis-Menten kinetics than by first-order kinetics. Thus, strictly speaking, it is inappropriate to refer to a half-life for phenytoin, at least in man. However, for comparative purposes data for different doses are given for various animal species and man

concentration (ALVAN et al. 1975). However, these data have become controversial. In such studies where the bioavailability of phenytoin sodium has been proven superior to that of the free acid, the product containing the free acid had an exceptionally poor bioavailability; thus, these results should not be generalized to all phenytoin acid products. Recent studies have shown that equivalent oral doses of either phenytoin acid or phenytoin sodium produce equivalent plasma concentrations, providing that high-quality formulations were administered (JOHANNESSEN and STRANDJORD 1975; TAMMISTO et al. 1976). It is now recognized that the size and form of phenytoin crystals exert a major influence on bioavailability, and major differences in bioavailability are likely related to such factors rather than to chemical form. Thus, phenytoin acid in a microcrystalline suspension has been shown to be completely absorbed after oral dosage (GLAZKO 1972 a), while the amorphous form may be poorly and erratically absorbed. In fact, several studies have demonstrated superior bioavailability for selected phenytoin acid formulations than for products containing the sodium salt (SANSOM et al. 1975; STEWART et al. 1975). A reasonable approximation of the absolute bioavailability of quality formulations, free acid or sodium salt, is in the order of 80%–95%.

The relatively alkaline contents of the small intestine (pH 7–8) permit greater solubility of phenytoin because of an increase in ionization (although the majority of drug is still unionized); and the presence of bile salts further enhances solubility. The considerably greater surface area available for absorption, and the higher vascularity and blood flow, are yet additional factors that combine to make the upper small intestine the major site of phenytoin absorption. Quantitative estimates of phenytoin absorption at different gastrointestinal sites were provided by DILL et al. (1956), who measured plasma concentrations in rats 4 h after placing 100 mg of the drug in isolated stomach and segments of the intestinal tract. Judged from plasma concentrations, absorption was greatest when phenytoin was placed in the isolated upper small intestine, and least when placed in the isolated stomach. Significant absorption also occurred from the lower small intestine, and less from the cecum and colon.

However, because phenytoin is relatively insoluble even at the higher pH of the intestinal fluid, its absorption from intestinal sites is often directly dependent upon the rate of dissolution of the remaining crystalline material. With the usual doses there may be substantial crystalline drug in the intestine. The solubility of phenytoin in intestinal fluid at pH 7.8 (37 °C) is about 100 μg/ml. Because the maximum volume of intestinal fluid available for solution is only 1,000 ml in humans, doses exceeding 100 mg may saturate the intestinal fluid and exceed the limit of phenytoin solubility. Because in reality the volume of distribution in intestinal fluid is much less than 1,000 ml, the limit of phenytoin solubility may be exceeded at doses much less than 100 mg. This has been demonstrated in rats given various oral doses of phenytoin (WOODBURY and SWINYARD 1972). Plasma concentrations increased with doses up to 66 mg/kg, but larger doses failed to produce further increases; hence, dissolution of crystalline phenytoin was rate-limiting with respect to absorption.

2. Intramuscular Administration

The absorption of phenytoin by the intramuscular route is limited by many of the properties which affect its gastrointestinal absorption. Because of its poor aqueous solubility, phenytoin at an intramuscular site acts as a repository preparation, and is absorbed only as fast as the free drug is cleared from the plasma by the disposition factors discussed above. However, unlike the gastrointestinal environment, the volume for dissolution and surface area for absorption are much less at the intramuscular site. Because phenytoin must be concentrated to a convenient volume for intramuscular injection, the solvent is made very alkaline; injection results in the precipitation of crystals which will dissolve slowly and erratically. In addition, because of capacity-limited metabolism (see Sect. F.III), the drop in plasma concentration in changing from oral to intramuscular administration would be more than proportional to the reduction in absorption at the intramuscular site. This was demonstrated by WILDER et al. (1974) when a change from oral to intramuscular administration resulted in an initial 40%–60% decrease in phenytoin plasma concentration, while metabolite excretion decreased by only 16%–20%. For these reasons, phenytoin is rarely recommended for intramuscular administration. If it is deemed necessary (e.g., for abdominal surgery or in a malabsorption syndrome), then it may require that dosage be increased by about 50%. On the other hand, intoxication may occur on resumption of oral therapy if dosage is not readjusted accordingly. When parenteral administration is necessary many consultants will prefer to give phenytoin by intravenous infusion rather than by the intramuscular route.

II. Distribution

1. Plasma Protein Binding

Following absorption, phenytoin distributes freely throughout the body because, at pH 7.4, it exists predominantly in the nonionized form, which permits the rapid penetration of membranes by passive diffusion. However, in man phenytoin is approximately 90% bound to plasma proteins (EHRNEBO et al. 1971; PORTER and LAYZER 1975), which, as already noted, increases its solubility in blood well above that in aqueous solution. The binding fraction in neonates is less (EHRNEBO et al. 1971; FREDHOLM et al. 1975), and in fetuses it is less still (EHRNEBO et al. 1971). Plasma binding in animals is generally less than in man (Table 3). The binding, which is reversible, is primarily to albumin (ODAR-CEDARLOF and BORGA 1976a), but secondary low-affinity sites on other proteins (alpha-globulins) bind the drug when it is displaced from albumin (MONKS et al. 1978).

The phenytoin-binding sites appear to be identical with those to which other drugs and endogenous substances bind. Phenytoin may compete with thyroxine and triiodothyronine for binding to albumin and alpha-globulin fractions, but not to prealbumin. Thus, phenytoin may displace the thyroid hormones onto prealbumin (WOODBURY and SWINYARD 1972). Bilirubin can cause displacement in the neonate (FREDHOLM et al. 1975); and free fatty acids have been reported to displace phenytoin in the rat (COLBURN and GIBALDI 1977). However, displacement by free fatty acids is not thought to represent an important interaction in neonates or adults (ODAR-CEDARLOF and BORGA 1976 b). Phenytoin can also be displaced from plasma protein-binding sites by valproic acid (MONKS et al. 1978), diazoxide (ROE et al. 1975), salicylic acid (ODAR-CEDARLOF and BORGA 1976a), phenylbutazone (LUNDE et al. 1970), sulfisoxazole (LUNDE et al. 1970), and other drugs (Sect. G). Because the displaced phenytoin is either redistributed in a larger body volume or metabolized more rapidly, the total serum phenytoin concentration will decrease. However, the lower total serum concentration reflects the amount of phenytoin displaced; the free phenytoin concentration at steady state does not change significantly. Therefore, the fraction of free drug concentration is now greater, and it may be possible to achieve the same therapeutic end point at lower total phenytoin concentration. It is important that allowance be made for this in therapeutic drug monitoring. It is also important to recognize that phenytoin can displace the above-mentioned drugs as well as being displaced itself. However, phenytoin is not readily displaced by other anticonvulsants that may be administered concomitantly.

There has been controversy on the significance of variability in protein binding among the population. While BOOKER and DARCEY (1973) reported that variability is considerable, their work has been criticized on technical grounds, and others (YACOBI et al. 1977) have indicated that the variation in free drug concentration is no greater than two fould, providing the albumin concentration is within the normal range. However, a two fold variation may indeed be significant. In man, for example, 10% of the serum phenytoin concentration is unbound; a factor that reduces binding by 10% (i.e., from 90% to 80%) produces a 100% increase in free drug concentration. Since the free drug is the pharmacologically and metabolically active form, there can be both pharmacodynamic and pharmacokinetic consequences of such interactions.

Other factors that might affect phenytoin binding to plasma protein include a variety of pathological changes. Because studies in humans have suggested a reciprocal relationship between the free phenytoin fraction and plasma albumin concentration (PORTER and LAYZER 1975), it is not surprising that phenytoin binding is reduced in hepatic diseases accompanied by hypoalbuminemia (HOOPER et al. 1974). Phenytoin binding to plasma proteins may also be reduced in uremic patients secondary to renal disease (REIDENBERG and AFFRIME 1973), and several mechanisms have been postulated to account for this phenomenon (LETTERI et al. 1971; BOOBIS 1977; KINNIBURGH and BOYD 1981; ODAR-CEDARLOF 1977).

Pregnancy (RUPRAH et al. 1980), age (HAYES et al. 1975), and severe burns (BOWDLE et al. 1980) have also been shown to affect phenytoin binding to plasma protein. In the latter study, rats exposed to severe experimental burns demonstrated an increase in clearance and volume of distribution, which the authors explained on the basis of decreased plasma protein binding; the decreased binding was in turn accounted for by a decrease in serum albumin.

2. Extravascular Distribution

Phenytoin which is not bound to plasma proteins readily enters cells and binds to subcellular fractions (see below). Within 15 min, the drug has reached its maximum volume of distribution (V_d), which in man ranges from about 1.6 to 2.5 liters/kg (Table 3) for measurements based upon the concentration of unbound phenytoin in plasma (WOODBURY and SWINYARD 1972). [Lower estimates of V_d are obtained in man if calculations are based upon total plasma concentration. See CRANFORD et al. (1977).] Estimates of V_d in experimental animals, when based on total plasma drug concentration, are generally greater than in man, an effect accounted for by the lower plasma protein binding in animals (Table 3). However, the difference is not as great in the dog as it is in cats and rats. Thus, it is apparent that phenytoin is distributed in a volume greater than total body water (about 41 liters), which suggests that the drug is bound in various cellular and tissue compartments as well as to plasma protein. According to NOACH et al. (1958) phenytoin in rats is present in liver, kidney, fat, muscle, and brain in greater amounts than in plasma. The same approximate relationships have been demonstrated for tissues from mice and cats (WOODBURY and SWINYARD 1972) and in man (HOUGHTON et al. 1975; MIRKIN 1971 b; SIRONI et al. 1980). The accumulation of phenytoin in tissues is due mainly to binding, since the concentration of unbound phenytoin in all tissues measured is approximately equal to that in plasma (WOODBURY and SWINYARD 1972).

Phenytoin in the unbound form also distributes into transcellular fluids, including CSF, saliva, gastrointestinal fluid, and bile (DILL et al. 1956; NOACH and VAN REES 1964; NOACH et al. 1958). Both CSF and saliva concentrations approximate the free phenytoin fraction (i.e., 10%–12%) in plasma (TROUPIN and FRIEL 1975). Because unbound drug concentration would represent a better guide for therapeutic monitoring than total serum concentration, some have advocated the use of saliva specimens to obtain this information. Because the salivary glands act as simple dialysis membranes across which free drug molecules in plasma are able to diffuse, the use of saliva would circumvent the cumbersome methods required to measure free drug in plasma. However, there is considerable interpatient variability in the relationship of plasma-free drug to saliva-free drug; and a consensus regarding the suitability of using saliva specimens in therapeutic monitoring has not yet evolved.

Most of an administered dose of phenytoin is metabolized in the liver and excreted in bile. After the metabolites enter the intestinal fluid they are reabsorbed into the blood and excreted in the urine. Approximately 60% of an administered dose in rats was excreted in a 48-h period; of this total, 46% was excreted in urine and 14% in feces (WOODBURY and SWINYARD 1972). If the bile duct was cannulated, approximately 72% of the administered dose in rats was excreted in a 48-h period; the bile contained 43% of the radioactivity, the urine 28%, and feces only 0.6% (WOODBURY and SWINYARD 1972). Thus, it is apparent that most of the metabolized phenytoin is excreted in bile, reabsorbed in the intestine, and ultimately excreted in urine.

After chronic administration, phenytoin concentrations in plasma from mother's blood, cord blood, and infant's blood are approximately equal at parturition (MIRKIN 1971 a; RANE et al. 1974; ISHIZAKI et al. 1981). Thus, phenytoin appears readily to cross the human placenta and reach equilibrium between mother and fetus. Available evidence suggests a similar distribution of phenytoin in experimental animals (WESTMORELAND and BASS 1971). In rhesus monkeys, placental transfer of the unconjugated metabolite 5-(p-hydroxyphenyl)-5-phenylhydantoin (*p*-HPPH) has also been demonstrated (GABLER and HUBBARD 1973).

MIRKIN (1971 b) studied the distribution of phenytoin in maternal and fetal tissues of rats on the 18th or 19th day of gestation. The animals were killed at varying times after intravenous or intraperitoneal administration, and maternal tissues (liver and brain) and fetal tissues (placenta, liver, and brain) analyzed for phenytoin. Peak phenytoin concentrations were observed in specimens of fetal liver (57 μg/g) and brain (47 μg/g) 1 h after a maternal injection of phenytoin (25 mg/kg, i.v.). Note that this peak time is significantly delayed in comparison with results from other studies (RAMSAY et al. 1979; NOACH et al. 1958). The ratio of fetal to maternal phenytoin concentration in liver and brain tissue demonstrated that phenytoin was more concentrated in the fetal tissues during the early periods following intravenous administration. In contrast, peak phenytoin concentrations were not achieved until 4 h after intraperitoneal administration, at which time the concentration in maternal liver was 213 μg/g, and 15 μg/g in fetal liver.

In the same investigation, MIRKIN (1971 b) reported the distribution of phenytoin in human maternal plasma, and in plasma and tissues from aborted fetuses 30 min after maternal injection (intravenous). Phenytoin was distributed widely in fetal tissues, with highest concentrations occurring in the liver. Lower concentrations occurred (in decreasing order) in the kidney, cerebral cortex, and plasma from cord blood. Maternal plasma phenytoin concentration 30 min after an intravenous dose was about 30% greater than that of umbilical cord plasma. Thus, the similarity of maternal and fetal plasma concentrations of phenytoin probably reflects an equilibrium established during long-term administration.

Breast milk obtained on various days postpartum from women on chronic phenytoin therapy contained from 15% to 69% of the concentration found in maternal plasma (MIRKIN 1971 b; RANE et al. 1974). Furthermore, increasing the maternal plasma concentration from 5.5 μg/ml to 8.4 μg/ml did not produce a corresponding increase in phenytoin concentration in breast milk (MIRKIN 1971 b). These data suggest a limited transport capacity of the mammary glands of phenytoin which is exceeded at relatively low plasma concentrations.

3. Brain and Cerebrospinal Fluid

According to RAMSAY et al. (1979), maximum phenytoin concentrations were attained in cat brain 6 min after a 2-min intravenous infusion was completed. This compares with 3 min for phenobarbital and 1 min for diazepam (RAMSAY et al. 1979). Thus penetration into the brain is rapid, and provides justification for its use in status epilepticus (although diazepam is currently considered the drug of choice). In the same experiments peak CSF concentration also occurred at 6 min, which is consistent with the idea that phenytoin enters the brain and CSF compartments by independent mechanisms. Others have also reported rapid equilibrium of unbound phenytoin between plasma, CSF, and brain water (FIREMARK et al. 1963; WILDER et al. 1977).

The rapid attainment of peak brain concentrations after intravenous administration is due to two factors: the high lipophilicity of the phenytoin molecule and the relatively high blood flow to the brain. These are factors which also contribute to the redistribution phenomenon; that is, the rapid termination of drug action due to a shift in concentration from the brain to peripheral binding or storage sites (e.g., muscle, fat). Intravenous administration of any drug will present initially high concentrations to the brain and other organs which receive a high blood flow. Because lipophilic molecules will rapidly enter the brain along the concentration gradient, a new gradient is quickly established from the brain to the periphery. Thus, the brain concentration rapidly declines as continued high blood flow discharges drug to the greater mass of less vascular peripheral tissue. However, redistribution kinetics are not as apparent with phenytoin as with some other more lipophilic molecules (e.g., thiopental, diazepam). This can be demonstrated using a conventional three-compartment model, as described by RAMSAY et al. (1979). The brain behaves as a rapidly equilibrating (shallow) compartment for most lipophilic molecules which readily penetrate membranes. A peripheral (deep) compartment communicates with the shallow compartment through the central (plasma) compartment. In this model the deep compartment equilibrates with the central compartment more slowly than does the shallow compartment. The constants k_{12} and k_{21} represent the rates of drug entry into the shallow (brain) compartment and its exit therefrom, respectively. Higher values for these constants indicate higher rates. RAMSAY et al. (1979) reported $k_{12}=0.539$/h for phenytoin and $k_{12}=1.092$/h for diazepam. Thus, diazepam enters cat brain much more rapidly than phenytoin, which is consistent with the very early onset of diazepam's action. The constants k_{21} for phenytoin and diazepam were 0.137/h and 0.194/h, respectively, which is consistent with the more rapid offset of diazepam's action. RAMSAY et al. (1979) acknowledge that k_{21} is unexpectedly low for diazepam, and attribute this to inaccuracy in the measurement of the initial plasma distribution phase. Thus, the rate of diazepam's distribution out of the brain is probably much greater in relation to phenytoin than the two values indicate. This is suggested by the much larger values for k_{21} cited by KAPLAN et al. (1973), who reported a mean k_{21} value of 3.89/h for diazepam in human experiments.

The ratio k_{21}/k_{12} reflects the net entry and return of drug from the shallow compartment. A ratio greater than unity indicates relatively free transfer of drug from the brain to the central compartment, whereas a value less than unity suggests slow equilibrium and binding of the drug in the shallow compartment. RAMSAY et al. (1979) reported k_{21}/k_{12} values of 0.389 and 0.547 for phenytoin and phenobarbital, respectively; the value for diazepam from KAPLAN et al. (1973) is 1.4. Thus, the relatively low ratio for phenytoin suggests that equilibrium of plasma with the shallow compartment is slow, probably due to tissue binding in the brain; phenobarbital equilibrates more rapidly, and diazepam faster still. These data correlate with the relatively stable phenytoin concentrations found in the brain for the 60-min experimental period described by RAMSAY et al. (1979). In contrast to diazepam, there was no significant difference between the brain phenytoin concentration at the 6-min peak time and 60 min postinfusion. Furthermore, the brain concentration remained stable even while the plasma concentration fell and the brain: plasma ratio increased. The brain: plasma concentration ratio peaked at 20 min and remained fairly constant for the duration of the experiment. The authors interpreted this as evidence for substantial binding of phenytoin in the brain. Other investigators have been led to the same conclusion. For example, FIREMARK et al. (1963) reported that phenytoin concentrations in 14 brain regions of the cat were only slightly lower at 24 h than 3 h, although plasma concentrations had fallen considerably. On the other hand, several studies have demonstrated much lower brain phenytoin concentrations at 24 h. NOACH et al. (1958) reported values near 0% at 16 h; YANAGIHARA and HAMBERGER (1971 c) reported values at 24 h which were only 10% of the maximum value; and LEE and BASS (1970) reported values 20%–25% of maximum at 24 h. The reasons for these discrepancies are not readily apparent.

The steady-state brain: plasma ratio has been reported by different investigators using different species at about 0.75 to 3.5 (SHERWIN et al. 1973; WOODBURY and SWINYARD 1972; VAJDA et al. 1974). If only the free concentrations are measured, the brain: plasma ratio is much less variable; estimates range from 0.91 to 1.0 (WOODBURY and SWINYARD 1972). Estimates of the brain: CSF ratio in various studies range from 0.88 to 1.0 for the unbound drug; and plasma: CSF ratios range from 0.96 to 1.0 (WOODBURY and SWINYARD 1972). Thus, the brain does bind phenytoin at least as well as plasma protein, and at equilibrium the concentrations of unbound phenytoin in plasma, CSF, and brain are approximately equal.

NAKAMURA et al. (1966) have shown that preferential accumulation of phenytoin occurs in the superior and inferior colliculus, amygdala, and hippocampus, as measured in dogs and cats. Measurements on human specimens taken at autopsy show that phenytoin concentrations in the midbrain were relatively high, while lower (and approximately equal) concentrations were found in both the cerebellum and cerebral cortex (SHERWIN et al. 1973). However, experiments in rats have shown that phenytoin accumulates in a perikaryon-enriched Purkinje-cell fraction isolated from cerebellar specimens, and that uptake in this fraction was about four times that in other cerebellar neurons and more than twice that in cerebral neurons (SAVOLAINEN et al. 1980). Although the functional significance remains unknown, it possibly relates to the action of phenytoin to increase cerebellar Purkinje-cell discharge rates. Its relationship to target-cell toxicity is questionable, especially since the cerebellar atrophy associated with Purkinje-cell loss is more likely the result of hypoxia or other changes associated with severe epilepsy than phenytoin toxicity (DAM 1972).

SIRONI et al. (1980) have reported on the distribution of phenytoin in the brain, plasma, and CSF in 12 surgically treated epileptic patients. They found that the brain: blood concentration ratios were highest in the temporal lobes, lower in the parietal lobes, and lowest in the frontal lobes, providing that white matter and gray matter were combined or if white matter only was measured. The concentration in the temporal lobes was about twice that in the frontal lobes, and about 20% greater than in the parietal lobes. If only gray matter was measured, the rank order was temporal lobes followed by frontal lobes and parietal lobes. The concentrations were higher in white matter than in gray matter, except in the frontal lobes.

Of considerable interest is the observation that the rank or of phenobarbital concentrations in the same brain regions was opposite that for phenytoin: highest concentrations were found in the frontal lobes, followed by the parietal lobes and the temporal lobes. This possibly has significance with respect to the relative selectivity of these drugs in the treatment of temporal lobe epilepsy. While phenytoin is quite effective against these seizures, phenobarbital is of only limited value. However, HOUGHTON et al. (1975) and SHERWIN et al. (1973) reported higher phenytoin concentrations in the frontal and parietal lobes.

SIRONI et al. (1980) also reported that the molar concentration of phenytoin in cerebral cortex was in the therapeutic range or higher for all of their medically refractory patients (i.e., those requiring surgery). This varies with the data of SHERWIN et al. (1977), which show that molar concentrations in cerebral cortex were significantly greater in patients whose seizures were well controlled medically than in those requiring surgery. Furthermore, SIRONI et al. (1980) reported that phenytoin concentration in epileptogenic scar tissue was not significantly different from that in normal tissue, while RAPPORT et al. (1975) and SHERWIN et al. (1977) found a marked decrease in phenytoin binding in such focal lesions. An explanation for these discrepancies is not apparent.

Another observation by SIRONI et al. (1980) was that phenytoin was slightly more concentrated in white matter than in gray matter. The brain: plasma ratio was 1.33 ± 0.48 in white matter, 1.13 ± 0.25 in gray matter, and 1.18 ± 0.35 in white plus gray matter. These data are in general agreement with those of SHERWIN et al. (1973, 1975, 1977), except that the latter authors reported a larger white matter: gray matter ratio (about 1.4–1.6). A similar distribution has been noted in the monkey (VAN DER KLEIJN et al. 1972), and other experimental observations also suggest a greater distribution of phenytoin in white matter (RAPPORT et al. 1975). FIREMARK et al. (1963) demonstrated that phenytoin accumulation in cat brain was greater in gray matter than in white matter during the first 30–60 min after a single 15 mg/kg intravenous dose. However, after 60 min cerebral and cerebellar white matter contained more phenytoin than the gray areas. They showed that the primary factor limiting the rate of accumulation in various brain regions is the blood flow and vascularity.

Several interpretations have been offered to account for a preferential distribution of phenytoin in white matter. Because phenytoin is highly lipophilic, it was suggested that the high lipid content of myelin (which is 2.5 times that of cerebral cortex) might be responsible (SHERWIN et al. 1973). The fact that white matter contains less water than gray matter might also improve the solubility of phenytoin. However, it has been shown by GOLDBERG and TODOROFF (1973) that phenytoin binding in the brain best correlates with protein content. Because the myelinated fibers in white matter contain more protein and proteolipid than the nerve-cell bodies and unmyelinated fibers of gray matter, such can possibly explain the observed distribution.

GOLDBERG and TODOROFF (1973) discussed methodological factors that might account for the apparent selective affinity of phenytoin for myelin. They suggested that such affinity might represent a redistribution phenomenon resulting in some of the drug being removed from other fractions during centrifugation. This is supported by the discrepancy in phenytoin binding observed when binding was studied in previously separated subcellular fractions versus binding after injection in vivo followed by subsequent separation. Using previously isolated fractions, GOLDBERG and TODOROFF (1973) demonstrated that binding to myelin could be related to protein content, as was true for all other brain fractions.

It has also been noted that the concentration of phenytoin in adipose tissue rises when the mobilization of fats from cells in stimulated, as in starvation- or epinephrine-induced lipolysis (ALVIN and BUSH 1977). This provides additional evidence that binding to cellular protein is quantitatively more important than solubility in fat. In fact, GOLDBERG and TODOROFF (1976) have shown that marked enhancement of phenytoin binding to the nonlipid material resulted when brain homogenates were extracted with cholorform-methanol. This was attributed to the possible unmasking of potential protein-binding sites by removing lipid normally associated with those sites (GOLDBERG 1980).

In order to characterize further the properties of phenytoin binding that lead to its prolonged retention in the brain, many investigators have studied various aspects of subcellular distribution. The apparent selective affinity of phenytoin for brain protein, as opposed to lipid, has already been noted. However, KEMP and WOODBURY (1971) found that [^{14}C]phenytoin associated with the nuclear fraction of rat brain shortly after administration and over a 12-h period declined in the nuclear fraction and increased in the microsomal fraction. They suggested that binding was covalent because it could only be released upon alkaline hydrolysis. On the basis of these observations they suggested that phenytoin was incorporated into messenger RNA, which might subsequently influence protein synthesis. Although phenytoin may inhibit protein synthesis in the brain (JONES and WOODBURY 1976; YANAGIHARA and HAMBERGER 1971 a, b), the possible mechanism suggested by KEMP and WOODBURY (1971) has been controversial. Other investigators have reported that phenytoin binding is neither irreversible nor time dependent (i.e., the concentrations decrease in all fractions at approximately equal rates) and that microsomes bind only a small percentage of total radioactivity (GOLDBERG and TODOROFF 1973; NIELSEN and COTTMAN 1971). YANAGIHARA and HAMBERGER (1971 c) found a significant fraction of drug associated with the microsomal fraction of rat brain, but in their study the microsomal binding decreased in unison with the decrease in total brain phenytoin. However, these authors did find a significant amount of phenytoin bound to the nuclear fraction at the earliest measurements (15 min), and the concentration decreased thereafter. On the other hand, the concentration in the microsomal fraction peaked at 30 min (as it did for brain slices and homogenates) and decreased thereafter. Therefore, it is conceivable that some transfer of phenytoin from the nuclear to the microsomal fractions occurs very early, but it is less certain that the transferred material might be covalently bound.

YANAGIHARA and HAMBERGER (1971 c) also reported a greater affinity of phenytoin for a neuronal fraction (nerve-cell bodies) than for a glial fraction. The phenytoin concentration in the glial fraction was only 5%–14% of that in the neuronal fraction. Most of the neuronal [^{14}C] phenytoin activity was associated with neuronal plasma membranes exclusive of the synaptosomal elements. Phenytoin concentrations were lowest in the synaptosomal fraction during the first 30 min of distribution; thereafter, phenytoin concentration in synaptosomes increased, but exceeded only that in the myelin and glial fractions. Much of the microsomal activity was thought to be due to phenytoin selectively bound to neuronal plasma membranes which were sheared from the neuronal structure during preparation. WILENSKY and LOWDEN (1972 b) also reported significant phenytoin binding to microsomes and concluded that the drug binds to all fractions containing plasma membranes. SEEMAN et al. (1972) reported that phenytoin also binds to synaptosomes in vitro.

Interpretation of data on subcellular distribution of phenytoin should be approached with caution. For example, GOLDBERG and TODOROFF (1973) have emphasized the possibility that the apparent selectivity of phenytoin for certain cellular and subcellular fractions might be due to isolation artifacts related to the redistribution of phenytoin during incubation, homogenization, and centrifugation. Another caution that should be applied to those studies that demonstrate a subcellular redistribution of phenytoin concentration is that anticonvulsant actions are often manifest much earlier than the time course of the proposed redistribution. A final caution relates to the false assumption that the active site must necessarily reside in the particular compartment where the drug concentrations are highest. Morphine, for example, does not concentrate in the neuronal tissue where it is thought to act (FISHMAN et al. 1976). Although a fundamental tenet in pharmacology is that dose and response are inextricably related, it is also established that only a very small fraction of the total dose is necessary to elicit a full response. Thus, it is conceivable that phenytoin concentrations in the active-site tissue may be so low as to preclude accurate measurement by sensitive methods.

III. Biotransformation

1. Phenytoin

Phenytoin is metabolized largely by the hydroxylase complex of hepatic endoplasmic reticulum. In man and most other species renal excretion of unchanged phenytoin accounts for less than 5% of an administered dose (BOCHNER et al. 1973). (Normal renal clearance was about 5.6 ml/min in a group of 16 patients.) The major metabolite in man is 5-(*p*-hydroxyphenyl)-5-phenylhydantoin (*p*-HPPH), but smaller amounts of 5-(*m*-hydroxyphenyl)-5-phenylhydantoin (*m*-HPPH), 5-(3,4-dihydroxy-1,5-cyclohexadien-1-yl)-5-phenylhydantoin (a dihydrodiol), diphenylhydantoic acid (DPHA), and catechol metabolites may be formed (Fig. 3) (ALVIN and BUSH 1977). The hydroxy metabolites (*p*-HPPH and *m*-HPPH) are mostly conjugated with glucuronic acid and excreted in urine. There is no evidence for the formation of other conjugates (e.g., sulfates), and other metabolic reactions involving *p*-HPPH (or *m*-HPPH) have not been demonstrated (CHANG and GLAZKO 1972). Renal excretion involves both filtration (free DPH) and tubular secretion. The conjugated metabolites are too polar to be reabsorbed, and are thus quantitatively eliminated from tubular volume. The *O*-glucuronidated metabolites are also secreted into the bile. However, in the intestine the conjugates are hydrolized by the bacterial flora, and the free hydroxy metabolites are then reabsorbed. In fact, such enterohepatic circulation is responsible for a major fraction of the metabolite delivered to the kidney for excretion. Only a very small fraction of an administered dose is normally excreted in feces. The metabolites of phenytoin have little or no anticonvulsant activity.

Metabolic hydroxylation of phenytoin presumably occurs via an arene oxide intermediate. Such intermediates are thought to be involved in all aromatic hy-

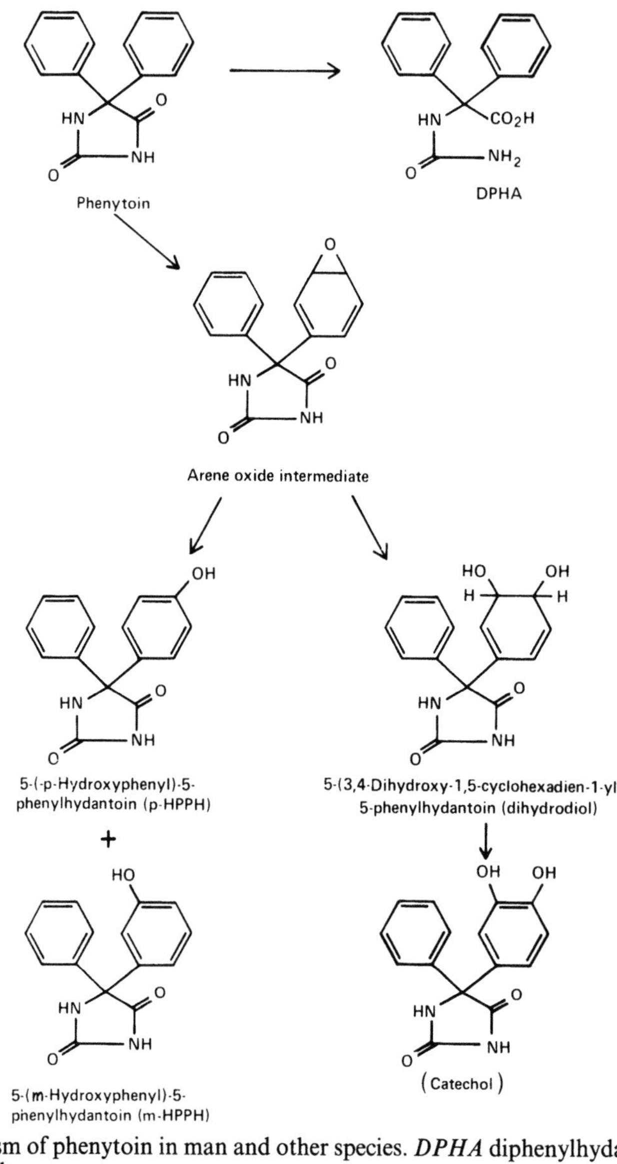

Fig. 3. Metabolism of phenytoin in man and other species. *DPHA* diphenylhydantoic acid. See text for details

droxylations, and may rearrange nonenzymatically in the presence of liver microsomes to phenols (DALY et al. 1969), or they may be enzymatically hydrated to dihydrodiols by epoxide hydrase. The dihydrodiol may be further oxidized to the corresponding catechol, which is then methylated to the 3-*O*-methylcatechol (CHANG et al. 1972). It has been suggested that the free catechol may compete with catecholamine neurotransmitters for 3-*O*-methylation and thereby potentiate the action of the latter (ALVIN and BUSH 1977). Other effects of the catechol metabolite might include the alteration of catecholamine uptake and binding (HADFIELD

1972) and inhibition of the oxidative deamination of catecholamines by monoamine oxidase (AZZARO and GUTRECHT 1973). Hydrolysis of the hydantoin ring (to form DPAH) is thought to be enzymatic, but the details of the reaction have not been established (DUDLEY et al. 1974).

The hydroxylated metabolite *p*-HPPH accounts for 50%–90% of an administered dose of phenytoin in man. As noted above, less than 5% is excreted unchanged; the remainder is excreted as various metabolites, which include *m*-HPPH, DPAH, and dihydrodiol and catechol derivatives. The dihydrodiol and DPAH metabolites are formed only in trace amounts in man, but larger amounts have been reported in urine from rats, mice, cats, rabbits, dogs, and monkeys (CHANG and GLAZKO 1972). HOPPEL et al. (1977) reported that steady-state plasma phenytoin concentrations of 5–30 μg/ml in man were associated with *p*-HPPH levels of 0.04–0.2 μg/ml and *p*-HPPH glucuronide levels of 1.2–4.5 μg/ml. Thus, the plasma *p*-HPPH glucuronide concentrations are about ten times greater than the unconjugated HPPH concentrations. Corresponding dihydrodiol levels were 0.02–0.45 μg/ml. As in man, the major metabolite found in urine from cats, mice, rats, rabbits, and monkeys was *p*-HPPH (CHANG and GLAZKO 1972). However, there is some species variation in the pattern of phenytoin metabolism. For example, the major hydroxylated metabolite in man is *p*-HPPH (about 90% of the total hydroxylated metabolite); *m*-HPPH accounts for only about 7% of the total hydroxylated metabolite (ATKINSON et al. 1970). The estimate for *m*-HPPH is probably high, since some investigators have reported only insignificant amounts of this metabolite. However, the major hydroxylated metabolite in dog is *m*-HPPH (75%), with smaller amounts (25%) of *p*-HPPH formed (ATKINSON et al. 1970).

The rate at which phenytoin is hydroxylated is "dose dependent". Other terms often applied to describe the same phenomenon include "capacity limited" and "saturation" elimination. This implies that metabolism is first-order (i.e., the rate is proportional to concentration) at very low plasma concentrations and zero-order (i.e., the rate is independent of concentration) at very high plasma concentrations. Because the calculation of half-life is based on the assumption that elimination is log linear for all concentrations, the usual concept of half-life cannot be used to describe the time course of plasma phenytoin concentrations. However, it is now known that "dose-dependent" metabolism can be conceptualized and adequately described in the context of Michaelis-Menten kinetics. Therefore, the pharmacokinetics of phenytoin can be characterized by (1) a K_m value (in units of concentration), which represents a whole-body Michaelis constant, and (2) a V_{max} paramater (in units of concentration per unit time), which represents the maximum metabolic rate. The Michaelis-Menten equation for enzyme kinetics can be modified by substituting drug concentration [*D*] for substrate concentration [*S*]. Thus:

$$v = \frac{V_{max}[D]}{K_m + [D]}. \tag{1}$$

At very low plasma phenytoin concentrations, where [*D*] is much smaller than K_m (the plasma concentration at which the enzyme complex is 50% saturated), Eq. (1)

simplifies to:

$$v = \frac{V_{\max}[D]}{K_m} \tag{2}$$

Because $V_{\max}/K_m$ is itself a constant, Eq. (2) clearly describes a first-order process; that is:

$$v = k[D]. \tag{3}$$

Under these conditions, concentration will decrease exponentially with time. The elimination half-life ($T_{1/2}$) is given by:

$$T_{1/2} = \frac{0.693\,K_m}{V_{\max}} \tag{4}$$

which is a simple rearrangement of the equation

$$T_{1/2} = \frac{0.693}{k_e}, \tag{5}$$

where k_e is the first-order elimination rate constant. Eq. (2) is useful when $[D] < 0.1\,K_m$.

On the other hand, at very high plasma phenytoin concentrations (e.g., $[D] > 10\,K_m$), the contribution of K_m becomes insignificant. Under these conditions the modified Michaelis-Menten equation simplifies to:

$$v = \frac{V_{\max}[D]}{[D]} = V_{\max} \tag{6}$$

which is the equation for a zero-order process. The rate, v, is simply $V_{\max}$; increasing the phenytoin concentration will not further increase the metabolic rate. Because concentration will decrease linearly with time under these conditions, the time required for the plasma concentration $[D]$ to decrease by half, T_{50}, is dependent upon the concentration.

$$T_{50} = \frac{[D]}{2 \cdot V_{\max}}. \tag{7}$$

As already noted, the usual concept of half-life cannot be strictly applied to describe the elimination of drugs which exhibit saturation kinetics, because the decay in plasma concentration is not log linear. Therefore, the term "effective half-life" will be used to distinguish T_{50} from a half-life ($T_{1/2}$) in the ordinary pharmacokinetic sense, which subsequently will be referred to simply as "half-life", or $T_{1/2}$. This should be remembered when referring to the experimental T_{50} values in Table 3.

Intermediate plasma concentrations (e.g., those with values in the range $0.1\,K_m < [D] < 10 K_m$) may be characterized by effective half-lives given by:

$$T_{50} = \frac{0.693\,K_m}{V_{\max}} + \frac{[D]}{2 \cdot V_{\max}}. \tag{8}$$

Statistically confident average values for K_m and V_{max} have not been established, but various estimates in different populations range from 1.2 to 24.2 μg/ml (4.8–96 μmol-liter) for K_m, and 155–818 mg/day for V_{max} (RAMBECK et al. 1979). Based upon these values for K_m, first-order kinetics will prevail at concentrations up to 0.12–2.42 μg/ml; nonlinear kinetics will apply at higher concentrations (to 12–242 μg/ml). Increases in plasma concentration up to 0.1 K_m (0.12–2.42 μg/ml) should produce reasonably proportionate increases in metabolic rate, with the result that half-life does not change. However, further increases in concentration (to 12–242 μg/ml) should produce less than proportionate increases in metabolic rate, with the result that effective half-life increases and clearance decreases. Increases in concentration greater than 10 K_m will result in effective half-lives that increase in direct proportion to concentration. Thus, phenytoin metabolism is saturable within the usual therapeutic range of plasma concentrations (10–20 μg/ml). The typical graphic appearance of such behavior is depicted in Fig. 4. A log-linear decline in serum concentration would be expected if the amount of phenytoin metabolized at any one time was determined by its concentration in serum (i.e., first-order kinetics). However, the nonlinear portion of the curve during the early periods of elimination show that the enzyme involved in phenytoin metabolism was saturated at higher concentrations. A gradual change from zero-order to first-order kinetics appears to occur as the concentration decreases.

Because the K_m is so low, the dose-concentration relationship for phenytoin is curvilinear in the therapeutic range of plasma concentrations (Chap. 24, this volume, Fig. 3). The most important clinical consequence of this relationship is that increases in dosage may produce disproportionate increases in plasma concentration, and the dose required to produce an acceptable concentration in the therapeutic range is very close that which will produce toxicity. Thus, a small increase in dose for a patient at the lower end of the therapeutic range might produce a large increase in plasma concentration, resulting in toxicity.

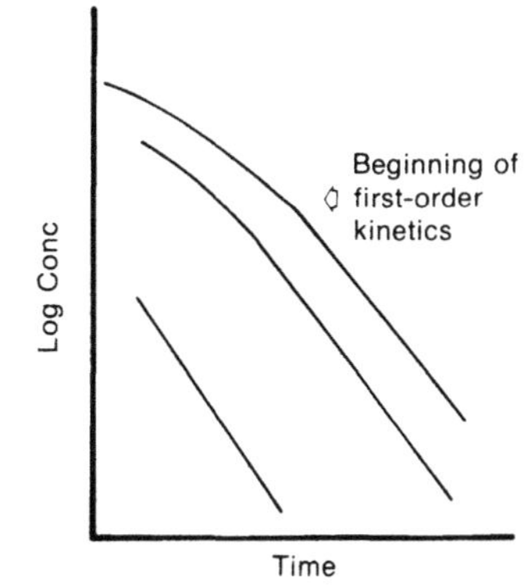

Fig. 4. The expected appearance of plasma decay curves for different concentrations of a drug that displays "dose-dependent" elimination. Low doses are expected to result in log-linear curves, as depicted; larger doses result in a progressive shift to more complex curves, the nonlinear portion of which is due to saturation of the drug-metabolizing enzymes. The depicted curves have been experimentally validated in numerous studies

This can be demonstrated by applying a revised form of Eq. (1), where the metabolic rate (v) is expressed as the daily dose or administration rate (R), and the drug concentration (D) is expressed as the average steady-state plasma concentration C_p:

$$R = \frac{V_{max}[C_p]}{K_m + [C_p]} . \tag{9}$$

This is permissible because the clearance of phenytoin from plasma occurs primarily by metabolism, and at steady state the rate of administration equals the rate of elimination. Assuming relatively low values of K_m and V_{max} of 2 μg/ml and 5 mg/kg per day, respectively, solution of Eq. (9) for daily doses of 200, 300, 320, and 330 mg gives 2.7, 12.0, 21.3, and 33.0 μg/ml plasma concentration, respectively. The calculations were based upon 70 kg body wt. Thus, an increase in dose of just 10% (30 mg/day) might result in an increase in plasma concentration from 12 μg/ml (low therapeutic range) to over 30 μg/ml (toxicity is normally associated with values greater than 30 μg/ml). Unfortunately, the clinical reality imposed by "dose-dependent" kinetics is not mitigated by the relatively narrow therapeutic range (i.e., low therapeutic index) of phenytoin.

The very sensitive relationship between dose and phenytoin concentration is further complicated by significant intersubject variability in the Michaelis-Menten parameters, V_{max} and K_m. The rate at which individual patients metabolize phenytoin appears to be determined genetically, probably by polygenic control (RICHENS 1975). Therefore, the variability in V_{max} and K_m possibly depends on genetic endowment. However, other factors might also contribute to intersubject variability in phenytoin metabolism. These include variables such as age, pregnancy, liver disease, and renal disease. Drug interactions may also be of considerable pharmacokinetic and clinical significance, due in large part to the very steep dose-concentration relationship and narrow therapeutic ratio of phenytoin. Drug interactions are discussed briefly in Sect. G of this chapter, and in further detail in a separate chapter of this volume (Chap. 28).

2. Mephenytoin

The basic and clinical pharmacology of mephenytoin and ethotoin have not been studied in nearly the same detail as for phenytoin. However, a considerable amount of information is now available on the metabolism of these agents. Mephenytoin (3-methyl-5-ethyl-5-phenylhydantoin) is metabolized by hydroxylation to 3-methyl-5-(*p*-hydroxyphenyl)-5-ethylhydantoin (*p*-OH-M) and by *N*-demethylation to the active anticonvulsant Nirvanol (5-ethyl-5-phenylhydantoin) (Fig. 5). Hydroxylation of the parent molecule is presumably achieved by the aromatic hydroxylase complex involved in the metabolism of phenytoin. Subsequent conjugation at the *p*-hydroxy group results in the rapid elimination of this metabolite in urine. The mean half-life of mephenytoin in man was reported by TROUPIN et al. (1979) to be 6.8 h. The mean half-life of the metabolite Nirvanol was shown in the same study to be 95.8 h. With long-term administration, me-

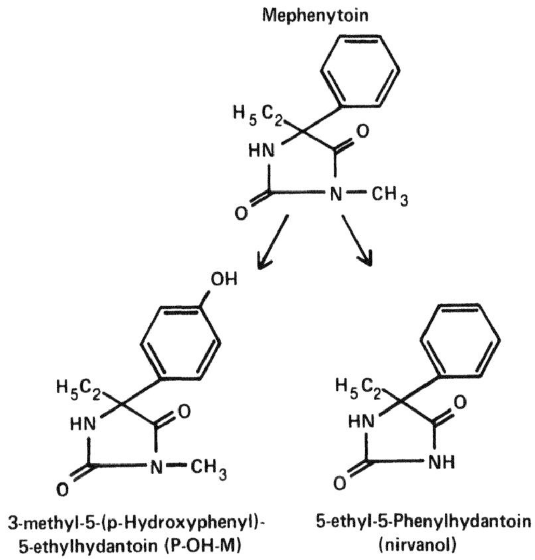

Fig. 5. Metabolism of mephenytoin. See text for details

phenytoin represents less than 10% of the total drug (including metabolites) in the serum. Thus, the clinical value of mephenytoin therapy is attributable to the metabolite Nirvanol. Although itself an anticonvulsant, unchanged mephenytoin has little relationship to the course of antiepileptic therapy or incidence of side effects (TROUPIN et al. 1976). The very long half-life of Nirvanol allows for ease in dosing, with very small fluctuations in plasma concentrations following once-daily administration.

Although it was formerly considered that mephenytoin was rapidly and nearly quantitatively demethylated prior to hydroxylation, recent studies have demonstrated that the major metabolites in dog and human urine are *p*-OH-M and Nirvanol (KUPFER and BIRCHER 1979; KUPFER et al. 1980, 1981); *p*-hydroxylated Nirvanol was not a significant metabolite. Furthermore, the above studies demonstrated a stereoselective basis for mephenytoin metabolism. Mephenytoin hydroxylation in the dog is stereoselective, but the demethylation reaction is not (KUPFER and BIRCHER 1979). In man, both metabolic reactions appear to be stereoselective (KUPFER et al. 1981).

In the human study (KUPFER et al. 1981), mephenytoin was administered as a racemic mixture of equal quantities of *S*- and *R*-enantiomers which were separately labeled with ^{14}C or ^{3}H, respectively. The urinary excretion of *p*-OH-M after a single oral dose of the racemix mixture was rapid, with a cumulative recovery of 45.8 ± 4.7% (mean ± SD) of the total dose in 72 h. In contrast, urinary excretion of Nirvanol was slow, and only 2.9 ± 1.4% of the administered dose was recovered in 72 h. Urinary recovery of the parent drug during the same period accounted for less than 0.5% of the dose. The cumulative recovery of ^{14}C (from the *S*-enantiomer) over the 72-h period was essentially complete (96.8 ± 5.4%). In contrast, the urinary excretion of ^{3}H from the *R*-enantiomer was slower, with only 25.2±4.5% being recovered in 72 h. Most (91%) of the *p*-OH-M present at 72 h was formed from *S*-mephenytoin; 9% was from *R*-mephenytoin. About 71% of the Nirvanol present at 72 h was formed from *R*-mephenytoin; 29% was from *S*-mephenytoin. The authors concluded from these data that the *S*-enantiomer was rapidly excreted, mainly as *p*-OH-M, whereas the *R*-enantiomer was slowly eliminated, mainly as Nirvanol. However, the combined contribution of tritium-labeled Nirvanol and *p*-OH-M during the first 72 h accounted for only 50% of the total tritium in urine. Thus, it is possible that smaller amounts of hydroxlated Nirvanol and other metabolites were also formed.

3. Ethotoin

Early studies demonstrated the existence of at least two distinct pathways for the metabolism of ethotoin (3-ethyl-5-phenylhydantoin). DUDLEY et al. (1970) reported that a major metabolic pathway in the dog involves *N*-deethylation followed by ring opening to form 2-phenylhydantoic acid (Fig. 6). A relatively minor pathway was reported to involve *p*-hydroxylation of the phenyl ring followed by conjugation with glucuronic acid, similar to that described for mephenytoin.

DUDLEY et al. (1970) further reported that racemic mixtures of 5-phenylhydantoin were metabolized in dogs by stereoselective ring-opening to form R(-)-2-phenylhydantoic acid. The enzyme responsible for this conversion was later iden-

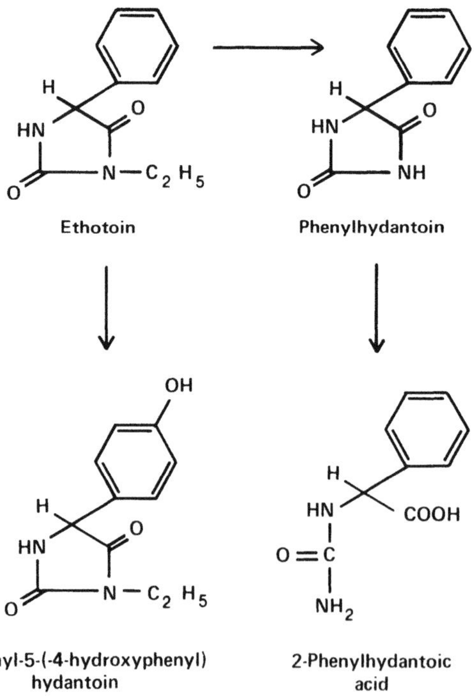

Fig. 6. Metabolism of ethotoin. See text for details

tified as dihydropyrimidinase, and shown to be selective for 5-monosubstituted hydantoins; 5,5-disubstituted and *N*-substituted hydantoins such as mephenytoin and ethotoin are not substrates for the enzyme (DUDLEY et al. 1974). Therefore, it was reasoned that *N*-deethylation of ethotoin must take place for the compound to be metabolized to 2-phenylhydantoic acid. It was also shown that only the R(-)-enantiomer of 5-phenylhydantoin is a substrate for the enzyme; the S(+)-enantiomer must undergo racemization before it can be metabolized by this enzyme (DUDLEY and BIUS 1976).

More recent studies by YONEKAWA et al. (1975) demonstrated the presence of an additional metabolite, *m*-hydroxyethotoin, in urine from epileptic patients. In other respects, their results in epileptic patients were consistent with the data for dog urine reported by DUDLEY et al. (1970). Both groups reported that only very small amounts of unchanged ethotoin appeared in urine.

NAESTOFT and LARSEN (1977) also studied ethotoin metabolism in epileptic patients. They found that *p*-hydroxylation is apparently a major pathway (14% –32% of daily dose) in the degradation of ethotoin; smaller amounts of 5-phenylhydantoin (5%–14%) and very small amounts of unchanged ethotoin (0.2%–2%) were also found. Four other unidentified metabolites were also detected. These were labeled as metabolites III, IV, V, and VI. Metabolite IV accounted for 17%–35% of the daily dose; the remaining metabolites combined accounted for about 0.8%–2% of the daily dose.

Most recently, BIUS et al. (1980) reported the detection in human urine of 11 metabolites of ethotoin. These included unchanged ethotoin, 5-phenylhydantoin, 2-phenylhydantoic acid, *p*-hydroxyethotoin, *m*-hydroxyethotoin, 5-hydroxyethotoin, 5-hydroxy-5-phenylhydantoin, 5-hydroxy-5-(*p*-hydroxyphenyl)-hydantoin, *O*-hydroxyethotoin, 3-methoxy-4-hydroxyethotoin, and a dihydrodiol. Careful analysis permitted the identification of metabolite III from the study of NAESTOFT and LARSEN (1977) as 5-hydroxyethotoin; metabolite IV was identified as 5-hydroxy-5-phenylhydantoin. Metabolites V and VI appeared to be the same as those to which BIUS et al. (1980) assigned the structures of dihydrodiol and 5-hydroxy-5-(*p*-hydroxyphenyl)hydantoin, respectively. There was no evidence for the presence in urine of 5-(*p*-hydroxyphenyl)hydantoin. The identification by BIUS et al. (1980) of the 5-hydroxylation products implies the existence of yet another major pathway for ethotoin metabolism in man, especially since 5-hydroxy-5-phenylhydantoin (metabolite IV) appeared to account for 17%–34% of the administered dose in the study reported by NAESTOFT and LARSEN (1977).

Thus, it would appear that the metabolism of ethotoin is considerably more complex than previously anticipated. Unlike mephenytoin, however, the anticonvulsant activity of ethotoin is apparently due only to the parent compound; the major metabolites lack anticonvulsant efficacy. Therefore, the half-life reported by TROUPIN et al. (1979), 5.1 h in man, can be used as a guide for therapeutic dosage schedules. With such a short half-life (less than 6 h), it will be necessary to administer ethotoin at least four times daily in order to maintain steady-state concentrations without excessive fluctuations in plasma concentration. Dose-dependent elimination kinetics were not observed by TROUPIN et al. (1979) despite an earlier report of such behavior (SJO et al. 1975).

IV. Excretion

Phenytoin is excreted primarily in the urine as the glucuronide conjugate of *p*-HPPH. Not more than 5% (and probably much less) of the drug is excreted unchanged in urine of experimental animals and man. Only small amounts (as free HPPH or HPPH glucuronide) are normally found in feces of all species. There is considerable variability in the values reported for urinary HPPH excretion. In one study in rats about 70% of the total phenytoin dose was excreted as HPPH, and about 25% as other metabolites (NOACH et al. 1958). In a study involving a single human subject, 75% of the dose was accounted for by urinary HPPH in a 5-day period following intravenous administration (GLAZKO et al. 1969). In another study, involving 12 normal human subjects receiving oral dosage, total HPPH recovery in the urine was 64% (GLAZKO and CHANG 1972). Other studies in humans have shown that the amount excreted as HPPH is dose dependent. Total urinary HPPH excretion was 60%–85% after oral administration of 100 mg; it was 76% at 250 mg and only 50% at a dose of 500 mg. In usual clinical doses, 60%–63% of the administered dose is excreted as HPPH (WOODBURY and SWINYARD 1972). However, values much higher and much lower have been reported. In yet another study (CHANG and GLAZKO 1972), the urinary excretion of free and conjugated HPPH, DPHA, and dihydrodiol were compared for six animal species. Whereas only trace amounts of dihydrodiol and DPHA are normally found in human urine, significant amounts of these metabolites may be found in certain species.

A significant fraction of an administered dose is metabolized in the liver and excreted in the bile as a conjugate of glucuronic acid. The conjugate is hydrolyzed by the bacterial flora in the gut, and the free HPPH is reabsorbed and ultimately eliminated in the urine (after being conjugated again in the liver). Evidence for this pathway was presented in Sect. C.II.2 for the rat. Similar evidence is available in rhesus monkeys and dogs (GLAZKO and CHANG 1972). A 5 mg/kg dose of phenytoin was administered intravenously to normal or bile fistula animals. The normal monkey excreted 88% of the dose in the urine and 6% in the feces over a 3-day period; in normal dogs, urinary and fecal excretion was 80.4% and 20.7%, respectively, during the same period. The presence of the drug in feces is evidence for excretion into the intestinal tract, since the drug was administered intravenously. The bile fistula monkey excreted 84% of the dose in the urine, about 10% in the bile, and only a trace in the feces during the 72-h period. The bile fistula dog excreted 54% of the dose in the urine, 34% in the bile, and 1% in the feces. Thus, it is apparent that significant amounts of phenytoin metabolites are excreted from the liver to bile, and the major fraction of the metabolite excreted in bile is reabsorbed from the intestinal tract.

The drug must be in its ionized form to be efficiently excreted. Although unchanged phenytoin might conceivably be excreted at the glomerulus, its extensive binding to plasma proteins will limit the amount filtered, and reabsorption of the lipophilic parent molecule will readily occur in the renal tubules. However, alkalinization of the urine should enhance phenytoin excretion because of a higher percentage of the drug in the ionized form. Active tubular secretion is probably responsible for the excretion of the bulk of phenytoin metabolites.

G. Drug Interactions

There are numerous experimental reports in the literature on drug interactions with hydantoins, especially phenytoin, but their significance for clinical treatment often remains equivocal, not least because the doses used were often clearly in excess of those used in the patient.

Drug interactions observed in patients have been reviewed often, most recently by PERUCCA and RICHENS (1981) and in the section on "Clinical Pharmacology" in this volume.

H. Toxicology

I. Acute Toxicity

1. Animal Studies

Animal data are summarized in Table 4 for the acute toxicity of phenytoin, mephenytoin, and ethotoin. The median toxic dose (TD_{50}) is that which elicits minimal neurological deficit in 50% of the test population. Such deficit was evaluated in most studies (in rodents) by the rotorod test of DUNHAM and MIYA (1957) and presumably reflects dysfunction of the cerebellar-vestibular system. Although Table 4 is not comprehensive, it should serve to illustrate approximate relationships among the drugs, between species, and for various routes of administration. For example, the oral LD_{50} for phenytoin in the mouse is reported to range from 367 to 1,800 mg/kg, while the intraperitoneal LD_{50} ranges from 310 to 360 mg/kg. The oral TD_{50} for phenytoin in the mouse ranges from 71 to 165 mg/kg; the intraperitoneal TD_{50} ranges from 66 to 74 mg/kg. The oral LD_{50} reported by RAINES et al. (1973) for phenytoin (1,800 mg/kg, mouse) contrasts significantly with values reported by FINK and SWINYARD (1959) or NAKAMURA et al. (1965), which were 490 and 367 mg/kg, respectively (Table 4). RAINES et al. (1973) suggested that the discrepancy between their value and that reported by FINK and SWINYARD (1959) might be due to differences in mouse strain (CFW versus CF1, respectively). Furthermore, it was noted that FINK and SWINYARD (1959) administered phenytoin as the sodium salt, while the study by RAINES et al. (1973) employed the free acid. Thus, significant differences in bioavailability might be responsible for the large variance in LD_{50} values. It should be emphasized that many factors other than species and route of administration might influence experimental TD_{50} and LD_{50} values. This was discussed in Sect. C.I.1 in the context of anticonvulsant potency in small rodents (Table 1).

2. Human Data

Although cases of phenytoin intoxication are not uncommon, relatively few deaths have occurred as a result of acute overdose. After acute ingestion of 2.8 g phenytoin by a $2^1/_2$-year-old child, a maximum blood concentration of 112 μg/ml was observed, at which time the patient was comatose (TENCKHOFF et al. 1968). A $4^1/_2$-year-old girl died 3 days after ingesting 2 g phenytoin. A blood sample drawn 24 h after the onset of symptoms revealed a phenytoin concentration of 94 μg/ml. Postmortem findings were: blood, 45 μg/ml; brain, 78 μg/ml; kidney,

Table 4. Acute and chronic toxicity of hydantoin derivatives in various animal species

Derivative	TD_{50}[a] (mg/kg)	LD_{50}[b] (mg/kg)	Species	Route of administration	Refs.
Phenytoin	74.3	–	Mouse	i.p.	WITIAK et al. (1972)
	65.5	–	Mouse	i.p.	KRALL et al. (1978b)
	ca. 95	–	Mouse	s.c.	SWINYARD et al. (1952)
	165	–	Mouse	p.o.	GESLER et al. (1961)
	110	–	Mouse	p.o.	WOLF et al. (1962)
	71	–	Mouse	p.o.	NAKAMURA et al. (1965)
	134	–	Rat	i.p.	HARNED et al. (1953)
	ca. 130	–	Rat	s.c.	SWINYARD et al. (1952)
	180	–	Rabbit	i.p.	TOMAN et al. (1946)
	40	–	Cat	i.p.	TOMAN et al. (1946)
	–	310	Mouse	i.p.	NAKAMURA et al. (1965)
	–	360	Mouse	i.p.	CARRAZ and EMIN (1967)
	–	490	Mouse	p.o.	FINK and SWINYARD (1959)
	–	1,000	Mouse	p.o.	GESLER et al. (1961)
	–	367	Mouse	p.o.	NAKAMURA et al. (1965)
	–	1,800	Mouse	p.o.	RAINES et al. (191973)
	–	350	Rat	i.p.	NAKAMURA et al. (1965)
	–	2,500	Rat	p.o.	NAKAMURA et al. (1965)
Mephenytoin	154	–	Mouse	i.p.	KRALL et al. (1978b)
	ca. 95	–	Mouse	p.o.	SWINYARD et al. (1952)
	ca. 80	–	Mouse	p.o.	BROWN et al. (1953)
	200	–	Mouse	p.o.	WOLF et al. (1962)
	50	–	Rat	i.p.	GOODMAN et al. (1948)
	ca. 140	–	Rat	p.o.	SWINYARD et al. (1952)
	–	317	Mouse	i.p.	NAKAMURA et al. (1965)
	–	1,460	Mouse	p.o.	SCHOEGL et al. (1961)
	–	475	Mouse	p.o.	NAKAMURA et al. (1965)
	–	560	Mouse	p.o.	BARNES and ELTHERINGTON (1966)
	–	300	Rat	i.p.	NAKAMURA et al. (1965)
	–	270	Rat	i.p.	BARNES and ELTHERINGTON (1966)
	–	2,500	Rat	p.o.	NAKAMURA et al. (1965)
	–	340	Rabbit	p.o.	BARNES and ELTHERINGTON (1966)
	–	190	Cat	p.o.	BARNES and ELTHERINGTON (1966)
Ethotoin	171	–	Mouse	i.p.	KRALL et al. (1978b)
	400	–	Mouse	p.o.	MILLICHAP (1972)
	–	2,000	Mouse	p.o.	MILLICHAP (1972)

[a] Median neutrotoxic dose, i.e., that dose eliciting minimal neurological deficit (rotorod) in 50% of the test population
[b] Median lethal dose

112 μg/ml; and liver, 272 μg/ml (LAUBSCHER 1966). The toxicity data available for mephenytoin and ethotoin are related primarily to chronic administration. Further descriptions of the human toxicology of antiepileptics are provided in a separate chapter in this volume.

II. Chronic Toxicity Studies

Because phenytoin received early clinical acceptance following its introduction by MERRITT and PUTNAM (1938 b), much of its toxicity was encountered for the first time in man. Consequently, most animal studies of hydantoin toxicology were undertaken to explain clinical observations reported in man. Similar to its acute toxicity, the most frequent toxicity associated with chronic phenytoin therapy is referable to the central nervous system and is dose related. Symptoms usually disappear soon after dosage is discontinued and can be correlated with plasma drug concentrations. The incidence of intoxication with increasing dosage is similar in both animals and man (DAM 1966). Nystagmus and ataxia have been investigated in pigs (DAM 1966), mice (DEL CERRO and SNIDER 1967), and cats and rats (KOKENGE et al. 1965). In these studies phenytoin dosage was increased until signs of toxicity appeared and dosage was continued for periods ranging from a few days to a month. In each case, the plasma phenytoin concentrations were 25–50 μg/ml when toxicity first appeared, which is similar to observations in man. In addition to these effects on the cerebellar-vestibular system, a syndrome termed "diphenylhydantoin encephalopathy" has been documented as a dose-related toxicity. This syndrome, which is thought to represent an action on "higher" cerebral activity, is described in more detail in the section on "Clinical Pharmacology" in this volume. Another toxic effect of chronic phenytoin therapy is the peripheral neuropathy that has been occasionally observed, especially in patients 40–50 years of age. This effect is also discussed in the section on "Clinical Pharmacology."

Although the above effects are generally regarded as dose related, and usually subside after withdrawal of the drug, there have been several reports of ataxia persisting for as long as 6 months after withdrawal (LIVINGSTON 1957; HABERLAND 1962; KOKENGE et al. 1965). UTTERBACK et al. (1958) reported that ataxia produced in cats given 8 mg/kg phenytoin for 10 days was irreversible and that doses of 30 mg/kg per day produced widespread loss of cerebellar Purkinje cells. Gliosis and other histological changes were also noted. KOKENGE et al. (1965) described a loss of Purkinje cells in both rats and cats receiving high doses of phenytoin; and also noted edema of Bergmann's glial layer. Similar losses of cerebellar Purkinje cells were reported in rats administered 10–40 mg phenytoin daily for 10 weeks (DEL CERRO and SNIDER 1967).

However, DAM (1972) provides evidence that phenytoin, in therapeutic or toxic doses, does not cause changes in Purkinje-cell density or glial-cell ultrastructure. Studies were conducted in pigs, monkeys, and rats, each receiving toxic doses of phenytoin for variable lengths of time. There was no difference in the density of Purkinje cells in treated and untreated animals in all three species. Furthermore, no gliosis was detected as was noted in previous studies (UTTERBACK et al. 1958). DAM (1972) noted that in the studies of KOKENGE et al. (1965) and

SNIDER and DEL CERRO (1967) many of the rats receiving high doses of phenytoin were comatose and died during the experimental period. Thus, the morphological changes described by these authors were probably secondary to hypoxia. DAM (1972) also performed studies in brains from autopsied epileptic patients. His findings were consistent with severe Purkinje-cell loss, but these changes were related to severe grand mal epilepsy rather than phenytoin toxicity.

Another well-documented effect of chronic phenytoin therapy in humans is gingival hyperplasia (Sect. H.V). DAM (1972) confirmed similar effects in both pigs and monkeys. This effect, which appears to be related more to duration of therapy than dose, is thought to be due to both inhibition of collagen catabolism (HOUCK 1970) and lowered defense mechanisms (via reduced folate and IgA levels) (HASSELL et al. 1979).

III. Teratogenic Effects

The frequency of malformation in progeny of mothers that received phenytoin during pregnancy has prompted concern over its possible teratogenic effects. The most consistent observations have involved mild to moderate retardation of both physical and mental indices, and dysmorphic facies, consisting of a short nose, low nasal bridge, and a mild ocular hypertelocism (HANSON et al. 1976; WAZIRI et al. 1976). The growth deficiency tends to be dysharmonic, of greater severity in the distal phalanges. Cleft lip and/or cleft palate, ptosis of the eyelid, and cardiac defects are also occasionally seen in this disorder, which has frequently been referred to as the "fetal hydantoin syndrome" (HANSON et al. 1976; PINTO et al. 1977). Although it is possible that the natural frequency of such defects in offspring of epileptic mothers might account for the apparent drug effects (SHAPIRO et al. 1976), HANSON et al. (1976) dispute this suggestion. Indeed, FRITZ et al. (1976) reported a 9.3% incidence of cleft palate in mice treated with 170 mg/kg phenytoin during the period of organogenesis (days 6–15 of gestation). The spontaneous incidence of this type of malformation in mice is about 0.13%. FRITZ et al. (1976) also reported lethal effects on the early postimplantation stages of embryonic development, but no significant effect on later embryonic deaths (resorptions). There was evidence for retardation of fetal growth following the 170 mg/kg dosage.

Others also dispute the idea that epilepsy per se is the decisive factor in the etiology of "fetal hydantoin syndrome". Using an animal model (inbred mice with spontaneous seizures controllable with phenytoin) thought to reproduce the malformations associated with the syndrome, FINNELL (1981) provided convincing evidence that phenytoin, not the presence of a maternal seizure disorder, is responsible for the increased incidence of congenital defects.

Phenytoin and/or its metabolite has been reported to bind covalently to maternal and fetal tissue (HASSELL et al. 1979). These investigators suggested that *p*-HPPH (via an epoxide intermediate) could bind covalently with critical molecules in the fetus and induce dysmorphic changes. This hypothesis has been supported by studies in pregnant mice treated with an inhibitor of epoxide hydratase. This group of animals demonstrated a high incidence of fetal anomalies when compared with appropriate controls.

IV. Mutagenic Effects

There is no substantive data to indicate that phenytoin produces significant mutagenicity.

V. Other Toxic Effects

Phenytoin may produce hypocalcemia and osteomalacia associated with alterations in vitamin D metabolism (ASHWORTH and HORN 1977; WINNACKER et al. 1977). The severity of this effect seems to be related in part to total drug dosage and duration of therapy. Enzyme induction by phenytoin results in increased metabolism of vitamin D and its active metabolites, which are essential for calcium absorption and disposition. In addition, phenytoin blocks the absorption of calcium from the intestine, resulting in significant alteration of the physiological disposition of calcium (CASPAR 1972). These processes are the presumed mechanisms for bone demineralization and related pathology associated with phenytoin therapy.

Hyperglycemia and glucosuria have been associated with phenytoin intoxication (SAID et al. 1968), but in the majority of patients this effect is associated with high plasma drug concentrations (MALHERBE et al. 1972). Plasma phenytoin concentrations of 75 μg/ml have been associated with hyperglycemia in animals and complete inhibition of insulin release from pancreatic islet cells in pancreatic perfusion studies (LEVIN et al. 1970). However, other studies have shown that plasma phenytoin levels of 5–22 μg/ml do not cause hyperglycemia, and that oral loading doses of glucose given subjects receiving phenytoin produced no difference in the blood sugar versus time curve when compared with a control group not receiving phenytoin (CUMMINGS et al. 1973). For further discussion of this effect, see Sect. E.IV.

It is well established that patients on phenytoin therapy demonstrate altered thyroid function tests while remaining euthyroid. The concentration of protein-bound iodine, total thyroxine, and free thyroxine are significantly reduced (CAPLAN et al. 1977). In some studies, triiodothyronine (T_3) concentrations and T_3 uptake have been found to be altered, while others have not demonstrated any significant change in these parameters; the same is true for thyrotropin (TSH) levels (HANSEN et al. 1974; HEYMA et al. 1977). While in vitro tests have demonstrated competitive displacement of thyroxine (T_4) to thyroxine-binding globulin by phenytoin, prospective studies have shown that total and free T_4 remain lower even 1 month after phenytoin had been discontinued (HEYMA et al. 1977). The latter study makes attractive the idea that lowered T_4 levels are the result of accelerated degradation of T_4 via increased glucuronidation and biliary, urinary, and fecal excretion, rather than direct displacement of thyroxine from the binding sites by phenytoin (MENDOZA et al. 1966).

Serum and cerebrospinal fluid folate levels may be reduced by as much as 50% in patients taking phenytoin or other antiepileptic medications (REYNOLDS 1975). However, folate-deficiency (megaloblastic) anemia occurs in less than 1% of patients taking phenytoin. Although the mechanism is not clear, impaired folate synthesis and/or impaired folate absorption is the most probable cause.

Other effects associated with phenytoin therapy include a possible coagulation deficiency (Solomon et al. 1975), lymphadenopathy (Rausing 1978), hirsutism (Merritt and Putnam 1939), gingival hyperplasia (Gardner et al. 1962), and various hypersensitivity and hematological reactions. While gingival hyperplasia may occur in as much as 20% of the population on chronic medication, the other effects are quite rare. Possible hypersensitivity reactions include skin rash (1%–5% of patients taking phenytoin), serum sickness (Mull and Mollinex 1966), Stevens-Johnson syndrome (Bianchine et al. 1968), lupus erythematosus, and hepatitis. Possible hematological reactions (most of which are thought to have an immunological basis) include aplastic anemia (Best 1963), pancytopenia (Chanarin 1969), leucopenia, agranulocytosis (Livingston 1966), thrombocytopenia (Weintraub et al. 1963), and erythroid aplasia (Yunis et al. 1967).

Toxicity or side effects generally occur less frequently with ethotoin than with phenytoin or mephenytoin. Those that do occur include skin rash, anorexia and vomiting, drowsiness, nystagmus, and occasionally lymphadenopathy. Ataxia occurs only with large doses of ethotoin, and gum hyperplasia and hirsutism are not reported. Mephenytoin causes less nausea and vomiting, less ataxia, and less gum hyperplasia than phenytoin, but these advantages are offset by a greater tendency to drowsiness and a higher incidence of serious dermatitis (Loscalzo 1952), blood dyscrasias (Abbott and Schwab 1954), and hepatitis, some reactions being fatal.

References

Abbott JA, Schwab RS (1954) Mesantoin in the treatment of epilepsy; a study of its effects on the leukocyte count in seventy-nine cases. N Engl J Med 250:197–199

Achari G, Sinha SP (1967) Anticonvulsant property of a new hydantoin derivative. J Indian Med Assoc 49:115–117

Agarwal P, Blake MI (1968) Determination of the pK_a' value for 5,5-diphenylhydantoin. J Pharm Sci 57:1434–1435

Alvan G, Bertler A, Eeg-Olofsson O, Karlsson E, Sjoqvist F, Tomson G (1975) Biological availability – a comparison of three phenytoin preparations. Läkartidningen 72:2621–2623

Alvin JD, Bush MT (1977) Physiological disposition of anticonvulsants. In: Vida JA (ed) Anticonvulsants. Medicinal chemistry, vol 15. Academic, New York, pp 113–150

Anderson RJ, Sternberg JC (1978) A rate nephelometer for immunoprecipitin measurement of specific serum proteins. In: Ritchie RF (ed) Automated immunoanalysis 2. Marcel Dekker, New York, pp 409–469

Atkinson AJ, MacGee J, Strong J, Garteiz D, Gaffney TE (1970) Identification of 5-*meta*-hydroxyphenyl-5-phenyl-hydantoin as a metabolite of diphenylhydantoin. Biochem Pharmacol 19:2483–2491

Ashworth B, Horn DB (1977) Evidence of osteomalacia in an outpatient group of adult epileptics. Epilepsia 18:37–43

Ayala GF, Johnston D (1980) Antiepileptic drugs: phenytoin: electrophysiological studies in simple neuronal systems. In: Glaser GH, Penry JK, Woodbury DM (eds) Antiepileptic drugs: mechanisms of action. Raven, New York, pp 339–351

Ayala GF, Lin G, Johnston D (1977a) The mechanism of action of diphenylhydantoin on invertebrate neurons: I. Effects on basic membrane properties. Brain Res 121:245–258

Ayala GF, Johnston D, Lin S, Dichter HN (1977b) The mechanism of action of diphenylhydantoin on invertebrate neurons. II. Effects on synaptic mechanisms. Brain Res 121:259–270

Azzaro AJ, Gutrecht JA (1973) The effect of diphenylhydantoin (DPH) on the in vitro accumulation and catabolism of H^3-*l*-norepinephrine (H^3-NE) in cerebral cortex slices. Neurology 23:431
Baker PF, Hodgkin AC, Ridgway EF (1971) Depolarization and calcium entry in squid giant axons. J Physiol (Lond) 218:709–755
Barnes CD, Eltherington LG (1966) Drug dosage in laboratory animals – a handbook. University of California Press, Berkeley
Barnes TC (1954) Effect of anticonvulsive drugs on electroencephalographic response to flickering light in unanesthetized rabbits. Fed Proc Fed Am Soc Exp Biol 13:333–334
Barth N, Alvan G, Borga O, Sjoqvist F (1976) Two fold interindividual variation in plasma protein binding of phenytoin in patients with epilepsy. Clin Pharmacokinet 1:444–452
Bashour FA, Jones RE, Edmonson R (1965) Ventricular tachycardia in acute myocardial infarction. Preliminary report on the prophylactic use of Dilantin. Clin Res 13:399
Baskin SI, Dutta S, Marks BH (1973) The effects of diphenylhydantoin and potassium on the biological activity of ouabain in the guinea pig heart. Br J Pharmacol 47:85–96
Bazemore RP, Zuckermann EC (1974) On the problem of diphenylhydantoin-induced seizures. Arch Neurol 31:243–249
Bernstein H, Gold H, Lang TW, Papelbaum S, Bazika V, Corday E (1965) Sodium diphenylhydantoin in the treatment of recurrent cardiac arrhythmias. JAMA 191:695–697
Best WR (1963) Drug associated blood dyscrasias. JAMA 185:286–290
Bianchi C, Beani L, Bertelli A (1975) Effects of some anti-epileptic drugs on brain acetylcholine. Neuropharmacology 14:327–332
Bianchine JR, Macaraeg PVJ Jr, Lasagna L, Azarnoff DL, Brunk SF, Hvidberg EF, Owen JA Jr (1968) Drugs as etiologic factors in the Stevens-Johnson syndrome. Am J Med 44:390–405
Biltz H (1908) Über die Konstitution der Einwirkungsprodukte von substituierten Harnstoffen auf Benzil und über einige neue Methoden zur Darstellung der 5,5-Diphenylhydantoine. Ber Dtsch Chem Ges 41:1379
Bius DL, Yonekawa WD, Kupferberg HJ, Cantor F, Dudley KH (1980) Gas chromatographic-mass spectrometric studies on the metabolic fate of ethotoin in man. Drug Metab Dispos 8:223–229
Bochner F, Hooper WD, Sutherland JM, Eadie MJ, Tyrer JH (1973) The renal handling of diphenylhydantoin and 5-(*p*-hydroxyphenyl)-5-phenylhydantoin. Clin Pharmacol Ther 14:791–796
Boobis SW (1977) Alteration of plasma albumin in relation to decreased drug binding in uremia. Clin Pharmacol Ther 22:147–153
Booker HE, Darcey B (1973) Serum concentrations of free diphenylhydantoin and their relationship to clinical intoxication. Epilepsia 14:177–184
Bowdle TA, Neal GD, Levy RH, Heimbach DM (1980) Phenytoin pharmacokinetics in burned rats and plasma protein binding of phenytoin in burned patients. J Pharmacol Exp Ther 213:97–99
Brodie DC, Huitric AC, Kumler WD (1958) Some anticonvulsant skeletal muscle relaxing, and toxic properties of a series of substituted cyclohexanones. J Am Pharm Assoc Sci Ed 47:240–244
Brodows RG, Campbell RG (1974) Control of refractory fasting hypoglycemia in a patient with suspected insulinoma with diphenylhydantoin. J Clin Endocrinol Metab 38:159–161
Brown WC, Schiffman DO, Swinyard EA, Goodman LS (1953) Comparative assay of antiepileptic drugs by "psychomotor" seizure test and minimal electroshock threshold test. J Pharmacol Exp Ther 107:273–283
Buchthal F, Lennox-Buchthal MA (1972) Relation of anticonvulsant effect to concentration in serum. In: Woodbury DM, Penry JK, Schmidt RP (eds) Antiepileptic drugs. Raven, New York, pp 193–209
Camerman A, Camerman N (1971 a) The stereochemical basis of anticonvulsant drug action. I. The crystal and molecular structure of diphenylhydantoin, a noncentrosymmetric structure solved by centric symbolic addition. Acta Crystallogr 27:2205–2211

Camerman A, Camerman N (1972a) The stereochemical basis of anticonvulsant drug action. II. Molecular structure of diazepam. J Am Chem Soc 94:268–272
Camerman A, Camerman N (1975) The stereochemical basis of anticonvulsant drug action. V. The crystal and molecular structure of sulthiame. Can J Chem 53:2194–2198
Camerman A, Camerman N (1977) Ethylphenacemide and phenacemide: conformational similarities to diphenylhydantoin and stereochemical basis of anticonvulsant activity. Proc Natl Acad Sci USA 74:1264–1266
Camerman A, Camerman N (1980) Stereochemical similarities in chemically different antiepileptic drugs. In: Glaser GH, Penry JK, Woodbury DM (eds) Antiepileptic drugs: mechanism of action. Raven, New York, pp 223–231
Camerman N, Camerman A (1971b) The stereochemical basis of anticonvulsant drug action. III. The structure of procyclidine hydrochloride. Mol Pharmacol 7:406–412
Camerman N, Camerman A (1972b) The stereochemical basis of anticonvulsant drug action IV. The crystal and molecular structure of trihexyphenidyl. J Am Chem Soc 94:8553–8556
Caplan RH, Mordon R, Kristoff K, Wickus G (1977) Diphenylhydantoin effects on thyroid function tests. Ann Neurol 1:603–604
Carraz G, Emin N (1967) Action anticonvulsivante du monouréide de l'acide di-*n*-propylacétique et du dérivé hydantoinique de cet acide. Therapie 22:641–652
Caspary WF (1972) Inhibition of intestinal calcium transport by diphenylhydantoin in rat duodenum. Naunyn Schmiedebergs Arch Pharmacol 274:146–153
Chanarin I (1969) The megaloblastic anaemias. Oxford, Blackwell
Chang T, Glazko AJ (1972) Diphenylhydantoin: biotransformation. In: Woodbury DM, Penry JK, Schmidt RP (eds) Antiepileptic drugs. Raven, New York, pp 149–162
Chang T, Okerholm RA, Glazko AJ (1972) A 3-*O*-methylated catechol metabolite of diphenylhydantoin (Dilantin) in rat urine. Res Commun Chem Pathol Pharmacol 4:13–23
Chen G, Ensor CR (1950) Evaluation of antiepileptic drugs. Arch Neurol Psychiatry 63:56–60
Chou CC, Kuiper DH, Hsieh CP (1972) Effects of diphenylhydantoin on motility and compliance of the canine ileum and colon. Gastroenterology 62:734
Clein NW (1945) New anticonvulsant in treatment of epilepsy (3-methyl 5,5-phenylethylhydantoin) (Hydantal). Preliminary report. Northwest Med 44:210–212
Close WJ, Spielman MA (1961) Anticonvulsant drugs. In: Hartung WH (ed) Medicinal chemistry, vol 5. Wiley, New York, pp 1–249
Cohen MS, Bower RH, Fidler SM, Hohnsonbaugh RE, Sode J (1973) Inhibition of insulin release by diphenylhydantoin and diazoxide in a patient with benign insulinoma. Lancet 1:40–41
Colburn WA, Gibaldi M (1977) Plasma protein binding and metabolic clearance of phenytoin in the rat. J Pharmacol Exp Ther 203:500–506
Collins AJ, Horlington M (1969) A sequential screening test based on the running component of audiogenic seizures in mice, including reference compound PD50 values. Br J Pharmacol 37:140–150
Collins RL (1972) Audiogenic seizures. In: Purpura DP, Penry JK, Tower DB, Woodbury DM, Walter RD (eds) Experimental models of epilepsy. A manual for the laboratory worker. Raven, New York, pp 347–372
Cook CE, Kepler JA, Christensen HD (1973) Antiserum to diphenylhydantoin: preparation and characterization. Res Commun Chem Pathol Pharmacol 5:767–774
Cook CE, Christensen HD, Amerson Ew, Kepler JA, Tallent CR, Taylor GF (1976) Radioimmunoassay of anticonvulsant drugs: phenytoin, phenobarbital and primidone. In: Kellaway P, Petersen I (eds) Quantitative analytic studies in epilepsy. Raven, New York, pp 39–58
Cranford RE, Leppik IE, Patrick B, Anderson CB, Kostick B (1977) Intravenous phenytoin: clinical and pharmacokinetic aspects. Neurology (Minneap) 27:376
Cummings NP, Rosenbloom AL, Kohler WC, Wilder BJ (1973) Plasma glucose and insulin response to oral glucose with chronic diphenylhydantoin therapy. Pediatrics 51:1091–1093

Daly J, Jerina D, Witkop B, Zaltzman-Nirenberg P, Udenfriend S (1969) Identification of 1,2-naphthalene oxide as an intermediate in the enzymatic conversion of naphthalene to naphthol and naphthalene-1,2-dihydrodiol. Fed Proc Fed Am Soc Exp Biol 28:546

Dam M (1966) Organic changes in phenytoin-intoxicated pigs. Acta Neurol Scand 42:491–494

Dam M (1972) Diphenylhydantoin: neurologic aspects of toxicity. In: Woodbury DM, Penry JK, Schmidt RP (eds) Antiepileptic drugs. Raven, New York, pp 227–235

Davis CM, Fenimore DC (1981) Rapid microanalysis of anticonvulsants by high performance thin layer chromatography. J Chromatogr 222:265–270

Dayton PG, Cucinell SA, Weiss M, Perel JM (1967) Dose-dependence of drug plasma level decline in dogs. J Pharmacol Exp Ther 158:305–316

Deisz RA, Lux HD (1977) Diphenylhydantoin prolongs post-synaptic inhibition and iontophoretic GABA action in the crayfish stretch receptor. Neurosci Lett 5:199–203

Del Cerro MP, Snider RS (1967) Studies on Dilantin intoxication. I. Ultrastructural analogies with the lipoidoses. Neurology (Minneap) 17:452–466

DeLorenzo RJ (1977) Antagonistic action of diphenylhydantoin and calcium on the level of phosphorylation of particular rat and human brain proteins. Brain Res 134:125–138

DeLorenzo RJ (1980) Antiepileptic drugs: phenytoin: calcium- and calmodulin-dependent protein phosphorylation and neurotransmitter release. In: Glaser GH, Penry JK, Woodbury DM (eds) Antiepileptic drugs: mechanism of action. Raven, New York, pp 399–414

Deupree JD (1977) The role or non-role of ATPase activation by phenytoin in the stabilization of excitable membranes. Epilepsia 18:309–315

DeWeer P (1980) Antiepileptic drugs: phenytoin: blockage of resting sodium channels. In: Glaser GH, Penry JK, Woodbury DM (eds) Antiepileptic drugs: mechanisms of action. Raven, New York, pp 353–361

Dill WA, Kazenko A, Wolf LM, Glazko AJ (1956) Studies of 5,5-diphenylhydantoin (Dilantin) in animals and man. J Pharmacol Exp Ther 118:270–279

Druckman R, Moore FJ (1955) Effects of sodium diphenylhydantoinate upon isolated small intestine of the rabbit. Proc Soc Exp Biol Med 90:173–176

Dudley KH, Bius DL (1976) Buffer catalysis of the racemization reaction of some 5-phenylhydantoins and its relation to the in vivo metabolism of ethotoin. Drug Metab Dispos 4:340–348

Dudley KH, Bius DL, Butler TC (1970) Metabolic fates of 3-ethyl-5-phenylhydantoin (ethotoin, Peganone),3-methyl-5-phenylhydantoin and 5-phenylhydantoin. J Pharmacol Exp Ther 175:27–37

Dudley KH, Butler TC, Bius DL (1974) The role of dihydropyrimidinase in the metabolism of some hydantoin and succinimide drugs. Drug Metab Dispos 2:103–112

Dunham NW, Miya TS (1957) A note on a simple apparatus for detecting neurological deficit in rats and mice. J Am Pharm Assoc Sci Ed 46:208–209

Ehrnebo M, Agurell S, Jalling B, Boreus LO (1971) Age differences in drug binding by plasma proteins: studies on human foetuses, neonates and adults. Eur J Clin Pharmacol 3:189–193

Esplin DW (1957) Effects of diphenylhydantoin on synaptic transmission in cat spinal cord and stellate ganglion. J Pharmacol Exp Ther 120:301–323

Fabrykant M, Pacella BL (1948) Labile diabetes: electroencephalographic status and effect of anticonvulsive therapy. Ann Intern Med 29:860–877

Fenimore DC, Davis CM (1978) Simultaneous determination of phenobarbital and diphenylhydantoin in blood plasma by high performance thin layer chromatography. J High Resolut Chromatogr Commun 1:105–106

Ferrendelli JA (1980) Antiepileptic drugs: phenytoin: cyclic nucleotide regulation in the brain. In: Gasler GH, Penry JK, Woodbury DM (eds) Antiepileptic drugs: mechanisms of action. Raven, New York, pp 429–433

Ferrendelli JA, Kinscherf DA (1977) Phenytoin: effects on calcium flux and cyclic nucleotides. Epilepsia: 18:331–336

Festoff BW, Appel SH (1968) Effect of diphenylhydantoin on synaptosome sodium-potassium-ATPase. J Clin Invest 47:2752–2758

Fichman MP, Kleeman CR, Bethune JE (1970) Inhibition of antidiuretic hormone secretion of diphenylhydantoin. Arch Neurol 22:45–53

Fink GB, Swinyard EA (1959) Modification of maximal audiogenic and electroshock seizures in mice by psychopharmacologic drugs. J Pharmacol Exp Ther 127:318–324

Finnell RH (1981) Phenytoin-induced teratogenesis: a mouse model. Science 211:483–484

Firemark H, Barlow CF, Roth LJ (1963) The entry, accumulation and binding of diphenylhydantoin-2-C^{14} in brain. Int J Neuropharmacol 2:25–38

Fishman J, Hahn EF, Norton BI (1976) N-Demethylation of morphine in rat brain is localized in sites with high opiate receptor content. Nature 261:64–65

Fredholm BB, Rane A, Persson B (1975) Diphenylhydantoin binding to proteins in plasma and its dependence on free fatty acid and bilirubin concentration in dogs and newborn infants. Pediatr Res 9:26–30

Frey HH, Löscher W (1980) Clinical pharmacokinetics of phenytoin in the dog: a reevaluation. Am J Vet Res 41:1635–1638

Frey HH, Löscher W, Reiche R, Schultz D (1981) Pharmacology of antiepileptic drugs in the gerbil I. Pharmacokinetics. Neuropharmacology 20:769–771

Fritz H, Müller D, Hess R (1976) Comparative study of the teratogenecity of phenobarbitone, diphenylhydantoin and carbamazepine in mice. Toxicology 6:323–330

Gabler WL, Hubbard GH (1973) The metabolism of 5,5-diphenylhydantoin (DPH) in non-pregnant and pregnant rhesus monkeys. Arch Int Pharmacodyn Ther 203:72–91

Gardner A, Gross S, Wunne L (1962) An investigation of gingival hyperplasia resulting from Dilantin therapy in 77 mentally retarded patients. Exp Med Surg 20:133–135

Gauldie J, Bienenstock J (1978) Automated nephelometric analysis of haptens. In: Ritchie RF (ed) Automated immunoanalysis 1. Marcel Dekker, New York, pp 321–333

Gayet-Hallion T (1944) Action de certains anticonvulsivants sur le muscle lisse. CR Soc Biol (Paris) 138:332–334

Gerich JE, Charles MA, Levin SR, Forsham PH, Grodsky GM (1972) *In vitro* inhibition of pancreatic glucagon secretion by diphenylhydantoin. J Clin Endocrinol Metab 35:823–824

Gesler RM, Lints CE, Swinyard EA (1961) Pharmacology of some substituted 2-thiohydantions with particular reference to anticonvulsant properties. Toxicol Appl Pharmacol 3:107–121

Gilbert JC, Wyllie MG (1976) Effects of anticonvulsant and convulsant drugs on the ATP-ase activities of synaptosomes and their components. Br J Pharmacol 56:49:57

Glazko AJ (1972a) Diphenylhydantoin. In Brodie BB, Heller WM (eds) Proceedings of the conference on bioavailability of drugs, Washington 1971. Karger, Basel, pp 163–177

Glazko AJ (1972b) Diphenylhydantoin: chemistry and methods for determination. In: Woodbury DM, Penry JK, Schmidt RP (eds) Antiepileptic drugs. Raven, New York, pp 103–112

Glazko AJ, Chang T (1972) Diphenylhydantoin: absorption, distribution and excretion. In: Woodbury DM, Penry JK, Schmidt RP (eds) Antiepileptic drugs. Raven, New York, pp 127–136

Glazko AJ, Chang T, Baukema J, Dill WA, Goulet JR, Buchanan RA (1969) Metabolic disposition of diphenylhydantoin in normal human subjects following intravenous administration. Clin Pharmacol Ther 10:498–504

Goldberg MA (1980) Antiepileptic drugs. phenytoin: binding. In: Glaser GH, Penry JK, Woodbury DM (eds) Antiepileptic drugs: mechanisms of action. Raven, New York, pp 323–337

Goldberg MA, Todoroff T (1973) Binding of diphenylhydantoin to brain protein. Biochem Pharmacol 22:2973–2980

Goldberg MA, Todoroff T (1976) Enhancement of diphenylhydantoin binding by lipid extraction. J Pharmacol Exp Ther 196:579–585

Goldstein RE, Penzotti C, Kuehl KS, Prindle HK Jr, Hall CA, Titus EO (1973) Correlation of antiarrhythmic effects of diphenylhydantoin with digoxin-induced changes in myocardial contractility, sodium-potassium adenosine triphosphatase activity, and potassium efflux. Circ Res 33:823–824

Goodman LS (1956) US Patent 2,744,852

Goodman LS, Grewal MS, Brown WC, Swinyard EA (1953) Comparison of maximal seizures evoked by pentylenetetrazol (Metrazol) and electroshock in mice, and their modification by anticonvulsants. J Pharmacol Exp Ther 108:168–176
Goodman LS, Swinyard EA, Brown WC, Schiffman DO (1954) Anticonvulsant properties of 5,5-diphenyltetrahydroglyoxaline-4-one (SKF 2599). J Pharmacol Exp Ther 110: 403–410
Goodman LS, Toman JEP, Swinyard EA (1948) Anticonvulsant properties of 5,5-phenyl thienyl hydantoin in comparison with Dilantin and Mesantoin. Proc Soc Exp Biol Med 68:584–587
Goodman LS, Toman JEP, Swinyard EA (1949) Anticonvulsant drugs: mechanism of action and methods of assay. Arch Int Pharmacol Ther 78:144–162
Greenly RH (1974) New approach to derivatization and gas-chromatographic analysis of barbiturates. Clin Chem 20:192–194
Gruber CM, Harry VG, Drake ME (1940) The toxic actions of sodium diphenylhydantoinate (Dilantin) when injected peritoneally and intravenously in experimental animals. J Pharmacol Exp Ther 68:433–436
Gruhzit OM (1939) Sodium diphenyl hydantoinate. Pharmacologic and histopathologic studies. Arch Pathol 28:761–762
Gugler R, Manion CV, Azarnoff DL (1976) Phenytoin: pharmacokinetics and bioavailability. Clin Pharmacol Ther 19:135–142
Gutman Y, Boonyaviroj P (1977) Mechanism of inhibition of catecholamine release from adrenal medulla by diphenylhydantoin and by low concentrations of ouabain (10^{-10} *M*). Naunyn Schmiedebergs Arch Pharmacol 296:293–296
Guzek JW, Russell JT, Thron NA (1974) Inhibition by diphenylhydantoin of vasopressin release from isolated rat neurohypophyses. Acta Pharmacol Toxicol 34:14
Haberland C (1962) Cerebellar degeneration with clinical manifestation in chronic epileptic patients. Psychiatr Neurol (Basel) 143:29–44
Hadfield MG (1972) Uptake and binding of catecholamines. Effect of diphenylhydantoin and a new mechanism of action. Arch Neurol 26:78–84
Hahn F (1960) Analeptics. Pharmacol Rev 12:447–530
Hansch C, Leo A (1979) Substituent constants for correlation analysis in chemistry and biology. John Wiley, New York
Hansen JM, Skovsted L, Lauridsen UB, Kirkegaard C, Siersbaek-Nielsen K (1974) The effect of diphenylhydantoin on thyroid function. J Clin Endocrinol Metab 39:785–789
Hanson JW, Myrainthopoulos NC, Harvey MAS, Smith DW (1976) Risks to the offspring of women treated with hydantoin anticonvulsants, with emphasis on the fetal hydantoin syndrome. J Pediatr 89:662–668
Harned BK, Cunningham RW, Clark MC, Hine CH, Kane MM, Smith FH, Vessey RE, Yuda NN, Zabransky FW (1953) The pharmacology of *N*-benzyl-*β*-chlorpropionamide (Hibicon), a new anticonvulsant. J Pharmacol Exp Ther 107:403–423
Hasbani M, Pincus J, Lee SH (1974) Diphenylhydantoin and calcium movement in lobster nerves. Arch Neurol 31:250–254
Hassell TM, Dudley KH, Hirsch PF, Hutchens LH, Johnston MC, Moriarty JD (1979) Summary of an international symposium on phenytoin-induced teratology and gingival pathology. JADA 99:652–655
Hauptmann A (1912) Luminal bei Epilepsie. Münch Med Wochenschr 59:1907–1909
Hawk GL, Franconi LC (1978) High-pressure liquid chromatography in quantitation of antiepileptic drugs. In: Pippinger CE, Penry JK, Kutt H (eds) Antiepileptic drugs: quantitative analysis and interpretation. Raven, New York, pp 153–162
Hayes MJ, Langman MJS, Short AH (1975) Changes in drug metabolism with increasing age: 2. Phenytoin clearance and protein binding. Br J Clin Pharmacol 2:73–79
Helfant RH, Scherlag BS, Damato AN (1967) The electrophysiological properties of diphenylhydantoin sodium (Dilantin) as compared to procainamide in the normal and digitalis intoxicated heart. Circulation 36:108–118
Heyma P, Larkins RG, Perry-Keene D, Peter CT, Ross O, Sloman JG (1977) Thyroid hormone levels and protein binding in patients on long-term diphenylhydantoin treatment. Clin Endocrinol (Tokyo) 6:369–376

Hofeldt FD, Dippe SE, Levin SR, Karam JH, Blum MR, Forshan PH (1974) Effects of diphenylhydantoin upon glucose-induced insulin secretion in three patients with insulinoma. Diabetes 23:192–198

Hooper WD, Bochner F, Eadie MJ, Tyrer JH (1974) Plasma protein binding of diphenylhydantoin. Effects of sex hormones, renal and hepatic disease. Clin Pharmacol Ther 15:276–282

Hoppel C, Garle M, Rane A, Sjöqvist F (1977) Plasma concentrations of 5-(4-hydroxyphenyl)-5-phenylhydantoin in phenytoin-treated patients. Clin Pharmacol Ther 21:294–300

Houck J (1970) Control of cutaneous collagenolysis. Adv Enzyme Regul 8:269–278

Houghton GW, Richens A, Toseland PA, Davidson S, Falconer MA (1975) Brain concentrations of phenytoin, phenobarbitone and primidone in epileptic patients. Eur J Clin Pharmacol 9:73–78

Isaacs H (1961) A syndrome of continuous muscle-fiber activity. J Neurol Neurosurg Psychiatry 24:319–325

Isaacs H (1964) Quantal squander. S Afr J Lab Clin Med 10:93–95

Isaacs H (1967) Continuous muscle fibre activity in an Indian male with additional evidence of terminal motor fiber abnormality. J Neurol Neurosurg Psychiatry 30:126–133

Ishizaki T, Tokochi K, Chiba K, Tabuchi T, Wagatsuma T (1981) Placental transfer of anticonvulsants (phenobarbital, phenytoin, valproic acid) and the elimination from neonates. Pediatr Pharmacol 1:291–303

Jailer JW (1951) Adrenocorticotropin content of immature rat pituitary gland. Endocrinology 49:826–827

Johannessen SJ, Strandjord RE (1975) Absorption and protein binding in serum of several anti-epileptic drugs. In: Schneider H, Janz D, Gardner-Thorpe C, Meinardi H, Sherwin AL (eds) Clinical pharmacology of antiepileptic drugs. Springer, Berlin Heidelberg New York, pp 262–273

Johnston D, Ayala GF (1975) Diphenylhydantoin: the action of a common anticonvulsant on bursting pacemaker cells in *Aplysia*. Science 189:1009–1011

Johnston D (1976) Voltage clamp reveals basis of calcium regulation of bursting pacemaker cells in *Aplysia*. Brain Res 107:418–423

Jones GL, Woodbury DM (1976) Effects of diphenylhydantoin and phenobarbital on protein metabolism in the rat cerebral cortex. Biochem Pharmacol 25:53–61

Jones GL, Amata RJ, Wimbish GH, Peyton GA (1981) Comparison of anticonvulsant potencies of cyheptamide, carbamazepine, and phenytoin. J Pharm Sci 70:618–620

Kaplan SA, Jack ML, Alexander K, Weinfeld RE (1973) Pharmacokinetic profile of diazepam in man following single intravenous and oral and chronic oral administration. J Pharm Sci 62:1789–1796

Kemp J, Woodbury D (1971) Subcellular distribution of 4-C^{14}-diphenylhydantoin in rat brain. J Pharmacol Exp Ther 177:342–349

Killam KF, Killam EK, Naquet R (1967) An animal model of light sensitive epilepsy. Electroencephalogr Clin Neurophysiol 22:497–513

Kinniburgh DW, Boyd ND (1981) Phenytoin binding to partially purified albumin in renal disease. Clin Pharmacol Ther 29:203–210

Kizer JS, Cordon MV, Brendel K, Bressler R (1970) The in vitro inhibition of insulin secretion by diphenylhydantoin. J Clin Invest 49:1942–1948

Kokenge R, Kutt H, McDowell F (1965) Neurological sequelae following Dilantin overdose in a patient and in experimental animals. Neurology (Minneap) 15:823–829

Kootstra A, Woodhouse SP (1974) The effect of diphenylhydantoin on the Na^+-K^+-stimulated ouabain inhibited ATPase. Proc Univ Otage Med Sch 52:6–7

Krall RL, Penry JK, Kupferberg HJ, Swinyard EA (1978a) Antiepileptic drug development. I. History and a program for progress. Epilepsia 19:393–408

Krall RL, Penry JK, White BG, Kupferberg HK, Swinyard EA (1978b) Antiepileptic drug development II. Anticonvulsant drug screening. Epilepsia 19:409–428

Kupfer A, Birchner J (1979) Stereoselectivity of differential routes of drug metabolism: the fate of the enantiomers of (^{14}C) mephenytoin in the dog. J Pharmacol Exp Ther 209:190–195

Kupfer A, Brilis GM, Watson JT, Harris TM (1980) A major pathway of mephenytoin metabolism in man. Aromatic hydroxylation to *p*-hydroxymephenytoin. Drug Metab Dispos 8:1–4
Kupfer A, Roberts RK, Schenker S, Branch RA (1981) Stereoselective metabolism of mephenytoin in man. J Pharmacol Exp Ther 218:193–199
Lal H, Davis WC, Ticku MK (1981) Specific H^3-pentylenetetrazol binding in the rat brain. Soc Neurosci Abstr 7:445
Landolt AM (1974) Treatment of acute postoperative inappropriate antidiuretic hormone secretion with diphenylhydantoin. Acta Endocrinol 76:625–628
Larsen NE, Naestoft J (1974) Quantitative determination of ethotoin in serum by gas chromatography. J Chromatogr 92:157–161
Laubscher FA (1966) Fatal diphenylhydantoin poisoning. JAMA 198:1120–1121
Laxer KD, Robertson LT, Julien RM, Dow RS (1980) Antiepileptic drugs: phenytoin: relationship between cerebellar function and epileptic discharges. In: Glaser GH, Penry JK, Woodbury DM (eds) Antiepileptic drugs: mechanisms of action. Raven, New York, pp 415–427
Lee SI, Bass NH (1970) Microassay of diphenylhydantoin: blood and regional brain concentrations in rats during acute intoxication. Neurology 20:115–124
Lee WY, Grumer HA, Bronsky D, Waldstein SS (1961) Acute water loading as a diagnostic test for the inappropriate ADH syndrome. J Lab Clin Med 58:937
Lepetit G (1977) Die pH-abhängige „Lipid-Löslichkeit“ von Arzneistoffen. Pharmazie 32:289–291
Letteri JM, Millk H, Louis S, Kutt H, Durante P, Glazko AJ (1971) Diphenylhydantoin metabolism in uremia. N Engl J Med 285:648–652
Levin SR, Booker J, Smith DF, Grodshy GM (1970) Inhibition of insulin secretion by diphenylhydantoin in the isolated perfused pancreas. J Clin Endocrinol Metab 30:400–401
Lewin E, Bleck V (1977) The effect of diphenylhydantoin administration on sodium-potassium-activated ATPase in cortex. Neurology 21:647–551
Leznicki AL, Dymecki J (1974) The effect of certain anticonvulsants in vitro and in vivo on enzyme activities in rat brain. Neurol Neurochir Pol 24:413–419
Lipicky RJ, Gilbert DK, Stilman IM (1972) Diphenylhydantoin inhibition of sodium conductance in squid giant axon. Proc Natl Acad Sci USA 69:1758–1760
Livingston S (1957) Drug therapy for childhood epilepsy. J Chronic Dis 6:46–80
Livingston S (1966) Drug therapy for epilepsy. Thomas, Springfield, Ill
Locock C (1857) Contribution to discussion on paper by E. H. Sieveking. Lancet 1:528
Löscher W (1979) A comparative study of the protein binding of anticonvulsant drugs in serum of dog and man. J Pharmacol Exp Ther 208:429–435
Loscalzo AE (1945) Treatment of epileptic patients with a combination of 3-methyl,5,5-phenylethylhydantoin and phenobarbital. J Nerv Ment Dis 101:537–544
Loscalzo AE (1952) Mesantoin in the control of epilepsy. Neurology (Minneap) 2:403–411
Lund L (1974) Clinical significance of generic inequivalence of three different pharmaceutical preparations of phenytoin. Eur J Clin Pharmacol 7:119–124
Lunde RKM, Rane A, Yaffe SJ, Lund L, Sjöqvist F (1970) Plasma protein binding of diphenylhydantoin in man: interaction with other drugs and the effect of temperature and plasma dilution. Clin Pharmacol Ther 11:844–855
Malherbe C, Burrill KC, Levin SR, Karam JH, Forsham PH (1972) Effect of diphenylhydantoin on insulin secretion in man. N Engl J Med 286:339–342
Marshall FJ (1958) Some 3,3-disubstituted-2-pyrrolidinones. J Org Chem 23:503–505
Mawer CE, Mullen PW, Rodgers M, Robins AJ, Lucas SB (1974) Phenytoin dose adjustment in epileptic patients. Br J Clin Pharmacol 1:163–168
McLennan H, Elliot KAC (1951) Effects of convulsant and narcotic drugs on acetylcholine synthesis. J Pharmacol Exp Ther 103:35–43
Mendoza DM, Flock EV, Oven CA, Paris J (1966) Effect of 5,5-diphenylhydantoin on the metabolism of L-thyroxine-^{131}I in the rat. Endocrinology 79:106–118
Mercer EN, Ziegler WG, Wickland GF, Dower GE (1976) The effect of diphenylhydantoin upon beating of heart cells grown in vitro. J Pharmacol Exp Ther 155:267–270

Merritt HH, Putnam TJ (1938a) A new series of anticonvulsant drugs tested by experiments on animals. Arch Neurol Psychiatry 39:1003–1015
Merritt HH, Putnam TJ (1938b) Sodium diphenyl hydantoinate in treatment of convulsive disorders. JAMA 111:1068–1073
Merritt HH, Putnam TJ (1939) Sodium diphenylhydantoinate in treatment of convulsive seizures. Toxic symptoms and their prevention. Arch Neurol Psychiatry 42:1053–1058
Mertens HG, Zschocke S (1965) Neuromytonie. Klin Wochenschr 43:917–925
Millichap JB (1972) Other hydantoins: mephenytoin, ethotoin, and albutoin. In: Woodbury DM, Penry JK, Schmidt RP (eds) Antiepileptic drugs. Raven, New York, pp 275–281
Mirkin BL (1971a) Placental transfer and neonatal elimination of diphenylhydantoin. Am J Obstet Gynecol 109:930–933
Mirkin BL (1971b) Diphenylhydantoin: placental transport, fetal localization, neonatal metabolism, and possible teratogenic effects. J Pediatr 79:329–337
Mittler JC, Glick SM (1972) Radioimmunoassayable oxytocin release from isolated neural lobes; responses to ions and drugs. IV International congress of endocrinolgy, Washington, 1972. Excerpta Medica Abstracts of Communications No. 117, p 46
Monks A, Boobis S, Wadsworth J, Richens A (1978) Plasma protein binding interaction between phenytoin and valproic acid in vitro. Br J Clin Pharmacol 6:487–492
Morell F, Bradley W, Ptashne M (1958) Effect of diphenylhydantoin on peripheral nerve. Neurology B:140–144
Mull JD, Mullinax F (1966) Diphenylhydantoin allergy: clinical and immunological studies. Arthritis Rheum 9:525–526
Musgrave FS, Purpura DP (1963) Effects of Dilantin on focal epileptogenic activity of cat neurocortex. Electroencephalogr Clin Neurophysiol 15:923
Naestoft J, Larsen N (1977) Mass fragmentographic quantitation of ethotoin and some of its metabolites in human urine. J Chromatogr 143C:161–169
Nakamura K, Masuda Y, Nakatsuji K, Hiroka T (1966) Comparative studies on the distribution and metabolic fate of diphenylhydantoin and 3-ethylcarbonyl-diphenylhydantoin (P-6127) after chronic administration to dogs and cats. Naunyn Schmiedebergs Arch Pharmacol 254:406–417
Nakamura K, O'Hashi K, Nakatsuji K, Hirooka T, Fujimoto F, Ose S (1965) The anticonvulsant activity of 3-ethoxycarbonyl-5,5-diphenylhydantoin (P-6127) in animals. Arch Int Pharmacodyn Ther 156:261–270
Neuman RA, Frank GB (1977) Effects of diphenylhydantoin and phenobarbital on voltage-clamped myelinated nerve. Can J Physiol Pharmacol 55:42–47
Nielsen T, Cottman C (1971) Binding of diphenylhydantoin to brain and subcellular fractions. Eur J Pharmacol 14:344–350
Nishikawa T, Kubo H, Saito M (1979) Competitive nephelometric immunoassay method for antiepileptic drugs in patient blood. J Immunol Methods 29:85–89
Noach EL, Van Rees H (1964) Intestinal distribution of intravenously administered diphenylhydantoin in the rat. Arch Int Pharmacodyn Ther 150:52–61
Noach EL, Woodbury DM, Goodman LS (1958) Studies on absorption, distribution, fate and excretion of 4-C^{14}-labeled diphenylhydantoin. J Pharmacol Exp Ther 122:301–314
Odar-Cederlof I, Borga O (1976a) Impaired protein binding of phenytoin in uremia and displacement effects of salicylic acid. Clin Pharmacol Ther 20:36–47
Odar-Cedarlof I, Borga O (1976b) Lack of relationship between serum free fatty acids and impaired plasma protein binding of diphenylhydantoin in chronic renal failure. Eur J Clin Pharmacol 10:403–405
Odar-Cederlof I (1977) Plasma protein binding of phenytoin and warfarin in patients undergoing renal transplantation. Clin Pharmacokinet 2:147–153
Oldendorf W (1974) Lipid solubility and drug penetration of the blood brain barrier Proc Soc Exp Biol Med 147:813–816
Oppenheimer JH, Tavernetti RR (1962) Studies on the thyroxine-diphenylhydantoin interaction: effect of 5,5-diphenylhydantoin on the displacement of L-thyroxine from thyroxine-binding globulin (TBG). Endocrinology 71:496–504

Pento JT (1976) Diphenylhydantoin inhibition of pentagastrin-stimulated calcitonin secretion in the pig. Horm Metab Res 8:399–401

Pento JT, Glick SM, Kagan A (1973) Diphenylhydantoin inhibition of calcitonin secretion induced by calcium and glucagon. Endocrinology 92:330–333

Perry JG, McKinney L, DeWeer P (1978) The cellular mode of action of antiepileptic drug 5,5-diphenylhydantoin. Nature 272:271–273

Perucca E, Richens A (1981) Drug interactions with phenytoin. Drugs 21:120–137

Petty WC, Karler R (1965) The influence of aging on the activity of anticonvulsant drugs. J Pharmacol Exp Ther 150:443–448

Pincus JH, Lee SH (1973) Diphenylhydantoin and calcium. Arch Neurol 29:239–244

Pinto W, Gardner LI, Rosenblum P (1977) Abnormal genitalia as a presenting sign in two male infants with hydantoin embryopathy syndrome. Am J Dis Child 131:452–455

Pippenger CE (1978) Pediatric clinical pharmacology of antiepileptic drugs: a special consideration. In: Pippenger CE, Penry JK, Kutt H (eds) Antiepileptic drugs: quantitative analysis and interpretation. Raven, New York, pp 315–319

Pippenger ED, Bastiani RJ, Schneider RS (1975) Evaluation of an experimental homogenous enzyme immunoassay for the quantitation of phenytoin and phenobarbitone in serum of plasma. In: Schneider H, Janz D, Gardner-Thorpe C, Meinardi H, Sherwin AL (eds) Clinical pharmacology of antiepileptic drugs. Springer, Berlin Heidelberg New York pp 331–335

Pippenger CE, Penry JK, Kutt H (eds) (1978) Antiepileptic drugs: quantitative analysis and interpretation. Raven, New York

Popelka SR, Miller DM, Holen JT, Kelso DM (1981) Fluorescence polarization immunoassay II. Analyzer for rapid, precise measurement of fluorescence polarization with use of disposable cuvettes. Clin Chem 27:1198–1201

Porter RJ, Layzer RB (1975) Plasma albumin concentration and diphenylhydantoin binding in man. Arch Neurol 32:298–303

Putnam TJ, Merritt HH (1941) Chemistry of anticonvulsant drugs. Arch Neurol Psychiatry 45:505–516

Raines A, Standaert FG (1967) An effect of diphenylhydantoin on post-tetanic hyperpolarization of intramedullary nerve terminals. J Pharmacol Exp Ther 156:591–597

Raines A, Niner JM, Pace DG (1973) A comparison of the anticonvulsant, neurotoxic and lethal effects of diphenylbarbituric acid, phenobarbital and diphenylhydantoin in the mouse. J Pharmacol Exp Ther 186:315–322

Rambeck B, Boenigk HE, Dunlop A, Mullen PW, Wadsworth J, Richens A (1979) Predicting phenytoin dose: a revised nomogram. Ther Drug Monit 1:325–333

Ramsay RE, Hammond EJ, Perchalski RJ, Wilder BJ (1979) Brain uptake of phenytoin, phenobarbital and diazepam. Arch Neurol 36:535–539

Rane A, Garle M, Borga O, Sjöqvist F (1974) Plasma disappearance of transplacentally transferred diphenylhydantoin in the newborn studied by mass fragmentometry. Clin Pharmacol Ther 15:39–45

Rapport RL II, Harris AB, Friel PN, Ojemann GA (1975) Human epileptic brain. Na, K-ATPase activity and phenytoin concentrations. Arch Neurol 32:549–554

Rausing A (1978) Hydantoin induced lymphadenopathies and lymphomas. In: Mathe G, Seligmann M, Tubiana M (eds) Recent results in cancer research, vol 64. Lymphoid neoplasias I. Classification, categorization, natural history. Springer, Berlin Heidelberg New York, pp 263–264

Reidenberg M, Affrime M (1973) Influence of disease on binding of drugs to plasma proteins. Ann NY Acad Sci 226:115–127

Rein R, Fukuda N, Win H, Clarke GA, Harris FW (1966) Iterative extended Huckel theory. Chem Phys 45:4743–4744

Reinhard JF, Reinhard JF Jr (1977) Experimental evaluation of anticonvulsants. In: Vida JA (ed) Anticonvulsants. Medicinal chemistry, vol 15. Academic, New York, pp 57–111

Reynolds EH (1975) Chronic antiepileptic toxicity: a review. Epilepsia 16:319–352

Richens A (1975) A study of the pharmacokinetics of phenytoin (diphenylhydantoin) in epileptic patients, and the development of a nomogram for making dose increments. Epilepsia 16:627–646

Rinne UK (1966) Effect of diphenylhydantoin treatment on the release of corticotropin in epileptic patients. Confin Neurol 27:431–440

Roe MD, Podosin RL, Blaskovics M (1975) Drug interaction: diazoxide and diphenylhydantoin. J Pediatr 87:480–484

Rümke CL (1967) Increased susceptibility of mice to seizures after some anticonvulsant drugs: Eur J Pharmacol 1:369–377

Ruprah M, Perucca E, Richens A (1980) Decreased serum protein binding of phenytoin in late pregnancy (letter). Lancet 2:316–317

Saad SF, El-Masry AM, Scott PM (1972) Influence of certain anticonvulsants on the concentration of gamma-aminobutyric acid in the cerebral hemisphere of mice. Eur J Pharmacol 17:386–392

Said DM, Fraga JR, Reichelderfer TE (1968) Hyperglycemia associated with diphenylhydantoin intoxication. Med Ann D C 37:170–172

Sansom LN, O'Reilly WJ, Wiseman CW, Stern LM, Derhan J (1975) Plasma phenytoin levels produced by various phenytoin preparations. Med J Austr 2:593–595

Savolainen H, Iivanainen M, Elovaara E, Tammisto P (1980) Distribution of ^{14}C-phenytoin in rat Purkinje cells, cerebellar and cerebral neuronal tissue after a single intraperitoneal injection. Eur Neurol 19:115–120

Scherf D, Blumenfeld S, Tanner D, Yildiz M (1960) The effect of diphenylhydantoin (Dilantin) on atrial flutter and fibrillation provoked by focal application of aconitine or delphinine. Am Heart J 60:936–947

Schlogl K, Wessely F, Kraupp O, Stormann H (1961) Synthese und Pharmakologie einiger 3,5-di- und trisubstituierter Hydantoine. J Med Pharm Chem 4:231–258

Schottelius DD (1978) Homogeneous immunoassay system (EMIT) for quantitation of antiepileptic drugs in biological fluids. In: Pippenger CE, Penry JK, Kutt H (eds) Antiepileptic drugs: quantitative analysis and interpretation. Raven, New York, pp 95–108

Schwade ED, Richards RK, Everett GM (1956) Peganone, a new antiepileptic drug. Dis Nerv Syst 17:155–158

Schwartz A, Lindenmayer GE, Allen JC (1975) The sodium-potassium adenosine triphosphatase: pharmacological and biochemical aspects. Pharmacol Rev 27:3–134

Schwartz JR, Vogel W (1977) Diphenylhydantoin: excitability reducing action in a single myelinated nerve fiber. Eur J Pharmacol 44:241–249

Schwartz PA, Rhodes CT, Cooper JW (1977) Solubility and ionization characteristics of phenytoin. J Pharm Sci 66:994–997

Seeman P, Chau-Wong M, Moyyen S (1972) The membrane binding of morphine, diphenylhydantoin and tetrahydrocannabinol. Can J Physiol Pharmacol 50:1193–1200

Selzer ME (1978) The action of phenytoin on a composite electrical-chemical synapse in the lamprey spinal cord. Ann Neurol 3:202–206

Shapiro S, Hartz SC, Siskind V, Mitchell AA, Slone D, Rosenberg L, Monson RR, Heinonen OP, Idanpaan-Heikkila J, Haro S, Saxen L (1976) Anticonvulsants and parental epilepsy in the development of birth defects. Lancet 1:272–275

Sherwin AL, Sokolowski CD (1975) Phenytoin and phenobarbitone levels in human brain and cerebrospinal fluid. In: Schneider H, Janz D, Gardner-Thorpe C, Meinardi H, Sherwin AL (eds) Clinical pharmacology of antiepileptic drugs. Springer, Berlin Heidelberg New York, pp 274–280

Sherwin AL, Eisen AA, Sokolowski CD (1973) Anticonvulsant drugs in human epileptogenic brain – correlation of phenobarbitone and primidone in epileptic patients. Arch Neurol 29:73–77

Sherwin AL, Harvey CD, Leppik IE (1977) Antiepileptic drugs in human cerebral cortex: clinical relevance of cortex: plasma ratios. In: Penry JK (ed) Epilepsy, eighth international symposium. Raven, New York, pp 103–108

Siegle GJ, Goodwin BB (1972) Sodium-potassium-activated adenosine triphosphatase of brain microsomes: modification of sodium inhibition by diphenylhydantoin. J Clin Invest 51:1164–1169

Sironi VA, Carbrini G, Porro MG, Ravagnati L, Marossero F (1980) Antiepileptic drug distribution in cerebral cortex, Ammon's horn, and amygdala in man. J Neurosurg 52:686–692

Sjo O, Hvidberg EF, Larsen NE (1975) Dose-dependent kinetics of ethotoin in man. Clin Exp Pharmacol Physiol 2:185–192

Slater IH, O'Leary JF, Leary DE (1950) The effect of 2,2-diethyl 1,3-propanediol (a new anticonvulsant) on spinal cord reflexes. J Pharmacol Exp Ther 100:316–324

Snider RS, Del Cerro MP (1967) Drug-induced dendritic sprouts on Purkinje cells in adult cerebellum. Exp Neurol 17:466–480

Sohn RS, Ferrendelli JA (1973) Inhibition of Ca^{++} transport into rat brain synaptosomes by diphenylhydantoin (DPH). J Pharmacol Exp Ther 185:272–275

Sohn RS, Ferrendelli JA (1976) Anticonvulsant drug mechanisms. Phenytoin, phenobarbital, and ethosuximide and calcium flux in isolated presynaptic endings. Arch Neurol 33:626–629

Solomon GE, Hilgartner MW, Kutt H (1975) Anticonvulsant induced depression of clotting factors in children. IV Panamerican congress of neurology, oct 1975, Mexico

Spain RC, Chidsey CA (1971) Myocardial Na/K adenosine triphosphatase activity during reversal of ouabain toxicity with diphenylhydantoin. J Pharmacol Exp Ther 179:594–598

Spiehler V, Sun L, Miyada DS, Sarandis SG, Walvick ER, Klein MW, Jordan DB, Jessen B (1976) Radioimmunoassay, enzyme immunoassay, spectrophotometry and gas-liquid chromatography compared for determination of phenobarbital and diphenylhydantoin. Clin Chem 22:749–753

Stambaugh JE, Tucker D (1974) Effect of diphenylhydantoin on glucose tolerance in patients with hypoglycemia. Diabetes 23:679–683

Stewart MJ, Ballinger BR, Devlin EH, Miller AY, Ramsay AC (1975) Bioavailability of phenytoin. A comparison of two preparations. Eur J Clin Pharmacol 9:209–212

Stille G, Brunckow I (1954) Die ganglioplegische Wirkung von 3-Alkylaminoalkyl-Hydantoinen. Arzneimittel-Forsch 4:723–725

Suzuki T, Saitoh Y, Nishihara K (1970) Kinetics of and diphenylhydantoin disposition in man. Chem Pharm Bull (Tokyo) 18:405–411

Swinyard EA, Toman JEP (1950) A comparison of the anticonvulsant actions of some phenylhydantoins and their corresponding phenylacetylureas. J Pharmacol Exp Ther 100:151–157

Swinyard EA (1949) Laboratory assay of clinically effective antiepileptic drugs. J Am Pharm Assoc 38:201–204

Swinyard EA (1972) Electrically induced convulsions. In: Purpura DP, Penry JK, Tower DB, Woodbury DM, Walter RD (eds) Experimental models of epilepsy. A manual for the laboratory worker. Raven, New York pp 433–458

Swinyard EA, Brown WC, Goodman LS (1952) Comparative assays of antiepileptic drugs in mice and rats. J Pharmacol Exp Ther 106:319–330

Swinyard EA, Castellion AW, Fink GB, Goodman LS (1963) Some neurophysiological and neuropharmacological characteristics of audiogenic-seizure-susceptible mice. J Pharmacol Exp Ther 140:375–384

Swinyard EA, Jolley JM, Goodman LS (1950) Anticonvulsant properties of Benadryl and Pyribenzamine. Proc Soc Exp Biol Med 75:239–242

Tammisto P, Kauko K, Viukari M (1976) Bioavailability of phenytoin. Lancet 1:254–255

Tenckoff H, Sherrard DJ, Hickman RO, Ladda RL (1968) Acute diphenylhydantoin intoxication. Am J Dis Child 116:422–425

Ticku MK, Ban M, Olsen RW (1978) Binding of [^{3}H]-dihydropicrotoxinin, a gamma-aminobutyric acid synaptic antagonist to rat brain membranes. Mol Pharmacol 14:391–402

Toman JEP (1951) Neuropharmacologic considerations in psychic seizures. Neurology 1:444–460

Toman JEP, Swinyard EA, Goodman LS (1946) Properties of maximal seizures and their alteration by anticonvulsant drugs and other agents. J Neurophys 9:231–240
Troupin AS, Friel P (1975) Anticonvulsant levels in saliva, serum and cerebrospinal fluid, Epilepsia 16:223
Troupin AS, Ojemann LM, Dodrill CB (1976) Mephenytoin: a reappraisal. Epilepsia 17:403–414
Troupin AS, Friel P, Lovely MP, Wilensky AJ (1979) Clinical pharmacology of mephenytoin and ethotoin. Ann Neurol 6:410–414
Utterback RA, Ojeman R, Malek J (1958) Parenchymatous cerebellar degeneration with Dilantin intoxication. J Neuropath Exp Neurol 17:516–519
Vajda F, Williams FM, Davidson S, Falconer MA, Breckenridge A (1974) Human brain, cerebrospinal fluid and plasma concentrations of diphenylhydantoin and phenobarbital. Clin Pharmacol Ther 15:597–603
Vanasin B, Bass DD, Mendeloff AI, Schuster MM (1973) Alteration of electrical and motor activity of human and dog rectum by diphenylhydantoin. Am J Dig Dis 18:403–410
Van Der Kleijn E, Rijntjes NVM, Guilen PJM, Wijffels CCG (1972) Systemic and brain distribution of diphenylhydantoin in the squirrel monkey. In: Woodbury DM, Penry JK, Schmidt RP (eds) Antiepileptic drugs. Raven, New York, p 124
Van Rees H, Woodbury DM, Noach EL (1969) Effects of ouabain and diphenylhydantoin on electrolyte and water shifts during intestinal absorption in the rat. Arch Int Pharmacodyn 182:437
Vernadakis A, Woodbury DM (1960) Effects of diphenylhydantoin and adenocortical steroids on free glutamic acid, glutamine and gamma-aminobutyric acid concentrations of rat cerebral cortex. In: Roberts E (ed) Inhibition in the nervous system and gamma-aminobutyric acid. Pergamon, Oxford, pp 242–248
Vernadakis A, Woodbury DM (1965) Effects of diphenylhydantoin on electroshock seizure thresholds in developing rats. J Pharmacol Exp Ther 148:144–150
Vernadakis A, Woodbury DM (1969) The developing animal as a model. Epilepsia 10:163–178
Verebely K, Kutt H, Sohn Y, Levitt B, Raines A (1970) Uptake and distribution of diphenylthiohydantoin (DPTH). Eur J Pharmol 10:106–110
Vida JA, Gerry EH (1977) Cyclic ureides. In: Vida JA (ed) Anticonvulsants. Medicinal chemistry, vol 15. Academic, New York, pp 151–291
Vida JA, O'Dea MH, Samour DM, Reinhard JF (1975) Anticonvulsants. 5. Derivatives of 5-ethyl-5-phenylhydantoin and 5,5-diphenylhydantoin. J Med Chem 18:383–385
Watson EL (1978) Effects of ionophores A23187 and X537A on vascular smooth muscle activity. Eur J Pharmacol 52:171–178
Watson EL, Seigel IA (1976) Diphenylhydantoin effects on salivary secretion and microsomal calcium accumulation and release. Eur J Pharmacol 37:207–211
Watson EL, Woodbury DM (1972) Effects of diphenylhydantoin on active sodium transport in frog skin. J Pharmacol Exp Ther 180:767–776
Watson EL, Woodbury DM (1973) The effect of diphenylhydantoin and ouabain, alone and in combination, on the electrocardiogram and on cellular electrolytes of guinea pig heart and skeletal muscle. Arch Int Pharmacodyn Ther 20:389–399
Waziri M, Ionasescu V, Zellweger H (1976) Teratogenic effects of anticonvulsant drugs. Am J Dis Child 130:1022–1023
Weinberger J, Nichlas WJ, Berl S (1976) Mechanism of action of anticonvulsants. Neurology (Minneap) 26:162–166
Weintraub RM, Pechet L, Alexander B (1963) Rapid diagnosis of drug-induced thrombocytopenia purpura. JAMA 180:528–532
Westmoreland B, Bass NH (1971) Diphenylhydantoin intoxication during pregnancy. A chemical study of drug distribution in the albino rat. Arch Neurol 24:158–164
Wilder BJ, Serrano EE, Ramsey E, Buchanan RA (1974) A method for shifting from oral to intramuscular diphenylhydantoin administration. Clin Pharmacol Ther 16:507–513
Wilder BJ, Ramsay E, Willmore LJ, Feussner GF, Perchalski RJ, Shumate JB (1977) Efficacy of intravenous phenytoin in the treatment of status epilepticus: kinetics of central nervous system penetration. Ann Neurol 1:511–519

Wilensky AJ, Lowden JA (1972a) The inhibitory effect of diphenylhydantoin on microsomal ATPase. Life Sci 11:319–327
Wilensky AJ, Lowden JA (1972b) Interaction of diphenylhydantoin-4-^{14}C with subcellular fractions of rat brain. Can J Physiol Pharmacol 50:346–353
Wilson WA, Wachtel H (1978) Prolonged inhibition in burst-firing neurons: synaptic inactivation of the slow regeneration inward current. Science 202:772–775
Winnacker JL, Yeager H, Saunders JA, Russell B, Anast CS (1977) Rickets in children receiving anticonvulsant drugs. Am J Dis Child 131:286–290
Withrow CD (1972) Systemic carbon dioxide derangements. In: Purpura DP, Penry JK, Tower DB, Woodbury DM, Walter RD (eds) Experimental models of epilepsy. A manual for the laboratory worker. Raven, New York, pp 477–494
Witiak DT, Seth SK, Baizman ER, Weibel SL, Wolf BH (1972) Para-substituted *N*-acetyl-L(*S*)- and -D(*R*)-α-amino-*N*-phenylsuccinimides and -glutarimides. Substituent effects on stereoselective anticonvulsant activity. J Med Chem 15:1117–1123
Wolf HH, Swinyard EA, Goodman LS (1962) Anticonvulsant properties of some *N*-substituted hydantoins. J Pharm Sci 51:74–76
Woodbury DM (1955) Effects of diphenylhydantoin on electrolytes and radiosodium turnover in brain and other tissues of normal, hyponatremic and postictal rats. J. Pharmacol Exp Ther 115:74–95
Woodbury DM (1969a) Mechanisms of action of anticonvulsants. In: Jasper HH, Ward AA, Pope A (eds) Basic mechanisms of the epilepsies. Little Brown, Boston, pp 647–681
Woodbury DM (1969b) Role of pharmacological factors in the evaluation of anticonvulsant drugs. Epilepsia 10:121–143
Woodbury DM (1972) Applications to drug evaluations. In: Purpura DP, Penry JK, Tower DB, Woodbury DM, Walter RD (eds) Experimental models of epilepsy. A manual for the laboratory worker. Raven, New York, pp 557–601
Woodbury DM, Karler R (1960) The role of carbon dioxide in the nervous system. Anesthesiology 21:686–703
Woodbury DM, Kemp JW (1971) Pharmacology and mechanisms of action of diphenylhydantion. Psychiatr Neurol Neurochir 74:91–115
Woodbury DM, Swinyard EA (1972) Diphenylhydantoin: absorption, distribution and excretion. In: Woodbury DM, Penry JK, Schmidt RP (eds) Antiepileptic drugs. Raven, New York, pp 113–123
Woodbury DM, Rollins LT, Gardner MD, Hirschi WL, Hogan JR, Rallison ML, Tanner GS, Brodie DA (1958) Effects of carbon dioxide on brain excitability and electrolytes. Am J Physiol 192:79–90
Wyke B (1963) Brain function and metabolic disorders. Butterworths, London
Yaari Y, Pincus JH, Argov Z (1977) Depression of synaptic transmission by diphenylhydantoin. Ann Neurol 1:334–338
Yacobi A, Lampman J, Levy G (1977) Frequency distribution of free warfarin and free phenytoin fraction values in serum of healthy human adults. Clin Pharmacol Ther 21:283
Yanagihara T, Hamberger A (1971a) Effect of diphenylhydantoin on protein metabolism in neuron and neuroglial fractions of central nervous tissue. Exp Neurol 32:152–162
Yanagihara T, Hamberger A (1971b) Effect of diphenylhydantoin on protein metabolism in the central nervous system. Study of subcellular fractions. Exp Neurol 31:87–99
Yanagihara T, Hamberger C (1971c) Distribution of diphenylhydantoin in rat organs: study with neuron-glia and subcellular fractions. J Pharmacol Exp Ther 179:611–618
Yonekawa W, Kupferberg H, Cantor F, Dudley KH (1975) Ethotoin distribution and metabolism in epileptic patients. Pharmacologist 17:193
Yunis AA, Arimura GH, Lutcher CL, Blasquez J, Halloran M (1967) Biochemical lesion in dilantin-induced erythroid aplasia. Blood 30:587–600
Zeft HJ, Whalen RE, Ratliff NB Jr, Davenport RT Jr, McIntosh HD (1968) Diphenylhydantoin therapy in experimental myocardial infarction. J Pharmacol Exp Ther 162:80–84

CHAPTER 14

Barbituric Acid Derivatives

B. B. GALLAGHER and L. S. FREER

A. Introduction

Recently, a number of reviews of various aspects of barbiturate pharmacology have appeared (PRICHARD 1980; VIDA 1977; HO and HARRIS 1981; NICOLL 1978). These books and reviews more than adequately cover the current understanding of barbiturate anticonvulsant, hypnotic, and tolerance activity at a cellular level and in the whole organism. In order to avoid, as much as possible, a recapitulation of this literature we will take a slightly different approach by focusing primarily upon the anticonvulsant barbiturates and in particular comparing the pharmacology of phenobarbital (PhB) with an experimental anticonvulsant barbituric acid derivative eterobarb (EtB; *N,N*-dimethoxymethyl phenobarbital). Where appropriate, and as information exists, we will consider the other anticonvulsant barbituric acid derivative, mephobarbital (MB).

B. Chemistry and Physicochemical Properties

The synthesis of barbital by FISCHER and VON MERING in 1903 provided the first practical method for the synthesis of the large series of barbiturates and resulted in the landmark discovery that barbital possessed hypnotic properties. Subsequently, the introduction of a second hypnotic barbiturate, phenobarbital, in 1912 (LOEWE 1912; HAUPTMANN 1912; JULIUSBURGER 1912) led to an awareness that certain barbiturate compounds exhibited anticonvulsant properties. As a result of these discoveries, systematic investigations describing the pharmacological activity of numerous barbiturate derivatives were carried out, many of which were directed toward discovering compounds which were active as anticonvulsants but devoid of sedative and toxic properties.

Analogous to the situation found with other classes of compounds which affect the central nervous system, both the qualitative and quantitative aspects of pharmacological activity demonstrated by barbituric acid derivatives are dependent upon: (1) the steric configuration of the molecules, which influences the ability of the compounds to interact with the "receptive" tissue; (2) the overall structural and electronic characteristics of the individual compounds, which dictate their ability to influence intrinsically the response of "receptive" tissue; and (3) the relative proportions of ionized or un-ionized molecules that exist at physiological pH, which influence the ability of a compound to cross the blood-brain barrier or other impeding membranes, thus determining access to sites of metabolism, tissue sites at which sequesterin occurs, or "receptive" tissue. For barbiturates many of the factors dictating the qualitative and quantitative aspects of pharmacological activity which would be predicted for an individual compound have been systematically investigated and are reviewed below.

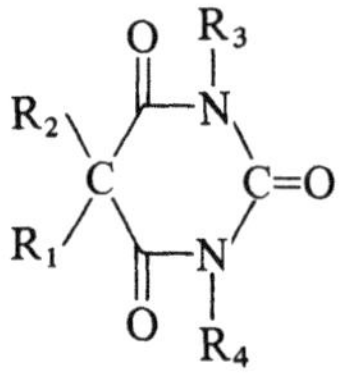

Barbiturate	R_1	R_2	R_3	R_4
Phenobarbital	Ethyl	Phenyl	H	H
Pentobarbital	Ethyl	1-Methylbutyl	H	H
Mephobarbital	Ethyl	Phenyl	Methyl	H
Eterobarb	Ethyl	Phenyl	Methoxymethyl	Methoxymethyl
Barbital	Ethyl	Ethyl	H	H

I. Relationship of Molecular Structure to Anticonvulsant Activity

As summarized by VIDA and GERRY (1977), the following structural features are required for anticonvulsant activity, based on maximal electroshock (MES) and pentylenetetrazol (PTZ) threshold testing.

1. Maximal anticonvulsant activity is obtained when one substituent attached to carbon-5 is a phenyl group.
2. Maximal anticonvulsant activity is obtained when the second substituent attached to carbon-5 is an alkyl group containing two to four carbon atoms (ethyl, propyl, or butyl groups).
3. Replacement of the ethyl group in 5-ethyl-5-phenylbarbituric acid by an alkyl group containing five carbon atoms decreases activity (5-amyl-5-phenylbarbituric acid is less active than 5-ethyl-5-phenylbarbituric acid).
4. Replacement of the ethyl group in 5-ethyl-5-phenylbarbituric acid by an alkyl group containing six or more carbon atoms destroys activity (5-hexyl-5-phenylbarbituric acid is inactive).
5. Replacement of the ethyl group in 5-ethyl-5-phenylbarbituric acid by a phenyl group decreases activity (5,5-diphenylbarbituric acid is less active than 5-ethyl-5-phenylbarbituric acid).
6. Replacement of the phenyl group in 5-ethyl-5-phenylbarbituric acid by an ethyl, butyl, isoamyl, *sec*-pentyl, amyl, or pentenyl group, in order, reduces activity in an increasing manner (5,5-diethylbarbituric acid is more active than 5-ethyl-5-amylbarbituric acid).
7. Replacement of the phenyl group in 5-ethyl-5-phenylbarbituric acid by a methyl or an alkyl group containing more than seven carbons destroys activity (5-ethyl-5-octylbarbituric acid is inactive).

8. Replacement of the phenyl group in 5-ethyl-5-phenylbarbituric acid by a benzyl or phenylethyl group greatly reduces (benzyl group) or destroys (phenylethyl group) anticonvulsant activity.

9. Replacement of both the ethyl and phenyl groups in 5-ethyl-5-phenylbarbituric acid by methyl groups destroys anticonvulsant activity (5,5-dimethylbarbituric acid is inactive).

10. Replacement of both ethyl and phenyl groups in 5-ethyl-5-phenylbarbituric acid by methyl groups coupled with methylation of one of the nitrogens retains some of the anticonvulsant activity of the parent compound (1,5,5-trimethylbarbituric acid is active in the PTZ but inactive in the MES test).

11. Replacement of the phenyl group in 5-ethyl-5-phenylbarbituric acid by an ethyl group coupled with methylation of one of the nitrogens produces a drug with satisfactory properties. Without methylation a less active compound is obtained (1-methyl-5,5-diethylbarbituric acid is more active than 5,5-diethylbarbituric acid).

12. Methylation of one of the nitrogens of 5-ethyl-5-phenylbarbituric acid does not significantly alter anticonvulsant activity.

13. Alkylation of one of the nitrogens in 5-ethyl-5-phenylbarbituric acid with the methoxymethyl group results in an anticonvulsant (3-mexthoxymethyl-5-ethyl-5-phenylbarbituric acid is as potent against MES as is 5-ethyl-5-phenylbarbituric acid).

14. Alkylation of both nitrogens in 5-ethyl-5-phenylbarbituric acid with small groups containing an electronegative atom produces potent anticonvulsants [e.g., 1,3-bis(methoxymethyl)-, 1,3-bis(acetoxymethyl)-, and 1,3-bis(bromomethyl)-5-ethyl-5-phenylbarbituric acids].

15. Introduction of polar groups (OH,NO_2, hydroxyalkyl, diazoamine, etc.) into the phenyl groups of 5-ethyl-5-phenylbarbituric acid decreases or destroys anticonvulsant activity.

II. Relationship of Acidic and Lipophilic Properties of Barbituric Acid Derivatives to CNS Activity

Following a series of studies on substituted barbituric acids, SANDBERG concluded that in order for a barbiturate to demonstrate definitive CNS activity two criteria must be met: (1) the compound must be a weak acid and (2) it must have a lipid/water partition coefficient within certain limits (SANDBERG 1949; ROSEN and SANDBERG 1950; HANSCH et al. 1968).

1. Acidic Properties

The acidic properties of barbituric acid derivatives result from the ability of these compounds to undergo lactim-lactam and keto-enol tautomerism. Unsubstituted barbituric acid is strongly acidic ($pK_a = 4.12$) and contains three sites at which tautomerism can occur. Under conditions of physiological pH (7.4), less than 0.1% is undissociated. The degree of acidity of substituted derivatives of barbituric acid in aqueous solution is determined by the number and position of the groups attached to the barbituric acid ring. Both the monosubstituted (1- or 5-substituted) and 1,5-disubstituted or 1,3-disubstituted barbituric acids are strong acids and at physiological pH are less than 0.1% undissociated. However, 5,5-disubstituted barbituric acid, the 5,5-disubstituted thiobarbiturates (with K_a ranging from 7.1 to 8.1), and the 1,5,5-trisubstituted barbituric acids (with K_a ranging from 8.0 to 9.0) are weak acids and at physiological pH exist approximately 40% –65% in the undissociated form. The 1,3,5,5-tetrasubstituted barbiturates exist totally in the undissociated form.

Based on the acidity characteristics or the degree of ionization at physiological pH, barbituric acid derivatives can be predicted to be either active or inactive compounds (DORAN 1959; VIDA 1977), Inactive compounds include barbituric acid, 1- and 5-monosubstituted barbituric acids, 1,3-, and 1,5-disubstituted barbituric acids, and 1,3,5,5-tetrasubstituted barbituric acids. The inactivity of some of these compounds has been logically attributed to their inability to cross the blood-brain barrier (BRODIE and HOGBEN 1957) due to their ionization characteristics. Active components include 5,5-disubstituted and 1,5,5-trisubstituted barbituric acids largely present in the un-ionized form. After the discovery of the hypnotic properties of barbital by FISCHER and VON MERING in 1903, a number of 5,5-dialkylbarbituric acids were shown to possess CNS activity (FISCHER and DILTHEY 1904). Notably all barbiturates currently in clinical use are disubstituted at the 5-position.

2. Lipophilic Properties

According to the theory of MEYER and OVERTON (HANSCH AND DUNN 1972), the potency of a depressant drug is proportional to its coefficient for distribution between lipid and water. The lipid/water partition coefficients of pharmacologically active barbiturates have also been found by SANDBERG (1951) to fall within a narrow range, suggesting that the relationship between the biological activity (i.e., biological response) of barbiturates and the relative lipophilic character of the drug is nonlinear (HANSCH et al. 1968; HANSCH and DUNN 1972; HANSCH and CLAYTON 1973). The relative drug response is defined in terms of the molar concentration of drug producing a standard response, and the lipophilic character of a compound is defined by its oil/water partition coefficient (P), where P equals the concentration in lipid phase/concentration in aqueous phase. The nonlinear relationship between drug response and P has been accurately described by HANSCH and CLAYTON (1973) to be a parabolic relationship. According to the parabolic model, as P for a given compound approaches zero, the compound will be so insoluble in lipid phases that it will not cross a lipid membrane and therefore will remain localized in the first aqueous phase it enters. Conversely, if P approaches infinity, the compound will be so insoluble in water that it will become sequestered in fatty tissue. An optimum P value would result in minimal inhibition of movement through the aqueous and lipophilic phases of living tissues (HANSCH and CLAYTON 1973). Although the partitioning process involved in a drug reaching its active site is dependent on lipophilic properties, the steric and electronic characteristics of the drug may also be rate limiting by influencing the actual interaction of drug with an active site (HANSCH and DUNN 1972). In general, structural changes that increase lipid solubility of barbiturates decrease latency of onset of activity, decrease duration of action, accelerate metabolic degradation, and may increase hypnotic potency (BREON et al. 1976).

Recent investigations have shown that 1,3-dialkoxymethyl derivatives of phenobarbital have marked activity against PTZ- and MES-induced seizures (SAMOUR and VIDA 1971). Several other derivatives of phenobarbital and mephobarbital have also been found to possess potent anticonvulsant activity (VIDA et al. 1973a, b). In the 1,3-dialkoxymethylphenobarbital series, the anticonvulsant activity decreased as the size of the alkoxy group increased. Eterobarb proved, therefore, to be the most effective of the series against PTZ- and MES-induced seizures and showed activity greater than phenobarbital against MES-induced seizures. Several of these derivatives including EtB were reported to be devoid of the hypnotic activity associated with the parent compound following oral administration in mice (SAMOUR and VIDA 1971). The pattern of toxicity observed was a progressive depression of the central nervous system, but loss of righting reflex did not occur except at lethal doses.

Based on the work of BUTLER (1955) and BREON et al. (1976) and its structure, EtB should be highly lipophilic. Determination of the partition coefficients of EtB, *N*-monomethoxymethyl-PhB (MMP), PhB, and *p*-OH-PhB between 1-chlorobutane and water revealed the high lipid solubility of EtB. The partition coefficients were EtB:MMP:PhB:*p*-OH-PhB = 50:12:0.4:0.02 (ALVIN and BUSH 1974a). In comparison, thiopental is ten times more lipid soluble than pentobarbital, which is about six times more lipophilic than PhB (MARK et al. 1949). These results suggest that EtB is approximately 125 times more lipid soluble than PhB and on a relative basis about two times more lipophilic than thiopental. The degree of lipid solubility of MMP lies between that of thiopental and pentobarbital.

Increasing lipid solubility of barbituric acid derivatives apparently has its limits as predicted by the parabolic model and as evidenced by the hypnotic activity of a series of 5-phenyl-5-alkyl barbituric acids determined in mice (ALLES et al. 1947). As the 5-alkyl group was increased in length, the hypnotic potency decreased. Although the increase in alkyl chain length increased lipid solubility, this was reflected in a decrease in water solubility; the latter characteristic probably is responsible for the decreased pharmacological activity. However, as emphasized by HO and HARRIS (1981) lipid solubility may govern access to sites of action but other factors such as hydrogen bonding may determine the molecular interactions leading to neurochemical changes.

Structure-activity relationships have been considered in more detail by SCHÄFER in this volume (Chap. 9).

C. Analytical Methods for Determination of Barbituric Acid Derivatives in Biological Fluids and Tissues

Although spectrophotometric and thin-layer chromatographic procedures have been described, they have been completely replaced by gas-liquid (GLC) and high-pressure liquid chromatography (HPLC) as well as by various immuno- and radioimmunoassay procedures.

Most of the GLC methods utilize flame ionization detection and pre- or on-column alkylation derivative formation. The procedures of BAYLIS et al. (1970)

and GREELEY (1974) are representative of these approaches. In agreement with GREELEY, we have found that pre-column butylation of barbiturates produces the greatest flame ionization sensitivity and we have utilized such a butylation procedure for all of the analytical data reported in this chapter. The problems associated with some derivatization procedures are discussed by KUPFERBERG (1978), and the interested reader should refer to this definitive text on antiepileptic drug determination.

SOLDIN and HILL (1976) have described the use of high-pressure liquid chromatography, and this procedure has been discussed in detail by HAWK and FRANCONI (1978). Similarly, the advantages and disadvantages of immunoassay (SCHOTTELIUS 1978) and radioimmunoassay (COOK 1978) have been considered in detail in the same volume.

D. Anticonvulsant Activity

Until relatively recently it was only possible to describe anticonvulsant compounds by their activity in certain experimental models of epilepsy or toxicity. While this served a useful descriptive and comparative purpose it revealed little or nothing about mechanism of action. Additionally, in part because the same battery of experimental models of epilepsy have been employed to screen new compounds for anticonvulsant activity, almost all anticonvulsant compounds currently in clinical use are variations of the molecular structure of the first modern anticonvulsant, phenobarbital. If more were known about the mechanism(s) of action of various anticonvulsant compounds it should be possible to synthesize new compounds more intelligently and to develop more specific tests for anticonvulsant activity.

Table 1 summarizes some data concerning anticonvulsant activity of phenobarbital and mephobarbital in different species and with varying test procedures. In the classical MES test, GOODMAN et al. (1953a) found that phenobarbital, as its sodium salt, and mephobarbital had about equal potency in mice on a molar basis. The ED_{50} for phenobarbital was 0.081 mmol/kg (95% confidence limits 0.077–0.087 mmol/kg) while that for mephobarbital was 0.085 mmol/kg (95% confidence limits, 0.069–0.105 mmol/kg). Rats are more effectively protected against MES than mice with phenobarbital but this species difference is less apparent with mephobarbital (SWINYARD et al. 1952). Additionally, with rats there is a direct correlation of age with efficacy for phenobarbital in the MES test (PETTY and KARLER 1965). In contrast, with threshold testing such as the PTZ test, minimal electroshock test, or hyponatremic electroshock threshold (HET) test, phenobarbital provides better protection for the mouse in comparison to rat (GOODMAN et al. 1953a, b). For both mouse and rat, phenobarbital and mephobarbital are about equally efficacious in threshold tests. In the audiogenic seizure model phenobarbital produces the same results as it does in the maximal and threshold tests, i.e., the maximal seizure is blocked at low doses while the minimal seizure (running component) requires much larger doses for inhibition (REINHARD and REINHARD 1977). In both mice and rats the time to peak effect is about 2 h with phenobarbital and 2.5 h (mice) to 3.5 h (rats with) mephobarbital (SWINYARD et al. 1952).

Table 1. Anticonvulsant activity of barbituric acid derivatives in standard experimental models of epilepsy utilizing various modes of drug administration. (Adapted from Table II of REINHARD and REINHARD 1977)

Test	Species	ED_{50} (mg/kg)	Route of administration	Refs.
Phenobarbital				
MES	Mouse (CF 1)	28.0 (24.8–31.6)[a]	p.o.	GOODMAN et al. (1953b)
	Mouse (CFW)	50 (27.5–90.9)	p.o.	RAINES et al. (1973)
	Mouse (CF #1)	20.6	s.c.	GOODMAN et al. (1953a)
	Mouse	13 (11–15)	p.o.	FREY and MAGNUSSEN (1971)
	Rat (young)	7.4	i.p.	PETTY and KARLER (1965)
	Rat (mature)	4.9 (3.7–6.5)	p.o.	GOODMAN et al. (1953b)
	Rat (mature)	12	i.p.	TOMAN et al. (1946)
	Rat (old)	1.4	i.p.	PETTY and KARLER (1965)
	Rabbit	15	i.p.	TOMAN et al. (1946)
	Cat	2	i.p.	TOMAN et al. (1946)
scPTZ	Mouse	9.8 (6.7–14.2)	p.o.	VIDA et al. (1973a)
	Mouse	15.5 (12.7–19.0)	p.o.	GOODMAN et al. (1953b)
	Mouse	11	s.c.	FERNGREN (1968)
	Rat	67 (48–93)	p.o.	GOODMAN et al. (1953b)
	Cat	30–60	i.m.	SPEHLMANN and COLLEY (1968)
MMS	Rat	9.5 (6.3–14.2)	s.c.	GOODMAN et al. (1953a)
MET (60-Hz EST)	Mouse	25 (18.5–34.0)	p.o.	GOODMAN et al. (1953b)
	Rat	62.5 (57–68)	p.o.	GOODMAN et al. (1953b)
HET	Mouse	29 (22–38)	p.o.	GOODMAN et al. (1953b)
	Rat	80 (70–91)	p.o.	GOODMAN et al. (1953b)
Audiogenic seizures	Mouse	2.3 (1.6–3.4)	i.p.	COLLINS and HORLINGTON (1969)
	Mouse	9.0 (5.5–14.8)	p.o.	ROBICHAUD et al. (1970)
	Mouse	4.6 (3.1–6.9)	p.o.	FINK and SWINYARD (1959)
Strychnine seizures	Mouse	25.0 (15.4–40.5)	p.o.	ROBICHAUD et al. (1970)
Bemegride seizures	Cat	30	s.c.	VAN DUIJN and VISSER (1972)
Picrotoxin seizures	Mouse	13–32	s.c.	FERNGREN (1968)
Focal seizures (cobalt)	Cat	Uneffectiv	s.c.	VAN DUIJN and VISSER (1972)
Intermittent photic stimulation	Baboon	15	i.m.	STARK et al. (1970)
Flurothyl seizures	Rat	20	i.p.	BAUMEL et al. (1973)
Alumina-induced seizures	Cat	10–15	i.m.	STEINMANN (1967)
Mephobarbital				
MES	Mouse	16 (11.4–22.4)	p.o.	VIDA et al. (1973b)
	Mouse	20.9	s.c.	GOODMAN et al. (1953a)
	Mouse	20	p.o.	SWINYARD et al. (1952)
	Rat	ca. 20	i.p.	CRAIG and SHIDEMAN (1971)
	Rat	10	s.c.	SWINYARD et al. (1952)
	Cat	12.5	p.o.	CHEN and ENSOR (1950)
scPTZ	Mouse	24 (16.9–34.1)	p.o.	VIDA et al. (1973)
	Mouse	25	p.o.	SWINYARD et al. (1952)
	Rat	40	p.o.	SWINYARD et al. (1952)
	Rat	15.3	s.c.	SWINYARD (1949)
MMS	Mouse	11.3	p.o.	GOODMAN et al. (1953a)
MET (60-Hz EST)	Mouse	ca. 30	p.o.	BROWN et al. (1953)
	Mouse	30	p.o.	SWINYARD et al. (1952)
	Rat	90	p.o.	SWINYARD et al. (1952)
HET	Mouse	26	p.o.	SWINYARD et al. (1952)
	Rat	80	p.o.	SWINYARD et al. (1952)

MES, maximal electroshock seizures; scPTZ, subcutaneous pentylenetetrazol seizure threshold test; MMS, maximal metrazole (pentylenetetrazol) seizure; MET (60-Hz EST), minimal electroshock seizure threshold; HET (60-Hz EST), hyponatremic electroshock seizure threshold

[a] Numbers in parentheses generally represent 95% fiducial limits

In the cat, phenobarbital raises the threshold for bemegride seizures but is ineffective in blocking focal cobalt seizures (VAN DUIJN and VISSER 1972) while it is quite effective (15 mg/kg i.m.) in blocking alumina-induced seizures. Photically induced seizures in the baboon are inhibited for as long as 24 h with phenobarbital (STARK et al. 1970).

With the kindling model of epilepsy in the rat, phenobarbital inhibits both cortical- and amygdala-kindled seizures with ED_{50}s of 12 mg/kg, respectively (ALBRIGHT and BURNHAM 1980). As with the standard experimental seizure models generalized seizures were controlled at lower doses of phenobarbital than threshold responses (focal amygdala seizures).

Investigation of the pharmacological activity of *p*-OH-PhB in mice by CRAIG and his associates (1960) revealed that it did possess significant anticonvulsant activity although it was less potent than phenobarbital. They report an ED_{50} of 20 mg/kg for PhB compared with 368 mg/kg for *p*-OH-PhB in the MES test; 25 vs 262 mg/kg in the MET test; 18 vs 160 mg/kg in the HET test, and 25 vs 445 mg/kg for pentylenetetrazol-induced seizures. Hypnotic potency (HD_{50}) was reported as 50 mg/kg for PhB and 1,275 mg/kg for *p*-OH-PhB. These data have not been reported other than in abstract form. While it is possible that some phenobarbital may have contaminated their preparation of *p*-OH-PhB, the varying protective indices for the two compounds and the differing ED_{50} ratios in different anticonvulsant models argue against this interpretation. The toxicity data are in close agreement with those found by BUTLER (1956), who observed that mice receiving 500 mg/kg (i.v.) were not noticeably affected, while 1,000 mg/kg caused sluggishness, tremor of the limbs, and some difficulty in righting. BUTLER (1956) has also shown that the plasma concentration of *p*-OH-PhB after a single dose declines rapidly ($t_{1/2}$, 22 min). Since in most species over half of the *p*-OH-PhB is conjugated, the disappearance from plasma is in all probability due mainly to conjugation. The relationship between the ratio of production and conjugation of *p*-OH-PhB is such that the plasma concentration of this substance as it arises from the metabolism of PhB probably remains low. Thus, it is unlikely that *p*-OH-PhB contributes to the pharmacological activity of PhB.

Some of the conventional estimates of anticonvulsant activity and toxicity have been compiled (REINHARD and REINHARD 1977; VIDA and GERRY 1977) for PhB, EtB, and MB (Table 2). In mice EtB was most effective for the MES test, PhB was least effective, and MB was intermediate. In contrast, in the threshold tests, PhB was most effective, EtB was least effective, and MB was again intermediate. In this species there was a striking difference in toxicity between EtB and PhB. Data relevant to this interesting observation will be presented later in this chapter. In these tests these three barbituric acid derivatives appear to behave as different compounds despite the fact that EtB and MB are completely metabolized to PhB. The difference between EtB and PhB in the MES is understandable in light of the findings of BAUMEL et al. (1976), who demonstrated the effectiveness of a metabolite of EtB in the MES test. This metabolite, *N*-monomethoxymethyl phenobarbital (MMP), was also shown to be ineffective in the PTZ test with this species, and consequently the differential activity in this test is undoubtedly a reflection of differences in the rate of phenobarbital accumulation in brain,

Table 2. Comparison of anticonvulsant activity and toxicity in mice for three barbituric acid derivatives. (REINHARD and REINHARD 1977; VIDA and GERRY 1977)

	ED_{50} (mg/kg) MES	ED_{50} (mg/kg) MET	ED_{50} (mg/kg) scPTZ	HD_{50} (mg/kg)
Phenobarbital	20 (13.8–29)	25 (18.5–34)	9.8 (6.7–14.2)	100 (72.5–138)
Eterobarb	13.5 (8–22.7)	57 (33.1–98)	47 (29.4–75.2)	None
Mephobarbital	16 (11.4–22.4)	30 (19.5–40)	24 (16.9–34.1)	180 (148.7–217.8)

MES, maximal electroshock, oral drug administration; MET, minimal electroshock threshold, oral drug administration; scPTZ, pentylenetetrazol threshold test; ED_{50}, effective dose required to induce effect in 50% of the animals; HD_{50}, hypnotic oral dose required to induce sleep (complete loss of fore- and hind-limb righting reflexes) in 50% of animals

Figures in parentheses are the 95% confidence limits

which is considerably slower when EtB is the source of PhB. The difference in hypnotic activity is now known to be due, at least in part, to a differential development of hypnotic tolerance between PhB and PhB derived from EtB. This will be elaborated upon later.

The neurophysiological effects of barbiturates are reviewed in detail by Jurna in this volume (Chap. 23).

E. Other CNS Effects

The principal other CNS effect of the anticonvulsant barbiturates is sedation. As noted previously, the anticonvulsant action of phenobarbital occurs at concentrations that are lower than those producing hypnosis. Recent work in our laboratory suggests that a differential tolerance to the hypnotic effect of phenobarbital occurs when eterobarb administration is compared with phenobarbital administration.

One of the most comprehensive studies on the factors altering the rate of tolerance to barbiturate has been carried out in cats by OKAMOTO and her colleagues. It has provided a quantitative assessment of the pharmacological parameters important in the development of tolerance to barbiturates (ROSENBERG and OKAMOTO 1974; OKAMOTO et al. 1975, 1977; BOISSE and OKAMOTO 1978 a, b, c, d). Basically the work relied on the development of a procedure termed the "chronically equivalent" barbiturate dosing method (based on the "maximally tolerable" dosing method in cats; OKAMOTO et al. 1975), which allowed a reproducible level of CNS depression to be maintained throughout a chronic treatment period. This permitted the direct quantitative comparison of the tolerance developed to a long-acting barbiturate, barbital, with the tolerance developed to the short-acting pentobarbital (ROSENBERG and OKAMOTO 1974; OKAMOTO et al. 1975; BOISSE and OKAMOTO 1978 a, b). From these studies the authors described several pharmacological parameters which in their opinion are critical to dispositional and functional tolerance development.

1. With short-acting barbiturates known to produce dispositional tolerance, the functional tolerance developed cannot be quantitatively characterized with changing brain concentrations and compared to a longer-acting minimally metabolized barbiturate, unless the challenge to the brain is stabilized throughout the treatment period.
2. The degree of barbiturate challenge to the brain can be individually adjusted to produce equi-effective peak CNS depression throughout chronic treatment and thus produce a constant barbiturate challenge for the development of functional tolerance.
3. The rate and extent of functional tolerance development to a short- and long-acting barbiturate were similar when induced by a dosing regimen which produced chronically equivalent levels of CNS depression.
4. The total time the CNS is challenged by depression is more important to functional tolerance development than the frequency of drug administration.
5. After 5 weeks of chronic barbiturate administration, functional tolerance developed slowly but continuously with no apparent maximum.

Although the specific biochemical or neurohumoral mechanism(s) underlying functional barbiturate tolerance have not been delineated (SMITH 1977; HO and HARRIS 1981), changes in CNS sensitivity have definitively been implicated in the development of tolerance to barbiturates.

Studies of EtB in animals (GALLAGHER et al. 1973; BAUMEL et al. 1976) and man (GALLAGHER and WOODBURY 1975; GALLAGHER et al. 1975) have confirmed its effective anticonvulsant activity and support the impression that hypnotic activity of this compound was attenuated in comparison to PhB in spite of the fact that EtB was completely metabolized to PhB (MATSUMOTO and GALLAGHER 1975; BAUMEL et al. 1976). More recently the hypnotic activity of EtB was extensively evaluated in acute and chronic animal studies (FREER 1978). Since these data have not yet been published they will be presented in part here because they are very relevant to an understanding of an important aspect of barbiturate pharmacology, tolerance.

Using loss of righting reflex (LRR) in the albino rat as an end point, orally administered PhB had an HD_{50} of 102 mg/kg (90–116 mg/kg), while EtB had an HD_{50} of 700 mg/kg (569–861 mg/kg). Latency to LRR over a range of oral doses of EtB was about 7 h while the same latency for PhB over a range of oral doses was about 1.5 h. In rat (BAUMEL et al. 1976) and man (MATSUMOTO and GALLAGHER 1975) oral EtB undergoes a rather complete first-pass metabolise so that little or no parent compound is detected in plasma, but its metabolites MMP and PhB do accumulate in plasma and tissues. Brain concentrations of PhB in rats receiving oral doses of PhB and MMP or oral doses of EtB were determined at LRR, and in a separate series of studies it was determined that the metabolite MMP had hypnotic activity equivalent to 0.7 of that of PhB. Consequently the total brain concentration at LRR averaged 192 nmol/g for the PhB-dosed animals and 308 nmol/g in phenobarbital equivalents for the EtB-dosed animals. Thus, a rather significant acute functional tolerance to the hypnotic activity of EtB was demonstrated. Further studies utilizing intravenous administration and oral combinations of MMP and PhB with and without metabolic blockade supported the conclusion that an interaction between the MMP and PhB metabolites resulted in the occurrence of acute functional tolerance.

Utilizing a modification, for the rat, of the chronically equivalent dosing technique of BOISSE and OKAMOTO (1978 a, b), rats were treated for 6 and 12 days with equivalently hypnotic doses of PhB or EtB. The doses were independently adjusted daily to compensate for tolerance (metabolic and functional). At the end of 6 days and 12 days PhB-treated animals were challenged with an oral dose of PhB (95 mg/kg) known to produce 100% LRR, and EtB-treated animals were challenged with a dose of EtB (120 mg/kg) known to produce 100% LRR. Brain concentrations of PhB and MMP were determined at LRR. In addition to the two chronic barbiturate-treated groups, vehicle-treated control animals also received the challenge doses and had brain concentrations of PhB and MMP determined at LRR.

When tolerance was assessed by the direct measurement of whole brain barbiturate concentration, a constant rate of functional tolerance development was observed with PhB treatment at 6 and 12 days so that 62% more brain PhB was found at LRR after 12 days of treatment. After 12 days of chronically equivalent doses of EtB, brain phenobarbital concentrations found at LRR were significantly greater than acute controls (121%) and chronically treated PhB rats (21%). Thus when PhB and EtB are administered in chronically equivalent doses to the rat, both the rate and magnitude of functional tolerance development to EtB are significantly increased over that developed to PhB.

Eterobarb, a 1,3,5,5-tetrasubstituted barbituric acid derivative, should be an inactive hypnotic compound (VIDA 1977). In addition, the pharmacokinetics of EtB are such that little or no EtB should reach or accumulate in brain because of the pronounced first-pass effect. Consequently, it is reasonable to assume that either MMP or more polar metabolites of EtB are involved in the development of functional hypnotic tolerance. With regard to acute functional tolerance it is most likely that MMP is the active compound because CNS concentrations of the polar metabolites would be negligible in the time required to reach LRR.

The functional tolerance that developed with chronic eterobarb treatment confirms the finding of others that functional tolerance develops slowly relative to metabolic tolerance (EBERT et al. 1964; KATO 1967; REMMER 1959; BELKNAP et al. 1977; BOISSE and OKAMOTO 1978 a, b). On the other hand, the differential rate and magnitude of tolerance developed with EtB in comparison to PhB suggests, in contrast to the finding of BOISSE and OKAMOTO (1978 a), that functional tolerance does not develop at the same rate to all barbiturates. It is not clear if this is a reflection of species differences or the different barbituric acid derivatives studied.

F. Pharmacodynamic Effects Outside the CNS

The ability of phenobarbital to induce increased activity in enzyme systems is the basis for numerous drug interactions and effects upon endogenous metabolic systems and hormones that are discussed subsequently in this chapter (drug interaction and toxicity section). Perhaps the most important nonepileptic use of phenobarbital is in the treatment of neonatal jaundice and the prevention of kernicterus (CRIGLER and GOLD 1969) as a result of its inducing properties.

G. Pharmacokinetics

The factors governing the movement of barbituric acid derivatives across membranes (solubility, percentage undissociated, acidity, and lipid solubility) have been discussed in relation to the physicochemical properties of these compounds and will not be repeated here in relation to absorption, distribution, and excretion.

I. Absorption

The calculations of BUTLER et al. (1954) and SVENSMARK and BUCHTHAL (1963) suggest that phenobarbital absorption in man is relatively complete. In contrast, mephobarbital is poorly absorbed by dog and man, with only 50%–60% of the dose accounted for following oral administration (BUTLER and WADDELL 1958; BUTLER et al. 1952). The absorption of anticonvulsant barbiturates has not been studied extensively. In the rat, intestinal absorption rate at pH 5.5 was calculated to be 1.57/h for phenobarbital in comparison to a rate of 1.12/h for mephobarbital (KAKEMI et al. 1967). The slower rate of absorption for mephobarbital was attributed to poorer protein binding of the methylated barbiturate. In addition to protein binding, the lipid solubility of the un-ionized barbiturate molecule is important for absorption at all gastrointestinal surfaces (SCHANKER 1961). Other factors may also influence the absorption of barbiturates. FREY and KAMPMANN (1966) have demonstrated in mice that DL-amphetamine is able to delay the absorption of phenobarbital and other anticonvulsants. In rats, ethanol increases the gastric but not the intestinal absorption of phenobarbital (MAGNUSSEN 1968).

II. Distribution

Following intravenous administration to mice, phenobarbital is found in the highest concentration in liver and blood, while about 5% of the dose administered is distributed to the brain within the first 6 h (GLASSON and BENAKIS 1961). In rabbits, intravenously administered phenobarbital was more evenly distributed between plasma, liver, brain, heart, kidney, lung, and muscle 1 h after administration (GOLDBAUM and SMITH 1954). Phenobarbital is relatively excluded from significant distribution to fat (SVENSMARK and BUCHTHAL 1963) while mephobarbital probably accumulates in fat (BUTLER et al. 1952). The volume of distribution (V_d) for intravenous phenobarbital in beagle dogs was found to be 0.6 ± 0.035 liters/kg in comparison to 2-phase elimination kinetics in mongrel dogs with a V_d of 0.68 ± 0.029 liters/kg (FREY et al. 1979). The same workers also found the ratio of CSF to plasma phenobarbital in the dog at steady state to be 0.565 with a permeability constant of 0.042/min.

One aspect of distribution which merits discussion is phenobarbital brain concentration. DOMEK et al. (1960) clearly demonstrated in adult cats that, although phenobarbital initially penetrates gray matter more effectively than white, distribution between gray and white matter is eventually equal. Furthermore, distribution within gray matter was uniform in the adult brain. They also found that phenobarbital distribution in newborn kittens was initially the reverse of that in adults and progressively evolved to the adult pattern as myelinization proceeded. In general, similar distribution has been found in human brain material obtained at the time of surgery for epilepsy (VAJDA et al. 1974; HOUGHTON et al. 1975; SHERWIN et al. 1976; HARVEY et al. 1977). Distribution of phenobarbital is equal between gray and white matter and, statistically, there is a good correlation between plasma and brain concentration with the latter uniformly the lower concentration. However, when one looks at individual brain to plasma ratios of phenobarbital concentration there is about a threefold variability in the ratio. Thus, for a given individual, plasma concentration of phenobarbital is not necessarily a good predictor of brain concentration.

Protein binding of phenobarbital is about 46% for the ionized and un-ionized forms and is rather independent of pH, concentration of the drug, and species (WADDELL and BUTLER 1957; GOLDBAUM and SMITH 1954; LOUS 1954; LÖSCHER 1979).

III. Metabolism

The general pathways by which the barbiturates are metabolized are known and have been extensively reviewed in animals and man (MAYNERT and VAN DYKE 1949; WILLIAMS and PARK 1964; MARK 1963; BUSH and SANDERS 1967; FREUDENTHAL and CARROLL 1973).

Since phenobarbital was first shown to be oxidized to *p*-hydroxy-PhB (BUTLER 1954), many studies have attempted to delineate the metabolic pathways of phenobarbital. These are still not fully understood. Although there are some species differences, radioactive tracer studies have indicated that 65%–85% of phenobarbital is excreted in the urine, with 18%–32% unchanged (EISENHARDT et al. 1977). The remaining 45%–65% is metabolized to *p*-hydroxy-PB, which then can be conjugated to glucuronide or sulfate (BUTLER 1956). It has been reported that CO_2 accounts for a small fraction of oxidized [^{14}C]PhB in the rat (GLASSON and BENAKIS 1961; EISENHARDT et al. 1977). A most unusual finding has been reported for phenobarbital metabolism in man. After oral administration of ^{14}C,^{15}N-labeled phenobarbital, the major metabolite recovered in urine was identified as *N*-hydroxy-PhB (31%). This compared to only 17% appearing as the *p*-OH derivative (TANG et al. 1977). However, subsequent studies of amobarbital *N*-hydroxylation established the *N*-metabolite as amobarbital-*N*-β-D-glucopyranoside rather than the originally identified metabolite *N*-hydroxyamobarbital (TANG et al. 1978). A recent review provides evidence that phenobarbital can potentially be biotransformed to several other minor metabolites, including 5-(l-hydroxyethyl)-5-phenylbarbituric acid, 5-(3,4-dihydroxyphenyl)-5-ethylbarbituric acid, and 5-(3,4-dihydroxycyclohexadien)-5-ethylbarbituric acid (FREUDENTHAL and CARROLL 1973). PhB is known to be slowly eliminated by rat ($t\frac{1}{2}$, 15 h) and man ($t\frac{1}{2}$, 3–6 days; MAYNERT 1972).

The importance of *N*-dealkylation of barbituric acids in vivo was first demonstrated by BUTLER and BUSH (1939). Following the intravenous administration of *N*-methylbarbital or *N*-methylphenobarbital to dogs, barbital or phenobarbital, respectively, were recovered in the urine. Subsequent studies in dogs (BUTLER 1952, 1953a, b) and rats (BUTLER et al. 1952) substantiated these early findings. When single doses of the methylated drugs were administered to dogs, complete demethylation required 1–2 days. The products of demethylation were eliminated very slowly and they persisted long after the parent drug was no longer detectable. Based on the plasma concentration of the products, estimates of the extent of demethylation indicated that conversion of the methylated drugs to the corresponding nonmethylated compounds was nearly complete. CRAIG and SHIDEMAN (1971) also demonstrated the rapid demethylation of MB by rats and presented data supporting significant induction of this dealkylation reaction with prior exposure to MB or PhB. BUTLER (1955) also studied demethylation of dimethylbarbital and methylbarbital in the rat and determined that the rate of removal of the first methyl group from dimethylbarbital was approximately six times greater than the second demethylation. BUTLER and WADDELL (1958) reported concentrations of demethylated products of MB and metharbital (MTB) in plasma of human subjects receiving the methylated drugs on a chronic dosage schedule. In three subjects receiving MB, PhB accumulated in concentrations two to six times higher than MB. A similar pattern was observed in four subjects receiving MTB, except that after approximately 1 week of chronic administration plasma MTB concentrations dropped to undetectable levels. This most likely occurred as a consequence of hepatic microsomal enzyme induction.

Initial studies in the rat and mouse have shown that EtB is metabolized to phenobarbital and an intermediate, MMP (GALLAGHER et al. 1973; RAPPORT and KUPFERBERG 1973). These results were supported and extended when it was shown that phenobarbital and its metabolites, *p*-OH-PhB and conjugated *p*-OH-PhB, accounted for 90% of a radioactive dose of [^{14}C] EtB excreted into the urine (ALVIN and BUSH 1974b). ALVIN and BUSH (1974b) also studied the in vitro metabolism of EtB and found that enzymatic removal of the first *N*-alkoxymethyl group was very rapid ($t\frac{1}{2}$, 12.5 min), while removal of the second methoxymethyl group took several hours. The rate of microsomal dealkoxylation of EtB in vitro was approximately 75 times that of its primary metabolite, MMP. In the in vitro study by ALVIN and BUSH (1974a), a minor metabolite, which accounted for about 8% of the radioactivity recovered from urine, also appeared as a metabolite of MMP in the liver homogenate studies. Based on partition coefficients it is comparable in lipid solubility to *p*-OH-PhB. It was suggested that this metabolite was hydroxylated MMP in free and conjugated form. Based on partition coefficients, MMP is considerably less polar than phenobarbital and therefore would be expected to penetrate rapidly into lipid tissue such as brain. In accordance one could expect a low renal clearance (BUTLER 1955) and, in fact, urine was devoid of MMP (ALVIN and BUSH 1974b).

The most extensive study evaluating the in vivo metabolism and tissue distribution of EtB in the rat also correlated brain concentrations of EtB, MMP, and PhB with anticonvulsant activity (BAUMEL et al. 1976). EtB (ethyl-1-[^{14}C], 24 mg/kg, i.p.) was rapidly metabolized to MMP and then converted at a slower rate to phenobarbital. It was no longer detectable in plasma after 30 min. Plasma concentrations of phenobarbital increased progressively during the 4 h of measurement. MMP declined at a slower rate from brain and liver than plasma, indicating that it is probably sequestered in these tissues. The observed accumulation of MMP and phenobarbital in the liver also suggested preferential binding in hepatic tissue. Baumel and associates demonstrated that MMP was effective against MES seizures but not PTZ seizures, at a time when brain concentrations of phenobarbital were too low to account for the protection. The data regarding the metabolism of EtB do suggest that the previously reported attenuated hypnotic properties of EtB (Samour and Vida 1971) could involve an interaction of MMP with phenobarbital.

A very polar, unidentified metabolite (s) also appears in liver, plasma, and brain. It shows two peaks in plasma, one at ½ h and the second at 2 h. The first peak coincides in time (in liver) with the EtB peak and the second coincides in time with the phenobarbital peak. Although not suggested by the authors, it seems possible these polar metabolites may represent *p*-OH-MMP and *p*-OH-PhB, respectively.

The most recent report on EtB metabolism in the rat (Jenden et al. 1978) is consistent with the EtB-MMP-PB metabolic sequence, each showing a later peak than the last, with the brain concentration following plasma concentrations. After intravenous administration there was a 2.5-min delay to peak plasma and brain concentrations of EtB. According to the authors this suggested very rapid tissue clearance and/or a substantial first-pass metabolism. Due to its very high lipid solubility, EtB appeared to be rapidly sequestered in the lipophilic regions of the liver and the brain. The MMP plasma and brain curves showed two peaks, at 2.5 and 30 min. This is consistent with its continued metabolic production at a time when tissues are approaching a steady state. An important finding by Jenden and his associates was that (in man) the rate of MMP formation occurred at zero-order kinetics, with its formation ending abruptly at a time when EtB metabolism was complete. Although these studies did not differentiate between the various possibilities for this, e.g., zero-order absorption or zero-order metabolism, the unusual metabolism of EtB is comparable to a sustained release preparation of MMP and PB. The combined results of these animal studies support a scheme of EtB metabolism as follows:

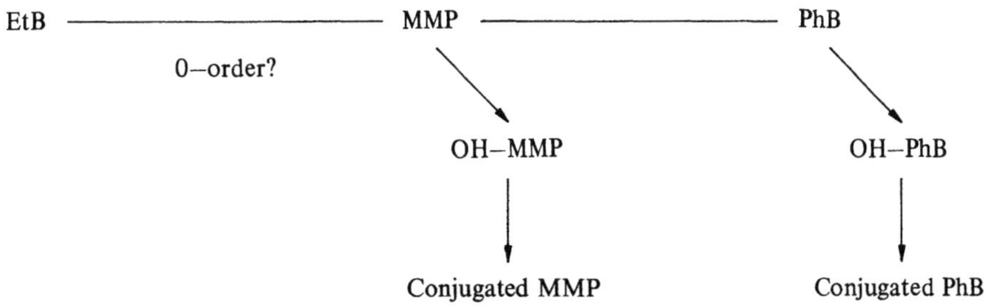

In man, two metabolites, MMP and PhB, appeared in plasma within 5 min after oral administration of [^{14}C] EtB (Matsumoto and Gallagher 1975) (Fig.

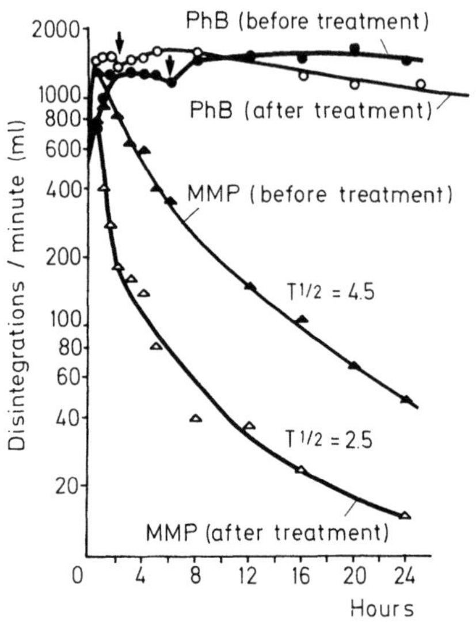

Fig. 1. Radioactivity in plasma associated with PhB and MMP following an oral dose of 4,6-[^{14}C]eterobarb (SA 10.5 μCi/mg). Study I (●, ▲) was performed before any anticonvulsant treatment and study 2 (○, △) was performed after 4 months of treatment with eterobarb at 360 mg/day (MATSUMOTO and GALLAGHER 1975)

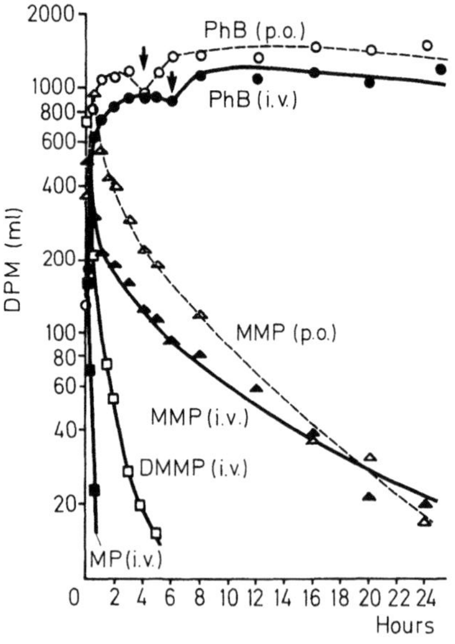

Fig. 2. Radioactivity in plasma associated with PhB, MMP, and eterobarb (EtB, DMMP) following an oral (○, △) or intravenous (●, ▲) dose of 4,6-[^{14}C]eterobarb (SA 10.5 μCi/mg). Study I (oral dose) performed during chronic treatment with phenytoin and eterobarb. Study 2 (intravenous) performed 3 months later during same treatment (MATSUMOTO and GALLAGHER 1975)

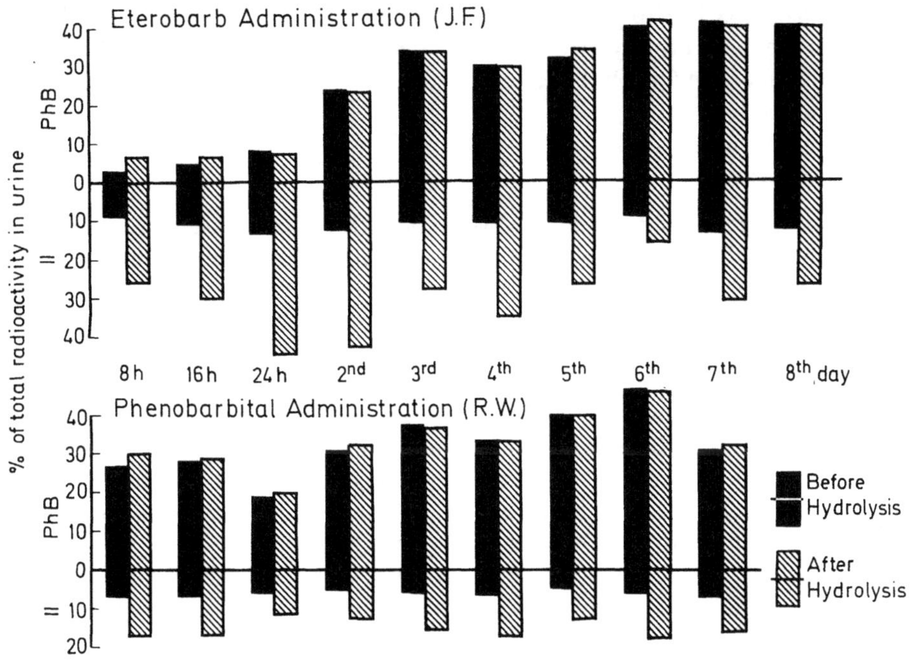

Fig. 3. Urinary excretion of PhB (*above the line*) and metabolite II (*p*-hydroxyphenobarbital) (*below the line*) following an oral dose of 4,6[^{14}C]eterobarb (SA 10.5 μCi/mg) in a patient not previously treated with anticonvulsant drugs (*top of figure*). Urinary excretion of the same compounds following an oral dose of [^{14}C]phenobarbital in a patient after 3 months of treatment with phenobarbital at 90 mg/day (*bottom of figure*) (MATSUMOTO and GALLAGHER 1975)

1). No EtB was found in the plasma at any time; a similar result has been reported by JENDEN and his colleagues (1978). MMP reached a peak plasma concentration at 30 min and declined with a half-life of 4–6 h after acute administration and 2–3 h after chronic (3 months) administration. Phenobarbital appeared rapidly in plasma and reached peak concentration within 4 h. A biphasic rise and fall in concentration was observed, with a second peak appearing at about 10 h after a slight decline. These data emphasize the extremely rapid absorption, distribution, and metabolism of EtB in man. Induction of metabolism was apparent for MMP when the study was repeated after chronic treatment with EtB. PhB derived from EtB was always cleared with a half-life varying from 4 to 6 days. When EtB was administered intravenously it was cleared with a half-life of 10 min and the distribution pattern of MMP and PhB strongly resembled oral administration of EtB (Fig. 2). Three polar metabolites, I, II, III, PhB, and as much as 50%–75% ether unextractable material were found free and as glucuronide conjugates in urine. Metabolite I and the ether unextractable material remain unidentified. Metabolite II was identified as *p*-OH-PB and metabolite III corresponds to the unidentified metabolite described by ALVIN and BUSH (1974a) and is probably *p*-OH-MMP. The pattern of excretion of phenobarbital and *p*-OH-PhB differed after EtB in comparison to phenobarbital administration (Fig. 3). With PhB administration the main urinary metabolite was unchanged phenobarbital. After EtB, larger amounts of *p*-OH-PhB were excreted.

IV. Excretion

The high lipid solubility of EtB, MMP, and MB assure efficient renal tubular reabsorption of these compounds. Consequently, the major excretion product in urine is phenobarbital and its metabolites. BUTLER (1952) found that the renal clearance of MB in dogs was 0.2 ml/min following a single dose of MB, while the renal clearance of the PhB metabolite was 0.9 ml/min. Similarly, in man, SVENDSON and BROCHMANN-HANNSEN (1962) demonstrated that following a single 150-mg dose of MB, 1.2 mg (0.8% of the dose) was excreted in urine during the first 9 h after the dose, with negligible amounts excreted subsequently. In contrast, unmetabolized phenobarbital amounted to 19.5 mg during 32 h of collection. Another individual given a single 200-mg dose of phenobarbital excreted 46.8 mg or 23.4% of the dose during the first 48 h after dosing.

FREY et al. (1979) measured renal clearance of phenobarbital after intravenous administration of a single dose of PhB in beagle and mongrel dogs. Beagles had a clearance rate of 13 ± 1.7 ml/kg per hour, while that for mongrel dogs was 7.0 ± 1.3 ml/kg per hour. The differences were statistically significant and related to different pharmacokinetic models in these dogs. FREY et al. (1981) have also measured some aspects of phenobarbital clearance in gerbils and found a clearance half-life of 10.6 h in this species after drug administration.

An important aspect of phenobarbital renal excretion is the effect of urine pH upon clearance rate. WADDELL and BUTLER (1957) found renal clearance of phenobarbital (expressed in terms of unbound drug) to be less than 1 ml/min with a urine flow of 0.2 ml/min in the dog. Diuresis of neutral or acidic urine produced linear increases in clearance up to at least 5 ml/min with urine flow of about 7 ml/min. Diuresis of alkaline (pH 7.8–8.0) urine produced linear increases in renal clearance up to about 45 ml/min with a flow of 7 ml/min. In man, with a urine pH of about 6 and a flow of 0.8–1.2 ml/min, clearance of phenobarbital ranged from 2.0 to 3.0 ml/min. Following alkalinization of urine, a flow of 2.3 ml/min was associated with a clearance of 9.8 ml/min, and a flow of 8.0 ml/min produced a clearance of 29.0 ml/min. These data emphasize the importance of the extent of ionization of renal tubular phenobarbital upon its excretion rate.

The kinetics of the excretion of hydroxylated and conjugated metabolites of phenobarbital have been less intensively studied. BUTLER (1956) demonstrated that the amount of phenobarbital that is hydroxylated increases with increased exposure to the drug. This is clearly demonstrated in the data discussed in the metabolism section above.

H. Drug Interactions

Phenobarbital is a classical inducing agent for the hepatic mixed function oxidase enzymes responsible for many drug oxidations. Inducing barbiturates also affect

Table 3. Barbituric acid derivative interactions with drugs: drugs which are cleared more rapidly as a result of barbiturate treatment

Compound	Ref.
Alprenolol	ALVAN et al. (1977)
Antipyrine	CONNEY (1967)
Bishydroxycoumarin	CUCINELL et al. (1965)
Clonazepam	KHOO et al. (1980)
DDT	DAVIES et al. (1969)
Digitoxin	CONNEY (1967)
Dipyrone	CONNEY (1967)
Griseofulvin	CONNEY (1967)
Isoniazid	LEVI et al. (1968)
Metoprolol	HAGLAND et al. (1979)
Phenylbutazone	LEVI et al. (1968)
Phenytoin	MORSELLI et al. (1971)
Propranolol	ROWLAND (1972)
Warfarin	CUCINELL (1972)
	O'REILLY et al. (1980)

numerous other hepatic and extrahepatic enzyme systems and consequently affect the metabolism of endogenous substances as well as xenobiotics. A number of compounds which have been documented as interacting with barbituric acid derivatives are listed in Table 3. This is not intended to be an exhaustive list of such compounds. Interactions in which barbiturates inhibit the metabolism of other drugs are less common as are interactions in which other drugs inhibit the metabolism of barbiturates. The interaction between valproic acid and phenobarbital is an important example of the latter interaction (KAPETANOVIC et al. 1981).

J. Toxicology

In the mouse, orally administered phenobarbital has a median neurotoxic dose (TD_{50}) of 51 mg/kg (44–60 mg/kg) (GOODMAN et al. 1953b). Subcutaneous administration increases the TD_{50} to about 100 mg/kg (SWINYARD et al. 1952). In the rat comparable TD_{50} values are 35 mg/kg (30–41 mg/kg) p.o. and 90 mg/kg s.c. (GOODMAN et al. 1953b; SWINYARD et al. 1952). The TD_{50} for rabbit is identical to that for rat, while the cat is much more sensitive to phenobarbital, with a TD_{50} of 5 mg/kg (TOMAN et al. 1946). The oral TD_{50} for mephobarbital is 60 mg/kg for mouse (SWINYARD et al. 1952). The same authors report a TD_{50} of 80 mg/kg for the rat with subcutaneous administration of mephobarbital.

VIDA et al. (1973a) did not find an HD_{50} in mice for EtB. In rats (FREER 1978) an oral HD_{50} of 102 mg/kg (90–116 mg/kg) was found for PhB and that for EtB was 700 mg/kg (569–861 mg/kg) when the HD_{50} was defined as 50% of the animals losing the righting reflex. The LD_{50} in mice with oral dosing is 270 mg/kg for PhB, 300 mg/kg for MB, and 470 mg/kg for EtB (VIDA and GERRY 1977).

The principal undesired side effect of the anticonvulsant barbiturates in man is sedation. This has been discussed extensively in this chapter and will not be further elaborated. Barbiturates do affect other organs directly and/or indirectly. Bone is affected by chronic barbiturate exposure. Vitamin D is metabolized by two hydroxylations which activate the vitamin. The first oxidation occurs in the liver, forming 25-hydroxyvitamin D, and the second in the kidney, forming 1,25-dihydroxyvitamin D (DELUCA 1979). Barbiturates induce the hepatic mixed function oxidase system that oxidizes vitamin D. In addition, anticonvulsant drugs have direct inhibitory effects on intestinal calcium transport as well as on parathyroid hormone or 1,25-dihydroxyvitamin-D-induced bone resorption (HAHN 1980).

Anticonvulsant treatment is also associated with decreased serum calcitonin concentration (KURSE et al. 1980). Because of the alterations and serum calcium in parathyroid hormone, secondary hyperparathyroidism can develop and further complicate bone pathology. It also seems likely that there are direct effects of anticonsulvant drugs upon calcium ion movement in bone. The net result of all of this is an incidence of severe osteopenia of at least 20% of epileptic patients (DYMLING et al. 1979; CHRISTIANSEN et al. 1973; HAHN et al. 1975; ZANZI et al. 1981).

Vitamin K deficiency has been noted in neonates born to mothers receiving phenobarbital treatment (VAN CREVELD 1958; DOUGLAS 1966). This may result in a potentially fatal bleeding disorder if it is not corrected with prophylactic vitamin K therapy. Serum folic acid concentration is also lowered during barbiturate treatment and, in some instances, this may produce a megaloblastic anemia (HAWKINS and MEYNELL 1956, 1958). The anemia is corrected with folic acid treatment (DRUSKIN et al. 1962); however, there is not benefit associated with treatment of the folate deficiency in the absence of anemia (MATTSON et al. 1973). Another effect of barbiturate treatment, again related to induction of hepatic enzymes, is the increased rate of metabolism of prophyrin precursors (GRANICK 1965). As a result, barbiturate treatment may precipitate attacks of acute porphyria in susceptible individuals. Anticonvulsant drug treatment, including barbiturates, has been associated with hypercortisolemia (GALLAGHER 1976) and an altered pattern of cortisol metabolism. The former effect may be a consequence of the epileptic process as well as anticonvulsant treatment (Gallagher, unpublished data) while the latter is a result of heptatic induction.

The teratogenicity of barbiturates has been suggested by some studies. NAKANE et al. (1980) found a correlation between PhB treatment and teratogenicity in humans. The association of teratogenicity with MB was less significant. However, the patients treated with either barbiturate may have been receiving other drugs and when the teratogenic influence of trimethadione was removed from the statistics the overall rate of congenital anomalies approximated that found in the nonepileptic population. Some of the complications in determining teratogenicity of anticonvulsant drugs in epileptic patients have been illustrated by FRIIS (1979).

All of the typical allergic reactions occur with barbiturates and these have frequently been discussed (BROWNING and MAYNERT 1972; MEINARDI and STOEL 1974) and thus will not be reenumerated here.

The last toxic effect to be considered is the effects of barbiturates upon higher mental functioning. When the appropriate psychological tests are employed, a positive correlation between impaired performance and rising phenobarbital concentration has been noted in normal subjects (Hutt et al. 1968). The susceptible tests required sustained attention, memory, and speed of thought. Similar results were obtained by Hartlage (to be published), again using a battery of tests selected for sensitivity to sedation. Interestingly, the only report in the literature comparing psychological performance of normal volunteers treated with phenobarbital with those treated with eterobarb found significantly less clinical toxicity in the eterobarb-treated group when blood concentrations of phenobarbital were comparable between groups (Smith et al. 1975; Smith, personal communication). This observation is consistent with the animal studies of Freer (1978) and suggests that further evaluation of eterobarb, as an alternative anticonvulsant to phenobarbital, may be warranted.

References

Albright PS, Burnham WM (1980) Development of a new pharmacological seizure model: effects of anticonvulsants on cortical- and amygdala-kindled seizures in the rat. Epilepsia 21:681–689

Alles G, Ellis C, Feigen G, Redemann M (1947) Comparative central depressant actions of some 5-phenyl-5-alkyl barbituric acids. J Pharmacol Exp Ther 89:356–367

Alvan G, Piafsky K, Lind M, Von Bahr (1977) Effect of pentobarbital on the disposition of alprenolol. Clin Pharmacol Ther 22:316–321

Alvin J, Bush M (1974a) Metabolic fate of dimethoxymethyl-phenobarbital in rat. J Pharmacol Exp Ther 188:8–14

Alvin J, Bush M (1974b) Metabolism of *N,N*-dimethoxymethyl-phenobarbital in the mouse. Pharmacologist 16:149

Baumel IP, Gallagher BB, DiMicco J, Goico H (1973) Metabolism and anticonvulsant properties of primidone in the rat. J Pharmacol Exp Ther 186:305–314

Baumel I, Gallagher B, DiMicco J, Dionne R (1976) Metabolism, distribution, and anticonvulsant properties of *N,N'*-dimethoxymethylphenobarbital in the rat. J Pharmacol Exp Ther 196:180–187

Baylis EM, Fry DE, Marks V (1970) Microdetermination of serum phenobarbitone and diphenylhydantoin by gas-liquid chromatography. Clin Chim Acta 30:93–103

Belknap J, Ondrusek G, Berg J, Waddingham S (1977) Barbiturate dependence in mice: effects of continuous versus discontinuous drug administration. Psychopharmacology 51:195–198

Boisse N, Okamoto M (1978a) Physical dependence to barbital compared to pentobarbital. I. Chronically equivalent dosing method. J Pharmacol Exp Ther 204:497–506

Boisse N, Okamoto M (1978b) Physical dependence to barbital compared to pentobarbital. II. Tolerance characteristics. J Pharmacol Exp Ther 204:507–513

Boisse N, Okamoto N (1978c) Physical dependence to barbital compared to pentobarbital. III. Withdrawal characteristics. J Pharmacol Exp Ther 204:514–525

Boisse N, Okamoto M (1978d) Physical dependence to barbital compared to pentobarbital. IV. Influence of elimination kinetics. J Pharmacol Exp Ther 204:526–540

Breon JL, Mauger J, Osborne G, Lausier J, Paruta A (1976) The aqueous solubility of variously substituted barbituric acids. I. Chemical effects. Drug Devel Comm 2:521–529

Brodie BB, Hogben C (1957) Some physiochemical factors in drug action. J Pharm Pharmacol 9:345–380

Brown WC, Schiffman DO, Swinyard EA, Goodman LS (1953) Comparative assay of antiepileptic drugs by "psychomotor" seizure test and minimal electroshock threshold test. J Pharmacol Exp Ther 107:273–283

Browning RA, Maynert EW (1972) Toxicity: phenobarbital, mephobarbital, and metharbital. In: Woodbury DM, Perry JK, Schmidt RP (eds) Antiepileptic drugs. Raven, New York, pp 345–351
Bush M, Sanders E (1967) Metabolic fate of drugs: barbiturates and closely related compounds. Ann Rev Pharmacol 7:57–76
Butler TC (1952) Quantitative studies on the metabolic fate of mephobarbital (*N*-methylphenobarbital). J Pharmacol Exp Ther 106:235–245
Butler TC (1953 a) Quantitative studies of the demethylation of *N*-methylbarbital (metharbital, Gemonil). J Pharmacol Exp Ther 108:474–480
Butler TC (1953 b) Further studies of metabolic removal of alkyl groups from nitrogen in barbituric acid derivatives. Proc Soc Exp Biol Med 84:105–108
Butler TC (1954) Metabolic oxidation of phenobarbital to *p*-OH-phenobarbital. Science 120:494
Butler TC (1955) The effects of *N*-methylation in 5,5-disubstituted derivatives of barbituric acid, hydantoin, and 2,4-oxazolidinedione. J Am Pharm Assoc Sci Ed 44:367–370
Butler TC (1956) The metabolic hydroxylation of phenobarbital. J Pharmacol Exp Ther 116:326–336
Butler TC, Bush MJ (1939) The metabolic fate of *N*-methylbarbituric acids. J Pharmacol Exp Ther 65:205–13
Butler TC, Waddell W (1958) *N*-Methylated derivatives of barbituric acid, hydantoin, and oxazolidinedione used in treatment of epilepsy. Neurology (suppl) 8:106–112
Butler TC, Mahafee D, Mahafee C (1952) Quantitative studies of the metabolic fate of mephobarbital. J Pharmacol Exp Ther 106:235–245
Butler TC, Mahafee C, Waddell WJ (1954) Phenobarbital: studies of elimination, accumulation, tolerance and dosage schedules. J Pharmacol Exp Ther 111:425–435
Chen G, Ensor CR (1950) Evaluation of antiepileptic drugs. Arch Neurol Psychiatry 63:55–60
Christiansen C, Rodbro P, Lund M (1973) Effect of vitamin D on bone mineral mass in normal subjects and in epileptic patients on anticonvulsants: a controlled therapeutic trial. Br Med J 2:208–209
Collins AJ, Horlington M (1969) A sequential screening test based on the running component of audiogenic seizures in mice, including reference compound PD_{50} values. Br J Pharmacol 37:140–150
Conney A (1967) Pharmacological implications of microsomal enzyme induction. Pharmacol Rev 19:317–366
Cook CE (1978) Radioimmunoassay. In: Pippenger CE, Penry JK, Kutt H (eds) Antiepileptic drugs: quantitative analysis and interpretation. Raven, New York, pp 163–173
Craig C, Hirano K, Shideman F (1960) Anticonvulsant activity of a metabolite of phenobarbital. Fed Proc 19:280
Craig CR, Shideman FE (1971) Metabolism and anticonvulsant properties of mephobarbital and phenobarbital in rats. J Pharmacol Exp Ther 176:35–41
Crigler JF, Gold NI (1969) Effect of sodium phenobarbital on bilirubin metabolism in an infant with congenital nonhemolytic unconjugated hyperbilirubinemia and kernicterus. J Clin Invest 48:42–55
Cucinell SA (1972) Phenobarbital: interactions with other drugs. In: Woodbury DM, Penry JK, Schmidt RP (eds). Raven, New York, pp 319–327
Cucinell SA, Coriney AH, Sansur MS, Burns JJ (1965) Drug interactions in man. I. Lowering effect of phenobarbital on plasma levels of bishydroxycoumarin (Dicumarol) and diphenylhydantoin (Dilantin). Clin Pharmacol Ther:420–429
Davies JE, Edmundson WF, Carter CH, Barquet A (1969) Effect of anticonvulsant drugs on dicophane (D.D.T.) residues in man. Lancet 2:7–9
DeLuca HF (1979) Vitamin D metabolism and function. Springer, Berlin Heidelberg New York
Domek N, Barlow C, Roth L (1960) An ontogenetic study of phenobarbital-^{14}C in cat brain. J Pharmacol Exp Ther 130:285–293

Doran W (1959) Barbituric acid hypnotics. In: Blicke J, Cos R (eds) Medicinal chemistry, vol 4. John Wiley, New York, pp 1–340
Douglas H (1966) Haemorrhage in the newborn. Lancet 1:816–817
Druskin MS, Wallen MH, Bonagura L (1962) Anticonvulsant-associated megaloblastic anemia response to 25 micrograms of folic acid administered by mouth daily. N Engl J Med 267:483–485
Dymling IR, Johnell D, Lindgren L, Niesson BE, Walloe A, Wiklund PE (1979) In: Norman AW, Schaefer K, Herrati DV, Grupoleit HG, Coburn JW, DeLuca HF, Mawer EB, Suda T (eds) Vitamin D basic research and its clinical applications. Walter de Gruyter, Berlin, pp 1193–1197
Ebert A, Yim G, Miya T (1964) Distribution and metabolism of barbital-^{14}C in tolerant and nontolerant rats. Biochem Pharmacol 13:1267–1274
Eisenhardt T, Levin S, Touchstone J, Cooper D (1977) Phenobarbital metabolism during chronic administration in rats. Fed Proc 36:844
Ferngren H (1968) Further studies on clinically induced seizures and their antagonism by anticonvulsants during postnatal development in the mouse. Acta Pharmacol Toxicol 26:177–188
Fink GB, Swinyard EA (1959) Modification of maximal audiogenic and electroshock seizures in mice by psychopharmacologic drugs. J Pharmacol Exp Ther 127:318–324
Fischer E, Dilthey A (1904) Justus Liebigs. Ann Chem 335:334
Freer LS (1978) Characterization of the functional tolerance development to *N,N'*dimethoxymethylphenobarbital. Unpublished doctoral thesis, Department of Pharmacology, Georgetown University, Washington DC
Freudenthal R, Carrol F (1973) Metabolism of certain commonly used barbiturates. Drug Metab Rev 2:265–278
Frey HH, Kampmann E (1966) Interaction of amphetamine with anticonvulsant drugs. II. Effect of amphetamine on the absorption of anticonvulsant drugs. Acta Pharmacol Toxicol (Kbh.) 24:310–316
Frey HH, Magnussen MP (1971) A hitherto undescribed feature in the anticonvulsant effect of phenobarbital. Pharmacology 5:1–8
Frey HH, Gobel W, Löscher W (1979) Pharmacokinetics of primidone and its active metabolites in the dog. Arch Int Pharmacodyn Ther 242:14–30
Frey HH, Löscher W, Reiche R, Schultz D (1981) Pharmacology of antiepileptic drugs in the gerbil – I. Pharmacokinetics. Neuropharmacol 20:769–771
Friis ML (1979) Epilepsy among parents of children with facial clefts. Epilepsia 20:69–76
Gallagher BB (1976) Adrenal hyperplasia in epileptic patients. In: Kellaway P, Petersen I (eds) Quantitative analytic studies in epilepsy. Raven, New York, pp 165–169
Gallagher B, Woodbury S (1975) A double-blind comparison of the anticonvulsant dimethoxymethyl phenobarbital and phenobarbital. In: Janz D (ed) Epileptology. Georg Thieme, Stuttgart, pp 117–122
Gallagher B, Baumel I, DiMicco J, Vida J (1973) Metabolism and distribution of dimethoxymethyl phenobarbital in the rat. Fed Proc 32:684
Gallagher B, Baumel I, Woodbury S, DiMicco J (1975) Clinical evaluation of eterobarb, a new anticonvulsant. Neurology 25:399–404
Glasson B, Benakis A (1961) Etude du phenobarbital-C^{14} dans l'organisme du rat. Helv Physiol Acta 19:324–334
Goldbaum LR, Smith PK (1954) The interaction of barbiturates with serum albumin and its possible relation to their disposition and pharmacological actions. J Pharmacol Exp Ther 111:197–209
Goodman LS, Grewal MS, Brown WC, Swinyard EA (1953 a) Comparison of maximal seizures evoked by pentylenetetrazol (Metrazol) and electroshock in mice and their modification by anticonvulsants. J Pharmacol Exp Ther 108:168–176
Goodman LS, Swinyard EA, Brown WC, Schiffman DO, Grewal MS, Bliss EL (1953 b) Anticonvulsant properties of 5-phenyl-5-ethyl hexahydropyrimidine-4, 6-dione (Mysoline), a new antiepileptic. J Pharmacol Exp Ther 108:428–436
Granick S (1965) Hepatic porphyria and drug-induced or chemical porphyria. Ann NY Acad Sci 123:188–197

Greeley RH (1974) New approach to derivatization and gas-chromatographic analysis of barbiturates. Clin Chem 20:192–194
Haglund K, Seideman P, Collote P, Borg KO, Von Bahr C (1979) Influence of pentobarbital on metoprolol plasma levels. Clin Pharmacol Ther 26:326–329
Hahn TJ (1980) Drug-induced disorders of vitamin D and mineral metabolism. Clin Endocrinol Metab 9:107–129
Hahn TJ, Hendin BA, Scharp CR, Boisseau VC, Haddad JG (1975) Serum 25-hydroxycalciferol levels and bone mass in children on chronic anticonvulsant therapy. N Eng J Med 292:550–554
Hansch C, Clayton J (1973) Lipophilic character and biological activity of drugs. II. The parabolic case. J Pharm Sci 62:1–21
Hansch C, Dunn W (1972) Linear relationships between lipophilic character and biological activity of drugs. J Pharm Sci 61:1–19
Hansch C, Steward A, Anderson S, Bentley D (1968) The parabolic dependence of drug action upon lipophilic character as revealed by a study of hypnotics. J Med Chem 11:1–11
Hartlage LC (to be published) Neuropsychological assessment of anticonvulsant drug toxicity. Clin Neuropsychol
Harvey CD, Sherwin AL, Van Der Kleijn E (1977) Distribution of anticonvulsant drugs in gray and white matter of human brain. Can J Neurol Sci 4:89–92
Hauptmann A (1912) Luminal bei Epilepsie. Münch Med Wochenschr 59:1907–1909
Hawk GL, Franconi LC (1978) High-pressure liquid chromatography in quantitation of antiepileptic drugs. In: Pippenger CE, Penry JK, Kutt H (eds) Antiepileptic drugs: quantitative analysis and interpretation. Raven, New York, pp 9–17
Hawkins CF, Meynell MJ (1956) Macrocytosis and megaloblastic anemia in epileptics on anticonvulsant drugs. Q J Med 25:567–568
Hawkins CF, Meynell MJ (1958) Macrocytosis and macrocytic anaemia caused by anticonvulsant drugs. Q J Med 27:45–63
Ho IK, Harris RA (1981) Mechanism of action of barbiturates. Ann Rev Pharmacol Toxicol 21:83–11
Houghton GW, Richens A, Toseland PA, Davidson S, Falconer MA (1975) Brain concentrations of phenytoin, phenobarbital and primidone in epileptic patients. Eur J Clin Pharmacol 9:73–78
Hutt SJ, Jackson PM, Belstram A, Higgins G (1968) Perceptual-motor behavior in relation to blood phenobarbitone level: a preliminary report. Dev Med Child Neurol 10:626–632
Jenden D, Cho A, Goldberg M, Steinborn J (1978) Study of the metabolism of demethoxymethyl phenobarbital. National Institutes of Health, Final Report. (Contract 1-NS-4-2330) pp 1–63
Juliusburger J (1912) Über Luminal, ein neues Hypnoticum and Sedatium. Berl Klin Wochenschr 49:940–942
Kakemi K, Takaichi A, Hori R, Konishi R (1967) Absorption of barbituric acid derivatives from rat small intestine. Chem Pharm Bull 15:1883–1887
Kapetanovic IM, Kupferberg HJ, Porter RJ, Theodore W, Schulwan E, Penry JK (1981) Mechanism of valproate-phenobarbital interaction in epileptic patients. Clin Pharmacol Ther 29:480–486
Kato R (1967) Analysis and differentiation of the mechanism in development of drug tolerance. Jpn J Pharmacol 17:499–508
Khoo KC, Mendels J, Rothhart M, Garland WA, Colburn WA, Min BH, Lucek R, Carbone JJ, Boxenbaum HG, Kaplan SA (1980) Influence of phenytoin and phenobarbital on the disposition of a single oral dose of clonazepam. Clin Pharmacol Ther 28:368–375
Kupferberg HJ (1978) Quantitative methods for antiepileptic drugs analysis: an overview. In: Pippenger CE, Penry JK, Kutt H (eds) Antiepileptic drugs: quantitative analysis and interpretation. Raven, New York, pp 9–17
Kurse K, Bartels H, Ziegler R, Dreller E, Kracht U (1980) Parathyroid function and serum calcitonin in children receiving anticonvulsant drugs. Eur J Pediatr 133:151–156

Levi AJ, Sherlock S, Walker D (1968) Phenylbutazone and isoniazid metabolism in patients with liver disease in relation to previous drug therapy. Lancet 2:1275–1279

Loewe S (1912) Clinical procedures with Luminal. Chem Abstr 6:2110

Löscher W (1979) A comparative study of the protein binding of anticonvulsant drugs in serum of dog and man. J Pharmacol Exp Ther 208:429–435

Lous P (1954) Blood, serum and cerebrospinal fluid levels and renal clearance of phenemal in treated epileptics. Acta Pharmacol Toxicol (Copenh) 10:166–177

Magnussen MP (1968) The effect of ethanol on gastrointestinal absorption of drugs in the rat. Acta Pharmacol Toxicol (Copenh) 26:130–144

Mark L (1963) Metabolism of barbiturates in man. Clin Pharmacol Ther 4:504–530

Mark L, Papper E, Brodie B, Rovenstine E (1949) Quantitative pharmacologic studies with penthothal. NY State J Med 49:1546–1549

Matsumoto H, Gallagher B (1975) Metabolism and excretion of C^{14}-eterobarb in epileptic patients. In: Janz D (ed) Epileptology. George Thieme, Stuttgart, pp 122–129

Mattson RH, Gallagher BB, Glass DH (1973) Folate therapy in epilepsy: a controlled study. Arch Neurol 29:78–81

Maynert E (1972) Phenobarbital, mephobarbital and metharbital: absorption, distribution and excretion. In: Woodbury D, Penry K, Schmidt R (eds) Raven, New York, pp 303–318

Maynert E, VanDyke H (1949) The metabolism of barbiturates. Pharmacol Rev 1:217–242

Meinardi H, Stoel LMK (1974) Side effects of anti-epileptic drugs. In: Vinker PJ, Bruyn GW (eds) Handbook of clinical neurology. American Elsevier, New York, pp 705–738

Morselli PL, Rizzo M, Garattini S (1971) Interaction between phenobarbital and diphenylhydantoin in animals and in epileptic patients. Ann NY Acad Sci 179:88–107

Nakane Y, Okuma T, Takahashi R, Sato R, Wada T, Sato T, Fukushima Y, Kumashiro H, Oho T, Takahasbi T, Aoki Y, Kazamatsuri H, Inami M, Komai S, Seino M, Miyakoshi M, Tanimura T, Hazama H, Kawahara R, Otsuki S, Hosokawa K, Inanaga K, Nakazawa Y, Yamamoto K (1980) Multi-institutional study on the teratogenicity and fetal toxicity of antiepileptic drugs: a report of a collaborative study group in Japan. Epilepsia 21:663–680

Nicoll R (1978) Selective action of barbiturates on synaptic transmission. In: Lipton MA, Dimascio A, Killam KF (eds) Psychopharmacology: a generation of progress. Raven Press, New York

Okamoto M, Rosenberg H, Boisse N (1975) Tolerance characteristics produced during the maximally tolerable chronic pentobarbital dosing in cat. J Pharmacol Exp Ther 192:555–569

Okamoto M, Boisse N, Rosenberg H (1977) Characteristics of functional tolerance during barbiturate physical dependency production. Pharmacologist vol:231

O'Reilly RA, Trager WF, Motley CH, Howald W (1980) Interaction of secobarbital with warfarin pseudoracemates. Clin Pharmacol Ther 28:187–195

Petty WC, Karler R (1965) The influence of aging on the activity of anticonvulsant drugs. J Pharmacol Exp Ther 150:443–448

Prichard JW (1980) Phenobarbital: proposed mechanisms of antiepileptic action. In: Glaser GH, Penry JK, Woodbury DM (eds) Antiepileptic drugs, mechanisms of action; Advances in neurology, vol 27. Raven Press, New York

Raines A, Niner JM, Pace DG (1973) A comparison of the anticonvulsant, neurotoxic and lethal effects of diphenylbarbituricadid, phenobarbital and diphenylhydantoin in the mouse. J Pharmacol Exp Ther 186:315–322

Rapport R, Kupferberg H (1973) Metabolism of dimethoxymethyl phenobarbital in mice: relationship between brain phenobarbital levels and anticonvulsant activity. J Med Chem 16:599–602

Reinhard JF, Reinhard JF Jr (1977) Experimental evaluation of anticonvulsants. In: Vida JA (ed) Medicinal chemistry, a series of monographs, vol 15. Academic, New York, pp 57–111

Remmer H (1959) Der beschleunigte Abbau von Pharmaka in den Lebermikrosomen unter dem Einfluß von Luminal. Naunyn-Schmiedebergs Arch Exp Pathol Pharmakol 235:279

Robichaud RC, Gylys JA, Sledge KL, Hillyard IW (1970) The pharmacology of prazepam. A new benzodiazepine derivative. Arch Int Pharmacodyn Ther 185:213–227

Rosen O, Sandberg I (1950) Studies on *N*-substituted barbituric acid derivatives II. Acta Chem Scand 4:675–687

Rosenberg H, Okamoto M (1974) A method for producing maximal pentobarbital dependence in cats: dependency characteristics. In: Singh L, Lal H (eds) Drug addiction. Experimental pharmacology, vol 3. Miami Symposium Specialist, Miami, pp 89–103

Rowland M (1972) Influence of route of administration on drug availability. J Pharm Sci 61:70–74

Samour C, Vida J (1971) Anticonvulsants 1. Alkoxymethyl derivatives of barbiturates and diphenylhydantoin. J Med Chem 14:187–189

Sandberg F (1949) Pharmacological properties of some new *N*-substituted barbituric acid derivatives. Acta Physiol Scand 18:204–217

Schanker LS (1961) Mechanisms of drug absorption and distribution. Ann Rev Pharmacol 1:29–44

Schottelius DD (1978) Homogenous immunoassay system (EMIT) for quantitation of antiepileptic drugs in biological fluids. In: Pippinger CE, Penry JK, Kutt H (eds) Antiepileptic drugs: quantitative analysis and interpretation. Raven, New York, pp 95–108

Sherwin AL, Harvey CD, Leppik IE (1976) Quantitation of antiepileptic drugs in human brain. In: Kellaway P, Petersen I (eds) Quantitative analytical studies in epilepsy. Raven, New York, pp 171–182

Smith CM (1977) The pharmacology of sedative hypnotics, alcohol and anesthetics: sites and mechanism of action. In: Martin WR (ed) Drug addiction I. (Handbook of experimental pharmacology, vol 45) Springer, Berlin Heidelberg New York, pp 413–587

Smith, DB, Golstein SG, Roomet A (1975) A comparison of the hypnotic effects of the anticonvulsant dimethoxymethylphenobarbital and phenobarbital in normal human volunteers. Epilepsia 16:201

Soldin SJ, Hill JG (1976) Rapid micromethod for measuring anticonvulsant drugs in serum by high performance liquid chromatography. Clin Chem 22:856–859

Spehlmann R, Colley B (1968) Effects of diazepam (Valium) on experimental seizures in unanesthetized cat. Neurology 18:52–59

Stark LG, Killam KF, Killam EK (1970) The anticonvulsant effects of phenobarbital, diphenylhydantoin and two benzodiazepines in the baboon, *Papio papio*. J Pharmacol Exp Ther 173:125–132

Steinmann HW (1967) Anfallsprophylaxe mit Phenobarbital im Tierexperiment. Dtsch Z Nervenheilkd 192:226–229

Svendsen A, Brochmann-Hannsen (1962) Gas chromatography of barbiturates: application to the study of their metabolism and excretion in humans. J Pharm Sci 51:494–495

Svensmark O, Buchthal F (1963) Accumulation of phenobarbital in man. Epilepsia 4:199–206

Swinyard EA (1949) Laboratory assay of clinically effective antiepileptic drugs. J Am Pharm Assoc Sci Ed 38:201–204

Swinyard EA, Brown WC, Goodman LS (1952) Comparative assays of antiepileptic drugs in mice and rats. J Pharmacol Exp Ther 106:319–330

Tang B, Inaba J, Kalow W (1977) *N*-Hydroxyphenobarbital – the major metabolite of phenobarbital in man. Fed Proc 36:966

Tang BK, Kalow W, Grey AA (1978) Amobarbital metabolism in man: *N*-glucoside formation. Res Commun Chem Pathol Pharmacol 21:45–53

Toman JEP, Swinyard EA, Goodman LS (1946) Properties of maximal seizures and their alteration by anticonvulsant drugs and other agents. J Neurophysiol 1:231–240

Vajda F, Williams FM, Davidson S, Falconer MA, Breckenridge A (1974) Human brain, cerebrospinal fluid and plasma concentrations of diphenylhydantoin and phenobarbital. Clin Pharmacol Ther 15:597–603

Van Creveld S (1958) Nouveax aspects de la maladie hemorragique du nouveax-ne'. Arch Fr Pediatr 15:721–735

Van Duijn H, Visser SL (1972) The action of some anticonvulsant drugs on cobalt induced epilepsy and on the bemegride threshold in alert cats. Epilepsia 13:409–420

Vida J (1977) Advances in anticonvulsant drug development. In: Vida JA (ed) Medicinal chemistry, a series of monographs, vol 15. Academic, New York, pp 1–9

Vida J, Gerry E (1977) Cyclic ureides. In: Vida JA (ed) Medicinal chemistry, a series of monographs, vol 15. Academic, New York, pp 157–193

Vida J, Hooker M, Reinhard J (1973a) Anticonvulsants 3: phenobarbital and mephobarbital derivatives. J Med Chem 16:602–605

Vida J, Hooker M, Samour C, Reinhard J (1973b) Anticonvulsants 4: metharbital and phenobarbital derivatives. J Med Chem 16:1378–1381

Waddell WJ, Butler TC (1957) The distribution and excretion of phenobarbital. J Clin Invest 36:1217–1226

Williams R, Parke D (1964) The metabolic fate of drugs. Ann Rev Pharmacol 4:85

Zanzi I, Roginsky MS, Rosen A, Cohn SH (1981) Skeletal mass in patients receiving chronic anticonvulsant therapy. Mineral Electrolyte Metab 5:240–248

CHAPTER 15

Primidone

H.-H. FREY

A. Chemistry and Physicochemical Properties

I. Physicochemical Properties

Primidone – 5-ethyldihydro-5-phenyl-4,6(1*H*,5*H*)-pyrimidinedione – is the 2-deoxy analogue of phenobarbital. It can be synthesized by electrolytic reduction of phenobarbital or by catalytic desulfuration of thiophenobarbital. The synthesis of ^{14}C- and ^{2}D-labeled primidone and its metabolite phenylethylmalondiamide has been described (ALVIN and BUSH 1975). Primidone has a molecular weight of 218.25 and a melting point of 281°–282 °C. It is a white, crystalline powder, is odorless, and has a slightly bitter taste. Primidone has no characteristic UV spectrum and no acidic properties. It is poorly soluble in water (0.6 g/liter at 37 °C), slightly more soluble in ethanol (5.88 g/liter), but nearly insoluble in most organic solvents. Low particle size is important for the rate of absorption of primidone formulations. A series of primidone analogues, substituted in the 1- and 3-positions, has been synthesized, but these compounds lacked the anticonvulsant activity of the parent drug (BÜCHI et al. 1966).

II. Analytical Methods for Determination from Biological Material

On account of its poor solubility in most solvents and its lack of characteristic UV spectrum, the determination of primidone proved difficult until the development of methods for thin-layer chromatography and more recently, highly sensitive methods for gas-liquid chromatography of the drug and its main metabolites. The simultaneous determination of the metabolite phenobarbital is indispensable since this metabolite is responsible for most of the antiepileptic activity of long-term primidone medication. Phenylethylmalondiamide (PEMA) is much less active as an anticonvulsant and its determination is thus of less importance for drug monitoring.

1. Thin-Layer Chromatography

Primidone and its metabolites can be extracted from serum or urine using chloroform/methylacetate (60:40), chloroform, or toluene (HUISMAN 1968; GARCEAU et al. 1973; WAD et al. 1977). HUISMAN (1968) nitrated the phenyl group of the drugs after extraction, separated the nitrated compounds by thin-layer chromatography (TLC), identified the spots under UV light, scratched them off the plate, and subsequently used a Bratton-Marshal reaction for quantitative photometric determination at 550 nm. Other authors made quantitative determinations by scanning the TLC plates at 215 or 220 nm with a spectrodensitometer (GARCEAU et al. 1973; WAD et al. 1977). The recovery was reported as 90%–100% for primidone, phenobarbital, and PEMA; the limit of detection was 1–2 µg. WIEGREBE and WEHRHAHN (1975) determined primidone, phenobarbital, and other antiepileptic drugs polarographically after separation by TLC, but this method was less sensitive (3.5–5.5 µg).

2. Gas-Liquid Chromatography

Numerous methods for gas-liquid chromatography (GLC) determination of primidone and its metabolites have been developed during the past 10 years. Most of these methods are equally reliable, differences being due to variations in equipment and the special requirements of the authors. The following citations are not intended to be a complete survey.

Most authors use flame ionization detectors, but the use of *N*-sensitive detectors (GOUDIE and BURNETT 1973; VANDEMARK and ADAMS 1976; SCHWEIZER et al. 1978) or electron-capture detectors (WALLACE et al. 1977) provides high sensitivity even when volumes of only 50–100 µl serum are extracted. Derivatization – mostly on-column methylation – is used in many methods (ABRAHAM 1976; ABRAHAM and JOSLIN 1976; BAUMEL et al. 1972; DAVIS et al. 1975; DORRITY and LINNOILA 1976; HILL and LATHAM 1877; KUPFERBERG 1970; LÖSCHER and GÖBEL 1978; NISHINA et al. 1976; PERCHALSKI et al. 1973; SCHWEIZER et al. 1978; VANDEMARK and ADAMS 1976; WALLACE et al. 1977), but also the determination of underivatized drug is recommended (COUCH ET AL. 1973; GUPTA et al. 1977; HEIPERTZ et al. 1977; SCHÄFER 1975; TOSELAND et al. 1972), though the latter methods are less sensitive on average. Most methods aim at the simultaneous determination of primidone and phenobarbital, and sometimes also PEMA and other antiepileptic drugs; but GUPTA et al. (1977) and LÖSCHER and GÖBEL (1978) separate the neutral drugs primidone and PEMA from two acidic phenobarbital by differential extraction, and determine both fractions in the subsequent runs.

NAU et al. (1980b) have combined mass spectrometry with GLC in the determination of primidone and its metabolites and reached limits of detection as low as 1.4–3.4 ng/ml from 100-µl serum samples.

3. High-Pressure Liquid Chromatography

High-pressure, liquid chromatography (HPLC) has been used for the simultaneous determination of primidone, phenobarbital, and other antiepileptic drugs, and is characterized by high sensitivity (100 ng/ml from 0.5-ml samples, or even the use of 25-µl samples). Quantification is by UV absorption and measuring of peak areas. Correlation with GLC is reported to be excellent (ADAMS and VANDEMARK 1976; KABRA et al. 1976; SOLDIN and HILL 1976).

4. Enzyme Immunoassay

Enzyme multiplied immunoassay technique (EMIT) assays for primidone and phenobarbital have been compared with GLC methods repeatedly, and high degrees of correlation between both methods have been reported (SUN and WALWICK 1976; BARTELS et al. 1977; DIETZLER et al. 1980). Kits for PEMA are not available. The method has the adventage of being simple and rapid, but it is rather expensive. Interference with other drugs seems to be minimal.

B. Anticonvulsant Activity

The anticonvulsant activity of primidone was described for the first time by BOGUE and CARRINGTON (1953) in rats. Since then its anticonvulsant activity has been studied in many experimental models and species.

Since primidone is metabolized to two metabolites with anticonvulsant activity, the question of whether the observed effect is dependent on primidone itself or partly, or even mostly, on its metabolite phenobarbital remains open in most studies. The time between drug administration and testing for anticonvulsant activity is crucial in this respect: the longer the interval the greater the share of the metabolites in the anticonvulsant effect observed.

I. Anticonvulsant Efficacy in Laboratory Animals

1. Standard Models in Mice and Rats

Primidone has been studied in the two standard tests for anticonvulsant activity, the maximal electroshock seizure (MES) test and the pentylenetetrazol seizure threshold (PTZ) test (SWINYARD et al. 1952), both in mice and rats. The drug was mostly administered orally, 3–8 h before testing. The results of these studies are summarized in Table 1. The data show that primidone is much more active against maximal electroconvulsions than against pentylenetetrazol-induced seizures. In the MES test, primidone was more potent than phenobarbital in most studies (BOGUE and CARRINGTON 1953; GOODMAN et al. 1953; SWINYARD et al. 1954; BOGUE et al. 1956), but some authors found both drugs equipotent (LÖSCHER 1975; BOURGEOIS et al. 1983a) or even phenobarbital considerably more potent than primidone (LEAL et al. 1979a). Against pentylenetetrazol-induced seizures, primidone was found to be two to ten times less potent than phenobarbital (BOGUE and CARRINGTON 1953; GOODMAN et al. 1953; BOGUE et al. 1956; FREY and HAHN 1960) or even ineffective, when the metabolism of the drug was inhibited by SKF 525-A (BOURGEOIS et al. 1983a). GOODMAN et al. (1953) compared primidone and phenobarbital 3 h after oral administration in the following models in rats and mice: minimal electroshock seizure threshold, hyponatremic electroshock seizure threshold, maximal pentylenetetrazol seizure pattern, and "psychomotor" seizures [for details of these methods see SWINYARD et al. (1952)]. The ED_{50} values in Table 2 show that primidone was the less potent drug in all procedures.

When the doses of primidone, phenobarbital, and PEMA elevating the electroconvulsive threshold in mice by 40 V were determined after oral administration, doses of 0.01 mmol/kg (2.4 mg/kg) phenobarbital, 0.017 mmol/kg (3.6 mg/

Table 1. Anticonvulsant effect of primidone and phenobarbital in standard models for antiepileptic activity in mice and rats

	Maximal electroshock seizure test		Pentylenetetrazol seizure threshold test		Refs.
	Primidone ED_{50} (mg/kg)	Pheno-barbital ED_{50} (mg/kg)	Primidone ED_{50} (mg/kg)	Pheno-barbital ED_{50} (mg/kg)	
Rat	~ 5 (6)	~10 (3)	~ 20 (4–6)	<10 (3)	BOGUE and CARRINGTON (1953)
	4.9 (6)	8.5 (3)	690 (6)	67 (3)	GOODMAN et al. (1953)
	~ 2 (3–6)	~ 7	20 (3–6)	10	BOGUE et al. (1956)
	4.0 (2), 4.9 (6)	7.1 (2–6)			SWINYARD et al. (1954)
Mouse	13 (3)	28 (3)	74 (3)	15.5 (3)	GOODMAN et al. (1953)
			79 (4–8)	17 (2)	FREY and HAHN (1960)
	18 (4)	15 (2)			LÖSCHER (1975)
	75 (7)	27 (3)			LEAL et al. (1979a)
	3.6 (3)[a]	2.4 (2)[a]			FREY et al. (1979)

Figures in parentheses are times of testing in hours after oral administration
[a] ED_{50} for elevation of the electroconvulsive threshold by 40 V

Table 2. Anticonvulsant effect of primidone and phenobarbital in different experimental models in mice and rats. The drugs were administered orally at the times indicated. (GOODMAN et al. 1953)

Test	Mouse		Rat	
	Primidone ED_{50} (mg/kg)	Phenobarbital sodium ED_{50} (mg/kg)	Primidone ED_{50} (mg/kg)	Phenobarbital sodium ED_{50} (mg/kg)
Time of testing	3 h	3 h	6 h	3 h
Minimal electroshock seizure test	86	25	560	62.5
Hyponatremic electroshock seizure	81	20	403	80
"Psychomotor" seizure test	1000	66		
Maximal pentylenetetrazol seizure pattern	16.5	9.5		

kg) primidone, and 0.37 mmol/kg (75 mg/kg) PEMA were found equipotent (FREY et al. 1979).

In mice sensitive to audiogenic seizures, COLLINS and HORLINGTON (1969) determined the following ED_{50} values 45 min after i.p. administration: primidone 1.3 mg/kg and phenobarbital 2.3 mg/kg. Since primidone has an LD_{50} three times higher than that of phenobarbital, a more favorable ratio, LD_{50}/ED_{100}, could be calculated for primidone.

In nephrectomized rats, the ED_{50} for primidone in the MES test was reduced from 4.9 mg/kg in the controls to 2.4 mg/kg, while that for phenobarbital was hardly changed (SWINYARD et al. 1954; GOODMAN et al. 1953). When the liver of rats was damaged by carbon tetrachloride, the ED_{50} of both drugs was reduced to about the same level (SWINYARD et al. 1954).

2. Special Experimental Models in Small Rodents

In mice isolated for long periods, a head twitch or even a convulsive movement can be elicited by touching the occiput. During a 7-h observation period, an oral dose of 200 mg/kg primidone inhibited the head twitch only slightly but reduced the incidence of convulsive movements by 30%. Fifty-six percent of the mice were considered sedated by this dose (BARNES 1960). MATIN et al. (1981) found primidone, 50 mg/kg i.p., without effect against convulsions elicited in mice by oral administration of 600 mg/kg chlorophenothane. Phenobarbital, with the same dose, suppressed the convulsions, but the time of only 1 h during which the animals were observed may have been too short to detect an effect of primidone.

In rats, GALLAGHER et al. (1970) determined the threshold of hexafluorodiethyl ether both for the first myoclonic jerk and for tonic-clonic convulsions. The elevation of the threshold for the first myoclonic jerk was clearly correlated with the phenobarbital plasma concentration, irrespective of whether the animals had been treated with phenobarbital or primidone. For tonic-clonic convulsions, the increase in the threshold at a given concentration of phenobarbital was more pronounced in animals treated with primidone. When rats were tested 4 h after administration of 32.5 mg/kg phenobarbital or 250 mg/kg primidone, the thresholds for tonic-clonic convulsions were identical in both groups, although the plasma concentration was 17.3 μg/ml phenobarbital or 11 μg/ml phenobarbital + 52 μg/ml primidone, respectively. In the same model, PEMA doses from 62.5 to 750 mg/kg raised both thresholds, with a maximal effect 1 h after oral administration. Given together with phenobarbital, doses from 31.25 mg/kg (tonic-clonic convulsion) or 62.5 mg/kg (myoclonic jerk) of PEMA clearly augmented the anticonvulsant effect of the barbiturate (BAUMEL et al. 1972).

In barbital-dependent rats, 50 mg/kg primidone suppressed audiogenically induced barbiturate withdrawal seizures. When primidone was withdrawn 6 days later, the animals became susceptible to audiogenic seizures (NORTON 1970).

Allylglycine-induced tonic convulsions of the limbs in rats could be antagonized by primidone given 2 h before allylglycine with an ED_{50} of about 15 mg/kg, but even the highest dose of 80 mg/kg only delayed the time to death (ASHTON and WAUQUIER 1979b).

In amygdaloid-kindled rats, doses of 400 and 800 mg/kg primidone were without effect on duration of afterdischarge and convulsion score after 30 min, had some positive effect at 2 h after administration, and showed the most pronounced reduction in seizure rank score and duration of afterdischarge at 48 h, when plasma concentrations of 5.9 μg/ml primidone together with 14 μg/ml phenobarbital and 7.7 μg/ml PEMA were determined at the highest dose level (ALBERTSON et al. 1980). In the same model, ASHTON and WAUQUIER (1979a) determined an ED_{50} for protection against the forepaw clonus of 82 mg/kg primidone

30 min after i.p. injection, but only 12 mg/kg 24 h after administration. Other components of the kindled seizure were less sensitive.

In gerbils, in which convulsions were elicited by a blast of compressed air, the maximal anticonvulsant effect was observed 6 h after oral administration (ED_{50} 9.5 mg/kg) (FREY et al. 1984).

3. Anticonvulsant Effect in Other Animal Species

In cats and rabbits, primidone provided long-lasting protection against minimal and maximal electroshock seizures and against convulsant doses of pentylenetrazol (15 mg/kg i.v.). In cats doses of 25–100 mg/kg protected for 3 days, and rabbits were protected for 24 h by 50 mg/kg and for 72 h by 100 mg/kg. However, all doses used in these species induced considerable side effects (GOODMAN et al. 1953). Treatment with 25 mg/kg primidone twice daily protected 70% of dogs against convulsions elicited by *dl*-methionine sulfoximine (BOGUE et al. 1956). Dogs could be protected against the convulsant effect of threshold doses of pentylenetetrazol (15–25 mg/kg i.v.) by daily oral doses of between 29 and 36 mg/kg primidone (FREY and HAHN 1960). Protection was complete in two out of three dogs on the 2nd day, when only traces of phenobarbital could be detected in the plasma of the one dog, and 8 μg/ml in that of the other. In the third dog full protection was only achieved after 11 days of treatment at a plasma concentration of 11 μg/ml phenobarbital. In parallel experiments with phenobarbital, protection was complete at plasma phenobarbital concentrations of 20–25 μg/ml (FREY and HAHN 1960). The authors concluded that at least 50% of the anticonvulsant effect of primidone must have been due to the metabolite phenobarbital. Later experiments (FREY et al. 1979) showed that the proportion of the effect due to phenobarbital is considerably higher when steady state has been achieved. In a clinical study in epileptic dogs, SCHWARTZ-PORSCHE et al. (1982) reported that 10 out of 30 dogs became free of fits at daily doses of 13–39 mg/kg primidone and at average phenobarbital plasma concentrations of 6–27 μg/ml. In a further ten dogs, the clinical condition was considerably improved by the administration of daily doses of 30–77 mg/kg.

Rhesus monkeys, in which focal seizures had been elicited by application of aluminum hydroxide gel beneath the pia of the left pre- and postcentral gyrus, seemd to fare better on a daily regimen of 15–60 mg/kg primidone than on 3–12 mg/kg phenobarbital. However, withdrawal reactions were more pronounced after primidone (LOCKARD et al. 1975).

Fits can be elicited by intermittent photic stimulation in seizure-susceptible chickens (CRAWFORD 1970). In the experiments by JOHNSON et al. (1978) 50% of these chickens were protected 1 h after i.p. injection of 69 mg/kg primidone. Plasma concentrations were 20–25 μg/ml primidone and 3.5 μg/ml phenobarbital at that time. Twelve hours after administration, primidone could no longer be detected in plasma, and phenobarbital concentrations averaged 10.7 μg/ml, but at that time 90% of the chickens were protected. A dose of 60 mg/kg PEMA had no anticonvulsant effect at plasma concentrations of 55 μg/ml.

II. Anticonvulsant Potency in Man

By treatment with daily oral doses of 0.75–3 g primidone, only three out of nine psychiatric patients were protected against the tonic phase of therapeutic electroshock, but side effects occurred in seven of the nine patients (GOODMAN et al. 1953). The period of treatment varied from 2.5 to 10 days so that steady-state conditions for phenobarbital had not been obtained. In patients with focal seizures, several groups have determined the doses of primidone and phenobarbital approximately equipotent in controlling the seizures. GRUBER et al. (1957) and WHITE et al. (1966) found primidone to have about one-fifth of the antiepileptic potency of phenobarbital, but in a later study GRUBER et al. (1962) found 30 mg phenobarbital equipotent with 200 mg primidone in focal epilepsies, and in a more recent review KUTT and LOUIS (1972) give average maintenance doses of 90 mg phenobarbital and 750 mg primidone for patients with grand mal or focal seizures. SCHMIDT (1981) even gives a dose ratio of 1 : 10.

III. Mechanism of Anticonvulsant Action

The exact mechanism of the anticonvulsant action of primidone is still unkown and few attempts have been made to elucidate it. One of the reasons is the still unsettled question of the importance of the active metabolites of primidone, especially phenobarbital, in the anticonvulsant effect of the parent drug. Therefore, attempts to elucidate the role of unmetabolized primidone, on the one hand, and of its metabolites phenobarbital and PEMA, on the other, for the total anticonvulsant effect of primidone will be reviewed before studies on the biochemical mechanism of action of the drug.

1. Importance of the Metabolites Phenobarbital and PEMA in the Anticonvulsant Effect of Primidone

The acute anticonvulsant activity of primidone and its metabolites has been compared by several authors. In rats, an ED_{50} of less than 4 mg/kg primidone, about 5 mg/kg phenobarbital, and about 62.5 mg/kg PEMA gave protection against maximal electroconvulsions, whereas the ratio of phenobarbital to PEMA with regard to protection against pentylenetetrazol-induced convulsions was about 1 : 10 in the study by BAUMEL et al. (1973). LEAL et al. (1979 a) determined ED_{50} values of 75 mg/kg primidone at 7 h after administration, 27 mg/kg phenobarbital at 3 h, and 840 mg/kg PEMA at 3 h in mice; and FREY et al. (1979) determined, also in mice, the doses of the three drugs which increased the electroconvulsive threshold by 40 V: 0.017 mmol/kg primidone at 3 h, 0.01 mmol/kg phenobarbital at 2 h, an 0.37 mmol/kg PEMA at 1 h after oral administration. At 3 h after primidone administration only negligible plasma concentrations of phenobarbital and PEMA could be detected. According to these studies, primidone has an activity in the same order of magnitude as phenobarbital, whereas PEMA only has about 1/20–1/40 of the anticonvulsant potency of primidone or phenobarbital. This metabolite must therefore be supposed to play a minor role in the total anticonvulsant effect of primidone, though BAUMEL et al. (1972) demonstrated that relatively small doses may potentiate the anticonvulsant effect of phenobarbital.

A true antiepileptic effect of primidone is beyond any doubt. Dogs treated with primidone were protected against pentylenetetrazol-induced convulsions at lower phenobarbital plasma concentrations than animals treated with phenobarbital (FREY and HAHN 1960). A similar observation has been reported in rats by GALLAGHER et al. (1970), and BAUMEL et al. (1973) found that their rats were protected against maximal electroconvulsions before the metabolites phenobarbital and PEMA could be detected in plasma and brain. On the other hand, the ED_{50} of primidone had to be raised from 75 to 110 mg/kg in order to protect mice against electroconvulsions when the metabolism of primidone had been inhibited by pretreatment with SKF 525-A (LEAL et al. 1979a). However, the effect of the drug against photically induced seizures in epileptic fowl seemed somewhat stronger after pretreatment with SKF 525-A (JOHNSON et al. 1978).

The study by BAUMEL et al. (1973) in rats is of special interest since the anticonvulsant effect against maximal electroconvulsions as well as against seizures induced by pentylenetetrazol or hexafluorodiethyl ether and the concentrations of primidone and its metabolites were followed for 24 h after administration. Primidone protected against electroconvulsions at a time when no metabolites could be detected, but protection against chemically induced convulsions required higher doses and occurred at a later point of time when considerable concentrations of the metabolites were detectable, and is thus dependent on transformation to phenobarbital. Similarly, epileptic fowl proved to be best protected at a time when phenobarbital plasma concentrations exceeded those of primidone (JOHNSON et al. 1978).

The main question is, of course, the role primidone and its metabolites play in the anticonvulsant effect during chronic treatment, i.e. under steady-state conditions. This has been studied by FREY et al. (1979) in dogs that were treated for 18 days with daily doses of 30–40 mg/kg primidone. When a steady state had been reached after about 1 week of treatment, phenobarbital had accumulated to an average plasma concentration of 65 nmol/ml, PEMA had accumulated to between 30 and 50 nmol/ml, and primidone levels fluctuated between 7 and 25 nmol/ml within one dosage interval (8 h) on account of its relatively short half-life. Transforming the steady-state concentrations of primidone and PEMA into phenobarbital equivalents on the basis of their anticonvulsant potencies in mice, the authors arrived at the conclusion that, during steady state, primidone accounts for only 11% and PEMA for 2% of the total anticonvulsant effect, thus leaving a share of more than 85% to phenobarbital. Since the pharmacokinetics of primidone are fairly similar in man and dog, comparable conditions can be taken to be valid during primidone treatment of human epilepsy. BOGAN and SMITH (1968) arrive at a similar conclusion by comparison of phenobarbital plasma levels during treatment with primidone or phenobarbital in man, and OLESEN and DAM (1967) even doubt a true antiepileptic effect of unmetabolized primidone in human epilepsy. OXLEY et al. (1980) see an advantage of primidone treatment over phenobarbital in a clinical study with control of phenobarbital plasma concentrations, but the statistical evaluation of their results is not very convincing.

FINCHAM and SCHOTTELIUS (1982) found primidone plasma concentrations in the same range as those for phenobarbital under steady-state conditions, and suppose that primidone plays a major role in the antiepileptic effect. The determinations were made 2–4 h after drug administration, i.e., when primidone values should be maximal. Determinations before drug administration might give a quite different concentration ratio.

In conclusion, phenobarbital must be considered to be responsible for the major part of the antiepileptic effect of treatment with primidone, although the parent drug has, in animal experiments, some properties clearly different from those of phenobarbital. These should, however, be more important for the acute effect of a single dose and less so under steady-state conditions, during which the concentrations of primidone show pronounced fluctuations (FREY and LÖSCHER 1980). The clinical consequence of only monitoring phenobarbital concentrations during treatment with primidone (EADIE 1974, 1979; RICHENS and WARRINGTON 1979) seems thus justified. However, BOURGEOIS et al. (1983 b) have shown that primidone is able to potentiate the effect of phenobarbital in the MES test, and at the same time, to increase the therapeutic index.

2. Biochemical Mechanism of Action

With regard to the part of the drug transformed to phenobarbital, its mechanism of action must be assumed to be identical to that known for barbituric acid derivatives. Studies into unique mechanisms by which unchanged primidone displays its anticonvulsant action are in fact lacking.

The well-known reduction of folic acid levels in serum, erythrocytes, cerebrospinal fluid, and brain during treatment with primidone (WOODBURY and KEMP 1970; REYNOLDS 1973) is a property the drug shares with phenobarbital and phenytoin. Since phenobarbital accumulates to therapeutically active concentrations during primidone treatment, this effect cannot be considered a unique property of primidone. The lowered concentrations of folate seem to be consequence of inhibition of intestinal absorption and interference with transport across the blood-brain barrier, and it has been suggested that they play a role in the anticonvulsant effect, but this opinion cannot be regarded as generally accepted (SINGH and HUOT 1973).

Interference of primidone with the cerebral gamma-aminobutyric acid (GABA) metabolism has been studied repeatedly. GABA concentrations in the hemispheres or the total brain were not influenced by i.p. or oral doses of up to 50 mg/kg primidone, both at 1 h and at 4 h after administration (SAAD et al. 1972; LÖSCHER 1975). The activity of glutamic acid decarboxylase (GAD) was not altered 4 h after oral administration of 44 mg/kg primidone in mice, but the activity of the degrading enzyme GABA-α-ketoglutarate transaminase (GABA-T) was slightly but significantly inhibited (LÖSCHER 1975). Doses of 25 or 50 mg/kg primidone given to mice 1 h before they were killed provided protection against the decline in cerebral GABA concentrations induced by insulin (SAAD 1970) or isoniazid (SAAD et al. 1972), and gave protection against the convulsions elicited by both drugs. Though primidone should not have been metabolized to a greater extent 1 h after administration, it shares this property with barbiturates and hydantoins, so that the effect on the metabolism of GABA cannot be regarded as a unique property of the drug. TICKU and OLSEN (1978) reported inhibition of the specific binding of [^{3}H]dihydropicrotoxinin to brain membranes by primidone. The drug had a median inhibitory concentration (IC_{50}) of 170 μM, and was thus more active than phenobarbital (400 μM), but less active than mephobarbital

(5 µ*M*), metharbital (10 µ*M*), and barbital (50 µ*M*), so that a correlation with its anticonvulsant effect seems hardly probable.

Both primidone and phenobarbital stimulated Na^+-independent GABA binding to bovine cortex membranes, but both drugs belonged to the less active among the barbiturates studied in this respect. For the whole group of barbiturates, the stimulation of GABA binding paralleled anesthetic activity better than anticonvulsant potency (ASANO and GASAWARA 1982).

C. Other Central Nervous System Effects

1. Sedative Effect

BARNES (1960) reported a sedative effect in 56% of mice given an oral dose of 200 mg/kg primidone. In the experiments of RÜMKE and BOUT (1960), the hexobarbital sleeping time was significantly prolonged 1 h after oral pretreatment with 100 mg/kg primidone. Also the metabolite PEMA prolonged the hexobarbital sleeping time in mice when injected i.p. 1 h before the anesthetic; the lowest dose with a significant effect was 62.5 mg/kg (BAUMEL et al. 1972).

2. Physical Dependence

Whereas pretreatment with primidone 1 h before hexobarbital prolonged the sleeping time, this was significantly shortened when primidone had been administered 24 or 48 h before hexobarbital (RÜMKE and BOUT 1960). At 72 h after pretreatment, no influence on sleeping time could be detected. In later experiments, RÜMKE (1967) reported a similar effect regarding the anticonvulsant action of the drug. The convulsive ED_{50} of bemegride was significantly increased 1 h after oral administration of 100 mg/kg primidone to mice, but was slightly but significantly depressed 48 h after administration. Similar results were obtained when pentylenetetrazol or dioxone was used as a convulsant, but not in the MES test. Primidone, at a daily dose of 50 mg/kg, suppressed audiogenically induced barbital withdrawal seizures in rats, but the incidence of convulsions was increased when primidone was withdrawn after 6 days of treatment (NORTON 1970). Also LOCKARD et al. (1975) saw an increased incidence of withdrawal seizures on termination of primidone treatment in monkeys made epileptic by cerebral implantation of aluminum hydroxide gel. This increase was more pronounced than after treatment with phenobarbital or phenytoin, and the authors speculate that the rapid elimination of unchanged primidone might be responsible for the phenomenon.

3. Brain Enzymes

A dose of 25 mg/kg primidone orally, which protected mice completely against audiogenic seizures 2 h after administration, was without effect on the activity of the following enzymes: cytochrome oxidase (E.C.1.9.3.1), alanine aminotransferase (E.C.2.6.1.2), aspartate aminotransferase (E.C.2.6.1.1), and monoamine oxidase (E.C.1.4.3.4) (CONSTANTINESCU et al. 1976).

D. Pharmacodynamic Actions Outside the Central Nervous System

There have been very few studies on the pharmacodynamic actions of primidone not related to its anticonvulsant effect.

1. Neuromuscular Junction

At the neuromuscular junction of the frog, primidone (0.2–1 m*M*)increased transmitter release presynaptically, but slightly decreased miniature end-plate potentials, whereas PEMA had no comparable effect (TALBOT and ALDERDICE 1982). Phenobarbital had a similar presynaptic effect, but a much stronger inhibitory postsynaptic effect (PROCTOR and WEAKLY 1976).

2. Antiarrhythmic Effect

In dogs in which ventricular tachycardia had been elicited by the two-stage coronary ligation technique, an i.v. dose of 15 mg/kg primidone reduced the ectopic activity by 75%–100% and was thus more potent than quinidine. The effect was maximal from 10 to 40 min after administration and disappeared after 2 h (ARORA and SHARMA 1958). BOSE et al. (1963) elicited atrial fibrillation in dogs by infusion of acetylcholine or by electrical stimulation. Primidone provided partial protection at a dose of 10 mg/kg and complete protection at 25 mg/kg. Since the acetylcholine content of the heart was reduced by 16% or 24% after doses of 4 or 8 mg/kg, the authors considered inhibition of acetylcholine uptake as the possible mechanism of action.

3. Thyroid Function

In children and adolescents treated with primidone for their epilepsy, protein-bound iodine, total and free thyroxine, thyroxine-binding globulin and thyrotropin were significantly reduced; however, the situation of the children was not clearly hypothyroid (FICHSEL and KNÖPFLE 1977). Interference with the hypothalamic-hypophyseal regulation of thyroid function was discussed.

E. Pharmacokinetics

I. Absorption

The absorption of primidone after oral administration has been studied in laboratory animals and in man.

In mice, an absorption rate constant, k_a, of 3.55 h^{-1} has been determined after oral administration of a suspension in carboxymethylcellulose; maximal plasma concentrations were reached at 36 min (LEAL et al. 1979 a, b). Maximal plasma concentrations were determined in rats 1–2 h after oral administration of suspensions of the drug (GALLAGHER et al. 1970; BAUMEL et al. 1973). After oral administration of commercial tablets of primidone to dogs, FREY et al. (1979) reported an average k_a of 0.0243 min^{-1} with extreme values of 0.011 and 0.046 min^{-1}. Maximal plasma concentrations of unchanged primidone were reached at 2.1 ± 0.63 h ($\bar{x} \pm SD$), which is in good agreement with the value of 2–4 h that can be read from the graphs of YEARY (1980).

After oral administration of 250–750 mg primidone to epileptic patients, peak plasma concentrations were reached at between 0.5 and 9 h (BAUMEL et al. 1972; GALLAGHER et al. 1972; GALLAGHER and BAUMEL 1972). The most concise data are given by GALLAGHER et al. (1972), 2.7±0.4 h, and by GALLAGHER and BAUMEL (1972), 3.2±1.0 h. MATZKE et al. (1981) have analyzed the pharmacokinetic data from an intoxication with phenytoin and primidone and for the latter drug found two distinct absorption phases characterized by absorption rate constants of 1.08 and 0.096 h^{-1}.

In children, KAUFFMAN et al. (1977) found maximal plasma concentrations 4–6 h after oral administration. These authors were able to recover an average of 92% of the total dose from the urine of their 12 patients within 24 h, either in the form of unchanged primidone or as one of the metabolites phenobarbital or PEMA. This high recovery permits the conclusion that the enteral absorption of primidone can be regarded as complete. In certain patients concomitant administration of acetazolamide suppressed or delayed the absorption of primidone (SYVERSEN et al. 1977).

After oral administration of 400 mg PEMA to human volunteers, peak plasma concentrations were reached within 2–4 h (COTTRELL et al. 1982).

II. Distribution

1. Apparent Volume of Distribution

A reliable determination of the apparent volume of distribution (V_d) for primidone is difficult on account of the insolubility of the drug in water. Whenever the drug has been injected i.v., solubilizers have had to be used, and these may have influenced the distribution of the drug. Following the i.v. injection of 10 mg/kg primidone to rabbits, a V_{dss} of 0.68 liters/kg and an apparent volume of the central compartment (V_c) of 0.2 liters/kg was calculated (HUNT and MILLER 1978). In the same study, V_c was 0.21 liters/kg and V_{dss} 0.58 liters/kg after administration of 10 mg/kg phenobarbital, and after administration of 10 mg/kg PEMA V_c was 0.3 liters/kg and V_{dss} 0.82 liters/kg. YEARY (1980) gives an apparent volume of distribution for the three compounds in the dog: primidone (10 mg/kg i.v.), 0.815 liters/kg; phenobarbital (15 mg/kg i.v.), 0.63 liters/kg; and PEMA (10 mg/kg i.v.), 0.73 liters/kg. In an experiment in a monkey, VAN DER KLEIJN et al. (1975) determined a value of 3.65 liters/kg, but only 0.6 liters/kg in a human subject. Since the authors calculated the pharmacokinetic data after infusion of the drug, it must be supposed that a greater share of it was transformed to phenobarbital or PEMA in the monkey, thus giving rise to the extraordinarily large apparent volume of distribution for unchanged primidone. During intoxication with primidone and phenytoin, MATZKE et al. (1981) calculated a V_d of 0.54 liters/kg, assuming complete absorption of the drug. For PEMA, a V_d of 0.71–0.86 liters/kg was calculated assuming complete absorption after oral administration (COTTRELL et al. 1982).

2. Binding to Serum Proteins

In the study by LEAL et al. (1979b), less than 10% of primidone and phenobarbital in mice were protein bound, while PEMA seemed to be totally in the free form. LÖSCHER (1979) found a fraction of a little less than 25% bound to serum proteins in the dog up to a concentration of 15 μg/ml; the binding percentage declined at higher concentrations. Corresponding values for phenobarbital and PEMA in the interesting range of concentrations were 40%–45%, and 6%–7%, respectively. Values determined in man range from 3%–22% binding for primidone, 42%–57% for phenobarbital and 7%–9% for PEMA (BAUMEL et al. 1972; LÖSCHER 1979).

3. Concentrations in Tissues and Body Fluids

In rats and mice primidone concentrations in brain were considerably lower than those in plasma and the peak concentration was delayed in some instances (BAUMEL et al. 1973; LEAL et al. 1979a). Also PEMA brain concentrations remained lower than the plasma concentration and were reached with delay, whereas phenobarbital concentrations in plasma and brain were practically equal (LEAL et al. 1979a). In samples from temporal lobectomies, HOUGHTON et al. (1975) found primidone concentrations only slightly lower than those in plasma.

FREY et al. (1979) determined an average permeability constant of 0.016/min for the penetration of primidone from plasma to CSF in dogs. CSF concentrations corresponded to about 80% of those in plasma, which agrees well with the fraction unbound to serum proteins. PEMA penetrated at about the same rate and reached 86%–88% of the plasma concentrations in CSF. In man, the CSF/serum ratio was in the range of 0.7–0.9 in most studies (HOUGHTON et al. 1975; SCHMIDT and KUPFERBERG 1975; TROUPIN and FRIEL 1975; MONACO et al. 1981), though earlier studies give lower or higher values (HUISMAN 1968; GALLAGHER and BAUMEL 1972; REYNOLDS et al. 1972).

The relation between primidone concentrations in plasma and saliva or tears has been studied in man. The saliva/plasma ratio ranges from 0.68 to 1.15 in these studies (SCHMIDT and KUPFERBERG 1975; TROUPIN and FRIEL 1975; BARTELS et al. 1979; MONACO et al. 1981). An explanation for the wide variation is given by BARTELS et al.: a high ratio of 1.15 was found under conditions of resting flow, but it declined to about 0.7 when secretion was stimulated by chewing gum. Drug monitoring by analysis of saliva concentrations seems justified when standard conditions are applied. The ratio between tears and plasma was 0.54 with wide variation (MONACO et al. 1981).

Transplacental passage of primidone has been shown by MARTINEZ and SNYDER (1973) and by NAU et al. (1980a), who determined the drug in maternal and cord serum. Especially the study of NAU et al. demonstrated complete equilibration: concentrations of primidone, phenobarbital, and PEMA were in fact equal in the plasma of the mother and that of the newborn infant.

In four patients milk/serum ratios of 0.72 for primidone, 0.76 for PEMA, and 0.41 for phenobarbital were determined (NAU et al. 1980a). In muscle samples from human patients, HOUGHTON et al. (1975) found the concentration of primidone on average was 57% of that in plasma. High primidone concentrations in ligaments have been reported from autoradiographic studies (VAN DER KLEIJN et al. 1975).

III. Metabolism

1. Qualitative Aspects (Fig. 1)

Phenylethylmalondiamide was the first metabolite of primidone to be identified (GOODMAN et al. 1953; BOGUE et al. 1956). This metabolite, which has only weak anticonvulsant activity (BOGUE et al. 1956; FREY et al. 1979; LEAL et al. 1979a), has now been found in all species in which primidone metabolism has been studied.

Of greater importance is phenobarbital, the second metabolite to be identified in man and dog (BUTLER and WADDELL 1956). It has since been found in all species studied and is thought to be mainly responsible for the anticonvulsant effect of primidone during prolonged treatment (see Sect. B.III.1).

Alpha-phenyl-gamma-butyrolactone has been identified in the urine of patients with primidone intoxication (ANDRESEN et al. 1976). This metabolite has also been found after administration of glutethimide and after intoxication with phenobarbital. No quantitative data are given. Further metabolites of minor importance are 2-phenyl-butyramide (FOLTZ et al. 1972) and hydroxyprimidone (HORNING et al. 1975).

In experiments with rat liver microsomes, relatively more *p*-hydroxyphenobarbital was found when primidone was used as the substrate than after phenobarbital (BOGAN and SMITH 1968). This opens the possibility that primidone is metabolized by aromatic hydroxylation before oxidation of the pyrimidine ring to a barbituric acid.

BOGUE et al. (1956) mention some other possible metabolites of primidone and give data for their anticonvulsant potency. These have, however, never been identified in animal or human studies. The metabolism of primidone can be inhibited by pretreatment with SKF 525-A, a known inhibitor of liver mixed function hydroxylases (JOHNSON et al. 1978; LEAL et al. 1979a).

2. Quantitative Aspects

From a practical point of view, the quantitative aspects of biotransformation of primidone, especially with regard to active metabolites, deserve much attention.

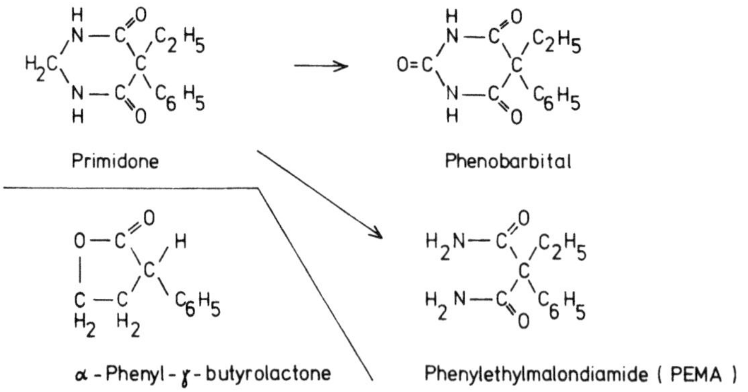

Fig. 1. Metabolic transformation of primidone. α-Phenyl-γ-butyrolactone has only been identified in the urine of patients with primidone intoxication (ANDRESEN et al. 1976)

In the following, the rates and percentages of biotransformation of phenobarbital and PEMA, as well as the steady-state concentrations of the three compounds with anticonvulsant activity, will be discussed for the different species that have been studied in this respect.

a) Mouse

In acute experiments, after oral doses of 50 or 100 mg/kg to normal or pregnant mice, peak concentrations of primidone in plasma were reached after 0.6–1 h, of PEMA at 4 or 6 h, and of phenobarbital at 4–8 h after administration (McElhatton et al. 1977b), but during chronic administration the plasma concentrations of all three compounds peaked at 2 h after administration (Leal et al. 1979b). In pregnant mice, plasma concentrations of primidone and PEMA, but not of phenobarbital, were lower than in nonpregnant mice (McElhatton et al. 1977a). When a dose of 50 mg/kg primidone was administered six times at 4-h intervals, steady-state concentrations of 4–5 μg/ml primidone, 11–13 μg/ml phenobarbital, and about 12.5 μg/ml PEMA were determined in plasma (Leal et al. 1979b).

b) Rat

Baumel et al. (1973) followed the concentrations of primidone and its metabolites in plasma and brain of rats for 24 h after oral administration of a wide range of primidone doses. Primidone concentrations peaked after 1–2 h, whereas the concentrations of the metabolites remained rather low, with maximal values after 4–6 h for PEMA and after 6–12 h for phenobarbital. In the isolated perfused rat liver, the metabolism of [^{14}C]primidone was studied by Alvin et al. (1975). During 2 h, 80% of the drug was converted to PEMA and 15% to phenobarbital. Pretreatment of the rats with phenobarbital accelerated both metabolic transformations, while addition of PEMA to the perfusion fluid reduced the rate of transformation.

c) Guinea Pig

Slow formation of phenobarbital and a correspondingly weak anticonvulsant effect of primidone has been reported for this species (Frey and Hahn 1960).

d) Gerbil

In gerbils the anticonvulsant effect was mostly born by unchanged drug at 1 h after oral administration, at 4 h phenobarbital concentrations exceeded those of primidone, and at 12 h unchanged primidone could no longer be detected (Frey et al. 1984).

e) Rabbit

After i.v. injection of primidone, 10 mg/kg, the metabolites phenobarbital and PEMA could be detected in plasma as soon as 5 min after administration. Peak concentrations of these metabolites were reached after 12 h or 6–8 h, respectively. About 20% of the primidone administered was excreted unchanged, whereas about 40% of the total dose was transformed to each of the two main metabolites (Hunt and Miller 1978). In another study in which the very high dose of 400 mg/kg was administered orally, Fujimoto et al. (1968) also found urinary excretion of 20% of the dose unchanged, 48% as PEMA, but only 10% as phenobarbital. The difference may be explained by saturation of the biotransformation to phenobarbital, but not to PEMA, when high doses are used (HUNT and MILLER 1978). Biotransformation was increased when rabbits were pretreated with phenytoin (FUJIMOTO et al. 1968).

f) Dog

BUTLER and WADDELL (1956) were the first to show biotransformation to phenobarbital in this species: during oral administration of 200 mg/kg primidone daily for 6 days, phenobarbital plasma concentrations rose to nearly 40 μg/ml. The authors concluded that 5% of the primidone dosed had been converted to phenobarbital. When dogs received daily primidone doses of 23–28 mg/kg orally for 30 days, phenobarbital plasma concentrations rose to final values of 12–15 μg/ml (FREY and HAHN 1960). A later study be FREY et al. (1979) showed that the appearance of phenobarbital can be delayed considerably: this metabolite could not be detected in the plasma of mongrel dogs after a single oral dose of 30 mg/kg, whereas in beagles phenobarbital could be detected as soon as 3 h after administration and remained at concentrations of 1–3 μg/ml from 6 to 30 h after administration. PEMA was rapidly formed both by mongrels and beagles, so that an apparent k_a for its appearance could be calculated: it averaged 0.0029 min^{-1} in the mongrels and 0.0047 min^{-1} in the beagles. During steady-state conditions after administration of daily doses of 30–40 mg/kg, plasma concentrations averaged 65 nmol/ml phenobarbital and 50 nmol/ml PEMA, whereas primidone, on account of its short half-life, showed great variations between 10 and 20 nmol/ml. A similar relation was found by YEARY (1980), and both authors agree that the role of unchanged primidone in the anticonvulsant effect of primidone should only be a minor one.

g) Fowl

In epileptic chickens treated with primidone i.p., primidone concentrations declined rapidly and were no longer detectable at 12 h, while phenobarbital concentrations were highest at 8 and 12 h after administration (JOHNSON et al. 1978).

h) Man

The appearance of phenobarbital plasma concentrations during treatment with primidone can be delayed for 2–4 days (BOOKER et al. 1970; GALLAGHER et al. 1972; CLOYD et al. 1981). HUISMAN (1969) mentions a single patient in whom phenobarbital could not be detected before the 7th day of treatment. Similar observations have been reported for PEMA (GALLAGHER et al. 1972; CLOYD et al. 1981). Combined treatment with other antiepileptic drugs seems to accelerate the appearance of the metabolites (CLOYD et al. 1981).

Rate constants for the conversion of primidone into the metabolites have been calculated in children (KAUFFMAN et al. 1977): 0.0424 h^{-1} for conversion to PEMA and 0.0045 h^{-1} to phenobarbital. MATZKE et al. (1981) calculated the rate constant for conversion to phenobarbital from a case of intoxication with phenytoin and primidone as 0.033 h^{-1}.

The degree to which primidone is converted to phenobarbital has been calculated by different authors and shows a fairly wide variation. ZAVADIL and

GALLAGHER (1976) estimated an overall conversion of 16%–17% of the total dose from [^{14}C]primidone studies in epileptic patients, whereas KAUFFMAN et al. (1977) found 1%–8% of the daily primidone dose excreted as phenobarbital or metabolites of phenobarbital in children. BUTLER and WADDELL (1956) mention a value of 15%; OLESEN and DAM (1967) calculated between 22% and 29% by comparing the phenobarbital steady-state concentrations during treatment with primidone or phenobarbital. The latter authors found the lowest conversion percentage with the highest doses of primidone. In the mentioned case of intoxication with phenytoin and primidone, a conversion rate of even 30% was calculated (MATZKE et al. 1981). BOGAN and SMITH (1967) calculated from a series of patients in steady state that 1 mg/kg phenobarbital/day resulted in a blood level of 5.2 µg/ml, and 1 mg/kg primidone/day gave a level of 1.1 µg/ml phenobarbital; a relation in agreement with the clinical potency ratio for both drugs (GRUBER et al. 1957). In the study of ZAVADIL and GALLAGHER (1976) about 40% of a single dose was excreted as unchanged primidone and 28% as PEMA over 5 days; in children KAUFFMAN et al. (1977) recovered 15%–66% of the daily dose as unchanged primidone and 16%–65% as PEMA from the urine. The degree of conversion may be different from different batches of primidone (BIELMANN et al. 1974).

The ratio between plasma concentrations of phenobarbital and primidone during steady state has been studied by many authors, with highly different results. Ratios of 1:1 to 2:1 have been reported (HUISMAN 1969; GALLAGHER et al. 1972; FINCHAM et al. 1974; CLOYD et al. 1981) for patients on monotherapy with primidone, but a value of 3 : 1 seems more common (BOOKER et al. 1970; WINDORFER et al. 1978; HEIPERTZ et al. 1979; LAMBIE and JOHNSON 1981). REYNOLDS et al. (1972) report a ratio of 4.4 : 1. The ratio may rise to values of up to 6 : 1 in cases of combined treatment (HUISMAN 1969; BOOKER et al. 1970; FINCHAM et al. 1974; REYNOLDS 1975; HEIPERTZ et al. 1979; LAMBIE and JOHNSON 1981), and even to 7 : 1 in cases of intoxication (HEIPERTZ et al. 1979). On account of the rapid elimination of unchanged primidone, this ratio must be highly dependent on the time after administration at which the blood sample is taken, and this may in part explain the differences. In neonates from mothers treated with primidone, phenobarbital/primidone ratios from less than 1.0 to about 3.0 were found (NAU et al. 1980 a).

PEMA has been reported as being found at about the same or slightly higher concentrations than primidone in the plasma of patients (KUTT 1974), but in another study, PEMA concentrations tended to be lower than those of primidone (CLOYD et al. 1981). Equal or even higher concentrations of primidone than of phenobarbital were reported in a patient with renal insufficiency and in children intoxicated with primidone (HEIPERTZ et al. 1979).

IV. Elimination

1. Renal Excretion

Primidone is excreted by the kidneys, partly unchanged and partly in the form of its active metabolites phenobarbital and PEMA, of which at least the former is mostly hydroxylated and conjugated with glucuronic acid. Quantitative data exist for the rabbit (FUJIMOTO et al. 1968), in which excretion in the urine was followed for 3–4 days after a single oral dose of 400 mg/kg. Of the total dose 20% was excreted as primidone, 48% as PEMA, but only 4% as unmetabolized phenobarbital. The proportion of the latter increases, however, to about 10% when account is taken of the part which is hydroxylated and conjugated. For man, BOGUE et al. (1956) stated that 60–80% of a single dose is excreted within 48 h, partly in the form of metabolic products. ZAVADIL and GALLAGHER (1976) followed the excretion of a single dose over 5 days: about 40% was excreted as primidone, 28% as PEMA, and 3,3% as unchanged phenobarbital. In children, an average of 92% of the daily dose could be recovered from the urine: 42% (15%–66%) as unchanged primidone, 45% (16%–65%) as PEMA, and 4.9% (1.1%–8.0%) as phenobarbital and metabolites of it (KAUFFMAN et al. 1977). NAU et al. (1980a) have given data for the renal clearance of primidone and its metabolites in neonates and their mothers (see Table 3).

2. Pharmacokinetic Parameters for Elimination

The elimination half-lives as well as data for the total body clearance of primidone and its metabolites from studies in laboratory animals and in humans have been compiled in Table 3. It is apparent from the data in the table that elimination kinetics in dogs is most similar to that in man. The studies of ZAVADIL and GALLAGHER (1976) and of CLOYD et al. (1981) show that the half-life of primidone is considerably shorter in patients also receiving other antiepileptic drugs than in patients on monotherapy with primidone. Prolonged treatment with primidone seems not to alter elimination kinetics significantly (GALLAGHER et al. 1972). Also the values determined in cases of primidone intoxications (BRILLMAN et al. 1974; MATZKE et al. 1981) were well within the range determined for nonintoxicated patients.

F. Drug Interactions

Interactions between primidone and other concomitantly administered drugs have been rarely studied in laboratory animals, and the clinical evidence is often equivocal. One chapter is devoted to clinical interactions in the section on "Clinical Pharmacology" in this volume (Chap. 28).

In rabbits the elimination of primidone and its active metabolites was considerably accelerated by pretreatment with 40 mg/kg phenytoin for 5 days (HUNT and MILLER 1974). This combination has been studied repeatedly in patients (FINCHAM et al. 1974; REYNOLDS 1975; CLOYD et al. 1981; LAMBIE and JOHNSON 1981), and an increased rate of elimination has been found in these studies. Also the ratio phenobarbital/primidone in plasma was increased. LAMBIE and JOHNSON (1981) also report an increase in the PEMA/primidone ratio. Pretreatment with high doses of nicotinamide inhibits the biotransformation of primidone and decreases the phenobarbital/primidone ratio (BOURGEOIS et al. 1982).

Acetazolamide has been reported to inhibit or delay absorption of primidone in some patients (SYVERSEN et al. 1977), and HUISMAN (1968) noted an increase in phenobarbital serum concentrations when acetazolamide was withdrawn. Valproate was reported to have no effect on primidone and phenobarbital plasma concentrations (BRUNI 1981) or to induce a transient increase in primidone plasma concentrations (WINDORFER et al. 1975).

Table 3. Elimination half-life and total body clearance for primidone and its metabolites phenobarbital and PEMA from studies in laboratory animals and from patients

Species	Elimination half-life (h)			Total body clearance (liters/kg/h)			Refs.
	Primidone	Phenobarbital	PEMA	Primidone	Phenobarbital	PEMA	
Mouse	2.2–2.9	2.75–4.3	1.2–2.3	2.26 ml/h			Leal et al. (1979a, b)
Rat	1.67						Gallagher et al. (1970)
Rabbit	2.3	31–51	8.8–9.8	0.23	0.013	0.067	Hunt and Miller (1978)
Dog							
Mongrel	10	70	14		0.007		Frey et al. (1979)
Beagle	5.1	32	7.4		0.013		
	1.85 (i.v.)	41	7.1				Yeary (1980)
Monkey	10			0.25			Van der Kleijn et al. (1975)
Man	3.3–5.8		29–36				Baumel et al. (1972)
	10–12						Booker et al. (1970)
	15±4.7[a]				0.035		Cloyd et al. (1981)
	8.3±2.9[b]				0,051		
	8 (3.3–19)	48, 84	17, 26				Gallagher et al. (1972)
	5–10		24–48				Kutt (1974)
	6.5				0.064		Van der Kleijn et al. (1975)
	14.4[a]		56				Zavadil and Gallagher (1976)
	8.3 (4.5–11)[b]	83 (42–138)	41 (28–81)				
			17–21			0.024–0.039	Cottrell et al. (1982)
Children	8.7 (4.5–11)						Kauffman et al. (1977)
Intoxications	15	108	20				Brillman et al. (1974)
	6.2				0.06		Matzke et al. (1981)
					Renal clearance	(mg/kg/h)	
Neonates	23 (8–80)	113±40	35±6	2–15	0.04–3.0	1–40	Nau et al. (1980a)
Mothers				10–30	0.8–16	20–70	

[a] Monotherapy, [b] Combined therapy

Clinical reports on interactions with carbamazepine or clonazepam are equivocal (for review see Eadie and Tyrer 1980). Elevated phenobarbital plasma concentrations during concomitant therapy with primidone and ethylphenacemide have been noted (Huisman 1968).

Pretreatment with primidone increased the activity of the mixed function hydroxylases in rat liver by 50% with a consequent increase in the elimination of meprobamate (Kato and Vassanelli 1962). A similar observation has been reported for griseofulvin (Kraml et al. 1966). Isoniazid decreased the biotransformation of primidone to phenobarbital in a patient so that suspiciously high primidone plasma concentrations could be measured (Sutton and Kupferberg 1975). Decreases in serum Ca^{++} during treatment with primidone were interpreted as the consequence of increased metabolic inactivation of vitamin D (Richens and Rowe 1970).

Some cases of failures of contraceptive medication during treatment with primidone are mentioned in the review of Back et al. (1981).

In many of these observations it cannot be excluded that the interaction was more dependent on the metabolite phenobarbital than on primidone itself.

G. Toxicology

I. Acute Toxicology

1. Animal Studies

An oral LD_{50} of 600–800 mg/kg was determined in mice; in rats of 100 g body weight the LD_{50} was 1.5 g/kg orally, but the LD_{50} was higher than 2 g/kg in rats weighing 200 g. The animals displayed ataxia and hypnosis; male rats were more resistant than females. Monkeys receiving 500 mg/kg orally for 4 days showed ataxia and torpor from the 2nd day; these symptoms lasted for several days after termination of treatment (Bogue and Carrington 1953). A neurotoxic dose (TD_{50}), i.e., the dose eliciting minimal neurological deficit, of 1.06 g/kg in mice and 630 mg/kg in rats was determined by Goodman et al. (1953). These authors noted crystalluria in animals treated with high doses; the crystals were identified as PEMA. Cats and rabbits showed signs of neurological impairment from doses as low as 25 or 50 mg/kg, respectively: ataxia; depression; impairment of placing, postural, corneal, and pinna reflexes; and decreased response to pain.

2. Human Data

After the first exposure to primidone, ataxia, drowsiness, and nystagmus were observed at primidone concentrations ranging from about 1 to 15 μg/ml and before any metabolites could be determined in plasma (Gallagher et al. 1973). Doses of up to 30 g primidone, even a dose of 400 mg/kg in a child, have been survived (Arnold and Ceranke-Höfermayer 1953; Kappy and Buckley 1969). A fatal dose of 32.5 g primidone was reported by Bogan et al. (1965). When this patient died after 33 h, phenobarbital concentrations of 93 μg/ml in plasma and 275 μg/g in liver were determined.

II. Chronic Toxicity Studies

Rats receiving daily oral doses of 125, 250, or 500 mg/kg primidone all showed pronounced ataxia, and, with the highest dose, torpor, but only six out of the ten females died between the 4th and 6th days of treatment. Newly weaned rats were treated for 9 weeks with daily doses of 100 or 250 mg/kg. The growth of these rats was somewhat retarded but all animals survived. The histological examination revealed swelling of the cells of the convoluted renal tubules as well as vacuolization and desquamation of these cells. In about half of the rats of both treated groups from the 9-week study, the thyroid epithelium was columnar and stained poorly (BOGUE and CARRINGTON 1953). Dogs survived daily oral doses of 50 mg/kg for 6 months and of 200 mg/kg for 4 months without signs of depression, ataxia, or hypnosis (BOGUE et al. 1956). Monkeys were treated with oral doses of 50, 100, or 250 mg/kg on 5 days of the week for 8 weeks. Only the largest dose provoked ataxia. Histologically, this group showed some alterations of the renal tubules but not of the thyroid. Blood counts were normal (BOGUE and CARRINGTON 1953). In an epileptic dog, treated with daily doses of 100–150 mg/kg for 3 months, JENNINGS et al. (1974) describe ataxia, incoordination, anorexia, tachycardia, and hyperventilation as well as an increase in the activity of serum alkaline phosphatase. Liver cirrhosis developed in dogs treated with primidone for 2–3 years, but the causal relationship remaines dubious since these dogs also received other antiepileptic drugs (BUNCH et al. 1982).

III. Teratogenic Effect

In pregnant mice receiving daily doses of 100–200 mg/kg primidone on days 12–16, 8.5%–10.5% of fetuses had a cleft palate. Concurrent administration of 3.75 mg/kg folic acid s.c. reduced the incidence of palatal defects from 10.9% to 3.4% in mice receiving 1.25 g/kg primidone in the diet on days 12–16 (SULLIVAN and MCELHATTON 1975). In a later study (SULLIVAN and MCELHATTON 1977), an increased incidence of cleft palate, enlarged cerebral ventricles, and clubfoot were noted in the offspring of mice treated on days 6–16 of pregnancy with doses of 90 or 180 mg/kg. The overall incidence of fetuses with major defects in all primidone-treated groups of the latter study was 4.8% compared with 1.3% for untreated controls. The same incidence of malformations was noted with equieffective doses of carbamazepine or phenobarbital, whereas a much higher number of malformations was seen in phenytoin-treated mice.

In two children, the mothers of whom had been treated with primidone and had extremely high serum concentrations of primidone and phenobarbital, RUDD and FREEDOM (1979) saw retarded growth, hirsutism, microencephaly, mental retardation, cardiac defects, and hypoplastic fingernails. In the collaborative study of NAKANE et al. (1980) primidone was judged to be significantly teratogenic.

IV. Mutagenic Effect

In cultures of human lymphocytes, primidone (2.5–375 μg/ml) and phenobarbital (22–388 μg/ml) caused a slight increase of aberrant mitoses, mostly gaps and breaks of the chromosomes. PEMA had no comparable effect up to a concentration of 750 µg/ml. The alterations were hardly dose dependent and remained within the borders of the normal range so that primidone and phenobarbital are considered not to be highly mutagenic (FOERST 1972). In the dominant lethal test system in mice, a treatment with twice 70 mg/kg primidone induced a significant dominant lethality in the postmeiotic stages, but chromosomal aberrations in spermatogonia were only slightly increased (BUCKEL 1975).

V. Other Toxic Effects

Megaloblastic anemias have repeatedly been reported during treatment with primidone (LÜLLMANN 1962). Treatment with vitamin B_{12} is ineffective, but folic acid has a curative action (GIRDWOOD and LENMAN 1956). In microorganisms primidone interfered with the following steps of folate metabolism: (1) reduction of folic acid to dihydrofolic acid, (2) metabolism of unconjugated pteridine, and (3) phosphorylation of thymidine to thymidilic acid. Only reactions (1) and (3) occur in man and interference at both these points may explain the megaloblastic anemia (BAKER et al. 1962). Enzymes of the folate metabolism from pigeon liver were not inhibited by high concentrations of primidone (HAMFELT and WILMANS 1965). Other authors think that interference of the drug with folic acid absorption and its transport into the CNS is the important step (WAXMAN et al. 1970; SINGH and HUOT 1973).

VI. Clinical Intoxications

Intoxications with primidone have been reported repeatedly (ARNOLD and CERANKE-HÖFERMAYER 1953; BOGAN et al. 1956; CARTELLIERI 1956; KAPPY and BUCKLEY 1969; WILSON and WILKINSON 1973; BRILLMAN et al. 1974; PLAA et al. 1974). In most cases the symptoms resemble those of barbiturate intoxication, and high phenobarbital concentrations have been determined in the plasma. However, especially in acute intoxications, primidone may be responsible for part of the symptomatology (ARNOLD and CERANKE-HÖFERMAYER 1953; BRILLMAN et al. 1974). Crystalluria has been reported; crystals consisted mostly of primidone (BRILLMAN et al. 1974). STERN (1977) found high concentrations of PEMA during intoxication with primidone and considers that this metabolite plays a significant role in the clinical picture. This conclusion does not seem convincing in view of the low pharmacological activity of PEMA and the high concentration of phenobarbital found in this case.

Particular attention will be paid to clinical intoxications in the section on "Clinical Pharmacology" in this volume.

References

Abraham CV (1976) Micromethod for the simultaneous analysis of phenobarbital, diphenylhydantoin, carbamazepine, and primidone in blood. Microchem. J. 21:272–278

Abraham CV, Joslin HD (1976) Simultaneous gas-chromatographic analysis for phenobarbital, diphenylhydantoin, carbamazepine, and primidone in serum. Clin Chem 22:769–771

Adams RF, Vandemark FL (1976) Simultaneous high-pressure liquid-chromatographic determination of some anticonvulsants in serum. Clin Chem 22:25–31

Albertson TE, Peterson SL, Stark LG, Baselt RC (1980) Barbiturate serum levels and protection against kindled amygdaloid seizures in the rat. Neuropharmacology 19:1141–1144

Alvin J, Goh E, Bush MT (1975) Study of the hepatic metabolism of primidone by improved methodology. J Pharmacol Exp Ther 194:117–125

Alvin JD, Bush MT (1975) Synthesis of millimole amounts of ^{14}C- and ^{2}D-labelled primidone, phenylethylmalonamide, and phenobarbital for high-sensitivity detection in biological materials. Microchim Acta 1:685–696

Andresen BD, Davis FT, Templeton JL, Hammer RH, Panzik HL (1976) Synthesis and characterization of alpha-phenyl-gamma-butyrolactone, a metabolite of glutethimide, phenobarbital and primidone in human urine. Res Commun Chem Pathol Pharmacol 15:21–30

Arnold OH, Ceranke-Höfermayer S (1953) Ein Fall von Suicidversuch mit Mysoline. Wien Med Wochenschr 103:692-693

Arora RB, Sharma PL (1958) Effectiveness of some anticonvulsant drugs in ventricular tachycardia resulting from acute myocardial infarction in the dog. Indian J Med Res 46:802–807

Asano T, Gasawara N (1982) Stimulation of GABA receptor binding by barbiturates. Eur J Pharmacol 77:355–357

Ashton D, Wauquier A (1979a) Behavioral analysis of the effects of 15 anticonvulsants in the amygdaloid kindled rat. Psychopharmacology 65:7–13

Ashton D, Wauquier A (1979b) Effects of some anti-epileptic, neuroleptic, and GABA-minergic drugs on convulsions induced by D,L-allylglycine. Pharmacol Biochem Behav 11:221–226

Back DJ, Breckenridge AM, Crawford FE, MacIver M, Orme ML'E, Rowe PH (1981) Interindividual variation and drug interaction with hormonal steroid contraceptives. Drugs 21:46–61

Baker H, Frank O, Hutner SH, Aaronson S, Ziffer H, Sobotka H (1962) Lesions in folic acid metabolism induced by primidone. Experientia 18:224–226

Barnes TC (1960) Relationship of chemical structure to central nervous system effects of tranquilizing and anticonvulsant drugs. J Am Pharm Assoc Sci Ed 49:415–417

Bartels H, Kruse K, Oldigs HD (1977) Zur Bestimmung der Serumspiegel von Phenobarbital, Primidon und Diphenylhydantoin. Erste Erfahrungen mit dem quantitativen Enzym-Immunoassay. Monatsschr Kinderheilk 125:572–573

Bartels H, Günther E, Wallis S (1979) Flow-dependent salivary primidone levels in epileptic children. Epilepsia 20:431–436

Baumel IP, Gallagher BB, Mattson RH (1972) Phenylethylmalonamide (PEMA). An important metabolite of primidone. Arch Neurol 27:34–41

Baumel IP, Gallagher BB, DiMicco J, Goico H (1973) Metabolism and anticonvulsant properties of primidone in the rat. J Pharmacol Exp Ther 186:305–314

Bielemann P, Levac TH, Langlois Y, Tetreault L (1974) Bioavailability of primidone in epileptic patients. Int J Clin Pharmacol 9:132–137

Bogan J, Smith H (1968) The relation between primidone and phenobarbital blood levels. J Pharm Pharmacol 20:64–67

Bogan J, Tentoul E, Smith H (1965) Fatal poisoning by primidone. J Forensic Sci Soc 5:97–98

Bogue JY, Carrington HC (1953) The evaluation of mysoline – a new anticonvulsant drug. Br J Pharmacol 8:230–236

Bogue JY, Carrington HC, Bentley S (1956) L'activité anticonvulsive de la mysoline. Acta Neurol Belg 56:640–650

Booker HE, Hosokowa K, Burdette RD, Darcey B (1970) A clinical study of serum primidone levels. Epilepsia 11:395–402

Bose BC, Saifi AQ, Sharma SK (1963) Studies on anticonvulsant and antifibrillatory drugs. Arch Int Pharmacodyn Ther 146:106–113

Bourgeois BFD, Dodson WE, Ferrendelli JA (1982) Interactions between primidone, carbamazepine, and nicotinamide. Neurology 32:1122–1126

Bourgeois BFD, Dodson WE, Ferrendelli JA (1983a) Primidone, phenobarbital, and PEMA. I. Seizure protection, neurotoxicity, and therapeutic index of individual compounds in mice. Neurology 33:283–290
Bourgeois BFD, Dodson WE, Ferrendelli JA (1983b) Primidone, phenobarbital, and PEMA. II. Seizure protection, neurotoxicity, and therapeutic index of varying combinations in mice. Neurology 33:291–295
Brillmann J, Gallagher BB, Mattson RH (1974) Acute primidone intoxication. Arch Neurol 30:255–258
Bruni J (1981) Valproic acid and plasma levels of primidone and derived phenobarbital. Can J Neurol Sci 8:91–92
Büchi J, Braunschweiger H, Kira M, Lauener H (1966) Synthese und pharmakologische Wirkung einiger 4,6-Dioxo-hexahydropyrimidin-Derivate. Helv Chim Acta 49:2337–2344
Buckel U (1975) Mutagenicity of Mysoline in spermatogenesis of mice. Mutat Res 29:204–205
Bunch SE, Castleman WL, Hornbuckle WE, Tennant BC (1982) Hepatic cirrhosis associated with long-term anticonvulsant drug therapy in dogs. J Am Vet Med Assoc 181:357–362
Butler TC, Waddell WJ (1956) Metabolic conversion of primidone (Mysoline) to phenobarbital. Proc Soc Exp Biol Med 93:544–546
Cartellieri L (1956) Klinische Erfahrungen mit dem Antiepileptikum Mylepsin. Med Klin 51:986–988
Cloyd JC, Miller KW, Leppik IE (1981) Primidone kinetics: effects of concurrent drugs and duration of therapy. Clin Pharmacol Ther 29:402–407
Collins AJ, Horlington M (1969) A sequential screening test based on the running component of audiogenic seizures in mice, including reference compound PD_{50} values. Br J Pharmacol 37:140–150
Constantinescu E, Hategan D, Tudor S, Volanschi D (1976) The influence of antiepileptic drugs on some enzymes. Activity in the brain of mice with audiogenic epilepsy. Note I. The action of phenobarbital, diphenylhydantoin and primidone. Rev Roum Méd Neurol Psychiatr (Bucur) 14:119–128
Cottrell PR, Streete JM, Berry DJ, Schäfer H, Pisani F, Perucca E, Richens A (1982) Pharmacokinetics of phenylethylmalonamide (PEMA) in normal subjects and in patients treated with antiepileptic drugs. Epilepsia 23:307–313
Couch MW, Greer M, Williams CM (1973) Determination of primidone and its metabolites in biological fluids by gas-chromatography. J Chromatogr 87:559–561
Crawford RD (1970) Epileptiform seizures in domestic fowl. J Hered 61:185–188
Davis HL, Falk KJ, Bailey DG (1975) Improved method for the simultaneous determination of phenobarbital, primidone, and diphenylhydantoin in patients' serum by gas-liquid chromatography. J Chromatogr 107:61–66
Dietzler DN, Hoelting CR, Leckie MP, Smith CH, Tieber VL (1980) Emit assays of five major anticonvulsant drugs. An evaluation of adaptations to two discrete kinetic analyzers. Am J Clin Pathol 74:41–50
Dorrity F, Linnoila M (1976) Rapid gas-chromatographic measurement of anticonvulsant drugs in serum. Clin Chem 22:860–862
Eadie MJ (1974) Laboratory control of anticonvulsant dosage. Drugs 8:386–397
Eadie MJ (1979) Which anticonvulsant drug? Drugs 17:213–218
Eadie MJ, Tyrer JH (1980) Anticonvulsant therapy. Pharmacological basis and practice, 2nd edn. Churchill-Livingstone, Edinburgh, p 198
Fichsel H, Knöpfle G (1977) Veränderungen im Schilddrüsenhormonsystem unter der Langzeitbehandlung mit Primidon bei epileptischen Kindern und Jugendlichen. Monatsschr Kinderheilkd 125:791–796
Fincham RW, Schottelius DD (1982) Primidone. Relation of plasma concentration to seizure control. In: Woodbury DM, Penry JK, Pippenger CE (eds) Antiepileptic drugs, 2nd edn. Raven, New York, pp 429–440
Fincham RW, Schottelius DD, Sahs AL (1974) The influence of diphenylhydantoin on primidone metabolism. Arch Neurol 30:259–262

Foerst D (1972) Chromosomenuntersuchungen nach der Einwirkung von Primidon (Mylepsinum) und seiner Abbauprodukte Phenobarbital und Phenylethylmalondiamide in vitro. Acta Genet Med Gemellol (Roma) 21:305–318

Foltz RL, Couch MW, Greer M, Scott KN, Williams CM (1972) Chemical ionization mass spectrometry in the identification of drug metabolites. Biochem Med 6:294–298

Frey HH, Hahn I (1960) Untersuchungen über die Bedeutung des durch Biotransformation gebildeten Phenobarbital für die antikonvulsive Wirkung von Primidon. Arch Int Pharmacodyn Ther 128:281–290

Frey HH, Löscher W (1980) Kann Primidon mehr als Phenobarbital? Versuch einer pharmakologischen Analyse. Nervenarzt 51:359–362

Frey HH, Göbel W, Löscher W (1979) Pharmacokinetics of primidone and its active metabolites in the dog. Arch Int Pharmacodyn Ther 242:14–30

Frey H-H, Löscher W, Reiche R, Schultz D (1984) Anticonvulsant effect of primdone in the gerbil. Time course and significance of the active metabolites. Pharmacology 28:329–335

Fujimoto JM, Mason WH, Murphy M (1968) Urinary excretion of primidone and its metabolites in rabbits. J Pharmacol Exp Ther 159:379–388

Gallagher BB, Baumel IP (1972) Primidone. Absorption, distribution, and excretion. In: Woodbury DM, Penry JK, Schmidt RP (eds) Antiepileptic drugs. Raven, New York, pp 357–359

Gallagher BB, Smith DB, Mattson RH (1970) The relationship of the anticonvulsant properties of primidone to phenobarbital. Epilepsia 11:293–301

Gallagher BB, Baumel IP, Mattson RH (1972) Metabolic disposition of primidone and its metabolites in epileptic subjects after single and repeated administration. Neurology 22:1186–1192

Gallagher BB, Baumel IP, Mattson RH, Woodbury SG (1973) Primidone, diphenylhydantoin and phenobarbital. Aspects of acute and chronic toxicity. Neurology 23:145–149

Garceau Y, Philopoulos Y, Hasegawa J (1973) Quantitative TLC determination of primidone, phenylethylmalonediamide, and phenobarbital in biological fluids. J Pharm Sci 62:2032–2034

Girdwood RH, Lenman JAR (1956) Megaboblastic anaemia occurring during primidone therapy. Br Med J 1:146–147

Goodman LS, Swinyard EA, Brown WC, Schiffman DO, Grewal MS, Bliss EL (1953) Anticonvulsant properties of 5-phenyl-5-ethyl-hexa-hydropyrimidine-4,6-dione(Mysoline), a new antiepileptic. J Pharmacol Exp Ther 108:428–436

Goudie JH, Burnett D (1973) A gas-chromatographic method for the simultaneous determination of phenobarbitone, primidone and phenytoin in serum using a nitrogen detector. Clin Chim Acta 43:423–429

Gruber CN, Mosier JM, Grant P (1957) Objective comparison of primidone and phenobarbital in epileptics. J Pharmacol Exp Ther 120:184–187

Gruber CM, Brock JT, Dyken M (1962) Comparison of the effectiveness of phenobarbital, mephobarbital, primidone, diphenylhydantoin, ethotoin, metharbital, and methylphenylethylhydantoin in motor seizures. Clin Pharmacol Ther 3:23–28

Gupta RN, Dobson K, Keane PM (1977) Gas-liquid chromatographic determination of primidone in plasma. J Chromatogr 132:140–144

Hamfelt A, Wilmanns W (1965) Inhibition studies on folic acid metabolism with drugs suspected to act on the myeloproliferative system. Clin Chim Acta 12:144–152

Heipertz R, Pilz H, Eickhoff K (1977) Evaluation of a rapid gas-chromatographic method for the simultaneous quantitative determination of ethosuximide, phenylethylmalonediamide, carbamazepine, phenobarbital, primidone and diphenylhydantoin in human serum. Clin Chim Acta 77:307–316

Heipertz R, Guthoff A, Bernhardt W (1979) Primidone metabolism in renal insufficiency and acute intoxication. J Neurol 221:101–104

Hill RE, Latham AN (1977) Simultaneous determination of anticonvulsant drugs by gas-liquid chromatography. J Chromatogr 131:341–346

Horning MG, Nowlin J, Buller CM, Lertratanangkoon K, Sommer K, Hill RM (1975) Clinical applications of gas chromatograph/mass spectrometer/computer systems. Clin Chem 21:1282–1287
Houghton GW, Richens A, Toseland PA, Davidson S, Falconer MA (1975) Brain concentration of phenytoin, phenobarbitone and primidone in epileptic patients. Eur J Clin Pharmacol 9:73–78
Huisman JW (1968) Metabolism and effect of the antiepileptic primidone in man (in Dutch) Pharm Weekbl 103:573–600
Huisman JW (1969) Disposition of primidone in man: an example of autoinduction of a human enzyme system. Pharm Weekbl 104:799–802
Hunt RJ, Miller KW (1978) Disposition of primidone, phenylethylmalonamide, and phenobarbital in the rabbit. Drug Metab Dispos 6:75–81
Jennings PB, Utter WF, Fariss BL (1974) Effects of long-term primidone treatment in a dog. J Am Vet Med Assoc 164:1123–1125
Johnson DD, Davis HL, Crawford RD (1978) Epileptiform seizures in domestic fowl. VIII. Anticonvulsant activity of primidone and its metabolites, phenobarbital, and phenylethylmalonamide. Can J Physiol Pharmacol 56:630–633
Kabra PM, Gotelli G, Stanfill R, Marton LJ (1976) Simultaneous measurement of phenobarbital, diphenylhydantoin, and primidone in blood by high-pressure liquid chromatography. Clin Chem 22:824–827
Kappy MS, Buckley J (1969) Primidone intoxication in a child. Arch Dis Child 44:282–284
Kato R, Vassanelli P (1962) Induction of increased meprobamate metabolism in rats pretreated with some neurotropic drugs. Biochem Pharmacol 11:779–794
Kauffman RE, Habersang R, Lansyk L (1977) Kinetics of primidone metabolism and excretion in children. Clin Pharmacol Ther 22:200–205
Kraml M, Marton AV, Dvornik D (1966) Effect of primidone (Mysoline) on tissular levels of griseofulvin in the rat. Proc Soc. Exp. Biol. Med 120:678–679
Kupferberg HJ (1970) Quantitative estimation of diphenylhydantoin, primidone, and phenobarbital in plasma by gas-liquid chromatography. J Chromatogr 29:283–288
Kutt H (1974) Pharmacodynamic and pharmacokinetic measurements of antiepileptic drugs. Clin Pharmacol Ther 16:243–250
Kutt H, Louis S (1972) Anticonvulsant drugs. II. Clinical pharmacological and therapeutic aspects. Drugs 4:256–282
Lambie DG, Johnson RH (1981) The effects of phenytoin on phenobarbitone and primidone metabolism. J Neurol Neurosurg Psychiatr 44:148–151
Leal KW, Rapport RL, Wilensky AJ, Friel PN (1979a) Single-dose pharmacokinetics and anticonvulsant efficacy of primidone in mice. Ann Neurol 5:470–474
Leal KW, Friel PN, Rapport RL, Wilensky AJ (1979b) Pharmacokinetics of primidone in mice after acute and chronic administration. Drug Metab Dispos 7:345
Lockard JS, Uhlir V, DuCharme LL, Farquhar JA, Huntsman BJ (1975) Efficacy of standard anticonvulsants in monkey model with spontaneous motor seizures. Epilepsia 16:301–317
Löscher W (1975) Einfluß klinisch gebräuchlicher Antikonvulsiva auf das γ-Aminobuttersäure-System bei der Maus. Dissertation, Freie Universität, Berlin
Löscher W (1979) A comparative study of the protein binding of anticonvulsant drugs in serum of dog and man. J Pharmacol Exp Ther 208:429–435
Löscher W, Göbel W (1978) Consecutive gas-chromatographic determination of phenytoin, phenobarbital, primidone, phenylethylmalondiamide, carbamazepine, trimethadione, dimethadione, ethosuximide, and valproate from the same serum specimen. Epilepsia 19:463–473
Lüllmann H (1962) Die Nebenwirkungen der Antiepileptika. Arzneimittelforsch 12:868–873
Martinez G, Snyder RD (1973) Transplacental passage of primidone. Neurology 23:381–383
Matin MA, Jaffery FN, Siddiqui RA (1981) A possible neurochemical basis of the central stimulatory effects of pp'DDT. J Neurochem 36:1000–1005

Matzke GR, Cloyd JC, Sawchuk RJ (1981) Acute phenytoin and primidone intoxication. A pharmacokinetic analysis. J Clin Pharmacol 21:92–99
McElhatton PR, Sullivan FM, Toseland PA (1977a) The metabolism of primidone in non-pregnant and 14-day pregnant mice. Xenobiotica 7:611–615
McElhatton PR, Sullivan FM, Toseland PA (1977b) Plasma level studies of primidone and its metabolites in the mouse at various stages of pregnancy. Xenobiotica 7:617–622
Monaco F, Piredda S, Mastropaolo C, Tondi M, Mutani E (1981) Diphenylhydantoin and primidone in tears. Epilepsia 22:185–189
Nakane Y, Okuma T, Takahashi R, Sori Y, Wada T, Sato T, Fukushima Y, Kumashiro H, Ono T, Takajashi T, Aoki Y, Kazamatsuri H, Inami M, Komai S, Seino M, Miyakoshi M, Tanimura T, Hazama T, Kawahara R, Otsuki S, Hosokawa K, Inanaga K, Nakazawa Y, Yamamoto K (1980) Multi-institutional study on the teratogenicity of antiepileptic drugs: a report of a collaborative study group in Japan. Epilepsia 21:663–680
Nau H, Rating D, Häuser I, Jäger E, Koch S, Helge H (1980a) Placental transfer and pharmacokinetics of primidone and its metabolites phenobarbital, PEMA and hydroxyphenobarbital in neonates and infants of epileptic mothers. Eur J Clin Pharmacol 18:31–42
Nau H, Jesdinsky D, Wittfoht W (1980b) Microassay for primidone and its metabolites phenylethylmalondiamide, phenobarbital and *p*-hydroxyphenobarbital in human serum, saliva, breast milk and tissues by gas chromatography-mass spectrometry using selected ion monitoring. J Chromatogr 182:71–79
Nishina T, Okoshi K, Kitamura M (1976) Improved method for measurement of serum levels of phenobarbital, carbamazepine, primidone and diphenylhydantoin by gas-liquid chromatography. Clin Chim Acta 73:463–468
Norton PRE (1970) The effect of drugs on barbiturate withdrawal convulsions in the rat. J Pharm Pharmacol 22:763–766
Olesen OV, Dam M (1967) The metabolic conversion of primidone (Mysoline[R]) to phenobarbitone in patients under long-term treatment. Acta Neurol Scand 43:348–356
Oxley J, Hebdige S, Laidlaw J, Wadsworth J, Richens A (1980) A comparative study of phenobarbitone and primidone in the therapy of epilepsy. In: Johannessen SI, Morselli PL, Pippenger CE, Richens A, Schmidt S, Meinardi H (eds) Antiepileptic therapy: advances in drug monitoring. Raven, New York, pp 237–242
Perchalski RJ, Scott KN, Wilder BJ, Hammer RH (1973) Rapid simultaneous GLC determination of phenobarbital, primidone, and diphenylhydantoin. J Pharm Sci 62:1735–1736
Plaa GL, Fujimoto JM, Hine CH (1958) Intoxication from primidone due to its biotransformation to phenobarbital. J Am Med Assoc 168:1769–1770
Proctor WR, Weakly JN (1976) A comparison of the presynaptic and post-synaptic actions of pentobarbitone and phenobarbitone in the neuromuscular junction of the frog. J Physiol (Lond) 258:257–268
Reynolds EH (1973) Anticonvulsants, folic acid, and epilepsy. Lancet I:1376–1378
Reynolds EH (1975) Longitudinal studies of serum antiepileptic drug levels. Preliminary observations: interaction of phenytoin and primidone. In: Schneider H, Janz D, Gardner-Thorpe C, Meinardi H, Sherwin AL (eds) Clinical pharmacology of anti-epileptic drugs. Springer, Berlin Heidelberg New York, pp 79–85
Reynolds EH, Mattson RH, Gallagher BB (1972) Relationships between serum and cerebrospinal fluid anticonvulsant drug and folic acid concentrations in epileptic patients. Neurology 22:841–844
Richens A, Rowe DJF (1970) Disturbance of calcium metabolism by anticonvulsant drugs. Br Med J 4:73–76
Richens A, Warrington S (1979) When should plasma drug levels be monitored? Drugs 17:488–500
Rudd NL, Freedom RM (1979) A possible primidone embryopathy. J Pediatr 94:835–837
Rümke CL (1967) Increased susceptibility of mice to seizures after some anticonvulsant drugs. Eur J Pharmacol 1:369–377

Rümke CL, Bout C (1960) Die Beeinflussung der Hexobarbitalnarkose durch vorher verabfolgte Pharmaka. Naunyn-Schmiedebergs Arch Exp Pathol Pharmakol 240:218–223
Saad SF (1970) The effect of isoniazid and some anticonvulsant drugs on the γ-aminobutyric acid content of mouse brain in insulin hypoglycaemia. J Pharm Pharmacol 22:372–374
Saad SF, El Masry AM, Scott PM (1972) Influence of certain anticonvulsants on the concentration of γ-aminobutyric acid in the cerebral hemispheres of mice. Eur J Pharmacol 17:386–392
Schäfer H (1975) Some problems concerning the quantitative assay of primidone and its metabolites. In: Schneider H, Janz D, Gardner-Thorpe C, Meinardi H, Sherwin AL (eds) Clinical pharmacology of anti-epileptic drugs. Springer, Berlin Heidelberg New York, pp 124–129
Schmidt D (1981) Behandlung der Epilepsien. Georg Thieme, Stuttgart, p 66, p 74
Schmidt D, Kupferberg HJ (1975) Diphenylhydantoin, phenobarbital, and primidone in saliva, plasma, and cerebrospinal fluid. Epilepsia 16:735–741
Schwartz-Porsche D, Löscher W, Frey HH (1982) Treatment of canine epilepsy with primidone. J Am Vet Med Assoc 181:592–595
Schweizer K, Wick H, Brechbühler T (1978) An improved method for preparation of samples for the simultaneous assay of some antiepileptic drugs by gas-liquid chromatography. Clin Chim Acta 90:203–208
Singh P, Huot J (1973) Neurochemistry of epilepsy and mechanism of action of anti-epileptics. In: Mercier J (ed) Anticonvulsant drugs, vol 2, Pergamon, Oxford, pp 427–504
Soldin SJ, Hill JG (1976) Rapid micromethod for measuring anticonvulsant drugs in serum by high-performance liquid chromatography. Clin Chem 22:856–859
Stern EL (1977) Possible phenylethylmalondiamide (PEMA) intoxication. Ann Neurol 2:356–357
Sullivan FM, McElhatton PR (1975) Teratogenic activity of the antiepileptic drugs phenobarbital, phenytoin and primidone in mice. Toxicol Appl Pharmacol 34:271–282
Sullivan FM, McElhatton PR (1977) A comparison of the teratogenic activity of the antiepileptic drugs carbamazepine, clonazepam, ethosuximide, phenobarbital, phenytoin, and primidone in mice. Toxicol Appl Pharmacol 40:365–378
Sun L, Walwick ER (1976) Primidone analyses: correlation of gas-chromatographic assay with enzyme immunoassay. Clin Chem 22:901–902
Sutton G, Kupferberg HJ (1975) Isoniazid as an inhibitor of primidone metabolism. Neurology 25:1179–1181
Swinyard EA, Brown WC, Goodman LS (1952) Comparative assay of antiepileptic drugs in mice and rats. J Pharmacol Exp Ther 106:319–330
Swinyard EA, Tedeschi DH, Goodman LS (1954) Effects of liver damage and nephrectomy on anticonvulsant activity of mysoline and phenobarbital. J Am Pharm Assoc Sci Ed 43:114–116
Syversen GB, Morgan JP, Weintraub M, Myers GJ (1977) Acetazolamide-induced interference with primidone absorption. Arch Neurol 34:80–84
Talbot PA, Alderdice MT (1982) Primidone but not phenylethylmalonamide, a major metabolite, increases nerve-evoked transmitter release at the frog neuromuscular junction. J Pharmacol Exp Ther 222:87–93
Ticku MK, Olsen RW (1978) Interaction of barbiturates with dihydropicrotoxinin binding sites related to the GABA receptor-ionophore system. Life Sci 22:1643–1652
Toseland PA, Grove J, Berry DJ (1972) An isothermal GLC determination of plasma levels of carbamazepine, diphenylhydantoin, phenobarbitone and primidone. Clin Chim Acta 38:321–328
Troupin AS, Friel P (1975) Anticonvulsant level in saliva, serum, and cerebrospinal fluid. Epilepsia 16:223–227
Vandemark FL, Adams RF (1976) Ultramicro gas-chromatographic analysis of anticonvulsants, with use of a nitrogen-selective detector. Clin Chem 22:1062–1065
Van der Kleijn E, Guelen PJM, Van Wijk C, Baars I (1975) Clinical pharmacokinetics in monitoring chronic medication with antiepileptic drugs. In: Schneider H, Janz D,

Gardner-Thorpe C, Meinardi H, Sherwin AL (eds) Clinical pharmacology of antiepileptic drugs. Springer, Berlin Heidelberg New York, pp 11–33

Wad N, Hanifl E, Rosenmund H (1977) Rapid thin-layer chromatographic method for the simultaneous determination of carbamazepine, diphenylhydantoin, mephenytoin, phenobarbital and primidone in serum. J Chromatogr 143:89–93

Wallace JE, Hamilton HE, Shimek EL, Schwertner HA, Blum K (1977) Determination of primidone by electron-capture gas-chromatography. Analyt Chem 49:903–906

Waxman S, Corcino JJ, Herbert V (1970) Drugs, toxins and dietary amino acids affecting vitamin B_{12} or folic acid absorption or utilization. Am J Med 48:599–608

White PT, Plott D, Norton J (1966) Relative anticonvulsant potency of primidone. A double blind comparison. Arch Neurol 14:31–35

Wiegrebe W, Wehrhahn L (1975) Polarographische Bestimmung einiger phenylsubstituierter Antikonvulsiva. Arzneimittelforsch 25:517–524

Wilson JT, Wilkinson GR (1973) Chronic and severe phenobarbital intoxication in a child treated with primidone and diphenylhydantoin. J Pediatr 83:484–489

Windorfer A, Sauer W, Gädeke R (1975) Elevation of diphenylhydantoin and primidone serum concentration by addition of dipropylacetate, a new anticonvulsant drug. Acta Paediatr Scand 64:771–772

Windorfer A, Stünkel S, Weinmann HM (1978) Bestimmung des Serumkonzentrationsverhältnisses von Primidon/Phenobarbital bei antikonvulsiver Primidonbehandlung als weiteres Kriterium bei der Therapiebeurteilung. Monatsschr Kinderheilk 126:507–511

Woodbury DM, Kemp JW (1970) Some possible mechanisms of action of antiepileptic drugs. Pharmakopsychiatr Neuro-Psychopharmakol 3:201–226

Yeary RA (1980) Serum concentrations of primidone and its metabolites, phenylethylmalonamide and phenobarbital, in the dog. Am J Vet Res 41:1643–1645

Zavadil P, Gallagher BB (1976) Metabolism and excretion of ^{14}C-primidone in epileptic patients. In: Janz D (ed) Epileptology. Proceedings of the 7th international symposium of epilepsy. Georg Thieme, Stuttgart, pp 129–139

CHAPTER 16

Carbamazepine

M. SCHMUTZ

A. Introduction

In the course of work on iminodibenzyl compounds in the laboratories of J. R. Geigy AG the first carbamoyl derivative was synthesized in 1953 and found to possess anticonvulsant properties. This discovery prompted the synthesis of related compounds of which the most promising turned out to be carbamazepine. It was synthesized by SCHINDLER and BLATTNER in 1957 and published in 1961. THEOBALD and KUNZ investigated the anticonvulsant activity of carbamazepine in the Geigy laboratories and reported on its characteristic spectrum of activity in 1963.

Clinical trials of carbamazepine had been in progress in several European countries since 1958 and the first results in epileptic patients were published in 1963 (BONDUELLE and SALLOU; MÜLLER; PAKESCH; RETT; TCHICALOFF and PENNETI). In the same year, the drug was introduced in Switzerland and Great Britain under the trade name of Tegretol. Carbamazepine has been used as drug of choice for the treatment of partial seizures as well as generalized tonic-clonic convulsions in adults and children (e.g., CEREGHINO et al. 1974; JEAVONS 1977; TROUPIN et al. 1977; JANZ 1978; PENIN 1978; EADIE 1979; HUF and SCHAIN 1980). As a rule it provokes no severe side effects; it can even bring about improvement in emotional difficulties and behavioral problems of epileptic patients. This "psychotropic effect" was first described by LORGE in 1963.

Besides its application in the epilepsies, carbamazepine has been useful also for other indications such as trigeminal neuralgia, glossopharyngeal neuralgia, postherpetic neuralgia, diabetic neuropathy, phantom-limb symptoms, causalgia, diabetes insipidus, delirium alcoholicum, alcohol withdrawal, antiarrhythmias, and manic-depressive psychosis (see SILLANPÄÄ 1981; AYD 1979; POST 1982).

B. Chemistry and Physicochemical Properties

The molecule of carbamazepine (5*H*-dibenz(b,f)azepine-5-carboxamide) consists of two benzene rings, one seven-membered ring, one double bond, and one amide group (see Fig. 1).

In contrast to the structure of other antiepileptic drugs, carbamazepine lacks a saturated carbon atom, its amide group is not part of a heterocyclic ring, and it is the only anticonvulsant compound having a tricyclic structure comparable to that of psychoactive drugs such as chlorpromazine or imipramine. The most

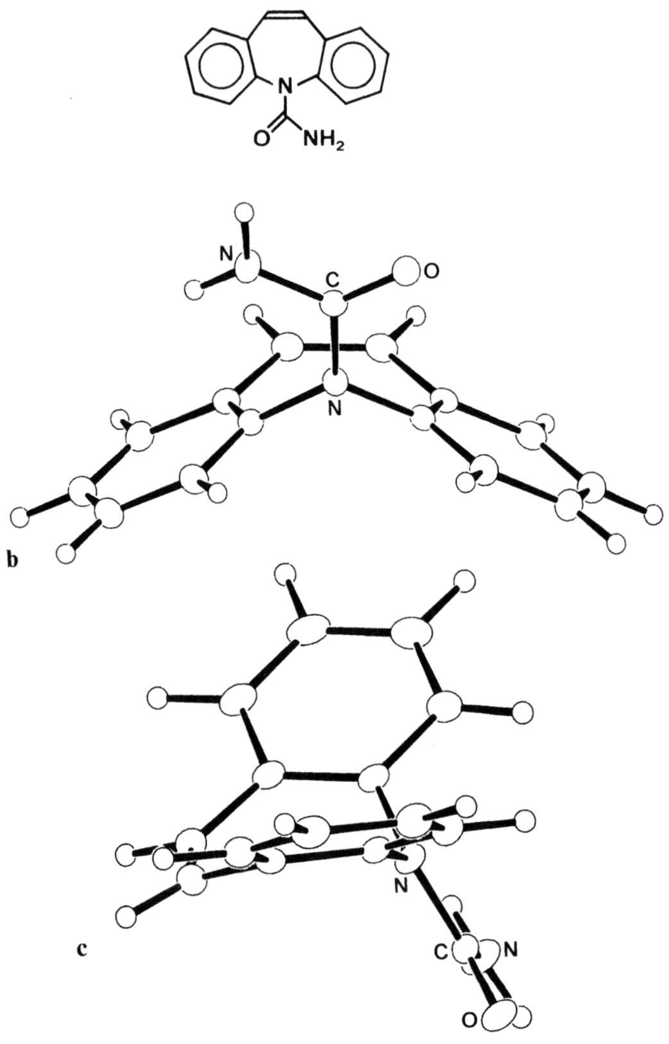

Fig. 1 a–c. Molecular structure of carbamazepine. **a** Structural formula of carbamazepine. **b**, **c**, Perspective view of the molecule (X-ray structure determination. Courtesy of Mrs. G. RIHS, Ciba-Geigy Ltd.)

reactive site of the carbamazepine molecule is the carbon-carbon double bond, which can undergo addition reactions (GAGNEUX 1976).

According to its chemical and physical properties, carbamazepine can be classified as a neutral, lipophilic compound (FAIGLE et al. 1976). It is soluble in acetone, alcohol, carbon tetrachloride, chloroform, dimethylformamide, dioxane, and propylene glycol but practically insoluble in water.

Gas-chromatographic methods have been developed for the quantitative determination of carbamazepine and its 10,11-epoxide metabolite in plasma and urine (e.g., GERARDIN and HIRTZ 1976). However, under these conditions neither compound is sufficiently stable (FRIGERIO et al. 1973), and high-performance liquid chromatography (HPLC) is therefore the best method for the simultaneous determination of the intact drug and its metabolites in blood and urine (e.g., EICHELBAUM and BERTILSSON 1975; WESTENBERG and DE ZEEUW 1976). For routine monitoring in clinical practice, a reliable enzyme immunoassay technique (EMIT) is available (e.g., SUN and SZAFIR 1977).

C. Anticonvulsant Activity

I. Anticonvulsant Activity in Rodent-Screening Tests

A number of authors have investigated the anticonvulsant activity of carbamazepine in *electroshock* and *chemoshock tests* in mice and rats (THEOBALD and KUNZ 1963; DAVIS et al. 1964; COYNE and CUSIC 1968; STILLE and SAYERS 1970; HOLLISTER and JULIEN 1974; JULIEN and HOLLISTER 1975; KOELLA et al. 1976; BALTZER and SCHMUTZ 1978; DAVIDSON et al. 1978; KRALL et al. 1978; MASUDA et al. 1979, 1980; JONES et al. 1981). As shown in Table 1, carbamazepine antagonizes electroshock-induced seizures in mice and rats, with ED_{50}s of 5–20 mg/kg p.o. or i.p. Effects of this nature are generally considered to be indicative of potential therapeutic activity against generalized tonic-clonic convulsions and also against partial seizures. In rats, the drug remains fully effective for at least 4 h after a single oral dose. No *"escape" phenomenon* occurs when rats are treated daily for a period of 28 days with carbamazepine (BALTZER et al. 1980). In pentylenetetrazol-induced seizures in mice, ED_{50}s of 16 mg/kg i.p. and 30 mg/kg p.o. were found, but occasionally the drug was also ineffective; more than 100 mg/kg carbamazepine is needed to protect 50% of the treated mice against picrotoxin-induced convulsions and strychnine-induced death (see Table 1). Differences in results in the chemoshock tests seem mainly due to variations in the experimental design. In rats susceptible to *audiogenic seizures,* the convulsions are suppressed by i.p. carbamazepine at an ED_{50} of 10 mg/kg (CONSROE et al. 1980).

II. Anticonvulsant Activity in Further Animal Models

There is evidence of a relationship between *temporal lobe epilepsy* and *the limbic system* (i.e., temporal lobe attacks are closely correlated to hippocampal sclerosis: SANO and MALAMUD 1953; MARGERISON and CORSELLIS 1966; SCHEIBEL et al. 1974). The demonstration of effects of anticonvulsants in this brain region (HERNANDEZ-PEON 1964, 1966; DOLCE 1969; HOLM et al. 1970; STILLE and SAYERS 1970; DAVID and GREWAL 1976; KOELLA et al. 1976; BALTZER and SCHMUTZ 1978; MARESOVA and MARES 1980; SCHMUTZ et al. 1981) may therefore be predictive, above all of therapeutic activity in complex partial seizures. In general, epileptic discharges elicited in limbic structures of monkeys, cats, or rabbits were shortened or completely suppressed by the drug. According to SCHMUTZ et al. (1981), in experiments on unrestrained cats, carbamazepine in doses within the clinically active range was somewhat more effective than phenytoin and distinctly more so than diazepam, valproate sodium, and ethosuximide in shortening electrically induced hippocampal afterdischarges.

Table 1. ED_{50} values (in mg/kg) of carbamazepine in various screening tests (for experimental details see references)

Test and species					Refs.
Electroshock test, mouse	Electroshock test, rat	Pentylenetetrazol test, mouse	Picrotoxin test, mouse	Strychnine test, mouse[a]	
	5.3 p.o.	>400.0 p.o.	>400.0 p.o.	100 p.o.	THEOBALD and KUNZ (1963)
19.0 i.p./20.5 p.o.		21.5 p.o.			DAVIS et al. (1964)
20.0 i.p.		Not effective			COYNE and CUSIC (1968)
6.1 p.o.		Not effective			STILLE and SAYERS (1970)
7.5 i.p.		16.0 i.p.			JULIEN and HOLLISTER (1975)
12.0 p.o.	10.0 p.o.	30.0 p.o.	>200.0 p.o.[b] ca. 60 p.o.[c]	150.0 p.o.	KOELLA et al. (1976)
11.0 p.o.	9.0 p.o.	30.0 p.o.	145.0 p.o.	150.0 p.o.	BALTZER and SCHMUTZ (1978)
8.8 i.p.		Not effective			KRALL et al. (1978)
13.3 p.o.		>500.0 p.o.			MASUDA et al. (1979)
9.7 i.p.					JONES et al. (1981)

[a] Protection from death
[b] Picrotoxin, 9–12 mg/kg i.p.
[c] Picrotoxin, 6 mg/kg i.p.

Cortical structures are thought to play an important role in the evolution and propagation of generalized tonic-clonic as well as of partial seizures. In cats and rabbits carbamazepine was mainly effective against seizures induced by electrical stimulation of the neocortex (HERNANDEZ-PEON 1964; STILLE and SAYERS 1970; ITO et al. 1977) and less so against chemically induced seizures (VAN DUIJN 1971; VAN DUIJN and VISSER 1972; HORI et al. 1979). In rhesus monkeys with aluminium hydroxide implants, beneficial effects of acutely and chronically administered carbamazepine have been reported. The drug controlled visible seizures and reduced intracortical spike propagation without completely normalizing the background EEG (LOCKARD et al. 1974; DAVID and GREWAL 1976) despite its short half-life and poor absorption in rhesus monkeys. With constant-rate infusion of carbamazepine, LOCKARD et al. (1979) obtained equivocal results probably because the levels reached in the serum were low (below 2 μg/ml). Carbamazepine had no appreciable effect on tonic-clonic convulsions induced by *infusion of bemegride* in cats; in fact, the seizure threshold was slightly lowered (VAN DUIJN and VISSER 1972). The drug did, however, decrease the frequency of occurence of such seizures induced by injection of *tungstic acid gel* into the thalamus of cats at doses of as little as 1.25 mg/kg i.v. (HORI et al. 1981).

Spike-wave discharges induced by penicillin and estrogen are thought to be indicative of absence-type epileptic activity. In these animal models, carbamazepine generally showed a slow onset of action. It was effective against penicillin-induced spike-wave discharges; in discharges produced by conjugated estrogens, the frequency of the spikes was more affected by the drug than their amplitude. In this latter model, carbamazepine was less effective than ethosuximide or clonazepam, but it did not intensify the spike-wave discharges as did phenytoin (JULIEN 1973; JULIEN et al. 1975; JULIEN and HOLLISTER 1975). However, according to BUSTAMENTE et al. (1981) carbamazepine, phenytoin, and phenobarbital, although they abolished penicillin-induced epileptic discharges in cats, increased the frequency of single spikes and decreased their duration at blood levels equivalent to the human therapeutic range. In experiments in which simultaneous microelectrode recordings were made from a penicillin focus in the sensorimotor cortex and from Purkinje cells in the cerebellum, JULIEN (1974) found that carbamazepine suppressed penicillin-induced epileptic discharges, but did not increase the firing rate of Purkinje cells. Phenytoin inhibited the penicillin-induced discharges and increased the firing rate of Purkinje cells. Thus, the anticonvulsant activity of carbamazepine does not seem to be based on increased Purkinje-cell discharge rates in the cerebellum. Carbamazepine was also effective in shortening the *electrically induced spike-wave afterdischarges* in unrestrained, freely moving cats in doses of 3 mg/kg p.o. and above. This animal model also seems related to absence-type clinical seizures, as is shown by the activity of drugs such as valproate sodium and ethosuximide in it (SCHMUTZ et al. 1980). As can be inferred from these experiments, carbamazepine also shows protective effects in animal models considered to be predictive of therapeutic activity in patients with absence-type seizures. Its activity was generally weaker than that of known antiabsence drugs, but, in contrast to phenytoin, cabamazepine did not intensify epileptic discharges. This is in accordance with the clinical profile of the above-mentioned drugs: carbamazepine, unlike phenytoin, is not contraindicated in absence-type seizures; in fact it has even shown some efficacy in that type of seizure (Grueter 1976).

A very informative model for the progressive development of epileptic seizures (and possibly, behavioral alterations) is provided by the *kindling experiment*. In this experiment carbamazepine has been shown to be effective in delaying the seizure development in cats (WADA et al. 1976b) and baboons (WADA 1977, 1980), whereas in rats it displayed no such activity (WADA 1977; BALTZER et al. 1981). When the compound was investigated in animals with fully developed limbic or cortical ("kindled") convulsions, it proved effective in cats and baboons (WADA et al. 1976a) and rabbits (EHLERS et al. 1979); in rats, on the other hand, positive results have been reported (BABINGTON and HOROWITZ 1973; ASHTON and WAUQUIER 1979; ALBRIGHT and BURNHAM 1980; HOWE et al. 1981; KAMEI et al. 1981) as well as negative or equivocal results (WADA 1977; ALBERTSON et al. 1980; HOWE et al. 1981; KAMEI et al. 1981). The findings in cats and monkeys demonstrate the ability of carbamazepine to suppress the development of seizures in, and the spread of seizures from, a given epileptic focus. This might be of importance when the use of carbamazepine in the prevention of post-traumatic seizures is discussed. As far as the equivocal results with carbamazepine in the rat kindling experiment are concerned, it is of interest to note that BALTZER et al. (1981) reported that mainly drugs active against absence-type seizures, such as valproate sodium (see also SCHMUTZ and KLEBS 1982), ethosuximide, and the benzodiazepines, were effective in their model.

Another interesting animal model is directed toward visual reflex epileptic seizures, i.e., seizures provoked by intermittent light or by the visual exploration of an intensely illuminated object. KILLAM et al. (1966) discovered the photosensitivity of the Senegalese baboon *Papio papio*. According to KILLAM (1976) and KILLAM et al. (1973), carbamazepine afforded protection against this photomyoclonic epileptoid response. In a large series of baboons, however, the effective dose varied considerably, probably owing to variability in absorption or metabolism of the drug, or both, in this species. In a modified model, in which the baboons were pretreated with allyglycine, MELDRUM et al. (1975 a, b) observed only weak protective activity of carbamazepine, associated with distinct side effects such as strabismus, nystagmus, and ataxia.

III. Pharmacological Effects Possibly Related to Anticonvulsant Activity

At 5 mg/kg i.p., carbamazepine slowed down the neocortical background activity in the *EEG* of cats, the rapid components, however, tending to be enhanced. In the hippocampus, hypersynchronization of theta waves was noted and the EEG of the reticular formation became more regular, showing higher amplitudes. Reticulocortical and thalamocortical projections as well as evoked potentials recorded in the formatio reticularis were hardly affected (DOLCE 1969). At 20 mg/kg i.p. the threshold of the efferent projections on the nervi ventrales anteriori thalami was raised. Simultaneously, inhibition of efferent connections of the centrum medianum and ventroanterior nucleus of the thalamus as well as of the afferent projections of the hippocampus was observed (HOLM et al. 1970). In baboons, carbamazepine in doses up to 40 mg/kg i.p. evoked dose-dependent increases in amplitude of the waves around 5/s and decreased the fast activity (15–30/s) over most of the cortex. An additional peak (9–10/s) at temporal derivations was noted, as were increases in overall power in the entire 0–60/s band (KILLAM 1976; SURIA and KILLAM 1980).

Electrophysiological studies with post-tetanic potentiation (KRUPP 1969a, b; THEOBALD et al. 1970; JULIEN and HOLLISTER 1975; KOELLA et al. 1976; HERSHKOWITZ et al. 1978), reflex discharges (THEOBALD and KUNZ 1963; KOELLA et al. 1976), muscle spindles (HERSHKOWITZ and RAINES 1978), neuromuscular junctions (ALDERDICE and TROMMER 1980), sciatic nerves (HONDA and ALLEN 1973), and giant axons (SCHAUF et al. 1974) indicate that carbamazepine exerts an inhibitory influence on certain neuronal tissues. But, compared with phenytoin, its effects are generally observed only at fairly high doses. For a more detailed description of electrophysiological data see Chap. 23, this volume.

IV. Neurobiochemical Effects Possibly Related to Anticonvulsant Activity

Biochemical disturbances such as an imbalance of central nervous transmitter substances or increased levels of cyclic nucleotides are thought to be of importance in the pathophysiology of epileptic seizures, and the action of anticonvulsants may to some degree be attributable to their corrective effect on such changes.

Since *gamma-aminobutyric acid (GABA)* levels were reported to be low in some experimental and clinical epilepsies, several authors investigated the influence of anticonvulsants on this important inhibitory neurotransmitter. BERNASCONI et al. (1982a, c) found that carbamazepine, as well as other anticonvulsants, reduced the GABA turnover rate in the cortex and hippocampus of mice, although only at relatively high doses (100 mg/kg p.o.). It did not change the steady-state concentrations of GABA in these structures. In the cerebellum of mice LUST et al. (1978) also observed no change in the steady-state levels of GABA after treatment with carbamazepine (25 mg/kg i.p.). On the other hand, VAROTTO et al. (1981) noted that carbamazepine and phenytoin markedly increased the cerebral GABA level in mice, whereas phenobarbital, diazepam, and clonazepam had no such effect. High concentrations of carbamazepine inhibited the activity of succinic semialdehyde dehydrogenase in mice by about 40% (SAWAYA et al. 1975). According to MINCHIN and IVERSEN (unpublished data cited in KOELLA et al. 1976), the drug did not influence the uptake of GABA into brain slices or into the satellite glial cells of dorsal-root ganglia. It did not alter the uptake of GABA and beta-alanine or tetanus labeling when added to cultures of fetal mouse cortex and maintained at a concentration of 24 μg/ml for 10 days (SHER et al. 1981). Moreover, the release of GABA in the rat brain was not influenced by carbamazepine or other anticonvulsants under in vivo (superfusion of sensorimotor cerebral cortex) or in vitro (superfusion of synaptosomes) conditions (ABDUL-GHANI et al. 1981). Only limited information exists on interactions between other amino acids (glutamate, glycine, alanine) and carbamazepine. In rat hippocampal slices the antiepileptic at 20 μM and above attenuated the excitatory influence of the Schaffer-commissural fiber input on CAI pyramidal cells. *Glutamate* is suggested to be the transmitter in these fibers: Since carbamazepine at 10 µm and above did not alter [^{3}H]glutamate binding but reduced [^{3}H]glutamate release it might act presynaptically to reduce glutamatergic transmission (OLPE, personal communication). YOUNG et al. (1974) failed to detect any influence of carbamazepine on the *glycine receptor* in strychnine-binding assays. Finally, BERNASCONI et al. (1982a, c) reported that carbamazepine and other anticonvulsants decrease the *alanine* content of the mouse cortex. This finding might be of importance, since electroshock-induced convulsions led to an increase in the content of this amino acid.

At doses of 15 mg/kg i.p. and above, carbamazepine increased *acetylcholine* levels selectivity in the striatum of rats, without affecting those in the mesence-phalon, diencephalon, hippocampus, cerebellum, and hemispheric residuum. It also decreased the *choline* level in the striatum; the enzymes involved in the synthesis and hydrolysis of acetylcholine, choline-O-acetyltransferase and cholinesterase, were not altered in vitro either by carbamazepine or by its main metabolite, carbamazepine-10, 11-epoxide. No tolerance to the action of carbamazepine on striatal acetylcholine was observed after treatment with 25 mg/kg i.p. twice per day for 6 days. Pimozide, a dopaminergic antagonist, did not prevent the increase in striatal acetylcholine by carbamazepine (CONSOLO et al. 1976). It is interesting to note that the 10,11-epoxide metabolite neither accumulated in the brain after chronic treatment, nor was present when the concentration of acetylcholine was maximal after acute treatment. The authors suggest that carbamazepine acts per se on the cholinergic system, and not via its main metabolite.

QUATTRONE and SAMANIN (1977) and QUATTRONE et al. (1978) assumed that catecholamines, in particular *norepinephrine*, may be preferentially involved in the mode of action of carbamazepine: when brain catecholamine concentrations were reduced by intraventricular injections of 6-hydroxydopamine, the seizure threshold was lowered and the anticonvulsant effect of carbamazepine, phenytoin, and phenobarbital diminished. However, in a later publication, QUATTRONE et al. (1981) reported that these drugs did not antagonize the decrease in norepinephrine concentrations induced by 6-hydroxydopamine, suggesting that in rats these anticonvulsants do not affect the brain norepinephrine uptake mechanism in vivo. On the other hand, PURDY et al. (1977) found that high concentrations of carbamazepine inhibited [^{3}H]norepinephrine uptake into brain synaptosomes and rabbit thoracic aorta. These activities were reported to be insufficient to account for the anticonvulsant action of the drug. In recent experiments carbamazepine at 100 mg/kg i.p. increased the content of MHPG-SO_4, an essential metabolite of norepinephrine, in the rat brain and, surprisingly, reduced the turnover of its amine (WALDMEIER, personal communication). Electrophysiological investigations also suggest interaction of carbamazepine with norepinephrine since at 3–30 mg/kg i.p. it dose-dependently activated the firing rate of presumed norepinephrinergic neurons in the rat locus coeruleus (OLPE and JONES 1983). In the study by KANEKO et al. (1981), carbamazepine did not influence norepinephrine levels in the mouse brain, but it increased the *dopamine* levels. In addition, a trend toward increased *serotonin* levels was observed. QUATTRONE and SAMANIN (1977) and QUATTRONE et al. (1978) made electrolytic lesions of the nucleus raphe medianus that selectively decreased brain serotonin; but this did not significantly modify seizure thresholds or the anticonvulsant activity of carbamazepine, phenytoin, or phenobarbital. They concluded that serotonin is not involved in the activity of the above anticonvulsants. After producing electrolytic lesions of the nucleus raphe dorsalis and administering intraventricular microinjections of serotonin neurotoxins (5,6- and 5,7-dihydroxytryptamine), CRUNELLI et al. (1979) also found no modification of the anticonvulsant activity of carbamazepine compared with that seen in control rats. These authors infer that serotoninergic neurons do not play a crucial role in modulating the anticonvulsant action of carbamazepine.

Pharmacological combinations of the benzodiazepine antagonists CGS 8216 and Ro 15-1788 with all major antiepileptic drugs provide evidence that *adenosine* may play a role in the anticonvulsant effect of carbamazepine (SCHMUTZ 1983; SCHMUTZ et al. 1983): the anticonvulsant activity of carbamazepine against electroshock- and pentylenetetrazol-induced seizures was diminished by CGS 8216, which interferes with benzodiazepine and adenosine receptors. On the other hand, Ro 15-1788, which binds to benzodiazepine but not to adenosine receptors, did not impair the anticonvulsant effect of carbamazepine. In addition, the adenosine antagonist theophylline interfered with in vivo and in vitro effects of the antiepileptic, and binding studies have shown that carbamazepine itself binds to adenosine receptors (MARANGOS et al. 1983; SKERRITT et al. 1983a, b).

All major anticonvulsants, including carbamazepine (WHITTLE and TURNER 1981 a), inhibit the activity of *aldehyde reductase* in vitro. Up to now there is little evidence of any direct association between this inhibitory effect and the prevention of seizures in animals. However, aldehyde reductase might be involved in the reduction of succinic semialdehyde to gamma-hydroxybutyrate, which was shown to elicit absence-like seizure activity in animals. This observation is quite consistent with data reported by WHITTLE and TURNER (1981 b) indicating that carbamazepine inhibits the formation of gamma-hydroxybutyrate to a slight extent in the rat.

In animals with induced seizures and in epileptic patients increases in cyclic AMP content have been observed. In mice, rats, and rabbits, carbamazepine inhibited the electrically or chemically evoked accumulation of *cyclic AMP* or *GMP* in vivo and in vitro (MYLLYLAE 1976; LEWIN and BLECK 1977; FERRENDELLI and KINSCHERF 1977, 1980; PALMER et al. 1979, 1981). On the one hand, it also depressed the steady-state levels of cyclic AMP (PALMER et al. 1979) and the cerebellar cyclic GMP concentration (LUST et al. 1978), or reduced the basal values of cyclic AMP in the cerebrospinal fluid of rabbits (MYLLYLAE 1976); on the other hand, FERRENDELLI and KINSCHERF (1979, 1980) reported that carbamazepine did not alter the basal levels of the cyclic nucleotides in the mouse. Thus, carbamazepine in general exerted a depressant effect on the concentrations of cyclic nucleotides and on the experimentally induced rise in cyclic AMP and GMP levels. However, there appears to be no unifying hypothesis in currency with regard to the central actions of various classes of anticonvulsants on cyclic AMP and GMP mechanisms.

High concentrations of K^+ and veratridine cause membrane depolarization which stimulates *Ca^{++} uptake*. FERRENDELLI and DANIELS-MCQUEEN (1982) noted that carbamazepine and phenytoin inhibit veratridine- and K^+-stimulated

Ca^{++} uptake in rat synaptosomes at approximately therapeutic concentrations. From these results it can be concluded that the therapeutic effects of the drugs may be due to their inhibitory action on Na^{+} and Ca^{++} conductances in nervous tissue (see also Sect. C. III).

V. Mechanisms of Action

Several hypotheses have been advanced to explain the mode of action of carbamazepine, but none that could satisfactorily account for all aspects of its unusually broad spectrum of activity. It seems improbable that its many different therapeutic properties could originate from a single mechanism of action and more reasonable to assume that they result from modulations within the brain caused by the aggregated effect of various central and peripheral mechanisms.

A number of investigators have attempted to explain the anticonvulsant effects of carbamazepine in terms of its effects on nerve conductance or interneuronal transmission. It was suggested that it might act by inhibiting Na^{+} or Ca^{++} uptake, or both. From the results of studies dealing with the influence of the drug on sciatic nerves or giant axons, it seems that a general depression of nerve excitability could form part of its mechanism of action. The inhibitory action of carbamazepine in post-tetanic potentiation points to its ability to prevent the spread of epileptic discharges from a given focus. The suppressant effect on the kindling phenomenon in cats and monkeys lends further support to this assumption. In addition, the results observed in kindling experiments may be indicative of a capacity to prevent the development of seizures in a given focus. An effect that may underlie the therapeutic activity of carbamazepine in complex partial seizures has been observed in cats, namely its ability to elevate the threshold of a reticulothalamic projection and that of efferent and afferent connections of thalamic nuclei and the hippocampus, respectively. Effects of this nature can result from direct actions on the nerve membrane, as described above, or from modulation of neurotransmission.

The inhibitory neurotransmitter GABA and catecholamines have been shown to interfere with various manifestations of epileptic seizures. In high doses, carbamazepine modifies the metabolism of GABA and probably also catecholaminergic transmission. Moreover a reduction of brain alanine levels, which are known to be increased in experimental seizures, has been reported. These effects on GABA turnover and alanine levels might be interpreted as being a consequence of a reduction in glucose metabolism due to the anticonvulsant. As the doses of carbamazepine needed to evoke these biochemical effects are distinctly higher than the anticonvulsant doses, the effects on the above-mentioned neurotransmitters probably do not reflect a primary mechanism of action of the compound. Convulsants are known to augment the spontaneous release and to lower the brain levels of acetylcholine; in the striatum of rats carbamazepine raised the acetylcholine content and decreased that of choline, without altering the enzymes involved in the synthesis and hydrolysis of acetylcholine. This suggests that the anticonvulsant has no direct action on the metabolism of acetylcholine. Since the effect of carbamazepine was not antagonized by pimozide, its influence on acetylcholine is most likely not mediated by dopaminergic neurons. With regard to other neurotransmitters, there is evidence that carbamazepine neither binds to the glycine receptor nor has any influence on the serotoninergic transmission in the brain. However, recent pharmacological and biochemical data suggest that adenosine may play a role in the mode of action of the antiepileptic, which might act as a partial agonist at adenosine receptors.

Several authors have reported that it lowers the content of cyclic AMP and also that of cyclic GMP in the brain. Since a rise in these cyclic nucleotides has been observed in experimental seizures, this effect might also contribute to the anticonvulsant properties of carbamazepine, provided that it is not merely consequential upon the suppression of seizures, as indeed might be true of the interference with cyclic GMP systems; here the actions of the drug seem more closely related to Na^{+}-induced depolarization of nerve tissue than to a direct influence on guanylate cyclase.

D. Behavioral, Neurological, and Autonomic Effects

I. Antiaggressive and/or Anxiolytic Effects

An antiaggressive or anxiolytic effect, probably related to the described psychotropic effect of carbamazepine in epileptic patients, was found in experiments in freely moving cats with electrodes implanted in the hypothalamus (KOELLA et al. 1976; BALTZER and SCHMUTZ 1978). After administration of carbamazepine the threshold current for the hissing reaction, induced by electrical stimulation of the perifornical area of the hypothalamus, was distinctly increased; the same observation has been made with benzodiazepine-like compounds, but not to any comparable degree with other antiepileptics. The fighting reaction of mice kept in isolation or subjected to electric foot-shocks was considerably less influenced by carbamazepine (KOELLA et al. 1976). These findings suggest that the antiagressive properties of the drug are selective and directed only against particular types of aggression.

II. Antineuralgic Effects

The inhibitory influence of carbamazepine upon the spinal nucleus of the trigeminal nerve as described by HERNANDEZ-PEON (1965), FROMM and KILLIAN (1967), FROMM (1969), and FROMM et al. (1981) may well explain the clinical antineuralgic properties of the drug (for details see Chap. 23, this volume). A further mechanism of action can be derived from the finding of HONDA and ALLEN (1973) that in rat sciatic nerves carbamazepine decreased or suppressed the action potentials of A-alpha and A-delta fibers and diminished the hyperexcitability produced by immersion in isotonic sodium oxalate or phosphate. The stabilization of the membrane of peripheral nerves may contribute to the therapeutic effect of the drug if one assumes that in the trigeminal neuralgia pools of activated neurons are built up in which an additional afferent, e.g., tactile stimulus, may trigger off an "epileptiform" discharge experienced in the form of an acute attack of pain (MUMENTHALER 1976). In peripheral nerves of streptozotocin diabetic rats carbamazepine normalized the lowered nerve conduction velocity and elevated the excitability threshold. It is suggested that increased excitability threshold of fast conducting peripheral nerves, presumably A-delta fibers, could be responsible for the effect of carbamazepine in diabetic neuropathy (DAVID and GREWAL, personal communication).

III. Antidiuretic Effects

The clinically well-known effect of carbamazepine against diabetes insipidus has proved difficult to explain on the basis of animal experiments. SUMMY-LONG et al. (1979) reported that in conscious rats systemic carbamazepine produced a decrease in nocturnal fluid intake as well as in the excretion of sodium and potassium. Furthermore, an increase in plasma vasopressin levels was observed. In rats with hereditary diabetes insipidus DUMAS et al. (1973) noted that both urinary output and fluid intake were rapidly diminished by carbamazepine, whereas food consumption was hardly influenced. On the other hand, UHLICH et al. (1972) found that neither carbamazepine alone nor carbamazepine together with antidiuretic hormone (ADH) increased urine osmolality or decreased urinary output in rats with hereditary diabetes insipidus. In normal rats, however, during water diuresis, carbamazepine induced a distinct reduction in urine flow and increased urine osmolality. The authors suggest that the drug may induce antidiuresis by a central mode of action (e.g., by stimulation of ADH production and/or release). As did MEIER and MENDOZA (1977), they also studied the effects of the drug on the water permeability of the toad bladder. When carbamazepine was added to the serosal or mucosal bath solution there was neither a change in osmotic water flow nor a potentiation of its increase caused by ADH. In a further study in osmotically stressed rats, HANEFELD et al. (1970) measured the effect of carbamazepine upon increased activity of the enzymes thiamine phosphatase, $NADPH_2$ diaphorase, and glucose-6-phosphate dehydrogenase. As carbamazepine had no influence on these enzyme activities, either in thirsting rats or in those fed regularly, the authors concluded that the antidiuretic effect of the drug did not result from stimulation of the supraoptic or paraventricular nucleus. The mechanism of action of carbamazepine in experimental diabetes insipidus remains unclear. In man, however, carbamazepine is known to augment vasopressin function; GOLD et al. (1980) believe that carbamazepine is a vasopressin receptor agonist since, compared with controls, lower doses of vasopressin are necessary to promote antidiuresis and maintain plasma osmolality when hypertonic saline is administered during carbamazepine treatment.

IV. Effects on Alcohol-Withdrawal Symptoms

CHU (1979) reported that chronic administration of carbamazepine to rats alleviated alcohol-withdrawal symptoms such as heightened spontaneous activity, the startle reflex in response to noise, stereotype chewing movements, and intermittent body stiffening. In addition, it prevented alcohol-withdrawal seizures when its serum levels were above 3 μg/ml (100 and 150 mg/kg via indwelling nasogastric tube). In this animal model carbamazepine appeared to be superior to valproate sodium, in that it exerted the above effects without producing sedation.

V. Antiarrhythmic Effects

STEINER et al. (1970) reported that carbamazepine displayed antiarrhythmic properties in vivo and in vitro. It restored sinus rhythm in dogs with ventricular arrhythmias provoked by digitalis, and ventricular tachycardia was similarly converted to normal sinus rhythm. Interatrial and intraventricular conduction was not affected by carbamazepine. In Purkinje fibers of dogs the drug was found to shorten the duration of the action potential as well as the relative refractory period. Unlike various antiarrhythmic agents, carbamazepine did not affect membrane responsiveness in "antiarrhythmic" concentrations. Ventricular arrhythmias are partly the result of an increase in the automaticity of the cells in the His-Purkinje system to the point where their firing rate exceeds that of the sinus node and they become the dominant pacemaker. The ventricles of dogs with complete heart block [destruction of the atrioventricular (AV) node or bundle of His] are driven by the automatic cells of the His-Purkinje system; the ability of carbamazepine to decrease the firing rate of these cells may therefore contribute to its mechanism of action in human arrhythmias. Besides these results in dogs, carbamazepine was also shown to suppress arrhythmias in anesthetized cats induced by epinephrine, ouabain, aconitine, and acute coronary ligation (PEREZ-OLEA et al. 1979).

VI. Antimaniacal Effects

If we assume that in its symptomatology mania seems related to aggressive behavior and that it probably originates from hyperexcitability of groups of neurons in the limbic system, the inhibitory influence of carbamazepine on limbic structures as outlined in Sect. C.II, C.III, and D.I may account for the antimaniacal properties of the drug. Of particular interest is the suppression of the kindling process, since kindling, a representative model for the development of seizures, might equally be a valuable tool for the investigation of long-lasting behavioral changes such as mania. As described in Sect. C.IV, at high doses carbamazepine interferes with the metabolism of catecholamines and GABA. Such effects may also account for the psychotropic and antimaniacal properties of the drug. It has been hypothesized that "GABA-ergic" anticonvulsants in general may possess antimaniacal properties (EMRICH et al. 1980; BERNASCONI et al. 1982b). According to POST et al. (1980), however, carbamazepine does not significantly alter GABA levels in the cerebrospinal fluid of patients with manic-depressive illness.

VII. Other Effects

The motor activity of mice is increased when they are systemically injected with morphine, whereas neither carbamazepine (10–50 mg/kg i.p.) nor phenytoin (5–20 mg/kg i.p.) induce such hyperactivity. However, KATZ and SCHMALTZ (1979) noted that pretreatment with the anticonvulsants facilitated this effect of morphine. Centrally injected D-Ala^2 leucine enkephalinamide, a long-acting analogue of leucine enkephalin, also increases motor activity in mice. Again, carbamazepine and phenytoin facilitated this effect. Both drugs are effective against various types of seizures and peripheral neuropathies. Since a relation between opioids and nonconvulsive limbic seizures has recently been postulated (HENRIKSEN et al. 1978) and the relation between opioids and pain is well known, closer studies of the effects on opioid functions might disclose important interactions. In mice, however, carbamazepine did not reveal *analgesic effects* at doses up to 200 mg/kg p.o.

Unlike other major anticonvulsants carbamazepine reduced the amnestic effect of cerebral electroshock in mice at doses lower than those evoking anticonvulsant activity (0,1 mg/kg i.p. and above; MONDADORI and CLASSEN, to be published). This property might be of clinical relevance as memory disturbances constitute a problem for a number of epileptic patients.

The most often observed *unwanted effects* of carbamazepine in rodents are sedation and ataxia, although doses well above the ED_{50} found in the electroshock test are needed to produce them. The ratio of the threshold dose of sedation to the ED_{50} in the electroshock test in mice and rats is about 3 (BALTZER and SCHMUTZ 1978). In *Papio papio* strabism and nystagmus were seen at doses as high as 20–40 mg/kg i.v. (MELDRUM et al. 1975 a, b).

E. Pharmacokinetics

I. Absorption

After oral administration, the absorption of carbamazepine in the rat is relatively slow, maximum concentrations in the brain and plasma being reached within 4–6 h (MORSELLI et al. 1971). After i.p. administration, however, peak plasma levels are demonstrable within 30–45 min (MORSELLI 1975). In gerbils given carbamazepine as a suspension, maximal plasma levels were observed 30 min after administration (FREY et al. 1981).

In cats, peak concentrations in cerebrospinal fluid and plasma were noted 90 min after i.p. application. Since the brain levels had already reached a steady state after 15 min, MONACO et al. (1982) suppose that carbamazepine enters the two compartments by way of independent mechanisms.

The absorption of orally administered carbamazepine in dogs is fairly rapid. The drug was found to be more readily absorbed from a liquid preparation than from tablets (peak plasma concentrations within average times of 1 and 2.1 h, respectively). Both formulations produced peak plasma levels of the epoxide metabolite after about 4 h (FREY and LÖSCHER 1980).

According to LEVY et al. (1975), plasma peak concentrations are detected within 1–2.5 h in rhesus monkeys given carbamazepine by mouth. After i.m. injection, PATEL and LEVY (1980) noted a biphasic absorption of the drug in this species: an initial rapid phase with plasma levels rising to peak values in less than 1 h was followed by a slower phase during which absorption seemed to be rate-limiting. In *Papio papio* i.v. administration led to maximum blood concentrations within 15 min (SURIA and KILLAM 1980).

Compared with these data, the absorption of carbamazepine in man is generally slow, maximum plasma levels of the unchanged drug being reached within 7–13 h (FAIGLE and FELDMANN, unpublished results).

II. Distribution

The distribution pattern in animals (mouse, rat, squirrel monkey) after i.v. administration of a single dose of ^{14}C-labeled carbamazepine indicates that the drug is rapidly and uniformly distributed throughout the body with no preferential affinity for particular organs or tissues (MORSELLI et al. 1971; FAIGLE et al. 1976;

WESTENBERG et al. 1977). Similar findings have been made in man (i.e., MORSELLI et al. 1977; FRIIS et al. 1978).

WAGNER (1982, personal communication) investigated the binding of [^{14}C]carbamazepine to serum proteins of healthy volunteers, dogs, rabbits, and rats in vitro by equilibrium dialysis. In man the drug was bound to serum protein to the extent of 73.6%. Similar values were obtained in rabbits (75.0%) and dogs (73.9%), while in rats a distinctly smaller portion of the dose was bound (68.4%). In dogs comparable results were reported by FREY and LÖSCHER (1980), who found the serum protein binding of carbamazepine and its epoxide metabolite to be 70% and 40%, respectively.

Placental transfer of carbamazepine has been demonstrated in pregnant rats (MORSELLI 1975), in pregnant women (PYNNOENEN et al. 1977), and in newborns of mothers treated continuously with carbamazepine during pregnancy (RANE et al. 1975; NIEBYL et al. 1979).

When ^{14}C-labeled carbamazepine was administered in a single dose to lactating rats, it penetrated immediately into the maternal milk, the milk levels exceeding the plasma levels by 15%–60% (STIERLIN and SCHUETZ 1981, personal communication). The concentrations of carbamazepine determined in human breast milk during chronic medication corresponded to about 40%–60% of the respective plasma value (PYNNÖNEN et al. 1977; KANEKO et al. 1979; NIEBYL et al. 1979; REITH and SCHÄFER 1979).

III. Metabolism

The metabolism of carbamazepine has been most thoroughly investigated in man. Biotransformation proceeds by four main pathways, as shown in Fig. 2 (FAIGLE and FELDMANN 1982):

1. Epoxidation of the 10,11-double bond of the azepine ring
2. Hydroxylation of the six-membered aromatic rings
3. Direct *N*-glucuronidation at the carbamoyl side chain
4. Substitution of the six-membered rings with sulfur-containing groups.

The rat is the only species on which an appreciable amount of information about the structures of the metabolites of carbamazepine has been accumulated. BAKER et al. (1973) and CSETENYI et al. (1973) described the occurrence of the metabolites I and II (see Fig. 2) and iminostilbene in the urine of rats after administration of carbamazepine. BAUER et al. (1976) identified a direct conjugate of carbamazepine, i.e., the *N*-glucuronide X, in rat bile. In a later communication, LYNN et al. (1977) mentioned hydroxy- and hydroxymethoxy derivatives as biliary metabolites. HORNING and LERTRATANANGKOON (1980) found the same type of phenolic compounds in the urine of rats. In most of these reports quantitative data on the metabolites or metabolic pathways are lacking, however. Unpublished results of a radiotracer study (DIETERLE 1980, unpublished work) indicate that rat bile and rat urine contain all the metabolites of carbamazepine previously identified in human urine (compounds I–XIV). In the rat also the greater part of the metabolites formed are excreted as conjugates. Hence, in spite of the widely differing rates of biotransformation in rat and man, the main pathways (1–4, Fig. 2) are qualitatively similar in both species. Some additional products were found in this rat study that were all derived from the known pathways; they include two

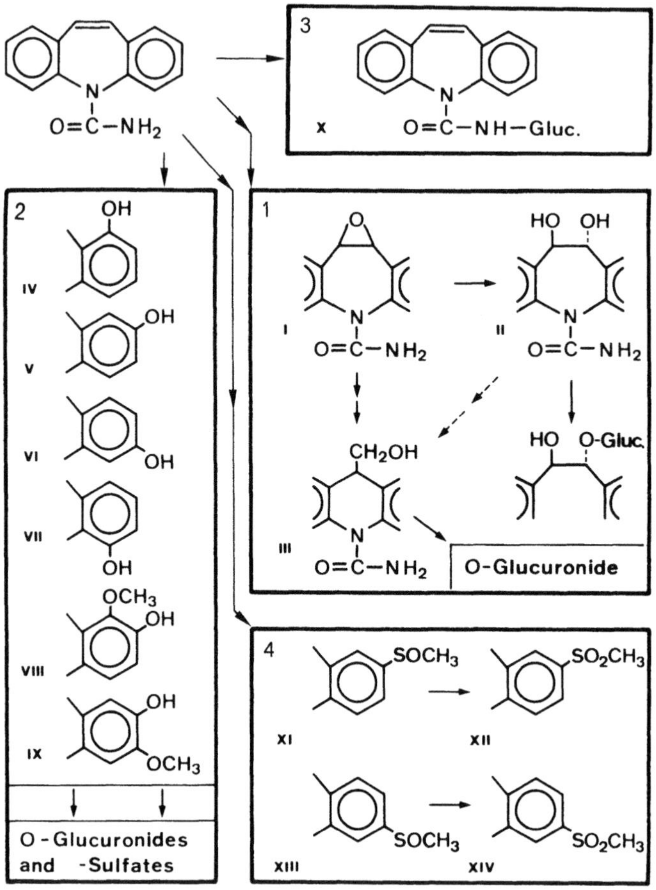

Fig. 2. Structures of metabolites of carbamazepine isolated from human urine and major pathways of biotransformation

further isomers of hydroxymethoxycarbamazepine, the 10-hydroxy-11-methylsulfonyl-10,11-dihydrocarbamazepine and some compounds carrying substituents introduced by more than one pathway. A few complementary metabolites formed by the pathways 1, 2, and 4 have been described recently by LERTRATANANGKOON and HORNING (1982).

Judging from the quantities and structures of the biliary and urinary metabolites in rats identified by DIETERLE (1980, unpublished), epoxidation of the 10,11-double bond of carbamazepine accounts for a higher percentage of the dose than does any of the other pathways. In the rat, however, further transformation of the epoxy intermediate to the diol metabolite occurs at a much slower rate than in man. The rat urine accordingly contains an appreciably greater amount of epoxycarbamazepine than human urine – about 10% of the dose compared with 1% – and less of the diol metabolite. The epoxide-hydrase activity in human liver homogenate was in fact found to be twice that demonstrable in the rat liver (OESCH 1973). The concentration profiles of carbamazepine and epoxycarbamazepine in plasma reflect the different rates of the metabolic reactions in rat and man (FAIGLE et al. 1976). Administration of a single oral dose of carbamazepine to the rat results in epoxide concentrations roughly equal to those of the unchanged drug; after repeated administration, the epoxide reaches even higher levels than carbamazepine. In healthy human subjects, on the other hand, the plasma concentrations of epoxycarbamazepine do not exceed 15% of those of the unchanged drug under similar experimental conditions. The occurrence of the epoxide metabolite of carbamazepine has also been observed in rhesus monkeys (PATEL et al. 1978) and in dogs (FREY and LÖSCHER 1980), whereas in gerbils this metabolite could not be detected (FREY et al. 1981).

Epoxycarbamazepine also possesses anticonvulsant properties. Its ED_{50}s in the electroshock test in mice and rats (12–18 mg/kg p.o.) and in the pentylenetetrazol test in mice (8–24 mg/kg p.o.) are similar to those of the parent drug (GAGNEUX 1976; FAIGLE and FELDMANN 1982; FREY and LÖSCHER 1980). However, in rats the anticonvulsant efficacy of carbamazepine was – on a blood concentration basis – higher than that of the epoxide metabolite (FAIGLE et al. 1977). The other metabolites of carbamazepine either display little anticonvulsant activity or are present in the plasma in low concentrations only and therefore hardly contribute toward the therapeutic effect of the parent compound.

IV. Elimination

In all animal species studied so far, carbamazepine is largely metabolized: At the most 2% of the dose can be recovered unchanged in urine or bile (FAIGLE and FELDMANN 1975; LEVY et al. 1975; PITLICK 1975; DIETERLE 1980, unpublished). In this respect, there is a close similarity between animals and man. The overall rate of biotransformation in man, however, differs greatly from that found in animals, as is evident from the elimination half-lives of carbamazepine determined in plasma: In rats, gerbils, dogs, rabbits, rhesus monkeys, and *Papio papio* the mean elimination half-lives after single doses of carbamazepine are between 0.9 and 1.9 h (LEVY et al. 1975; PITLICK 1975; FARGHALI-HASSAN et al. 1976; RIMERMAN et al. 1979; FREY and LÖSCHER 1980; SURIA and KILLAM 1980; FREY et al. 1981); in healthy volunteers, the mean half-life is 36 h. The metabolic clearance of carbamazepine in the above animal species is consequently more than one power of ten higher than in man. Hence, to maintain a given concentration of carbamazepine in plasma, correspondingly higher doses would be required in animals. Thus, although possibly equal in pharmacological activity, the same plasma concentration of carbamazepine may toxicologically impose a greater burden on animals than on man.

It should be noted that male rats eliminate carbamazepine more rapidly than females, in which the half-life is about 50% longer (FARGHALI-HASSAN et al. 1976). Clinical data indicate that the kinetics of carbamazepine in male and female patients are not significantly different (HOOPER et al. 1974).

The phenomenon whereby carbamazepine accelerates its own metabolism when given repeatedly has been observed in rats, dogs, and monkeys (FAIGLE et al. 1976; FARGHALI-HASSAN et al. 1976; LOCKARD et al. 1979; FREY and LÖSCHER 1980). The compound primarily induces the microsomal mono-oxygenase system (WAGNER and SCHMID 1980, unpublished results); the induction pattern in rats is similar to that produced by phenobarbital, although the effects of carbamazepine are generally less marked. These results are in accordance with data on human volunteers and epileptic patients indicating that multiple-dose treatment reduces the half-life of carbamazepine through autoinduction of drug-metabolizing enzymes (FAIGLE and FELDMANN 1982).

F. Drug Interactions

SCHMUTZ et al. (1979) investigated the combination of *carbamazepine and valproate sodium* in mice, rats (electroshock test), and cats (hippocampal afterdischarge). In all species tested, seizure protection afforded by the two drugs combined in various dose-ratios exceeded the additive effects of the same doses of each alone. Additionally, in the hippocampal afterdischarge experiments, some dose combinations prolonged the anticonvulsant activity. No potentiation of undesired effects or of acute oral toxicity (rat) resulted from the combination. In the electroshock test in mice, especially at lower doses, the combination of *carbamazepine and phenytoin* potentiated the anticonvulsant activity of carbamazepine less than did the combination of carbamazepine and valproate sodium.

The mode of action underlying this potentiating effect on the anticonvulsant activity of carbamazepine is not clear. SCHUETZ et al. (1982, unpublished results) noted that the concomitant administration of valproate sodium and carbamazepine in rats increased the integrated blood concentrations (0–24 h) of [^{14}C]carbamazepine and its epoxide metabolite by 26% and 38%, respectively, without altering the elimination half-life of the parent drug. Thus, valproate sodium does not seem to inhibit the hepatic enzymes metabolizing carbamazepine, but rather to cause its redistribution. Augmented absorption can be excluded, since carbamazepine, given alone, is completely absorbed from the gastrointestinal tract of the rat. Finally, in dogs, valproate sodium had no effect on the serum protein binding of carbamazepine (LÖSCHER 1979).

SCHMUTZ et al. (1982) and MONDADORI et al. (to be published) also investigated the influence of vincamine and piracetam on the anticonvulsant effect of carbamazepine in the electroshock test in the rat. The protection against seizures afforded by several dose combinations of *carbamazepine with vincamine and piracetam*, respectively, exceeded the additive effects of the components, indicating potentiation. As in the above-mentioned study, potentiation of unwanted effects or of acute oral toxicity (combination with vincamine) was not observed.

Further studies may reveal whether some modes of action of the drugs combined are complementary, whether the serum protein binding of carbamazepine is influenced, or whether these drugs show agonistic activities at the as yet unknown receptor sites of carbamazepine.

SCHUETZ et al. (1982, unpublished results) also found that simultaneous administration of *carbamazepine and the analgesic propoxyphene* increased the integrated blood concentrations (0–24 h) of [^{14}C]carbamazepine by up to 105% and decreased those of its epoxide metabolite. In addition, the mean elimination half-life of the parent compound was prolonged. These effects of propoxyphene are similar to, though weaker than, those of the enzyme inhibitor *SKF-525-A*, indicating that the analgesic has an inhibitory effect on the enzymes metabolizing carbamazepine.

G. Toxicology[1]

I. Acute Toxicity Studies

In mice, rats, rabbits, and guinea pigs, the LD_{50} of orally administered carbamazepine was found to be in the range of 1,000 mg/kg, or above. Dogs tolerated single doses of more than 5,000 mg/kg; higher doses could not be given without causing emesis. The principal preterminal toxic effects in the mouse, rat, rabbit, and guinea pig were labored respiration, ataxia, clonic and tonic convulsions, and coma.

II. Subacute and Chronic Toxicity Studies

Toxic manifestations after treatment of rats and dogs with carbamazepine for periods up to 12 months were found predominantly in the central nervous systems, gonads, and liver.

Signs of encephalopathy, occurring at doses not lower than 150 mg/kg daily, formed part of the symptoms of systemic toxicity appearing at lethal or sublethal doses.

At doses of 400 mg/kg, which proved lethal in about half of the animals, testicular changes were detected in approximately one-third of the treated male rats. Spermatogenesis was inhibited in rats that were debilitated and had markedly lost condition. In dogs, inhibition of spermatogenesis was only seen sporadically and was unrelated to the dose administered.

Hepatic changes occurred in both species and were approximately dose related. The livers were enlarged, and, upon, histological examination, hypertrophy of centrilobular hepatocytes was visible, accompanied by reduced basophilia of the cytoplasm and low glycogen contents. The changes were reversible, as demonstrated in a 3-month dietary study in the rat including a 1-month post-treatment observation period. The threshold dose required to elicit hepatic changes in subacute and chronic studies is estimated to be 50 mg/kg. The effect of carbamazepine on the rat liver after repeated oral administration was examined in a combined biochemical and electron-microscopic study. It was concluded that the drug induces a reversible, adaptive response of rat hepatocytes closely resembling the non-specific type of liver induction produced by a large variety of drugs (e.g., phenobarbital). No particular toxicological significance is attached to this finding, which is considered to represent an adaptive response to metabolic load.

III. Reproduction Studies

Reproduction and teratology studies have been performed at different research centers after both oral and parenteral administration of the drug to rats, mice, and rabbits. Analysis of all the teratological data obtained since 1963 furnishes no unequivocal evidence of any potential teratogenic action of carbamazepine in laboratory animals. More recent studies have in fact, confirmed that, in contrast

---

1 This section is based on unpublished data from toxicity tests conducted between 1958 and 1981 by or for Ciba-Geigy Ltd., Basel, Switzerland, where all reports are on file

to certain other antiepileptic agents, carbamazepine does not appear to possess teratogenic properties in several breeds of mice, i.e., the species considered most susceptible to this type of drug reaction. Rare malformations (e.g., cleft palate) were invariably associated with a high rate of maternal and/or fetal toxicity of the administered doses. It is nevertheless recommended that if pregnancy should occur in a woman receiving carbamazepine, or if the question of initiating treatment with carbamazepine should arise during pregnancy, the potential benefits of the drug should be carefully weighed against its possible hazards, particularly in the first trimester. This applies also to nursing mothers, as carbamazepine passes into the breast milk.

IV. Mutagenicity Studies

Carbamazepine was found to be devoid of any mutagenic activity in the Ames test, performed with and without microsomal activation, in the nucleus anomaly test (2 days and 12 weeks), in the dominant lethal test, in chromosome studies in somatic cells (bone marrow) and male germinal epithelial cells (mouse spermatogonia and spermatocytes), and in the mouse lymphoma assay (in vitro and host mediated).

V. Carcinogenicity Studies

In rats treated with carbamazepine for 2 years, the incidence of tumors of the liver was found to be increased. There is, however, no evidence to indicate that this observation has any significant bearing on the therapeutic use of carbamazepine in man.

Acknowledgments. The author wishes to thank Dr. Peter Graepel for preparing Sect. G, Drs. Hans Allgeier and Karl F. Feldmann for revising Sects. B and E, Chantal Portet for her technical assistance, and, especially, Yvonne Kessler for her efficient secretarial help.

References

Abdul-Ghani AS, Coutinho-Netto J, Druce D, Bradford HF (1981) Effects of anticonvulsants on the in vivo and in vitro release of GABA. Biochem Pharmacol 30:363–368

Albertson TE, Peterson SL, Stark LG (1980) Anticonvulsant drugs and their antagonism of kindled amygdaloid seizures in rats. Neuropharmacology 19:643–652

Albright PS, Burnham WM (1980) Development of a new pharmacological seizure model: effects of anticonvulsants on cortical- and amygdala-kindled seizures in the rat. Epilepsia 21:681–689

Alderdice MT, Trommer BA (1980) Differential effects of the anticonvulsants phenobarbital, ethosuximide and carbamazepine on neuromuscular transmission. J Pharmacol Exp Ther 215:92–96

Ashton D, Wauquier A (1979) Behavioral analysis of the effects of 15 anticonvulsants in the amygdaloid kindled rat. Psychopharmacology 65:7–13

Ayd FJ (1979) Carbamazepine: a potential alternative for lithium therapy for affective disorders. Intern Drug Ther Newsletter 14:29–31

Babington RG, Horovitz ZP (1973) Neuropharmacology of SQ 10996. A compound with several therapeutic indications. Arch Int Pharmacodyn Ther 202:106–118

Baker KM, Csetenyi J, Frigerio A, Morselli PL, Parravacini F, Pfifferi G (1973) 10,11-Dihydro-10,11-dihydroxy-5*H*-dibenz(b,f)azepine-5-carboxamide, a metabolite of carbamazepine isolated from human and rat urine. J Med Chem 16:703–705

Baltzer V, Schmutz M (1978) Experimental anticonvulsive properties of GP 47680 and of GP 47779, its main human metabolite; compounds related to carbamazepine. In: Meinardi H, Rowan AJ (eds) Advances in epileptology: 9th Epilepsy international symposium. Raven, New York, pp 295–299

Baltzer V, Baud J, Degen P, Koella WP (1980) A procedure to detect development of tolerance ("escape") to antiepileptic drugs: first results. In: Wada JA, Penry JK (eds) Advances in epileptology. 10th Epilepsy international symposium. Raven, New York, pp 315–320

Baltzer V, Klebs K, Schmutz M (1981) Effects of oxcarbazepine, a compound related to carbamazepine, and of GP 47779, its main metabolite in man, on the evolution of amygdaloid-kindled seizures in the rat. 13th Epilepsy international symposium, Kyoto, Sept 17–21, 1981, Abstracts p 151

Bauer JE, Gerber N, Lynn RK, Smith RG, Thompson RM (1976) A new N-glucuronide metabolite of carbamazepine. Experientia 32:1032–1033

Bernasconi R, Martin P, Schmutz M (1982a) Effects of antiepileptic drugs on amino acid concentrations in mouse brain as a function of time: correlation with anticonvulsant activity. In: The brain in health and disease. The 1st world congress of IBRO (Lausanne, 31. March – 6. April 1982). Pergamon Press, Oxford, p 24 (= Neuroscience, Supplement to Vol. 7, 1982)

Bernasconi R, Bittiger H, Martin P, Schmutz M (1982b) Effects of chronic treatment with lithium and other antimanic drugs on GABA turnover. 13th CINP Congress, Tel Aviv, June 20–25, 1982, Abstracts

Bernasconi R, Klein M, Martin P, Schmutz M (1982c) The influence of anticonvulsant drugs on GABA-turnover and amino acid levels in mice. In: Giuffrida Stella AM, Gombos G, Benzi G, Bachelard HS (eds) Basic and clinical aspects of molecular neurobiology. 4th meeting of the European society for neurochemistry. Fondazione Internazionale Menarini, Milano, p 394

Bonduelle M, Sallou C (1963) Tegretol (Geigy). Thérapie 18:543–548

Bustamente L, Lueders H, Pippenger C, Goldensohn ES (1981) Quantitative evaluation of anticonvulsant effects on penicillin-induced spike foci in cats. Neurology 31:1163–1166

Cereghino JJ, Brock JT, Van Meter JC, Penry JK, Smith LD, White BG (1974) Carbamazepine for Epilepsy. A controlled prospective evaluation. Neurology 24:401–410

Chu NS (1979) Carbamazepine: prevention of alcohol withdrawal seizures. Neurology 29:1397–1401

Consolo S, Bianchi S, Ladinski H (1976) Effect of carbamazepine on cholinergic parameters in rat brain areas. Neuropharmacology 15:653–657

Consroe P, Kudray K, Schmitz R (1980) Acute and chronic drug effects in audiogenic seizure-susceptible rats. Exp Neurol 70:626–637

Coyne WE, Cusic JW (1968) Anticonvulsant semicarbazides. J Med Chem 11:1158–1160

Crunelli V, Bernasconi S, Samanin R (1979) Evidence against serotonin involvement in the tonic component of electrically induced convulsions and in carbamazepine anticonvulsant activity. Psychopharmacology 66:79–85

Csetenyi J, Baker KM, Frigerio A, Morselli PL (1973) Iminostilbene – a metabolite of carbamazepine isolated from rat urine. J Pharm Pharmacol 25:340-341

David J, Grewal RS (1976) Effect of carbamazepine (Tegretol[R]) on seizure and EEG patterns in monkeys with alumina-induced focal motor and hippocampal foci. Epilepsia 17:415–422

Davidson DLW, Tsukada Y, Barbeau A (1978) Ouabain induced seizures. Site of production and response to anticonvulsants. Can J Neurol Sci 5:405–411

Davis MA, Winthrop SO, Thomas RA, Herr F, Charest MP, Gaudry R (1964) Anticonvulsants. I. Dibenzo(a,d)cycloheptadiene-5-carboxamide and related compounds. J Med Chem: 88–94

Dolce G (1969) Über den antiepileptischen Aktionsmechanismus von 5-Carbamoyl-5*H*-dibenzo(b,f)azepin. Neurophysiologische Untersuchungen an Katzen. Arzneimittelforsch 19:1257–1263

Dravet C, Mesdjian E, Cenrand B, Roger J (1977) Interaction between carbamazepine and triacetyloleandomycine. Lancet 1:810–811

Dumas JC, Traves J, Auriac A, Roux G (1973) Action de la carbamoyl-dibenzo-azepine sur le metabolisme hydrique des rats en diabete insipide. C R Soc Biol (Paris) 167:161–164
Eadie MJ (1979) Which anticonvulsant drug? Curr Therapeutics: 29–37
Ehlers C, Chappus P, Whitmoyer P, Sawyer C (1979) Experiments on hippocampal "kindling" in the rabbit. Neurosci Abstr 5:192
Eichelbaum M, Bertilsson L (1975) Determination of carbamazepine and its epoxide metabolite in plasma by high speed liquid chromatography. J Chromatogr 103:135–140
Emrich HM, Zerssen D, Kissling W, Moeller HJ, Windorfer A (1980) Effect of sodium valproate on mania. Arch Psychiatr Nervenkr 229:1–16
Faigle JW, Feldmann KF (1975) Pharmacokinetic data of carbamazepine and its major metabolites in man. In: Schneider H, Janz D, Gardner-Thorpe C, Meinardi H, Sherwin AL (eds) Clinical pharmacology of anti-epileptic drugs. Springer, Berlin Heidelberg New York, pp 159–165
Faigle JW, Feldmann KF (1982) Carbamazepine: biotransformation. In: Woodbury DM, Penry JK, Pippenger CE (eds) Antiepileptic drugs, 2nd edn. Raven, New York, pp 483–495
Faigle JW, Feldmann KF, Baltzer V (1977) Anticonvulsant effect of carbamazepine. An attempt to distinguish between the potency of the parent drug and its epoxide metabolite. In: Gardner-Thorpe C, Janz D, Meinardi H, Pippenger CE (eds) Antiepileptic drug monitoring. Pitman Medical, Tunbridge Wells, pp 104–109
Faigle JW, Brechbuehler S, Feldmann KF, Richter WJ (1976) The biotransformation of carbamazepine. In: Birkmayer E (ed) Epileptic siezures-behavior-pain. Huber, Bern, pp 127–140
Farghali-Hassan, Assael BM, Bossi L, Gerna M, Garattini S, Gomeni G, Morselli PL (1976) Carbamazepine pharmacokinetics in young, adult and pregnant rats. Relation to pharmacological effects. Arch Int Pharmacodyn Ther 220:125–139
Ferrendelli JA, Daniels-McQueen S (1982) Comparative actions of phenytoin and other anticonvulsant drugs on potassium- and veratridine-stimulated calcium uptake in synaptosomes. J Pharmacol Exp Ther 220:29–34
Ferrendelli JA, Kinscherf DA (1979) Inhibitory effects of anticonvulsant drugs on cyclic nucleotide accumulation in brain. Ann Neurol 5:533–538
Ferrendelli JA, Kinscherf DA (1980) Comparative effects of phenytoin, phenobarbital and carbamazepine on cyclic nucleotide regulation in brain. In: Wada JA, Penry JK (eds) Advances in epileptology: 10th Epilepsy international symposium. Raven, New York, pp 477–484
Frey HH, Löscher W (1980) Pharmacokinetics of carbamazepine in the dog. Arch Int Pharmacodyn Ther 243:180–190
Frey HH, Löscher W, Reiche R, Schultz D (1981) Pharmacology of antiepileptic drugs in the gerbil – I. Pharmacokinetics. Neuropharmacology 20:769–771
Frigerio A, Baker KM, Belvedere G (1973) Gas chromatographic degradation of several drugs and their metabolites. Analyt Chem 45:1846–1851
Friis ML, Christiansen J, Hvidberg E (1978) Brain concentrations of carbamazepine and carbamazepine-10,11-epoxide in epileptic patients. Eur J Clin Pharmacol 14:47–51
Fromm GH (1969) Pharmacological consideration of anticonvulsants. Headache 9:35–41
Fromm GH, Killian JM (1967) Effect of some anticonvulsant drugs on the spinal trigeminal nucleus. Neurology 17:275–280
Fromm GH, Chattha AS, Terrence CF, Glass JD (1981) Role of inhibitory mechanisms in trigeminal neuralgia. Neurology 31:683–687
Gagneux AR (1976) The chemistry of carbamazepine. In: Birkmayer W (ed) Epileptic seizures–behaviour–pain. Huber, Bern, pp 120–126
Gérardin A, Hirtz J (1976) The quantitative assay of carbamazepine in biological material and its application to basic pharmacokinetic studies. In: Birkmayer W (ed) Epileptic seizures–behaviour–pain. Huber, Bern, pp 151–164
Gold PW, Goodwin FK, Ballenger JC, Weingartner H, Robertson GL, Post RM (1980) Central vasopressin function in affective illness. In: De Wied D, Van Keep PA (eds) Hormones and the brain. MTP Press, pp 241–252

Grueter W (1976) Discussion contribution. In: Birkmayer W (ed) Epileptic seizures–behaviour–pain. Huber, Bern, pp 205–206
Hanefeld F, Levsen I, Stefan H (1970) Untersuchungen zur Wirkung von Carbamazepine auf die neurosekretorischen Kerne der Ratte. Z Ges Exp Med 153:95–98
Henriksen SJ, Bloom FE, McCoy F, Ling N, Guillemin R (1978) Beta endorphin induces nonconvulsive limbic seizures. Proc Natl Acad Sci USA 75:5221–5225
Hernandez-Peon R (1964) Anticonvulsive action of G 32883. In: Bradley PB, Fluegel F, Hoch PH (eds) Neuropsychopharmacol 3. Elsevier, Amsterdam, pp 303–311
Hernandez-Peon R (1965) Central action of G 32883 upon transmission of trigeminal pain impulses. Med Pharmacol Exp 12:73
Hernandez-Peon R (1966) Acciones del G-32883 sobre descargas neuronales convulsivogenas y sobre la transmission de impulsos nociceptivos trigeminales. Sem Med Mex 50:391–393
Hershkowitz N, Raines A (1978) Effects of carbamazepine on muscle spindle discharges. J Pharmacol Exp Ther 204:581–591
Hershkowitz N, Dretchen KL, Raines A (1978) Carbamazepine suppression of post-tetanic potentiation at the neuromuscular junction. J Pharmacol Exp Ther 207:810–816
Hollister RP, Julien RM (1974) Studies on the mode of the antiepileptic action of carbamazepine. Proc West Pharmacol Soc 17:103–106
Holm E, Kelleter R, Heinemann H, Hamann KF (1970) Elektrophysiologische Analyse der Wirkungen von Carbamazepin auf das Gehirn der Katze. Pharmakopsychiatr Neuro-Psychopharmakol 3:187–200
Honda H, Allen MB (1973) The effect of an iminostilbene derivative (G 32883) on peripheral nerves. J Med Assoc Ga 62:38–42
Hooper WD, Dubetz DK, Eadie MJ, Tyrer JH (1974) Preliminary observations on the clinical pharmacology of carbamazepine (TEGRETOL[R]). Proc Aust Assoc Neurol 11:189–198
Hori M, Ito T, Yoshida K, Shimizu M (1979) Effect of anticonvulsants on spiking activity induced by cortical freezing in cats. Epilepsia 20:25–36
Hori M, Ito T, Shimizu M (1981) Thalamic generalized seizure induced by tungstic acid gel in cats and its suppression by anticonvulsants. Jpn J Pharmacol 31:771–779
Horning MG, Lertratanangkoon K (1980) High-performance liquid chromatographic separation of carbamazepine metabolites excreted in rat urine. J Chromatogr 181:59–65
Howe SJ, Salt TE, Tulloch I, Walter DS (1981) Effect of anti-grand mal drugs on kindled epilepsy in the rat. Br J Pharmacol 72:501P–502P
Huf R, Schain RJ (1980) Long-term experiences with carbamazepine (Tegretol) in children with seizures. J Pediatr 97:310–312
Ito T, Hori M, Yoshida K, Shimizu M (1977) Effect of anticonvulsants on cortical focal seizure in cats. Epilepsia 18:63–71
Janz D (1978) Was muß der praktische Arzt von Epilepsiebehandlung wissen? Tempo Medical 9:37–40
Jeavons PM (1977) Choice of drug therapy in epilepsy. Practitioner 219:542–556
Jones GL, Amato RJ, Wimbish GH, Peyton GA (1981) Comparison of anticonvulsant potencies of cyheptamide, carbamazepine and phenytoin. J Pharm Sci 70:618–620
Julien RM (1973) Effect of carbamazepine on experimental epilepsy in the cat. Proc West Pharmacol Soc 16:126–128
Julien RM (1974) Experimental epilepsy: cerebro-cerebellar interactions and antiepileptic drugs. In: Cooper IS, Riklan M, Snider RS (eds) The cerebellum, epilepsy and behavior. Plenum, New York, pp 97–117
Julien RM, Hollister RP (1975) Carbamazepine: mechanism of action. Adv Neurol 11:263–277
Julien RM, Fowler GW, Danielson MG (1975) The effects of antiepileptic drugs on estrogen-induced electrographic spike-wave discharge. J Pharmacol Exp Ther 193:647-656
Kamei C, Oka M, Masuda Y, Yoshida K, Shimizu M (1981) Effects of 3-sulfamoylmethyl-1,2-benzisoxazole (AD 810) and some antiepileptics on the kindled seizures in the neocortex, hippocampus and amygdala in rats. Arch Int Pharmacodyn Ther 249:164–176

Kaneko S, Sato T, Suzuki K (1979) The levels of anticonvulsants in breast milk. Br J Clin Pharmacol 7:624–627

Kaneko S, Fukushima Y, Sato T, Hiramatsu M, Mori A (1981) Effects of carbamazepine on catecholamine level in mouse brain. IRCS J Med Sci 9:80–81

Katz RJ, Schmaltz K (1979) Facilitation of opiate and enkephaline-induced motor activity in the mouse by phenytoin sodium and carbamazepine. Psychopharmacology 65:65–68

Killam EK (1976) Measurement of anticonvulsant activity in the *Papio papio* model of epilepsy. Fed Proc 35:2264–2269

Killam KF, Naquet R, Bert J (1966) Paroxysmal responses to intermittent light stimulation in a population of baboons (*Papio papio*). Epilepsia 7:215–219

Killam EK, Matsuzaki M, Killam KF (1973) Studies of anticonvulsant compounds in the *Papio papio* model of epilepsy. In: Sabelli MC (ed) Chemical modulation of brain function. Raven, New York, pp 161–171

Koella WP, Levin P, Baltzer V (1976) The pharmacology of carbamazepine and some other antiepileptic drugs. In: Birkmayer W (ed) Epileptic seizures–behaviour–pain. Huber, Bern, pp 23–48

Krall RL, Penry JK, White BG, Kupferberg HJ, Swinyard EA (1978) Antiepileptic drug development: II. Anticonvulsant drug screening. Epilepsia 19:409–428

Krupp P (1969a) Elektrophysiologische Untersuchungen über den Angriffsmechanismus von Antiepileptika im Tierversuch. Helv Paediatr Acta 24:270–277

Krupp P (1969b) The effect of Tegretol on some elementary neuronal mechanisms. Headache 9:42–46

Lertratanangkoon K, Horning MG (1982) Metabolism of carbamazepine. Drug Metab Dispos 10:1–10

Levy RH, Lockard JS, Green JR, Friel P, Martis L (1975) Pharmacokinetics of carbamazepine in monkeys following intravenous and oral administration. J Pharm Sci 64:302–307

Lewin E, Bleck V (1977) Cyclic AMP accumulation in cerebral cortical slices: effect of carbamazepine, phenobarbital and phenytoin. Epilepsia 18:237–242

Lockard JS, Levy RH, Uhlir V, Farquhar JA (1974) Pharmacokinetic evaluation of anticonvulsants prior to efficacy testing exemplified by carbamazepine in epileptic monkey model. Epilepsia 15:351–359

Lockard JS, Levy RH, DuCharme LL, Congdon WC, Patel IH (1979) Carbamazepine revisited in a monkey model. Epilepsia 20:169–173

Löscher W (1979) A comparative study of the protein binding of anticonvulsant drugs in serum of dog and man. J Pharmacol Exp Ther 208:429–435

Lorgé M (1963) Klinische Erfahrungen mit einem neuen Antiepileptikum, Tegretol (G 32883), mit besonderer Wirkung auf die epileptische Wesensveränderung. Schweiz Med Wochenschr 93:1042

Lust WD, Kupferberg HJ, Yonekawa WD, Penry JK, Passonneau JV, Wheaton AB (1978) Changes in brain metabolites induced by convulsants or electroshock: effects of anticonvulsant agents. Mol Pharmacol 14:347–356

Lustig B (1964) Über Behandlungsergebnisse mit dem neuen Antiepileptikum G 32883. Med Welt 4:203–204

Lynn RK, Bowers JL, Gerber N (1977) Identification of glucuronide metabolites of carbamazepine in human urine and in bile from the isolated perfused rat liver. Fed Proc 36:961

Marangos PJ, Post RM, Patel J, Zander K, Parma A, Weiss S (1983) Specific and potent interactions of carbamazepine with brain adenosine receptors. Eur J Pharmacol 93:175–182

Maresova D, Mares P (1980) Influence of carbamazepine on thalamo-cortical and hippocampocortical self-sustained after-discharges in rats. Act Nerv Super 22:217–218

Margerison JH, Corsellis JA (1966) Epilepsy and the temporal lobes. A clinical, electroencephalographic and neuropathological study of the brain in epilepsy, with particular reference to the temporal lobes. Brain 89:499–530

Masuda Y, Utsui Y, Shiraishi Y, Karasawa T, Yoshida K, Shimizu M (1979) Relationships between plasma concentrations of diphenylhydantoin, phenobarbital, carbamazepine and 3-sulfamoylmethyl-1,2-benzisoxazole (AD 810), a new anticonvulsant agent and their anticonvulsant or neurotoxic effects in experimental animals. Epilepsia 20:623–633

Masuda Y, Shiraishi Y, Karasawa T, Yoshida K, Shimizu M (1980) Differential antagonisms of anticonvulsants to various components of maximal seizures induced by electroshock or pentylenetetrazole in mice. J Pharm Dyn 3:526–531

Meier KE, Mendoza SA (1977) Effects of carbamazepine on the water permeability and short-circuit current of the urinary bladder of the toad and the response to vasopressin, adenosine 3,5-cyclic phosphate and theophylline. J Pharmacol Exp Ther 200:95–100

Meldrum BS, Anlezark G, Balzamo E, Horton RW, Trimble M (1975a) Photically induced epilepsy in *Papio papio* as a model for drug studies. Adv Neurol 10:119–128

Meldrum BS, Horton RW, Toseland PA (1975b) A primate model for testing anticonvulsant drugs. Arch Neurol 32:289–294

Monaco F, Mutani R, Piredda S, Traccis S, Ramsay RE (1982) Brain uptake of carbamazepine in the cat. Epilepsia 23:19–22

Mondadori C, Classen W (to be published) The effect of various antiepileptic drugs on E-shock-induced amnesia in mice: Dissociability of effects on convulsions and effects on memory. Acta Neurol Scand

Mondadori C, Schmutz M, Baltzer V (to be published) Potentiation of the anticonvulsant effects of antiepileptic drugs by "nootropics"; a potential new therapeutic approach. Acta Neurol Scand

Morselli PL (1975) Carbamazepine: absorption, distribution and excretion. Adv Neurol 11:279–293

Morselli PL, Gerna M, Garattini S (1971) Carbamazepine plasma and tissue levels in the rat. Biochem Pharmacol 20:2043–2047

Morselli PL, Baruzzi A, Gerna M, Bossi L, Porta M (1977) Carbamazepine and carbamazepine-10,11-epoxide concentrations in human brain. Br J Clin Pharmacol 4:535–540

Müller HA (1963) Ein neuartiges Antiepilepticum bei chronisch anstaltsbedürftigen Epileptikern. Nervenarzt 34:463–464

Mumenthaler M (1976) The pathophysiology of pain. In: Birkmayer W (ed) Epileptic seizures–behaviour–pain. Huber, Bern, pp 275–312

Myllylae VV (1976) Effect of convulsions and anticonvulsant drugs on cerebrospinal fluid cyclic AMP in rabbits. Eur Neurol 14:97–107

Niebyl JR; Blake DA, Freeman JM, Luff RD (1979) Carbamazepine levels in pregnancy and lactation. Obstet Gynecol 53:139–140

Oesch F (1973) Mammalian epoxide hydrase: inducible enzymes catalysing the inactivation of carcinogenic and cytotoxic metabolites derived from aromatic and olefinic compounds. Xenobiotica 3:305–340

Olpe HR, Jones RSG (1983) The action of anticonvulsant drugs on the firing of locus coeruleus neurons: selective activating effect of carbamazepine. Europ J Pharmacol 91:107–110

Pakesch E (1963) Untersuchungen über ein neuartiges Antiepileptikum. Wien Med Wochenschr 113:794–796

Palmer GC, Jones DJ, Medina MA, Stavinoha WB (1979) Anticonvulsant drug actions on in vitro and in vivo levels of cyclic AMP in the mouse brain. Epilepsia 20:95–104

Palmer GC, Palmer SJ, Legendre JL (1981) Guanylate cyclase-cyclic GMP in mouse cerebral cortex and cerebellum: modification by anticonvulsants. Exp Neurol 71:601–614

Patel IH, Levy RH (1980) Intramuscular absorption of carbamazepine in rhesus monkeys. Epilepsia 21:103–109

Patel IH, Levy RH, Trager WF (1978) Pharmacokinetics of carbamazepine-10,11-epoxide before and after autoinduction in rhesus monkeys. J Pharmacol Exp Ther 206:607–613

Penin H (1978) Antiepileptische Langzeitmedikation. Nervenarzt 49:497–506

Perez-Olea J, Mordoh I, Quevedo M (1979) Efectos antiarritmicos de la carbamazepina. Estudio experimental y clinico. Rev Med Chile 107:203–209

Pitlick WH (1975) Investigation of the pharmacokinetics of carbamazepine. Including dose and time dependency in dogs, monkeys and humans. Thesis, University of Washington, Seattle

Post RM (1982) Carbamazepine's acute and prophylactic effects in manic and depressive illness: an update. Intern Drug Ther Newsletter 17:5–10

Post RM, Ballenger JC, Hare TA, Bunney WE (1980) Lack of effect of carbamazepine on gamma-aminobutyric acid levels in cerebrospinal fluid. Neurology 30:1008–1011

Purdy RE, Julien RM, Fairhurst AS, Terry MD (1977) Effect of carbamazepine on the in vitro uptake and release of norepinephrine in adrenergic nerves of rabbit aorta and in whole brain synaptosomes. Epilepsia 18:251–257

Pynnönen S, Kanto J, Sillanpää M, Erkkola R (1977) Carbamazepine: placental transport, tissue concentrations in foetus and newborn, and level in milk. Acta Pharmacol Toxicol 41:244–253

Quattrone A, Samanin R (1977) Decreased anticonvulsant activity of carbamazepine in 6-hydroxydopamine-treated rats. Eur J Pharmacol 41:333–336

Quattrone A, Crunelli V, Samanin R (1978) Seizure susceptibility and anticonvulsant activity of carbamazepine, diphenylhydantoin and phenobarbital in rats with selective depletions of brain monoamines. Neuropharmacology 17:643–647

Quattrone A, Annunziato L, Aguglia U, Preziosi P (1981) Carbamazepine, phenytoin and phenobarbital do not influence brain catecholamine uptake, in vivo, in male rats. Arch Int. Pharmacodyn Ther 252:180–185

Rane A, Bertilsson L, Palmer L (1975) Disposition of placentally transferred carbamazepine (TEGRETOL[R]) in the newborn. Eur J Clin Pharmacol 8:283–284

Reith M, Schäfer H (1979) Antiepileptika während Schwangerschaft und Stillzeit. Dtsch Med Wochenschr 104:818–823

Rett A (1963) Zur Beurteilung der Wirkung von Antikonvulsiva im Kindesalter – ein klinisches und entwicklungsphysiologisches Problem. Neue Oesterr Z Kinderheilkd 7:178–191

Rimerman RA, Taylor SM, Lynn RK, Rodgers RM, Gerber N (1979) The excretion of carbamazepine in the semen of the rabbit and man: comparison of the concentration in semen and plasma. Pharmacologist 21:264

Sano K, Malamud N (1953) Clinical significance of sclerosis of cornu ammonis; ictal "psychic phenomena". Arch Neurol Psychiatr 70:40–53

Sawaya MCB, Horton RW, Meldrum BS (1975) Effects of anticonvulsant drugs on the cerebral enzymes metabolizing GABA. Epilepsia 16:649–655

Schauf CL, Davis FA, Marder J (1974) Effects of carbamazepine on the ionic conductances of myxicola giant axons. J Pharmacol Exp Ther 189:538–543

Scheibel ME, Crandall PH, Scheibel AB (1974) The hippocampal-dentate complex in temporal lobe epilepsy. Epilepsia 15:55–80

Schindler W, Blattner H (1961) Über Derivate des Iminodibenzyls: Iminostilben-Derivate. Helv Chim Acta 44:753–762

Schmutz M (1983) Benzodiazepines, GABA, and epilepsy – the animal evidence. In: Trimble MR (ed) Benzodiazepines divided: a multidisciplinary review. Wiley, Chichester, pp 149–166

Schmutz M, Klebs K (1982) Effects of valproate sodium on amygdaloid kindling and amygdaloid kindled seizures in the rat. In: Klee MR, Lux HD, Speckmann EF (eds) Physiology and pharmacology of epileptogenic phenomena. Raven, New York, p 391

Schmutz M, Baltzer V, Koella WP (1979) Combination of carbamazepine and valproate sodium in mice, rats and cats. 11th Epilepsy international symposium, Firenze, Sept 30–Oct 3, 1979, Abstracts, p 148

Schmutz M, Klebs K, Koella WP (1980) A chronic petit mal model. In: Wada JA, Penry JK (eds) Advances in epileptology: 10th Epilepsy international symposium. Raven, New York, pp 311–314

Schmutz M, Buerki H, Koella WP (1981) Electrically induced hippocampal afterdischarge in the freely moving cat: an animal model of focal (possibly temporal lobe) epilepsy. In: Dam M, Gram L, Penry JK (eds) Advances in epileptology: 12th Epilepsy international symposium. Raven, New York, pp 59–65

Schmutz M, Bernasconi R, Baltzer V (1983) Benzodiazepine antagonists, GABA and the mode of action of antiepileptic drugs. In: Baldy-Moulinier M, Ingvar DH, Meldrum BS (eds) Cerebral blood flow, metabolism and epilepsy. Libbey, London, pp 378–383

Schmutz M, Mondadori C, Portet C, Baltzer V (1982) Potentiation of the anticonvulsant effect of carbamazepine by vincamine and piracetam in rats. 14th Epilepsy international symposium, London, Aug 15–18, 1982. Abstracts, pp 104–105

Schneider H, Berenguer J (1977) CSF and plasma concentrations of carbamazepine and some metabolites in steady state. In: Gardner-Thorpe C, Janz D, Meinardi H, Pippenger CE (eds) Antiepileptic drug monitoring. Pitman Medical, Tunbridge Wells, pp 264–273

Sher PK, Neale EA, Nelson PG (1981) The effects of anticonvulsants on fetal mouse cerebral cortex in culture. Ann Neurol 10:290

Sillanpää M (1981) Carbamazepine. Pharmacology and clinical uses. Acta Neurol Scand 64 (suppl 88):1–202

Skerritt JH, Davies LP, Johnston GAR (1983 a) Interactions of the anticonvulsant carbamazepine with adenosine receptors. 1. Neurochemical studies. Epilepsia 24:634–642

Skerritt JH, Johnston GAR, Chen Chow S (1983 b) Interactions of the anticonvulsant carbamazepine with adenosine receptors. 2. Pharmacological studies. Epilepsia 24:643–650

Steiner C, Wit AL, Weiss MB, Damato AN (1970) The antiarrhythmic actions of carbamazepine. J Pharmacol Exp Ther 173:323–335

Stille G, Sayers A (1970) Problems involved in the pharmacological investigation of anticonvulsant drugs by electroshock methods. Pharmakopsychiatr Neuro-Psychopharmakol 3:176–187

Summy-Long JY, Keil LC, Crawford IL (1979) Effect of carbamazepine on salt-water balance, plasma and urine vasopressin in unanaesthetized rats. Fed Proc 38:754

Sun L, Szafir J (1977) Enzyme immunoassay compared to gas chromatography for determination of carbamazepine and ethosuximide in human serum. Clin Chem 23:1125

Suria A, Killam EK (1980) Carbamazepine. In: Glaser GH, Penry JK, Woodbury DM (eds) Antiepileptic drugs: mechanisms of action. Raven, New York, pp 563–575

Tchicaloff M, Penneti F (1963) Résultats thérapeutiques d'un nouvel antiépileptique le Tegretol. Schweiz Med Wochenschr 93:1664–1666

Theobald W, Kunz HA (1963) Zur Pharmakologie des Antiepileptikums 5-Carbamyl-5*H*-dibenzo(b,f)azepin. Arzneimittelforsch 13:122–125

Theobald W, Krupp P, Levin P (1970) Neuropharmacological aspects of the therapeutic action of carbamazepine in trigeminal neuralgia. In: Hassler R, Walker AE (eds) Trigeminal neuralgia. Pathogenesis and pathophysiology. Thieme, Stuttgart, pp 107–114

Troupin A, Ojemann LM, Halpern L, Dodrill C, Wilkus R, Friel P, Feigl P (1977) Carbamazepine – a double-blind comparison with phenytoin. Neurology 27:511–519

Uhlich E, Loeschke K, Eigler J (1972) Zur antidiuretischen Wirkung von Carbamazepine bei Diabetes insipidus. Klin Wochenschr 50:1127–1133

Van Duijn H (1971) Eine elektrocorticographische Untersuchung des Einflusses einzelner Antikonvulsiva auf die experimentelle fokale und primär generalisierte Epilepsie der Katze. Proefschrift, Amsterdam, 86 pp

Van Duijn H, Visser SL (1972) The action of some anticonvulsant drugs on cobalt-induced epilepsy and on the bemegride threshold in alert cats. Epilepsia 13:409–420

Varotto M, Roman G, Battistin L (1981) Influenze farmacologiche sul livello e trasporto cerebrale del GABA. Boll Soc It Biol Sper 57:904–908

Wada JA (1977) Pharmacological prophylaxis in the kindling model of epilepsy. Arch Neurol 34:389–395

Wada JA (1980) Kindling, antiepileptic drugs, seizure suspectibility and a warning. In: Robb P (ed) Epilepsy updated: causes and treatment. Year Book Medical Publishers, Chicago, pp 51–69

Wada JA, Osawa T, Sato M, Wake A, Corcoran ME, Troupin AS (1976 a) Acute anticonvulsant effects of diphenylhydantoin, phenobarbital and carbamazepine: a combined electroclinical and serum level study in amygdaloid kindled cats and baboons. Epilepsia 17:77–88

Wada JA, Sato M, Wake A, Green JR, Troupin AS (1976b) Prophylactic effects of phenytoin, phenobarbital, and carbamazepine examined in kindling cat preparations. Arch Neurol 33:426-434
Westenberg HGM, De Zeeuw RA (1976) Rapid and sensitive liquid chromatographic determination of carbamazepine suitable for use in monitoring multiple drug anticonvulsant therapy. J Chromatogr 118:217–224
Westenberg HGM, Jonkman JHG, Van der Kleijn E (1977) The distribution of carbamazepine and its metabolites in squirrel monkey and mouse. Acta Pharmacol Toxicol 41 (Suppl. 1):136–137
Whittle SR, Turner AJ (1981a) Anti-convulsants and brain aldehyde metabolism. Biochem Pharmacol 30:1191–1196
Whittle SR, Turner AJ (1981b) Biochemical actions of sodium valproate. Biochem Soc Trans 9:313–314
Young AB, Zukin SR, Snyder SH (1974) Interactions of benzodiazepines with central nervous system receptors: possible mechanism of action. Proc Natl Acad Sci USA 71:2246–2250

CHAPTER 17

Valproic Acid

W. LÖSCHER

A. Chemistry and Physicochemical Properties

Valproic acid was first synthesized by Burton in 1881. There were no reported investigations into its anticonvulsant properties until 1963, when MEUNIER et al. noted that several compounds dissolved in valproic acid protected mice and rabbits from pentylenetetrazol-induced seizures. Valproic acid is the trivial name for 2-propylpentanoic acid (also called *n*-dipropylacetic acid). As a simple branched-chain carboxylic acid it differs markedly in structure from other antiepileptic drugs. Its structural formula is as follows:

$$\begin{matrix} CH_3{-}CH_2{-}CH_2 \searrow \\ \qquad\qquad\qquad\qquad CH{-}COOH\,. \\ CH_3{-}CH_2{-}CH_2 \nearrow \end{matrix}$$

Valproic acid (molecular weight, 144.21; mp, 120°–121 °C) is a colorless liquid with a pK_a value of 4.56 (LÖSCHER and ESENWEIN 1978). Valproic acid is usually used as its sodium salt, which has a molecular weight of 166.198. Valproate sodium is a hygroscopic white powder which dissolves readily in polar solvents (e.g., water, ethanol, methanol) but is poorly soluble in solvents of lower polarity (e.g., acetone, chloroform, diethylether, benzene).

The partition coefficients of valproic acid between organic solvents and buffer at pH 7.4 have been reported as <0.01 for heptane and benzene and 0.23 for chloroform (LÖSCHER and ESENWEIN 1978). As for most short-chain fatty acids, gas chromatography is the most obvious method for determination of valproic acid. The analysis of valproic acid following other methods appears to be more intricate. Difficulties as to the proper detection of valproic acid from biological material may arise because of its volatility during enrichment.

Early gas chromatographic methods required derivatization of valproic acid to the methyl ester (ALARY et al. 1972) or to the trimethylsilyl derivative (FERRANDES and EYMARD 1973). MEIJER and HESSING-BRAND (1973) were the first to describe the analysis of underivatized valproic acid using a 5% free fatty acid phase (FFAP) column (Carbowax mixed with 2-nitroterephthalic acid) with 3,3,5-trimethyl-caproic acid as internal standard. Valproic acid was concentrated from plasma by microdiffusion following the Conway method. Several laboratories have simplified the analysis by the use of microextraction methods, i.e., valproic acid is extracted from acidified plasma into a small volume of solvent, usually chloroform or carbon tetrachloride, and 1–2 μl of the organic solvent is directly injected into the gas chromatography (e.g., DIJKHUIS and VERVLOET 1974;

SCHOBBEN and VAN DER KLEIJN 1974a, LÖSCHER 1977; OELKERS et al. 1977). Most of these methods use a liquid phase traditionally used for the analysis of fatty acids such as Carbowax 6000. The internal standard should have physical properties similar to those of valproic acid. 3,3,5-Trimethylcaproic acid, 2-methylcaproic acid, or other analogues of valproic acid may be used. For the simultaneous measurement of valproic acid and other antiepileptic drugs such as ethosuximide, gas chromatographic assays using the weakly polar stationary phase OV 17 have been described (KLOTZ 1977; LÖSCHER and GÖBEL 1978).

Valproic acid is rapidly metabolized in different species including man (see Sect. E), and several methods for the quantitative analysis of valproic acid metabolites have been reported (SCHÄFER and LÜHRS 1978; KOCHEN and SCHEFFNER 1980; SCHÄFER et al. 1980; LÖSCHER 1981a; NAU et al. 1981). In these methods either gas chromatography or combined gas chromatography-mass spectrometry is used for determination. However, in contrast to valproic acid, several difficulties impede the isolation, identification, and quantification of valproic acid metabolites (GUGLER and VON UNRUH 1980). Especially the chemical lability of these compounds can lead to erroneous results since degradation products may coincide with other metabolites in the gas chromatogram (LÖSCHER 1981a). The problem of such interference can be resolved by the use of differential extraction (LÖSCHER 1981a). More recently, the evaluation of a new enzyme immunoassay (EMIT) for the determination of valproic acid in plasma has been reported (BRAUN et al. 1981; DONNIAH and BUCHANAN 1981).

B. Antiepileptic Activity

Since the antiepileptic properties of valproic acid were serendipitously discovered by MEUNIER et al. in 1963 and CARRAZ et al. reported the first clinical trial of the drug in 1964, numerous investigations have asserted its antiepileptic effect in both experimental and clinical epilepsy. Valproic acid is now widely used for the treatment of absence seizures but also shows promise in the management of partial and generalized tonic-clonic seizures. Two major reviews have summarized its therapeutic efficacy (SIMON and PENRY 1975; PINDER et al. 1977). In the following, the anticonvulsant properties of valproic acid in various seizure models will be reviewed.

I. Valproic Acid in Experimental Models of Epilepsy

The anticonvulsant properties of valproic acid are summarized in Table 1. Only those reports have been considered in which dose-response relationships were presented. In general, valproic acid displays a broad spectrum of moderate activity against several types of chemically or electrically induced convulsions in a variety of species. As shown in Table 1, valproic acid also protects against audiogenic seizures in mice and against photic seizures in the baboon, *Papio papio*. Furthermore, it blocks kindled amygdaloid seizures in different species and is active in preventing seizures induced by sensory stimulation in the Mongolian gerbil.

Table 1. The anticonvulsant activity of valproic acid in various seizure models. The doses refer to the sodium salt of valproic acid

Species	Seizure model			Anticonvulsant activity, of valproic acid			Refs.
	Convulsant	Dose (mg/kg)	Route	Premedication interval (h)	Route	ED_{50} (mg/kg)	
Mice	Pentylene-	85	s.c.	0.5	p.o.	265	Swinyard (1964)
	tetrazol	100	s.c	0.5	p.o.	220	Shuto and Nishigaki (1970)
		100	s.c	0.75	p.o.	420	Frey and Löscher (1976)
		125	s.c.	0.5	p.o	273	Lacolle et al. (1978)
		100	s.c.	0.5	p.o.	430	Löscher (1979a)
		85	s.c.	1.0	p.o.	388	Kupferberg (1980)
		85	s.c.	0.25	i.p.	120	Swinyard (1964)
		100	s.c.	0.25	i.p.	120	Shuto and Nishigaki (1970)
		85	s.c.	0.25	i.p.	150	Krall et al. (1978)
		100	s.c.	0.5	i.p.	340	Löscher (1980a)
		35	i.v.	0.5	i.p.	42	Worms and Lloyd (1981)
Rats	Pentylene-	70	s.c.	1.0	p.o.	1020	Swinyard (1964)
	tetrazol	70	s.c.	0.5	p.o.	179	Kupferberg (1980)
		70	s.c.	0.5	i.p.	263	Swinyard (1964)
		70	s.c.	0.5	i.p.	74	Kupferberg (1980)
Mice	Maximal	50 mA	Corneal	0.5	p.o.	605	Swinyard (1964)
	electroshock	50 mA	elec-	0.5	p.o.	315	Shuto and Nishigaki (1976)
		250 V	tro-	1.0	p.o.	490	Frey and Löscher (1976)
		50 mA	des	1.0	p.o.	664	Kupferberg (1980)
		50 mA		0.25	i.p.	260	Swinyard (1964)
		50 mA		0.25	i.p.	235	Shuto and Nishigaki (1970)
		50 mA		0.25	i.p.	270	Krall et al. (1978)
		250 V		0.5	i.p.	290	Löscher (1980a)
Rats	Maximal	150 mA		1.0	p.o.	318	Swinyard (1964)
	electroshock	150 mA		1.0	p.o.	489	Kupferberg (1980)
		150 mA		0.5	i.p.	140	Swinyard (1964)
		150 mA		0.5	i.p.	169	Kupferberg (1980)
Rabbits	Maximal			0.5	i.p.	235	Swinyard (1964)
Cats	electroshock			0.5	i.p.	67	Swinyard (1964)
Mice	Picrotoxin	4	s.c.	0.75	p.o.	200	Frey and Löscher (1976)
		6.5	s.c.	0.5	p.o.	165	Lacolle et al. (1978)
		4	s.c.	0.75	p.o.	430	Löscher (1979a)
		3.2	s.c.	0.25	i.p	387	Kupferberg (1980)
		1.6	i.v.	0.5	i.p.	240	Worms and Lloyd (1981)
Mice	Bicuculline	5.5	s.c.	0.75	p.o.	600	Frey and Löscher (1976)
		2.7	s.c.	0.25	i.p.	359	Kupferberg (1980)
		0.45	i.v.	0.5	i.p.	35	Worms and Lloyd (1981)
Mice	3-Mercapto-	40	i.p.	0.5	p.o.	118	Lacolle et al. (1978)
	propionic	60	s.c.	0.75	p.o.	370	Löscher (1979a)
	acid	66	s.c.	0.5	i.p.	290	Löscher (1980a)
Mice	Allylglycine	400	i.v.	0.5	i.p.	200	Worms and Lloyd (1981)
		250	i.p.	0.5 after allylglycine	p.o.	350	Schultz (1983)

Table 1 (continued)

Species	Seizure model			Anticonvulsant activity, of valproic acid			Refs.
	Convulsant	Dose (mg/kg)	Route	Premedication interval (h)	Route	ED_{50} (mg/kg)	
Mice	Isoniazid	200	s.c.	None	p.o.	280	LÖSCHER and FREY (1977a)
Mice	Strychnine	1.2	s.c.	0.75	p.o.	700	FREY and LÖSCHER (1976)
		1.2	s.c.	0.25	i.p.	292	KUPFERBERG (1980)
		1.2	s.c.	0.5	i.p.	>900	LÖSCHER (1980a)
Mice	Audiogenic seizures			0.75	i.p.	~300	ANLEZARK et al. (1976)
				0.5	i.p.	55	WORMS and LLOYD (1981)
Rats	Amygdaloid kindling			0.5	i.p.	200	ALBERTSON et al. (1980)
Baboons	Photosensitive epilepsy				i.v.	100–200	MELDRUM et al. (1977)
Gerbils	Reflex epilepsy						
	Myoclonic seizures			0.75	p.o.	210	FREY et al. (1983)
				0.75	p.o.	290	FREY et al. (1983)
	Clonic-tonic seizures			0.5	i.p.	84	LÖSCHER et al. (1983)

The absence of concordance among different investigators testing valproic acid in the same seizure model is most likely accounted for by a different sensitivity of the animal strain used and methodological differences such as route of administration, the time at which the tests were carried out after the administration of valproic acid, and different test parameters.

The prevention of maximal electroshock seizures in mice is considered the classical animal model for evaluating agents potentially useful in the treatment of generalized tonic-clonic seizures (SWINYARD 1969). Comparative studies have shown that valproic acid has only a weak effect in this model, at least when compared with drugs useful in the treatment of grand mal epilepsy such as phenobarbital and phenytoin (FREY and LÖSCHER 1976; KRALL et al. 1978).

The prevention of pentylenetetrazol-induced seizures in mice is generally considered the classical animal model with the most predictive value for evaluating agents potentially useful in absence seizures (SWINYARD 1969). Actually, in this seizure model the anticonvulsant ED_{50} of valproic acid is in the same range as that of trimethadione or ethosuximide, which are considered standard drugs in the therapy of absence seizures (FREY and LÖSCHER 1976; KRALL et al. 1978). In dogs, MARTINEK and ARBEITER (1980) found that i.p. or i.v. administration of 80–180 mg/kg valproic acid protected 47% of the animals from seizures induced by i.p. pentylenetetrazol, whereas orally administered valproic acid was ineffective in this regard.

VAN DUIJN and BECKMANN (1975) investigated the effect of valproic acid on bemegride-induced tonic-clonic convulsions in cats. Forty-five minutes after sc.

administration of 200 mg/kg valproic acid no significant effect was obtained, whereas 5 min after the same dose given i.v., marked protection was observed.

Several investigators have evaluated the effect of valproic acid on seizures induced by drugs which impair the function of the inhibitory neurotransmitter gamma-aminobutyric acid (GABA) in the brain. Thus, valproic acid has been shown to prevent seizures induced by picrotoxin and bicuculline, two specific and selective GABA antagonists (FREY and LÖSCHER 1967; LACOLLE et al. 1978; LÖSCHER 1979a; KUPFERBERG 1980; LÖSCHER 1980a; WORMS and LLOYD 1981). In a similar dose range valproic acid proved active against seizures caused by 3-mercaptopropionic acid, isoniazid, and allylglycine, which are potent inhibitors of GABA synthesis (LÖSCHER and FREY 1977a; LACOLLE et al. 1978; LÖSCHER 1979a, 1980a; WORMS and LLOYD 1981; SCHULTZ 1983). At least in our laboratory, valproic acid was clearly more effective against picrotoxin-,3-mercaptopropionic acid-, or isoniazid-induced convulsions than against seizures caused by strychnine, a specific antagonist of glycine (FREY and LÖSCHER 1976; LÖSCHER and FREY 1977a; LÖSCHER 1979a, 1980a). These results were considered to point to a role of GABA in the mediation of the anticonvulsant effect of valproic acid.

Similar to the pentylenetetrazol-induced seizure test, the ability of a drug to prevent EEG and clinical seizure manifestations induced by photic stimulation of the baboon is considered to be of value in evaluating agents potentially useful against absence seizures (WOODBURY 1972). PATRY and NAQUET (1971) and MELDRUM et al. (1977) found valproic acid effective in this model after i.v. administration of doses up to 200 mg/kg. Several investigators have shown valproic acid to prevent audiogenic seizures in mice and carbon dioxide withdrawal seizures in rats, also useful models of absence seizures (SWINYARD 1964; SIMLER et al. 1973; ANLEZARK et al. 1976).

HILLBOM (1975) studied the effects of valproic acid on ethanol withdrawal seizures in rats. Chronically administered valproic acid decreased the number of withdrawal seizures; however, seizures were not prevented if valproic acid was given 12 h after the withdrawal of ethanol. The anticonvulsant effect of valproic acid against ethanol withdrawal seizures was confirmed by NOBLE et al. (1976) and GOLDSTEIN (1979).

In the Mongolian gerbil, seizures can be reliably initiated by sensory stimulation and evaluated by a standardized rating system (LOSKOTA et al. 1974). Valproic acid has recently been shown effective in this model of reflex epilepsy (LÖSCHER et al. 1983; FREY et al. 1983; Table 1).

Another genetic animal model of epilepsy is the mutant mouse *tottering*, which displays, in the young homozygote, abnormal bursts of bilaterally synchronous spike waves in electrocorticograms recorded from awake, unrestrained animals (NOEBELS and SIDMAN 1979). In addition to these "absence seizures" focal motor seizures occur. Valproic acid in oral doses up to 600 mg/kg did not influence these focal seizures (SCHULTZ 1983). Similar results were obtained with ethosuximide (ineffective up to 500 mg/kg), whereas diazepam proved highly active in this model (oral ED_{50}, 1.15 mg/kg).

In dogs in which epileptic seizures were induced by emotional excitement, valproic acid was anticonvulsantly active following parenteral administration but showed no effect when administered orally on a chronic basis (MARTINEK and ARBEITER 1980).

LEVIEL and NAQUET (1977) studied the action of valproic acid on kindling induced by repeated stimulation of the amygdala in cats. Daily i.p. doses of 50 mg/kg prevented the progressive establishment of generalized seizures. Higher doses (75–150 mg/kg) were necessary to protect the animals against generalized tonic-clonic seizures when kindling was established. Similarly, WADA (1977) and ALBERTSON et al. (1980) reported that in rats, cats, and baboons valproic acid had anticonvulsant effects in the kindling model and prophylaxis was demonstrated in cats. More recently, LÖSCHER (1983) studied the effect of valproic acid on the decrease in seizure threshold and progressive intensification of motor seizures developing in the time course of repeated administration of pentylenetetrazol in dogs. Daily oral administration of valproic acid in doses up to 180 mg/kg exerted no effect on the development of these kindling-like phenomena. Actually, a certain anticonvulsant effect was only determined 1.5–2 h after the daily administration of valproic acid.

In cats with cortical cobalt or alumina lesions, the experimental model for partial focal seizures with elementary symptomatology (WOODBURY 1972), valproic acid did not decrease focal discharges in the cortex but rather inhibited the spread of seizure activity from the focus (FARIELLO and MUTANI 1970; VAN DUIJN and BECKMANN 1975). It was about as effective as phenobarbital in suppressing ictal and interictal EEG phenomena. In a study by EMSON (1976), valproic acid did not affect either the behavioral or EEG manifestations of an intracortical cobalt lesion in the rat. However, with respect to the short half-life of valproic acid in this species (LÖSCHER 1978), the dose regimen of the chronic treatment was not suited to maintain active drug levels. LOCKARD and LEVY (1976) evaluated the anticonvulsant activity of valproic acid in monkeys following intracortical injection of aluminum hydroxide. Constant-rate i.v. infusion of valproic acid attenuated the bursts of seizure activity caused by alumina and reduced focal motor seizures at higher plasma levels. Interestingly, these authors reported a decrease in electrographic seizure activity for a period of 2 weeks after valproic acid was withdrawn.

Carry-over effects of the drug's anticonvulsant action have also been reported in mice, after both acute and chronic administration of valproic acid (LACOLLE et al. 1978; LÖSCHER and NAU 1982; NAU and LÖSCHER 1982). Thus, the anticonvulsant activity of valproic acid against seizures induced by pentylenetetrazol, 3-mercaptopropionic acid, or electroshock persisted after the drug had disappeared from the brain. Actually, delayed postdrug effects of valproic acid have also been described in patients (HARDING et al. 1978). The possibility that valproic acid metabolites could account for these findings will be discussed in Sect. E.III.3.

JULIEN and FOWLER (1977) evaluated valproic acid for its ability to alter the pattern of febrile convulsions induced in mice by microwave diathermy. Doses of valproic acid up to 400 mg/kg i.p. failed to raise the temperature threshold for febrile convulsions, but reduced seizure severity at 200 and 400 mg/kg and depressed the rate of rise of temperature at 400 mg/kg. This effect was comparable to that observed in phenobarbital-treated animals. Indeed, CAVAZUTTI (1975) noted a comparable efficacy of valproic acid and phenobarbital in the clinical prevention of febrile convulsions.

II. Mechanism of Anticonvulsant Action of Valproic Acid

1. Effects on GABA Metabolism

The role of GABA as an inhibitory neurotransmitter and the relationship between neuronal excitability and GABA are beyond the scope of this chapter, but it seems generally accepted that impairment of the GABA system can lead to convulsions whereas enhancement of its effectiveness has an anticonvulsant effect (MELDRUM 1979). SIMLER et al. (1968) were the first to describe that valproic acid raises brain GABA levels. Following i.p. administration of 400 mg/kg in mice a maximum GABA increase of 37% was observed after 30 min. Since then, most reports dealing with the mechanism of action of valproic acid refer to its ability to raise brain GABA levels. Actually, the increase in whole brain GABA of mice correlates temporally with the onset and duration of the anticonvulsant activity of valproic acid (SIMLER et al. 1973; LUST et al. 1976; LACOLLE et al. 1978; LÖSCHER 1981 b). GABA levels determined in mouse and rat brain regions after valproic acid, 200–400 mg/kg i.p., show increases varying from 0% (caudate nucleus, temporal cortex) to 80%–100% (hypothalamus and olfactory bulb) (SIMLER et al. 1978; IADAROLA et al. 1979). However, since GABA concentrations were determined in homogenates of whole brain or brain regions, it is not certain what portion of the increase in GABA produced by valproic acid is associated with nerve endings concerned with neurotransmission. GABA is present in many cells including glial cells and neurons which do not use this amino acid as a neurotransmitter (BALÁSZ et al. 1970). Thus, the cellular compartmentation of GABA makes it difficult to correlate elevation of whole brain GABA concentrations and neuropharmacological effects such as anticonvulsant action. IADAROLA and GALE (1979) have shown in rats that after section of the striatonigral pathway the increase in nigral GABA seen after valproic acid was abolished. This observation has been interpreted as showing that increases in GABA content after valproic acid occur specifically in GABAergic terminals. Indeed, SARHAN and SEILER (1979), who examined GABA levels in subcellular fractions of brain tissue obtained from mice treated with valproic acid (400 mg/kg), found a pronounced GABA increase in a crude fraction of synaptosomes, i.e., discrete particles which have been derived from nerve endings. However, this finding was limited by the fact that the fraction used (P2) contains a significant amount of nonsynaptic mitochondria in addition to the synaptosomes. More recently, LÖSCHER (1981 c) studied the effects of valproic acid, 125–250 mg/kg i.p., on GABA metabolism in purified synaptosomes from mouse brain. In all doses valproic acid produced significant increases of synaptosomal GABA levels of about 20%–30% which were comparable to the relative increases determined in whole brain. The enzymic basis for the rise in brain GABA following valproic acid remains subject to controversy. Before considering in detail the mechanisms by which valproic acid might increase GABA levels, it is pertinent to illustrate the routes by which GABA is formed and catabolized. As shown in Chap. 7, this volume, Fig. 1, GABA is synthesized by decarboxylation of glutamate and is degraded by transamination to succinic semialdehyde (SSA). SSA can either be oxidized to succinate or it can be reduced to gamma-hydroxybutyrate. The relative importance of these two degradative pathways in vivo is unclear, although it appears that the reduction to gamma-hydroxybutyrate is generally a minor route of metabolism. All the enzymes of GABA metabolism have been extensively characterized with the exception of SSA reductase. This latter enzyme may be similar or identical to NADPH-dependent aldehyde reductases (EC 1.1.1.2), which act as general aldehyde-metabolizing enzymes in brain and other tissues and can reduce SSA in vitro (TURNER and WHITTLE 1980). The GABA-elevating action of valproic acid was originally attributed to inhibition of GABA transaminase (GABA-T; EC 2.6.1.19) (GODIN et al. 1969; SIMLER et al. 1973). However, more recent studies have shown that this inhibition by valproic acid is extremely weak ($K_i > 20$ mM) and not likely to be of any significance for the action of the drug in vivo (FOWLER et al. 1975; LÖSCHER and FREY 1977 b; Whittle and TURNER 1978; VAN DER LAAN et al. 1979; LÖSCHER 1980 b). Actually, following administration of therapeutic dose levels of valproic acid in man, brain concentrations of only 0.04–0.2 mM have been determined (VADJA et al. 1981). Several authors have reported a more potent inhibitory effect against SSA dehydrogenase (SSADH; EC 1.2.1.16), the enzyme responsible for the subsequent stage in the GABA shunt pathway (HARVEY et al. 1975; ANLEZARK et al. 1976; VAN DER LAAN et al. 1979), but studies by SIMLER et al. (1981) suggest that it is apparently not possible to raise brain GABA levels even with near total inhibition of SSADH by *p*-hydroxybenzaldehyde. Recently, WHITTLE and TURNER (1978) have shown that valproic acid is a potent inhibitor of aldehyde reductase purified from ox brain, with a K_i of 38–85 μM. The physiological significance of inhibition of aldehyde reductase has not been established. Its possible involvement in the conversion of SSA into gamma-hydroxybutyrate has been discussed above. In fact, inhibition of this pathway by valproic acid has recently been demonstrated in rat brain homogenates, 67% inhibition occurring at 1 mM (WHITTLE and TURNER 1982). Tentatively, inhibition of gamma-hydroxybutyrate formation by valproic acid could be of considerable interest since this metabolite of GABA has been shown to produce epileptogenic effects in monkeys and rats (MARCUS et al. 1976; SNEAD 1978). Besides effects of valproic acid on GABA degradation, an activation of GABA synthesis could be a likely explanation for the GABA-elevating action of this drug. GODIN et al. (1969) measured the relative incorporation of ^{14}C into GABA in rat brain following the s.c. injection of [^{14}C]glucose. Thirty minutes after administration of valproic acid, 400 mg/kg i.p., the incorporation of ^{14}C into the GABA molecule was increased by 29%, which, however, was not significant on account of the small number of animals studied. In similar experiments in mice, TABERNER et al. (1980) found that valproic acid, 80 mg/kg i.p., produced a significant increase in the rate of production of GABA by 90%, whereas after 160 mg/kg the incorporation of ^{14}C into GABA was elevated by 40%. Actually, LÖSCHER (1981 c) showed that valproic acid, 125–205 mg/kg i.p., significantly increased the activity of the GABA-synthesizing enzyme glutamic acid decarboxylase (GAD; EC 4.1.1.15) both in the whole brain and brain synaptosomes of mice. The time course of this effect matched that of the GABA increase (LÖSCHER 1981 b). Increase of GAD activity was confirmed by PHILLIPS and FOWLER (1982), who demonstrated significant increases in the medulla, pons cerebellum, and midbrain regions of rats. Higher, sedative doses of valproic acid seem to depress GAD activity (LÖSCHER and FREY 1977 b) and to decrease the rate of incorporation of ^{14}C from glutamate into GABA (CHAPMAN et al. 1982). Accordingly, these findings may be interpreted in that at least in part valproic acid raises brain GABA levels by elevation of GABA synthesis, but this effect seems to occur only within a certain dose range. Irrespective of the mechanisms causing the rise in brain GABA concentrations, is it sufficient to explain the anticonvulsant action of valproic acid? The GABA increases after the administration of valproic acid are small in comparison to the five- to tenfold increases seen after potent inhibitors of GABA-T, such as gamma-acetylenic GABA and gabaculine (JUNG 1978). However, since decreases in GABA concentrations in nerve terminals of only 28% have been demonstrated to impair the function of the inhibitory transmitter to such an extent that seizures occur (WOOD et al. 1979), the modest potency of valproic acid to increase synaptosomal GABA seems sufficient to predict anticonvulsant activity (LÖSCHER 1981c). It has been repeatedly objected that the valproic acid doses used in most rodent studies to demonstrate GABA increases were far above those used for clinical treatment (20–60 mg/kg). Actually, in dogs valproic acid, 60 mg/kg, was recently shown to increase brain GABA levels by about 100% (LÖSCHER 1982a). This effect was reflected by similar relative increases in GABA levels of plasma and CSF. Accordingly, in volunteers and patients under chronic treatment with valproic acid, a pronounced increase in plasma and CSF GABA levels has been recently described (LÖSCHER and SCHMIDT 1980, 1981; ZIMMER et al. 1980; LÖSCHER and SIEMES 1984). However, in two other clinical studies CSF measurements showed no significant change in GABA levels of patients with schizophrenia and Parkinson's disease (NUTT et al. 1979; LAUTIN et al. 1980).

2. Effects on Release, Receptors, and Uptake of GABA

Recent biochemical studies have examined the effects of valproic acid on GABA-linked mechanisms other than metabolism as a possible site of action, namely (a) the release of GABA from nerve terminals, (b) the sodium-independent binding of GABA to postsynaptic receptors, and (c) the sodium-dependent high-affinity GABA reuptake system which removes GABA from the synaptic cleft and thereby terminates its action (for illustration see Chap. 7, this volume, Fig. 2).

Valproic acid at concentrations up to 1 mM had no effects on the release of preloaded radiolabeled GABA from rat brain synaptosomal preparations (ABDUL-GHANI et al. 1981). In the same study it was shown that valproic acid, 200–400 mg/kg i.p., caused no detectable efflux of GABA from rat cerebral cortex in vivo.

The effect of valproic acid on sodium-independent GABA binding to postsynaptic receptors has been determined with a crude synaptic membrane fraction from rat brain (LÖSCHER 1979b, 1980b). Up to 10 mM the drug produced no perceptible changes in GABA binding. Similarly, valproic acid did not interfere with [^{3}H]muscimol binding (KERWIN et al. 1980; LÖSCHER et al. 1981).

The effect of valproic acid on the sodium-dependent uptake of [^{3}H]GABA has been measured with a crude mitochondrial fraction from rat brain (KULIG et al. 1977; LÖSCHER 1980b). Valproic acid had very little affinitiy to GABA-uptake sites, producing 20%–25% inhibition at 10 mM.

Recent studies of TICKU and OLSEN (1978) have shown that several convulsants and anticonvulsants interact with a site in the GABA receptor-ionophore complex distinct from the GABA recognition sites to which the neurotransmitter attaches. This site seems directly associated with the GABA-linked chloride ionophore and can be labeled by radioactive dihydropicrotoxinin (DHP). Actually, a number of barbiturates which have been shown to activate GABA-linked Cl^- channels are potent inhibitors of DHP binding to rat brain membranes (OLSEN et al. 1979). Preliminary experiments in this laboratory suggest that valproic acid is a weak inhibitor of DHP binding ($IC_{50} > 1$ mM), whereas TICKU and DAVIS (1981) found valproic acid to inhibit DHP binding in a Lubrol-solubilized fraction from rat brain with an IC_{50} of 0.5 mM.

3. Neurophysiological Effects

Although binding experiments did not indicate a potent action of valproic acid on GABA receptor function, there are several neurophysiological studies which suggest direct postsynaptic effects of valproate leading to potentiation of GABA-mediated neurotransmission independent of alterations in GABA metabolism (reviewed by JURNA in Chap. 23, this volume). Recent experiments on the neurophysiological effects of 2-en-valproic acid, the major metabolite of valproic acid, are described in this chapter in Sect. E.III.3.

4. Effects on Glycine Metabolism

There is considerable evidence that glycine acts as an inhibitory transmitter in the spinal cord and brain stem (WERMAN et al. 1968). Its postsynaptic action is blocked by strychnine and related alkaloids and this effect appears to be responsible for the convulsant action of these drugs.

There have been several studies which have reported elevated CSF, plasma, and urine glycine concentrations in patients on medication with valproic acid (JAECKEN et al. 1977; SIMILAE et al. 1979, 1980; MORTENSEN et al. 1980). Hyperglycinemia and hyperglycinuria have also been determined following valproic acid treatment in rats and have been accounted for by inhibition of the glycine cleavage enzyme complex (MORTENSEN et al. 1980). Though the physiological significance of these findings is not yet evident, the weak anticonvulsant effect of valproic acid against strychnine seizures does not suggest that the glycinergic system is a primary site of action of the drug (FREY and LÖSCHER 1976; LÖSCHER 1979a, 1980a).

5. Effects on Aspartate

Evidence has accumulated to indicate that aspartate may be the excitatory transmitter at some central synapses (CURTIS and WATKINS 1963; CURTIS and JOHNSTON 1974). Following i.p. administration of valproic avid, 400 mg/kg in mice, decreases of brain aspartate levels have been reported which correlated temporally with the anticonvulsant activity against audiogenic seizures (SCHECHTER et al. 1978). Similar decreases in brain aspartate have been determined in rats after i.p. injection of 400 mg/kg, whereas subchronic oral treatment (315–365 mg/kg per day) proved ineffective in this regard (KUKINO and DEGUCHI 1977; PERRY and HANSEN 1978). Subcellular studies of SARHAN and SEILER (1979) indicate that the decrease in brain aspartate induced by valproic acid is confined to nonsynaptosomal compartments, thus suggesting that this effect is not related to a neurotransmitter role of the amino acid.

6. Effects on Cyclic Nucleotides

LUST and associates (1976, 1978) studied the relationship of cyclic nucleotides to anticonvulsant activity in mice. In general, cyclic 3′,5′-GMP concentrations in the cerebellum were elevated by convulsants and diminished by anticonvulsant agents, whereas the levels of cyclic 3′,5′-AMP remained unchanged by either treatment. Following administration of valproic acid, 400 mg/kg i.p., the decrease in cyclic GMP was accompanied by an increase in cerebellar GABA. Interestingly, the increase in cerebellar cyclic GMP induced by isoniazid was suppressed in the presence of valproic acid. Similar results were obtained by MCCANDLESS et al. (1979) in discrete layers of mouse cerebellum. The authors speculated that the decreased cerebellar cyclic GMP level after valproic acid could lead to an increase in Purkinje-cell activity, which in turn could then have an inhibitory influence on various cortical and subcortical areas.

7. Effects on Monoamine Metabolism

An involvement of norepinephrine, dopamine, and 5-hydroxytryptamine in the mechanism of action of anticonvulsants has repeatedly been suggested (MELDRUM 1978; LÖSCHER 1981 d). Following administration of valproic acid (400–600 mg/kg i.p.) in rodents, changes have been reported in the brain concentrations of these amines and their principal acid metabolites, which, however, did not correlate with the anticonvulsant effect (HORTON et al. 1977; HWANG and VAN WOERT 1979; KUKINO and DEGUCHI 1977). When mice were pretreated with inhibitors of monoamine synthesis, the anticonvulsant action of valproic acid was not altered (HORTON et al. 1977). Thus, changes in activity in monoaminergic systems would not appear to play a major part in the anticonvulsant action of valproic acid.

In conclusion, enhancement of GABA-mediated inhibition by a presynaptic effect on GABA metabolism and/or a direct postsynaptic action remains the strongest hypothesis concerning the mechanism of action of valproic acid. However, several important questions need a more detailed examination before this hypothesis can be accepted as definitive evidence.

C. Central Nervous System Effects Besides the Anticonvulsant Effect

Because of the effects of valproic acid on pre- and postsynaptic GABA-ergic function, there have been attempts to use it in the treatment of neurological disorders which are thought to involve impairment of GABA-mediated transmission, such as Huntington's disease, Parkinsons's disease, schizophrenia, tardive dyskinesia, and manic-depressive psychosis. In general, the results have not been as promising as in the treatment of epilepsy, but there have been reports of ameliorization of symptoms with higher dosages of valproic acid (see HAMMOND et al. 1981). In rats with kainic acid-induced lesions of the striatum, a model for Huntington's disease, valproic acid (400 mg/kg i.p.) only partially corrected the GABA deficiency in the striatum, whereas low doses of the GABA-T inhibitor gamma-acetylenic GABA completely restored the decreased GABA levels (SCHWARCZ et al. 1977). The hyperactivity induced by the bilateral injection of dopamine into the nucleus accumbens of rats can be inhibited by valproic acid (KURUVILLA and URETSKY 1981), which is consistent with findings of NAGAO et al. (1979) that valproic acid seems to reduce dopaminergic hyperactivity in schizophrenics with tardive dyskinesia. Accordingly, a reduction of dopamine synthesis after valproic acid was reported by WALTERS et al. (1979). On the other hand, valproic acid, 100–400 mg/kg i.p., caused only inconsistent effects in the dyskinesia model using 2-(*N*,*N*-dipropyl)amino-5,6-dihydroxytetralin to induce perioral movements in guinea pigs (COSTALL et al. 1978). Furthermore, valproic acid failed to inhibit amphetamine-induced stereotyped behaviour, which is considered as a screening test for antipsychotic compounds with antidopaminergic effect (PATEL et al. 1975).

LAL and SHEARMAN (1980) recently reported that valproic acid exerts anxiolytic activity similar to that of the benzodiazepines in a rat model, and it was suggested that this action might be due to the effects of valproic acid on the GABA system.

Sedative effects have been noted in patients receiving valproic acid alone but are found most often in patients receiving valproic acid in addition to other antiepileptic drugs, especially phenobarbital (PINDER et al. 1977; see also Sect. F). NORONKA and BEVAN (1976) calculated an overall incidence of drowsiness and sedation of 5.1%, of which only 0.2% could be attributed directly to valproic acid. Animal studies have shown that valproic acid per se is more sedative than trimethadione or phenacemide but less so than phenobarbital or phenytoin (SWINYARD 1964). Decreases of spontaneous motor activity do not occur until doses of 400–600 mg/kg (i.p.) are reached (e.g., MISSLIN et al. 1972; LÖSCHER 1980 a). In mice, valproic acid, 10–50 mg/kg i.p., has been reported to potentiate the hypnotic activity of chloral hydrate and, less markedly, hexobarbital and phenobarbital (LEBRETON et al. 1964).

SHUTO and NISHIGAKI (1970) found that valproic acid in s.c. doses of 300–500 mg/kg exerted antinociceptive action in mice and potentiated the antinociceptive effect of morphine. Actually, the antinociceptive effect of 400 mg/kg valproic acid was of the same order as that of morphine, 8 mg/kg s.c.

More recently, acute administration of valproic acid in drug-naive rats has been found to evoke a behavioral syndrome which was designated as "quasi-morphine abstinence behavior" (as defined by COLLIER 1974) since it resembled the behavioral syndrome observed during morphine abstinence (DE BOER et al. 1977, 1980; COWAN and WATSON 1978; COWAN 1981). The syndrome is characterized by a high incidence of shaking behavior ("wet dog shaking"), digging, hunchback posture, and piloerection occurring within minutes following i.p. injection of valproic acid, 200–300 mg/kg. Swallowing and teeth chattering were less frequently observed, and so were ptosis and catalepsy, which have also been described in mice after high doses of the drug (LÖSCHER 1981 a). Most behavioral symptoms induced by valproic acid could also be evoked by other branched chain fatty acids (VAN DER LAAN et al. 1980). The quasi-abstinence effects were suppressed by bicuculline, picrotoxin, and 3-mercaptopropionic acid, whereas strychnine was ineffective. Thus it was suggested that valproic acid-induced quasi-abstinence behavior may be evoked by an increase of GABA levels at its receptor sites (DE BOER et al. 1977, 1980; VAN DER LAAN et al. 1980). The behavioral syndrome was further suppressed by amino-oxyacetic acid, lysergic acid diethylamine, and morphine, whereas naloxone had no effect (COWAN and WATSON 1980; COWAN 1980; DE BOER et al. 1980). When rats were injected twice daily with valproic acid for 7 days, marked tolerance developed to the behavioral components of the syndrome (COWAN 1981).

D. Pharmacodynamic Properties Outside the Central Nervous System

Despite the widespread use of valproic acid, there have been very few reports of studies on the pharmacodynamic effects of the drug outside the CNS (see also Sect. G). Following acute and subacute administration in rats, valproic acid was shown to exert a moderate diuretic effect (CARRAZ et al. 1965; SHUTO and NISHIGAKI 1970).

A number of studies indicate that valproic acid has an immunostimulant action. Thus, administration of the drug to rabbits during immunization doubled the quantity of antibodies formed and opposed the depression of antibody formation induced by cortisone (CARRAZ and FIORINA 1967; CARRAZ et al. 1970). Subsequent studies in mice showed that valproic acid enhances humoral immunity in vivo, but is uneffective in vitro, suggesting the involvement of metabolites in the immunostimulant action of the drug (DE SOUZA-QUEIROZ and MULLEN 1980).

According to studies of SHUTO and NISHIGAKI (1970), valproic acid hardly affected the cardiovascular system. Recently, a more detailed study on the cardiovascular activity of valproic acid has been carried out in dogs and rats (LÖSCHER 1982b). In dogs, valproic acid was injected i.v. in a priming dose followed by maintenance infusion to compensate the rapid elimination of valproic acid in this species (see Sect. E). Doses up to 40 mg/kg plus infusion produced only transient reduction of blood pressure. A decrease in heart rate was observed in two of ten dogs studied. At 60 mg/kg with subsequent infusion the transient fall in blood pressure was followed by sustained hypertension. In rats, valproic acid up to 50 mg/kg i.v. induced a temporary fall in blood pressure and heart rate. Administration of 100–400 mg/kg provoked prolonged cardiovascular depression which, at doses of 300–400 mg/kg, was very similar to that observed with high i.v. doses of GABA and inhibitors of GABA-T. Both hypotension and bradycardia induced by valproic acid could be counteracted by the GABA antagonist bicuculline, whereas manipulation of other transmitter systems exerted inconsistent effects. Interestingly, the dopamine agonist apomorphine led to a considerable intensification of the cardiovascular depression provoked by valproic acid.

In rats which were made hypertensive by removing the right kidney and by implanting a 50-mg pellet of desoxycorticosterone acetate, the daily i.p. administration of 100 mg/kg valproic acid for 6 weeks was very effective in reducing the development of hypertension, but did not prevent suppression of renin activity (ROTIROTI et al. 1982). The antihypertensive effect of valproic acid seemed not to include interference with peripheral vascular noradrenergic activity or arterial baroreflex control.

E. Pharmacokinetics

The main pharmacokinetic data for valproic acid in different species are summarized in Table 2.

I. Absorption and Bioavailability

Valproic acid is rapidly absorbed in man following single oral doses in conventional tablet form, peak plasma concentrations being attained 1–4 h after administration. A mean absorption half-time of 0.42 h has been calculated (see GUGLER and VON UNRUH 1980). With enteric-coated preparations, a lag time of absorption of 1–2 h is observed. Bioavailability studies have shown that valproic acid is almost completely absorbed from solution, tablet, or enteric-coated preparations (KLOTZ and ANTONIN 1977).

Following oral administration in mice and dogs, valproic acid is even more rapidly absorbed than it is in man (LÖSCHER and ESENWEIN 1978). In dogs, the bioavailability from solutions, tablets, and enteric-coated preparations is similar to that determined in humans, whereas poor absorption was noted in mice (LÖSCHER and ESENWEIN 1978; LÖSCHER 1981 e). Absorption of valproic acid from the small intestine has been studied by perfusing drug solutions through the intestine of anesthetized rats and by varying the pH (SCHNITGER 1984). Absorption decreased when the pH was raised from 6 to 8. Furthermore, the relative intestinal absorption significantly declined with increasing drug concentrations. Actually, experiments in rats and dogs may indicate the existence of a probenecid-sensitive transport of valproic acid from the intestine into the circulation (SCHNITGER 1984; LÖSCHER 1981 e).

II. Distribution and Protein Binding

Following i.v. administration of valproic acid in man, an apparent volume of distribution of 0.085–0.203 liters/kg has been determined (KLOTZ and ANTONIN 1977). These values are small compared with most other antiepileptic drugs and suggest that distribution of valproic acid is almost restricted to the extracellular compartment. Similar figures have been reported for rhesus monkeys, whereas higher values were determined in other species (Table 2). This may be explained at least in part by the striking species differences in the degree of plasma protein binding. At "therapeutic" plasma concentrations of 50–80 μg/ml the proportion bound varies from about 90% in man to 60% in rat and 10% in mice (Table 2). In man and dog, binding is saturable so that a higher proportion of valproic acid is unbound at high plasma levels (JORDAN et al. 1976; LÖSCHER 1979 c).

Tissue distribution studies with radiolabeled valproic acid in rodents have shown that the drug is rapidly distributed in various tissues, maximum concentrations being reached within 10–30 min after i.v., i.p., or oral administration (EYMARD et al. 1971; SCHOBBEN and VAN DER KLEIJN 1974 b; DICKINSON et al. 1979; ALY and ABDEL-LATIF 1980). Large amounts of activity were found in the liver and kidney whereas the radioactivity in brain was only about 20%–30% of that in the blood. Valproic acid seems to be relative homogeneously distributed in the brain of mice and rats (SCHOBBEN and VAN DER KLEIJN 1974 b; ALY and

Table 2. Pharmacokinetics of valproic acid in different species

Species	Approximate volume of distribution[a] (liters/kg)	Half-life[b] (h)	Bioavailability (%)	Plasma protein binding[c] (%)	Brain/plasma ratio[c]	CSF/Plasma-ratio[c]	Refs.
Man	0.085–0.203	9.3–18.4	70–100	80–95	0.07–0.28	0.08–0.25	KLOTZ and ANTONIN (1979); WULFF et al. (1977); LÖSCHER (1978); VAJDA et al. (1981)
Rhesus monkey	0.17	0.66		80	0.22	0.3	LEVY (1980; WILENSKY (1980)
Dog	0.21–0.77	1.2–3.7	80–90	70–80	0.28–0.39	0.2–0.4	FREY and LÖSCHER (1978); LÖSCHER (1978); LÖSCHER and ESENWEIN (1978); LÖSCHER (1979c); LÖSCHER (1982a)
Cat	0.38	8.5			0.2–0.7		VAN DUIJN and BECKMANN (1975); HAMMOND et al. (1981)
Rat	0.66	4.6		63	0.18–0.32		LÖSCHER (1978); DICKINSON et al. (1979)
Mouse	0.33	0.8	34–47	12	0.15–0.2		LÖSCHER (1978); LÖSCHER and ESENWEIN (1978); NAU and LÖSCHER (1982)

[a] $V_d(\beta)$ or $V_d(ss)$
[b] $t_{0.5}(\beta)$
[c] At "therapeutic" plasma concentrations of 50–80 μg/ml

ABDEL-LATIF 1980). Studies on the subcellular distribution of the drug showed that it is associated mostly with the soluble and mitochondrial brain fractions, with little radioactivity in the myelin and synaptosomal fractions.

In human brain tissue obtained from patients during neurosurgery, valproic acid levels were 6.8% to 27.9% of those in plasma (VAJDA et al. 1981). Though the concentration in brain seemed related to the free fraction of drug in plasma, very similar plasma/brain concentration ratios have been determined in other species despite the marked species differences in plasma protein binding (Table 2). In fact, there is evidence for carrier-mediated transport of valproic acid into and out of CSF and brain, most probably utilizing the common monocarboxylic acid carrier (FREY and LÖSCHER 1978; LEVY 1980). The clearance out of the CNS is twice as large as the entry and can be inhibited by probenecid. Thus valproic acid appears to behave like other relatively strong acids, such as salicylic acid and penicillin, for which active transport has been demonstrated in several species.

Valproic acid apparently does not bind to brain proteins (GOLDBERG and TODOROFF 1980). Accordingly, acute and subacute studies in mice showed no retention of valproic acid in brain tissue (LÖSCHER and NAU 1982; NAU and LÖSCHER 1982). However, a gradual accumulation of radioactivity was observed in the olfactory bulb in mice following i.v. injection as well as in monkeys after long-term infusion of radiolabeled valproic acid (SCHOBBEN et al. 1980).

During steady-state therapy with valproic acid in pregnancy, an increase in apparent volume of distribution has been determined in the third trimester by means of ^{13}C-labeled valproic acid (WITTFOHT et al. 1982). Concomitantly, hepatic and renal clearance increased, resulting in a drop of serum levels.

Transfer of ^{14}C-labeled valproic acid across the placenta of pregnant rodents was reported by EYMARD et al. (1971). Placental transfer has also been demonstrated in humans (NAU et al. 1981 b). Valproic acid is excreted into breast milk, but milk concentrations did not exceed 5% of those in plasma (ESPIR et al. 1976; NAU et al. 1981 b).

The excretion of valproic acid into semen has been demonstrated in rabbit and man (SWANSON et al. 1978). In semen of rabbits 17%–30% of the concurrent levels in plasma were found, whereas these figures were 11%–17% in man.

Whereas for most antiepileptics the concentration in human saliva equals the free drug concentration in plasma, salivary levels of valproic acid were only 0.5% –4.5% of total plasma concentration (SCHMIDT 1976; GUGLER et al. 1977).

III. Elimination

1. Elimination Half-life

Following single-dose administration to volunteers or epileptic patients, plasma half-lives of 9–18 h have been reported (see GUGLER and VON UNRUH 1980). The plasma concentration decay in man is obviously biphasic, indicating that a two-compartment open model should be applied to describe its pharmacokinetics adequately. No difference in plasma half-life was found when determined in the same subject after a single dose and after multiple dosing, which suggests that neither autoinduction nor saturation of the metabolism of valproic acid occurs (GUGLER et al. 1977).

In animals, half-lives of valproic acid are considerably lower than in man, ranging from about 8 h in cats to 40 min in rhesus monkeys (Table 2). Studies by LÖSCHER (1978) suggest that the protein binding of valproic acid is rate-limiting for its clearance by the liver and may be responsible for the striking differences in the half-lives of the drug in different species. More recently, DICKINSON et al. (1979, 1980) have described that the decline in concentration of valproic acid in blood of rats and cynomolgus monkeys was dose dependent and did not follow linear first-order kinetics. In rats, enterohepatic recirculation was demonstrated. No evidence of dose-dependent kinetics was found in man, mouse, rabbit, and dog (LÖSCHER and ESENWEIN 1978; DICKINSON et al. 1979).

2. Renal Excretion

In general, the renal excretion of unchanged valproic acid is of minor importance for the elimination of the drug. In humans, only 1.8% following a single oral dose and 3.2% of one dose during chronic treatment are excreted as the unchanged drug (GUGLER et al. 1977). Similar figures have been reported in dog, rat, rabbit, and monkey (MERITS 1977; DICKINSON et al. 1979, 1980).

3. Metabolism

Biotransformation ist the major route of elimination of valproic acid in man and animals. Several metabolites have been identified which indicate four main metabolic pathways, namely glucuronidation, β-oxidation, and ω-oxidation (ω_1 and ω_2) (GUGLER and VON UNRUH 1980). These pathways appear to be as shown in Fig. 1.

Studies with ^{14}C-labeled valproic acid (MERITS 1977) have shown that the glucuronide of the drug ist the dominating metabolite in dog, monkey, and rabbit, comprising 75%–90% of the total radioactivity in urine, whereas about half of the urinary radioactivity in rat and man was due to other metabolism products. 5-Hydroxy-valproic acid was responsible for 27%–34% of urinary radioactivity in man; its content in animal urine was 1.4%–8.6%. During long-term treatment with valproic acid in man, besides valproic acid glucuronide, 3-keto-valproic acid was determined as a major metabolite in urine (KOCHEN et al. 1977; SCHÄFER and LÜHRS 1978; SCHÄFER et al. 1980). In addition, 2-*n*-propylglutaric acid was found to be a major metabolite in the urine of rabbit, rat, and man (KUHARA and MATSUMOTO 1974; FERRANDES and EYMARD 1977; KOCHEN et al. 1977).

Despite extensive work on the identification and quantification of valproic acid metabolites in urine, quantification of these compounds in plasma has only just begun. In the plasma of 26 epileptic patients, mostly adults, undergoing chronic therapy with valproic acid, the metabolic products of β-oxidation were found to be the major metabolites, averaging 9.5% (2-en-), 2,8% (3-hydroxy-), and 8.1% (3-keto-valproic acid) of the corresponding valproic acid concentrations (LÖSCHER 1981a). Besides, minor levels of 4-hydroxy- and 5-hydroxy-valproic acid were found. Accordingly, KOCHEN and SCHEFFNER (1980) reported the 2-en compound to be the major metabolite in plasma of epileptic children.

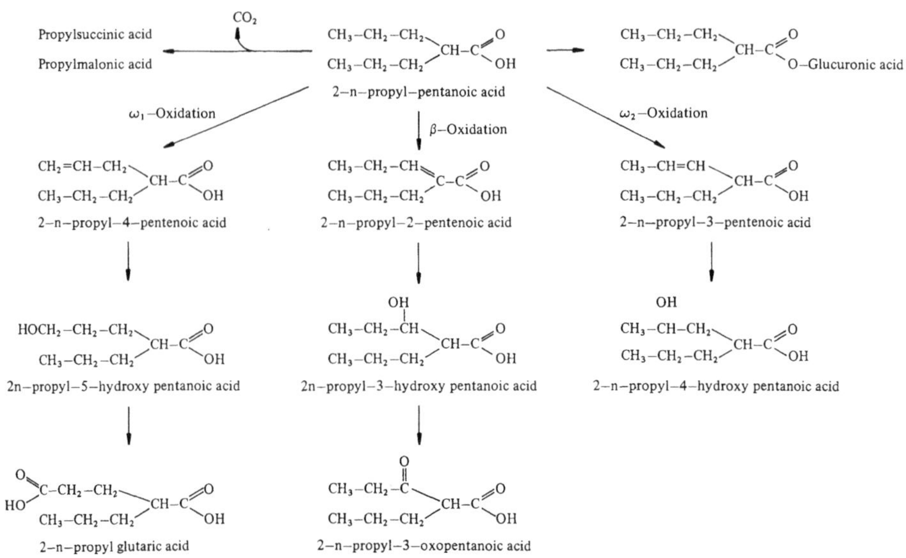

Fig. 1. Proposed metabolic pathways of valproic acid (2-*n*-propyl-pentanoic acid). All metabolites shown have been identified in urine and/or plasma following valproic acid administration in different species, including man

During continued treatment with valproic acid in dogs, plasma concentrations of 2-en-valproic acid and 3-keto-valproic acid averaged 81% and 51% of the corresponding plasma concentrations of the parent compound determined prior to the morning administration (LÖSCHER 1981e). Interestingly, accumulation of both metabolites occurred during the first days of treatment.

An open question is the contribution of valproic acid metabolites to the antiepileptic activity of the parent drug. The anticonvulsant activity of these compounds has recently been determined by studying their effects on electro- and chemoconvulsive thresholds in mice (LÖSCHER 1981f). All metabolites gave rise to significant threshold elevations but were less potent than valproic acid itself. The 2-en and 4-en unsaturated metabolites were the most active compounds, showing 50%–90% of the potency of valproic acid. However, these calculations did not account for possible differences in tissue distribution. Investigations on the concentration-time course of metabolites of valproic acid in plasma and brain of mice after acute and subacute administration of valproic acid have shown that, besides valproic acid itself, only 2-en-valproic acid occurred in the brain in significant concentrations, although other metabolites were present in plasma (LÖSCHER and NAU 1982; NAU and LÖSCHER 1982). After both acute and subacute administration, delayed (post-drug) effects on seizure threshold were observed which extended to time periods when valproic acid could no longer be detected in the brain, but the 2-en metabolite was still present.

The effects of valproic acid metabolites on brain GABA metabolism have recently been studied in mice (WEISSMAN et al. 1978; LÖSCHER et al. 1981). Administered in anticonvulsant doses, the respective compounds caused elevations in both whole brain and synaptosomal GABA levels, and a linear relationship was found between anticonvulsant potency and the relative increase in GABA concentrations of synaptosomes (LÖSCHER et al. 1981). WEISSMAN et al. (1978) have shown that 2-en-valproic acid, 350 mg/kg i.p., causes differential increases in GABA levels in discrete areas of mouse brain, varying from 10% in the hippocampus to 90% in the substantia nigra.

Neurophysiological studies have shown that inhibitory responses of single neurons in rat cortex to iontophoretic application of GABA are strikingly intensified by iontophoretically applied 2-en-valproic acid, which in this respect is more potent than valproic acid (W. LÖSCHER and D. FELIX, personal communication).

F. Drug Interactions

Clinical drug interactions with valproic acid have been reviewed by LEVY and KOCH (1982) and by PERUCCA and RICHENS (Chap. 28, this volume). In the following, only experimental data will be reviewed.

I. Effect of Valproic Acid on Other Drugs

Several authors have reported that valproic acid may alter the plasma levels of other antiepileptic drugs. Thus, valproic acid caused a remarkable elevation of phenobarbital concentrations in plasma, brain, and liver of rats (HULSHOF et al. 1977). MESDJIAN et al. (1980) studied the interaction of valproic acid and phenobarbital in rabbits and found a lower phenobarbital urinary excretion when both drugs were administered. Other studies have pointed to inhibition of phenobarbital metabolism as a mechanism of interaction (e.g., KAPETANOVIC and KUPFERBERG 1980).

In rats, valproic acid has been shown to lower plasma levels but raise brain levels of phenytoin (PATSALOS and LASCELLES 1977). This effect has been attributed at least in part to the finding that valproic acid displaces phenytoin from plasma protein binding sites, thus favoring a higher distribution of the drug with subsequent lower total plasma levels of phenytoin (PATSALOS and LASCELLES 1977; LÖSCHER 1979c). Besides effects on plasma protein binding, studies in rhesus monkeys suggest that valproic acid may inhibit phenytoin metabolism (KOCH et al. 1981). In rats, higher plasma concentrations of the principal phenytoin metabolite 5-(*p*-hydroxyphenyl)-5-phenyl-hydantoin (HPPH) were observed following administration of valproic acid (O'LEARY and SAMSOM 1981). This finding was related to inhibition by valproic acid of the glucuronidation of HPPH, whereas the half-life of phenytoin itself remained unchanged.

Besides interactions with the metabolism or protein binding of other antiepileptic drugs, marked competitive inhibition by valproic acid of aminophenazone *N*-demethylation and codeine *O*-demethylation have been determined in rat liver homogenates (BORCHERT et al. 1980).

Contrary to other antiepileptic drugs, especially the barbiturates, valproic acid has no enzyme-inducing properties. Administration to rats of daily oral doses of 100 mg/kg for 7 days did not affect the activity of hepatic enzymes, and the enzyme-inducing effects of phenobarbital were unaltered by concomitant administration of valproic acid (JORDAN et al. 1976).

II. Effect of Other Drugs on Valproic Acid

In dogs phenobarbital has been found to increase the elimination of valproic acid by a factor of 2.5–3 (VREE et al. 1977), and it was suggested that phenobarbital induces metabolism of valproic acid via the cytochrome-P 450 system. 3-Methyl cholanthrene was also active in this regard. Glucuronidation of valproic acid was not altered by phenobarbital. Similar observations were described in rats and rabbits (HULSHOF et al. 1977; MESDJIAN et al. 1980; HEINEMEYER and GUNDLACH 1981). On the other hand, phenytoin in rats did not exert a clear effect on valproic acid elimination (HULSHOF et al. 1977).

In therapeutic concentrations, phenytoin, phenobarbital, and carbamazepine were shown not to affect the binding of valproic acid to plasma proteins in dog and man (LÖSCHER 1979c).

G. Toxicity

The incidence of toxicity associated with the clinical use of valproic acid is remarkably low compared with other antiepileptic drugs. The most common side effects are transient gastrointestinal symptoms, namely anorexia, nausea, and vomiting (see SIMON and PENRY 1975; PINDER et al. 1977). Effects on the CNS, such as sedation, ataxia, and incoordination, occur very infrequently. There is, however, increasing evidence that the drug is associated with serious hepatotoxicity. To date, about 60 patients, mostly children on multiple drug therapy, are known to have died with hepatic failure in the first 6 months of treatment (JEAVONS 1984). Thus it was suggested that in all patients liver function tests should be performed before therapy is started and then repeated at frequent intervals particularly during the first 6 months of therapy, and always before increasing the dose. Raised liver transaminase levels occur in up to 44% of patients on valproic acid. They are usually transient and often occur without clinical manifestations (PINDER et al. 1977). However, studies by KINGSLEY et al. (1980) with rat hepatocyte cultures suggest that valproic acid is a hepatotoxin at concentrations ranging from 10 to 320 μg/ml.

More recently, at least seven cases of pancreatitis, including two with fatal hemorrhagic pancreatitis, have been attributed to valproic acid (PARKER et al. 1981).

Valproic acid can inhibit the secondary phase of platelet aggregation, and this may be reflected in increased bleeding times (e.g., SUTOR and JESDINSKY-BUSCHER 1974). Furthermore, relative lymphocytosis and thrombocytopenia have occasionally been reported.

The acute toxicity of valproic acid in animals is low; LD_{50} values range from 565 mg/kg (i.p.) in cats to 1 700 mg/kg (p.o.) in mice (see Table 3). Human subjects have recovered from doses as high as 36 g (PILLEN 1973). According to studies of CONINE et al. (1976), the oral LD_{50} appears to increase with animal size (surface area), that is toxicity was least in dogs (LD_{50} 28.7 g/m^2) and greatest in mice (3.54 g/m^2) and newborn male rats (0.82 g/m^2). Signs of toxicity in rodents included ataxia, sedation, hypothermia, catalepsy, and ptosis, and in dogs sedation, loss of coordination, sleep, tremors, and/or emesis (CONINE et al. 1976; LÖSCHER 1980a). Deaths usually occurred within the first 24 h following administration. In long-term studies, mice treated for 160 days with 400 mg/kg valproic acid showed a significantly higher incidence of fatalities (30%) than did control animals (PINDER et al. 1977). Studies of DIAZ and SHIELDS (1978) in young rats suggested that chronic administration of valproic acid early in life may have adverse consequences on brain development and behaviour.

Table 3. Acute toxicity of valproic acid in different species

Species	TD_{50} (mg/kg)[a]		LD_{50} (mg/kg)			Refs.
	i.p.	p.o.	i.v.	i.p.	p.o.	
Mice	415	1,165		1,060	1,700	SWINYARD (1964)
	290	580	766	838	1,197	SHUTO and NISHIGAKI (1970)
		290	750			FREY and LÖSCHER (1976)
	425	1,264		1,104		KUPFERBERG (1980)
	480			960		LÖSCHER (1980a)
Rats	188	570		790	1,530	SWINYARD (1964)
			946	1,045	1,519	SHUTO and NISHIGAKI (1970)
	365	280				KUPFERBERG (1980)
Rabbits	216			1,200		SWINYARD (1964)
	1,100	1,750			1,650	SHUTO and NISHIGAKI (1970)
Cats	105			565		SWINYARD (1964)

[a] Dose producing minimal evidence of neurotoxicity (rotorod or chimney test) in 50% of animals at time of peak drug effect

Valproic acid has been shown to produce dose-related dysmorphogenic effects in mice, rats, and rabbits, principally kidney defects, cleft palates, encephaloceles, ablepharia, and fusion of ribs and vertebrae (WHITTLE 1976). Their incidence at intermediate doses (150–200 mg/kg) was about the same as that observed with phenytoin at similar dose levels. However, because of the marked differences in pharmacokinetics of valproic acid between rodents and humans (see Table 2), embryotoxicity testing with conventional procedures, i.e., administration to pregnant animals once a day throughout organogenesis, may yield erraneous information on the embryotoxic potential of this drug. Actually, when human therapeutic levels of valproic acid were maintained in mice throughout the organogenesis period by means of constant-rate application by implanted osmotic pumps, embryotoxicity was drastically reduced from that found after conventional multiple administration of comparable drug doses (NAU et al. 1981c). Nevertheless, evidence is now accumulating that valproic acid causes teratogenic effects in humans (e.g., HURD et al. 1983).

References

Abdul-Ghani AS, Coutinho-Netto J, Druce D, Bradford HF (1981) Effects of anticonvulsants on the in vivo and in vitro release of GABA. Biochem Pharmacol 30:363–368

Alary J, Cantin D, Coeur A, Carraz G (1972) Dosage de l'acide dipropylacétique et du dipropylacétamide par chromatographie gaz-liquide. Bull Trav Soc Pharm Lyon 16:53–64

Albertson TE, Peterson SL, Stark LG (1980) Anticonvulsant drugs and their antagonism of kindled amygdaloid seizures in rats. Neuropharmacology 19:643–652

Aly MI, Abdel-Latif AA (1980) Studies on distribution and metabolism of valproate in rat brain, liver, and kidney. Neurochem Res 5:1231–1242

Anlezark G, Horton RW, Meldrum BS, Sawaya MCB (1976) Anticonvulsant action of ethanolamine-*0*-sulphate and di-*n*-propylacetate and the metabolism of γ-aminobutyric acid (GABA) in mice with audiogenic seizures. Biochem Pharmacol 25:413–417

Balázs R, Machiyama Y, Hammond BJ, Julian T, Richter D (1970) The operation of the γ-aminobutyrate bypath of the tricarboxyclic acid cycle in brain tissue in vitro. Biochem J 116:445–467

Borchert HH, Schuster S, Pfeifer S (1980) Metabolische Wechselwirkungen von Valproinsäure. Pharmazie 34:313–314

Braun SL, Tausch A, Vogt W, Jakob K, Knedel M (1981) Evaluation of a new valproic acid enzyme immunoassay and comparison with a capillary gas-chromatographic method. Clin Chem 27:169–172

Carraz G, Fiorina S (1967) Activation de la formation d'anti corps par le système réticulo-endothelial. Ann Biol Clin (Paris) 76:187

Carraz G, Fau R, Chateau R, Bonnin J (1964) Communication à propos des premiers essais cliniques sur l'activité anti-épileptique de lacide n-dipropylacétique (sel de Na). Ann Med Psychol 122:577–585

Carraz G, Bériel H, Luu-Duc H, Lebreton S (1965) Approches dans la pharmacodynamie biochimique de la structure *N*-dipropylacétique. Thérapie 20:419–426

Carraz G, Eymard P, Benel H, Lebreton S, Biotard M (1970) Structure dipropylacétique et potentialisation de l'immunité. J Pharmacol (Paris) 1:313–322

Cavazutti GB (1975) Prevention of febrile convulsions with dipropylacetate (Depakine). Epilepsia 16:647–648

Chapman AG, Riley K, Evans MC, Meldrum BS (1982) Acute effects of sodium valproate and γ-vinyl GABA on regional amino acid metabolism in the rat brain: incorporation of 2-(^{14}C)glucose into amino acids. Neurochem Res 7:1089–1105

Collier HOJ (1974) The concept of the quasi-abstinence effect and its use in the investigation of dependence mechanisms. Pharmacology 11:58–61

Conine DL, Majors KR, Lehrer S, Becker BA (1976) Acute toxicity of sodium 2-propylpentenoate, a compound whose toxicity decreases as animal size increases. Toxicol Appl Pharmacol 37:144

Costall B, Naylor RJ, Owen RT (1978) GABAminergic and serotonergic modulation of the antidyskinetic effects of tiaproide and oxiperomide in the model using 2-(*N*,*N*-dipropyl)amino-5,6-dihydroxytetralin. Eur J Pharmacol 49:407–413

Cowan A (1980) Interactional studies with sodium valproate and naloxone. Ann Neurol 7:388

Cowan A (1981) RX 366-M, a new chemical tool in the analysis of the quasi-morphine withdrawal syndrome. Fed Proc 40:1497–1501

Cowan A, Watson T (1978) Lysergic acid diethylamide antagonizes shaking induced in rats by five chemically different compounds. Psychopharmacology 57:43–46

Curtis DR, Johnston GAR (1974) Amino acid transmitters in the mammalian central nervous system. Ergeb Physiol 69:97–188

Curtis DR, Watkins JC (1963) Acidic amino acids with strong excitatory actions on mammalian neurones. J Physiol (Lond) 166:1–14

De Boer T, Metselaar HJ, Bruinvels J (1977) Suppression of GABA-induced abstinence behaviour in naive rats by morphine and bicuculline. Life Sci 20:933–942

De Boer T, Bartels K, Metselaar HJ, Bruinvels J (1980) Di-*n*-propylacetate-induced abstinence behaviour as a possible correlate of increased GABA-ergic activity in the rat. Psychopharmacology 71:257–267

De Souza Queiroz ML, Mullen PW (1980) The effects of phenytoin, 5-(para-hydroxyphenyl)-5-phenylhydantoin, and valproic acid on humoral immunity in mice. Int J Immunopharmacol 2:224–225

Diaz J, Shields WD (1978) Chronic administration of dipropylacetate early in life: effects on brain development and behavior. Ann Neurol 4:198

Dickinson RG, Harland RC, Ilias AM, Rodgers RM, Kaufman SN, Lynn RK, Gerber N (1979) Disposition of valproic acid in the rat: dose-dependent metabolism, distribution, enterohepatic recirculation and choleretic effect. J Pharmacol Exp Ther 211:583–595

Dickinson RG, Taylor SM, Kaufman SN, Rodgers RM, Lynn RL, Gerber N, Baughman WL (1980) Nonlinear elimination and choleretic effect of valproic acid in the monkey. J Pharmacol Exp Ther 213:38–48

Dijkhuis IC, Vervloet E (1974) Rapid determination of the antiepileptic drug di-*n*-propylacetic acid in serum. Pharm Weekblad [Sci] 109:42–45

Donniah P, Buchanan N (1981) Serum sodium valproate assays: comparison between EMIT and GLC methodologies. Med J Aust 1:192

Emson PC (1976) Effects of chronic treatment with amino-oxyacetic acid or sodium *n*-dipropylacetate on brain GABA levels and the development and regression of cobalt epileptic foci in rats. J Neurochem 27:1489–1494

Espir MLE, Benton P, Will E, Hayes MJ, Walker G (1976) Sodium valproate (epilim) – some clinical and pharmacological aspects. In: Legg NJ (ed) Clinical and pharmacological aspects of sodium valproate (epilim) in the treatment of epilepsy. MCS Consultants, Tunbrigde Wells, pp 145–151

Eymard P, Simiand J, Teoule R, Polverelli M, Werbenec JP, Broll M (1971) Etude de la répartition et de la resorption de dipropylacétate de sodium marque au ^{14}C chez le rat. J Pharmacol (Paris) 2:359–368

Fariello R, Mutani R (1970) Modificazioni dell'attivita del focus epilettogeno corticomotorio da allumina indotte dal sale di sodo dell'acido *n*-dipropilacetico (DPA). Acta Neurol (Napoli) 25:116–122

Ferrandes B, Eymard P (1973) Methode rapide de analyse quantitative du dipropylacetate de sodium dans le serum ou le plasma. Ann Pharm Fr 31:279–282

Ferrandes B, Eymard P (1977) Metabolism of valproate sodium in rabbit, rat, dog, and man. Epilepsia 18:169–182

Fowler LJ, Beckford J, John RA (1975) An analysis of the kinetics of the inhibition of rabbit brain γ-aminobutyrate aminotransferase by sodium *n*-dipropylacetate and some other simple carboxylic acids. Biochem Pharmacol 24:1267–1270

Frey HH, Löscher W (1976) Di-*n*-propylacetic acid – profile of anticonvulsant activity in mice. Arzneimittelforsch 26:299–301

Frey HH, Löscher W (1978) Distribution of valproate across the interface between blood and cerebrospinal fluid. Neuropharmacology 17:637–642

Frey HH, Löscher W, Reiche R, Schultz D (1983) Anticonvulsant potency of common antiepileptic drugs in the gerbil. Pharmacology 27:330–335

Godin Y, Heiner L, Mark J, Mandel P (1969) Effects of di-*n*-propylacetate, an anticonvulsive compound, on GABA metabolism. J Neurochem 16:869–873

Goldberg MA, Todoroff T (1980) Brain binding of anticonvulsants: carbamazepine and valproic acid. Neurology 30:826–831

Goldstein DB (1979) Sodium bromide and sodium valproate: effective suppressants of ethanol withdrawal reactions in mice. J Pharmacol Exp Ther 208:223–227

Gugler R, Von Unruh GE (1980) Clinical pharmacokinetics of valproic acid. Clin Pharmacokinet 5:67–83

Gugler R, Schell A, Eichelbaum M, Fröscher W, Schulz HU (1977) Disposition of valproic acid in man. Eur J Clin Pharmacol 12:125–132

Hammond EJ, Wilder BJ. Bruni J (1981) Central actions of valproic acid in man and in experimental models of epilepsy. Life Sci 29:2561–2574

Harding GFA, Herrick CE, Jeavons PM (1978) A controlled study of the effect of sodium valproate on photosensitive epilepsy and its prognosis. Epilepsia 19:555–565

Harvey PKP, Bradford HF, Davison AN (1975) The inhibitory effect of sodium *n*-dipropyl acetate on the degradative enzymes of the GABA shunt. FEBS Lett 52:251–254

Heinemeyer G, Gundlach J (1981) Modification of valproic acid metabolism by phenobarbital and clofibrate. Naunyn-Schmiedebergs Arch Pharmacol 316:[Suppl 1] R4

Hillbom ME (1975) The prevention of ethanol withdrawal seizures in rats by dipropylacetate. Neuropharmacology 14:755–761

Horton RW, Anlezark GM, Sawaya MCB, Meldrum BS (1977) Monoamine and GABA metabolism and the anticonvulsant action of di-*n*-propylacetate and ethanolamine-*O*-sulphate. Eur J Pharmacol 41:387–397

Hulshof JAM, Schobben F, Van Der Kleijn E (1977) The interactions of 2-propyl pentanoate with phenobarbital and with phenytoin in rat. Pharm Weekblad [Sci] 112:326–329

Hurd RW, Wilder BJ, Van Rinsvelt HA (1983) Valproate, birth defects, and zinc. Lancet II:181

Hwang EC, Van Woert MH (1979) Effect of valproic acid on serotonin metabolism. Neuropharmacology 18:391–397

Iadarola MJ, Gale K (1979) Dissociation between drug-induced increases in nerve terminal and non-nerve terminal pools of GABA in vivo. Eur J Pharmacol 59:125–129

Iadarola MJ, Raines A, Gale K (1979) Differential effects of *n*-diprophylacetate and amino-oxyacetic acid on γ-aminobutyric acid levels in discrete areas of rat brain. J Neurochem 33:1119–1123

Jaekeen J, Corbeel L, Carchon H, Casaer P, Eeckels R, Eggermon E (1977) Dipropylacetate (valproate) and glycine metabolism. Lancet II:617

Jeavons PM (1984) Non-dose related side effects of valproate. Epilepsia 25 [Suppl. I]:50–55

Jordan BJ, Shillingford JS, Steed KP (1976) Preliminary observations on the protein-binding and enzyme-inducing properties of sodium valproate (epilim). In: Legg (NJ (ed) Clinical and pharmacological aspects of sodium valproate (epilim) in the treatment of epilepsy. MCS Consultants, Tunbridge Wells, pp 112–118

Julien RM, Fowler GW (1977) A comparative study of the efficacy of newer antiepileptic drugs on experimentally-induced febrile convulsions. Neuropharmacology 16:719–724

Jung MJ (1978) In vivo biochemistry of GABA transaminase inhibition. In: Seiler N, Jung MJ, Koch-Weser J (eds) Enzyme-activated irreversible inhibitors. Elsevier, Amsterdam, pp 135–148

Kapetanovic IM, Kupferberg HJ (1980) Inhibition of microsomal phenobarbital metabolism by valproic acid. Fed Proc 39:1099

Kerwin RW, Olpe HR, Schmutz M (1980) The effect of sodium-n-dipropyl acetate on γ-aminobutyric acid dependent inhibition in the rat cortex and substantia nigra in relation to its anticonvulsant activity. Br J Pharmacol 71:545–551

Kingsley E, Tweedale R, Tolman KG (1980) Hepatotoxicity of sodium valproate and other anticonvulsants in rat hepatocyte cultures. Epilepsia 21:699–704

Klotz U (1977) Pharmacokinetic studies with valproic acid in man. Arzneimittelforsch 27:1085–1088

Klotz U, Antonin KH (1977) Pharmacokinetics and bioavailability of di-*n*-propylacetate (sodium valproate) in man. Clin Pharmacol Ther 21:736–743

Koch KM, Ludwick BT, Levy RH (1981) Phenytoin-valproic acid interaction in rhesus monkey. Epilepsia 22:19–25

Kochen W, Scheffner H (1980) On unsaturated metabolites of the valproic acid (VPA) in serum of epileptic children. In: Johannessen SI, Morselli PL, Pippenger CE, Richens A, Schmidt D, Meinardi H (eds) Antiepileptic therapy: advances in drug monitoring. Raven, New York, pp 111–117

Kochen W, Imbeck H, Jakobs C (1977) Untersuchungen über die Ausscheidung von Metaboliten der Valproinsäure im Urin der Ratte und des Menschen. Arzneimittelforsch 27:1090–1099

Krall RL, Penry JK, White BG, Kupferberg HJ, Swinyard EA (1978) Antiepileptic drug development. II. Anticonvulsant drug screening. Epilepsia 19:409–428
Krogsgaard-Larsen P (1980) Inhibitors of the GABA uptake systems. Mol Cell Biochem 31:105–121
Kuhara T, Matsumoto I (1974) Metabolism of branched medium chain length fatty acid. I. Oxidation of sodium dipropylacetate in rats. Biomed Mass Spectrom 1:291–294
Kukino K, Deguchi T (1977) Effects of sodium dipropylacetate on γ-aminobutyric acid and biogenic amines in rat brain. Chem Pharm Bull (Tokyo) 25:2257–2262
Kulig BM, Gonzales-Portal C, Somoza E, DeFeudis FV (1977) Effect of di-*n*-propylacetate on the "binding" of GABA to a synaptosome-enriched fraction of rat cerebral cortex. Psychopharmacology 53:255–257
Kupferberg HJ (1980) Sodium valproate. In: Glaser GH, Penry JK, Woodbury DM (eds) Antiepileptic drugs: mechanism of action. Raven, New York, pp 643–654
Kuruvilla A, Uretsky NJ (1981) Effect of sodium valproate on motor function regulated by the activation of GABA receptors. Psychopharmacology 72:167–172
Lacolle JY, Ferrandes B, Eymard P (1978) Profile of anticonvulsant activity of sodium valproate. Role of GABA. In: Meinardi H, Rowan AJ (eds) Advances in epileptology. Psychology, pharmacotherapy and new diagnosic approaches. Swets and Zeitlinger, Amsterdam, pp 162–167
Lal H, Shearman GT (1980) Effect of valproic acid on anxiety-related behaviours in the rat. Brain Res Bull 5:[Suppl 2] 575–577
Lautin A, Angrist B, Stanley M, Gershon S, Heckl K, Karobath M (1980) Sodium valproate in schizophrenia: some biochemical correlates. Br J Psychiatr 137:240–244
Lebreton S, Carraz G, Beriel H, Meunier H (1964) Propriétés pharmacodynamiques de l'acide *N*-dipropylacétique. Thérapie 19:457–467
Leviel V, Naquet R (1977) A study of the action of valproic acid on the kindling effect. Epilepsia 18:229–234
Levy RH (1980) CSF and plasma pharmacokinetics: relationship to mechanisms of action as exemplified by valproic acid in monkey. In: Lockard JS, Ward AA (eds) Epilepsy: a window to brain mechanisms. Raven, New York, pp 191–200
Levy RH, Koch KM (1982) Drug interactions with valproic acid. Drugs 24:543–556
Lockard JS, Levy RH (1976) Valproic acid: reversibly acting drug? Epilepsia 17:477–479
Löscher W (1977) Rapid determination of valproate sodium in serum by gas chromatography. Epilepsia 18:225–227
Löscher W (1978) Serum protein binding and pharmacokinetics of valproate in man, dog, rat, and mouse. J Pharmacol Exp Ther 204:255–261
Löscher W (1979a) 3-Mercaptopropionic acid: convulsant properties, effects on enzymes of the γ-aminobutyrate system in mouse brain and antagonism by certain anticonvulsant drugs, aminooxyacetic acid and gabaculine. Biochem Pharmacol 28:1397–1407
Löscher W (1979b) GABA in plasma and cerebrospinal fluid of different species. Effects of γ-acetylenic GABA, γ-vinyl GABA and sodium valproate. J Neurochem 32:1587–1591
Löscher W (1979c) A comparative study of the protein binding of anticonvulsant drugs in serum of dog and man. J Pharmacol Exp Ther 208:429–435
Löscher W (1980a) A comparative study of the pharmacology of inhibitors of GABA-metabolism. Naunyn-Schmiedebergs Arch Pharmacol 315:119–128
Löscher W (1980b) Effect of inhibitors of GABA transaminase on the synthesis, binding, uptake, and metabolism of GABA. J Neurochem 34:1603–1608
Löscher W (1981a) Concentration of metabolites of valproic acid in plasma of epileptic patients. Epilepsia 22:169–179
Löscher W (1981b) Correlation between alterations in brain GABA metabolism and seizure excitability following administration of GABA aminotransferase inhibitors and valproic acid – a re-evaluation. Neurochem Int 3:397–404
Löscher W (1981c) Valproate induced changes in GABA metabolism at the subcellular level. Biochem Pharmacol 30:1364–1366
Löscher W (1981d) Zum Wirkungsmechanismus der Antiepileptika. Tierexperimentelle Befunde zur Bedeutung von Neurotransmittern. Nervenarzt 52:61–67

Löscher W (1981e) Plasma levels of valproic acid and its metabolites during continued treatment in dogs. J Vet Pharmacol Ther 4:111–119
Löscher W (1981f) Anticonvulsant activity of metabolites of valproic acid. Arch Int Pharmacodyn Ther 249:158–163
Löscher W (1982a) GABA in plasma, CSF and brain of dogs during acute and chronic treatment with γ-acetylenic GABA and valproic acid. In: Okada Y, Roberts E (eds) Problems in GABA research. From brain to bacteria. Excerpta Medica, Amsterdam, pp 102–109
Löscher W (1982b) Cardiovascular effects of GABA, GABA aminotransferase inhibitors and valproic acid following systemic administration in rats, cats, and dogs. Arch Int Pharmacodyn Ther 257:32–58
Löscher W (1983) Alterations in CSF GABA levels and seizure susceptibility developing during repeated administration of pentetrazole in dogs. Effects of γ-acetylenic GABA, valproic acid and phenobarbital. Neurochem Int 5:405–412
Löscher W, Esenwein H (1978) Pharmacokinetics of sodium valproate in dog and mouse. Arzneimittelforsch 28:782–787
Löscher W, Frey HH (1977a) Effect of convulsant and anticonvulsant agents on level and metabolism of γ-aminobutyric acid in mouse brain. Naunyn-Schmiedebergs Arch Pharmacol 296:263–269
Löscher W, Frey HH (1977b) Zum Wirkungsmechanismus von Valproinsäure. Arzneimittelforsch 28:1081–1082
Löscher W, Göbel W (1978) Consecutive gas chromatographic determination of phenytoin, phenobarbital, primidone, phenylethylmalondiamide, carbamazepine, trimethadione, dimethadione, ethosuximide, and valproate from the sam serum specimen. Epilepsia 21:611–615
Löscher W, Nau H (1982) Valproic acid: metabolite concentrations in plasma and brain, anticonvulsant activity, and effects on GABA metabolism during subacute treatment in mice. Arch Int Pharmacodyn Ther 257:20–31
Löscher W, Schmidt D (1980) Increase of human plasma GABA by sodium valproate. Epilepsia 21:611–615
Löscher W, Schmidt D (1981) Plasma GABA levels in neurological patients under treatment with valproic acid. Life Sci 28:2383–2388
Löscher W, Siemens H (1984) Valproic acid increases γ-aminobutyric acid in CSF of epileptic children. Lancet II:225
Löscher W, Böhme G, Schäfer H, Kochen W (1981) Effect of metabolites of valproic acid on the metabolism of GABA in brain and brain nerve endings. Neuropharmacology 20:1187–1192
Löscher W, Frey HH, Reiche R, Schultz D (1983) High anticonvulsant potency of GABA-mimetic drugs in gerbils with genetically determined epilepsy. J Pharmacol Exp Ther 226:839–844
Loskota WJ, Lomax P, Rich ST (1974) The gerbil as a model for the study of the epilepsies. Epilepsia 15:109–119
Lust WD, Kupferberg HJ, Passonneau JV, Penry JK (1976) On the mechanism of action of sodium valproate: the relationship of GABA and cyclic GMP in anticonvulsant activity. In: Legg NJ (ed) Clinical and pharmacological aspects of sodium valproate (epilim) in the treatment of epilepsy. MCS Consultants, Tunbrigde Wells, pp 123–129
Lust WD, Kupferberg HJ, Yonekawa WD, Penry JK, Passoneau JV, Wheaton AB (1978) Changes in brain metabolites induced by convulsants or electroshock: effects of anticonvulsant agents. Molec Pharmacol 14:347–356
Marcus RJ, Winters WD, Hultin E (1976) Neuropharmacological effects induced by butanol, 4-hydroxybutyrate, 4-mercaptobutyric acid, thiolactone, tetrahydrofuran, pyrrolidone, 2-deoxy-*d*-glucose and related substances in the rat. Neuropharmacology 15:229–238
Martinek Z, Arbeiter E (1980) Beitrag zur antikonvulsiven Wirkung von Dipropylessigsäure (DPA) bei Hunden. Kleintier-Praxis 25:275–280
McCandless DW, Feussner GK, Lust WD, Passoneau JV (1979) Metabolite levels in brain following experimental seizures: the effects of isoniazid and sodium valproate in cerebellar and cerebral cortical layers. J Neurochem 32:755–760

Meijer JW, Hessing-Brand L (1973) Determination of lower fatty acids, particularly the anti-epileptic dipropyl-acetic acid, in biological materials by means of micro diffusion and gas chromatography. Clin Chim Acta 43:215–222

Meldrum B (1978) Neurotransmitters and epilepsy. In: Legg NJ (ed) Neurotransmitter systems and their clinical disorders. Academic, London, pp 167–181

Meldrum B (1979) Convulsant drugs, anticonvulsants and GABA-mediated neuronal inhibition. In: Krogsgaard-Larsen P, Scheel-Krüger J, Kofod H (eds) GABA-neurotransmitters. Munksgaard, Copenhagen, pp 309–405

Meldrum BS, Anlezark GM, Ashton CG, Horton RW, Sawaya CB (1977) Neurotransmitters and anticonvulsant drug action. In: Majkowski J (ed) Epilepsy. ILEA, Warsaw, pp 139–153

Merits I (1977) Metabolic fate of valproate sodium in dog, rat, rabbit, monkey, and human. Epilepsia 18:289–290

Mesdjian E, Valli M, Bruguerolle B, Jadot G, Bouyard P, Mandel P (1980) Phenobarbitone and sodium valproate interaction: an experimental study. Prog Neuropsychopharmacol 4:247–252

Meunier H, Carraz G, Meunier Y, Eymard P, Aimard M (1963) Propriétés pharmacodynamiques de l'acide *n*-dipropylacétique. ler memoire: propriétés antiépileptiques. Thérapie 18:435–438

Misslin R, Ropartz P, Mandel P (1972) Effets du di *n*-propylacétate sur l'activité spontanée et conditionée de la souris. CR Seances Acad Sci (III.) 275:1279–1281

Mortensen PB, Kolvraa S, Christensen E (1980) Inhibition of the glycine cleavage system: hyperglycinemia and hyperglycinuria caused by valproic acid. Epilepsia 21:563–569

Nagao T, Ohshimo T, Mitsunobo K, Sato M, Otsuki S (1979) Cerebrospinal fluid monoamine metabolites and cyclic nucleotides in chronic schizophrenic patients with tardive dyskinesia or drug-induced tremor. Biol Psychiatry 14:509–523

Nau H, Löscher W (1982) Valproic acid: brain and plasma levels of the drug and its metabolites, anticonvulsant effects and GABA metabolism in the mouse. J Pharmacol Exp Ther 220:654–659

Nau H, Wittfoht W, Schäfer H, Jakobs C, Rating D, Helge H (1981 a) Valproic acid and several metabolites: quantitative determination in serum, urine, breast milk and tissues by gas chromatography-mass spectrometry using selected ion monitoring. J Chromatogr 226:69–78

Nau H, Rating D, Koch S, Häuser I, Helge H (1981 b) Valproic acid and its metabolites: placental transfer, neonatal pharmacokinetics, transfer via mother's milk and clinical status in neonates of epileptic mothers. J Pharmacol Exp Ther 219:768–777

Nau H, Zierer R, Spielmann H, Neubert D, Gansau C (1981 c) A new model for embryotoxicity testing: teratogenicity and pharmacokinetics of valproic acid following constant-rate administration in the mouse human therapeutic drug and metabolite concentrations. Life Sci 29:2803–2814

Noble EP, Gillies R, Vigran R, Mandel P (1976) The modification of the ethanol withdrawal syndrome in rats by di-*n*-propylacetate. Psychopharmacology 46:127–131

Noebels JL, Sidman RL (1979) Inherited epilepsy: spike wave and focal motor seizures in the mutant mouse tottering. Science 204:1334–1336

Noronha MJ, Bevan PLT (1976) A literature review of unwanted effects with epilim. In: Legg NJ (ed) Clinical and pharmacological aspects of sodium valproate (epilim) in the treatment of epilepsy. MCS Consultants, Tunbridge Wells, pp 61–65

Nutt J, Williams A, Plotkin C, Eng N, Ziegler M, Calne DB (1979) Treatment of Parkinson's disease with sodium valproate: clinical, pharmacological and biochemical observations. Can J Neurol Sci 6:337–343

Oelkers W, Stoffels G, Schäfer H, Reith H (1977) Zur enteralen Resorption von Valproinsäure. Arzneimittelforsch 27:1088–1090

O'Leary TD, Sansom LN (1981) Interaction between phenytoin, 5-(*p*-hydroxyphenyl)-5-phenylhydantoin and valproate in the rat. J Pharmacol Exp Ther 216:613–616

Olsen RW, Ticku MK, Greenlee D, Van Ness P (1979) GABA receptor and ionophore binding sites: interaction with various drugs. In: Krogsgaard-Larsen P, Scheel-Krüger J, Kofod H (eds) GABA-neurotransmitters. Munksgaard, Copenhagen, pp 165–178

Parker PH, Helinek GL, Gishan FK, Greene HL (1981) Recurrent pancreatitis induced by valproic acid. A case report and review of the literature. Gastroenterology 80:826–828
Patel BC, Crosset P, Klawans HL (1975) Failure of increased brain γ-aminobutyric acid levels to influence amphetamine-induced stereotyped behavior. Res Commun Chem Pathol Pharmacol 12:635–643
Patry G, Naquet R (1971) Action de l'acide dipropylacetique chez le *Papio papio* photosensible. Can J Physiol Pharmacol 49:568–572
Patsalos PN, Lascelles PT (1977) Effect of sodium valproate on plasma protein binding of diphenylhydantoin. J Neurol Neurosurg Psychiatr 40:570–574
Perry T, Hansen S (1978) Biochemical effects in man and rat of three drugs which can increase brain GABA content. J Neurochem 30:679–684
Phillips NI, Fowler LJ (1982) The effects of sodium valproate on γ-aminobutyrate metabolism and behavior in naive and ethanolamine-*O*-sulphate pretreated rats and mice. Biochem Pharmacol 31:2257–2261
Pillen E (1973) Case report on file. Labaz, Paris
Pinder RM, Brogden RN, Speight TM, Avery GS (1977) Sodium valproate: a review of its pharmacological properties and therapeutic efficacy in epilepsy. Drugs 13:81–123
Rotiroli D, Palella B, Losi E, Nistico G, Caputi AP (1982) Evidence that a GABAergic mechanism influences the development of DOCA-salthypertension in the rat. Eur J Pharmacol 83:153–154
Sarhan S, Seiler N (1979) Metabolic inhibitors and subcellular distribution of GABA. J Neurosci Res 4:399–421
Schäfer H, Lührs R (1978) Metabolite pattern of valproic acid. Part I: Gas chromatographic determination of the valproic acid metabolite artifacts, heptanone-3, 4- and 5-hydroxyvalproic acid lactone. Arzneimittelforsch 28:657–662
Schäfer H, Lührs R, Reith H (1980) Chemistry, pharmacokinetics, and biological activity of some metabolites of valproic acid. In: Johannessen SI, Morselli PL, Pippenger CE, Richens A, Schmidt D, Meinardi H (eds) Antiepileptic therapy: advances in drug monitoring. Raven, New York, pp 103–110
Schechter PJ, Tranier Y, Grove J (1978) Effect of *n*-dipropylacetate on amino acid concentrations in mouse brain: correlations with anti-convulsant activity. J Neurochem 3:1325–1327
Schmidt D (1976) Salivary concentrations of antiepileptic drugs. Lancet II:639
Schnitger G (1984) Versuche an Ratten zur gastroenteralen Resorption von Valproinsäure. Dissertation, Freie Universität Berlin, Fachbereich Veterinärmedizin
Schobben F, Van Der Kleijn E (1974a) Determination of sodium di-*n*-propylacetate in plasma by gas-liquid chromatography. Pharm Weekblad [Sci] 109:30–33
Schobben F, Van Der Kleijn E (1974b) Pharmacokinetics of distribution and elimination of sodium di-*n*-propylacetate in mouse and dog. Pharm Weekblad [Sci] 109:33–41
Schobben F, Van Der Kleijn E, Vree TB (1980) Therapeutic monitoring of valproic acid. Ther Drug Monit 2:61–67
Schultz D (1983) Versuche mit einfachen tierexperimentellen Modellen der Petit-mal Epilepsien. Dissertation, Freie Universität Berlin, Fachbereich Veterinärmedizin
Schwarcz R, Bennett JP, Coyle JT (1977) Inhibitors of GABA metabolism: implications for Huntington's disease. Ann Neurol 2:299–303
Shuto K, Nishigaki T (1970) The pharmacological studies on sodium dipropylacetate anticonvulsant activities and general pharmacological actions (in Japanese). Pharmacometrics 4:937–949
Similae S, Von Wendt L, Linna SL, Saukkonen AL, Huhtaniemi I (1979) Dipropylacetate and hyperglycemia. Neuropaediatrie 1:158–160
Similae S, Von Wendt L, Linna SL (1980) Dipropylacetate and aminoaciduria. J Neurol Sci 45:83–86
Simler S, Randrianarisoa H, Lehmann A, Mandel P (1968) Effets du di-*n*-propylacétate sur les crises audiogènes de la souris. J Physiol (Paris) 60:547
Simler S, Ciesielski L, Maitre M, Randrianarisoa H, Mandel P (1973) Effect of sodium *n*-dipropylacetate on audiogenic seizures and brain γ-aminobutyric acid level. Biochem Pharmacol 22:1701–1708

Simler S, Gensburger C, Ciesielski L, Mandel P (1978) Time course of the increase in GABA level in different mice brain regions following *n*-dipropylacetate treatment. Commun Psychopharmacol 2:123–130

Simler S, Ciesielski L, Klein M, Gobaille S, Mandel P (1981) Sur le mécanisme d'action d'un anticonvulsivant, le dipropylacétate de sodium. C R Soc Biol (Paris) 175:114–119

Simon D, Penry JK (1975) Sodium di-*n*-propylacetate (DPA) in the treatment of epilepsy. Epilepsia 16:549–573

Snead OC (1978) Gamma-hydroxybutyrate in the monkey. I. Electroencephalographic, behavioral, and pharmacokinetic studies. Neurology 28:636–642

Sutor AH, Jesdinky-Buscher C (1974) Coagulation changes caused by dipropylacetic acid. Med Welt 25:447–448

Swanson BN, Harland RC, Dickinson RG, Gerber N (1978) Excretion of valproic acid into semen of rabbits and man. Epilepsia 19:541–546

Swinyard EA (1964) The pharmacology of dipropylacetic acid sodium with special emphasis on its effects on the central nervous system. University of Utah, College of Pharmacy, Salt Lake City, Utah, pp 1–25

Swinyard EA (1969) Laboratory evaluation of antiepileptic drugs. Review of laboratory methods. Epilepsia 10:107–119

Taberner PV, Charington CB, Unwin JW (1980) Effects of GAD and GABA-T inhibitors on GABA metabolism in vivo. Brain Res Bull 5 [Suppl 2]:621–625

Ticku MK, Davis WC (1981) Effect of valproic acid on (^{3}H)diazepam and (^{3}H)dihydroxypicrotoxinin binding sites at the benzodiazepine-GABA receptor-ionophore complex. Brain Res 223:218–222

Ticku MK, Olsen RW (1978) Interaction of barbiturates with dihydropicrotoxinin binding sites related to the GABA receptor-ionophore system. Life Sci 22:1643–1652

Turner AJ, Whittle SR (1980) Sodium valproate, GABA and epilepsy. Trends Pharmacol Sci 1:257–260

Vadja FJ, Donnan GA, Phillips J, Bladin PF (1981) Human brain, plasma, and cerebrospinal fluid concentration of sodium valproate after 72 hours of therapy. Neurology 31:486–487

Van Der Laan JW, De Boer T, Bruinvels J (1979) Di-*n*-propylacetate and GABA degradation. Peferential inhibition of succinic semialdehyde dehydrogenase and indirect inhibition of GABA-transaminase. J Neurochem 32:1769–1780

Van Der Laan JW, Jakobs AWC, Bruinvels J (1980) Effects of branched-chain fatty acids on GABA-degradation and behavior: further evidence for a role of GABA in quasi-morphine abstinence behavior. Pharmacol Biochem Behav 13:843–849

Van Duijn, Beckmann MKF (1975) Dipropylacetic acid (depakine) in experimental epilepsy in the alert cat. Epilepsia 16:83–88

Vree TB, Damsma J, Van Der Kleijn E (1977) Increase of the clearance of 2-propyl pentenoate in dogs undergoing concomitant administration of phenobarbital and 3-methyl cholanthrene. Pharm Weekblad [Sci] 112:316–319

Wada JA (1977) Pharmacological prophylaxis in the kindling model of epilepsy. Arch Neurol 34:389–395

Walters JR, Lakoski JM, Eng N, Waszcak BL (1979) Effect of muscimol, AOAA and Na valproate on the activity of dopamine neurons and dopamine synthesis. In: Krogsgaard-Larsen P, Scheel-Krüger J, Kofod H (eds) GABA-neurotransmitters. Munksgaard, Copenhagen, pp 118–134

Weissman D, Simler S, Ciesielski L, Mandel P (1978) Variations de la teneur en GABA de certaines zones du cerveau de la souris sous l'effet de l'acide propyl-2-pentène-2 oique. C R Soc Biol (Paris) 172:707–712

Werman R, Davidoff A, Aprison MH (1968) Inhibitory actions of glycine on spinal neurons in the cat. J Neurophysiol 31:81–87

Whittle BA (1976) Pre-clinical teratological studies on sodium valproate (epilim) and other anticonvulsants. In: Legg NJ (ed) Clinical and pharmacological aspects of sodium valproate (epilim) in the treatment of epilepsy. MCS Consultants Tunbridge Wells, pp 105–110

Whittle SR, Turner AJ (1978) Effects of the anticonvulsant sodium valproate on γ-aminobutyrate and aldehyde metabolism in ox brain. J Neurochem 31:1453–1459
Whittle SR, Turner AJ (1982) Effects of anticonvulsants on the formation of γ-hydroxybutyrate from γ-aminobutyrate in rat brain. J Neurochim 38:848–851
Wilensky AJ (1980) Antiepileptic drugs in the central nervous system. In: Lockard JS, Ward AA (eds) Epilepsy: a window to brain mechanisms. Raven, New York, pp 201–213
Wittfoht W, Nau H, Rating D, Helge H (1982) ^{13}C-labeled valproic acid pulse dosing during steady state antiepileptic therapy for pharmacokinetic studies during pregnancy. In: Schmidt HL, Förstel H, Heinzinger K (eds) Stable isotopes. Elsevier, Amsterdam, pp 265–270
Wood JD, Russell MP, Kurylo E, Newstead JD (1979) Stability of synaptosomal GABA levels and their use in determining the in vivo effects of drugs: convulsant agents. J Neurochem 33:61–68
Woodbury DM (1972) Applications to drug evaluation. In: Purpura DP, Penry JK, Tower D, Woodbury DM, Walter R (eds) Experimental models of epilepsy. Raven, New York, pp 557–583
Worms P, Lloyd KG (1981) Functional alterations of GABA synapses in relation to seizures. In: Morselli PL, Lloyd KG, Löscher W, Meldrum BS, Reynolds EH (eds) Neurotransmitters, seizures, and epilepsy. Raven, New York, pp 37–46
Wulff K, Flachs H, Würtz-Jörgensen A, Gram L (1977) Clinical pharmacological aspects of valproate sodium. Epilepsia 18:149–157
Zimmer R, Teelken AW, Gündürewa M, Rüther E, Cramer H (1980) Effect of sodium-valproate on CSF GABA, cAMP, cGMP and homovanillic acid levels in man. Brain Res Bull 5 [Suppl 2]:585–588

CHAPTER 18

Oxazolidinediones

R. KRETZSCHMAR and H. J. TESCHENDORF

A. Introduction

Until the introduction of succinimides for therapeutic use in 1960, oxazolidinediones were the drugs of choice in the treatment of petit mal epilepsy. They had been used since 1946. Now the oxazolidinediones are merely of historical interest since their clinical tolerance is unequivocally inferior to that of the succinimides. Nevertheless, their pharmacology deserves detailed consideration since they were the first relatively selective petit mal antiepileptics on which intensive experimental investigations of the type and mechanisms of action were carried out. Several reviews have dealt with oxazolidinediones (WOODBURY et al. 1972, 1982; WITHROW 1980). For structure-activity relationship see Chap. 9, this volume.

Two oxazolidinediones were used in therapy and are sometimes still used today: trimethadione and paramethadione:

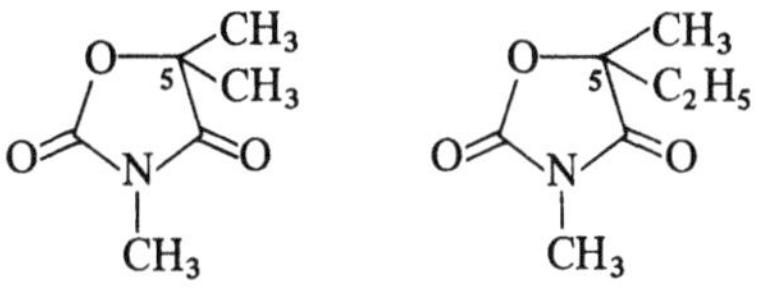

Trimethadione Paramethadione

This chapter reports on the pharmacological and toxicological properties of the oxazolidinediones mainly in the light of results obtained with trimethadione, supplemented by results obtained with paramethadione and dimethadione, the metabolite of trimethadione.

B. Anticonvulsant Effects

Trimethadione and paramethadione have a distinct anticonvulsant action in the majority of the various experimental seizure models mentioned below. The most important effect, however, is pentylenetetrazol antagonism, with inhibition of clonic-tonic seizures. On the other hand, efficacy in electroshock is less pronounced. It has been the aim of numerous experiments to find an experimental equivalent of petit mal seizures or a method for predicting anti-petit mal effects of new compounds. According to the available literature, this seems to be only true of two recently described models: the syndrome similar to petit mal epilepsy, induced by gamma-hydroxybutyrate or leucine enkephalin (GODSCHALK et al. 1976; SNEAD and BEARDEN 1980; SNEAD et al. 1980).

Since the investigations of BUTLER (1953), only a surprisingly small number of studies have become available on the anticonvulsant effect of dimethadione, the main metabolite of trimethadione. According to the results available the anticonvulsant effect of dimethadione is not in doubt. It is to be assumed that, with chronic administration necessary for therapeutic use, a large part of the trimethadione effect is due to dimethadione.

The ED_{50} values found in the various test models show that the efficacy of dimethadione is lower than that of trimethadione when given orally. In a direct comparison of the two substances given i.v. FREY (1969) found trimethadione to be more effective by a factor of 1.25. Taking central availability into account, however, dimethadione has been shown to be more effective (THUESON et al. 1974; WITHROW 1980).

I. Chemically Induced Convulsions

1. Pentylenetetrazol

EVERETT and RICHARDS (EVERETT and RICHARDS 1944; RICHARDS and EVERETT 1944) were the first to report on the effect of trimethadione on convulsions elicited by pentylenetetrazol. The capacity of trimethadione for antagonizing the effects of pentylenetetrazol has since been confirmed by numerous authors and described in detail for many effects of pentylenetetrazol. Clonic-tonic convulsions produced by pentylenetetrazol are inhibited in mice, rats, rabbits, cats, monkeys, and chickens by trimethadione, with ED_{50} values of 240–600 mg/kg, depending on species, age of the experimental animals, route of administration, and dose of pentylenetetrazol needed to elicit convulsions (GOODMAN and MANUEL 1945; GOODMAN et al. 1946a, b; RICHARDS 1946; TOMAN and GOODMAN 1948; SWINYARD 1949; TOMAN 1949, CHEN and ENSOR 1950; SWINYARD 1952a; GOODMAN et al. 1953; SANDERS 1967; FERNGREN 1968; BONNEVAUX et al. 1968; AHMAD and DHAWAN 1969; SWINYARD 1969; BAXTER et al. 1973; IORIO et al. 1973; DESMEDT et al. 1976; LÖSCHER and FREY 1977; GO et al. 1978a; KRALL et al. 1978; LAHAN et al. 1979; STONE and JAVID 1979).

Paramethadione is more potent than trimethadione in clonic-tonic convulsions induced by pentylenetetrazol. ED_{50} values of 64–150 mg/kg are found, the corresponding values for trimethadione being two to five times higher (SWINYARD 1949; CHEN et al. 1951; SWINYARD et al. 1952a; BROWN et al. 1953; GOODMAN et al. 1953; DESMEDT et al. 1976; KRALL et al. 1978). For dimethadione FREY (1969) reported ED_{50} values of between 360 and 790 mg/kg in mice with i.v. administration, depending on the latency period between administration of the drug and pentylenetetrazol. According to FERNGREN (1968), the ED_{50} values of dimethadione in 1- to 21-day-old mice vary between 200 and 1,200 mg/kg.

The interdependence of the anticonvulsant dose of trimethadione and the convulsant dose of pentylenetetrazol is very clearly demonstrated by the finding that the convulsant threshold dose of pentylenetetrazol can be augmented up to 15-fold by 100–1,600 mg/kg trimethadione (CHEN and PORTMAN 1952). This dependency was also shown by LOEWE et al. (1955) with isobolic graphs of the combination of trimethadione and pentylenetetrazol. As was demonstrated by DESMEDT et al. (1976), the various components in the course of convulsions after a fixed dose of pentylenetetrazol can be inhibited by different doses of trimethadione.

The tonic convulsion of the hindlimbs in rats can be suppressed by lower doses of trimethadione or paramethadione, whereas higher doses are required to inhibit tonic convulsions of the forelimbs and clonic convulsions; and for the inhibition of tremor, doses twice as high are needed.

By the repeated administration of pentylenetetrazol in a dose eliciting clonic seizures when given as a single dose, violent seizures, which can be referred to as a kindling phenomenon, can be elicited (ITO et al. 1977 a). For inhibition of these seizures higher doses of trimethadione are required than with a single administration of pentylenetetrazol.

Convulsant patterns in the EEG provoked by pentylenetetrazol are abolished by trimethadione (BIRCHER et al. 1963; GARDNER and WEBSTER 1973, 1977), and the threshold doses of pentylenetetrazol required to produce EEG changes (dysrhythmias, paroxysms) are increased by trimethadione (GOODMAN et al. 1946 a, b; FAINGOLD and BERRY 1973 b).

Trimethadione also abolishes biochemical changes associated with pentylenetetrazol-induced EEG changes or convulsions, such as increased release of acetylcholine from the cortical surface in rats (GARDNER and WEBSTER 1973, 1977), an increase of 5-hydroxytryptamine (5-HT) and a decrease of 5-hydroxyindoleacetic acid (5-HIAA) in the brain of rats (DIAZ 1974), and an increase of prostaglandins ($PgF_{2\alpha}$ and PgE_2) and of thromboxan (TBX_2) in the brain of mice (STEINHAUER et al. 1979).

2. Other Convulsant Substances

Tonic-clonic convulsions in mice (RÜMKE 1961; GO et al. 1978 a) and seizure patterns in the EEG of rabbits (GO et al. 1978 b) elicited by bemegride are abolished by trimethadione in doses which are effective against pentylenetetrazol.

Trimethadione increases the convulsant dose of picrotoxin (STONE and JAVID 1979) and eliminates the convulsive discharges in the EEG of dogs (BIRCHER et al. 1963). Convulsions in mice after low doses (LÖSCHER and FREY 1977) but not after higher doses of picrotoxin (GO et al. 1978 a) are inhibited. Trimethadione suppresses strychnine convulsions in mice (EVERETT and RICHARDS 1944; LÖSCHER and FREY 1977) and in chickens (LAHAN et al. 1979) and delays death after the i.v. infusion of strychnine in mice (IORIO et al. 1973). According to GO et al. (1978 a) trimethadione is ineffective, but compared with other authors higher doses of strychnine were given. Convulsions elicited by bicuculline (LÖSCHER and FREY 1977; STONE and JAVID 1979) or by 3-mercaptopropionic acid (LÖSCHER 1979 a) are inhibited by trimethadione. The effects of 3-mercaptopropionic acid on the metabolism of GABA are reduced or abolished. The main metabolite of trimethadione, dimethadione, surprisingly is ineffective against 3-mercaptopropionic acid (LÖSCHER 1979 a).

Trimethadione eliminates convulsions and counteracts in part the changes of GABA metabolism induced by isoniazid (LÖSCHER and FREY 1977). The pattern of EEG changes and behavior similar to petit mal provoked in rats by high doses of gamma-hydroxybutyrate is inhibited by trimethadione and other drugs clinically effective in petit mal epilepsy (GODSCHALK et al. 1976; SNEAD et al. 1980). Similarly, the symptoms induced by intracerebroventricular (i.c.v.) administration of leucine enkephalin in rats are inhibited by trimethadione, ethosuximide, and valproate sodium (SNEAD and BEARDEN 1980). The authors suggest using these models for testing petit mal drugs, since other anticonvulsants such as phenobarbital or diphenylhydantoin are not effective in these models.

In addition, trimethadione inhibits convulsions produced by thujone in mice (EVERETT and RICHARDS 1944), procaine in guinea pigs and mice (EVERETT and RICHARDS 1944; SANDERS 1967), folic acid in dogs (BAXTER et al. 1973), deslanoside in dogs (BIRCHER et al. 1963), 4-aminopyridine in mice (LEMEIGNAN 1971), 3-*tert*-butylsydnone in rats (BULGER et al. 1976) *N*-sulfamoyl-hexahydroazepine in mice (GO et al. 1978a), amino-oxacetic acid in chickens (OSUIDE 1972), kainic acid in mice (STONE and JAVID 1980), high doses of methadone in mice (SHANNON and HOLTZMAN 1976), chlorinated hydrocarbon insecticides (dieldrin and DDT) in mice (JOY 1973), and diisopropylfluorophosphate (DFP) in rabbits (HIMWICH et al. 1950).

Trimethadione is active in convulsant models, too, in which convulsions are produced by topical application of penicillin (GOGERTY and GUNN 1964), conjugated estrogens (JULIEN et al. 1975; WILKINSON and HALPERN 1974), tungstic acid gel (ELAZAR and BLUM 1971; ITO et al. 1979), or metallic cobalt (CRAIG et al. 1976; CHIU et al. 1979) to certain regions of the brain. However, besides the suppression of convulsions or seizure equivalents by higher doses of trimethadione, augmentation of convulsions by lower dose ranges has also been reported (CRAIG et al. 1976; WILKINSON and HALPERN 1974).

II. Electrically Induced Convulsions

Oxazolidinediones show marked effects on electrically elicited convulsions. Generally the doses required for these effects are higher than those counteracting chemically induced convulsions. Thus, for trimethadione various authors report ED_{50} values of 400–900 mg/kg p.o. for the inhibition of tonic-clonic convulsions after maximal electroshock in mice and rats (SWINYARD 1949; CHEN and ENSOR 1950; GOODMAN et al. 1953; FERNGREN and PAALZOW 1969; BAXTER et al. 1973; IORIO et al. 1973; CONSROE and WOLKIN 1973; GO et al. 1978; KRALL et al. 1978) and for paramethadione ED_{50} values of 150–250 mg/kg p.o. (SWINYARD 1949; SWINYARD et al. 1952a; GOODMAN et al. 1953; KRALL et al. 1978). With ED_{50} values of 700 (rat) and approximately 2,000 mg/kg (mouse) dimethadione is clearly less effective (WITHROW et al. 1968; CAHEN et al. 1971).

Tonic-clonic convulsions elicited by maximal electroshock lead to a rapid reduction of ATP, phosphocreatine, and glucose, and to an increase of lactate in the cerebral cortex. The changes are eliminated if the convulsion is inhibited by trimethadione or phenobarbital, but not by diphenylhydantoin (KING and CARL 1969).

Convulsions produced by minimal electroshock are also inhibited by trimethadione, paramethadione, and dimethadione. The duration and severity of the convulsions are more easily affected than the convulsant threshold. But the convulsant threshold can be increased particularly if the sensitivity of the animals to convulsion is raised by appropriate pretreatment (e.g., by hydration) (EVERETT and RICHARDS 1944; GOODMAN and MANUEL 1945; GOODMAN and TOMAN 1945; GOODMAN et al. 1946a; SWINYARD 1949; CHEN and ENSOR 1950; SWINYARD et al. 1952a; BROWN et al. 1953; WITHROW et al. 1968).

Effects of trimethadione were also found on stimulating defined structures of the brain. When stimulating the dorsal hippocampus of conscious rats, trimethadione raises the threshold of minimal seizures (YEOH and WOLF 1970). According to ASHTON and WAUQUIER (1979), the forelimb clonus of amygdaloid-kindled rats is inhibited by moderate doses, but in the same model, ALBERTSON et al. (1980) found trimethadione to be effective only in the toxic dose range. Afterdischarge experiments are described by Jurna (Chap. 23, this volume).

III. Convulsions Produced by Other Methods

Convulsions evoked by positive pressure oxygen respiration are delayed by trimethadione (PATON 1967; NOLTE and SCHNAKENBURG 1973). The threshold of convulsions elicited in mice by helium pressures $9.6–11.3 \times 10^6$ Pa is markedly raised by trimethadione (BRAUER et al. 1979). Trimethadione inhibits clonic seizures in rats induced by abrupt withdrawal from a high, anesthetic concentration of CO_2 (WOODBURY et al. 1958).

Epileptic seizures provoked in rabbits by freezing a small area of the cortex are completely suppressed by trimethadione 2 h after 100 mg/kg i.p., following an initial stage of primary focus activation and augmentation of spread (MORELL 1959). Trimethadione (160 mg/kg i.v.) fails to have an effect on the spiking activity induced by cortical freezing in the cat (HORI et al. 1979), but suppresses secondary generalized seizures elicited by pentylenetetrazol or thiosemicarbazide (ITO et al. 1977b).

In experiments performed to measure the acetylcholine release from the cerebral cortex of guinea pigs with permanently implanted epidural cups, focal seizures can be elicited by heating the superfused Ringer solution to 40 °C. These seizures as well as the simultaneously increased cortical acetylcholine outflow are inhibited by trimethadione (BIANCHI et al. 1975).

Trimethadione is effective in mice (SWINYARD et al. 1963) and rats (CONSROE and WOLKIN 1977; CONSROE et al. 1979) susceptible to audiogenic seizures. The tonic extensor component of the audiogenic seizure is inhibited by lower doses than the initial ocurrence of running.

Seizures elicited by intermittent light stimulation in baboons (*Papio papio*) with genetically high seizure susceptibility are not completely eliminated even by toxic doses of trimethadione (KILLAM 1976), whereas in domestic fowl both convulsions and the electrographic signs of photic stimulation are abolished by nonsedative doses (JOHNSON et al. 1974).

Trimethadione was also effective in convulsions during withdrawal in barbiturate-dependent cats. Most of the withdrawal symptoms are suppressed by trimethadione. Dimethadione was less effective in reversing withdrawal and caused greater acute toxicity (OKAMOTO et al. 1977).

C. Central Nervous System Effects Besides the Anticonvulsant Effect

Neurophysiological effects of the oxazolidinediones are described by Jurna in Chap. 23, this volume.

I. Influence on the Electroencephalogram

There have been no systematic investigations either with or without the use of computer-aided methods of analysis of the influence of trimethadione on the EEG. GOODMAN et al. (1946a) found changes in rabbits, such as bursts of fast waves and irregular slow waves, only with high doses (700 mg/kg i.p.). CAHEN et al. (1971) reported, however, that dimethadione induces marked EEG changes such as increase in amplitude, decrease in frequency, and spindles in rabbits when given i.v. in doses of 50–75 mg/kg. Guinea pigs showed no effects after 100 mg/kg i.p. trimethadione (BIANCHI et al. 1975), while fast cortical frequencies were increased in cats and monkeys (DELGADO and MIHAILOVIĆ 1956). In the cortex of curarized cats, augmented synchronization and raised arousal thresholds were observed after 200 or 500 mg/kg i.p. (MCMILLEN and ISAAC 1978; FAINGOLD and BERRY 1973a).

II. Influence on Behavior

Doses of trimethadione with an antagonistic effect on pentylenetetrazol seizures affect the behavior of experimental animals only slightly. Doses approximately 1.3–3.1 times higher produce neurotoxic signs (SWINYARD 1949; SWINYARD et al. 1952a; SWINYARD and CASTELLION 1966; KRALL et al. 1978). Disturbed coordination and ataxia have been reported for mice, rats, and rabbits after doses of 445–900 mg/kg (s.c., i.p., or oral administration) (GOODMAN et al. 1946a; SWINYARD 1949; BASTIAN 1961; CONSROE and WOLKIN 1977; GO et al. 1978a; KRALL et al. 1978), whereas in cats as little as 200 mg/kg i.p. produces sedation and ataxia (MCMILLEN and ISAAC 1978). CHEN and ENSOR (1950) described a hypnotic effect in rats after 700 mg/kg and an anesthetic effect after 1,200 mg/kg i.p.

Anticonvulsant doses have analgesic effects in mice, rats, and rabbits (RICHARDS and EVERETT 1944). In the same dose range anesthesia with barbital (GO et al. 1978a) or hexobarbital (RÜMKE and BOUT 1960) is potentiated, which may be considered an expression of a sedative action. After a latency of 24 h the hexobarbital sleeping time is slightly shortened (RÜMKE 1963), possibly as the consequence of an enzyme-inducing effect.

There are few reports on the influence of trimethadione on operant behavior. Rats with electrodes implanted into the medial forebrain bundle showed a tendency toward an increased self-stimulation rate after 325 mg/kg i.p. (ST. LAURENT 1971). Pentylenetetrazol-induced impaired retention in a passive avoidance situation is counteracted by trimethadione (CLINCKE and WAUQUIER 1979). In mice bulbectomy does not lead (unlike benzodiazepines) to a changed sensitivity to trimethadione in maximal electroshock or in pentylenetetrazol shock (UEKI et al. 1977).

Dimethadione, in contrast to trimethadione, displays a conspicuous effect on the CNS in doses which have no anticonvulsant effects (CAHEN et al. 1971). Doses of 165–200 mg/kg have an antiaggressive effect; 500 mg/kg inhibit motility and exploration in mice and prolong hexobarbital-induced sleeping time; and 100 mg/kg (i.p.) inhibit yohimbine-induced effects such as anxiety. On the basis of these findings the authors suggest that dimethadione possesses anxiolytic properties.

D. Biochemical Effects

I. Transmitter

Trimethadione scarcely affects the concentration or metabolism of gamma-aminobutyric acid (GABA) in the brain. FERRARI and ARNOLD (1961) reported that the GABA level in the whole brain of rats is reduced by approximately 20% after 1,000 mg/kg i.p.; lower doses are ineffective (LUST et al. 1978; NAHORSKI 1972). The influence on glutamate decarboxylase has not been investigated. The activity of GABA transaminase in brain homogenates is moderately diminished by high doses ($>10^{-3}M$) of trimethadione (LÖSCHER 1980; NAKAMURA and BERNSTEIN 1961).

Trimethadione, like ethosuximide, changes the concentration of gamma-hydroxybutyric acid (GHB) in the brain of rats. GHB occurs endogenously as a metabolite of GABA. Its function, if any, is unclear. After a single dose of trimethadione (300 mg/kg) GHB concentration increases, but is reduced after 7 days of treatment (150 mg/kg daily). The authors (SNEAD et al. 1980) postulate a relationship between the anti-petit mal effects of trimethadione and ethosuximide and their effects on the concentration of GHB.

Trimethadione and paramethadione (4×150 and 4×200 mg/kg, respectively) increase the 5-HT content in the brain of rats, but not in the periphery (BONNYCASTLE et al. 1957). According to DIAZ (1974), the content of 5-HT and 5-HIAA in the rat brain is not affected by a single dose but the rate of synthesis is altered. The level of 5-HIAA in the cerebrospinal fluid of cats is not changed by trimethadione, and the content of homovanillic acid (HVA) decreases (MCMILLEN and ISAAC 1978).

II. Other Effects

In high concentration, which can be attained therapeutically in vivo, trimethadione inhibits oxygen uptake by brain slices of dogs (motor cortex) (STRUCK et al. 1950) and mice (TAYLOR et al. 1950). Increased respiration in brain slices of guinea pigs, rats, or rabbits produced by high-frequency electrical stimulation was abolished by trimethadione; an increase produced by low-frequency stimulation, KCl, or dinitrophenol was not affected (GREENGARD and MCILWAIN 1955; FORDA and MCILWAIN 1953).

Cytochromoxidase from brain or liver was not inhibited by concentrations of $\leq 10^{-3}$ M trimethadione (TORDA and WOLFF 1950).

Whereas convulsant drugs raise the concentration of cyclic nucleotides in the brain, trimethadione reduces the concentration of 3′,5′-cyclic GMP in the cerebellum of mice (LUST et al. 1978).

After administering 500 mg/kg trimethadione i.p. to rats, NAHORSKI (1972) found no changes in concentrations of glycolytic intermediates, ATP, ADP, AMP, and phosphocreatine. Of the intermediates of the tricarboxylate cycle, alpha-oxoglutarate, malate, fumarate, and glutamate were reduced. The cerebral glucose level slightly increased, while the blood glucose content decreased significantly. This results in an increased brain/blood glucose ratio, which is considered by the author as an expression of augmented glucose transportation to the brain.

The uptake of xylose by cerebral cortex slices, as a model of glucose transportation, is augmented (GILBERT et al. 1966).

In synaptic vesicles of rat cortex magnesium-activated ATPase is inhibited by trimethadione and dimethadione as well as by other anticonvulsant drugs. The relative efficacies of the substances in this test correspond to the order of potencies against experimental convulsions in mice, so that the authors postulate that the effect on the magnesium-activated ATPase might play a part in the mechanism of action of anticonvulsant drugs (GILBERT and WYLLIE 1976).

The NADPH-linked aldehyde reductase of the bovine brain is inhibited by anticonvulsant drugs; in this test trimethadione and paramethadione had only weak effects, whereas that of dimethadione was markedly stronger (ERWIN and DEITRICH 1973).

After subchronic treatment with trimethadione (125–150 mg/kg for 12–23 days) the amino acid content (alanine, glutamic acid, glycine, methionine, tyrosine, phenylalanine) in pyramidal-cell layers in the hippocampus of rats was diminished (ENDRÖCZI and PEKETE 1967).

Trimethadione and paramethadione lead to a moderate induction of delta-amino-levulinic acid synthetase in liver cells of the chicken embryo, a model for testing a possible porphyria-inducing effect (GRANICK 1966; RIFKIND 1973).

E. Pharmacodynamic Properties Outside the Central Nervous System

Few investigations have been carried out on the peripheral effects of trimethadione, and, in particular, there are no studies in the literature on the influence of the oxazolidinediones on cardiovascular functions.

RICHTER (1964) found that the skin temperature of the forepaws of mice was raised after trimethadione, a fact suggesting peripheral vasodilation. A weak local anesthetic effect (infiltration or surface anesthesia) corresponding to about one-tenth of the effect of lidocaine has been reported for trimethadione (GANDHI et al. 1976). In addition, the authors reported a neuromuscular-blocking effect which they partly ascribed to a curare-like effect and partly to the above-mentioned local anesthetic effect.

A series of investigations dealt with antiarrhythmic effects, which are to be expected owing to the local anesthetic action. Arrhythmias elicited by aconitine, by petroleum ether in combination with epinephrine, or by coronary ligation are not affected by trimethadione or paramethadione (SINGH et al. 1971). A weak effect against ouabain arrhythmias was found in rabbits (DRESSLER et al. 1972); in cats, however, trimethadione was ineffective (ADAMSKA-DYNIEWSKA et al. 1970). According to BIRCHER et al. (1963), arrhythmias induced in dogs by the i.v. or i.c.v. administration of pentylenetetrazol, picrotoxin, or deslanoside are abolished by trimethadione (300–500 mg/kg i.v.).

F. Pharmacokinetics

I. Absorption

Oxazolidinediones are rapidly absorbed. Using a manometric analytical method, TAYLOR and BERTCHER (1952) found peak blood levels 15 min after i.p. trimethadione in mice and rabbits. Similar results were obtained by THUESON et al. (1974) in rats injected i.p. with radioactively labeled trimethadione. In dogs, FREY and SCHULZ (1970) observed peak serum concentrations 1–3 h after oral administration of trimethadione, with a rapid initial increase. Trimethadione is believed to be absorbed in the upper duodenum. RICHARDS and EVERETT (1946) reported that the effect of trimethadione, given by the oral route, is markedly delayed by pyloric ligation. Dimethadione, a weak acid, is absorbed rapidly from the stomach, but slowly from the small intestine (WITHROW 1982). The absorption of paramethadione is similar to that of trimethadione (SWINYARD et al. 1952a).

II. Distribution

In mice, the volume of distribution of trimethadione is 60% of body weight, a value approximately equal to the total body water (FREY and SCHULZ 1970). In dogs, the volume of distribution was found to be 60%–90% of body weight (FREY and SCHULZ 1970) and in rats 82% (THUESON et al. 1974). The smaller volume of distribution of dimethadione [58% of body weight in rats (THUESON et al. 1974) and 40% in dogs (WADDELL and BUTLER 1957)] is due to the higher ionization of dimethadione at physiological pH (BUTLER 1953). At a pH of 7.4 dimethadione is ionized to 94% and trimethadione not at all (BUTLER 1955b). TAYLOR and BERTCHER (1952) determined the relative distribution of trimethadione in the organs of mice and, 30 min after i.p. injection, found tissue/plasma ratios of 0.61 for the brain, 0.94 for muscles, 0.62 for the liver, and 0.75 for the kidneys. The concentration of trimethadione declines rapidly in blood and brain, but decreases more slowly in the kidney, and very slowly in muscle and liver. According to THUESON et al. (1974), trimethadione is distributed passively into the cerebrospinal fluid and into the tissue water of the cerebral cortex, muscle, and gastrointestinal tract within 1 h after i.p. administration to rats.

Serum protein binding of trimethadione is very low, with values of 8%–11% in humans and 6.5%–9% in dogs (LÖSCHER 1979). Dimethadione also shows virtually no binding to plasma and tissue proteins (WADDELL and BUTLER 1957).

Distribution of dimethadione is slow and pH dependent. Because of this property dimethadione can be used to measure intracellular pH (WADDELL and BUTLER 1957). Constant plasma/tissue or plasma/cerebrospinal fluid ratios were measured 1–4 h after i.v. injection of dimethadione (KIBLER et al. 1964; ROLLINS and REED 1970; ROOS 1965). The relative concentrations of dimethadione in the brain and in other tissues are lower (50%) than those of trimethadione (THUESON et al. 1974). After i.p. administration of trimethadione to rats the authors found a brain/plasma ratio of 0.8 for trimethadione and about 0.4 for dimethadione. In pregnant rats, which were given trimethadione for several days, MIDHA et al. (1979) found large accumulations of dimethadione in the organs, placenta, and fetuses, but low concentrations of trimethadione.

The distribution of paramethadione has not yet been investigated. The demethylation product of paramethadione behaves similarly to dimethadione (e.g., volume of distribution 37%; BUTLER and WADDELL 1955).

III. Metabolism

In the mammalian organism, *N*-alkylated oxazolidinediones are metabolized at different rates but in an identical manner to *N*-dealkylated products (rat: THUESON et al. 1974; MIDHA et al. 1979; mouse: FREY and SCHULZ 1970; FREY and BUTLER 1955a; BUTLER and WADDELL 1957; human: SCHULZ 1970; BUTLER and WADDELL 1958; dog: BUTLER et al. 1952). Evidently, the stereoisomers of the racemic substances are metabolized at different rates, D-enantiomers being metabolized more rapidly (BUTLER and WADDELL 1955). The *N*-dealkylated products are ionized to a greater extent at physiological pH values, have a lower volume of distribution, penetrate more slowly, and display similar pharmacological activity to the parent compounds (BUTLER and WADDELL 1955; WITHROW et al. 1968; FREY 1969). They are eliminated slowly without further biotransformation, so that marked accumulation results with multiple dosing (BUTLER and WADDELL 1958; BUTLER 1953, BUTLER 1955a).

FREY and SCHULZ (1970) examined the time course of the demethylation of trimethadione in mice and dogs after high i.v. doses. They determined plasma half-lives of 45 min and 8 h, respectively, for trimethadione and of 30 h and 50–80 h, respectively, for dimethadione. The authors suggested that the longer half-lives for trimethadione in dogs are the results of self-inhibition of metabolism following high doses. This effect had already been presumed by CONNEY (1967). Paramethadione is also more rapidly metabolized in mice than in dogs (BUTLER 1955a; BUTLER and WADDELL 1955). For rats the demethylation half-life of trimethadione is reported to be 2.6 h (THUESON et al. 1974) and for rabbits 2–2.5 h (TAYLOR and BERTCHER 1952).

The liver plays a major role in the metabolism of the oxazolidinediones (BUTLER and WADDELL 1954). Impaired oxidative metabolism in the liver leads to increased potency and duration of the effect of oxazolidinediones (SWINYARD et al. 1952b, 1954; BUTLER and WADDELL 1954). Metabolism corresponding to that in vivo can be obtained in vitro by enzymes of hepatic microsomes. Trimethadione metabolism in hepatic microsomes occurs slowly and is not saturable; it is performed exclusively by demethylation (BUTLER et al. 1965). Increasing concentrations of dimethadione inhibit demethylation of trimethadione. There appears to be no induction of microsomal enzymes of the liver by trimethadione, but by paramethadione (CONNEY 1967). Possibly, metabolism also occurs in other organs. According to TAYLOR and BERTCHER (1952), trimethadione is metabolized in vitro by rat tissue slices in the following order of decreasing effectiveness: intestinal mucosa > kidney > liver = muscle > brain.

IV. Excretion

Trimethadione is excreted primarily in the form of its metabolite dimethadione. In rats 1.5% of the dose is eliminated in the 24-h urine as trimethadione and 8% as dimethadione (THUESON et al. 1974). The plasma half-life of trimethadione corresponds to the metabolic half-life. The elimination half-lives from less lipophilic tissues are markedly longer. Thus, Taylor and Bertcher (1952) measured elimination half-lives in mice; these were 3 h for the kidneys, 5 h for the muscle, and 8 h for the liver. The elimination of dimethadione is far slower than that of trimethadione. Dimethadione is also excreted primarily by the kidney (BUTLER et al. 1952; WADDELL and BUTLER 1957). The elimination of dimethadione in dogs can be shortened from 2 weeks to 2 days by alkalinization of the urine (WADDELL and BUTLER 1957), since, at a pH value of 7, a large proportion of dimethadione in the primary urine is reabsorbed. Bilateral nephrectomy prolongs the pharmacodynamics of trimethadione in mice and rats (RICHARDS and EVERETT 1946).

All these facts point to a marked accumulation of dimethadione in the organism after administration of trimethadione or dimethadione (FREY and KRETZSCHMER 1971). In mice which were offered trimethadione in the drinking water (0.5% –1.0%) for 7 days, the serum level of dimethadione increased from 200 μg/ml on the 1st day to 1,800 μg/ml, whereas the serum level of trimethadione remained constant at 20–30 μg/ml. According to CHAMBERLIN et al. (1965) dimethadione is accumulated in humans until the body contains 14.3 times the daily dose. More than 30 days of treatment would be required in order to attain this equilibrium.

Elimination of the demethylation product of paramethadione is even slower than that of dimethadione (BUTLER 1955a).

G. Interactions

The combination of trimethadione and the hydantoin derivative albutoin (allylisobutylthiohydantoin) results in synergistic effects in the pentylenetetrazol test and additive effects in maximal electroshock (WALLIN et al. 1970). In the pentylenetetrazol threshold test, the ED_{50} of trimethadione remains unchanged when 2–30 mg/kg diphenylhydantoin is added (WEAVER et al. 1958). The convulsant threshold dose of pentylenetetrazol is increased by administration of trimethadione and can be reduced by administration of reserpine, corresponding to the known lowering of convulsant thresholds by the depletion of monoamines (DIAZ 1974). Concurrent administration of trimethadione (or paramethadione) and iproniazide, which has a weak anticonvulsant effect, potentiates the anticonvulsant effect of both oxazolidinediones, an effect considered to be due to increased monoamine levels in the brain (YEN et al. 1962). The anticonvulsant ED_{50} values of trimethadione are increased by simultaneously administering amphetamine, amphetamine alone having no distinct influence on convulsant thresholds (FREY 1964). Trimethadione antagonizes the anticonvulsant effects of cannabidiol in seizures induced by maximal electroshock and in audiogenic seizures (CONSROE and WOLKIN 1977).

H. Toxicity

The pattern of toxicity of the oxazolidinediones is well known from many years of clinical use in epileptic patients (GALLAGHER 1972; BOOKER 1982). The most important clinical symptoms such as hemeralopia, dermatological manifestations, decrease in white cell count and platelets, and the nephrotic syndrome have not been described for animals. In a chronic (9-month) toxicity study in rats, trimethadione was admixed to the feed in concentrations of 0.25%, 0.5%, and 1.0%. The animals tolerated the substance without severe organic damage. Doses of 0.5% and 1.0% only led to weight loss and 1.0% to a slight decrease of red-cell count (RICHARDS and EVERETT 1946). With high doses toxic responses of the CNS such as sedation, ataxia, and sleep became obvious, as described by RICHARDS and EVERETT (1946). Corresponding findings were reported for mice, rabbits, cats, and dogs. Respiratory and circulatory depression also occurred in the acute pattern of intoxication. Neurotoxic symptoms have been reported to occur with trimethadione doses of 250–500 mg/kg. Ataxia is observed after 400–750 mg/kg and mortality at 1,500–2,000 mg/kg (RICHARDS and EVERETT 1946). The following LD_{50} values have been given: mice, 2,200–3,200 mg/kg orally (RICHARDS and EVERETT 1944; AHMAD and DHAWAN 1969; WALLIN et al. 1970; GO et al. 1978a); rats, 2,000 mg/kg s.c.; and rabbits, 1,500 mg/kg i.v. (RICHARDS and EVERETT 1944).

There is some clinical evidence of potential teratogenicity of trimethadione and paramethadione (BOOKER 1982). POSWILLO (1972) examined the effect of trimethadione and paramethadione on embryonal development of monkeys (*Macaca irus*) by giving 300–900 mg from the 25th to 46th day of gestation. He found no malformed fetuses, but spontaneous resorption of the embryos beginning with a dose of 600 mg; 900 mg was toxic to the females. The slight effect of oxazolidinediones on embryonal development of monkeys is in contrast to the apparent teratogenic findings in other animal species. RIFKIND (1974) found teratogenic effects in chicken embryos when injecting trimethadione or dimethadione into the egg during the early phase of embryonal development. Malformations were observed in the heart (globular heart), eyes (micro-oranophthalmia), lower extremities (missing thigh, missing toes) as well as hernias and celosomia. In Wistar rats, BUTTAR et al. (1976) found fetotoxic effects and anomalies (additional ribs, delayed ossification of the skull and sternum, curved radius, ulna, tibia, and fibula as well as umbilical hernias and subcutaneous edema) after trimethadione and paramethadione doses as high as eight times the therapeutic doses. Dimethadione provoked similar effects (BUTTAR et al. 1976, 1978). Trimethadione also has a teratogenic effect in mice. In CD-1 mice the substance caused numerous malformations of the skeleton, cardiovascular system (atresia of the aortic arch, truncus arteriosus), and kidneys (aplasia), as well as hydrocephalus and cleft palate (SHULL and FABRO 1978; BROWN et al. 1979). Teratogenic doses are well below those causing maternal toxicity. With a daily dose of 1,045 mg/kg in the early phase of organogenesis, embryonal mortality is 80% and malformation 100% (BROWN et al. 1979). According to GORDON (1981), the relative teratogenicity of the oxazolidinediones is markedly higher than that of the hydantoins and succinimides. Thus, the teratogenic effect of trimethadione in mice is more than ten times, that of paramethadione more than four times, greater than that of ethosuximide. BROWN et al. (1980) found valproic acid to have similar teratogenic effects to trimethadione in rabbits, rats, and mice.

References

Adamska-Dyniewska H, Czernek Z, Goch JH, Rosiek S (1970) Anticonvulsants in treatment of ouabain-induced ectopic heart activity in cats. Pol Tyg Lek 25:1205–1207

Ahmad A, Dhawan BN (1969) Metrazol test for rapid screening of anticonvulsants. Jpn J Pharmacol 19:472–474

Albertson TE, Peterson SL, Stark LG (1980) Anticonvulsant drugs and their antagonism of kindled amygdaloid seizures in rats. Neuropharmacology 19:643–652

Ashton D, Wauquier A (1979) Behavioral analysis of the effects of 15 anticonvulsants in the amygdaloid kindled rat. Psychopharmacology 65:7–13

Bastian JW (1961) Classification of CNS drugs by a mouse screening battery. Arch Int Pharmacodyn Ther 133:347–364

Baxter MG, Miller AA, Webster RA (1973) Some studies on the convulsant action of folic acid. Br J Pharmacol 48:350–351

Bianchi C., Beani L, Bertelli A (1975) Effects of some anti-epileptic drugs on brain acetylcholine. Neuropharmacology 14:327–332

Bircher R, Kanai T, Wang SC (1963) Action of anticonvulsants (pentobarbital, trimethadione and 3-methyl-5,5-phenylethyl hydantoin) on the EEG, ECG and blood pressure changes induced by pentylenetetrazol, picrotoxin and deslanoside in dogs. Arch Int Pharmacodyn Ther 141:357–376

Bonnevaux De SC, Diez Altares MC, Carrillo L (1968) Autonomic response to pentamethylenetetrazol following trimethadione and benzodiazepines administration. Arch Int Pharmacodyn Ther 173:34–43

Bonnycastle DD, Giarman NJ, Paasonen MK (1957) Anticonvulsant compounds and 5-hydroxy-tryptamine in rat brain. Br J Pharmacol 12:228–231

Booker HE (1982) Trimethadione, toxicity. In: Woodbury DM, Penry JU, Pippenger CE (eds) Antiepileptic drugs. Raven, New York, pp 701–703

Brauer RW, Mansfield WM, Beaver RW, Gillen HW (1979) Stages in development of high-pressure neurological syndrome in the mouse. J Appl Physiol 46:756–765

Brown NA, Shull G, Fabro S (1979) Assessment of the teratogenic potential of trimethadione in the CD-1 mouse. Toxicol Appl Pharmacol 51:59–71

Brown NA, Kao J, Fabro S (1980) Teratogenic potential of valproic acid. Lancet I:660–661

Brown WC, Schiffman DO, Swinyard EA, Goodman LS (1953) Comparative assay of antiepileptic drugs by "psychomotor" seizure test and minimal electroshock threshold test. J Pharmacol Exp Ther 107:273–283

Bulger WH, Wells PR, Roche EB (1976) Pharmacological assessment of 3-tert-butylsydnone. J Pharm Sci 65:109–111

Butler TC (1953) Quantitative studies of the demethylation of trimethadione (tridione). J Pharmacol Exp Ther 108:11–17

Butler TC (1955a) Metabolic demethylation of 3,5-dimethyl-5-ethyl 2,4-oxazolidinedione (paramethadione, paradione). J Pharmacol Exp Ther 113:178–185

Butler TC (1956b) The effects of N-methylation in 5,5-disubstituted derivatives of barbituric acid, hydantoin, and 2,4-oxazolidinedione. J Am Pharm Assoc Sci Ed 44:367–370

Butler TC, Waddell WJ (1954) The role of the liver in the demethylation on *N*-methyl derivatives of hydantoin and of 2,4-oxazolidinedione. J Pharmacol Exp Ther 110:241–243

Butler TC, Walddell WJ (1955) A pharmacological comparison of the optical isomers of 5-ethyl-5-methyl-2,4-oxazolidinedione and of 3,5-dimethyl-5-ethyl-2,4-oxazolidinedione (paramethadione, paradione). J Pharmacol Exp Ther 113:238–240

Butler TC, Waddell WJ (1957) Metabolic deethylation of 5,5-dimethyl-3-ethyl-2,4 oxazolidinedione (Dimedion). Arch int Pharmacodyn Ther 111:308–313

Butler TC, Waddell WJ (1958) N-Methylated derivatives of barbituric acid, hydantoin and oxazolidinedione used in the treatment of epilepsy. Neurology (Minneap.) 8:106–112

Butler TC, Mahaffee D, Mahaffee C (1952) Metabolic demethylation of 3,5,5-trimethyl-2,4-oxazolidinedione (trimethadione, Tridione). Proc Soc Exp Biol Med 81:450–452

Butler TC, Waddell WJ, Poole DT (1965) Demethylation of trimethadione and metharbital by rat liver microsomal enzymes: substrate concentration-yield relationships and competition between substrates. Biochem Pharmacol 14:937–942

Buttar HD, Dupuis I, Khera KS (1976) Fetotoxicity of trimethadione and paramethadione in rats Toxicol Appl Pharmacol 37:126

Buttar HS, Dupuis I, Khera KS (1978) Dimethadione-induced fetotoxicity in rats Toxicology 9:155–164

Cahen R, Boucard M, Faurre L, Vedel Y (1971) Effet de la 5,5-diméthyl 2-4 oxazolidinedione sur le comportement d'anxiété et d'aggression chez l'animal de laboratoire. C R Soc Biol (Paris) 165:1035–1040

Chamberlin HR, Waddell WJ, Butler TC (1965) A study of the product of demethylation of trimethadione in the control of petit mal epilepsy. Neurology 15:449–454

Chen G, Ensor CR (1950) Evaluation of antiepileptic drugs. Arch Neurol Psychiatry 63:56–60

Chen G, Portman R (1952) Titration of central-nervous-system depression. AMA Arch Neurol Psychiatry 68:498–505

Chen G, Ensor CH R, Clarke IG (1951) Central nervous action of hydantoins, oxazolidinediones and thiazolidones. AMA Arch Neurol Psychiatry 66:329–337

Chiu P, Olsen DM, Borys HK, Karler R, Turkanis SA (1979) The influence of cannabidiol and Δ^9-tetrahydrocannabinol on cobalt epilepsy in rats. Epilepsia 20:365–375

Clincke G, Wauquier A (1979) Metrazol-produced impairment of passive avoidance retention specifically antagonized by anti-petit mal drugs. Psychopharmacology 66:243–246

Conney AH (1967) Pharmacological implications of microsomal enzyme induction. Pharmacol Rev. 19:317–366

Consroe P, Wolkin A (1977) Cannabidiol-antiepileptic drug comparisons and interactions in experimentally induced seizures in rats. J Pharmacol Exp Ther 201:26–32

Consroe P, Picchioni A, Chin L (1979) Audiogenic seizure susceptible rats. Fed Proc 38:2411–2416

Craig CR, Chiu P, Colasanti BK (1976) Effects of diphenylhydantoin and trimethadione on seizure activity during cobalt experimental epilepsy in the rat. Neuropharmacology 15:485-489

Delgado JMR, Mihailović L (1956) Use of intracerebral electrodes to evaluate drugs that act on the central nervous system. Ann NY Acad Sci 64:644–666

Desmedt LKC, Niemegeers CJE, Lewi PJ, Janssen PAJ (1976) Antagonism of maximal Metrazol seizures in rats and its relevance to an experimental classification of antiepileptic drugs. Arzneimittelforsch 26:1592–1603

Diaz PM (1974) Interaction of pentylenetetrazol and trimethadione on the metabolism of serotonin in brain and its relation to the anticonvulsant action of trimethadione. Neuropharmacology 13:615–621

Dressler WE, Rossi GV, Orzechowski RF (1972) Effect of several anticonvulsant drugs and procainamide against ouabain-induced cardiac arrhythmias in rabbits. J Pharm Sci 61:133–134

Elazar Z, Blum B (1971) Effect of drugs on interictal spikes and afterdischarges in experimental epilepsy. Arch Int Pharmacodyn Ther 189:310–318

Endröczi E, Fekete T (1967) Amino acid composition of the ammon's horn and the effect of anticonvulsant drugs. Acta Physiol Hung 32:389–398

Erwin VG, Deitrich RA (1973) Inhibition of bovine brain aldehyde reductase by anticonvulsant compounds in vitro. Biochem Pharmacol 22:2615–2624

Everett GM, Richards RK (1944) Comparative anticonvulsants action of 3,5,5-trimethyloxazolidine-2,4-dione (tridione), dilantin and phenobarbital. J Pharmacol Exp Ther 81:402–407

Faingold CL, Berry CA (1973 a) Anticonvulsant modification of tripelennamine effects on the electrographic activity of the cat brain. Neuropharmacology 12:383–390

Faingold CL, Berry CA (1973 b) Quantitative evaluation of the pentylenetetrazol-anticonvulsant interaction on the EEG of the cat. Eur J Pharmacol 24:381–388

Ferngren H (1968) Further studies on chemically induced seizures and their antagonism by anticonvulsants during postnatal development in the mouse. Acta Pharmacol Toxicol 26:177–188

Ferngren H, Paalzow L (1967) Studies on electrically induced seizures and their antagonism by anticonvulsants during neonatal development in the mouse. Acta Pharmacol Toxicol 25 (Suppl 4):60

Ferngren H, Paalzow L (1969) High frequency electro-shock seizures and their antagonism during postnatal development in the mouse. II. Effects of phenobarbital sodium, mephobarbital, trimethadione, dimethadione, ethosuximide and acetazolamide. Acta Pharmacol Toxicol 27:249–261 (1969)
Ferrari RA, Arnold A (1961) The effect of central nervous system agents on rat-brain γ-aminobutyric acid level. Biochim Biophys Acta 52:361–367
Forda O, McIlwain H (1953) Anticonvulsants on electrically stimulated metabolism of separated mammalian cerebral cortex. Br J Pharmacol 8:225–229
Frey HH (1964) Note on the interactions of amphetamine with anticonvulsant drugs. Acta Pharmacol Toxicol 21:290–298
Frey HH (1969) Determination of the anticonvulsant potency of unmetabolized trimethadione. Acta Pharmacol Toxicol 27:295–300
Frey HH, Kretschmer B-H (1971) Anticonvulsant effect of trimethadione in mice during continued treatment via the drinking water. Arch Int Pharmacodyn Ther 193:181–190
Frey HH, Schulz R (1970) Time course of the demethylation of trimethadione. Acta Pharmacol Toxicol 28:477–483
Gallagher BB (1972) Trimethadione and other oxazolidinediones: toxicity. In: Woodbury DM, Penry JK, Schmidt P (eds) Antiepileptic drugs. Raven, New York, pp 409–411
Gandhi IC, Jindal MN, Patel VK (1976) Mechanism of neuromuscular blockade with some antiepileptic drugs. Arzneimittelforsch 26:258–261
Gardner CR, Webster RA (1973) The effect of some anticonvulsant drugs on leptazol and bicuculline induced acetylcholine efflux from rat cerebral cortex. Br J Pharmacol 47:652
Gardner CR, Webster RA (1977) Convulsant-anticonvulsant interactions on seizure activity and cortical acetylcholine release. Eur J Pharmacol 42:247–256
Gilbert JC, Wyllie MG (1976) Effects of anticonvulsant and convulsant drugs on the ATP-ase activities of synaptosomes and their components. Br J Pharmacol 56:49–57
Gilbert JC, Ortiz WR, Millichap JG (1966) The effects of anticonvulsant drugs on the permeability of brain cells to D-xylose. J Neurochem 13:247–255
Go K, Tsurumi K, Fujimura H (1978a) Anti-convulsant effect of phthalazino-2,3-b-phthalazine-5(14*H*), 12(7*H*)-dione (L-5418). I. Behavioral effect. Jpn J Pharmacol 28:1–12
Go K, Tsurumi K, Fujimura H (1978b) Anti-convulsant effect of phthalazino-[2,3b]-phthalazine-5 (14*H*), 12 (7*H*)-dione (L-5418). II. Electroencephalographic study. Jpn J Pharmacol 28:93–104
Godschalk M, Dzoljic MR, Bonta IL (1976) Antagonism of gamma-hydroxybutyrate-induced hypersynchronization in the ECoG of the rat by anti-petit mal drugs. Neurosci Lett 3:145–150
Gogerty JH, Gunn CG (1964) Effects of various centrally acting agents on penicillin-induced temporal lobe seizures in cats. Fed Proc 23:349
Goodman L, Manuel C (1945) The anticonvulsant properties of dimethyl-*N*-methyl barbituric acid and 3,5,5-trimethyloxazolidine-2, 4-dione (tridione). Fed Proc 4:119
Goodman LS, Toman EP (1945) Experimental indices for comparing the efficacy of compounds with anticonvulsant and antiepileptic properties. Fed Proc 4:120
Goodman LS, Toman JEP, Swinyard EA (1946a) The anticonvulsant properties of tridione. Am J Med 1:213–228
Goodman LS, Swinyard EA, Toman JEP (1946b) Further studies on the anticonvulsant properties or tridione (3,5,5-trimethyloxazolidinedione). Fed Proc 5:179–180
Goodman LS, Singh Grewal M, Brown WC, Swinyard EA (1953) Comparison of maximal seizures evoked by pentylenetetrazol (Metrazol) and electroshock in mice, and their modification by anticonvulsants. J Pharmacol Exp Ther 108:168–176
Gordon SR (1981) Anticonvulsants found to have teratogenic potential. JAMA 245:36
Granick S (1966) The induction in vitro of the synthesis of δ-aminolevulinic acid synthetase in chemical prophyria: a response to certain drugs, sex hormones and foreign chemicals. J Biol Chem 241:1359–1375
Greengard O, McIlwain H (1955) Anticonvulsants and the metabolism of separated mammalian cerebral tissues. Biochem J 61:61–68

Gross GJ, Woodbury DM (1972) Effects of pentylenetetrazol on ion transport in the isolated toad bladder. J Pharmacol Exp Ther 181:257–272

Himwich HE, Essig CF, Hampson JL, Bales PD, Freedman AM (1950) Effect of trimethadione (tridione) and other drugs on convulsions caused by di-isopropyl fluorophosphate (DFP). Am J Psychiatry 106:816–820

Hori M, Ito T, Yoshida K, Shimizu, M (1979) Effect of anticonvulsants in spiking activity induced by cortical freezing in cats. Epilepsia 20:25–36

Iorio LC, Ryan EA, Gogerty JH (1973) Anticonvulsant testing with a new analeptic convulsant: *N*-sulfamoyl-hexahydro-azepine (Sah 41–178). Arch Int Pharmacodyn Ther 206:282–287

Ito T, Hori M, Yoshida K, Shimizu M (1977a) Effect of anticonvulsants on seizures developing in the course of daily administration of pentetrazol to rats. Eur J Pharmacol 45:165–172

Ito T, Hori M, Yoshida K, Shimizu M (1977b) Studies on freezing-induced experimental epilepsy: II. Effect of anticonvulsants on secondary generalized seizures in cats. Jpn J Pharmacol 27 (Suppl):35

Ito T, Hori M, Yoshida K, Shimizu M (1979) Effect of anticonvulsants on experimental cortical epilepsy induced by tungstic acid gel in rats. Arch Int Pharmacodyn Ther 241:287–299

Johnson DD, Crichlow EC, Crawford RD (1974) Epileptiform seizures in domestic fowl IV. The effects of anticonvulsant drugs. Can J Physiol Pharmacol 52:991–994

Joy RM (1973) Electrical correlates of preconvulsive and convulsive doses of chlorinated hydrocarbon insecticides in the CNS. Neuropharmacology 12:63–76

Julien RM, Fowler GW, Danielson MG (1975) The effects of antiepileptic drugs on estrogen-induced electrographic spike-wave discharge. J Pharmacol Exp Ther 193:647–656

Kibler RF, O'Neill RP, Robin ED (1964) Intracellular acid-base relations of dog brain with reference to the brain extracellular volume. J Clin Invest 43:431–443

Killam EK (1976) Measurement of anticonvulsant activity in the *Papio papio* model of epilepsy. Fed Proc 35:2264–2269

King LJ, Carl J (1969) Effects of antiepileptic drugs on brain energy reserves during convulsions. J Neurochem 16:637–643

Krall RL, Penry JK, White BG, Kupferberg HJ, Swinyard EA (1978) Antiepileptic drug development. II. Anticonvulsant drug screening. Epilepsia 19:409–428

Lahan GD, Osuide G., Stansfield F (1979) Anticonvulsant properties of ethyl-*N*-phtalimidoxy acetate. Br J Pharmacol 67:441–442

Lemeignan M (1971) Abord pharmacologique de l'étude du mécanisme de l'action convulsivante de l'amino-4 pyridine. Thérapie 26:927–940

Löscher W (1979a) 3-Mercaptopropionic acid: convulsant properties, effects on enzymes of the γ-aminobutyrate system in mouse brain and antagonism by certain anticonvulsant drugs, aminooxyacetic acid and gabaculine. Biochem Pharmacol 28:1397–1407

Löscher W (1979b) A comparative study of the protein binding of anticonvulsant drugs in serum of dog and man. J Pharmacol Exp Ther 208:429–435

Löscher W (1980) Comparative study of the inhibition of GABA aminotransferase by different anticonvulsant drugs. Arch Int Pharmacodyn Ther 243:48–55

Löscher W, Frey HH (1977) Effect of convulsant and anticonvulsant agents on level and metabolism of γ-aminobutyric acid in mouse brain. Naunyn-Schmiedebergs Arch Pharmacol 296:263–269

Loewe S, Aldous RA, Fox SR, Johnson DG, Perkins W (1955) Isobols of dose-effect relations in the combination of pentylenetetrazole and trimethadione. J Pharmacol Exp Ther 113:475–480

Lust WD, Kupferberg HJ, Yonekawa WD, Penry JK, Passonneau JV, Wheaton AB (1978) Changes in brain metabolites induced by convulsants or electroshock: effects of anticonvulsant agents. Mol Pharmacol 14:347–356

McMillen B, Isaac L (1978) Effects of pentylenetetrazol and trimethadione on feline brain monoamine metabolism. Biochem Pharmacol 27:1815–1820

Midha KK, Buttar HS, Rowe M, Dupuis J (1979) Metabolism and disposition of trimethadione in pregnant rats. Epilepsia 20:417–423

Morrell F, Bradley W, Ptashne M (1959) Effect of drugs on discharge characteristics of chronic epileptogenic lesions. Neurology 9:492–498
Nahorski SR (1972) Biochemical effects of the anticonvulsants trimethadione, ethosuximide and chlordiazepoxide in rat brain. J Neurochem 19:1937–1946
Nakamura K, Bernheim F (1961) Effects of some drugs on the γ-aminobutyric acid transaminase and the succinic semialdehyde dehydrogenase of rat brain. Jpn J Pharmacol 11:37–45
Nolte H, Von Schnakenburg K (1973) Morphologische und pharmakologisch-toxikologische Aspekte der Hyperoxie. Int J Clin Pharmacol 74:340–347
Okamoto M, Rosenberg HC, Boisse NR (1977) Evaluation of anticonvulsants in barbiturate withdrawal. J Pharmacol Exp Ther 202:479–489
Osuide G (1972) Pharmacological properties of amino-oxyacetic acid in the chicken. Br J Pharmacol 44:31–44
Paton WDM (1967) Experiments on the convulsant and anaesthetic effects of oxygen. Br J Pharmacol 29:350–366
Poswillo DE (1972) Tridione and paradione as suspected teratogens. Ann R Coll Surg Engl 50:367–370
Richards RK (1946) Tridione: a new experimental drug for treatment of convulsive and related disorders. I. Pharmacologic aspects. Arch Neurol Psychol 55:164
Richards RK, Everett GM (1944) Analgesic and anticonvulsive properties of 3,5,5-trimethyloxalidine-2,4-dione (tridione). Fed Proc 3:39
Richards RK, Everett GM (1946) Tridione: a new anticonvulsant drug. J Lab Clin Med 31:1330–1336
Richter W (1964) Estimation of vasodilator drug effects in mice by measurements of paw skin temperature. Acta Pharmacol Toxicol 21:91–104
Rifkind AB (1974) Teratogenic effects of trimethadione and dimethadione in the chick embryo. Toxicol Appl Pharmacol 30:452–457
Rifkind AB, Gilette PN, Song CS, Kappas A (1973) Drug stimulation of δ-aminolevulinic acid synthetase and cytochrome P-450 in vivo in chick embryo liver. J Pharmacol Exp Ther 185:214–225
Rollins DE, Reed DJ (1970) Transport of DMO out of cerebrospinal fluid of rats. Am J Physiol 219:1200–1204
Roos A (1965) Intracellular pH and intracellular buffering power of the cat brain. Am J Physiol 209:1233–1246
Rümke CL (1961) Beeinflussung der Krampfwirkung des Bemegrids. Naunyn-Schmiedebergs Arch Exp Pathol Pharmacol 241:511–512
Rümke CL (1963) The influence of drugs on the duration of hexobarbital and hydroxydione narcosis in mice. Naunyn-Schmiedebergs Arch Exp Pathol Pharmakol 244:519–530
Rümke CL, Bout J (1960) Die Beeinflussung der Hexobarbitalnarkose durch vorher verabfolgte Pharmaka. Naunyn-Schmiedebergs Arch Exp Pathol Pharmakol 240:218–223
Sanders HD (1967) A comparison of the convulsant activity of procaine and pentylenetetrazol. Arch Int Pharmacodyn Ther 170:165–177
Shannon HE, Hotzmann SG (1976) Blockade of the specific lethal effects of narcotic analgesics in the mouse. Eur J Pharmacol 39:295–303
Shull EG, Fabro SE (1978) The teratogenicity of trimethadione in the CD-1 mouse. Pharmacologist 20:263
Singh N, Sinha JN, Rastogi SK, Dua PR, Kohli RP (1971) An experimental investigation on the antiarrhythmic activity of antiepileptic agents. Jpn J Pharmacol 21:755–761
Snead OC, Bearden LJ (1980) Anticonvulsants specific for petit mal antagonize epileptogenic effect of leucin encephalin. Science 210:1031–1033
Snead III OC, Bearden LJ, Pegram V (1980) Effect of acute and chronic anticonvulsant administration on endogenous γ-hydroxybutyrate in rat brain. Neuropharmacology 19:47–52
St-Laurent J (1971) Effect of trimethadione on the self-stimulation phenomenon. Can J Physiol Pharmacol 49:850–853 (1971)
Steinhauer HB, Anhut H, Hertting G (1979) The synthesis of prostaglandins and thromboxane in the mouse brain in vivo. Naunyn-Schmiedebergs Arch Pharmacol 310:53–58

Stone WE, Javid MJ (1979) Quantitative evaluation of the actions of anticonvulsants against different chemical convulsants. Arch Int Pharmacodyn Ther 240:66–78

Stone WE, Javid MJ (1980) Effects of anticonvulsants and glutamate antagonists on the convulsive action of kainic acid. Arch Int Pharmacodyn Ther 243:56–65

Struck HC, Stumpff DL, Caffrey RJ (1950) Effect of tridione (3,3,5-trimethyl oxazolidine-2,4-dione) on the oxygen uptake of motor and sensory cortex of dog brain. Fed Proc 9:123

Swinyard EA (1949) Laboratory assay of clinically effective antiepileptic drugs. J Am Pharm Ass Sci Ed 38:201–204

Swinyard EA (1969) Laboratory evaluation of antiepileptic drugs. Epilepsia 10:107–119

Swinyard EA, Castellion AW (1966) Anticonvulsant properties of some benzodiazepines. J Pharmacol Exp Ther 151:369-375

Swinyard EA, Brown WC, Goodman LS (1952a) Comparative assays of antiepileptic drugs in mice and rats. J Pharmacol Exp Ther 106:319–330

Swinyard EA, Schiffman DO, Goodman LS (1952b) Effects of liver injury and nephrectomy on the anticonvulsant activity of oxazolidine-2,4-diones. J Pharmacol Exp Ther 105:365–370

Swinyard EA, Madsen JA, Goodman LS (1954) The effect of β-diethylaminoethyldiphenylpropylacetate (SKF No. 525 A) on the anticonvulsant properties of antiepileptic drugs. J Pharmacol Exp Ther 111:54–63

Swinyard EA, Castellion AW, Fink GB, Goodman LS (1963) Some neurophysiological and neuropharmacological characteristics of audiogenic-seizure-susceptible mice. J Pharmacol Exp Ther 140:375–384

Taylor JD, Bertcher EL (1952) The determination and distribution of trimethadione (Tridione) in animal tissues. J Pharmacol Exp Ther 106:277–285

Taylor JD, Richards RK, Everett GM, Bertcher EL (1950) Effect of tridione (3,3,5-trimethyloxazolidine-2,4-dione) on the oxygen uptake of mouse brain. J Pharmacol Exp Ther 98:392–399

Taylor JD, Davin JC, Richards RK (1956) Duration of anticonvulsant action of trimethadione and some demethylated oxazolidinediones against pentylenetetrazol in mice. Fed Proc 15:491

Thueson DO, Withrow CD, Giam CS, Woodbury DM (1974) Uptake, distribution, metabolism, and excretion of trimethadione in rats. Epilepsia 15:563–578

Toman JEP (1949) The neuropharmacology of antiepileptics. Electroencephalogr Clin Neurophysiol 1:33–44

Toman JEP, Goodman LS (1948) Anticonvulsants. Physiol Rev 28:409–432

Torda C, Wolff HG (1947) Effect of convulsant and anticonvulsant agents on acetylcholine metabolism (activity of choline acetylase, cholinesterase) and on sensitivity to acetylcholine of effector organs. Am J Physiol 151:345-354

Torda C, Wolff HG (1950) Effect of convulsant and anticonvulsant agents on the activity of cytochrome oxidase. Proc Soc Exp Biol Med 74:744–746

Ueki S, Araki Y, Watanabe S (1977) Changes in sensitivity of mice to anticonvulsant drugs following bilateral olfactory bulb ablations. Jpn J Pharmacol 27:183–192

Waddell WJ, Butler TC (1957) Renal excretion of 5,5-dimethyl-2,4-oxazolidinedione (product of demethylation of trimethadione). Proc Soc Exp Biol Med 96:563–565

Wallin RF, Blackburn WH, Napoli MD (1970) Pharmacologic interactions of albutoin with other anticonvulsant drugs. J Pharmacol Exp Ther 174:276–282

Weaver LC, Swinyard EA, Goodman LS (1958) Anticonvulsant drug combinations: diphenylhydantoin combined with other antiepileptics. J Am Pharm Assoc Sci Ed 47:645–648

Wilkison DM, Halpern LM (1974) Effects of selected anticonvulsants on conjugated estrogen-induced epileptiform activity. Proc West Pharmacol Soc 17:87–91

Withrow CD (1980) Oxazolidinediones. In: Glaser GH, Penry JK, Woodbury DM (eds) Antiepileptic drugs: mechanism of action. Raven, New York, pp 577–586

Withrow CD (1982) Trimethadione: absorption, distribution and excretion. In: Woodbury DM, Penry JK, Pippenger CE (eds) Antiepileptic drugs. Raven, New York, pp 681–687

Withrow CD, Stout RJ, Barton LJ, Beacham WS, Woodbury DM (1968) Anticonvulsant effects of 5,5-dimethyl-2,4-oxazolidinedione (DMO). J Pharmacol Exp Ther 161:335–341

Woodbury DM (1952) Effects of chronic administration of anticonvulsant drugs, alone and in combination with desoxycorticosterone, on electroshock seizure threshold and tissue electrolytes. J Pharmacol Exp Ther 105:46–57
Woodbury DM, Rollins LT, Gardner MD, Hirschi WL, Hogan JR, Rallison ML, Tanner GS, Brodie DA (1958) Effects of carbon dioxide on brain excitability and electrolytes. Am J Physiol 192:79–90
Woodbury DM, Penry JK, Schmidt RP (eds) (1972) Antiepileptic drugs. Raven, New York
Woodbury DM, Penry JK, Pippenger CE (eds) (1982) Antiepileptic drugs. Raven, New York
Yen HCY, Silverman AJ, Salvatore A (1960) Iproniazid reinforcement of anticonvulsants. Fed Proc 19:278
Yen HCY, Salvatore AT, Silverman AJ, King TO (1962) A study of the effect of iponiazid on anticonvulsants in mice. Arch Int Pharmacodyn Ther 140:631–645
Yeoh PN, Wolf HH (1970) Pharmacological evaluation of seizures induced by electrical stimulation of the hippocampus. J Pharm Sci 59:950–954

CHAPTER 19

Succinimides

H. J. TESCHENDORF and R. KRETZSCHMAR

A. Introduction

Succinimides were introduced for the therapy of petit mal epilepsy in 1951, gradually replacing the oxazolidinediones because of their superior clinical tolerance. The first succinimide employed clinically was phensuximide, followed by methsuximide. Ethosuximide, which like trimethadione has a relatively strong efficacy against experimental pentylenetetrazol-induced seizures and is weaker against electrically induced seizures, was introduced somewhat later. The experimental pharmacological profile of these compounds as well as their pharmacokinetics and toxicity will be described in this chapter. The substances have already been reviewed by different authors (WOODBURY et al. 1972, 1982; FERRENDELLI and KUPFERBERG 1980).

The structure-response relationships of succinimides have been reported in reviews by HARGREAVES et al. (1970), VIDA and GERRY (1977), FERRENDELLI and KUPFERBERG (1980), and SCHÄFER (Chap. 9, this volume).

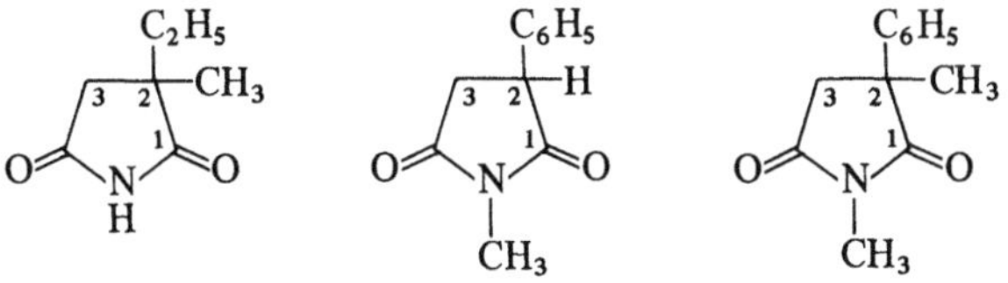

Ethosuximide Phensuximide Methsuximide

Ethosuximide has a molecular weight of 141.17; its melting point is 64°–65 °C. The substance is highly soluble in water. The molecular weight of phensuximide is 189.21 and that of methsuximide 203.23. Their melting points are 71°–73 °C and 52°–53 °C, respectively. Phensuximide is slightly soluble and methsuximide is insoluble in water.

Various procedures have been developed for the quantitative determination of these substances from body fluids or organs. Earlier methods based on colorimetry, thin-layer or gas-liquid chromatography were often not adequately sensitive. For a review of these methods see GLAZKO and DILL (1972a, b). Gas-liquid chromatography (GLC) was improved by the use of modern columns, more sensitive detectors, and derivatization of succinimides so that adequately sensitive methods, enabling other antiepileptics to be determined at the same time, are now available (HORNING et al. 1973b, 1974). High-performance liquid chromatography techniques were also developed and are equal to GLC procedures (SOLDIN and

HILL 1976; KABRA et al. 1977). Ethosuximide can also be determined with an immunoassay (MALKUS et al. 1978; SCHOTTELIUS 1978). A survey of today's procedures is given by GLAZKO (1982).

B. Anticonvulsant Effects

The majority of animal experiments on the anticonvulsant effects of the succinimides have been carried out with ethosuximide, whereas only few experiments with methsuximide and phensuximide have been reported. The reason seems to be that clinically ethosuximide has proven to be the most specific substance of the group of succinimides for the treatment of petit mal epilepsy. According to clinical experience methsuximide and phensuximide are effective in psychomotor attacks and also in grand mal epilepsy (CHEN et al. 1963).

I. Chemically Induced Convulsions

1. Pentylenetetrazol

The antagonistic effect of succinimides against pentylenetetrazol-induced convulsions was first described by CHEN et al. (1951, 1963). In doses of 63 and 250 mg/kg, respectively, methsuximide and phensuximide completely suppressed convulsions elicited by pentylenetetrazol (95 mg/kg s.c.) in rats. These doses brought about slight ataxia, whereas the effective dose of ethosuximide, 125 mg/kg, had no neurotoxic effects. As reported by the same authors there is no difference between methsuximide and phensuximide if the increase of the convulsant dose of pentylenetetrazol in mice is taken into account (the dose is doubled by approximately 100 mg/kg of either substance), whereas the effect of ethosuximide is markedly less pronounced (effective dose ~300 mg/kg). This dose relation of methsuximide and ethosuximide was also found by DESMEDT et al. (1976) and by KRALL et al. (1978), whose experiments make a direct comparison of the two substances in mice and rats possible.

The ED_{50} values reported in the literature for the antagonistic effect of ethosuximide to pentylenetetrazol are between 130 and 180 mg/kg with i.p. administration and between 190 and 420 mg/kg with oral doses, depending on animal species and the dose of pentylenetetrazol used (FREY 1964; MEYER and FREY 1973; KRALL et al. 1978; LÖSCHER 1979a; MASUDA et al. 1980). According to STONE and JAVID (1979), the mean convulsant dose (CD_{50}) of pentylenetetrazol and bemegride is increased threefold by 450 mg/kg ethosuximide. The ED_{50} values of i.p. methsuximide are reported to be 60 and 68 mg/kg (DESMEDT et al. 1976; KRALL et al. 1978). The CD_{50} of pentylenetetrazol is increased by 50–200 mg/kg methsuximide (BASTIAN 1961; NICHOLLS and SCOULAR 1975; STONE and JAVID 1979). ED_{50} values of phensuximide are between 50 and 150 mg/kg (DESMEDT et al. 1976; KRALL et al. 1978; RUMP et al. 1979).

When ethosuximide was admixed to the drinking water of mice, daily intake of 400–1000 mg/kg, not more than a 40% protection against pentylenetetrazol could be obtained (FREY and KAMPMANN 1965), which is due to the very rapid metabolism of the substance in mice.

EEG changes induced by pentylenetetrazol are suppressed by ethosuximide. As outlined by WENZEL et al. (1971) 30 mg/kg pentylenetetrazol administered s.c. to rats led to spindle activity in the cortical and subcortical EEG, which is completely suppressed by 200 mg/kg ethosuximide (i.p.). Likewise the facilitation of photic recruitment and of photic afterdischarges elicited by pentylenetetrazol is abolished.

2. Other Convulsant Substances

Picrotoxin-induced convulsions in mice are inhibited by ethosuximide, with ED_{50} values of 330–350 mg/kg (LÖSCHER and FREY 1977; LÖSCHER 1979a); the CD_{50} of picrotoxin is doubled by administration of 450 mg/kg ethosuximide (STONE and JAVID 1979). According to LÖSCHER and FREY (1977) and RUMP et al. (1979), strychnine-induced convulsions are inhibited by similar doses. MASUDA et al. (1980), however, found that mice were not protected against the lethal effect of strychnine by 1 000 mg/kg ethosuximide.

Investigations by LÖSCHER and FREY (1977) which showed that isoniazid led to a decreased GABA level in the brain and to inhibited glutamate decarboxylase (GAD) and gamma-aminobutyrate-alpha-oxoglutarate aminotransferase (GABA-T) activity suggest that GABA is involved in the anticonvulsant effect of ethosuximide. Ethosuximide counteracts convulsions induced by isoniazid and diminishes the fall of GABA levels and the inhibition of GAD. The inhibition of GABA-T is not affected.

The following findings contradict the relation of ethosuximide to the GABA system: LÖSCHER and FREY (1977) as well as STONE and JAVID (1979) found oral doses of 450–1 000 mg/kg to be ineffective against bicuculline. Ethosuximide is also ineffective against kainic acid, the convulsant effect of which the authors (STONE and JAVID 1980) attribute also to the GABA system. Convulsions induced by 3-mercaptopropionic acid are not antagonized either (LÖSCHER 1979; STONE and JAVID 1979). Neither are changes of GABA metabolism (inhibition of GAD, activation of GABA-T) induced by 3-mercaptopropionic acid influenced by ethosuximide. With methsuximide in an oral dose of 135 mg/kg, however, the mean convulsant dose of 3-mercaptopropionic acid is almost doubled (STONE and JAVID 1979).

Ethosuximide is effective in some other convulsant models, which the authors consider to be specific for substances effective in petit mal epilepsy. A pattern similar to petit mal epilepsy is induced in monkeys and rats by high doses (200 mg/kg i.v.) of gamma-hydroxybutyric acid, an endogenous metabolite of GABA. Bursts of hypersynchronous waves progressing to continuous hypersynchrony are found in the EEG. The bursts are accompanied by phases of immobility resembling stupor (GODSCHALK et al. 1976; SNEAD 1978; SNEAD et al. 1980). In the same manner as trimethadione and valproic acid, ethosuximide eliminates these changes. Phensuximide is inefficacious and even aggravates gamma-hydroxybutyric acid (GHB)-induced symptoms (GODSCHALK et al. 1976).

In a different model described by SNEAD and BEARDEN (1980) in which a pattern similar to petit mal epilepsy is induced by intracerebroventricular injection of leucine enkephalin, ethosuximide, trimethadione, and valproic acid all have an effect, whereas phenobarbital, diphenylhydantoin, diazepam, and clonazepam are ineffective. Generalized epileptic activity induced in cats by high parenteral doses of penicillin is a syndrome similar to petit mal epilepsy, which is inhibited by ethosuximide and not distinctly influenced by diphenylhydantoin (GUBERMAN et al. 1975).

Ethosuximide inhibits seizures induced by procaine (RUMP et al. 1979), by chlorinated hydrocarbon insecticides (dieldrin) in mice (JOY 1973), and by Δ^9-tetrahydrocannabinol in a population of New Zealand White rabbits (CONSROE et al. 1977); it raises the convulsive threshold of fluorothyl (bis-2,2,2-trifluoro-ethyl ether) in rats (ADLER 1972) and of enflurance in dogs (SCHETTINI and WILDER 1974). The LD_{50} of fluostigmine, increased in mice and rats by atropine and obidoxime, can be further increased by phensuximide. EEG changes determined in rabbits by fluostigmine are transiently suppressed by phensuximide (GRUDZINSKA et al. 1978, 1979).

Further investigations have been made on the effect of ethosuximide in models of acute or chronic epilepsy with convulsions elicited by the topical cortical application of drugs. In cats, topical application of conjugated estrogens to the sensorimotor cortex leads to epileptiform spike and slow-wave discharges in the EEG, which can be inhibited by ethosuximide, benzodiazepines, and trimethadione, but not by diphenylhydantoin (WILKINSON and HALPERN 1974; JULIEN et al. 1975). Convulsant discharges produced in rats by the cortical implantation of metallic cobalt are suppressed by 200–400 mg/kg ethosuximide (KÄSTNER et al. 1970; DOW et al. 1973; SCUVEE-MOUREAU et al. 1977; CHIU et al. 1979), secondary foci being more easily affected than primary ones (KÄSTNER et al. 1970).

Weak anticonvulsant or even proconvulsion effects have been demonstrated for ethosuximide in chronic epilepsy induced in rhesus monkey by implants of aluminum hydroxide gel (LOCKARD et al. 1977).

II. Electrically Induced Convulsions

In the maximal electroshock test, marked differences have been found between the effects of methsuximide and phensuximide, on the one hand, and ethosuximide on the other. The following ED_{50} ranges for protection from tonic convulsions induced by maximal electroshock have been reported in the literature: methsuximide 70–84 mg/kg (CHEN et al. 1963; KRALL et al. 1978) and phensuximide 47–313 mg/kg, depending on animal species and route of administration (CHEN et al. 1951, 1963; STILLE and SAYERS 1967; KRALL et al. 1978; RUMP 1979). The values for the two substances reported by CHEN et al. (1963) and KRALL et al. (1978) are somewhat higher than those required for protection against pentylenetetrazol. With ethosuximide, however, these values are far higher than those effective against pentylenetetrazol. The doses suppressing electroshock seizures are as high as 1,000–2,000 mg/kg, thus being in the neurotoxic range. With lower dosed ethosuximide (260 mg/kg s.c.) FERNGREN and PAALZOW (1969) observed effects against electrically induced convulsions in 3- to 15-day-old mice, but these were absent in 21-day-old mice.

STILLE and SAYERS (1967) reported that phensuximide does not alter seizure pattern in the cortical EEG after maximal electroshock, although convulsions are stopped. As in the controls, there is an afterdischarge after stimulation, followed, after an exhaustion phase, by spikes or multiple spikes and sharp waves on the EEG.

In amygdaloid-kindled rats weak effects have been found for ethosuximide, but marked effects for methsuximide. ALBERTSON et al. (1980) found that ethosuximide did not lower seizure rank scores or afterdischarge duration until toxic doses were used. ASHTON and WAUQUIER (1979) showed methsuximide, ED_{50} values of 17–21 mg/kg i.p., to be effective against the various components of these seizures (foreleg clonus, rearing-up, falling-down). The doses were slightly lower than those producing ataxia.

There have been varying reports on the effect of succinimides on afterdischarges after local stimulation of individual brain regions. STEINMANN (1964) found that ethosuximide raised the convulsant threshold in the hippocampus, but not in the cortex, of rabbits. LITTROW et al. (1970) observed that the electrically evoked self-sustaining hippocampal afterdischarge in rats is not eliminated by ethosuximide. On the contrary, the spike frequency of the initial afterdischarge is increased and its duration is prolonged, suggesting seizure facilitation.

Ethosuximide reduced evoked responses in the sensorimotor cortex after stimulation of the ventrolateral thalamus, and diminished (like valproic acid) in particular the responses to stimulation, at a rate of 3/s (ENGLANDER et al. 1975; NOWAK et al. 1979). The authors find this of particular interest in view of the good therapeutic results obtained with the substances in absence attacks with repetitive activity occurring at a rate of 3/s.

III. Convulsions Induced by Other Methods

In models based on, often genetically determined, hypersensitivity to visual or acoustic stimuli, ethosuximide shows minor effects. DAVIS et al. (1978) have shown ethosuximide to have no effect in fowl with high susceptibility to seizures after intermittent photic stimulation. In the model of photomyoclonic seizures of the baboon (*Papio papio*) ethosuximide has only weak effects. NAQUET et al. (1975) and KILLAM (1979) found the effect to be age dependent; thus, the doses required for inhibiting the epileptic response are two to three times higher in adult than in young animals. In both cases the animals show marked central side effects (RINNE et al. 1978). When susceptibility to seizures is augmented by allylglycine, the anticonvulsant effect of ethosuximide on photically induced seizures in baboons is also weak (MELDRUM et al. 1975).

Afterdischarge potentials of the visually evoked response in rats are diminished in number and amplitude by ethosuximide (TURKANIS et al. 1977; KÄSTNER et al. 1968). These afterdischarges, which can only be triggered in the relaxed state of arousal by photic stimulation, can also be suppressed by activating the animals. Thus, the effect of ethosuximide is possibly mediated by a reticular activation. Topical application of ethosuximide to the lateral geniculate body had no effect on afterdischarges (KÄSTNER and ROUGERIE 1978).

In rats susceptible to audiogenic seizures, 100 mg/kg ethosuximide is ineffective (CONSROE and WOLKIN 1977). Convulsions elicited by acoustic stimuli in barbiturate-dependent rats during withdrawal are attenuated by ethosuximide (NORTON 1970).

C. Central Nervous System Effects Besides the Anticonvulsant Effect

Neurophysiological effects of the succinimides are described by Jurna in Chap. 23, this volume.

I. Influence on the EEG

KÄSTNER et al. (1968) found the amplitude in the cortical EEG of rats to be decreased after 100–500 mg/kg i.p. Sleep spindles were absent and the hippocampus showed a theta rhythm of 5–7 s corresponding to the activated state of arousal. With higher doses, the animals were relaxed or showed a loss of the righting reflex. GODSCHALK et al. (1976) also reported desynchronization of the cortical EEG of rats after administratiion of ethosuximide or phensuximide. In the baboon, RINNE et al. (1978) found a reduction of spectral power in frequencies around 15 s, with a simultaneous dose-dependent increase of slow activity (4–8 s).

II. Influence on Behavior

In mice, ethosuximide and methsuximide in the anticonvulsant dose range lead to increased motor activity (BASTIAN 1961; KEHRHAHN 1973). Higher doses of the succinimides produce ataxia (CHEN et al. 1951; 1963; KRALL et al. 1978; MASUDA et al. 1980). The dose intervals between anticonvulsant effects on pentylenetetrazol convulsions and neurotoxic effects (ataxia or inhibition of performance at the rotarod) are 2.8–4.6 (KRALL et al. 1978). As described by MASUDA et al. (1980), high doses of ethosuximide lead to a loss of righting reflex and prolonged sleeping time after hexobarbital.

In rats, ASHTON and WAUQUIER (1979) observed ataxia with methsuximide doses as low as 28 mg/kg i.p. KÄSTNER et al. (1968) reported diminished startle response and muscle relaxation with ethosuximide doses of 50 mg/kg i.p. or more and a loss of righting reflex with 500 mg/kg. According to GUBERMAN et al. (1975), cats show mild muscular rigidity and a paucity of spontaneous movements at an ethosuximide plasma level of 140 µg/ml, i.e., a level double that required for significant anticonvulsant effects. Dystonic posture was observed after 200 mg/kg. Chronic administration of ethosuximide (15–60 mg/kg daily i.p. for 8 weeks) to baboons led to a dose-related decrease of learning performance, which was not related to motor difficulties (PAULE and KILLAM 1979). This disruption of learning performance was evident for up to 4 months after cessation of ethosuximide administration. LOCKARD et al. (1977) reported a reduced duration of sleep and a depression of REM stages in rhesus monkeys with cortical aluminum hydroxide implantation during the chronic administration of ethosuximide. According to CLINCKE and WAUQUIER (1979), pentylenetetrazol impaired passive avoidance retention in rats. This effect of pentylenetetrazol could be suppressed by ethosuximide.

III. Effects on Neurochemical Processes

1. Neurotransmitters

No changes in the concentration or metabolism of neurotransmitters have become known for succinimides which might explain the anticonvulsant effect. The following individual findings are described in the literature:

In the brain of rats (NAHORSKI 1972) or mice (LUST et al. 1978) ethosuximide does not change the concentration of GABA. LÖSCHER and FREY (1977) indicate that GAD is slightly activated, while LEZNICKI and DYMECKI (1974) observed no effect of the substance. Of the enzymes degrading GABA, GABA-T, measured in mouse brain homogenates, is inhibited to a small extent by ethosuximide in concentrations of 0.1–10 m*M* (SAWAYA et al. 1975), but is slightly activated by phensuximide (10 m*M*). LÖSCHER (1980) has also shown ethosuximide to inhibit GABA-T slightly. Succinic semialdehyde dehydrogenase is activated by ethosuximide (10 m*M*), but slightly inhibited by phensuximide (10 m*M*). The relevance of these findings is questionable since in most cases the concentrations were higher than the expected therapeutic blood levels.

The concentration of GHB in the total brain and, in particular, in the subcortex and cerebellum of rats is increased by a single dose of ethosuximide, but decreased after subchronic administration for 7 days (SNEAD et al. 1980). The physiological significance of GHB, an endogenous metabolite of GABA, has not yet been determined. But the findings are of interest in view of the epileptiform changes which can be produced experimentally by high doses of GHB and which can be specifically inhibited by drugs acting on petit mal epilepsy.

In the study by BONNYCASTLE et al. (1957) phensuximide in three i.p. doses as high as 450 mg/kg increased the concentration of 5-hydroxytryptamine (5-HT) in the brain of rats, but not in the periphery. No protection against the convulsant or lethal effects of pentylenetetrazol is obtained by increasing the 5-HT level in the brain by monoamine oxidase (MAO) inhibitors (iproniazid) or 5-hydroxytryptophan. As described by MEYER and FREY (1973), any such increase has a synergistic effect when ethosuximide is given simultaneously.

Ethosuximide increases dopamine metabolism, as measured in the dihydroxyphenylacetic acid (DOPAC) and homovanillic acid (HVA) concentrations in mesolimbic structures, but not in the striatum. The relevance of these findings for anticonvulsant action appears doubtful. In the model of GHB-induced epileptoid changes, the anticonvulsant effect of ethosuximide depends on intact dopaminergic function. According to KLUNK and FERRENDELLI (1980), dopamine receptor blockers or inhibitors of dopamine synthesis abolish the anticonvulsant effect of ethosuximide against GHB. No data are available on the influence of succinimides on the norepinephrine level or metabolism.

2. Effects on Other Nervous Tissue Systems

Ethosuximide inhibits oxygen uptake by brain slices (LEZNICKI and DYMECKI 1974). Glucose concentration in the brain is increased by ethosuximide, the blood glucose level remaining unchanged (GILBERT et al. 1971; NAHORSKI 1972). This is explained, as was shown by GRAY and GILBERT (1970), in the model of the xylose uptake by guinea pig brain slices, by increased glucose uptake, not by reduced degradation. By investigating energy metabolism in the rat brain, NAHORSKI (1972) found that glucose-6-phosphate and fructose-6-phosphate of the glycolytic intermediates were increased and that fructose-1,6-phosphate was decreased. Among the tricarboxylate cycle intermediates, citrate and alpha-oxoglutarate were reduced. Other intermediates or high-energy phosphates were not changed. The findings signify a reduced metabolic rate, which, however, cannot be considered to be a causative factor in the anticonvulsant action of the succinimides. Like most other anticonvulsant drugs, ethosuximide lowers the concentration of cyclic 3,5-GMP in the cerebellum, but not in the cerebral cortex (LUST et al. 1978).

Ethosuximide inhibits Na^+K^+-ATPase (GILBERT et al. 1974a; LEZNICKI and DYMECKI 1974) in the microsomal and synaptosomal fractions of the rat brain (GILBERT et al. 1974), but not Mg^{++}-ATPase. As outlined by GILBERT and WYLLIE (1974), Mg^{++}-ATPase located in synaptosomal vesicles can be inhibited by ethosuximide in concentrations of 0.25–25 m*M*, the higher concentrations being higher than those necessary for the anticonvulsant effect. Conversely, LEZNICKA and DYMECKI (1974) found Na^+K^+-ATPase to be activated, on in vivo administration of ethosuximide. A number of other enzymes (acetylcholine esterase, monoamine oxidase, arylsulfatase) are not affected (LEZNICKA and DYMECKI 1974).

Two enzymes of the polyol pathway, aldose reductase and hexonate dehydrogenase, isolated from human brain are inhibited by ethosuximide (O'BRIAN and SHOFIELD 1980). These enzymes seem to correspond to the aldehyde reductases described earlier (ERWIN and DEITRICH 1973; RIS et al. 1975), which, isolated from bovine and human brain, can also be inhibited by succinimides. In these cases, ionizable ethosuximide has a stronger inhibitory effect than methsuximide or phensuximide.

D. Pharmacodynamic Properties Outside the Central Nervous System

Animal experiments on the peripheral effects of succinimides have not been performed. Neither have there been systematic investigations of the cardiac and circulatory functions. There is some evidence that ethosuximide in doses of 100–500 mg/kg lowers heart and respiratory rates in rats (KÄSTNER et al. 1968). GANDHI et al. (1976) reported a weak local anesthetic effect of ethosuximide which was 8% of the effect of lidocaine. In addition, they found a dose-related blocking of neuromuscular transmission, which is not only due to the local anesthetic effect, but also to a curare-like effect. No antiarrhythmic effect was observed in the model of ouabain-induced arrhythmia in rabbits (DRESSLER et al. 1972).

Several authors investigated the porphyria-inducing activity of succinimides: marked activation of porphyrin synthesis in chick embryo livers and in livers of chicks aged 5–7 weeks induced by methsuximide and phensuximide was observed (RACZ and MARKS 1969; CREIGHTON and MARKS 1972; ORTON and NICHOLLS 1972a, b; RIFKIND et al. 1973). Ethosuximide was ineffective. The effects were dependent on the animal species used. In livers of mice a porphyria-inducing effect was not found (CREIGHTON and MARKS 1972).

In rats, ethosuximide, methsuximide, and phensuximide lead to the induction of hepatic microsomal enzyme activity (ORTON and NICHOLLS 1972; GILBERT et al. 1974b). The administration of 0.5–2 mmol/kg daily for 3 days significantly reduced the hexobarbital sleeping time, increased oxidation of hexobarbital, and augmented hydroxylation of aniline. Morphologically, the animals showed increased weight of the liver and proliferation of the hepatic smooth endoplasmatic reticulum. Microsomal cytochrome-P-450 activity was also augmented. In guinea pigs, corresponding effects were not observed for ethosuximide (GILBERT et al. 1974b).

Ethosuximide did not inhibit the binding of hexobarbital to cytochrome P-450 (LATHAM and SWEENEY 1976). PATSALOS and LASCELLES (1977, 1980) describe ethosuximide as showing a competitive, but weak, inhibition of the hydroxylation of diphenylhydantoin by a liver microsomal enzyme preparation.

E. Pharmacokinetics

The results of many experiments on animals to investigate the pharmacokinetics of ethosuximide are available in the literature. In addition, there have been a few investigations performed with methsuximide and phensuximide.

I. Absorption

Using a gas-chromatographic technique, DILL et al. (1965) found that ethosuximide is rapidly absorbed by rats after oral administration and attains a maximum plasma level after 1 h. In dogs approximately 90% is absorbed from the gastrointestinal tract. The peak plasma levels were measured after 0.8–4 h (EL SAYED et al. 1978).

In rhesus monkeys, the bioavailability of ethosuximide from a syrup preparation was $96 \pm 12\%$ (PATEL et al. 1975). In the dose range examined bioavailability was dose independent.

Methsuximide is also rapidly absorbed by rats. The absorption half-life from the duodenum was 17.4 min (NICHOLLS and ORTON 1972).

II. Distribution

In rats ethosuximide is very evenly distributed in all tissues except for adipose tissue (DILL et al. 1965; BURKETT et al. 1971). The relative distributions in organs related to the plasma (DILL et al. 1965) are 1.04 for the brain, 0.94 for the muscles, 1.04 for the kidneys, but only 0.11 for the liver. Ethosuximide crosses the placental barrier and penetrates the fetal tissue of rats (CHANG et al. 1972). In dogs and monkeys the kinetics can be described by a one-compartment open model (EL SAYED et al. 1978; PATEL et al. 1975). The distribution volume was 67% of the body weight in dogs (EL SAYED et al. 1978) and 80% in monkeys (PATEL et al. 1975). In the cerebrospinal fluid of the dog the steady state was reached within 30 min (EL SAYED et al. 1978).

Plasma protein binding of ethosuximide is very low; 90%–98% is found unbound in the dog plasma (EL SAYED et al. 1978). LÖSCHER (1979b) determined the protein binding of ethosuximide in dogs by using equilibrium dialysis; he found 7%–12% at 37 °C. This value largely corresponds to that of protein binding in humans (LUNDE et al. 1970).

Anticonvulsant plasma levels of ethosuximide are approximately 50–100 μg/ml (LOCKARD et al. 1977). After chronic oral administration in rhesus monkeys (initial dose 40–60 mg/kg and maintenance dose 16–24 mg/kg every 24 h) steady-state plasma levels of 30–50 μg/ml were measured after 5 days (PATEL and LEVY 1975). With constant zero-order infusion of ethosuximide in rhesus monkeys, PATEL et al. (1975) found variations of the plasma levels which were probably caused by circadian metabolic changes.

Using mass fragmentography, YONEKAWA and KUPFERBERG (1976) determined equal plasma levels and cerebral concentrations of phensuximide and its *N*-demethylated degradation product in mice. With methsuximide and its *N*-demethylated metabolite the concentrations are equal only during the 1 st h after administration. Later on, the concentration of *N*-demethylmethsuximide declines far more slowly than that of the unchanged substance.

In contrast to ethosuximide, DOBRINSKA and WELLING (1977) described the kinetics of methsuximide by a two-compartment open model. Organ distribution of methsuximide is relatively uniform, brain included, and protein binding is very low (GLATZKO et al. 1953). With ^{14}C-labeled substance, NICHOLLS and ORTON (1972) found maximum blood and tissue values 1 h after oral administration to rats.

III. Metabolism

After administration of ethosuximide, DILL et al. (1963) detected more than five metabolites in rats. In the urine of rats after administration of [^{14}C]ethosuximide, BURKETT et al. (1971) recovered 78% of the radioactivity administered: 12% as unchanged substance, 40% as 2-(1-hydroxyethyl)-2-methylsuccinimide, and a further 48% as nonidentified metabolites. HORNING et al. (1973 b) determined various glucuronides of hydroxyethosuximides in the urine of rats after administration of ethosuximide. Similar findings were established in monkeys by CHANG and GLAZKO (1982). In addition to 2-(1-hydroxyethyl)-2-methylsuccinimide, the analogous 2-hydroxyethyl compound and a 3-hydroxy derivative of ethosuximide were identified.

The demethylation product 2-methyl-2-phenylsuccimide was identified in rats and dogs as the main metabolite of methsuximide, which, unlike ethosuximide, is *N*-methylated (NICHOLLS and ORTON 1972; DOBRINSKA and WELLING 1977); this compound is pharmacologically active. Unlike the parent compound, distribution of the metabolite complies with a one-compartment model; the elimination half-life from the plasma of dogs is 15 h. Moreover, DUDLEY et al. (1974 a) found 7%–20% of glucuronides of derivatives *p*-hydroxylated at the 2-phenylic ring (2-(*p*-hydroxyphenyl)-2-methylsuccinimide and *N*-methyl-2-(*p*-hydroxyphenyl)-2-methylsuccinimide) in the urine of dogs collected for 48 h. According to HORNING et al. (1973 a), methsuximide metabolism follows an epoxide-diol pathway. Three characteristic metabolites detected by gas chromatography (GC) and GC mass spectrometry in rats, guinea pigs, and humans (3,4-dihydroxycyclohexadiene-1-yl; 3- or 4-hydroxyphenyl derivatives) support this fact. Small quantities of nonepoxidic metabolites were also determined (*N*-methyl-2-hydroxymethyl-2-phenylsuccinimide, *N*,2-dimethyl-3-hydroxy-2-phenylsuccinimide, and *N*,2-dimethyl-2(4-hydroxyphenyl)-3-hydroxy succinimide).

HORNING et al. (1976) reported that the metabolism of the stereoisomers of methsuximide differs quantitatively. After administration of racemic methsuximide the metabolites *N*-methyl-2-(*p*-hydroxyphenyl)-2-methylsuccinimide and 2-(*p*-hydroxyphenyl)-2-methylsuccinimide are found to occur in a ratio of 1:1.2 in the urine of rats, whereas after administration of the corresponding *l*- or *d*-compound the ratio of the metabolites is 0.6:1 and 1:5.9, respectively. There is no evidence that methsuximide or ethosuximide is metabolized to succinamic acid by opening of the ring (DUDLEY et al. 1974b). In contrast, phensuximide appears to be metabolized to the acid by ring-opening. In the urine of dogs, DUDLEY and BUTLER (1971) and DUDLEY et al. (1974b) detected 14% of *l*-2-phenyl-succinamic acid and 5% of *p*-hydroxyphenyl metabolites (*N*-methyl-2-(*p*-hydroxyphenyl)-succinimide) in the form of glucuronides and trace amounts of unchanged substance. Corresponding stereospecific ring metabolism is also known for a hydantoin which has a related structure (DUDLEY et al. 1974b). These metabolites were found by DUDLEY et al. (1974b) in rat liver homogenate after incubation with phensuximide. The hydrolyzation of the ring of enantiomers is effected by dihydropyrimidinase (MAGUIRE and DUDLEY 1978).

IV. Elimination

The elimination of ethosuximide has been investigated repeatedly in various animal species, but only a few investigators have studied the elimination of methsuximide and phensuximide. The elimination half-lives of ethosuximide were found to differ greatly in the examined species. They were 1 h in mice (EL SAYED et al. 1978), 16, 12, and 10 h in rats (DILL et al. 1965; CHANG et al. 1972; EL SAYED et al. 1978), 18 h in dogs (EL SAYED et al. 1978), and 28, 22, and 22.4–35.6 h in monkeys (DILL et al. 1965; CHANG et al. 1972; PATEL et al. 1975). The elimination half-life of ethosuximide in humans is 30–60 h (SHERWIN et al. 1971; EL SAYED et al. 1978). Elimination occurs monoexponentially by first-order kinetics over four to five elimination half-lives (PATEL et al. 1975). Saturable elimination of ethosuximide was reported for the dog (EL SAYED et al. 1978).

Ethosuximide is excreted primarily by the kidneys; in the rat excretion with the feces accounts for only 4%. Thus external bile duct fistulae in monkeys did not affect the plasma half-life of ethosuximide (CHANG et al. 1972).

Methsuximide is more rapidly excreted than ethosuximide. The plasma half-life in the dog was reported to be 1–3.5 h (DOBRINSKA and WELLING 1977). In the 24-h urine of rats, two-thirds of the amount administered was recovered almost exclusively in the form of metabolites (GLATZKO et al. 1953). After administration of [^{14}C]methsuximide, NICHOLLS and ORTON (1972) found 26% of the radioactivity in the urine and 29% in the expired air.

From the plasma of mice, phensuximide is eliminated twice as quickly as methsuximide (YONEKAWA and KUPFERBERG 1976).

F. Interactions

FREY (1964) and FREY and KAMPMANN (1966) investigated the influence of amphetamine on the anticonvulsant action of ethosuximide in the pentylenetetrazol threshold test. Amphetamine doses not affecting the threshold dose of pentylenetetrazol led to an increase in the ED_{50} values of ethosuximide. Simultaneously, plasma levels were found to be lowered, which was attributable to reduced absorption of ethosuximide, so that central effects could not account for the antagonism.

For cannabidiol CONSROE and WOLKIN (1977) reported dose-related protective effects against maximal electroshock-induced and audiogenic seizures. When administering ethosuximide simultaneously, graded dose-response effects are no longer obtained.

MEYER and FREY (1973) investigated how changes in the central level and metabolism of norepinephrine, dopamine, and 5-HT and how receptor-blocking drugs interfere with the anticonvulsant effect of ethosuximide against pentylenetetrazol convulsions. The effect of ethosuximide was potentiated by 5-HT, whereas *p*-chloro-phenylalanine and cyproheptadine attenuated the effect. The effect of ethosuximide was also reduced by all substances interfering with norepinephrine and dopamine.

G. Toxicity

CHEN et al. (1963) examined the acute and chronic toxicity of ethosuximide and phensuximide in animal experiments. The acute toxicities of the succinimides in mice differ only slightly. The LD_{50} with oral dosing was determined to be between 1,400 and 1,550 mg/kg. The lethal doses were larger by more than one decimal power than the anticonvulsant doses. In pentylenetetrazol-induced convulsions and maximal electroshock, CHEN et al. determined anticonvulsant ED_{50} values of 40–65 mg/kg and 80–210 mg/kg, respectively. The dose interval between anticonvulsant and toxic doses was smaller for phensuximide than for ethosuximide and methsuximide. The toxic symptoms observed were disturbed coordination and loss of righting and grasping reflexes, indicating neurotoxicity, and dyspnea. The chronic toxicity of the succinimides was determined in mice and rats by admixture to the feed, in dogs by oral administration in capsules, and in monkeys by gavage. Ethosuximide was administered to mice, rats, dogs, and monkeys for 5 weeks, 26 weeks, 6 months, and 6 months; methsuxinimide for 4 weeks, 26 weeks, and 1 year; phensuximide for 8 weeks, 8 weeks, and 6 months (monkeys excluded). The hematological or laboratory parameters were not affected in any study. Weight loss was the only symptom observed. Daily amounts of 1,206 mg/kg ethosuximide, 806 mg/kg methsuximide, and 770 mg/kg phensuximide were well tolerated by mice. Admixture of only 1% of phensuximide to the feed, corresponding to 1,328 mg/kg daily, caused reduced food intake; weight loss was produced by admixing as little as 0.125% of succinimides to the feed.

Rats tolerated doses of about 650–750 mg/kg, corresponding to 1% admixture to the feed, without weight loss. Histologically the organs revealed mild liver cell necroses after 567 mg/kg ethosuximide, 600 mg/kg methsuximide, and 284 mg/kg phensuximide, which, however, were not accompanied by any functional disturbance. Dogs tolerated 12.5–50 mg/kg ethosuximide, 10–40 mg/kg methsuximide, and 75 mg/kg phensuximide administered twice daily for a period of 45 days to 1 year. Impaired coordination was observed with doses exceeding 100 mg/kg. Single daily doses of 50–100 mg ethosuximide and methsuximide had no adverse effects in monkeys. Doses of approximately 200 mg/kg led to ataxia.

Various investigators studied the question of a potential teratogenicity of succinimides. McElhatton and Sullivan (1977) and Sullivan and McElhatton (1977) administered CD–1 mice ethosuximide in doses of up to 360 mg/kg from the 6th to the 16th day of gravity and detected malformations in only 3.2% of the fetuses. There was no significant difference versus the controls. By contrast, diphenylhydantoin produced malformations in 20.9% of fetuses. Gordon (1981) reported that succinimides exert a distinctly smaller teratogenic effect in mice than do oxazolidinediones. Fabro et al. (1976) have determined that non-substituted succinimide is not teratogenic in CD–1 mice, the corresponding anhydride (succinic anhydride), like other anhydrides (e.g. phthalic anhydride) being teratogenic, however.

References

Adler MW (1972) The effect of single and multiple lesions of the limbic system on cerebral excitability. Psychopharmacologia 24:218–230

Albertson TE, Peterson SL, Stark LG (1980) Anticonvulsant drugs and their antagonism of kindled amygdaloid seizures in rats. Neuropharmacology 19:643–652

Ashton D, Wauquier A (1979) Behavioral analysis of the effects of 15 anticonvulsants in the amygdaloid kindled rat. Psychopharmacology 65:7–13

Bastian JW (1961) Classification of CNS drugs by a mouse screening battery. Arch Int Pharmacodyn Ther 133:347–364

Bonnycastle DD, Giarman NJ, Paasonen MK (1957) Anticonvulsant compounds and 5-hydroxy-tryptamine in rat brain. Br J Pharmacol 12:228–231

Burkett AR, Chang T, Glazko AJ (1971) A hydroxylated metabolite of ethosuximide (Zarontin®) in rat urine. Fed Proc 30:391

Chang T, Glatzko AJ (1982) Ethosuximide. Biotransformation In: Woodbury DM, Penry JK, Pippenger CE (eds) Antiepileptic drugs. Raven, New York, pp 631–635

Chang T, Burkett AR, Glazko AJ (1972) Ethosuximide. Biotransformation. In: Woodbury DM, Penry JK, Schmidt RP (eds) Antiepileptic drugs. Raven, New York, pp 425–429

Chen G, Portman R, Ensor CR, Bratton AC (1951) The anticonvulsant activity of α-phenyl succinimides. J Pharmacol Exp Ther 103:54–61

Chen G, Weston JK, Bratton AC (1963) Anticonvulsant activity and toxicity of phensuximide, methsuximide and ethosuximide. Epilepsia 4:66–76

Chiu P, Olsen DM, Borys HK, Karler R, Turkanis SA (1979) The influence of cannabidiol and Δ^9-tetrahydrocannabinol on cobalt epilepsy in rats. Epilepsia 20:365–375

Clincke G, Wauquier A (1979) Metrazol-produced impairment of passive avoidance retention specifically antagonized by anti-petit mal drugs. Psychopharmacology 66:243–246

Consroe P, Wolkin A (1977) Cannabidiol-antiepileptic drug comparisons and interactions in experimentally induced seizures in rats. J Pharmacol Exp Ther 201:26–32

Consroe P, Martin P, Eisenstein D (1977) Anticonvulsant drug antagonism of Δ^9-tetrahydrocannabinol-induced seizures in rabbits. Res Commun Chem Pathol Pharmacol 16:1–13

Creighton JM, Marks GS (1972) Drug-induced porphyrin biosynthesis. VII. Species, sex, and developmental differences in the generation of experimental porphyria. Can J Physiol Pharmacol 50:485–489

Davis HL, Johnson DD, Crawford RD (1978) Epileptiform seizures in domestic fowl. IX. Implications of the absence of anticonvulsant activity of ethosuximide in a pharmacological model of epilepsy. Can J Physiol Pharmacol 56:893–896
Desmedt LKC, Niemegeers CJE, Lewi PJ, Janssen PAJ (1976) Antagonism of maximal metrazol seizures in rats and its relevance to an experimental classification of antiepileptic drugs. Arzneimittelforsch 26:1592–1603
Dill WA, Peterson L, Chang T, Glazko AJ (1965) Physiological disposition of α-methyl-α-ethyl succinimide (ethosuximide; Zarontin®) in animals and in man. Abstracts of the 149th National Meeting of the American Chemical Society. Detroit, Michigan, p 30N. American Chemical Society, Washington
Dobrinska MR, Welling PG (1977) Pharmacokinetics of methsuximide and a major metabolite in dogs. J Pharm Sci 66:688–692
Dow RC, Forfar JC, McQueen JK (1973) The effects of some anticonvulsive drugs on cobalt-induced epilepsy. Epilepsia 14:203–212
Dressler WE, Rossi GV, Orzechowski RF (1972) Effect of several anticonvulsant drugs and procainamide against ouabain-induced cardiac arrhythmias in rabbits. J Pharm Sci 61:133–134
Dudley KH, Butler TC (1971) Metabolic fates of *N*-methyl-α-phenylsuccinimide (phensuximide, milontin) and of α-phenylsuccinimide in the dog. Pharmacologist 13:221
Dudley KH, Bius DL, Waldrop CD (1974a) Urinary metabolites of *N*-methyl-α-methyl-α-phenylsuccinimide (methsuximide) in the dog. Drug Metab Dispos 2:113–122
Dudley KH, Butler TC, Bius DL (1974b) The role of dihydropyrimidinase in the metabolism of some hydantoin and succinimide drugs. Drug Metab Dispos 2:103–112
El Sayed MA, Löscher W, Frey HH (1978) Pharmacokinetics of ethosuximide in the dog. Arch Int Pharmacodyn Ther 234:180–192
Englander RN, Johnson RN, Hanna GR (1975) A comparison of the effects of anticonvulsant drugs and cerebellar stimulation on the thalamocortical motor system. Arch Neurol 32:348
Erwin VG, Deitrich RA (1973) Inhibition of bovine brain aldehyde reductase by anticonvulsant compounds in vitro. Biochem Pharmacol 22:2615–2624
Fabro S, Shull G, Dixon R (1976) Further studies on the mechanism of teratogenic action of thalidomide. Pharmacologist 18:231
Ferngren H, Paalzow L (1967) Studies on electrically induced-seizures and their antagonism by anticonvulsants during neonatal development in the mouse. Acta Pharmacol Toxicol (Copenh) 25 (Suppl) 4:60
Ferngren H, Paalzow L (1969) High frequency electro-shock seizures and their antagonism during postnatal development in the mouse. II. Effects of phenobarbital sodium, mephobarbital, trimethadione, dimethadione, ethosuximide and acetazolamide. Acta Phamacol Toxicol (Copenh) 27:249–261
Ferrendelli JA, Kupferberg HJ (1980) Succinimides. In: Glaser JH, Penry JK, Woodbury DM (eds) Antiepileptic drugs: mechanism of action. Raven, New York, 587–596
Frey HH (1964) Note on the interactions of amphetamine with anticonvulsant drugs. Acta Pharmacol Toxicol (Copenh) 21:290–298
Frey HH, Kampmann E (1965) Tolerance to anticonvulsant drugs. Acta Pharmacol Toxicol (Copenh) 22:159–171
Frey HH, Kampmann E (1966) Interaction of amphetamine with anticonvulsant drugs. II. Effect of amphetamine on the absorption of anticonvulsant drugs. Acta Pharmacol Toxicol (Copenh) 24:310–316
Gandhi IC, Jinda MN, Patel VK (1976) Mechanism of neuromuscular blockade with some antiepileptic drugs. Arzneimittelforsch 26:258–261
Glazko AJ (1982) Ethosuximide. Chemistry and methods of determination. In: Woodbury DM, Penry JK, Pippenger CE (eds) Antiepileptic drugs. Raven, New York, pp 617–622
Glazko AJ, Dill WA (1972a) Ethosuximide. Chemistry and methods for determination. In: Woodbury DM, Penry JK, Schmidt RP (eds) Antiepileptic drugs. Raven, New York, pp 413–415
Glazko AJ, Dill WA (1972b) Other succinimides. Methsuximide and phensuximide. In: Woodbury DM, Penry JK, Schmidt RP (eds) Antiepileptic drugs. Raven, New York, pp 455–464

Glazko AJ, Dill WA, Wolf LM, Miller CA (1953) The determination and physiological disposition of milontin (*N*-methyl-α-phenylsuccinimide). J Pharmacol Exp Ther 111:413–424
Gilbert JC, Wyllie MG (1974) The effects of the anticonvulsant ethosuximide on adenosine triphosphatase activities of synaptosomes prepared from rat cerebral cortex. Br J Pharmacol 52:139–140
Gilbert JC, Gray P, Heaton CM (1971) Anticonvulsant drugs and brain glucose. Biochem Pharmacol 20:240–243
Gilbert JC, Scott AK, Wyllie MG (1974a) Effects of ethosuximide on adenosine triphosphatase activities of some subcellular fractions prepared from rat cerebral cortex. Br J Pharmacol 50:452–453
Gilbert JC, Scott AK, Galloway DB, Petrie JC (1974b) Ethosuximide: liver enzyme induction and D-glucaric acid excretion. Br J Clin Pharmacol 1:249–252
Godschalk M, Dzoljic MR, Bonta IL (1976) Antagonism of gamma-hydroxybutyrate-induced hypersynchronization in the ECoG of the rat by anti-petit mal drugs. Neurosci Lett 3:145–150
Gordon RS (1981) Anticonvulsants found to have teratogenic potential. JAMA 245:36
Gray P, Gilbert JP (1970) Anticonvulsant drugs and xylose uptake by cerebral cortex slices. Biochem J 120:27–28
Grudzińska E, Lechowska-Postek M, Ilczuk I, Rump S (1978) Vergleich der therapeutischen Wirkung von Trimethadion und Phensuximid bei akuter Organophosphatvergiftung. Ther Hung 26:126–130
Grudzińska E, Gidyńska T, Rump S (1979) Therapeutic value of anticonvulsant drugs in poisonings with an organophosphate. Arch Int Pharmacodyn Ther 238:344–350
Guberman A, Gloor P, Sherwin AL (1975) Response of generalized penicillin epilepsy in the cat to ethosuximide and diphenylhydantoin. Neurology 25:758–764
Hargreaves MK, Pritchard JG, Dave HR (1970) Cyclic carboxylic monoimides. Chem Rev 70:439–469
Horning MG, Butler C, Harvey DJ, Hill RM, Zion TE (1973a) Metabolism of *N*,2-dimethyl-2-phenylsuccinimide (methsuximide) by the epoxide-diol pathway in rat, guinea pig and human. Res Commun Chem Pathol Pharmacol 6:565–578
Horning MG, Stratton C, Nowlin J, Harvey DJ, Hill RM (1973b) Metabolism of 2-ethyl-2-methylsuccinimide in the rat and human. Drug Metab Dispos 1:569–576
Horning MG, Lertratanangkoon K, Nowlin J, Stillwell WG, Zion TE, Kellaway P, Hill RM (1974) Anticonvulsant drug monitoring by GC-MS-COM techniques. J Chromatogr Sci 12:630–635
Horning MG, Butler CM, Glazko AJ (1976) GC-MS studies of the metabolism of methsuximide enantiomers. Pharmacologist 18:155
Joy RM (1973) Electrical correlates of preconvulsive and convulsive doses of chlorinated hydrocarbon insecticides in the CNS. Neuropharmacology 12:63–76
Julien RM, Fowler GW, Danielson MG (1975) The effects of antiepileptic drugs on estrogen-induced electrographic spike-wave discharge. J Pharmacol Exp Ther 193:647–656
Kabra PM, Stafford BE, Marton LJ (1977) Simultaneous measurement of phenobarbital, phenytoin, primidone, ethosuximide and carbamazepine in serum by high-pressure liquid chromatography. Clin Chem 23:1284–1288
Kästner I, Rougerie A (1978) Photisch ausgelöste Potentialfolgen nach lokaler Applikation von Ethosuximid ins Corpus geniculatum laterale. Acta Biol Med Ger 37:677–679
Kästner I. Klingberg F, Müller M (1968) Untersuchungen zur zentralnervösen Wirkung des Ethosuximids. Arch Psychiatr Nervenkr 211:365–376
Kästner I, Klingberg F, Müller M (1970) Zur Wirkung des Ethosuximids auf die Kobalt-induzierte Epilepsie der Ratte. Arch Int Pharmacodyn Ther 186:220–226
Kehrhahn OH (1973) Das Verhalten männlicher Albinomäuse im Laufrad-Versuch. Arzneimittelforsch 23:981–991
Killam EK (1979) Photomyoclonic seizures in the baboon, *Papio papio*. Fed Proc 38:2429–2433

Klunk WE, Ferrendelli JA (1980) Reversal of the anticonvulsant action of ethosuximide by drugs that diminish CNS dopaminergic neurotransmission. Neurology (Minneap) 30:421

Krall RL, Penry JK, White BG, Kupferberg HJ, Swinyard EA (1978) Antiepileptic drug development. II. Anticonvulsant drug screening. Epilepsia 19:409–428

Latham AN, Sweeney GD (1976) Binding of anticonvulsant drugs to cytochrome P-450: correlation with evidence of induction of hepatic microsomal enzymes. Can J Physiol Pharmacol 54:844–849

Levy RH, Lockard JS, Patel IH, Lai AA (1977) Efficacy testing of valproic acid compared to ethosuximide in monkey model. I. Dosage regimen design in the presence of diurnal oscillations. Epilepsia 18:191–203

Leźnicki AL, Dymecky J (1974) The effect of certain anticonvulsants in vitro and in vivo on the activity of enzymes in rat brain. Neurol Neurochir Pol 24:413–420

Littrow CV, Klingberg F, Müller M (1970) Die Wirkung von Ethosuximid auf die Schwelle und den Ablauf der durch elektrische Reizung im Hippokampus ausgelösten generalisierten Nachentladungen. Arch Int Pharmacodyn Ther 186:213–219

Lockard JS, Levy RH, Congdon WC, DuCharme LL, Patel IH (1977) Efficacy testing of valproic acid compared to ethosuximide in monkey model II. Seizure, EEG, and diurnal variations. Epilepsia 18:205–224

Löscher W (1979a) 3-Mercaptopropionic acid: convulsant properties, effects on enzymes of the γ-aminobutyrate system in mouse brain and antagonism by certan anticonvulsant drugs, aminooxyacetic acid and gabaculine. Biochem Pharmacol 28:1397–1407

Löscher W (1979b) A comparative study of the protein binding of anticonvulsant drugs in serum of dog and man. J Pharmacol Exp Ther 208:429–435

Löscher W (1980) Comparative study of the inhibition of GABA aminotransferase by different anticonvulsant drugs. Arch Int Pharmacodyn Ther 243:48–55

Löscher W, Frey HH (1977) Effect of convulsant and anticonvulsant agents on level and metabolism of γ-aminobutyric acid in mouse brain. Naunyn-Schmiedebergs Arch Pharmacol 296:263–269

Lunde PKM, Rane A, Yaffe SJ, Lund L, Sjöqvist F (1970) Plasma protein binding of diphenylhydantoin in man. Interaction with other drugs and the effect of temperature and plasma dilution. Clin Pharmacol Ther 11:846–855

Lust WD, Kupferberg HJ. Yonekawa WD, Penry JK, Passonneau JV, Wheaton AB (1978) Changes in brain metabolites induced by convulsants or electroshock: effects of anticonvulsant agents. Mol Pharmacol 14:347–356

Malkus H, Dicesare JL, Meola JM, Pippenger CE, Ibanez J. Castro A (1978) Evaluation of EMIT methods for the determination of the five major antiepileptic drugs on an automated kinetic analyzer. Clin Biochem 11:139–142

Masuda Y, Karasawa T, Shiraishi Y, Hori M, Yoshida K, Shimizu M (1980) 3-Sulfamoylmethyl-1,2-benzisoxazole, a new type of anticonvulsant drug. Arzneimittelforsch. 30:477–483

Maguire JH, Dudley KH (1978) Partial purification and characterization of dihydropyrimidinases from calf and rat liver. Drug Metab Dispos 6:601–605

McElhatton PR, Sullivan FM (1977) Comparative teratogenicity of six antiepileptic drugs in the mouse. Br J Pharmacol 59:494–495

Meldrum BS, Horton RW, Toseland PA (1975) A primate model for testing anticonvulsant drugs. Arch Neurol 32:289–294

Meyer H, Frey HH (1973) Dependence of anticonvulsant drug action on central monoamines. Neuropharmacology 12:939–947

Nahorski SR (1972) Biochemical effects of the anticonvulsants trimethadione, ethosuximide and chlordiazepoxide in rat brain. J Neurochem 19:1937–1946

Naquet R, Catier J, Menini C (1975) Neurophysiology of photically induced epilepsy in *Papio papio*. Adv Neurol 10:107–118

Nicholls PJ, Orton TC (1972) The physiological disposition of ^{14}C-methsuximide in the rat. Br J Pharmacol 45:48–59

Nicholls PJ, Scoular IT (1975) Preliminary pharmacological study of *N*,2-dimethyl, 2-(*p*-aminophenyl) succinimide. Br J Pharmacol 54:242

Norton PRE (1970) The effects of drugs on barbiturate withdrawal convulsions in the rat. J Pharm Pharmacol 22:763–766
Nowack WJ, Johnson RN, Englander RN, Hanna GR (1979) Effects of valproate and ethosuximide on thalamocortical excitability. Neurology (Minneap) 29:96–99
O'Brien MM, Schofield PJ (1980) Partial purification and properties of aldose reductase and hexonate dehydrogenase. Biochem J 187:21–30
Orton TC, Nicholls PJ (1972a) Effect in rats of subacute administration of ethosuximide, methosuximide, and phensuximide on hepatic microsomal enzymes and porphyrin turnover. Biochem Pharmacol 21:2253–2261
Orton TC, Nicholls PJ (1972b) Porphyrogenic activity of methsuximide and its demethylated metabolite. J Pharm Pharmacol 24:151–152
Patel IH, Levy RH (1975) Pharmacokinetic properties of ethosuximide in monkeys. II. Chronic intravenous and oral administration. Epilepsia 16:717–730
Patel IH, Levy RH, Bauer TG (1975) Pharmacokinetic properties of ethosuximide in monkeys. I. Single-dose intravenous and oral administration. Epilepsia 16:705–716
Patsalos PN, Lascelles PT (1977) In vitro hydroxylation of diphenylhydantoin and its inhibition by other commonly used anticonvulsant drugs. Biochem Pharmacol 26:1929–1933
Patsalos PN, Lascelles PT (1980) Diphenylhydantoin substrate induced difference spectra: inhibition by other anticonvulsant drugs. Res Commun Chem Pathol Pharmacol 27:31–43
Paule MG, Killiam EK (1979) Disruption of learning performance of chronic ethosuximide administration in the baboon. Fed Proc 38:862
Racz WJ, Marks GS (1969) Drug-induced porphyrin biosynthesis. II. Simple procedure for screening drugs for porphyria-inducing activity. Biochem Pharmacol 18:2009–2018
Rifkind AB, Gilette PN, Song CS, Kappas A (1973) Drug stimulation of δ-aminolevulinic acid synthetase and cytochrome P-450 in vivo in chick embryo liver. J Pharmacol Exp Ther 185:214–225
Rinne SP, Bowyer JF, Barrows EB, Killiam EK (1978) EEG effects of ethosuximide in *Papio papio*. Pharmacologist 20:161
Ris MM, Deitrich RA, Von Wartburg JP (1975) Inhibition of aldehyde reductase isoenzymes in human and rat brain. Biochem Pharmacol 24:1865–1869
Rump S, Ilczuk I, Walczyna K (1979) Anticonvulsant properties of some new derivates of phensuccinimide. Arzneimittelforsch 29:290–292
Sawaya MCB, Horton RW, Meldum BS (1975) Effects of anticonvulsant drugs on the cerebral enzymes metabolizing GABA. Epilepsia 16:649–655
Schettini A, Wilder BJ (1974) Effects of anticonvulsant drugs on enflurane cortical dysrhythmias. Anesth Analg (Cleve) 53:951–962
Schottelius DD (1978) Homogenous immunoassay system (EMIT) for quantitation of antiepileptic drugs in biological fluids. In: Pippenger CE, Penry JK, Kutt H (eds) Antiepileptic drugs: quantitative analysis and interpretation. Raven, New York, pp 95–108
Scuvee-Moreau J, Lepot M, Brotchi J, Gerebtzoff MA, Dresse A (1977) Action of phenytoin, ethosuximide and of the carbidopa-L-dopa association in semi-chronic cobalt-induced epilepsy in the rat. Arch Int Pharmacodyn Ther 230:92–99
Sherwin AL, Lechter M, Marlin AE, Robb JP (1971) Plasma ethosuximide (Zarontin) levels: a new aid in the management of epilepsy. Ann R Coll Physicians Surg Can 4:48–49
Snead OC (1978) Gamma hydroxybutyrate in the monkey III. Effect of intravenous anticonvulsant drugs. Neurology 28:1173–1178
Snead OC, Bearden LJ (1980) Anticonvulsants specific for petit mal antagonize epileptiogenic effect of leucin enkephalin. Science 210:1031–1033
Snead III OC, Bearden LJ, Pegram V (1980) Effect of acute and chronic anticonvulsant administration on endogenous γ-hydroxybutyrate in rat brain. Neuropharmacology 19:47–52
Soldin SJ, Hill JG (1976) Rapid micromethod for measuring anticonvulsant drugs in serum by high-performance liquid chromatography. Clin Chem 22:856–859

Steinmann HW (1964) Succinimide und Krampferregbarkeit. Naunyn-Schmiedebergs Arch Exp Pathol Pharmacol 247:316–317
Stille G, Sayers A (1967) Motor convulsions an EEG during maximal electroshock in the rat. Int J Neuropharmacol 6:169–174
Stone WE, Javid MJ (1979) Quantitative evaluation of the actions of anticonvulsants against different chemical convulsants. Arch Int Pharmacodyn Ther 240:66–78
Stone WE, Javid MJ (1980) Effects of anticonvulsants and glutamate antagonists on the convulsive action of kainic acid. Arch Int Pharmacodyn Ther 243:56–65
Sullivan FM, McElhatton PR (1977) A comparison of the teratogenic activity of the antiepileptic drugs carbamazepine, clonazepam, ethosuximide, phenobarbital, phenytoin, and primidone in mice. Toxicol Appl Pharmacol 40:365–378
Turkanis SA, Chiu P, Borys HK, Karler R (1977) Influence of Δ^9-tetrahydrocannabinol and cannabidiol on photically evoked after-discharge potentials. Psychopharmacology 52:207–212
Vida JA, Gerry EH (1977) Cyclic ureides. In: Vida JA (ed) Anticonvulsants, vol 15. Medical chemistry – a series of monographs. Academic, New York, pp 152–291
Wenzel J, Krüger E, Müller M (1971) Hemmung Pentetrazol-induzierter hypersynchroner Aktivität im thalamo-kortikalen System durch Ethosuximid. Acta Biol Med Ger 26:567–572
Westerink BHC, Lejeune B, Korf J, Van Praag HM (1977) On the significance of regional dopamine metabolism in the rat brain for the classification of centrally acting drugs. Eur J Pharmacol 42:179–190
Wilkinson DM, Halpern LM (1974) Effects of selected anticonvulsants on conjugated estrogen-induced epileptiform activity. Proc West Pharmacol Soc 17:87–91
Woodbury DM, Penry JK, Schmidt RP (eds) (1972) Antiepileptic drugs. Raven, New York
Woodbury DM, Penry JK, Pippenger CE (eds) (1982) Antiepileptic drugs. Raven, New York
Yonekawa W, Kupferberg HJ (1976) Relationship between the metabolism and anticonvulsant activity of methsuximide and phensuximide in mice. Pharmacologist 18:155

CHAPTER 20

Benzodiazepines

S. CACCIA and S. GARATTINI

A. Introduction

Drugs of the benzodiazepine class have been introduced in several areas of clinical practice over the past years (ZBINDEN and RANDALL 1967; GREENBLATT and SHADER 1974; BELLANTUONO et al. 1980). Among their various valuable properties is their potent effect against experimental convulsions and various forms of epilepsy in man (BANZIGER 1965; GASTAUT et al. 1971; BROWNE and PENRY 1973). This property was noted during early animal and clinical studies with chlordiazepoxide and diazepam (RANDALL et al. 1960, 1968; ZBINDEN and RANDALL 1967), the prototype drugs of this class (STERNBACH and REEDER 1961). Subsequent studies with newly developed benzodiazepines revealed similar anticonvulsant activities, differing mainly in quantitative rather than qualitative aspects (GREENBLATT and SHADER 1974; GARATTINI et al. 1981).

A number of reviews have focused entirely or in part on the anticonvulsant properties of benzodiazepines (SCHALLEK et al. 1972; RANDALL and KAPPELL 1973; PINDER et al. 1976; VAN DER KLEIJN et al. 1977; MATTSON 1972; KILLAM and SURIA 1980). The general pharmacology and neuropharmacology (HAEFELI et al. 1981), biochemical effects (BRAESTRUP 1981), pharmacokinetics and metabolism (KAPLAN and JACK 1981), and toxicology and side effects (HINES 1981) of the benzodiazepines have been reviewed in a recent volume of this handbook. Therefore, the present review is confined to the anticonvulsant effects of this class of drugs.

B. Chemical Structure of Benzodiazepines

On the basis of present knowledge the benzodiazepines appear to fall into three main classes: the 1,4 benzodiazepines, 1,5-benzodiazepines, and *s*-triazolo derivatives. Chemically the 1,5-benzodiazepines differ from the well-known 1,4 derivatives only in the carbon and nitrogen in the isomeric position 4 and 5 of the diazepine ring. The *s*-triazolo derivatives were prepared later by fusing a five-membered heterocyclic ring into the diazepine ring of 1,4 or 1,5-benzodiazepines.

At the other end of the spectrum of anticonvulsant potency is the convulsant benzodiazepine RO-3663 (SCHLOSSER and FRANCO 1979) (Fig. 1). This derivative elicits convulsions in mice at a dose of 30 mg/kg i.p. and is antagonized by diazepam at a dose (ED_{50}) of 1.5 mg/kg p.o. (SCHLOSSER et al. 1973). Structure-activity relationships are reviewed by SCHÄFER in Chap. 9, this volume.

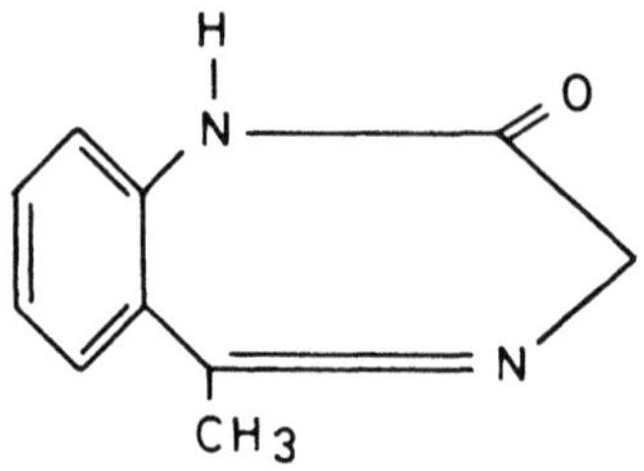

Fig. 1. Chemical structure of RO 5-3663 (1,3-dihydro-5-methyl-2*H*-1,4-benzodiazepine-2-one)

C. Methods of Determination

The analysis of benzodiazepines in body fluids requires highly sensitive, specific techniques since the usual therapeutic doses produce very low levels and there is extensive tissue distribution and biotransformation (GREENBLATT and SHADER 1974; GARATTINI et al. 1977). Spectrophotometry, ^{14}C-labeled compounds, and polarography have been mainly used in animal studies but they are still not sufficiently sensitive for kinetic studies in humans and often fail to differentiate between drugs and metabolites. Gas-liquid chromatography (GLC) and, more recently, high-pressure liquid chromatography (HPLC) are therefore the most suitable techniques for quantitation of benzodiazepines.

Most of the GLC methods are very simple and rapid and are suitable for routine analysis in biological samples containing as little as 10 ng/ml of benzodiazepines or metabolites (GARATTINI et al. 1969). They involve initial solvent extraction (diethylether, *n*-hexane, benzene, etc.) and the extract is then directly injected into the GLC column. The use of a selective electron capture detector (ECD) significantly improves the sensitivity for compounds containing electronegative groups (halogens, nitro groups). Detection is also possible by nitrogen-phosphorus detection (NPD) (BARAZI and BONINI 1980). The thermally unstable benzodiazepines such as 3-hydroxy and *N*-4-oxide derivatives (SADÉE and VAN DER KLEIJN 1971) must be converted to trimethylsilyl derivatives (BELVEDERE et al. 1972) or to their respective aminobenzophenones by acid hydrolysis (DE SILVA and KAPLAN 1966) before chromatography. With the latter approach, however, hydrolysis products of the parent compounds may coincide with its metabolite(s) (VAN DER KLEIJN et al. 1977).

The direct measurement of other derivatives mainly unsubstituted at the N1 position often does not yield optimal sensitivity and reproducibility because they are avidly absorbed into the stationary phase of GLC column packings. Again, acid hydrolysis of these compounds to form the corresponding benzophenones improves the sensitivity (CANO et al. 1975), but specificity may be lost. Another approach is methylation of these compounds to *N*-methyl derivatives. This has been successful in the analysis of clonazepam, nitrazepam, flunitrazepam (DE SILVA and BEKERSKY 1974), and bromazepam (KLOTZ 1981).

Some of these problems can be overcome by using HPLC methods, which provide adequate separation of benzodiazepines at room temperature with quantitation of the parent compounds and their metabolites at the nanogram level. These methods have been successfully applied to the analysis of the thermally labile chlordiazepoxide (SKELLERN et al. 1978), diazepam and its metabolites (VREE et al. 1979), and various nitrobenzodiazepines (VREE et al. 1977; CANO et al. 1977).

D. Kinetics

I. Absorption and Distribution

All the benzodiazepines are rapidly and almost completely absorbed from the gastrointestinal tract after ingestion of therapeutic doses. Maximum blood concentrations appear within 30–180 min, the duration of absorption varying in different studies and with the various benzodiazepines (for a review see GARATTINI et al. 1982). Following absorption of benzodiazepines there is evidence of considerable protein binding (> 90%), with the possible exception of flurazepam, whose binding appears to be very low (GREENBLATT et al. 1975).

At physiological pH, all benzodiazepines are highly lipid soluble and are readily distributed in body tissues. Animal and human studies suggest benzodiazepines reach higher concentrations in liver, lungs, and adipose tissue (for a review see MANDELLI et al. 1978). These drugs enter the brain very rapidly from the bloodstream, maximum concentrations being reached within minutes of parenteral injection (GARATTINI et al. 1973). This could explain the rapid anticonvulsant effects in man (GASTAUT et al. 1965). Distribution in the brain is uneven as indicated by observations in various animal species, with maximal concentrations found initially in gray matter and later in white matter (MORSELLI et al. 1973; VAN DER KLEIJN et al. 1977).

II. Metabolism and Elimination Half-lives

Benzodiazepines are lipophilic compounds which are almost entirely eliminated from the body after biotransformation (SCHWARTZ 1973). Their main metabolic pathways have been discussed in detail in a number of reviews (SCHWARTZ 1973; GREENBLATT and SHADER 1974; GARATTINI et al. 1977). Here it is interesting to report how changes in the basic structure may result in a different metabolism of the benzodiazepine concerned, thus providing a basis for further classification of the benzodiazepines as long acting, intermediate, or short acting (see Table 1).

Long-acting compounds are characterized by the formation of nor-derivatives, mostly nordiazepam (see Fig. 2 for the general metabolic pathways of some of these compounds), which have a very long half-life in man (MANDELLI et al. 1978). The rate and extent of hepatic *N*-dealkylation vary for the different benzodiazepines and in relation to states affecting hepatic metabolism (liver disease, age, smoking). Chlordiazepoxide is first metabolized to desmethylchlordiazepoxide and demoxepam, both of which are pharmacologically active. The latter is then partly inactivated and partly converted to *N*-desmethyl-diazepam (GREENBLATT et al. 1978). Prazepam can be considered a pro-drug of *N*-desmethyl diazepam as it undergoes almost complete first-pass metabolism in the liver with removal of the cyclopropylmethyl side chain (GREENBLATT and SHADER 1978).

Table 1. Elimination half-lives of benzodiazepines

Classification	Common characteristic	Bezodiazepines
Long-acting	Pro-nordiazepam compounds	Chlordiazepoxide
		Diazepam
	Elimination half-life longer than 48 h	Chlorazepate
		Prazepam
		Pinazepam
		Flurazepam
		O-Chloro-*N*-desmethyl-diazepam
		Phenazepam
		Medazepam
		Clobazam
Intermediate	Nitro compounds	Nitrazepam
	Elimination half-life 24–48 h	Flunitrazepam
		Nimetazepam
		Clonazepam
Short-acting	Elimination half-life shorter than 24 h	Oxazepam
		Lorazepam
		Camazepam
		Tamazepam
		Estazolam
		Triazolam
		Midazolam

Chlorazepate, on the other hand, is quickly hydrolyzed to *N*-desmethyl-diazepam in the acid gastric fluid before the absorption. Pinazepam, diazepam, and medazepam are metabolized to *N*-desmethyl-diazepam (GARATTINI et al. 1977).

Similarly, flurazepam (a 2′-halogenated derivative) is partly converted to *N*-desalkyl-flurazepam (SCHWARTZ and POSTMA 1970). *N*-Dealkylation does not differ for the 1,4 and 1,5-benzodiazepines. For clobazam it results in the formation of the active metabolite *N*-desmethyl-clobazam (VOLZ et al. 1979; CACCIA et al. 1980c). The formation of nor derivatives may have specific clinical relevance, as they accumulate during repeated treatment (well documented mainly in studies with diazepam, prazepam, flurazepam, and clobazam) and may well account for a substantial part of the effects (GREENBLATT et al. 1975; MANDELLI et al. 1978; RUPP et al. 1979). The second important common step is hydroxylation in position-3, as in the case of the conversion of *N*-desmethyl-diazepam to oxazepam (GARATTINI et al. 1973), *O*-chloro-*N*-desmethyl-diazepam to lorazepam (LANZONI et al. 1979), phenazepam to 3-hydroxyphenazepam (EKONOMOV et al. 1979), and *N*-desalkyl-flurazepam to its corresponding 3-hydroxy derivative (GARATTINI et al. 1977). Unlike the 1,4 derivatives, the 1,5-benzodiazepines are not hydroxylated at the 3-position (VOLZ et al. 1979; GRIMES et al. 1973). Nitrobenzodiazepines have a different metabolic pathway with no important known active metabolites. The biotransformation pathways of these derivatives are presented in Fig. 3. After *N*-desmethylation flunitrazepam follows the same inactivation pathway as nitrazepam and clonazepam via reduction of the nitro group and its further acetylation (BARTOSEK et al. 1970).

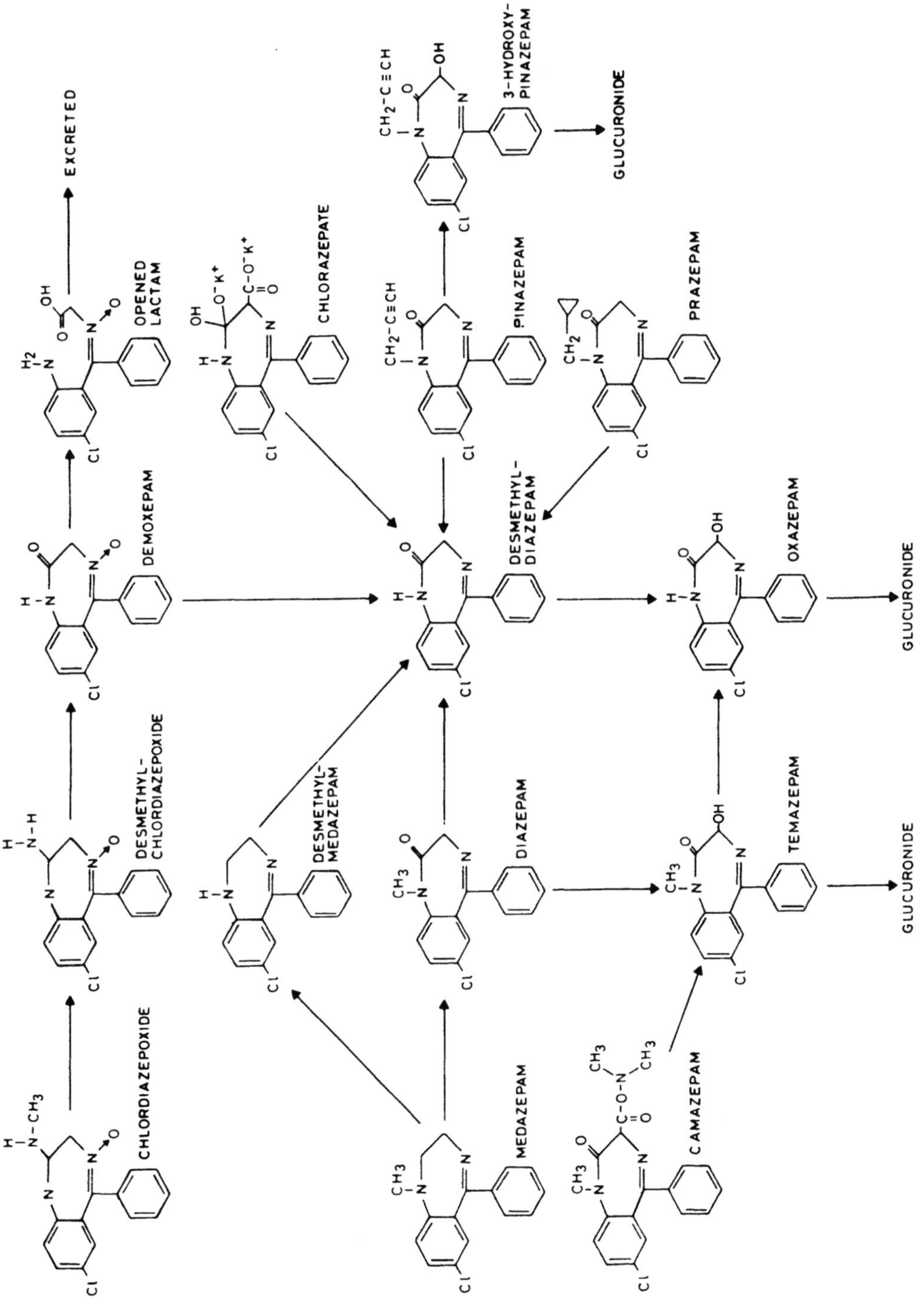

Fig. 2. Metabolic pathways of 7-chloro-1,4-benzodiazepines

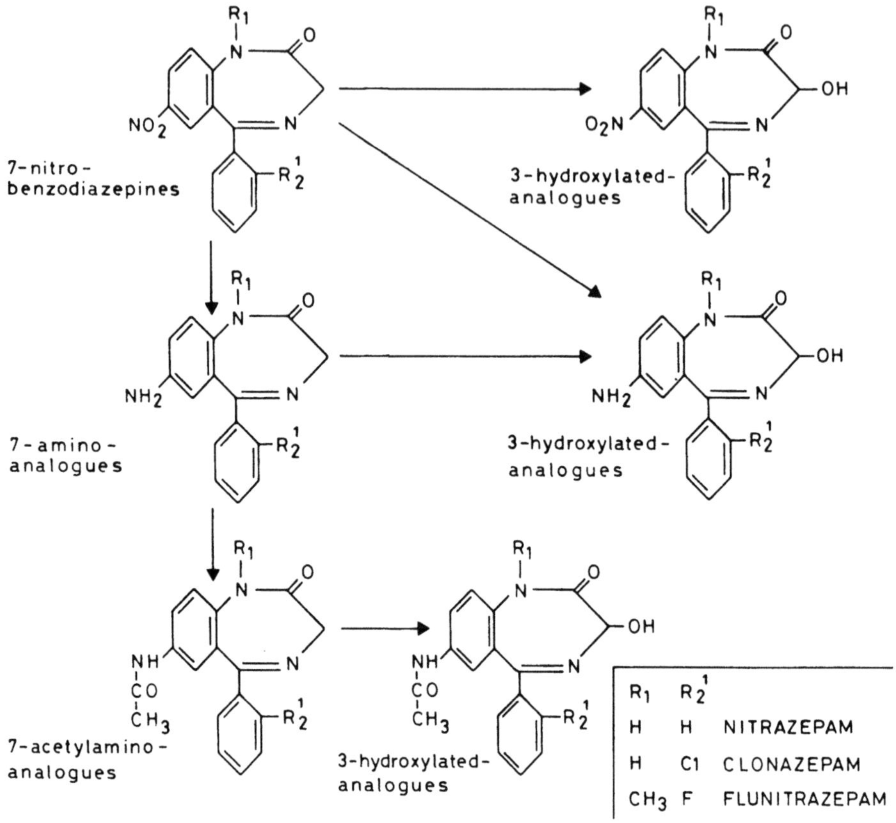

Fig. 3. Metabolic pathways for the 7-nitrobenzodiazepines

The elimination kinetics of nitrobenzodiazepines can be classified as intermediate, with T½ values between 24 and 48 h, longer than those of the rapidly eliminated benzodiazepines (T½ less than 24 h) but shorter than the pro-nordiazepam compounds.

Within the short-acting group, lorazepam and oxazepam have no active metabolites and are directly conjugated with glucuronic acid while camazepam and temazepam are partly metabolized respectively to temazepam and/or oxazepam and partly directly conjugated and excreted (GARATTINI et al. 1977; CACCIA et al. 1981). The kinetic profiles of these compounds appear interesting because of the absence of active metabolites – no clinically relevant plasma concentrations of temazepam and oxazepam are detectable after camazepam (GARATTINI et al. 1977) and temazepam (FUCCELLA et al. 1977) – and because of the short elimination half-life, suggesting potential advantages for their use in routine practice. Triazolobenzodiazepines are relatively new. The best known of this series, triazolam (RUDZIK et al. 1973) and estazolam (NAKAJIMA et al. 1971 a, b), reportedly have elimination half-lives of about 4 h (GREENBLATT et al. 1981) and 16 h (ALLEN et al. 1979), respectively. The main metabolic pathway of these derivatives resembles those of other 1,4-benzodiazepines and leads to the formation of similar metabolites arising from oxidation and/or hydroxylation of the parent compounds (KITAGAWA et al. 1979; KANAI 1974). An oxidated metabolite of estazolam, 1-oxo-estazolam (KITAGAWA et al. 1979), has been shown to possess anti-pentylenetetrazol activity (CACCIA et al., unpublished results) and antimuricidal effects in olfactory-bulbectomized rats as potent as the parent compound (NAKAJIMA et al. 1973), but its contribution to the clinical effects of estazolam remains to be established.

The imidazo derivative midazolam can be considered the shortest-acting benzodiazepine available; its elimination half-life has been reported to be about 2 h (SMITH et al. 1981) and no known active metabolites are formed.

E. Anticonvulsant Properties

Benzodiazepines are the most potent drugs in preventing or interrupting various forms of experimental convulsions. Action against convulsions induced by pentylenetetrazol is particularly notable and widely used but these drugs antagonize most other convulsants too. In this respect they are much more potent than tranquilizers of the meprobamate type and more active than the standard anticonvulsants such as diphenylhydantoin, trimethadione, or phenobarbital (BANZIGER 1965; SCHALLEK et al. 1972; ZBINDEN and RANDALL 1967). Benzodiazepines are also effective against electroshock convulsions but only at relatively high doses.

The mechanism of their anticonvulsant action has so far proved hard to characterized because of the different types of convulsions they antagonize. Moreover, benzodiazepines produce other pharmacological effects, unrelated to their anticonvulsant action (i.e., anxiolytic effect), within the same dose range as the anticonvulsant action. Thus it has not been possible to determine which biochemical mechanisms are responsible for the anticonvulsant activity and which for the other pharmacological effects. Different theories and hypothesis involving serotonergic (STEIN et al. 1973, 1975), cholinergic (for a review see LADINSKY et al. 1981), GABAergic (COSTA et al. 1975a; HAEFELY et al. 1975), and glycinergic (YOUNG et al. 1974; YOUNG and SNYDER 1973) mechanisms have been proposed for the powerful anticonvulsant, antianxiety, and muscle relaxant action of the benzodiazepines. The hypothesis of the involvement of GABA receptors in most of the central effects of benzodiazepines is widely accepted. Biochemical studies provide evidence that benzodiazepines exert their action by indirect potentiation of GABA neurons (COSTA et al. 1975a, b) and that benzodiazepines and GABA receptors can be functionally linked to form a GABA-benzodiazepine receptor unit (BRILEY and LANGER 1978; MARTIN and CANDY 1978, 1980). Evidence (SPETH et al. 1978; TALMAN et al. 1981) of abnormal functioning of the GABAergic mechanism in the brain in convulsive states has been put forward on the basis of the convulsive states induced by drugs that interfere with the GABAergic system. Blockade of GABA receptors by the selective antagonist bicuculline or of GABA-mediated chloride channels by picrotoxin (TICKU et al. 1978; OLSEN and LEEB-LUNDBERG 1981) or by penicillin (MACDONALD and BARKER 1978) produce convulsions which are prevented by various benzodiazepines at dose levels substantially lower than those required to antagonize convulsions by other convulsants with different modes of action (MAO et al. 1975; DINGLEDINE et al. 1978; BUCKETT 1980). Similarly, convulsions elicited by high doses of naloxone, perhaps via GABA-receptor blockade (BILLINGSLEY and KUBENA 1978) or by bemegride, are antagonized or prevented by diazepam (DINGLEDINE et al. 1978; SOUBRIE and SIMON 1978) and other less well-known benzodiazepine derivatives (KAMIOKA et al. 1972). Benzodiazepines were also effective against convulsions induced by isoniazid, which depletes GABA by inhibiting glutamic acid decarboxylase (GAD) (MAO et al. 1975; LEMBECK and BEUBLER 1977) or by other GAD inhibitors such as thiozemicarbazide (RUDZIK et al. 1973; BANZIGER and HANE 1967; HAEFELY et al. 1981), 3-mercaptopriopionic acid (LÖSCHER 1979; HAEFELY et al. 1981), and allylglycine (MELDRUM and HORTON 1979; ASHTON and WAUQUIER 1979). However, benzodiazepines also antagonize convulsions induced by

Table 2. Anticonvulsant properties of diazepam in mice

Convulsants	(mg/kg)	Time[a]	Anticonvulsant ED_{50} of diazepam (mg/kg)	Refs.
Pentylenetetrazol	(125 i.p.)	5	0.28 i.v.	GARATTINI et al. (1973)
	(85 s.c.)	30	0.70 p.o.	RUDZIK et al. (1973)
	(100 s.c.)	60	1.40 p.o.	KAMIOKA et al. (1972)
	(125 s.c.)	60	1.37–2.00 p.o.	BANZIGER and HANE (1967); RANDALL and KAPELL (1973)
Bicuculline	(0.55 i.v.)	2	0.038 i.v.	BUCKETT (1980)
Bemegride	(30 s.c.)	60	0.32 p.o.	KAMIOKA et al. (1972)
	(40 s.c.)	30	0.56 p.o.	RUDZIK et al. (1973)
Picrotoxin	(4 p.o.)	60	1.60 p.o.	LÖSCHER (1979)
Nicotine	(2 i.p.)	30	0.28 i.p.	RUDZIK et al. (1973)
	(5 i.v.)	60	4.50 p.o.	FIELDING and HOFFMANN (1979)
Isoniazid	(0.5 s.c.)	25	0.78 i.p.	LEMBECK and BEUBLER (1977)
Thiosemicarbazide	(20 i.p.)	S	0.70 i.p.	RUDZIK et al. (1973)
3-Mercapto-propionic acid	(60 s.c.)	60	1.70 p.o.	LÖSCHER (1979)
2,4-Dimethyl-*S*-hydroxymethyl-pyridine	(10 i.p.)	S	4.00 p.o.	BANZIGER and HANE (1967)
Strychnine	(0.75 s.c.)	60	14.00 p.o.	LÖSCHER (1979)
	(1.2 p.o.)	60	66.00 p.o.	KAMIOKA et al. (1973)
Maximal electroshock		60	6.50–22.00 p.o.	BANZIGER and HANE (1967); Randall and KAPPELL (1973)

S, diazepam and convulsant administered simultaneously
[a] Minutes between diazepam administration and challenge with convulsants

mechanisms unrelated to dysfunction of GABA neurons, for example, the epileptiform syndrome evoked by strychnine, a glycine antagonist (ZBINDEN and RANDALL 1967; LEMBECK and BEUBLER 1977; FIELDING and HOFFMANN 1979).

The benzodiazepines are by far the most powerful anti-pentylenetetrazol drugs known. The mechanism of action of this convulsant is still not clear, although it does affect the GABA mechanism to some degree (JOHNSTON and MITCHELL 1971; MACDONALD and BARKER 1978). Pentylenetetrazol, however, may induce convulsions partly through its action on cholinergic neurons (for a review see LADINSKY et al. 1981). Anticonvulsant activities of diazepam in mice are summarized in Table 2, which includes anticonvulsant effect against both chemically and electrically induced convulsions. The data vary somewhat, depending on the experimental conditions used, dose and route of administration, and time elapsed between diazepam administration and challenge with convulsant.

F. Relationship Between Anti-Pentylenetetrazol Activity and Brain Concentrations of Benzodiazepines

All the benzodiazepines prevent pentylenetetrazol-induced convulsions in laboratory animals, but their potency differs considerably depending on the species considered, the route of administration, and the time elapsed between administration and the pentylenetetrazol challenge. However, the brain concentrations achieved by an effective dose of benzodiazepines (ED_{50}) are consistent when the drug does not give rise to active metabolites. Table 3 shows for instance that oxazepam protects 50% of rats from pentylenetetrazol convulsions when the brain concen-

Table 3. Brain concentrations of camazepam (CZ), temazepam (TMZ), and oxazepam (OX) after administration of the ED_{50}s against pentylenetetrazol-induced convulsions

Species	Drugs	Time[a]	Route	ED_{50} (95%confidence limits) (mg/kg)	Brain concentrations (nmol/g ± SEM) CZ	TMZ	OX
Rat	CZ	5	i.v.	5.19 (7.03–3.83)	9.92 ± 1.47	<0.10	<0.10
		30	p.o.	55.08 (73.54–41.30)	0.74 ± 0.17	0.60 ± 0.13	0.38 ± 0.10
		180	p.o.	33.65 (41.69–27.16)	0.68 ± 0.22	0.69 ± 0.23	0.41 ± 0.17
	TMZ	5	i.v.	0.18 (0.23–0.14)		0.80 ± 0.13	<0.10
		30	p.o.	4.12 (5.06–3.36)		0.50 ± 0.09	0.38 ± 0.10
		180	p.o.	10.33 (13.30–8.02)		0.50 ± 0.19	0.30 ± 0.03
	OX	5	i.v.	0.21 (0.27–0.17)			0.80 ± 0.13
		30	p.o.	6.74 (9.46–4.81)			0.91 ± 0.24
		180	p.o.	10.30 (12.84–8.31)			0.94 ± 0.21
Mouse	CZ	30	p.o.	9.84 (12.58–7.69)	0.08 ± 0.02	0.39 ± 0.09	0.14 ± 0.03
	TMZ	30	p.o.	0.50 (0.63–0.40)		0.36 ± 0.09	0.24 ± 0.03
	OX	30	p.o.	0.52 (0.66–0.41)			0.59 ± 0.10

[a] Minutes between drug pretreatment and pentylenetetrazol (120 mg/kg i.p.). Each ED_{50} was calculated on at least five doses with eight animals for each dose (CACCIA et al. 1981). Brain concentrations are the mean of five animals

trations are around 0.9 nmol/g. This concentration remains constant regardless of the dose used to obtain the anticonvulsant effect, the variables being the route of administration and the time between oxazepam and pentylenetetrazol administration.

In mice oxazepam appears to be more active, the anticonvulsant effect being achieved at lower concentrations than in rats (GARATTINI et al. 1973). However, depending on the animal species and the experimental conditions a benzodiazepine may be active per se or through the formation of active metabolities. Camazepam, for instance, is anticonvulsant per se when injected into rats at shorter intervals before the pentylenetetrazol challenge (see Table 3), but at longer intervals temazepam and oxazepam are present in the brain of rats and mice at concentrations similar to those observed when temazepam and oxazepam are given at their ED_{50} (CACCIA et al. 1981). Temazepam is converted to oxazepam (GARATTINI et al. 1973), and therefore its effect in rats and mice is partially related to the presence of this metabolite in the brain. In rats the *N*-desmethylated metabolite is present in the brain only in trac amounts whereas in mice and guinea pigs it is a major metabolite (MARCUCCI et al. 1970, 1971; CACCIA et al. 1979; BALLABIO et al. 1981).

Table 4 shows the different ED_{50} of clobazam and its metabolite for the anti-pentylenetetrazol effect in these animal species, lower in mice than in guinea pigs or rats. The brain concentrations corresponding to the ED_{50} are also not similar; in rats the concentrations of *N*-desmethyl-clobazam are negligible, whereas this metabolite accumulates in the brain of guinea pigs and mice. The concentrations of *N*-desmethyl-clobazam attained in the latter two species when the compound was given at effective anticonvulsant doses is in the range of the concentrations

Table 4. Brain concentrations of clobazam (CBZ) and *N*-desmethyl-clobazam (DCBZ) in rats, mice, and guinea pigs after administration of the ED_{50} against pentylenetetrazol

Species	Compound	Time[a]	ED_{50} against pentylenetetrazol (95% confidence limits) mg/kg	Route	Brain concentrations (nmol/g ± SEM)	
					CBZ	DCBZ
Rat	CBZ	30	10.28 (12.30–8.59)	i.p.	1.46 ± 0.15	0.14 ± 0.01
		90	32.73 (38.18–28.06)	i.p.	1.20 ± 0.15	<0.06
Mouse	CBZ	30	1.37 (1.59–1.19)	i.p.	0.36 ± 0.08	1.71 ± 0.17
		90	2.00 (2.32–1.68)	i.p.	<0.03	2.72 ± 0.25
	DCBZ	30	12.20 (15.40–9.70)	i.p.	–	2.23 ± 0.22
		90	13.00 (17.38–11.37)	i.p.	–	2.44 ± 0.24
Guinea pig	CBZ	30	2.72 (3.36–2.20)	i.p.	1.53 ± 0.10	2.20 ± 0.27
		90	5.78 (6.80–4.91)	i.p.	1.00 ± 0.04	5.82 ± 0.36
	DCBZ	360	22.60 (29.30–17.42)	i.p.	–	6.73 ± 0.44
		60	6.97 (8.57–5.66)	i.v.	–	5.86 ± 0.48

[a] Minutes between drug pretreatment and pentylenetetrazol administration (100–120 mg/kg, i.p.). Each ED_{50} was calculated on at least five doses, with ten animals for each dose (CACCIA et al. 1980b; BALLABIO et al. 1981). Brain concentrations are the mean of eight animals

Table 5. Brain concentrations of various benzodiazepines in rats after oral administration of the ED_{50} against pentylenetetrazol

Drug	ED_{50} (95% confidence limits) (mg/kg p.o.)	Brain concentrations (nmol/g ± SEM)
Lorazepam	0.43 (0.57–0.32)	<0.01
Clonazepam	1.12 (1.37–0.92)	0.06 ± 0.01
O-Chloro-*N*-desmethyl diazepam	1.48 (1.75–1.26)	0.06 ± 0.01
Niflurazepam	1.30 (1.60–1.05)	0.12 ± 0.03
Estazolam	0.63 (0.75–0.54)	0.17 ± 0.03
N-Desalkyl-flurazepam	2.31 (3.07–1.73)	0.17 ± 0.02
Phenazepam	1.38 (1.68–1.14)	0.19 ± 0.05
1-oxo-Estazolam	3.71 (4.78–2.88)	0.22 ± 0.04
Diazepam	1.89 (2.46–1.45)	0.42 ± 0.07
N-Desmethyl-diazepam	2.46 (3.25–1.86)	0.92 ± 0.06

Each ED_{50} was calculated on at least five doses with eight to ten rats for each dose. Benzodiazepines were administered orally 30 min before pentylenetetrazol (120 mg/kg i.p.). Brain concentrations are the mean of four to eight rats

present at certain times after administration of clobazam. *N*-Desmethyl-clobazam may therefore be responsible for the activity of clobazam in certain experimental conditions (Caccia et al. 1980 b). It is interesting to note that in guinea pigs *N*-desmethyl-clobazam is probably very poorly absorbed after i.p. injection as indicated by the higher anti-pentylenetetrazol activity when it is injected i.v. (Ballabio et al. 1981). The "active" brain concentrations of other benzodiazepines after administration to rats at the ED_{50} against pentylenetetrazol are summarized in Table 5. The measurement times and routes of administration were selected to minimize the contribution of known active metabolites. There are large differences with ED_{50} (almost ten times), but there is an even larger range for the active brain concentrations (more than 90 times). In addition, the rank order for the ED_{50} is not the same as for brain concentrations. In some cases, for example diazepam, the brain concentration is higher than would be expected on the basis of the ED_{50}, while in other cases, e.g., lorazepam, it is lower. These data indicate that for various benzodiazepines the in vivo disposition (absorption, metabolism, clearance, partition between plasma and brain) show individual characteristics which are important in determining the ED_{50}.

G. Relationship Between Benzodiazepine Concentrations in the Brain and High-Affinity Drug-Binding Sites

There is considerable evidence that benzodiazepines exert their action in the central nervous system by indirect potentiation of GABA neurons (Costa et al. 1975 b). This specific enhancing effect is initiated by the combination of benzodiazepines with high-affinity binding sites (receptors) (Braestrup and Squires 1977, 1978; Chang and Snyder 1978; Möhler and Okada 1977; Möhler et al. 1978). This may be important in view of the possibility that benzodiazepines may compete in vivo with endogenous ligands involved in the mechanism of convul-

Table 6. Distribution of bound [^{3}H]-diazepam in various parts of rat brain and displacement by the ED_{50} against pentylenetetrazol (1.3 mg/kg i.p. of diazepam given 15 min before)

Brain area	% [^{3}H]-diazepam bound	Effect of diazepam (% displacement)
Forebrain	37.0	46
Hippocampus	25.0	32
Brain stem	25.0	32
Striatum	21.0	40
Cerebellum	16.0	40

[^{3}H]-Diazepam binding in vivo was determined according to the method of WILLIAMSON et al. (1978)

sions. Furthermore the nature of the mechanism involving the coupling of the benzodiazepine and GABA receptors may reveal important biochemical reactions. Significant correlations have been observed between the pharmacological potencies of several benzodiazepines and their ability to displace [^{3}H]-benzodiazepine binding in vitro and in vivo (BRAESTRUP and SQUIRES 1978; CHANG and SNYDER 1978; SQUIRES and BRAESTRUP 1977). Correlations have also been found between the inhibitory effect of benzodiazepine pretreatment on [^{3}H]diazepam binding in vitro and these drugs' anticonvulsant (PAUL et al. 1979, 1980) and anticonflict (LIPPA et al. 1978) activity. The authors were interested in investigating the relationship between the anti-pentylenetetrazol activity of some benzodiazepines and their ability to displace [^{3}H]diazepam binding in vivo, considering the actual brain concentrations of drugs and of their known active metabolites (MENNINI et al. 1982).

Table 6 shows that the distribution of bound [^{3}H]diazepam is higher in the forebrain followed by hippocampus, brain stem, and striatum and finally by cerebellum. Irrespective of the degree of bound [^{3}H]diazepam, an effective dose of diazepam (ED_{50} against pentylenetetrazol given i.p.) displaces the labeled compound from high-affinity binding sites preferentially from the forebrain, and a lower percentage in the other brain areas. The cerebellum seems to be the least sensitive, although this dosage of diazepam displaces [^{3}H]diazepam binding to about the same extent in all the brain areas considered (40%); a larger dose of diazepam (ED_{50} effective on rotarod) produces about the same displacement in the cerebellum (46%) but about 75% in the other brain regions.

Other benzodiazepines (see Table 7) cause less displacement of [^{3}H]diazepam bound to the cerebellum than to the brain. The effect of oxazepam and CP 1414 S[1] in displacing [^{3}H]diazepam bound to cerebellum is negligible. It is noteworthy that all the benzodiazepines tested displace brain [^{3}H]diazepam in vivo by about 50% when utilized at the ED_{50} against pentylenetetrazol regardless of the fact that the actual doses have a range of about 40 times. The fact that the ED_{50} against pentylenetetrazol displaces similar amounts of [^{3}H]diazepam from the brain but not from the cerebellum suggests that the high-affinity binding sites for benzodiazepines located in the cerebellum are not an important factor in explain-

1 7-nitro-2-amino-S-phenyl-3H-1,5-benzodiazepine

Table 7. Displacement of [^{3}H]-diazepam bound to rat brain and cerebellum by several benzodiazepines given at the ED_{50} against pentylenetetrazol

Benzodiazepines	Injected dose (mg/kg)	Time of pretreatment (min)	% Displacement of [^{3}H]-diazepam in vivo	
			Brain	Cerebellum
Diazepam	1.31 i.p.	15	44.3	31.0
Clobazam	8.70 i.p.	30	49.9	17.2
Camazepam	55.00 p.o.	30	45.5	17.2
Temazepam	4.10 p.o.	30	59.9	10.3
Oxazepam	6.70 p.o.	30	50.2	2.0
CP 1414 S	11.40 i.p.	15	39.4	3.4

CP 1414S, 7-nitro-2-amino-5-phenyl-3H-1,5-benzodiazepine

Table 8. Correlation between anti-pentylenetetrazol activity and brain high-affinity binding for several benzodiazepines in rats

Benzodiazepine	ED_{50} (mg/kg)	Brain concentrations (pmol/g)		[^{3}H]-Diazepam	
				% Displacement in vitro	IC_{50} in vitro (pmol/ml)
Diazepam	1.31 (i.p.)	DZ	596	45.7	6.4
		DDZ	185		5.7
Camazepam	55.00 (p.o.)	CZ	740		950.0
		TMZ	600	46.4	24.0
		OX	385		43.0
Temazepam	4.10 (p.o.)	TMZ	500	59.0	24.0
		OX	385		43.0
Oxazepam	6.70 (p.o.)	OX	910	50.2	43.0
Clobazam	9.70 (i.p.)	CBZ	4,266	50.2	260.0
		DCBZ	210		580.0
CP 1414 S	11.40 (i.p.)	CP	7,857	39.4	490.0

DZ, diazepam; DDZ, *N*-desmethyl-diazepam; CZ, camazepam; TMZ, temazepam; OX, oxazepam; CBZ, clobazam; DCBZ, *N*-desmethyl-clobazam; CP, CP 1414 S

ing the effect of these drugs against pentylenetetrazol-induced convulsions. As suggested by other authors (KLEPNER et al. 1979), this may be related to different properties of the benzodiazepine receptors in the cerebellum.

Table 8 is an attempt to correlate pharmacological effects, brain levels, and high-affinity binding sites of several benzodiazepines. In the case of clobazam the anticonvulsant and anticonflict activities in rats are probably related much more to the presence of brain clobazam than *N*-desmethylclobazam, because the latter is less effective than the former in displacing [^{3}H]diazepam in vitro. In the case of diazepam it is more difficult to decide whether the parent compound or its metabolite is of importance for the anticonvulsant and anticonflict activities. In the case of camazepam it can probably be excluded that the parent compound is effective, the metabolites temazepam and oxazepam probably being responsible for its anticonvulsant effect.

No conclusions about the mechanism of action of benzodiazepines can be drawn at present. Many of the data are difficult to explain only on the basis of benzodiazepine receptors. For instance, several compounds including norharmane (MORIN et al. 1981), harmane and other beta-carbolines (ROMMELSPACHER et al. 1981), and the imidazodiazepine RO 15-1788 [8-fluoro-5,6-dihydro-5-methyl-6-oxo-4H-imidazo-[1,5.a] [1,4]benzodiazepine-3-carboxylate(flumazepil)] (HUNKELER et al. 1981) are able to displace [^{3}H]diazepam from binding sites but they do not show anticonvulsant activity.

In summary, benzodiazepines are among the most powerful anticonvulsant agents, showing a broad spectrum of activity against a large variety of convulsant agents supposedly acting through different mechanisms. Depending on the animal species, the intensity and duration of action of benzodiazepines may be quite different. For instance, benzodiazepines show longer-lasting anticonvulsant activity in mice than in rats. This is partly related to the formation of active metabolites which in several cases play a crucial role in sustaining the duration of action of the parent compound.

Because of the formation of such metabolites careful consideration must be given to any extrapolation from in vitro (high-affinity benzodiazepine receptor binding) to in vivo (anticonvulsant) activities. For several benzodiazepines equal anticonvulsant effects correspond in vivo to equal binding to benzodiazepine receptors. However, further studies on the mechanism of action of benzodiazepines are still required.

References

Allen MD, Greenblatt DJ, Arnold JD (1979) Single- and multiple-dose kinetics of estazolam, a triazolo benzodiazepine. Psychopharmacology 66:267–274

Ashton D, Wauquier A (1979) Effects of some anti-epileptic, neuroleptic and gabaminergic drugs on convulsions induced by *d,l*-allylglycince. Pharmacol Biochem Behav 11:221–226

Ballabio M, Caccia S, Garattini S, Guiso G, Zanini MG (1981) Antileptazol activity and kinetics of clobazam and *N*-desmethyl-clobazam in the guinea-pig. Arch Int Pharmacodyn Ther 253:192–199

Banziger RF (1965) Anticonvulsant properties of chlordiazepoxide, diazepam and certain other 1,4-benzodiazepines. Arch Int Pharmacodyn Ther 154:131–136

Banziger RF, Hane D (1967) Evualation of a new convulsant for anticonvulsant screening. Arch Int Pharmacodyn Ther 167:245–249

Barazi S, Bonini M (1980) Determination de onze dérivés des benzodiazépines en solution acétonique par chromatographie en phase gaseuse utilisant un detecteur specifique azote. J Chromatogr 202:473–477

Bartosek I, Kvetina J, Guaitani A, Garattini S (1970) Comparative study of nitrazepam metabolism in perfused isolated liver of laboratory animals. Eur J Pharmacol 11:378–382

Bellantuono C, Reggi V, Tognoni G, Garattini S (1980) Benzodiazepines: clinical pharmacology and therapeutic use. Drugs 19:195–219

Belvedere G, Tognoni G, Frigerio A, Morselli PL (1972) A specific, rapid and sensitive method for gas-chromatographic determination of methyl-oxazepam in small samples of blood. Anal Lett 5:531–541

Billingsley ML, Kubena RK (1978) The effects of naloxone and picrotoxin on the sedative and anti-conflict effects of benzodiazepines. Life Sci 22:897–906

Braestrup C (1981) Biochemical effects of anxiolytics. In: Hoffmeister F, Stille G (eds) Psychotropic agents. Springer, Berlin Heidelberg New York, pp 293–319 (Handbook of experimental pharmacology, vol 55/2)
Braestrup C, Squires RF (1977) Specific benzodiazepine receptors in rat brain characterized by high-affinity (3H) diazepam binding. Proc Natl Acad Sci USA 74:3805–3809
Braestrup C, Squires RF (1978) Brain specific benzodiazepine receptors. Br J Psychiatry 133:249–260
Briley MS, Langer SZ (1978) Influence of GABA receptor agonists and antagonists on the binding of ^{3}H-diazepam to the benzodiazepine receptor. Eur J Pharmacol 52:129–132
Browne TR, Penry JK (1973) Benzodiazepines in the treatment of epilepsy. A review. Epilepsia 14:277–310
Buckett WR (1980) Intravenous bicuculline in mice facilitates in vivo evaluation of drugs affecting GABA like mechanisms. Br J Pharmacol 68:177–178
Caccia S, Ballabio M, Guiso G, Zanini MG (1979) Gas-liquid chromatographic determination of clobazam and *N*-desmethyl-clobazam in plasma. J Chromatogr 164:100–105
Caccia S, Carli M, Garattini S, Pogessi E, Rech R, Samanin R (1980a) Pharmacological activities of clobazam and diazepam in the rat. Relation to drug brain levels. Arch Int Pharmacodyn Ther 243:275–283
Caccia S, Guiso G, Garattini S (1980b) Brain concentrations of clobazam and *N*-desmethyl-clobazam and antileptazol activity. J Pharm Pharmacol 32:295–296
Caccia S, Guiso G, Samanin R, Garattini S (1980c) Species differences in clobazam metabolism and antileptazol effect. J Pharm Pharmacol 32:101–103
Caccia S, Ballabio M, Garattini S (1981) Relationship between camazepam, *N*-methyl-oxazepam and oxazepam brain concentration and antileptazol effect in the rat. J Pharm Pharmacol 33:185–187
Cano JP, Baille AM, Viala A (1975) Determination of bromazepam in plasma with an internal standard by gas liquid chromatography. Arzneimittelforsch 25:1012–1016
Cano JP, Guintrand J, Aubert C, Viala A (1977) Determination of flunitrazepam, desmethylflunitrazepam and clonazepam in plasma by gas liquid chromatography with an internal standard. Arzneimittelforsch 27:338–342
Chang RSL, Snyder SH (1978) Benzodiazepine receptors: labeling in intact animals with [^{3}H] flunitrazepam. Eur J Pharmacol 48:213–218
Costa E, Guidotti A, Mao CC (1975a) Evidence for involvement of GABA in the action of benzodiazepines. Studies on rat cerebellum. In: Costa E, Greengard PG (eds) Mechanism of action of benzodiazepines. Raven, New York, pp 113–130
Costa E, Guidotti A, Mao CC, Suria A (1975b) New concepts on the mechanism of action of benzodiazepines. Life Sci 17:167–186
De Silva JAF, Bekersky I (1974) Determination of clonazepam and flunitrazepam in blood by electron-capture gas-liquid chromatography. J Chromatogr 99:447–460
De Silva JAF, Kaplan J (1966) Determination of 7-bromo-1,3-dihydro-5-(2-pyridyl)-2*H*-1,4-benzodiazepine-2-one (RO-5-3350) in blood by gas-liquid chromatography. J Pharm Sci 55:1278–1283
Dingledine R, Iversen LL, Breuker E (1978) Naloxone as a GABA antagonist: evidence from iontophoretic, receptor binding and convulsant studies. Eur J Pharmacol 47:19–27
Ekonomov AL, Rodionov AP, Zherdev VP, Vikhlyaev YUI (1979) 7-Bromo-5-(2′-chlorophenyl)-1,3-dihydro-2*H*-1,4-benzodiazepin-2-one(1), a new tranquillizing agent: metabolism in rats. Xenobiotica 9:503–510
Fielding S, Hoffmann I (1979) Pharmacology of anti-anxiety drugs with special reference to clobazam. Br J Clin Pharmacol 7:7–15
Fuccella LM, Bolcioni G, Tamassia V, Ferrario L, Tognoni G (1977) Human pharmacokinetics and bioavailability of temazepam administered in soft gelatin capsules. Eur J Clin Pharmacol 12:383–386
Garattini S, Marcucci F, Mussini E (1969) Gas chromatographic analysis of benzodiazepines. In: Porter R (ed) Gas chromatography in biology and medicine. Churchill, London, pp 161–172

Garattini S, Mussini E, Marcucci F, Guaitani A (1973) Metabolic studies on benzodiazepines in various animal species. In: Garattini S, Mussini E, Randall LO (eds) The benzodiazepines. Raven, New York, pp 75–97
Garattini S, Marcucci F, Mussini E (1977) The metabolism of pharmacokinetics of selected benzodiazepines. In: Usdin E, Forrest IS (eds) Psychotherapeutic drugs, part 2. Applications. Dekker, New York, pp 1039–1087
Garattini S, Caccia S, Mennini T (1981) Pharmacological and biochemical studies on benzodiazepines. In: De Las Heras FG, Vega S (eds) Medicinal chemistry advances. Pergamon, Oxford, pp 171–178
Garattini S, Caccia S, Carli M, Mennini T (1981) Notes on kinetics and metabolism of benzodiazepines. Adv Biosci 31:351–364
Gastaut H, Naquet R, Poiré R, Tassinari CA (1965) Treatment of status epilepticus with diazepam (valium). Epilepsia 6:167–182
Gastaut H, Courjon J, Poiré R, Weber M (1971) Treatment of status epilepticus with a new benzodiazepine more active then diazepam. Epilepsia 12:197–214
Greenblatt DJ, Shader RI (1974) Benzodiazepines in clinical practice. Raven, New York
Greenblatt DJ, Shader RI (1978) Prazepam and lorazepam, two new benzodiazepines. N Engl J Med 299:1342–1344
Greenblatt DJ, Shader RI, Koch-Weser J (1975) Flurazepam hydrochloride. Clin Pharmacol Ther 17:1–14
Greenblatt DJ, Shader RI, MacLeod SM, Sellers EM (1978) Clinical pharmacokinetics of chlordiazepoxide. Clin Pharmacokinet 3:381–394
Greenblatt DJ, Divoll M, Moschitto LJ, Shader RI (1981) Electron-capture gas chromatographic analysis of the triazolobenzodiazepines, alprazolam and triazolam. J Chromatogr 225:202–207
Grimes RM, Alton KB, Shaw C (1973) Metabolism of a 1,5-benzodiazepine ORF 8063 in man. Pharmacologist 15:254
Haefely W, Kulcsàr A, Möhler H, Pieri L, Polc P, Schaffner R (1975) Possible involvement of GABA in the central actions of benzodiazepines. In: Costa E, Greengard P (eds) Mechanism of action of benzodiazepines. Raven, New York, pp 131–151
Haefely W, Pieri L, Polc P, Schaffner R (1981) General pharmacology and neuropharmacology of benzodiazepine derivatives. In: Hoffmeister F, Stille G (eds) Psychotropic agents. Springer, Berlin Heidelberg New York, pp 13–262 (Handbook of experimental pharmacology, vol 55/2)
Hines LR (1981) Toxicology and side-effects of anxiolytics. In: Hoffmeister F, Stille G (eds) Psychotropic agents. Springer, Berlin Heidelberg New York, pp 359–393 (Handbook of experimental pharmacology, vol 55/2)
Hunkeler W, Möhler H, Pieri L, Polc P, Bonetti EP, Cumin R, Schaffner R, Haefely W (1981) Selective antagonists of benzodiazepines. Nature 290:514–516
Johnston GA, Mitchell JF (1971) The effect of bicuculline, metrazol, picrotoxin and strychnine on the release of [^{3}H]GABA from rat brain slices. J Neurochem 18:2441–2446
Kamioka T, Nakayoma I, Akijama S, Takagi H (1972) Pharmacological studies on 10-chloro-11b-(2-chlorophenyl)-2,3,5,6,7,11b-hexahydrobenzo-[6,7]-1,4-diazepino[5,4-b] oxazol-6-one(CS-370), a new psychosedative agent. Arzneimittelforsch 22:884–891
Kanai Y (1974) The biotransformation of 8-chloro-6-phenyl-4*H*-*S*-triazolo[4,3,9] [1,4]benzodiazepine(D-40TA) a new central depressant, in man, dog and rat. Xenobiotica 4:441–456
Kaplan SA, Jack ML (1981) Pharmacokinetics and metabolism of anxiolytics. In: Hoffmeister F, Stille G (eds) Psychotropic agents. Springer, Berlin Heidelberg New York, pp 321–358 (Handbook of experimental pharmacology, vol 55/2
Killam EK, Suria A (1980) Antiepileptic drugs. Benzodiazepines. In: Glaser GH, Penry JK, Woodbury DM (eds) Antiepileptic drugs: mechanisms of action. Raven, New York, pp 597–615
Kitagawa H, Esumi Y, Kurosawa S, Sekine S, Yokoshima T (1979) Metabolism of 8-chloro-6-(*O*-chlorophenyl)-1-methyl-4*H*-*S*-triazolo[4,3-a] [1,4]benzodiazepine, triazolam, a new central depressant. II. Identification and determination of metabolites in rats and dogs. Xenobiotica 9:429–439

Klepner CA, Lippa AS, Benson DI, Sano MC, Beer B (1979) Resolution of two biochemically and pharmacologically distinct benzodiazepine receptors. Pharmacol Biochem Behav 11:457–462
Klotz U (1981) Determination of bromazepam by gas-liquid chromatography and its application for pharmacokinetic studies in man. J Chromatogr 222:501–506
Ladinsky H, Consolo S, Bellantuono C, Garattini S (1981) Interaction of benzodiazepines with known and putative neurotransmitter in the brain. In: Van Praag HM (ed) Brain mechanisms and abnormal behavior-chemistry. Dekker, New York, pp 825–858 (Handbook of biological psychiatry, part 4)
Lanzoni J, Airoldi L, Marcucci F, Mussini E (1979) Gas Chromatographic determination of chlorodesmethyldiazepam and lorazepam in rats and mice. J Chromatogr 168:260–265
Lembeck F, Beubler E (1977) Convulsion induced by hyperbaric oxygen: inhibition by phenobarbital, diazepam and baclofen. Naunyn Schmiedebergs Arch Pharmacol 297:47–51
Lippa AS, Klepner CA, Yunger L, Sano MC, Smith WV, Beer B (1978) Relationship between benzodiazepine receptors and experimental anxiety in rats. Pharmacol Biochem Behav 9:853–856
Löscher W (1979) 3-Mercaptopropionic acid: Convulsant properties, effects on enzymes of the γ-aminobutyrate system in mouse brain and antagonism by certain anticonvulsant drugs, aminooxyacetic acid and gabaculine. Biochem Pharmacol 28:1397–1407
Macdonald RL, Barker JL (1978) Specific antagonism of GABA-mediated postsynaptic inhibition in cultured mammalian spinal cord neurons. A common mode of convulsant action. Neurology 28:325–330
Mandelli M, Tognoni G, Garattini S (1978) Clinical pharmacokinetics of diazepam. Clin Pharmacokinet 3:72–91
Möhler H, Okada T (1977) Properties of 3*H*-diazepam binding to benzodiazepine receptors in rat cerebral cortex. Life Sci 20:2101–2110
Möhler H, Okada T, Heitz P, Ulrich J (1978) Biochemical identification of the site of action of benzodiazepines in human brain by ^{3}H-diazepam binding. Life Sci 22:985–996
Morin AM, Tanaka IA, Wasterlain CG (1981) Norharman inhibition of [^{3}H] diazepam binding in mouse brain. Life Sci 28:2257–2263
Morselli PL, Cassano GB, Placidi GF, Muscettola GB, Rizzo M (1973) Kinetics of the distribution of ^{14}C-diazepam and its metabolites in various areas of cat brain. In: Garattini S, Mussini E, Randall LO (eds) The benzodiazepines. Raven, New York, pp 129–143
Nakajima R, Hattori C, Nagawa Y (1971 a) Structure-activity relationship of *S*-triazolo-1,4-benzodiazepines in central nervous depressant action. Jpn J Pharmacol 21:489–495
Mao CC, Guidotti A, Costa E (1975) Evidence for an involvement of GABA in the mediation of the cerebellar cGMP decrease and the anticonvulsant action of diazepam. Naunyn Schmiedebergs Arch Pharmacol 289:369–378
Marcucci F, Fanelli R, Mussini E, Garattini S (1970) Further studies on species difference in diazepam metabolism. Eur J Pharmacol 9:253–256
Marcucci F, Guaitani A, Fanelli R, Garattini S (1971) Metabolism and anticonvulsant activity of diazepam in guinea pigs. Biochem Pharmacol 20:1711–1713
Martin IL, Candy JM (1978) Facilitation of benzodiazepine binding by sodium chloride and GABA. Neuropharmacology 17:993–998
Martin IL, Candy JM (1980) Facilitation of specific benzodiazepine binding in rat brain membrane fragments by a number of anions. Neuropharmacology 19:175–179
Mattson RH (1972) Other antiepileptic drugs. The benzodiazepines. In: Woodbury DM, Penry JK, Schmidt RP (eds) Antiepileptic drugs. Raven, New York, pp 497–516
Meldrum BS, Chapman AG, Horton RW (1979) Clobazam: anticonvulsant action in animal models of epilepsy. Br J Clin Pharmacol 7:59–60
Mennini T, Cotecchia S, Caccia S, Garattini S (1982) Benzodiazepines: relationship between pharmacological activity in the rat and in vivo receptor binding. Pharmacol Biochem Behav 16:529–532

Nakajima R, Take Y, Moriya R, Saji Y, Yui T, Nagawa Y (1971 b) Pharmacological studies on new potent central depressants, 8-chloro-6-phenyl-4*H*-*s*-triazolo[4,3a] [1,4] benzodiazepine (D-40 TA) and its 1-methyl analogue (D-65 MT). Jpn J Pharmacol 21:497–516

Nakajima R, Saji Y, Kozato Y, Mikoda R, Tanayama S, Nagawa Y (1973) Dissociative change in anti-aggressive and muscle relaxant actions of *S*-triazolobenzodiazepine (D-40 TA) by repeated administration and phenobarbital pretreatment and its relation to metabolism. J Takeda Res Lab 32:264–274

Olsen RW, Leeb-Lundberg F (1981) Convulsant and anticonvulsant drug binding sites related to GABA-regulated chloride ion channels. In: Costa E, Di Chiara G, Gessa GL (eds) GABA and benzodiazepine receptors. Raven, New York, pp 93–102

Paul SM, Syapin PJ, Paugh BA, Moncada V, Skolnick P (1979) Correlation between benzodiazepine receptor occupation and anticonvulsant effect of diazepam. Nature 281:688–689

Paul SM, Marangos PJ, Skolnick P, Goodwin FK (1980) Brain-specific benzodiazepine receptors and putative endogenous "benzodiazepine-like" compounds. Psychopharmacol Bull 16:9–20

Pinder RM, Brogden RN, Speight TM, Avery GS (1976) Clonazepam: a review of its pharmacological properties and therapeutic efficacy in epilepsy. Drugs 12:321–361

Randall LO, Kappell B (1973) Pharmacological activity of some benzodiazepines and their metabolites. In: Garattini S, Mussini E, Randall LO (eds) The benzodiazepines. Raven, New York, pp 27–51

Randall LO, Schallek W, Heise GA, Keit EF, Bagdon RE (1960) The psychosedative properties of methaminodiazepoxide. J Pharmacol Exp Ther 129:163–171

Randall LO, Schallek W, Scheckel C, Banziger R, Moe RA (1968) Zur Pharmakologie des neuen Psychopharmakons 7-chlor-2,3-dihydro-1-methyl-5-phenyl-1*H*-1,4-benzodiazepin (RO-5-4556). Arzneimittelforsch 18:1542–1545

Rommelspacher H, Nanz C, Borbe HO, Fehske KJ, Müller WE, Wollert U (1981) Benzodiazepine antagonism by hormone and other β-carbolines in vitro and in vivo. Eur J Pharmacol 70:409–416

Rudzik AD, Hester JB, Tang AH, Straw RN, Friis W (1973) Triazolobenzodiazepines, a new class of central nervous system-depressant compounds. In: Garattini S, Mussini E, Randall LO (eds) The benzodiazepines. Raven, New York, pp 285–297

Rupp W, Badian M, Christ O, Hajdù P, Kulkarni RD, Taeuber K, Uihlein M, Bender R, Vanderbeke O (1979) Pharmacokinetics of single and multiple doses of clobazam in humans. Br J Clin Pharmacol 7:51–57

Sadée W, Van Der Kleijn E (1971) Thermolysis of 1,4-benzodiazepines during gas chromatography and mass spectroscopy. J Pharm Sci 60:135–137

Schallek W, Schlosser W, Randall LO (1972) Recent developments in the pharmacology of the benzodiazepines. Adv Pharmacol Chemother 10:119–183

Schlosser W, Franco S (1979) Reduction of γ-aminobutyric acid (GABA)-mediated transmission by a convulsant benzodiazepine. J Pharmacol Exp Ther 211:290–295

Schlosser W, Zavatsky E, Kappell B, Sigg EB (1973) Antagonism of bicuculline and RO-5-3663 by diazepam. Pharmacologist 15:162

Schwartz MA (1973) Pathways of metabolism of the benzodiazepines. In: Garattini S, Mussini E, Randall LO (eds) The benzodiazepines. Raven, New York, pp 53–74

Schwartz MA, Postma E (1970) Metabolism of flurazepam, a benzodiazepine, in man and dog. J Pharm Sci 59:1800–1806

Skellern GG, Meier J, Knight BI, Whiting B (1978) The application of HPLC to the determination of some 1,4-benzodiazepines and their metabolites in plasma. Br J Clin Pharmacol 5:483–487

Smith MT, Eadi MJ, O'Rourke Brophy T (1981) The pharmacokinetics of midazolam in man. Eur J Clin Pharmacol 19:271–278

Soubrie P, Simon P (1978) Comparative study of the antagonism of bemegride and picrotoxin on behavioural depressant effects of diazepam in rats and mice. Neuropharmacology 17:121–125

Speth RC, Wastek GJ, Johnson PC, Yamamura HI (1978) Benzodiazepine binding in human brain: characterization using [^{3}H]flunitrazepam. Life Sci 22:859–866

Squires RF, Braestrup C (1977) Benzodiazepine receptors in rat brain. Nature 266:732–734

Stein L, Wise CD, Berger BD (1973) Antianxiety action of benzodiazepines: decrease in activity of serotonin neurons in the punishment systems. In: Garattini S, Mussini E, Randall LO (eds) The benzodiazepines. Raven, New York, pp 299–326

Stein L, Wise CD, Belluzzi JD (1975) Effects of benzodiazepines on central serotonergic mechanisms. In: Costa E, Greengard P (eds) Mechanism of action of benzodiazepines. Raven, New York, pp 29–44

Sternbach LH, Reeder E (1961) Quinazolines and 1,4-benzodiazepines. II. The rearrangement of 6-chloro-2-chloromethyl-4-phenylquinazoline-3-oxide into 2-amino derivatives of 7-chloro-5-phenyl-3*H*-1,4-benzodiazepine-4-oxide. J Organic Chem 26:1111–1118

Tallman JF, Mallorga P, Thomas JW, Gallager DW (1981) Benzodiazepine binding sites: properties and modulation. In: Costa E, Di Chiara G, Gessa GL (eds) GABA and benzodiazepine receptors. Raven, New York, pp 9–18

Ticku MK, Van Ness PC, Haycock JW, Levy WB, Olsen RW (1978) Dihydropicrotoxinin binding sites in rat brain: comparison to GABA receptors. Brain Res 150:642–647

Van Der Kleijn E, Vree TB, Guelen PJM (1977) 7-Chloro-1,4-benzodiazepines: diazepam, desmethyldiazepam, oxydiazepam, oxydesmethyldiazepam (oxazepam) and chlordiazepoxide. In: Usdin E, Forrest IS (eds) Psychotherapeutic drugs, part 2. Application. Dekker, New York, pp 997–1037

Volz M, Christ O, Kellner HM, Kuch H, Fehlhaber HW, Gantz D, Hajdu P, Cavagna F (1979) Kinetics and metabolism of clobazam in animals and man. Br J Clin Pharmacol 7:41–50

Vree TB, Lenselink B, Van Der Kleijn E (1977) Determination of flunitrazepam in body fluids by means of high-performance liquid chromatography. J Chromatogr 143:530–534

Vree TB, Baars AM, Hekster YA, Van Der Kleijn E (1979) Simultaneous determination of diazepam and its metabolites *N*-desmethyldiazepam, oxydiazepam and oxazepam in plasma and urine of man and dog by means of high-performance liquid chromatography. J Chromatogr 162:605–614

Williamson MJ, Paul SM, Skolnick P (1978) Demonstration of [^{3}H]diazepam binding to benzodiazepine receptors in vivo. Life Sci 23:1935–1940

Young AB, Snyder SG (1973) Strychnine binding associated with glycine receptors of the central nervous system. Proc Natl Acad Sci USA 70:2832–2836

Young AB, Zukin SR, Snyder SH (1974) Interaction of benzodiazepines with central nervous glycine receptors: possible mechanism of action. Proc Natl Acad Sci USA 71:2246–2250

Zbinden G, Randall LO (1967) Pharmacology of benzodiazepines: laboratory and clinical correlations. Adv Pharmacol 5:213–251

CHAPTER 21

Carbonic Anhydrase Inhibitors

J. E. RIGGS and R. C. GRIGGS

A. Introduction

Inhibitors of carbonic anhydrase presently have a limited role in the treatment of epilepsy. Inorganic anions, such as I^-, CN^-, SH^-, CNO^-, SCN^-, and Br^-, and sulfonamides are inhibitors of the enzyme carbonic anhydrase (MAREN 1967). Both bromides and sulfonamides have been used in the treatment of epilepsy in man. Bromide therapy for epilepsy was introduced in the nineteenth century (LOCOCK 1857). Bromides are presently rarely used as an anticonvulsant because of their potential toxicity (MOSES and KLAWANS 1979). For example, bromides are occasionally used in patients with acute intermittent porphyria and a coexistent seizure disorder (MAGNUSSEN et al. 1975). Interestingly, the bromide concentration required to inhibit carbonic anhydrase significantly (MAREN 1967) is remarkably similar to the bromide concentration required to produce an anticonvulsant effect (MOSES and KLAWANS 1979). The mechanism by which bromides exert their anticonvulsant effect remains unknown.

Sulfonamide use in epilepsy was initially reported in the 1930s (YEOMAN 1938). Shortly thereafter, azosulfamide was found to have an anticonvulsant effect (COHEN and COBB 1941). These investigators speculated on the possibility that azosulfamide's anticonvulsant effect might be related to the recently described carbonic anhydrase-inhibiting property of sulfonamides (MANN and KEILIN 1940). The use of acetazolamide in the treatment of epilepsy was initially reported in the early 1950s (BERGSTROM et al. 1952), and subsequently by MERLIS (1954), LOMBROSO et al. (1956), ANSELL and CLARKE (1956), and MILLICHAP (1956). This chapter will focus on the anticonvulsant properties of carbonic anhydrase inhibitors, and acetazolamide in particular, since this agent has been the most extensively studied and frequently used carbonic anhydrase inhibitor in epilepsy (WOODBURY 1980). The general chemical properties of carbonic anhydrase inhibitors, including their pharmacokinetics and pharmacodynamic properties outside the central nervous system, have been reviewed in a previous volume of the *Handbook of Experimental Pharmacology* (MAREN 1969) and will not be reviewed further in this chapter.

B. Anticonvulsant Effect

Early investigators attributed the anticonvulsant effect of acetazolamide to its induction of a systemic metabolic acidosis, akin to the acidosis and anticonvulsant effect of starvation or a ketogenic diet (LOMBROSO et al. 1956). The existence of carbonic anhydrase in the brain has been known since the 1940s (ASHBY 1944).

Subsequent investigations showed that the anticonvulsant effect of acetazolamide in experimental animals correlated directly with the degree of inhibition of brain carbonic anhydrase and was independent of the systemic metabolic acidosis produced by inhibition of kidney carbonic anhydrase (MILLICHAP et al. 1955; GRAY et al. 1957). The consequence of the inhibition of brain carbonic anhydrase activity is decreased facilitated transport of carbon dioxide away from neurons with a resultant accumulation in the brain of carbon dioxide in the form of carbonic acid (KOCH and WOODBURY 1960; WOODBURY and KARLER 1960; KJALLQUIST et al. 1969; HEUSER 1975). Brain carbonic anhydrase is concentrated in glial cells (GIACOBINI 1962), particularly oligodendrocytes (DELAUNOY et al. 1980; LANGLEY et al. 1980). A significant proportion of brain carbonic anhydrase is membrane bound and associated with myelin (SAPIRSTEIN et al. 1978; LEES et al. 1980).

Animal studies on the anticonvulsant mechanism of carbonic anhydrase inhibitors have suggested that their therapeutic effect may involve the monoaminergic neurotransmitter system. Much of this work was done in mouse and rat animal models; see Table 1 for ED_{50} values of methazolamide and acetazolamide in mice and rats. Pretreatment of mice with reserpine will abolish the anticonvulsant effect of methazolamide in a noncompetitive manner (GRAY et al. 1958; TORCHIANA et al. 1973). Prior treatment of mice with monoamine oxidase inhibitors prevents the reserpine antagonism of the anticonvulsant effect of carbonic anhydrase inhibitors (GRAY et al. 1963). In related studies, treatment with catecholamine precursors also restored the anticonvulsant activity of carbonic anhydrase inhibitors in mice (GRAY et al. 1963). Similar results were obtained by other investigators using mouse animal models (RUDZIK and MENNEAR 1966). Further studies in mice suggested that norepinephrine was the most significant brain amine required for the anticonvulsant effect of carbonic anhydrase inhibitors (GRAY and RAUH 1967). Subsequent work, however, in the rat animal model has shown that antagonism of the anticonvulsant effect by reserpine is surmountable by increasing doses of carbonic anhydrase inhibitor (GRAY and RAUH 1968; BROWNING and SIMONTON 1978). As in the mouse, investigators concluded that reserpine antagonism of the anticonvulsant potency of carbonic anhydrase inhibitors in the rat is via the monoaminergic system (KOSLOW and ROTH 1971). In addition to adrenergic systems, serotonergic systems are also involved in the anticonvulsant action of carbonic anhydrase inhibitors in the rat (GRAY and RAUH 1971, 1974). Finally, a recent study in mice has suggested that the noradrenergic mechanism required for the anticonvulsant action of carbonic anhydrase inhibitors is extracerebral (GRAY and RAUH 1974).

The role of catecholamines in the anticonvulsant activity of carbonic anhydrase inhibitors remains undefined. There may be some species variation in the mechanism by which carbonic anhydrase inhibition decreases brain excitability since reserpine is a competitive antagonist in rats and a noncompetitive antagonist in mice. Additional evidence for species variation is the observation that ED_{50} values for carbonic anhydrase inhibitors against maximal electroshock seizures increase with age in mice and decrease in rats (Table 1).

In conclusion, the precise molecular mechanism by which carbonic anhydrase inhibition decreases brain excitability, particularly in man, remains unsolved (WOODBURY 1980).

Table 1. Potencies of methazolamide and acetazolamide against maximal electroshock seizures in rats and mice

		ED_{50} (mg/kg)		Refs.
		Rats	Mice	
Methazolamide				
oral		2.4 (1.7–3.4)[a]	14 (12–16)	GRAY et al. (1958)
i.v.			19 (15–22)	GRAY et al. (1957)
i.v.			19 (15–22)	GRAY et al. (1957)
i.v.			15 (11–22)	GRAY et al. (1963)
i.v.		4.3 (2.9–6.1)		GRAY and RAUH (1971)
i.v.	Young	4.2 (3.5–5.0)	18.3 (14–23)	RAUH and GRAY (1968)
	Adult	2.1 (1.4–3.2	60 (44–83)	
Azetazolamide				
oral		6.0 (3.9–9.3)	49 (37–65)	GRAY et al. (1958)
oral			74 (60–91)	MILLICHAP et al. (1955)
i.v.			77 (66–90)	GRAY et al. (1957)
i.v.	Young	4.5 (2.5–7.2)	93 (69–127)	RAUH and GRAY (1968)
	Adult	2.1 (2.1–3.4)	259 (186–360)	
i.p.	Young	10.0 (6.6–15.1)	64 (49–83)	PETTY and KARLER (1965)
	Aged	5.2 (4.5–6.0)	690 (345–1,379)	

[a] Numbers in parentheses are 95% confidence limits

C. Clinical Use and Limitations

Although its use is limited, acetazolamide has been shown to be most effective in patients with petit mal epilepsy (LOMBROSO et al. 1956). Long-term use of acetazolamide in patients with epilepsy and laboratory animals has shown that tolerance to the anticonvulsant effect develops (ANSELL and CLARKE 1956; MILLICHAP 1956; LOMBROSO and FORXYTHE 1959; CHAO and PLUMB 1961; KOCH and WOODBURY 1958). The tolerance that develops during chronic acetazolamide treatment limits its clinical utility. Evidence suggests that tolerance develops consequent to an adaptive increase in carbonic anhydrase activity in glial tissue (WOODBURY 1980).

Because of the development of tolerance, intermittent use of acetazolamide is theoretically more effective. Catamenial epilepsy is a clinical situation where intermittent therapy has been considered (NEWMARK and PENRY 1980). Although acetazolamide in catamenial epilepsy has been reported to be efficacious in some patients (ANSELL and CLARKE 1956; LIVINGSTON 1972; POSER 1974), controlled studies have not been done. Interestingly, bromides, which as previously noted are also carbonic anhydrase inhibitors, were initially used in the treatment of patients with catamenial epilepsy (LOCOCK 1857). The current use of acetazolamide in epilepsy is limited to an adjuvant role in the treatment of catamenial epilepsy and otherwise refractory cases of petit mal epilepsy (FORSTER and BOOKER 1975).

Acetazolamide is dramatically effective in the treatment of certain forms of paroxysmal ataxia (GRIGGS et al. 1978); however, an epileptic basis for this disorder is not likely. The mechanism of action of acetazolamide in paroxysmal ataxia is not established.

D. Toxicity

Clinically, acetazolamide is usually administered in dosages of 3–20 mg/kg per 24 h in divided doses, but can be tolerated in much larger amounts by both man and animals (MAREN 1967). Toxicity resulting from carbonic anhydrase inhibition is usually slight, including dysgeusia (MAREN 1967), hypokalemia (RIGGS et al. 1981), and paresthesias. Carbonic anhydrase inhibitors are hazardous in patients with pulmonary disease and carbon dioxide retention, despite the fact that they were advocated in the past as "respiratory stimulants" (BLOCK and ROSTAND 1978). Renal calculi have occurred not infrequently with long-term acetazolamide use in patients with periodic paralysis (RIGGS and GRIGGS 1979). Acetazolamide may be teratogenic (MAREN 1971), perhaps discouraging its use in catamenial epilepsy. Acetazolamide may aggravate osteoporosis occurring during the treatment of epilepsy (MALLETTE 1977). Acetazolamide increases urinary calcium and phosphate and may also interfere with the synthesis of 1,25-dihydroxy vitamin D_3 (MALLETTE 1977). Finally, acetazolamide may interfere with the absorption of other anticonvulsants, complicating the management of epileptic patients (SYVERSEN et al. 1977).

References

Ansell B, Clarke E (1956) Acetazolamide in treatment of epilepsy. Br Med J 1:650–654
Ashby W (1944) A parallelism between the quantitative incidence of carbonic anhydrase and functional levels of the central nervous system. J Biol Chem 152:235–240
Bergstrom WH, Carzoli RF, Lombroso C, Davidson DT, Wallace WM (1952) Observations on the metabolic and clinical effects of carbonic-anhydrase inhibitors in epileptics. Am J Dis Child 84:771–772
Block ER, Rostand RA (1978) Carbonic anhydrase inhibition in glaucoma: hazard or benefit for the chronic lunger? Surv Ophthalmol 23: 169–172
Browning RA, Simonton RL (1978) Antagonism of the anticonvulsant action of phenytoin, phenobarbital and acetazolamide by 6-hydroxydopamine. Life Sci 22:1921–1930
Chao DHC, Plumb RL (1961) Diamox in epilepsy. J Pediatr 58:211–218
Cohen ME, Cobb S (1941) Anticonvulsive action of azosulfamide in patients with epilepsy. Arch Neurol Psychiatry 46:676–694
Delaunoy JP, Hog F, Devilliers G, Bansart M, Mandel P, Sensenbrenner M (1980) Developmental changes and localization of carbonic anhydrase in cerebral hemispheres of the rat and in rat glial cell cultures. Cell Mol Biol 26:235–240
Forster FM, Booker HE (1975) The epilepsies and convulsive disorders. In: Baker AB, Baker LH (eds). Clinical neurology. Harper and Row, Philadelphia, pp 1–45
Giacobini E (1962) A cytochemical study of the localization of carbonic anhydrase in the nervous system. J Neurochem 9:169–177
Gray WD, Rauh CE (1967) The anticonvulsant action of inhibitors of carbonic anhydrase: relation to endogenous amines in brain. J Pharmacol Exp Ther 155:127–134
Gray WD, Rauh CE (1968) The anticonvulsant action of carbon dioxide: interaction with reserpine and inhibitors of carbonic anhydrase. J Pharmacol Exp Ther 163:431–438
Gray WD, Rauh CE (1971) The relation between monoamines in brain and the anticonvulsant action of inhibitors of carbonic anhydrase. J Pharmacol Exp Ther 177:206–218

Gray WD, Rauh CE (1974) The anticonvulsant action of the carbonic anhydrase inhibitor methazolamide: possible involvement of a noradrenergic mechanism. Eur J Pharmacol 28:42–54

Gray WD, Maren TH, Sisson GM, Smith FH (1957) Carbonic anhydrase inhibition. VII. Carbonic anhydrase inhibition and anticonvulsant effect. J Pharmacol Exp Ther 121:160–170

Gray WD, Rauh CE, Osterberg AC, Lipchuck LM (1958) The anticonvulsant actions of methazolamide (a carbonic anhydrase inhibitor) and diphenylhydantoin. J Pharmacol Exp Ther 124:149–160

Gray WD, Rauh CE, Shanahan RW (1963) The mechanism of the anticonvulsant effect of inhibitors of carbonic anhydrase. J Pharmacol Exp Ther 139:350–360

Griggs RC, Moxley RT, LaFrance RA, McQuillen J (1978) Hereditary paroxysmal ataxia: response to acetazolamide. Neurology 28:1259–1264

Heuser D, Astrup J, Lassen NA, Betz E (1975) Brain carbonic acid acidosis after acetazolamide. Acta Physiol Scand 93:385–390

Kjallquist A, Nardini M, Siesjo BK (1969) The effect of acetazolamide upon tissue concentrations of bicarbonate, lactate, and pyruvate in the rat brain. Acta Physiol Scand 77:241–251

Koch A, Woodbury DM (1958) Effects of carbonic anhydrase inhibition on brain excitability. J Pharmacol Exp Ther 122:335–342

Koch A, Woodbury DM (1960) Carbonic anhydrase inhibition and brain electrolyte composition. Am J Physiol 198:434–440

Koslow SH, Roth LJ (1971) Reserpine and acetazolamide in maximum electroshock seizure in the rat. J Pharmacol Exp Ther 176:711–717

Langley OK, Ghandour MS, Vincendon G, Gombos G (1980) Carbonic anhydrase: an ultrastructural study in rat cerebellum. Histochem J 12:473–483

Lees MB, Sapirstein VS, Reiss DS, Kolodny EH (1980) Carbonic anhydrase and 2′, 3′ cyclic nucleotide 3′-phosphohydrolase activity in normal human brain and in demyelinating diseases. Neurology 30:719–725

Livingston S (1972) Comprehensive management of epilepsy in infancy, childhood and adolescence. CC Thomas, Springfield

Locock C (1857) Discussion of paper by Sieveking EH. Analysis of fift-two cases of epilepsy observed by the author. Lancet 2:138

Lombroso CT, Forxythe I (1959) A long-term follow-up of acetazolamide (Diamox) in the treatment of epilepsy. Epilepsia 1:493–500

Lombroso CT, Davidson DT, Grossi-Bianchi ML (1956) Further evaluation of acetazolamide (diamox) in treatment of epilepsy. JAMA 160:268–272

Magnussen CR, Doherty JM, Hess RA, Tschudy DP (1975) Grand mal seizures and acute intermittent porphyria: the problem of differential diagnosis and treatment. Neurology 25:1121–1125

Mallette LE (1977) Acetazolamide-accelerated anticonvulsant osteomalacia. Arch Intern Med 137:1013–1017

Mann T, Keilin D (1940) Sulphanilamide as a specific inhibitor of carbonic anhydrase. Nature 146:164–165

Maren TH (1967) Carbonic anhydrase: chemistry, physiology, and inhibition. Physiol Rev 47:595–781

Maren TH (1969) Renal carbonic anhydrase and the pharmacology of sulfonamide inhibitors. In: Eichler E, Farah A, Herken H, Welch AD (eds) Diuretica. Springer, Berlin Heidelberg New York, pp 195–256 (Handbook of experimental pharmacology, vol 24)

Maren TH (1971) Teratology and carbonic anhydrase inhibition. Arch Ophthalmol 85:1–2

Merlis S (1954) Diamox: a carbonic anhydrase inhibitor. Its use in epilepsy. Neurology 4:863–868

Millichap JG (1956) Anticonvulsant action of diamox in children. Neurology 6:552–559

Millichap JG, Woodbury DM, Goodman LS (1955) Mechanism of the anticonvulsant action of acetazolamide, a carbonic anhydrase inhibitor. J Pharmacol Exp Ther 115:251–258

Moses H, Klawans HL (1979) Bromide intoxication. In: Vinken PJ, Bruyn GW (eds) Handbook of clinical neurology, vol 36. Elsevier North-Holland Biomedical, Amsterdam, pp 291–318
Newmark ME, Penry JK (1980) Catamenial epilepsy: a review. Epilepsia 21:281–300
Petty WC, Karler R (1965) The influence of aging on the activity of anticonvulsant drugs. J Pharmacol Exp Ther 150:443–448
Poser CM (1974) Modification of therapy for exacerbation of seizures during menstruation. J Pediatr 84:779
Rauh CE, Gray WD (1968) The anticonvulsant potency of inhibitors of carbonic anhydrase in young and adult rats and mice. J Pharmacol Exp Ther 161:329–334
Riggs JE, Griggs RC (1979) Diagnosis and treatment of the periodic paralyses. In: Klawans HL (ed) Clinical neuropharmacology, vol 4. Raven, New York, pp 123–138
Riggs JE, Griggs RC, Moxley RT, Lewis ED (1981) Acute effects of acetazolamide in hyperkalemic periodic paralysis. Neurology 31:725–729
Rudzik AD, Mennear JH (1966) The mechanism of action of anticonvulsants. II. Acetazolamide. Life Sci 5:747–756
Sapirstein VS, Lees MB (1978) Purification of myelin carbonic anhydrase. J Neurochem 31:505–511
Syversen GB, Morgan JP, Weintraub M, Myers GJ (1977) Acetazolamide-induced interference with primidone absorption: case reports and metabolic studies. Arch Neurol 34:80–84
Torchiana ML, Lotti VJ, Stone GA (1973) The anticonvulsant effect of carbonic anhydrase inhibitors in mice – a noradrenergic mechanism of action. Eur J Pharmacol 21:343–349
Woodbury DM (1980) Carbonic anhydrase inhibitors. In: Glaser GH, Penry JK, Woodbury DM (eds) Antiepileptic drugs: mechanisms of action. Raven, New York, pp 617–633
Woodbury DM, Karler R (1960) The role of carbon dioxide in the nervous system. Anesthesiology 21:686–703
Yeoman JC (1938) Sulphonamide for epilepsy. Br Med J 2:261

CHAPTER 22

Acetylurea Derivatives

E. A. SWINYARD

A. Introduction

Phenacemide (Phenurone, phenylacetylurea) was the prototype of the first group of anticonvulsant substances to depart from the traditional barbiturate, hydantoin, and oxazolidinedione ring structures characteristic of antiepileptic drugs in use prior to 1948. These noncyclic ureides may be considered analogues of their corresponding ring structures. Thus, phenacemide is a straight-chain analogue of 5-phenylhydantoin (opened between the number-5 carbon and the adjacent nitrogen). Other antiepileptic straight-chain analogues of hydantoins, available in various countries, include pheneturide (Benuride), chlorphenacemide (Comitiadon), and acetylpheneturide (Crampol).

The chemistry, experimental pharmacology, and toxicity of phenacemide and the other three clinically employed acetylureas will be reviewed briefly in this chapter. The data considered are largely based upon animal studies. However, clinical results have occasionally been included when considered appropriate to a more definitive interpretation of the laboratory results.

B. Chemistry

I. Synthesis and Physicochemical Properties

The acetylureas are usually synthesized by allowing an acid halide (VOLWILER and TABERN 1936; STOUGHTON 1938) or anhydride (WERNER 1916) to react with an excess of urea, or by condensing an ester with urea in the presence of a base (SPIELMAN et al. 1948). A large number of acetylureas have been synthesized; however, only four will be considered in this review: phenacemide, 1-(2-phenylacetyl) urea (mol. wt., 178.19; mp, 212°–216 °C), pheneturide, (2-phenylbutyryl) urea (mol. wt., 206.24; mp, 149°–150 °C), acetylpheneturide, 1-acetyl-3-(2-phenylbutyryl) urea (mol. wt., 248.27, mp, 100°–101 °C), and chlorphenacemide, α-chlorophenacetyl urea (mol. wt., 248.77; mp, 200 °C). Pheneturide possesses an asymmetrical carbon atom, and its optical isomers (mp: *d*-form, 168°–169 °C; *l*-form, 162°–163 °C) have been separated (FROMMEL et al. 1959).

II. Structure-Activity Relations

The structure-activity relations of the phenylacylureas are summarized in Table 1. The branched-chain aliphatic acid derivatives of urea are the most active, with

Table 1. Structure-activity relationship of the phenylacylureas (MERCIER 1973)

R_1	R_2	R_3	R_4	Results
Phenyl-	H–	H–	H–	Maximum activity for all types of experimental epileptic seizures, MES or Met
Phenyl-	H–	CH_3–	H–	Met protection increased
Phenyl-	CH_3–	H–	H–	Increased sedation; no change in anticonvulsant activity over phenacemide
Phenyl-	H–	H–	CH_3–	Reduced anticonvulsant activity
Phenyl-	H–	CH_3–	CH_3–	Elimination of Met protection
Phenyl-	C_2H_5–	H–	H–	Increased MES protection, decreased Met protection, and increased sedation
Phenyl-	Phenyl-	H–	H–	No activity

optimal activity at seven carbon atoms. Further increases in molecular weight decrease the anticonvulsant potency and induce hypnotic activity (MERCIER 1973). The inactivity of diphenylacetylurea suggests that diphenylhydantoin is not transformed metabolically to diphenylacetylurea (SWINYARD and TOMAN 1950; HAZARD et al. 1951). Conversely, single-crystal X-ray diffraction studies show that the acetylurea portion of phenacemide and ethylphenacemide folds back upon itself to form a six-atom ring with the open end closed by an intramolecular hydrogen bond between a hydrogen atom on the terminal nitrogen and a carbonyl oxygen atom (CAMERMAN and CAMERMAN 1977). For a more detailed structure-activity analysis the reader is referred to three excellent reviews (CLOSE and SPIELMAN 1961; MERCIER 1973; MURRAY and KIER 1977).

C. Experimental Pharmacology

I. Anticonvulsant Activity

Phenacemide was initially considered an "all-purpose" antiepileptic drug, particularly effective in psychomotor seizures (GIBBS et al. 1949; ZEIFERT 1949; DAVIDSON and LENNOX 1950; LIVINGSTON and KAJDI 1950; and others), however, a reevaluation of the clinical literature does not support this notion. Indeed, a review of 250 clinical studies indicates that phenacemide is toxic and relatively ineffective; it should be a drug of last resort if used at all (COATSWORTH and PENRY 1972). Laboratory studies show that, although phenacemide is not especially potent, it does possess a broad profile of anticonvulsant activity (SPIELMAN 1948; SPIELMAN et al. 1948; EVERETT 1949; SWINYARD 1949; EVERETT and RICHARDS 1952). The minimal neurotoxic (TD_{50}) and anticonvulsant doses (ED_{50}) of phenacemide by various laboratory tests in mice and rats are summarized in Table 2. Phenacemide also prevents thujone- and *d*-desoxyephedrine-induced convulsions in mice (EVERETT and RICHARDS 1952), abolishes the tonic component of maximal electroshock seizures in rabbits and cats (EVERETT and RICHARDS 1952), and inhibits the violent phase of maximal electroshock seizures in salamanders (PETERS and VONDERAHE 1953). It also obtunds the seizures induced by the

Table 2. Minimal neurotoxic and anticonvulsant doses of phenacemide in mice and rats

Anticonvulsant test (classification)	Route of administration	Mice				Rats			
		TD_{50} (mg/kg)	Anticonvulsant ED_{50} (mg/kg)	PI	Ref.	TD_{50} (mg/kg)	Anticonvulsant ED_{50} (mg/kg)	PI	Ref.
Seizure spread									
MES	i.p.	421	87	4.8	1				
	p.o.	640	109	5.9	3	730	41	17.7	2
MMS	p.o.	640	58	11.0	3	740	212	3.5	4
Strychnine	p.o.	600	<400	> 1.5	4				
Seizure threshold									
60-Hz EST	p.o.	640	118	5.5	3	730	39	18.7	2
60-Hz HET	p.o.	640	140	4.6	3	730	225	3.2	2
6-Hz EST	p.o.	640	420	1.5	3				
Metrazol	i.p.	421	116	3.6	1				
Metrazol	p.o.	640	125	5.1	3	730	200	3.7	2
Picrotoxin	p.o.	600	<400	> 1.5	4				

MMS, maximal Metrazol (pentylenetetrazol); EST, minimal electroshock; HET, hyponatremic electroshock; PI, protective index
Refs.: 1, KRALL et al. (1978); 2, SWINYARD (1949); 3, SWINYARD et al. (1952); 4, EVERETT and RICHARDS (1952)

intracerebellar injection of ouabain (DAVIDSON et al. 1978), prevents audiogenic seizures in rats (CONSROE et al. 1980), and antagonizes kindled amygdaloid seizures in rat (BABBINGTON and WEDEKING 1973; ASHTON and WAUQUIER 1979; ALBERTSON et al. 1980).Pheneturide also exhibits a broad profile of anticonvulsant activity. Its maximal electroshock seizure and subcutaneous pentylenetetrazol ED_{50}s in mice (i.p.) are 77 and 42 mg/kg, respectively (KRALL et al. 1978). It also protects mice against seizures induced by the timed intravenous infusion of ammonium acetate and strychnine; however, it does not prevent seizures induced by the timed intravenous infusion of pentylenetetrazol, although it modifies the convulsions and protects the animals from death (ORLOFF et al. 1951). The optical isomers of pheneturide also possess anticonvulsant activity, despite differences in their overt central effects; the *d*-isomer is a central stimulant, whereas the *l*-isomer is a central depressant. However, there are no appreciable differences in the anticonvulsant activity of either of the isomers or of the parent substance (FROMMEL et al. 1959).

Acetylpheneturide is reportedly more potent, has a longer duration of action, and has higher protective indices by the MES and scMet tests than phenacemide (NAKAMURA et al. 1968). It does not obtund hippocampal after discharges evoked in unanesthetized spinal cats (NAKAMURA and KUREBE 1962).

Chlorphenacemide is also said to be more potent than phenacemide against MES and scMet seizures and clinically superior to phenacemide, both in terms of lack of toxicity and usefulness in the three major types of epilepsy (JOB et al. 1954; STROTZKA 1955).

II. Other Pharmacodynamic Properties

A number of acetylureas and their amide derivatives have been shown to possess sedative-hypnotic, analgesic, local anesthetic, and, on oral administration, convulsant properties (VOLWILER and TABERN 1936). Phenacemide induces mild diuresis and analgesia in dogs, but does not alter body temperature (normal or elevated), heart rate, or blood pressure (either normal or ischemic kidney type hypertension) in rats (EVERETT and RICHARDS 1952).

Pheneturide induces liver enzyme activity in man and is considerably more potent in this respect than phenobarbital; chronic studies in rats show it does not produce perturbations in vitamin D_3 metabolism (RISING 1979). Moreover, its concentration-dependent inhibition of hexobarbital binding to cytochrome P-450 type 1 sites in rats correlates directly with its ability to enhance the excretion of glucaric acid (LATHAM and SWEENEY 1967).

III. Pharmacokinetics

Phenacemide, orally administered to mice, is rapidly and completely absorbed from the small intestine (EVERETT and RICHARDS 1952). Pheneturide follows first-order kinetics when administered to healthy human volunteers either in single doses of 750–2,000 mg or 500 mg twice daily for 10.5 days (GALEAZZI et al. 1979). The single-dose half-life is 54 h (range, 31–90 h), and total body clearance (100% nonrenal) is 2.6 liters/h (range, 1.73–3.59 h). After repetitive administration, the half-life is 40 h, but clearance remains unchanged because of a lower volume of distribution (GALEAZZI et al. 1979).

The acetylureas are metabolized by the liver and the metabolites excreted by the kidneys (ASHER et al. 1953; GLASSON et al. 1960; TATSUMI et al. 1967, 1969). Two different pathways are involved in the metabolism of phenacemide. The first involves successive hydroxylation at the 4-position and then at the 3-position of the benzene nucleus, followed by methylation of the 3-OH group. The second involves hydrolysis of the ureide group and conjugation with glycine. Three metabolites are common to mice, rats, guinea pigs, and rabbits: 4-hydroxyphenylacetylurea, phenaceturic acid, and phenylacetic acid. Rabbits and guinea pigs also excrete 3-methoxy-4-hydroxyphenylacetylurea. A small amount of unchanged phenylacetylurea is excreted in all four animal species and man (TATSUMI et al. 1967, 1969).

Pheneturide is also metabolized by the liver (GLASSON et al. 1960). Studies in rats given ^{14}C-labeled pheneturide indicate that some unchanged drug and two metabolites are excreted in the urine, but their chemical structures have not been determined (GLASSON et al. 1960).

From 62% to 68% of a single oral dose (160 mg/kg) of ^{14}C-labeled phenacemide administered to mice can be recovered from the urine within the first 24 h after administration (TATSUMI et al. 1969). Assay of mice excreta indicates that the major portion of the radioactivity (59.2%–62.9%) is present in the urine; only 1.4%–4.8% of the administered ^{14}C was found in the feces (TATSUMI et al. 1969).

IV. Drug Interactions

Relatively few drug interactions involving phenacemide and/or its congeners have been described. In mice, SKF No. 525A has no significant effect on anticonvulsant potency, protective indices, or duration of anticonvulsant action of phenacemide; however, it significantly increases (14%) minimal neurotoxicity (SWINYARD et al. 1954). A combination of phenacemide (83.3%) and phenytoin (16.7%) has greater anti-pentylenetetrazol potency in mice than phenacemide alone (ED_{50} for the combination, 74.1 mg/kg vs ED_{50} for phenacemide alone, 119.7 mg/kg; WEAVER et al. 1958). In contrast, pheneturide has been shown to inhibit the anti-pentylenetetrazol activity of clonazepam in mice (ROLDAN et al. 1977). Pheneturide also increases serum phenytoin and phenobarbital concentrations in man (HUISMAN et al. 1970; HOUGHTON and RICHENS 1974). The long-term administration of pheneturide increases the serum level of phenytoin by an average of 25% (LATHAM and RICHENS 1973). Obviously, the sedative-hypnotic acylureas (carbromal, bromisovalum, etc.) will increase the depressant effect of other sedative-hypnotic agents.

V. Effects on Clinical Laboratory Tests

Phenacemide increases the serum values in the alanine aminotransferase, alkaline phosphatase, aspartate aminotransferase, bilirubin, BSP (bromosulfophthalein sodium) retention, cephalin flocculation, thymol turbidity, and urea nitrogen tests (YOUNG et al. 1975). It also increases the levels of bile and protein in urinalysis tests. In contrast, it decreases the blood hematocrit, hemoglobin, platelet count, red-cell count, and white-cell count. The changes in the serum tests may be related to abnormal liver function, those in urine tests to possible nephropathy, and those in blood tests to aplastic anemia, agranulocytosis, or leukopenia (YOUNG et al. 1975).

D. Toxicity

I. Acute Administration

The toxicity profiles induced in mice, cats, and dogs by a single oral dose of phenacemide are shown in Table 3. The symptoms and lethal doses are essentially the same after intraperitoneal administration in mice. A similar toxicity profile is also observed in rats (EVERETT and RICHARDS 1952). The toxicity profile in cats is remarkably similar to that observed in mice, except for a somewhat expanded dose range. Dogs, however, appear to react differently to high doses of phenacemide. For example, three dogs given 4.0 g/kg orally of phenacemide and 24 h later an additional 2 g/kg became ataxic and one was unable to walk; nevertheless, no marked sedative effects were induced. All three dogs were normal within 48 h of the second dose of phenacemide (EVERETT and RICHARDS 1952). The acute fatal doses of phenacemide in mice, rats, and cats range from 3–5 g/kg (EVERETT and RICHARDS 1952).

Three patients under treatment with phenacemide for uncontrollable psychomotor epilepsy were found to have greatly increased serum creatinine levels

Table 3. Phenacemide toxicity and symptoms (EVERETT and RICHARDS 1952)

Species	Number	Oral dose (mg/kg)	Drug effect
Mouse	10	200	None
	20	400	Slight ataxia
	20	600	Ataxia
	20	800	Light sleep
	10	1,000	Sleep
	10	3,000	Sleep, slow respiration
	10	5,000	Sleep, respiratory depression, fatal in 24–48 h
Cat	1	100	Slightly depressed
	1	200	Very slight ataxia
	2	500	Slight ataxia
	1	750	Ataxia, impaired placing and righting reflexes
	2	1,000	Marked ataxia, slight placing reflexes, depressed righting reflexes
	1	2,000	Light sleep, withdrawal reflex present, pupillary and wink reflex maintained. Heart and respiration slow, but strong recovery in 48 h
Dog	1	200	None
	1	400	Slight ataxia
	2	600	Ataxia, slight depression
	2	700	Ataxia, slight depression
	2	2,000	One marked ataxia and slight depression, one unable to stand up, slight depression
	2	4,000	Dogs vomit part of dose and become very ataxic, one unable to stand

(indication of impaired renal function) with normal blood urea nitrogen (BUN) values (RICHARDS et al. 1978). Subsequently, it was shown that phenacemide increased the serum creatinine levels in rabbits and to a lesser extent in rats (RICHARDS 1979). Further investigation in rabbits revealed that this is a common property of acylureas with an aromatic ring substituent; however, phenacemide had the greatest effect on the serum level of creatinine (RICHARDS 1980).

The laboratory toxicity profile of pheneturide is similar to that of phenacemide. The acute minimal toxic dose in mice (i.p.) is 355 mg/kg (KRALL et al. 1978). Administered orally to dogs, 250 mg/kg is nontoxic; 500 mg/kg produces slight ataxia of 30-min duration; and 1.14 g/kg induces vomiting and slight ataxia for about 2 h (ORLOFF et al. 1951).

The acute oral lethal dose of acetylpheneturide is less than that for pheneturide but greater than that for phenacemide (NAKAMURA et al. 1968).

II. Chronic Administration

Early enthusiasm for the clinical effectiveness of phenacemide was markedly tempered by reports of fatalities in patients on the drugs, hepatic and/or renal disorder (DAVIDSON and LENNOX 1950; LEVY et al. 1950; LIVERSEDGE et al. 1952; FIELD and JUSTI 1954), and aplastic anemia (FORSTER and FRANKEL 1949; SIMPSON et al.

Table 4. Frequency of side effects in 1,539 cases (TYLER and KING 1951)

		No. of cases	%
Psychic changes		263	17
Hepatitis		31	2
Deaths	4		
Gastrointestinal symptoms		130	8
Anorexia	78		
Nausea and vomiting	36		
Abdominal distress	15		
Diarrhea	1		
Rash		79	5
Exfoliative dermatitis	1		
Drowsiness		58	4
Blood changes		36	2
Leukopenia	22		
Leucocytosis	6		
Low platelet count	4		
Aplastic anemia with death	2		
Granulocytopenia	2		
Headache		24	2
Abnormal urinary findings		21	1
Transient albuminuria	8		
Acetone	10		
Sugar	2		
Nephritis	1		
Insomnia		15	1
Fatigue		14	–
Fever		14	–
Dizziness		11	–
Paresthesia		5	–
Muscle pain		5	–
Weight loss		5	–
Palpitation		3	–
Pruritus		1	–

1950). Table 4 summarizes the frequency of clinical side effects in 1539 cases reviewed by TYLER and KING (1951).

Phenacemide given daily to rats (0.25%, 0.5%, and 1% in food) for 30 months, to dogs (100–700 mg/kg) for 18–24 months, and to cats (100–150 mg/kg) for over 1 year induced no significant changes in the various organs beyond those in control animals (EVERETT and RICHARDS 1952).

Pheneturide, given orally to mice (200 mg/kg) for 3 weeks, did not induce any signs or symptoms of toxicity (ORLOFF et al. 1951).

Four weeks' chronic feeding of acetylpheneturide, pheneturide, and phenacemide (0.2%, 0.5%, and 1.0% in laboratory food) suppressed growth in all rats fed 1% of the drugs and in rats fed 0.5% pheneturide and phenacemide. Pheneturide and phenacemide significantly increased plasma glutamate pyruvate transaminase and glutamate oxalate transaminase. All three drugs induced hypocholesterolemia; it was most marked in male rats. Phenacemide-treated female rats exhibited signs of interstitial nephrosis (NAKAMURA et al. 1968).

E. Conclusions

The antiepileptic acetylureas, although not particularly potent, exhibit a broad profile of experimental anticonvulsant activity in laboratory animals. Some acetylureas also exhibit hypnotic, analgesic, and anesthetic activity. They are metabolized by the liver and excreted by the kidneys. Pheneturide is a potent liver enzyme inducer. The original phenacemide chronic toxicity studies in rats and dogs failed to reveal the potential toxicity of this drug, largely because of the doses selected and the fact that sophisticated tests capable of detecting early signs of liver and kidney damage were not available. Moreover, little if any attention has been directed to the effect of phenacemide and other acetylureas on laboratory animal behavior. More recent chronic toxicity studies in rats show that phenacemide and pheneturide induce liver damage and phenacemide some renal damage. These observations are in agreement with the adverse effects noted in clinical studies 30 years earlier and lend support to the recommendation that phenacemide be used only as a drug of last resort.

References

Albertson TE, Peterson SL, Stark LG (1980) Anticonvulsant drugs and their antagonism of kindled amygdaloid seizures in rats. Neuropharmacology 19:643–652

Asher DT, Taylor JD, Richards RK (1953) Excretion of radioactive C^{14} by rats given C^{14}-phenurone (phenacetylurea). Fed Proc 12:299

Ashton D, Wauquier A (1979) Behavioral analysis of the effects of 15 anticonvulsants in the amygdaloid kindled rat. Psychopharmacology 65:7–13

Babington RG, Wedeking PW (1973) The pharmacology of seizures induced by sensitization with low intensity brain stimulation. Pharmacol Biochem Behav 1:461–467

Camerman A, Camerman N (1977) Ethylphenacemide and phenacemide: Conformational similarities to diphenylhydantoin and stereochemical basis of anticonvulsant activity. Proc Natl Acad Sci USA 74:1264–1266

Close WJ, Spielman MA (1961) Anticonvulsant drugs. In: Hartung WH (ed) Medicinal chemistry, vol 5. Wiley, New York, pp 1–349

Coatsworth JJ, Penry KJ (1972) General principles: clinical efficacy and use. In: Woodbury DM, Penry KJ, Schmidt RP (eds) Antiepileptic drugs. Raven, New York, pp 87–96

Consroe P, Kudray K. Schmitz R (1980) Acute and chronic antiepileptic drug effects in audiogenic seizure-susceptible rats. Exp Neurol 70:626–637

Davidson DLW, Tsukada Y, Barbeua A (1978) Quabain induced seizures: site of production and response to anticonvulsants. J Can Sci Neurol 5:405–411

Davidson DT, Lennox WG (1950) Phenacetylurea – phenurone – in epilepsy. Dis Nerv Syst 11:167–173

Everett GM (1949) Pharmacological studies on phenacetylurea (phenurone), an anticonvulsant drug. Fed Proc 8:289

Everett GM, Richards RK (1952) Pharmacological studies of phenacetylurea (phenurone), an anticonvulsant drug. J Pharmacol Exp Ther 106:303–311

Field JB, Justi RA (1954) Fatal hepatitis after phenurone therapy for epilepsy. N Engl J Med 251:147–149

Forster FM, Frankel K (1949) Fatal aplastic anemia during anti-convulsant therapy. Dis Nerv Syst 10:108–111

Frommel E, Gold-Aubert P, Fleury C (1959) Pharmacological study of dextrorotatory and levorotatory pheneturide. Arch Int Pharmacodyn Ther 122:15–31
Galeazzi RL, Egli M, Wad N (1979) Pharmacokinetics of phenylethylacetylurea (pheneturide), an old antiepileptic drug. J Pharmacokinet Biopharm 7:453–462
Gibbs FA, Everett GM, Richards RK (1949) Phenurone in epilepsy. Dis Nerv Syst 10:2–4
Glasson B, Lerch P, Benakis A (1960) Métabolisme et excrétion comparée de quelque médicaments anticonvulsant. Thérapie 18:1483–1491
Hazard R, Cheymol J, Chabrier P, Smarzewska K (1951) Action anticonvulsivante et structure moleculaire de quelques composes heterocycliques pentagonaux. VIII. Influence de pouserture du noyau. Comptes Rendus Hebdomadaires des Seances de l'Academie des Science 232:658–660
Houghton GW, Richens A (1974) The effect of benzodiazepines and pheneturide on phenytoin metabolism in man. Br J Clin Pharmacol 1:344–345
Huisman JW, Van Heycop Ten Ham MW, Van Zijl CHW (1970) Influence of ethylphenacemide on serum levels of other antiepileptic drugs. Epilepsia 11:207–215
Job C, Lindinger H, Zellner H (1954) Phenyl-alpha-chloracetylharnstoff (Comitiadon) ein neues Antiepileptikum bei psychomotorischen und petit-mal-Anfällen. Wien Med Wochenschr 104:911–917
Krall RL, Penry JK, White BG, Kupferberg HJ, Swinyard EA (1978) Antiepileptic drug development. II. Anticonvulsant drug screening. Epilepsia 19:409–428
Latham AN, Richens A (1973) Pheneturide, a more potent liver enzyme inducer in man than phenobarbitone? Br J Clin Pharmacol 47:615
Latham AN, Sweeney GD (1967) Binding of anticonvulsant drugs to cytochrome P-450: Correlation with evidence of induction of hepatic microsomal enzymes. Can J Physiol Pharmacol 54:844–849
Levy RW, Simons DJ, Aronson S (1950) Fatal hepatorenal syndrome associated with phenurone therapy. N Engl J Med 243:933–936
Liversedge LA, Yates PO, Lempert H (1952) Acute yellow atrophy of the liver following treatment with phenylacetylurea. Lancet 1:242–243
Livingston S, Kajdi L (1950) The use of phenurone in the treatment of epilepsy. J Pediatr 36:159–164
Mercier J (1973) Chemical compounds possessing anticonvulsant activity. Structure-activity relationships. International Encyclopedia of Pharmacology and Therapeutics:203–238
Murray WJ, Kier LB (1977) Noncyclic anticonvulsants. In: Vida JA (ed) Medicinal chemistry, vol 15. Wiley, New York, pp 577–619
Nakamura K, Kurebe M (1962) Differential effects of anti-epileptic drugs on hippocampal and pallidal after-discharge in cats. Jpn J Pharmacol 12:180–190
Nakamura K, Murai K, Nakatsuji K, Kobayashi M, Masuda Y, Kadokawa T, Soji Y, Nakamura H, Hirooka T, Senda H (1968) Neuropharmacological and toxicological studies on a new anti-epileptic, *N*-α-ethyl-phenylacetyl-*N*-acetyl urea, in experimental animals. Arzneimittelforsch 18:524–529
Orloff MK, Feldman PE, Shaiova CH, Pfeiffer CC (1951) Anticonvulsant and toxic effects of alpha-phenyl-butyryl urea. Neurology 1:377–385
Peters JJ, Vonderahe AR (1953) Effect of themisone and phenurone on electrically-induced seizures in salamander. Neurology 3:890–895
Richards RK (1979) Effects of phenacemide and primidone on plasma creatinine in humans and experimental animals. Naunyn Schmiedebergs Arch Pharmacol 308:(Suppl)R25
Richards RK (1980) Structure-activity relationships in the effects of phenacemide analogs on serum creatinine and anticonvulsant activity. Arch Int Pharmacodyn Ther 244:107–112
Richards RK, Bjornsson TD, Waterbury LD (1978) Rise in serum and urine creatinine after phenacemide. Clin Pharmacol Ther 23:430–437
Rising TJ (1979) Effects of hepatic microsomal enzyme inducers on the endogenous substrates vitamin D_3 and folate in rat. Biochem Pharmacol 28:63–67

Roldan CM, Rabadan FP, Galan J (1977) Modification of clonazepam anticonvulsive activity by its association with other anti-epileptic drugs. Experientia 33:640–642
Simpson TW, Wilson EB, Zimmerman SL (1950) Fatal aplastic anemia occurring during anticonvulsant therapy: probable idiosyncrasy to phenurone. Ann Intern Med 32:1224–1228
Spielman MA (1948) Some anticonvulsants. First National Medicinal Chemistry Symposium of the American Chemical Society, Ann Arbor, Michigan, p 119
Spielman MA, Geiszler AO, Close WJ (1948) Anticonvulsant drugs. II. Some acylureas. J Am Chem Soc 70:4189–4191
Stoughton RW (1938) Diacylureas. I. Preparation and properties of diacylureas derived from normal aliphatic acids. J Org Chem 2:514–521
Strotzka VH (1955) Ein neues Antiepileptikum (Comitiadon). Wien Med Wochenschr 105:137–139
Swinyard EA (1949) Laboratory assay of clinically effective antiepileptic drugs. J Am Pharm Assoc Sci Ed 38:201–204
Swinyard EA, Brown WC, Goodman LS (1952) Comparative assays of antiepileptic drugs in mice and rats. J Pharmacol Exp Ther 106:319–330
Swinyard EA, Toman JEP (1950) A comparison of the anticonvulsant actions of some phenylhydantoins and their corresponding phenylacetylureas. J Pharmacol Exp Ther 100:151–157
Swinyard EA, Madsen JA, Goodman LS (1954) The effect of β-diethylaminoethylpropylacetate (SKF No. 525A) on the anticonvulsant properties of antiepileptic drugs. J Pharmacol Exp Ther 111:54–63
Tatsumi K, Yoshimura H, Tsukamoto H (1967) Metabolism of drugs – LVI. The metabolic fate of phenacetylurea. Chem Pharm Bull (Tokyo) 16:1941–1951
Tatsumi K, Yoshihara S, Yamato C, Yoshimura H, Tsukamoto H (1969) Metabolism of drugs. LXIV. Species differences of metabolism of phenacetylurea. Chem Pharm Bull (Tokyo) 17:1629–1635
Tyler MW, King EQ (1951) Phenacemide in treatment of epilepsy. JAMA 147:17–21
Volwiler EH, Tabern DL (1936) Some alkyl and aryl amides and ureides as hypnotics. J Am Chem Soc 58:1352–1354
Weaver LC, Swinyard EA, Goodman LS (1958) Anticonvulsant drug combinations: Diphenylhydantoin combined with other antiepileptics. J Am Pharm Assoc Sci Ed 47:645–648
Werner EA (1916) The constitution of carbamides. Part III. The reaction of urea and thiourea with acetic anhydride. J Chem Soc 109:1127
Young DS, Pestaner LC, Gibberman V (1975) Effects of drugs on clinical laboratory tests. Clin Chem 21:1–3
Zeifert M (1949) Phenurone in epilepsy. Dis Nerv Syst 10:245–248

CHAPTER 23

Electrophysiological Effects of Antiepileptic Drugs

I. JURNA

A. Introduction

This chapter will attempt to correlate the anticonvulsant action of antiepileptic agents with the effects of these drugs on electrophysiological parameters. Effects of antiepileptic or anticonvulsant drugs have been determined in neurons showing both normal behavior and abnormal activity due to direct or transsynaptic activation at high frequencies, treatment with different convulsant agents, or localization within or in the vicinity of an epileptogenic focus produced by local lesioning or application of cobalt or penicillin.

There are various models of experimental epilepsy which have been extensively studied for electrophysiological processes occurring in the neuronal systems involved. Unfortunately, however, not all the important anticonvulsants have been included in rigorous studies conducted on these models. Therefore, the description of drug effects on neurons and neuron systems in this chapter is not arranged on the basis of the electrophysiological test which may be employed (e.g., determination of membrane resting and action potential, membrane conductance of neurons outside and inside an epileptogenic focus, reflex activation, evoked potentials), but is arranged according to chemical group.

Changes in electrophysiological parameters can reflect direct action of an anticonvulsant on the neuron membrane, but they may also result from interference by the drug with ion-exchange mechanisms, cell metabolism, or transmitter function. To avoid redundancy, reference to other chapters in this volume (e.g., Chap. 10, "Biochemistry", by JONES and WOODBURY) will be made throughout this chapter.

It is well established that convulsions may result from either enhanced excitatory or reduced inhibitory processes in neuronal circuits. Since convulsant agents such as strychnine, picrotoxin, bicuculline, pentylenetetrazol, and bemegride produce seizure activity by reducing inhibitory or/and facilitating excitatory processes (for reviews see ESPLIN and ZABLOCKA-ESPLIN 1969; WOODBURY 1980), anticonvulsants may produce their effects not only by reducing neuron excitation or hyperexcitability, but also by increasing inhibitory influences. It seems, however, that none of the anticonvulsant agents depresses seizure activity by only one mode of action.

It should be borne in mind that an anticonvulsant action is not a corollary to the general central depression such as that produced by general anesthetics. In fact, seizure activity will be suppressed by ether or halothane in concentrations that are nearly fatal. Moreover, some depressant barbiturates inhibit seizure activity only in hypnotic doses while other depressant barbiturates will prevent seizure generation in doses which may not cause drowsiness. Some benzodiazepines may produce a potent anticonvulsant action in a dose range in which they are devoid of any sedative action. And, finally, phenytoin is an anticonvulsant agent with no sedative or hypnotic properties.

B. Phenytoin

I. Neuronal Membranes

Phenytoin is often apostrophized as a "stabilizer" of excitable membranes, because it prevents or depresses repetitive electrical activity. However, in about 60% of *Helix aspersa* neurons, phenytoin produced burst-like activity, but in about 30% neurons of this species it reduced pentylenetetrazol-induced bursts (FAUGIER-GRIMAUD 1978).

Phenytoin ($4 \times 10^{-4} M$) reduced the excitability of frog sciatic nerve that responded to supramaximal and frequent electrical stimulation with considerable increase in excitability, as signaled by a 50% lowering of the threshold (TOMAN 1949, 1952). After supramaximal and frequent stimulation, single electrical stimuli evoked repetitive discharges in the nerve fibers which were depressed by the drug. Phenobarbital ($10^{-3} M$) also prevented hyperexcitability from developing, while trimethadione (in concentrations of up to $10^{-2} M$) was ineffective. Similarly, phenytoin (1.8×10^{-5} to $1.8 \times 10^{-4} M$) and phenobarbital (5×10^{-4} and $10^{-3} M$) were found to suppress spontaneous activity in myelinated nerve fibers of the frog in which excitability had been increased by lowering the concentration of calcium ions in the suspension medium (NEUMAN and FRANK 1977).

Adding phenytoin to the perfusion with artificial seawater did not affect the electrical activity of isolated giant axons of the squid, but it reduced the spontaneous impulse discharge that occurred when the concentration of calcium and magnesium ions was reduced in the medium (KOREY 1951; ROSENBERG and BARTELS 1967). Like calcium ions, phenytoin at 10^{-6} to $5 \times 10^{-4} M$ prevented repetitive firing at the frog neuromuscular junction kept in media either deficient of calcium ions or containing germine monoacetate, an alkaloid which facilitates repetitive excitation. It also accelerated the postjunctional receptor desensitization of the end-plate region depolarized by carbamyl choline in a calcium-deficient medium (CARNAY and GRUNDFEST 1974).

Supramaximal tetanic stimulation of the cat vagus nerve produced a post-tetanic enhancement of the compound action potential of the nonmyelinated nerve fibers, which was reduced by an i.v. administration of phenytoin, 10–40 mg/kg (FRANZ and ESPLIN 1965). The post-tetanic enhancement of the compound action potential has been ascribed to a summation of afterpotentials which increases with the frequency of stimulation because of an accumulation of potassium ions in the extracellular space (RITCHIE and STRAUB 1957). Consequently, this effect of phenytoin was explained by a reduction of the extracellular potassium concentration (FRANZ and ESPLIN 1965). Indeed, stimulation by phenytoin, $10^{-4} M$, of potassium influx has been observed in motor axons of the lobster [(FERTZIGER et al. 1971); for description of activation of the potassium transport by phenytoin see Chap. 10, this volume].

Chronic administration of phenytoin (5–20 mg/kg i.p., three times daily for 5 days) to rabbits markedly shortened the period of decreased excitability which followed repetitive electrical stimulation of nonmyelinated fibers in the isolated vagus nerve (JULIEN and HALPERN 1970). This period of decreased excitability correlated with the time course of post-tetanic hyperpolarization, which is essential for the post-tetanic potentiation of synaptic transmission. The reduction by phenytoin of the recovery period was interpreted in terms of the membrane stabilization which is responsible for the suppression of epileptiform activity (JULIEN and HALPERN 1970). A decrease in post-tetanic hyperpolarization also occurred after administration of phenytoin in the crayfish stretch receptor neuron (AYALA et al. 1977b). RAINES and STANDAERT observed that systemic administration of phenytoin in doses from 0.5 to 50 mg/kg dose dependently reduced the post-tetanic hyperpolarization established in the central terminals of dorsal root fibers of spinal cats (RAINES and STANDAERT 1967). They also reported that phenytoin, 20 mg/kg i.v., depressed the repetitive activity generated in cat motor nerve endings by tetanic stimulation and the post-tetanic potentiation of skeletal muscle contraction (RAINES and STANDAERT 1969); they concluded that these depressant effects are due to abolition by the drug of post-tetanic hyperpolarization. Repetitive activity established by physiological stimulation, e.g., by muscle stretch, may equally be influenced by the drug. ANDERSON and RAINES (1974) observed that phenytoin (5–40 mg/kg i.v.) depressed the discharge from deefferented muscle spindles in the triceps surae muscle of anesthetized cats.

Numerous findings indicate that the effects of phenytoin on excitable membranes might be due to an action on the movement of sodium and calcium ions (see also Chap. 10, this volume). Phenytoin (5×10^{-5} to $10^{-4} M$) decreased the bursting pacemaker activity which appeared spontaneously or after the administration of pentylenetetrazol in cells of *Aplysia*, and the sodium-dependent negative resistance characteristic which is essential for this bursting behavior (JOHNSTON and AYALA 1975).

In voltage-clamp experiments performed on squid axons, phenytoin (5×10^{-6}, 10^{-5}, and $5 \times 10^{-5} M$) dose dependently and reversibly decreased the early transient sodium current; it was therefore proposed that phenytoin reduced the number of open sodium channels (LIPICKY et al. 1972). This is in agreement with the observation that, in a concentration of $10^{-4} M$, the drug reduced the influx of sodium ions in stimulated but not in resting walking nerves of the lobster (PINCUS 1972). In concentrations between 10^{-4} and $5 \times 10^{-4} M$, the drug prevented the depolarization of neurons and reduced sodium influx in slices of guinea pig cerebral cortex stimulated electrically at high frequencies (CRANE and SWANSON 1970; SWANSON and CRANE 1970, 1972). Phenytoin and desoxycorticosterone reduced sodium concentration in neurons of the rat cerebral cortex and in processes of astrocytes that adjoin synaptic terminals (HARTMANN 1966). On the other hand, the sodium transport in frog skin was enhanced by phenytoin (100 µg/ml) and by vasopressin (WATSON and WOODBURY 1972). When phenytoin (33 µg/ml) was added to the medium bathing the external side of the frog skin, it produced a sustained rise in potential difference and short circuit current, which both were abolished by amiloride, a drug that decreases sodium transport (DESOUSA and GROSSO 1973).

In voltage-clamped single nerve fibers of the frog kept in Ringer solution at a normal calcium concentration, phenytoin (1.8×10^{-5} and $1.8 \times 10^{-4} M$) reduced sodium permeability without affecting potassium conductance, voltage-dependent time constants of sodium activation and inactivation, and potassium activation (NEUMAN and FRANK 1977). When the calcium concentration in the medium was lowered, the curves relating the time constants of sodium activation and inactivation to the membrane potential were shifted in the direction of hyperpolarization. Phenytoin (and phenobarbital) prevented this shift. From this it was concluded that phenytoin stabilizes the hyperexcitable membrane by influencing sodium inactivation (NEUMAN and FRANK 1977).

In neurons and peripheral nerves, phenytoin hyperpolarized the resting membrane potential (SCHWARZ and VOGEL 1977; PERRY et al. 1978), raised the threshold (MORRELL et al. 1958; SCHWARZ and VOGEL 1977), reduced the conduction velocity (MORRELL et al. 1958; SCHWARZ and VOGEL 1977) and the amplitude of the action potential (MORRELL et al. 1958; KRUPP 1969; AYALA and JOHNSTON 1977; AYALA et al. 1977b; SCHWARZ and VOGEL 1977), and decreased or abolished repetitive impulse discharges (TOMAN 1949; KOREY 1951; MORRELL et al. 1958; RAINES and STANDAERT 1966; ROSENBERG and BARTELS 1967; AYALA et al. 1977b). SCHWARZ and VOGEL (1977) also found that phenytoin, $8 \times 10^{-5} M$, reduced the peak of the sodium current in current and voltage-clamp experiments performed on myelinated nerve fibers of *Xenopus laevis* and ascribed the excitability-reducing effect of the drug to a potential-dependent blockage of the sodium channel by the phenytoin molecule. They proposed that phenytoin and procaine bind to sites in the sodium channel which are different from those to which tetrodotoxin or saxitoxin bind. On account of results obtained with isolated giant axons of the squid preloaded with radiolabeled sodium, PERRY et al. (1978) arrived at the conclusion that phenytoin (7.5×10^{-5} to $10^{-5} M$) blocks passive resting sodium channels in much the same way as tetrodotoxin. According to DE WEER (1980), phenytoin interferes with the gating mechanism of the sodium channel.

There are also indications of an involvement of calcium ions in the effects exerted by phenytoin. Both phenytoin ($2 \times 10^{-4} M$) and procaine hydrochloride ($2 \times 10^{-2} M$) reduced the uptake and outflow of radiolabeled calcium in resting lobster axons (HASBANI et al. 1974).

DRETCHEN et al. (1977) observed that phenytoin in doses of 5–20 mg/kg i.v. reduced the repetitive afterdischarges evoked in motor nerve endings of the cat by tetanic stimulation, administration of dibutyryl cyclic AMP, or adenylate cyclase activation with sodium fluoride. The inhibitory effect of phenytoin was antagonized by theophylline or the calcium current antagonist verapamil. These authors proposed therefore that phenytoin blocks a calcium influx which is mediated by cyclic nucleotides, controls the slow potassium current responsible for post-tetanic hyperpolarization, and is also associated with the release of transmitter substances (see also PINCUS et al. 1980).

PINCUS (1977) noted that phenytoin, although having previously been found to decrease synaptic transmission at the neuromuscular junction, augments transmitter release when synaptic transmission is depressed by a lowered calcium ion concentration on the outside. He proposed that phenytoin antagonizes both the calcium influx into the presynaptic terminals and the intracellular sequestration of calcium.

The reports on the various effects exerted by phenytoin on different excitable membranes agree remarkably well. It seems justified to assume that the anticonvulsant action of the drug is largely due to the abolition of hyperexcitability evoked in neurons and nerve fibers. However, it is only fair to state that the biochemical mechanisms underlying the drug-induced changes of electrophysiological parameters are still not fully understood, as is evident from the reviews of WOODBURY and KEMP (1970), AYALA and JOHNSTON (1977), LA MANNA et al. (1977), DELGADO-ESCUETA and HORAN (1980), and JONES and WOODBURY in Chap. 10, this volume.

II. Synaptic Transmission

1. Ganglia and Neuromuscular Junctions

In the abdominal ganglion of *Aplysia,* phenytoin, $10^{-4}M$, decreased the amplitude of the excitatory postsynaptic potential; it was ineffective on the "short" acetylcholine-mediated chloride-dependent inhibitory postsynaptic potential (IPSP) and facilitated the "long" acetylcholine-mediated potassium-dependent IPSP (AYALA et al. 1977a). Moreover, the drug prolonged the time course of the gamma-aminobutyric acid (GABA)-mediated, chloride-dependent IPSP in the crayfish stretch receptor neuron about ten times (AYALA et al. 1977a). This latter result was also obtained by DEISZ and LUX (1977), who observed that phenytoin, $10^{-4} M$, prolonged the IPSP evoked in the crayfish stretch receptor neuron as well as the conductance and potential changes produced by GABA. Moreover, these authors reported that phenytoin prevented the blockade by picrotoxin of postsynaptic inhibition and responses to GABA.

ESPLIN (1957) observed that phenytoin, 30 mg/kg i.v., reduced the post-tetanic potentiation (PTP) of impulse transmission through the stellate ganglion of the cat. Similarly, SURIA and COSTA (1973) found that the drug dose dependently (10^{-6} and $10^{-5}M$) reduced the PTP of the transmission in sympathetic ganglia of the bullfrog.

PINCUS et al. (1980) noted that transmission at the frog neuromuscular junction is depressed by phenytoin (10^{-4} and $2 \times 10^{-4}M$), and they concluded from further findings that the drug exerts its primary action on the calcium mechanism at the membrane of the motoneuron terminals; it reduced the quantal content of transmitter released and the effect of acetylcholine at the postsynaptic membrane.

2. Spinal Cord

a) Depressant Effects

In spinal cats, phenytoin, 30 mg/kg i.v., reduced the monosynaptic reflex (MSR) by about 10% and polysynaptic reflexes (PSR) by about 20% (ESPLIN 1957). The most prominent effect of phenytoin on the impulse transmission in spinal reflex paths is the depression of PTP of the MSR, which shows dose dependence after i.v. administration in doses of 10–40 mg/kg (ESPLIN 1957). Several mechanisms are discussed as being responsible for the development of PTP (for details see Es-

PLIN and ZABLOCKA 1969), such as (1) post-tetanic hyperpolarization of presynaptic terminals (ECCLES and KRNJEVIĆ 1959); (2) increased transmitter release from tetanically stimulated presynaptic terminals (see also WEINREICH 1971); and (3) opening-up of new afferent paths which will lead to recruitment of postsynaptic neurons and thus to spread of excitation. Indications for an influence of phenytoin on factors (1) and (2) have been presented in the preceding sections.

Synaptic recovery after impulse transmission in spinal reflex pathways of the cat is not influenced by phenytoin (ESPLIN 1963).

Continuous maximal high-frequency stimulation of the cervical spinal cord in decapitated animals (cat, rabbit, hamster, and mouse) resulted in a sequence of hindlimb movements which are identical to those seen in the maximal electroshock seizure in intact animals; this spinal seizure activity was not depressed by phenytoin in doses which were effective on maximal electroconvulsions in the intact animal (ESPLIN and FRESTON 1960). The same was true for phenobarbital and trimethadione with the exception that trimethadione prolonged the spinal postictal depression. These results were taken as evidence for a supraspinal site of the therapeutic action of the anticonvulsant agents. However, in an attempt to demonstrate that phenytoin can depress seizure activity in the absence of the cerebellum (see also Sect. B. III.4), LOTHMAN and SOMJEN (1976) showed that spinal seizure activity evoked in functionally decapitated cats by local or systemic administration of penicillin (KAO and CRILL 1972a, b; DAVENPORT et al. 1977) was suppressed by an i.v. injection of phenytoin (20–40 mg/kg), phenobarbital (15–35 mg/kg), and pentobarbital (20–30 mg/kg), while diazepam was ineffective when administered cumulatively in doses up to 7 mg/kg.

b) Excitatory Effects

Phenytoin differs markedly from all other anticonvulsants in that it does not produce central depression; it distinguishes itself by signs of central excitation in animals and man.

During early postnatal development, the drug has been found to exert excitatory effects by blocking both pre- and postsynaptic inhibition. At later stages of development and in adulthood this excitatory effect was counteracted by the activation by phenytoin of inhibitory systems (VERNADAKIS and WOODBURY 1965).

The thioderivative of phenytoin diphenylthiohydantoin (DPTH) has a spectrum of anticonvulsant activity which is similar to that of phenytoin (SOHN et al. 1970). In cats with the spinal cord left intact or transected at the cervical level, DPTH depressed mono- and polysynaptic reflex activity (RAINES et al. 1971; GROSSMANN et al. 1974c) like phenytoin (ESPLIN 1957). In cats with spinalization performed at the lumbar level, DPTH enhanced mono- and polysynaptic reflex activity (GROSSMANN et al. 1974c), amplitude of the action potential, afterhyperpolarization in motoneurons activated by antidromic stimulation, membrane resistance, and excitatory and inhibitory postsynaptic potentials in spinal motoneurons (GROSSMANN et al. 1974b). In decerebrate cats, DPTH enhanced ascending and descending inhibition of spinal reflex activity (GROSSMANN et al. 1974a). From these results it was concluded that DPTH, by exerting an excitatory effect on neurons, enhances inhibitory processes and that such a mode of action might also explain part of the anticonvulsant action of phenytoin (for phenytoin and activation of inhibitory Purkinje cells in the cerebellum see below).

In experiments performed on isolated spinal cords of the frog, DAVIDOFF (1972a) observed that phenytoin, in concentrations of 10^{-6} to $10^{-4}M$, depressed monosynaptic reflex activity and enhanced PSRs. Presynaptic inhibition of PSRs resulting from primary afferent depolarization by GABA was consistently augmented by phenytoin. Perfusion of the cord with phenytoin had no influence on the action of glycine, glutamate, or aspartate.

3. Spinal Trigeminal Nucleus

In experiments conducted to find an explanation for the therapeutic effect of phenytoin in trigeminal neuralgia in terms of neurophysiological data, FROMM and co-workers (FROMM and LANDGREN 1963; FROMM and KILLIAN 1967; FROMM 1969) found that the drug (10–15 mg i.v.) increased the latency of the synaptic response of single neurons in the cat trigeminal nucleus to stimulation of the maxillary nerve with single electrical impulses. Cells responding to single stimuli with more than one spike showed a decrease in the number of spike discharges after the injection of phenytoin. Since the amplitude of the spike evoked by antidromic stimulation and that of the spike in the afferent nerve remained unchanged, it was concluded that phenytoin depressed synaptic transmission in a more specific way than phenobarbital (0.75 mg/kg), which progressively decreased the amplitude of the spike evoked in the trigeminal neuron by both orthodromic and antidromic stimulation (for further details see Chap. 13 this volume).

III. Brain

1. Synaptic Transmission

The synaptic activation of pyramidal tract neurons produced by electrical stimulation of the motor cortex or ventrolateral nucleus of the thalamus in unanesthetized cats was reduced by i.v. injection of phenytoin in doses from 10 to 25 mg/kg, while the effect on the response of these neurons was markedly weaker (BLUM 1964). A similar effect was observed when paired electrical stimuli were delivered to the ventrolateral thalamus and the responses evoked by the stimulation were recorded from the sensorimotor cortex of the cat; phenytoin, 15 mg/kg i.v., depressed the synaptic excitability of the cortical neurons (ENGLANDER et al. 1977).

2. Afterdischarges

When a group of neurons in the brain is stimulated electrically, afterdischarges following the response to the stimulus may occur in these neurons and in distant second groups of neurons to which the first group of neurons projects. These afterdischarges are regarded as an indicator of the tendency to develop epileptogenic activity.

SCHALLEK and KUEHN (1963) noted that systemic administration of phenytoin, 10 mg/kg, decreased the duration of the afterdischarges evoked in the cortex and hippocampus in response to electrical stimulation of the thalamus of the cat, but not in the thalamus. Later, it was found that phenytoin increased the threshold of stimulation to evoke afterdischarges in both the cortex and thalamus (SCHALLEK et al. 1964). This agrees with the early observation of GANGLOFF and MONNIER (1957) that phenytoin exerted an effect only on the afterdischarges evoked in the rabbit by stimulation of the thalamus. The drug also raised the threshold of the afterdischarges to stimulation of the cat nucleus centralis lateralis of the thalamus and the rat nucleus reticularis (ITO et al. 1977). Although elevation by phenytoin of the threshold to stimulation of the cat hippocampus and ectosylvian nucleus has been reported (STROBOS and SPUDIS 1960; ALBERTSON et al. 1977), the main site of action of phenytoin in depressing afterdischarges seems to be the diencephalon.

Recording with potassium-sensitive electrodes from the extracellular space of the cat cerebral cortex revealed that during intense electrical stimulation or repetitive epileptiform discharges of cortical neurons the extracellular potassium ion concentration increased to reach values which could both increase transmitter release from terminals and have a significant depolarizing effect on neurons (PRINCE et al. 1973). Phenytoin 15 or 25 mg/kg i.v. reduced this increase in the extracellular potassium concentration (HEINEMANN and LUX 1973).

3. Seizure Activity and Its Spread

Generally phenytoin does not depress activity in epileptogenic foci but limits spread of activity from the foci (MUSGRAVE and PURPURA 1963; LOUIS et al. 1968). SHERWIN (1973) also found that phenytoin had little effect on the seizure activity in the focus produced by an injection of penicillin into the cerebral cortex of the cat, and that the accompanying relayed pyramidal tract response was consistently and dose-dependently reduced in amplitude by phenytoin. Moreover, this author demonstrated that the activity in the epileptogenic focus could be triggered by stimulation in the ventrolateral nucleus of the thalamus and that the triggering effect was suppressed by phenytoin which acted on the cortex, not on the thalamus.

LOUIS et al. (1971) produced an epileptogenic focus by applying ampicillin to the cat cortex. By electrical stimulation in the periphery or applying touch stimuli, they could either drive the activity or produce afterdischarges in the focus. Phenytoin, 20–25 mg/kg, abolished peripheral manifestations (jerking of limbs), cortical afterdischarges, and receptivity of the focus to triggering by sensory stimuli.

MORRELL et al. (1959) failed to observe a depressant effect of phenytoin on the activity in a cortical focus produced in rabbits by local freezing, nor was the spread of this activity to the basal diencephalon limited by the drug. Phenytoin did not decrease epileptogenic activity induced by injection of penicillin into the rat cortex in situ (EDMONDS et al. 1974), but depressed the seizure afterdischarges evoked by electrical stimulation in chronically and neuronally isolated slabs of the cat cerebral cortex (KRIP and VAZQUEZ 1971). It may be that phenytoin, by way of facilitating inhibitory influences, increases the "surround" inhibition which builds up like a protective zone around the epileptogenic focus produced by local application of penicillin (PRINCE and WILDER 1967; PRINCE 1968).

Cortical application of tungstic acid gel to rats produced spikes, spike-and-wave complexes and secondary generalized seizure activity in the brain;

phenytoin shortened the duration of the secondary generalization and prolonged the interictal period (ITO et al. 1979).

4. Activation of Cerebellar Inhibition by Excitatory Effects

It has been mentioned above (Sect. B.II.2.b) that phenytoin may produce excitation of neurons. Electroencephalographic evidence has been obtained that during acute or chronic intoxication with phenytoin seizure-like activity may appear in various animal species (BAZEMORE and ZUCKERMANN 1974).

When one of the first descriptions of the clinical effects of phenytoin was given by MERRIT and PUTNAM (1939), this included a syndrome of cerebellar dysfunction consisting of ataxia, tremor, diplopia, and nystagmus. Experimental data illustrating the role of the cerebellum in seizure activity have been reviewed by JULIEN (1974) and LAXER et al. (1980). The incidence of phenytoin-induced cerebellar degeneration including loss of the Purkinje-cell layer has been critically evaluated by VERNADAKIS and PARKER (1980), who also give an account of the neurotoxicity of other anticonvulsant agents.

Cerebellar stimulation, particularly stimulation of the vermis, depresses seizure activity in animal models (LAXER et al. 1980). JULIEN and LAXER (1974) observed in rats that after local injection of penicillin into the cerebral cortex, high-frequency discharges appeared in cerebellar Purkinje cells which were evoked by focal spike activity in the cerebral cortex. The discharges of Purkinje cells could outlast epileptiform cortical bursts of short duration. However, when the discharge of Purkinje cells ceased during periods of sustained focal discharge, seizure activity appeared in the electroencephalogram of both hemispheres, and convulsive episodes became manifest. Discharge of Purkinje cells did not appear again unless seizure activity had subsided.

Extracellular microelectrode recordings made from cerebellar Purkinje cells of the cat revealed that after an i.v. injection of phenytoin, 10 mg/kg, the random activity of the cells was replaced by a sustained high-frequency discharge persisting for hours (JULIEN and HALPERN 1971; HALPERN and JULIEN 1972). Simultaneously, phenytoin reduced the spreading of epileptiform activity from a penicillin-induced cortical focus (JULIEN and HALPERN 1971). These results suggest that an activation by phenytoin of inhibitory influences from the cerebellum may be involved in the anticonvulsant action of the drug (but see PURO and WOODWARD 1973).

IV. Summary

Suppression of hyperexcitability and limitation of the spread of hyperactivity by reducing post-tetanic potentiation and facilitating inhibitory processes seem to be the main factors by which phenytoin produces its anticonvulsant effect. However, none of the changes in electrophysiological parameters can explain why the drug effectively increases the threshold of maximal electroseizure in normal and hyponatremic animals (MERRITT and PUTNAM 1938; TOMAN et al. 1946; WOODBURY 1955), but fails to increase the threshold for pentylenetetrazol-induced seizures, to prevent "petit mal"-like EEG dysrhythmias elicited in animals by subconvulsive pentylenetetrazol doses, and to elevate the electroseizure threshold to low-frequency stimulation (GOODMAN et al. 1946a; WOODBURY and ESPLIN 1959).

C. Barbiturates

I. General Remarks

Since the beginning of this century, barbiturates have been widely used as sedatives and hypnotics. The anticonvulsant property of phenobarbital was recognized very early (HAUPTMANN 1912). It soon became evident that phenobarbital could show anticonvulsant properties in a dose range that did not produce sleep, while with other barbiturates such as pentobarbital suppression of seizure activity was not achieved unless hypnotic doses of the drug were administered. From this it may be concluded that the anticonvulsant action of barbiturates is a specific one which is not correlated to a general depressant or anesthetic action.

It seems to be generally recognized that barbiturates act by affecting either membrane excitability or synaptic transmission. Most of the data obtained in experiments carried out on single neurons or synapses do not enable the distinction to be made between barbiturates acting primarily as anticonvulsants and those exerting a predominantly hypnotic or general anesthetic effect, nor do they point toward a particular effect which might be considered as essential for the anticonvulsant action. Information relevant to a specific effect associated with the suppression of seizure activity may thus be expected from experiments conducted on supraspinal neuron populations.

Mephobarbital is demethylated in the liver into phenobarbital, and a major part of the anticonvulsant property of mephobarbital may be ascribed to its metabolite phenobarbital, but the unchanged molecule also exerts an anticonvulsant effect (CRAIG and SHIDEMAN 1971). Primidone is metabolized in man to phenobarbital and phenylethylmalonamide (GALLAGHER and BAUMEL 1972). Phenobarbital, mephophenobarbital, and primidone have widely overlapping spectra of anticonvulsant action and will therefore be treated as belonging to the group of substances of which the prototype is phenobarbital.

II. Membrane Excitability

Barbiturates block action potentials in nerve preparations in concentrations which are likely to be above those present in the central nervous system during anesthesia, and which are substantially above those which affect synapses (LARRABEE and POSTERNAK 1952). HEINBECKER and BARTLEY (1940) noted that pentobarbital and ether blocked the generation of action potentials in nerve fibers. This block produced by pentobarbital in single nerve fibers is similar to that resulting from procaine (KRUPP et al. 1969) and is, like the procaine-induced block, removed by anodal depolarization (SCHOEPFLE 1957). The blocking effect of pentobarbital on frog nerve action potentials was enhanced by epinephrine, while that of phenobarbital and procaine was antagonized by epinephrine (SABELLI et al. 1977); however, the effect of phenobarbital differed from that of procaine in that it was not dependent on calcium ions. On account of these results and additional findings obtained with beta-adrenoceptor blockers, SABELLI et al. (1977) conclude that pentobarbital and phenobarbital exert specific effects on excitable membranes.

Differential effects of these two barbiturates are also evident from the results obtained by VAZQUEZ et al. (1975) in experiments carried out on isolated cat sciatic nerves. In these preparations, both pentobarbital and phenobarbital, in concentrations from 1 to $5 \times 10^{-3} M$, raised the threshold and lowered the spike amplitude, and the action of the two barbiturates was increased by reducing the sodium concentration or increasing the pH in the suspension medium. Exchange of H_2O by D_2O in the medium enhanced the depressant effect of pentobarbital like that of ether or halothane, but did not modify the effect of phenobarbital or procaine.

In frog nerve fibers which were made hyperexcitable by repetitive electrical stimulation, phenobarbital, $10^{-3} M$, reduced repetitive spike discharges (TOMAN 1949, 1952). Similarly, NEUMAN and FRANK (1977) observed that phenobarbital (5×10^{-4} and $10^{-3} M$) diminished the hyperexcitability induced in voltage-clamp experiments performed on frog nerve fibers by lowering the extracellular calcium. These authors suggest that phenobarbital (and phenytoin) stabilize hyperexcitable membranes by acting on sodium activation. On the other hand, SEEMAN et al. (1974) and STAIMAN and SEEMAN (1974) noted that calcium antagonized the block of impulse conduction produced by pentobarbital and barbital in the isolated rat phrenic nerve.

In voltage-clamp experiments carried out on lobster axons, the maximum conductances for sodium and potassium ions were reduced by pentobarbital, $6 \times 10^{-3} M$, and thiopental $2 \times 10^{-3} M$ (BLAUSTEIN 1968); both barbiturates also slowed the rate at which the sodium conductance turns on. When pentobarbital (1 and $3 \times 10^{-3} M$) was applied to either side of the giant axon of the squid, it reduced the sodium and potassium conductances (NARAHASHI et al. 1969), but more effectively on the inside (NARAHASHI et al. 1971).

In neurons of *Aplysia* and *Helix,* phenobarbital suppressed spontaneous activity (TAKEUCHI and CHALAZONITIS 1968). In *Aplysia* neurons, phenobarbital hyperpolarizes the membrane like halothane, diminishes the excitability and resistance of the membrane and blocks the generation of an action potential (TAKEUCHI 1969). In this type of neuron, pentobarbital increased the resting potassium conductance (SATO et al. 1967). WILSON et al. (1980) observed that superfusion of *Aplysia* neurons with pentobarbital and phenobarbital in concentrations ranging from 5×10^{-5} to $5 \times 10^{-4} M$ enhanced the adaptation of neurons to depolarizing stimuli (before the administration the neurons discharged repetitively as long as the depolarizing pulse lasted; during barbiturate administration the neuron ceased to fire before the end of the depolarizing pulse). Voltage-clamp studies revealed that this enhanced adaptation was due to a barbiturate-induced slow, potassium-dependent outward current in response to depolarization. Amobarbital increased the membrane potential of *Helix aspersa* neurons; it prevented burst-like activity elicited by administration of pentylenetetrazol but not the one due to intracellularly applied depolarizing currents (FAUGIER-GRIMAUD 1978).

III. Synaptic Transmission

1. Ganglia and Neuromuscular Junctions

Pentobarbital has been reported to block the frog neuromuscular junction (THESLEFF 1956; BARKER and GAINER 1973; BARKER 1975a, b, c; SEYAMA and NARAHASHI 1975). Phenobarbital dose-dependently reduced the amplitude of miniature end-plate potentials at the frog neuromuscular junction but did not affect that of the end-plate potential; it increased the quantal content of transmitter released (ALDERDICE and TROMMER 1980). Synaptic transmission through the ganglia of *Limulus polyphemus* was inhibited by pentobarbital and ether (HEINBECKER and BARTLEY 1940). In the sympathetic ganglion of the bullfrog, pentobarbital reduced the fast nicotinic excitatory postsynaptic potential of B cells without affecting the slow muscarinic excitatory and inhibitory postsynaptic potentials, the presynaptic spike, the number of transmitter quanta released, or the membrane properties of the postsynaptic ganglion cell (NICOLL 1978; NICOLL and IWAMOTO 1978). In the perfused stellate ganglion of the cat, pentobarbital depressed synaptic transmission more readily than impulse conduction along any type of axon (LARRABEE and POSTERNAK 1952). Unfortunately, information about the effect exerted by an anticonvulsant barbiturate in these preparations is lacking.

Pentobarbital (4×10^{-4} and $7.5 \times 10^{-4} M$) and thiopental ($3 \times 10^{-4} M$) blocked the uptake of radiolabeled calcium into stimulated or potassium-depolarized isolated superior cervical ganglia of the rat (BLAUSTEIN 1976). This is in accord with an earlier observation made by BLAUSTEIN and ECTOR (1975), who had found that pentobarbital ($4–5 \times 10^{-4} M$) and thiopental reduced the extra uptake of calcium which was induced by depolarizing agents in synaptosomes isolated from the rat brain. These results have been interpreted in terms of an interference of these barbiturates with the release of transmitters (see also GOLDRING and BLAUSTEIN 1980). However, it seems unlikely that inhibition of transmitter release is an important mode of action of the anticonvulsant barbiturates because phenobarbital in concentrations up to $9 \times 10^{-4} M$ had little effect on the extra uptake of calcium, while the convulsant isomer of 5-(1,3-dimethylbutyl)-5-ethylbarbituric acid [(+)-DMBB] reduced it (BLAUSTEIN and ECTOR 1975).

2. The GABA Receptor Complex and Glutamate-Mediated Transmission

Much evidence has accumulated in support of the view that barbiturates interact with the inhibitory transmitter GABA at various synapses. Detailed accounts of the interaction between barbiturates, benzodiazepine derivatives, and the convulsant agents picrotoxin and bicuculline at the GABA receptor complex are given in the reports and reviews by OLSEN and co-workers (OLSEN 1981 a, b; OLSEN et al. 1978, 1979, 1980; TICKU and OLSEN 1978; LEEB-LUNDBERG et al. 1980; OLSEN and LEEB-LUNDBERG 1981; IADAROLA and GALE 1981) and MELDRUM in Chap. 7, this volume.

NICOLL (1975 a) observed that frog motoneurons which were hyperpolarized by GABA were also hyperpolarized by pentobarbital in a concentration of $10^{-4} M$ or more, and that the hyperpolarization produced by either substance was antagonized by the GABA antagonists picrotoxin or bicuculline, but not by strychnine, the antagonist of the inhibitory transmitter glycine. Moreover, pentobarbital in low concentrations (from 2×10^{-5} to $10^{-4} M$) increased the amplitude and duration of the GABA-induced hyperpolarization. In a later study, NICOLL and WOJTOWICZ (1980) confirmed the results obtained with pentobarbital and, in addition, found that phenobarbital had the same effects but was only one-fifth as potent as pentobarbital.

Likewise, RANSOM and BARKER (1975, 1976) found that pentobarbital prolonged the postsynaptic inhibition and conductance changes induced by GABA in the membrane of mouse spinal neurons in tissue cultures. The drug did not affect the postsynaptic action of glycine but blocked the postsynaptic excitation produced by glutamate. Identical results were obtained somewhat later with phenobarbital and mephobarbital by MACDONALD and BARKER (1979a).

When comparing the effects of anticonvulsant barbiturates (phenobarbital and mephobarbital) and anesthetic barbiturates (pentobarbital, secobarbital) in cultured spinal neurons of the mouse, it was found that all barbiturates augmented the membrane response to GABA and inhibited that to glutamate; anesthetic barbiturates differed from anticonvulsant barbiturates in that they were more potent (MACDONALD and BARKER 1979b).

BOWERY and DRAY (1976, 1978) noted that, in the isolated cervical ganglion of the rat, pentobarbital at concentrations higher than $8 \times 10^{-5} M$ produced membrane depolarization, as did GABA at concentrations greater than $10^{-6} M$, and that the depolarizations produced by either pentobarbital or GABA were abolished by bicuculline. These authors also report that the anticonvulsant barbiturates phenobarbital and mephobarbital were less effective than pentobarbital. EVANS (1979) observed that pentobarbital potentiated GABA-induced responses in isolated superior cervical ganglia and in dorsal and ventral root fibers of immature isolated spinal cords of the rat. Moreover, he found that pentobarbital did not significantly alter the antagonism between GABA and bicuculline.

SAAD et al. (1972) reported that phenobarbital and mephobarbital increased the GABA content in the cerebral hemisphere of mice. However, TAPPAZ and PACHECO (1973) failed to detect an accumulation of radiolabeled GABA in rat brain slices. Likewise, PECK et al. (1976) could not detect an effect of pentobarbital in concentrations exceeding $10^{-3} M$ on GABA uptake into synaptosomes of the rat cerebral cortex and hippocampus. Thus, it is more likely that the anticonvulsant effect of barbiturates involves an action of the GABA receptor complex than on GABA synthesis, uptake, or metabolism (see also Chaps. 7, 10, this volume)

IV. Spinal Cord

1. Depression of Excitatory Transmission

Numerous investigators have reported that phenobarbital, pentobarbital, and other barbiturates depress monosynaptic and polysynaptic reflexes in the spinal cord of frogs and cats (SOMJEN 1943, 1963; WIKLER 1945; ECCLES 1946; BROOKS and ECCLES 1947; DE SALVA and OESTER 1960; SHAPOVALOV 1964). The reflex depression has mostly been attributed to a "stabilization" of the motoneuron membrane. However, barbiturates producing general anesthesia have been found to reduce the excitability of primary afferents and transmitter release and, hence, diminish excitatory postsynaptic potentials (SOMJEN and GILL 1963; LØYNING et al. 1964; WEAKLY 1969). It has therefore been concluded that these barbiturates act mainly on the afferent terminals (but see also Sect. C.III.1).

Barbiturates probably exert an effect at presynaptic and postsynaptic sites. GROSSMANN et al. (1974d) observed that the (+)-isomer of 1-methyl-5-phenyl-5-

propyl barbituric acid (MPPB) increased the monosynaptic reflex in spinal rats while (−)-MPPB depressed it; (+)-MPPB lowered the membrane resistance and the firing level of cat motoneurons and increased the amplitude of the excitatory postsynaptic potential, while (−)-MPPB increased membrane resistance and firing level and reduced the amplitude of the monosynaptic excitatory postsynaptic potential. These authors concluded that the excitatory and depressant isomer of MPPB acted both pre- and postsynaptically (see also RICHARDS 1974) and that the two isomers produced opposite effects at one and the same membrane site. This agrees well with the observation made by DOWNES and WILLIAMS (1969) that depression of the monosynaptic reflex produced in the spinal cat by i.v. administration of pentobarbital was antagonized by i.v. injection of the convulsant barbiturate 5-(2-cyclohexylideneëthyl)-5-ethyl barbituric acid (CHEB). A postsynaptic site of action of barbiturates is suggested by the finding that pentobarbital progressively reduced the amplitude of the spike evoked in single neurons of the cat spinal trigeminal nucleus by orthodromic and antidromic stimulation (FROMM and KILLIAN 1967). In a study carried out with the microelectrode technique on mouse spinal neurons growing in tissue culture, it was found that the (+)-isomer of pentobarbital predominantly produced excitatory effects, while the (−)-isomer was an inhibitory drug that was more effective in potentiating the effects of GABA than the excitatory isomer (HUANG and BARKER 1980).

In contrast to phenytoin, pentobarbital has little effect on the post-tetanic potentiation of monosynaptic reflex activity (ESPLIN 1963). On the other hand, pentobarbital prolonged the synaptic recovery of the reflex like trimethadione (ESPLIN 1963).

2. Facilitation of Presynaptic Inhibition

Depressant barbiturates including pentobarbital and phenobarbital facilitate presynaptic inhibition like GABA, the transmitter mediating this type of inhibition in the spinal cord (ECCLES et al. 1963; ECCLES 1965; SCHMIDT 1963, 1964; MIYAHARA et al. 1966; NICOLL 1975b). NICOLL (1975b) assumes that the primary afferent depolarization produced by pentobarbital should reduce the amount of (excitatory) transmitter released at the first synapse of the reflex pathway.

3. Reflex Activity in Long Loops and Influence on the Brain Stem Reticular Formation

Electrical stimulation of peripheral nerves carried out in anesthetized cats with an intact neuraxis produce a reflex discharge with a relatively short latency and sometimes a second reflex discharge with a remarkably longer latency. The first or early reflex is based on events in segmental-spinal paths, while the second or late reflex discharge is brought about by activity in so-called long loops, i.e., that which ascends to the brain stem and, after having been relayed there, descends to spinal neurons. Phenobarbital (10–40 mg/kg i.v.) was equally potent in reducing both spinal and long-loop reflexes (SCHLOSSER et al. 1975a, b); phenytoin (10–40 mg/kg i.v.) predominantly depressed the spinal reflex, while diazepam (0.01–1.4 mg/kg) markedly depressed the long-loop reflex but was considerably less effective on the spinal reflexes.

Cutting the brain of cats at the intercollicular level results in rigidity and enhancement of stretch reflexes due to an increased excitatory impulse flow from the brain stem reticular formation causing hyperactivity of the spinal γ-motoneurons. These changes in spinal motor activity were depressed by pentobarbital (CHIN and SMITH 1962; SCHALLEK et al. 1964). It seems that barbiturates exclusively depress excitatory influences on spinal reflexes from the brain stem reticular formation, while inhibitory influences remain unaffected by the barbiturates (BROOKS et al. 1956; MANDELL and BACH 1957).

4. Seizure Activity

In decapitated animals (cat, rabbit, hamster, mouse), electrical stimulation of the spinal cord resulted in motor convulsions of the hindlimbs which were similar to those seen in electroconvulsions produced in intact animals (ESPLIN and FRESTON 1960). Phenobarbital had only a weak effect in a dose (8 mg/kg) which suppressed convulsions in the intact animal, while pentobarbital (8 mg/kg) markedly depressed the spinal seizure activity.

LOTHMAN and SOMJEN (1976) noted that i.v. injections of phenobarbital (10 mg/kg), pentobarbital (20–30 mg/kg), and thiamylal (2 mg/kg) suppressed the seizure activity which appeared after local or systemic administration of penicillin in the recordings from the spinal cord in decapitated cats.

V. Brain

1. Neuron Activity and Synaptic Transmission

Various barbiturates depressed the spontaneous activity of cortical neurons in the intact brain (HERZ and FUSTER 1964) and the *cerveau isolé* (CRAWFORD 1970) of cats and reduced the activity evoked by microiontophoretic administration of the excitatory substances acetylcholine and DL-homocysteic acid in the *cerveau isolé* preparation (CRAWFORD 1970).

In neurons of the rabbit olfactory bulb, pentobarbital in relatively high doses (40–70 mg/kg i.v.) depressed the synaptic excitatory potentials evoked by lateral olfactory tract (LOT) stimulation (NICOLL 1972); antidromic activation of these neurons was only slightly less sensitive or, in other words, pentobarbital acted pre- and postsynaptically. Postsynaptic inhibition was prolonged by pentobarbital and hexobarbital (NICOLL 1972), and this prolongation was not enhanced by aminooxyacetic acid, an inhibitor of GABA metabolism. Prolongation of the inhibitory postsynaptic potential was also observed by NICOLL et al. (1975) in cat hippocampal neurons after pentobarbital. In slices prepared from the guinea pig olfactory cortex containing the LOT, stimulation of this bundle produced a summed action potential in the activated afferent fibers of the LOT as well as a monosynaptic and a polysynaptic response in the cortex; pentobarbital consistently depressed the synaptic transmission while the summed action potential was relatively resistant to the action of the drug (RICHARDS 1972; SCHOLFIELD and HARVEY 1975; SCHOLFIELD 1977), indicating that the barbiturate mainly acted presynaptically.

In agreement with observations made in peripheral nerves (see Sect. C.III.1), phenobarbital was found to inhibit the calcium influx into synaptosomes of the rabbit neocortex which was produced by depolarizing potassium concentrations in the suspension medium (SOHN and FERRENDELLI 1976).

2. Afterdischarges

Afterdischarges as a sign set up by neurons to signal imminent seizure activity were depressed by phenobarbital when they were evoked from the thalamus and rhinencephalon of the rabbit (GANGLOFF and MONNIER 1957). Intraperitoneal injections of phenobarbital (7.5, 15, und 30 mg/kg) also depressed the afterdischarges evoked in the rat cortex by electrical stimulation of the hippocampus (ALBERTSON et al. 1977); it was more effective than diazepam (1.4–15 mg/kg). The threshold for eliciting afterdischarges in the thalamus of cats and rats was raised by systemic administration of phenobarbital, 5–40 mg/kg (ITO et al. 1977). It was raised in the cat caudate nucleus, septum, amygdala, and septum by phenobarbital, 10 mg/kg i.v. (SCHALLEK and KUEHN 1965; SCHALLEK et al. 1964).

Epileptiform afterdischarges evoked by repetitive electrical stimulation of chronically isolated slabs of the cat cortex were shortened by a low dose of 5 mg/kg phenobarbital i.p.; they were not affected by a hypnotic dose of pentobarbital (5 mg/kg i.p.). This model seems to be able to distinguish between the actions of anticonvulsant and hypnotic barbiturates.

3. Focal Seizure Activity

The results concerning the effect of barbiturates on focal epileptiform activity in the cortex are controversial. Phenobarbital (5–15 mg/kg) increased the frequency and duration of spike discharges from a cobalt-induced focus in the rat cortex and also produced bilateral bursts of discharges in control animals after oral administration (DOW et al. 1973). Likewise, enhancement by phenobarbital (5–40 mg/kg i.v.) of spike discharges was observed in foci produced by freezing of the visual cortex (HORI et al. 1979).

EDMONDS et al. (1974) observed no significant effect of phenobarbital (15 and 30 mg/kg orally) on the spike discharge from a penicillin-induced focus in the rat cortex. MORRELL et al. (1959), on the other hand, noted that phenobarbital, 50 mg/kg i.p., slightly suppressed the activity in the primary focus produced by freezing of the visual cortex of the rabbit, and markedly depressed the spread of seizure activity to the basal diencephalon. VASTOLA and ROSEN (1960) observed a clear depression by 4 mg/kg i.v. phenobarbital (and phenytoin) on focal activity evoked in the visual cortex of the decerebrate cat by electrical stimulation.

STRASBERG et al. (1967) reported that focal epileptiform activity produced by local freezing in the cat developed only in the awake animal, not under pentobarbital or ether anesthesia. Intravenous injection of GABA depressed the focal epileptiform activity; radiolabeled GABA administered by i.v. injection passed rapidly from the blood into the brain at the site of the freezing lesion.

In experiments performed on epileptiform activity produced by local administration of penicillin to the rat cortex, MAREŠ et al. (1977) found that three subsequent i.p. injections of pentobarbital (5, 15, and 40 mg/kg) increased the intervals between seizure bursts in the primary as well as in the mirror focus. The shape of the primary and the projected focal discharges after administration of pentobarbital and local application of GABA to the mirror focus were similar.

ROLDÁN et al. (1971) noted that allobarbital or thiopental (10–20 mg/kg) markedly reduced the incidence of the motor manifestations induced by chronic cobalt implantation into the rat hippocampus and/or thalamic nuclei.

Kindled seizure activity recorded from the hippocampus or sensory cortex in response to repeated stimulation of the rat hippocampus were not suppressed by phenobarbital 30 mg/kg; however, when the same dose was given before kindling, it prevented the appearance of seizure activity (ALBERTSON et al. 1978). Phenobarbital (15, 30, and 60 mg/kg i.p.) and, more effectively, pentobarbital (3.75, 7.5, and 15 mg/kg i.p.) reduced the duration of the seizure discharges in the cortex and amygdala, and attenuated the motor manifestations of kindled amygdaloid seizures in rats (ALBERTSON et al. 1980); diazepam and clonazepam were also very effective in this model, while phenytoin and other anticonvulsants (oxazolidines, ethosuximide, and valproic acid) exerted only very weak effects. Phenobarbital, diazepam, and the GABA transaminase inhibitor ethanolamine-*o*-sulfate prevented the motor manifestation of kindling induced by electrical stimulation of the frontal cortex in rats without suppressing the clonus evoked by nonkindling stimulation (GOFF et al. 1978); folic acid in subconvulsive doses facilitated the kindling response.

VI. Summary

The anticonvulsant action of phenobarbital may be ascribed primarily to a reduction of membrane excitability. In contrast to phenytoin, it does not selectively affect hyperexcitability of neurons but depresses normal excitatory synaptic transmission. Facilitation of GABA-mediated transmission will also contribute to the depression of the spread of excitation along neuron paths. In general, the anesthetic pentobarbital is more potent than the anticonvulsant phenobarbital, and there are only very few examples where phenobarbital is more effective than pentobarbital. Thus, it is not possible to demonstrate the specific action on neuronal membranes (or neuron populations) which makes a barbiturate more an anticonvulsant than a hypnotic-anesthetic agent.

D. Carbamazepine

I. Nerve Fibers

In voltage-clamp experiments performed on *Myxicola* giant axons, SCHAUF et al. (1974) found that carbamazepine (from 2.5×10^{-4} to $10^{-3} M$) dose dependently and reversibly reduced the sodium and potassium conductances. The reduction of the sodium conductance was slightly more marked than that of the potassium conductance. The leakage current for hyperpolarizing voltage steps was reduced by the drug, and the membrane was reversibly depolarized. It must be noted that the concentrations used in this preparation were relatively high compared with therapeutic plasma levels (23.6 μg/ml in contrast to about 10 μg/ml).

HONDA and ALLEN (1973) noted that carbamazepine increased the threshold of the frog sciatic nerve, reduced conduction velocity and amplitude of compound action potentials (especially Aδ fibers), and prevented hyperexcitability following high-frequency stimulation or reduced calcium concentration. JULIAN and HOLLISTER (1975), however, did not observe significant changes in excitability and conduction velocity of myelinated or nonmyelinated sciatic nerve fibers after administration of carbamazepine (2.1×10^{-5} to $8.5 \times 10^{-5} M$). In the rabbit sciatic nerve, KRUPP (1969) observed a reduction in amplitude and an increase in latency and duration of action potentials after i.v. administration of carbamazepine 20 mg/kg, the same result was obtained with phenytoin.

Carbamazepine, 300 mg/kg i.p., inhibited repetitive afterdischarges caused by high-frequency (tetanic) stimulation of the cat sural nerve in situ without changing conduction velocity or the capacity of the nerve fibers to follow high-frequency stimulation (HERSHKOWITZ et al. 1978). Likewise, carbamazepine (9–45 µg/ml plasma) produced a concentration-dependent depression of repetitive discharge (post stretch, tonic stretch, spontaneous) from deefferented muscle spindles of spinal and chloralose-anesthetized cats (HERSHKOWITZ and RAINES 1978).

II. Synaptic Transmission

1. Neuromuscular Junctions

At the frog neuromuscular junction, carbamazepine decreased the quantal content of transmitter released and reduced the amplitude of the end-plate potential more than the amplitude of the miniature end-plate potential (ALDERDICE and TROMMER 1980). The drug depressed the post-tetanic potentiation of muscle contraction in the in vivo neuromuscular preparation of the cat soleus; the depression was proportional to the plasma concentration of carbamazepine (HERSHKOWITZ et al. 1978). Contractions elicited by single stimuli were not influenced by the drug.

2. Spinal Cord

Carbamazepine depressed polysynaptic reflexes in spinal cats in doses (10–30 mg/kg i.v.) which did not reduce the amplitude of monosynaptic reflex responses; moreover, carbamazepine reduced the post-tetanic potentiation of the monosynaptic reflex as did phenytoin (KRUPP 1969). Similar results were obtained by THEOBALD and co-workers (THEOBALD and KUNZ 1963; THEOBALD et al. 1970), who noted that carbamazepine (32 mg/kg i.v.) reduced polysynaptic reflexes in spinal and anesthetized cats and slightly enhanced monosynaptic reflexes. The drug reduced post-tetanic potentiation of monosynaptic reflex activity in a dose (10 mg/kg i.v.) which did not change the monosynaptic reflex amplitude. JULIEN and HOLLISTER (1975) failed to produce depression of post-tetanic potentiation in spinal nonanesthetized cats when administering 10 mg/kg, while doses of 30–40 mg/kg markedly depressed post-tetanic potentiation.

3. Spinal Trigeminal Nucleus

In awake cats with chronic electrodes implanted in the spinal trigeminal nucleus and in the center median of the thalamus, HERNÁNDEZ-PEÓN (1965) observed that carbamazepine (15 mg/kg) produced a partial but significant depression of the response evoked in the trigeminal nucleus by stimulation of the infraorbital nerve. The evoked potentials recorded from the center median were almost completely or totally abolished by the drug.

Recordings made from single neurons of the cat spinal trigeminal nucleus revealed that carbamazepine in very low doses (4 to 6 mg/kg i.v.) increased the latency and reduced the number of impulse discharges in response to electrical stimulation of the afferent maxillary nerve, while the response to antidromic stimulation remained unchanged (FROMM and KILLIAN 1967; FROMM 1969). Phenytoin (3 mg/kg i.v.) exerted an identical effect. When the response of trigeminal neurons was inhibited by conditioning stimulation of the maxillary nerve (to which also the test stimulus was applied), carbamazepine (5–20 mg/kg i.v.) and phenytoin (5–20 mg/kg i.v.) increased the inhibition (FROMM et al. 1981 a). Carbamazepine and phenytoin had no effect on the inhibition produced by stimulation in the periaqueductal gray matter (FROMM et al. 1981 b).

The depression of impulse transmission in the trigeminal nucleus is assumed to be the cause for the beneficial effect of both carbamazepine and phenytoin in the trigeminal neuralgia.

III. Brain

1. Evoked Responses and Afterdischarges

Carbamazepine (10–15 mg/kg i.p.) depressed or abolished the afterdischarges evoked by electrical stimulation in the nucleus amygdala and hippocampus of cats, and limited the propagation of this hyperactivity to the hypothalamus (HERNÁNDEZ-PEÓN 1964). The threshold of afterdischarges in parts of the limbic system of unanesthetized cats was markedly increased by carbamazepine (5–10 mg/kg); the elevation of the threshold by carbamazepine in the corticothalamic system was less marked and no effect was exerted by the drug on the afterdischarge threshold in the lenticular nucleus (KOBAYASHI et al. 1967).

HOLM et al. (1970) observed in the *encéphale isolé* preparation of the cat (i.e., in the brain transected at the upper cervical segment) that carbamazepine (20 mg/kg) raised the threshold of evoked responses in reticulothalamic projections, in efferent projections from the center median and ventroanterior nucleus of the thalamus, and in efferent connections of the hippocampus; carbamazepine, 60 mg/kg and above, raised the threshold of several responses to stimulation of the brain stem reticular formation, and evoked responses in efferent amygdaloid projections were inhibited at a dose of 120 mg/kg. DOLCE (1969) observed that carbamazepine (5–10 mg/kg i.v.) did not influence the evoked responses in reticulocortical and thalamocortical projections (arousal and recruitment); however, the afterdischarges evoked in the hippocampus and neocortex by electrical stimulation in the amygdala pars basolateralis was effectively blocked.

Carbamazepine (10 mg/kg) increased the threshold and reduced the duration of afterdischarges evoked by electrical cortical stimulation in the cat (JULIEN and HOLLISTER 1975).

2. Focal Seizure Activity

DOLCE (1969) noted that chronic administration of carbamazepine (2 × 30 mg/day for 1 week) did not depress focal cortical seizure activity induced by chronic epileptogenic lesions with aluminum oxide gel applied to the nucleus amygdala.

DAVID and GREWAL (1976) produced focal cortical seizure activity in rhesus monkeys by implanting alumina gel in the sensorimotor cortex of hippocampus and observed that carbamazepine (10 mg/kg i.m.) reduced intracortical spike propagation. The aggressivity and other behavioral manifestations in monkeys with hippocampal foci were markedly reduced by carbamazepine.

JULIEN and HOLLISTER (1975) reported that the drug (5 mg/kg i.p.) reduced or abolished focal cortical seizure activity evoked by applying penicillin to the cat cortex.

IV. Summary

Carbamazepine depresses post-tetanic potentiation as does phenytoin. This effect may largely account for the usefulness of the drug in the treatment of grand mal epilepsy, and focal and psychomotor seizures. Very likely, the effect of carbamazepine on the limbic system also contributes to the anticonvulsant action of the drug.

E. Valproic Acid

I. Ganglia and Spinal Cord Neurons

Valproic acid (5–30 m*M*) produced a dose-dependent hyperpolarization of *Aplysia* neurons which was associated with an increased potassium conductance (SLATER and JOHNSTON 1978). MACDONALD and BERGEY (1979) noted that microiontophoretic application of valproic acid to neurons of the mouse spinal cord grown in cell culture dose-dependently enhanced the membrane responses (hyperpolarization, increase in conductance) following microiontophoretically applied GABA, whereas the effect of glycine or glutamate was not influenced. Valproic acid was ineffective when applied alone and directly to neuron somata. These authors conclude that valproic acid (like barbiturates or benzodiazepine derivatives) acts on a "modulator site" in the GABA receptor complex and thereby increases either the affinity of the receptor for GABA or the unitary GABA-coupled chloride conductance.

GABA-induced depolarization of dorsal root ganglion cells of the cat, which are devoid of synapses, was increased by phenobarbital but not by valproic acid (GALLAGHER et al. 1981). This finding suggests that valproic acid is effective only at the GABA receptor sites in the synaptic region where this inhibitory transmitter is released.

II. Brain

1. Spontaneous Activity of Single Neurons

In two reports, microiontophoretically applied valproic acid has been described to produce either a slight excitatory effect on neurons in the cerebral cortex (SCHMUTZ et al. 1979) or even a marked enhancement of the activity of cortical and hippocampal neurons (BLUME et al. 1979) of the rat. In view of the anticonvulsant property of valproic acid, its interaction with GABA is of particular interest.

SCHMUTZ et al. (1979) and KERWIN et al. (1980) observed that microiontophoretical application of valproic acid to neurons in the rat neocortex increased and prolonged the inhibitory effect of microiontophoretically applied GABA, while the inhibitory effect of glycine was not changed. Intraperitoneal injection of valproic acid (100–400 mg/kg) dose-dependently depressed the spontaneous activity of neocortical neurons, the time course of this effect being similar to that of the anticonvulsant effect of the drug in electroseizures. However, the synaptic (presumably GABA-mediated) inhibition of neurons in the substantia nigra or Deiter's nucleus of the rat was generally not affected by systemic or local application of valproic acid. BALDINO and GELLER (1981) also report that valproic acid enhanced GABA-induced inhibition of neurons in the rat cerebral cortex without influencing glycine-induced inhibition. The effect of combined microiontophoretic application of valproic acid and GABA was abolished by bicuculline.

In similar experiments using microiontophoretic drug application to neurons in the rat brain stem, GENT and PHILLIPS (1980) found that valproic acid enhanced the inhibitory effect of GABA and the GABA agonist muscimol but did not affect glycine-induced inhibition or glutamate-induced excitation. The effect of microiontophoretically applied GABA or muscimol was also enhanced by intravenous injections of valproic acid, 200 and 400 mg/kg. These authors assume that valproic acid acts on the GABA receptor complex.

When the response to maxillary nerve stimulation of single neurons in the spinal trigeminal nucleus of the cat was inhibited by conditioning stimulation in the periaqueductal gray matter, valproic acid reduced the inhibition as was signalled by a decrease in the latency of the response (FROMM et al. 1981 b). It should be borne in mind, however, that stimulation in the periaqueductal gray matter produces morphine-like depression of nociceptive activity, and that 5-hydroxytryptamine rather than GABA plays an important role in this type of inhibition (BESSON et al. 1978).

2. Evoked Responses and Afterdischarges

VOSKUYL et al. (1975) recorded field potentials evoked in the piriform cortex by electrical stimulation of the lateral olfactory tract in slices prepared from the guinea pig brain. Valproic acid (6×10^{-3} to $1.2 \times 10^{-2} M$) slightly depressed excitatory synaptic transmission and prevented the appearance of penicillin-induced spikes.

Valproic acid (200 mg/kg i.p.) suppressed afterdischarges in the hippocampus of the cat evoked by electrical stimulation of this brain area (MUTANI et al. 1968). The drug (400 and 600 mg/kg orally) significantly decreased the duration of afterdischarges in the rat amygdala and elevated the threshold (SALT et al. 1980). Valproic acid (40–160 mg/kg) also raised the threshold of thalamic afterdischarges induced by electrical stimulation of the cat nucleus centralis lateralis and the rat nucleus reticularis without changing the duration of the afterdischarges in both species (ITO et al. 1977).

3. Focal Seizures and Kindling

Valproic acid (200 mg/kg i.p.) suppressed the epileptogenic activity generated by a cobalt focus in the cat hippocampus (MUTANI et al. 1968); it blocked the spreading of spontaneous as well as electrically induced seizure discharges from the hippocampus to the neocortex. MUTANI and FARIELLO (1969) noted that valproic acid (200 mg/kg i.p.) suppressed the ictal and interictal seizure discharges in cats with an epileptogenic cobalt focus in the cruciate cortex. After administration of the drug, electrical stimulation of the cobalt focus failed to produce seizure activity. The same authors (FARIELLO and MUTANI 1970) observed that subcortical injection of aluminum gel into the sensorimotor cortex of cats produced focal cortical seizure discharges and myoclonic jerks of the head. This focal seizure activity could generalize, and valproic acid prevented this secondary generalization without influencing the epileptogenic focus. Also VAN DUJN and BECKMANN (1975) noted that valproic acid (200 mg/kg s.c.) did not decrease the focal discharge in the sensorimotor cortex of the awake cat produced by topical cobalt administration, but effectively inhibited the spread of seizure activity from the focus; protection against seizure spread was about the same as after administration of phenobarbital (30 mg/kg s.c.) and somewhat less than after administration of diazepam (2 mg/kg s.c.).

ELAZAR and GOTTESFELD (1975) found that aminooxyacetic acid (20 and 30 mg/kg) and valproic acid (200 and 400 mg/kg) produced a significant increase of the GABA level in the vicinity of a penicillin-induced cortical focus in rats, but did not prevent the fall in GABA concentration in the focus or reduce focal epileptogenic activity. Local administration of GABA to the focus, however, produced a short-lasting depression of seizure activity. The authors suppose that the increase in the GABA level produced by aminooxyacetic acid (AOAA) or valproic acid may be insufficient to overcome the effect of penicillin.

Forelimb clonus and full convulsions kindled by repeated stimulation of the rat amygdala were reduced by valproic acid (400 and 600 mg/kg orally) (SALT et al. 1980); the drug was found to have a depressant effect on a kindled epileptogenic focus and a prophylactic effect on the development of kindled seizures. However, ALBERTSON et al. (1980) think that valproic acid has only a poor effect on kindled amygdaloid seizures in rats.

III. Summary

At present, the most plausible explanation for the anticonvulsant action of valproic acid is a facilitation of GABA-ergic inhibition in the central nervous system. Thus, the drug acts like the benzodiazepines. Its indications in the treatment of the epilepsies overlap with those of the benzodiazepine derivatives, but it is well known that there are fundamental differences in the actions of both groups of substances which need consideration.

F. Oxazolidinediones

I. Nerve Fibers and Ganglia

Trimethadione at concentrations of up to $10^{-2} M$ had no effect on impulse conduction and hyperexcitability produced in the isolated frog sciatic nerve by supramaximal and frequent electrical stimulation; nor did it reduce calcium concentration in the suspension medium (TOMAN 1952). In *Helix aspersa* neurons it increased the membrane potential, reduced the rate of pentylenetetrazol-induced burst-like discharges, and prevented bursts elicited by depolarizing currents (FAUGIER-GRIMAUD 1978).

II. Spinal Cord

Trimethadione (400 mg/kg i.v.) did not affect monosynaptic reflex activity and its post-tetanic potentiation, but slightly depressed polysynaptic reflexes (GOODMAN et al. 1946b; ESPLIN and CURTO 1957; ESPLIN 1963). In anesthetized cats, trimethadione (200 mg/kg) reduced the spontaneous activity of spinal interneurons as well as the activation of the interneurons by electrical stimulation of the dorsal roots, ipsi- and contralateral motor cortex, and various parts of the reticular formation (ARUSHANYAN et al. 1967).

The most conspicuous effect of trimethadione on spinal reflex activity is the increase by the drug (400 mg/kg i.v.) of the time of synaptic recovery of monosynaptic reflexes determined by testing with two supramaximal stimuli delivered at varying intervals (ESPLIN and CURTO 1957; ESPLIN 1963; ESPLIN and ZABLOCKA 1969), and this effect is antagonized by pentylenetetrazol (ESPLIN and CURTO 1957). It is in agreement with this result that ARUSHANYAN et al. observed that trimethadione (200 mg/kg i.v.) markedly reduced the number of monosynaptic responses of single spinal motoneurons of the cat to high-frequency stimulation of primary afferents and, moreover, prolonged the duration of afterhyperpolarization. Prolongation of synaptic recovery will also be the reason why trimethadione depresses polysynaptic reflex activity, because the drug will reduce the frequency of the impulse discharges from the interneurons in the polysynaptic reflex path. However, trimethadione at doses of 200–400 mg/kg i.v. has also been found to enhance presynaptic inhibition of a monosynaptic reflex in spinalized cats (MIYAHARA et al. 1966).

ESPLIN and FRESTON (1960) noted that continuous high-frequency stimulation of the cervival spinal cord in decapitated animals (cat, rabbit, hamster, mouse) produced a sequence of hindlimb movements identical to those seen in the maximal electroshock seizure in intact animals; at low stimulus frequencies either tonic flexion or phasic movements occur. Postictal depression, declining exponentially with time, was seen following spinal cord stimulation, and trimethadione (400 mg/kg i.v.) markedly prolonged spinal postictal depression.

III. Synaptic Transmission in the Spinal Trigeminal Nucleus

The latency of the response and number of impulses evoked by stimulation of the maxillary nerve in single spinal trigeminus nucleus neurons of the cat was reduced by low doses of trimethadione, whereas doses required to produce an anticonvulsant effect facilitated the response (FROMM and KILLIAN 1967). Inhibition by conditioning cortical stimulation of the trigeminal neuron response to maxillary nerve stimulation was reduced by the drug in doses of 10–40 mg/kg (FROMM and KOHLI 1972).

IV. Brain

1. Afterdischarges

In the unanesthetized rabbit, trimethadione in an exceptionally high dose (1.5–2.0 g/kg) raised the threshold and prolonged the cortical afterdischarges; it exerted a similar but weaker effect on afterdischarges in the rhinencephalon and elevated the threshold of thalamic afterdischarges without changing their duration (GANGLOFF and MONNIER 1957).

In acute and chronic experiments carried out on cats, trimethadione (120 mg/kg) lowered the threshold of afterdischarges in the ectosylvian cortex and produced only a weak reduction in the duration and spread of afterdischarges in the hippocampus, amygdala, and septum (STROBOS and SPUDIS 1960). SCHALLEK and KUEHN (1963) noted that the drug (100 mg/kg i.v.) elevated the threshold of afterdischarges evoked from the central lateral nucleus of the cat thalamus, while it did not exert an effect on the threshold of the dorsomedial thalamic nucleus, cortex, or hippocampus.

2. Focal Seizure Activity

Trimethadione (100 mg/kg i.p.) suppressed the primary epileptogenic focus produced by local freezing of the rabbit visual cortex and limited the spread of seizure activity to the basal diencephalon (MORRELL et al. 1959); transcortical spread was not effectively limited by the drug until the primary focus itself was suppressed. HORI et al. (1979) found that trimethadione (160 mg/kg i.v.) was ineffective in suppressing spike activity in the neighborhood of local freezing of the cat visual cortex and in limiting cortical spread. Administered at a lower dose (14 mg/kg i.v.), trimethadione failed to influence focal cortical seizure activity evoked in the visual cortex of intercollicularly decerebrate cats by electrical stimulation in the neighboring cortex (VASTOLA and ROSEN 1960). Trimethadione (400 mg/kg i.p.) depressed the cortical epileptogenic activity produced by cobalt implantation into the cortex of rats (CHIU et al. 1979).

Seizure activity elicited by electrical stimulation in isolated cerebral cortex slabs of the suprasylvian gyrus was not influenced by trimethadione or ethosuximide, while phenytoin reduced the duration of seizure discharges (KRIP and VAZQUEZ 1971).

Trimethadione (from 100 to 800 mg/kg i.p.) and paramethadione (from 50 to 200 mg/kg i.p.) showed only a weak effect in attenuating kindled amygdaloid seizures in rats (ALBERTSON et al. 1980).

V. Summary

Nearly all the studies presented here have made use of trimethadione instead of 5,5-dimethyl-2,4-oxazolidinedione (DMO), which is an active metabolite of the drug. One might feel safer in interpreting the results in terms of an anticonvulsant action if crucial experiments had also been carried out with DMO, but a comparison of the doses of trimethadione and DMO which provide protection against electroconvulsion in rats makes it unlikely that trimethadione is a pre-drug; the protective dose of trimethadione in rats is 500 mg/kg (GOODMAN et al. 1946c) while that of DMO is 610 mg/kg (WITHROW et al. 1968). WITHROW et al. (1968) and FREY (1969) also state that trimethadione is a better antagonist of pentylenetetrazol than DMO. Thus, trimethadione may be judged as an anticonvulsant agent of its own (but see also WITHROW 1980), and most likely its effect derives from the slowing of synaptic recovery. However, this particular action does not explain per se why oxazolidinediones are specifically effective in petit mal epilepsy. Predilective sites of action do not become apparent from studies on afterdischarges evoked in various brain areas or on focal seizure activity.

G. Succinimides

Remarkably few electrophysiological studies have been carried out on the succinimides (ethosuximide, methsuximide, phensuximide).

I. Synaptic Transmission

1. Neuromuscular Junction

At the frog neuromuscular junction, ethosuximide decreased the amplitudes of miniature end-plate potentials and end-plate potentials in a proportional manner, while it had no effect on the quantal content of transmitter released (ALDERDICE and TROMMER 1980). PINCUS (1977) noted that ethosuximide ($2 \times 10^{-4} M$) markedly increased the end-plate potential and quantal content at the partially curarized frog neuromuscular junction and in some instances abolished the effect of curare. In a medium with a low calcium concentration, the drug was ineffective. The author concluded that ethosuximide may augment transmitter release by increasing the influx of calcium ions into the presynaptic terminal.

2. Spinal Cord and Spinal Trigeminal Nucleus

CAPEK and ESPLIN (1973, 1977) observed in experiments performed on monosynaptic reflexes in spinal cats that the decline in reflex amplitude occurring during repetitive stimulation was enhanced by ethosuximide (200 and 400 mg/kg i.v.). They conclude that the decline is due to depletion of the excitatory transmitter released at the endings of primary afferent terminals and that ethosuximide enhances transmitter release, thereby intensifying depletion. But it is not clear why the first response evoked by a train of stimuli was not increased by drug-induced enhancement of transmitter release but, instead, remained unchanged.

Ethosuximide (10–25 mg/kg i.v.) reduced both the latency of the response of single neurons of the cat spinal trigeminal nucleus to maxillary nerve stimulation and inhibition by conditioning cortical stimulation of this response (FROMM and KOHLI 1972).

3. Brain

In unrestrained rats with chronically implanted recording electrodes in the visual and sensorimotor cortex, olfactory bulb, and hippocampus, photic stimulation produced afterdischarges which were reduced by i.p. injections of ethosuximide (from 50 mg/kg to 500 mg/kg), while the primary components of the evoked potentials were enhanced by the drug (KÄSTNER et al. 1968).

When paired electrical stimuli were delivered to the ventrolateral thalamus and the evoked responses were recorded from the ipsilateral sensorimotor cortex of cats, ethosuximide (40 mg/kg i.v. or more) did not change or increased the excitability (i.e., lowered the threshold) of the thalamic neurons at short stimulus intervals, while it reduced the excitability and raised the threshold at longer stimulus intervals (ENGLANDER et al. 1977).

II. Brain: Focal Seizure Activity

KÄSTNER et al. (1970) observed that epileptiform focal activity produced by cobalt implantation into the sensorimotor cortex of the rat is reduced by ethosuximide in doses higher than 200 mg/kg. Likewise, DOW et al. (1973) and CHIU et al. (1979) noted that ethosuximide (50–200 mg/kg) suppressed spike activity in cobalt-induced epileptogenic foci in the rat cortex.

Succinimides exerted only a weak depressant effect on kindled amygdaloid seizures in rats (ALBERTSON et al. 1980). Ethosuximide reduced burst activity in the electroencephalogram of penicillin-induced generalized convulsions in cats (GUBERMAN et al. 1975). Seizures evoked in domestic epileptic fowl by photic stimulation were not depressed by either acute or chronic administration of ethosuximide (DAVIS et al. 1978).

III. Summary

In view of the strikingly scarce information on the effects of the succinimides on single neurons and neuron populations, it is hard even to speculate on the mechanisms by which these drugs might produce their anticonvulsant action. Since succinimides are more effective against pentylenetetrazol convulsions than against maximal electroseizure, it has been proposed that they might act like the oxazolidinediones. There are some more resemblances in the effects of the two groups of drug on neuron responses (effectiveness on afterdischarges, ineffectiveness on amygdaloid kindling), but it must be admitted that the mode of action of the succinimides is less clear than that of the oxazolidinediones.

H. Benzodiazepines

I. Facilitation of GABAergic Transmission

Benzodiazepines bind to specific receptor sites (BRAESTRUP and SQUIRES 1977, 1978; MÖHLER and OKADA 1977, 1978) which are part of the gamma-aminobutyric acid (GABA) receptor-ionophore complex, to which also barbiturates and the convulsants picrotoxin and bicuculline bind (OLSEN et al. 1978, 1979; TICKU and OLSEN 1978; OLSEN 1981 a, b; IADAROLA and GALE 1981; OLSEN and LEEB-LUNDBERG 1981). GABA is the inhibitory transmitter mediating presynaptic inhibition by depolarization of primary afferents in the spinal cord, while in the brain it is one of the transmitters producing postsynaptic inhibition; glycine is the transmitter which mediates postsynaptic inhibition by hyperpolarization (for a short review on GABA and glycine as inhibitory transmitters see COSTA et al. 1975b). The GABA receptor is closely associated with the chloride ionophore, while the benzodiazepines seem to interact with a modulator protein which changes the recognition sites for GABA and thus enhances the effect of the inhibitory transmitter (COSTA and GUIDOTTI 1979). Barbiturates enhance the binding of diazepam to the benzodiazepine receptor site (LEEB-LUNDBERG et al. 1980). Bicuculline inhibits the binding of GABA to the receptor sites (ZUKIN et al. 1974). Picrotoxin blocks the chloride ionophore (TICKU and OLSEN 1977; OLSEN et al. 1979; OLSEN and LEEB-LUNDBERG 1981). Both agents antagonize the inhibitory effect of GABA and, by disinhibition, produce convulsions. The role of GABA in convulsive disorders is discussed by MELDRUM in Chap. 7, this volume, and in the review of STRAUGHAN (1974) and ROBERTS (1980). Although phenobarbital acts (like picrotoxin) at the chloride ionophore of the GABA receptor complex (TICKU 1980; for further literature see above), diazepam was about nine times more effective against picrotoxin convulsions (LÖSCHER and FREY 1977).

Reference to an involvement of the GABA receptor complex in the effect of benzodiazepines on neuronal membranes or neuron pools will be made in the following sections whenever information is available. Examples of facilitation of GABAergic transmission by benzodiazepines, barbiturates, and various other drugs are given in the reviews of HAEFELY et al. (1975, 1979). The effect of benzodiazepines on GABA uptake, synthesis, and metabolism are dealt with by JONES and WOODBURY in Chap. 10, this volume.

II. Excitable Membranes and Synaptic Transmission in the Periphery

CHEYMOL et al. (1967) observed that diazepam (3.5–10 mg/kg i.v.) increased the amplitude of muscle contraction of the tibialis anterior muscle evoked by electrical stimulation of the sciatic nerve in the rabbit; moreover, diazepam (4 mg/kg) enhanced the partial block produced by *d*-tubocurarine or gallamine triethiodide at the neuromuscular junction, antagonized a total gallamine-induced block, and did not change the effect of succinylcholine. HAMILTON (1967), on the other hand, noted that both diazepam (0.4 and 0.8 mg/kg) and chlordiazepoxide reduced the nonreflex contraction of the tibialis anterior muscle of the cat to stimulation of the sciatic nerve and, more effectively, the reflex contraction evoked by stimulation of the peroneal nerve. This author also carried out experiments on the isolated rat phrenic nerve-diaphragm preparation and found that the two compounds produced a dose-dependent inhibition of directly and indirectly elicited muscle contractions; diazepam was about five times more potent than chlordiazepoxide. HUDSON and WOLPERT (1970) did not observe an effect of i.v. diazepam (0.125–8 mg/kg) at the neuromuscular junction of the cat tibialis anterior muscle in vivo.

SURIA and COSTA (1975a, b) reported that diazepam ($10^{-6}M$), dibutyryl cyclic guanosinetriphosphate ($10^{-6}M$), and GABA ($10^{-4}M$) depolarized the preganglionic nerve terminals in bullfrog sympathetic ganglia without affecting the interganglionic nerve trunk membrane potential; the depolarization was blocked by picrotoxin. These authors assumed that diazepam might release GABA from glia cells. They also found that chlordiazepoxide (10^{-8} and $10^{-6}M$) dose-dependently reduced the post-tetanic potentiation of impulse transmission in the ganglion (SURIA and COSTA 1973). Since prostaglandins of the E series also reduced the post-tetanic potentiation (SURIA and COSTA 1974), it was suggested that diazepam might act by increasing the synthesis of the prostaglandins, an assumption that would have included an antagonism between benzodiazepines and corticosteroids or nonsteroidal antiinflammatory drugs. BOWERY and DRAY (1978) found that GABA and pentobarbital depolarized the superfused isolated superior ganglion of the rat; however, they failed to detect a depolarization after the administration of chlordiazepoxide and other benzodiazepines.

III. Spinal Cord

1. Reflex Activity

In intact chloralose-anesthetized cats, an i.v. injection of diazepam, 0.1 mg/kg, or chlordiazepoxide, 10 mg/kg, had no effect on the monosynaptic patellar reflex but reduced polysynaptic reflex activity (CRANKSHAW and RAPER 1970). Likewise, SCHLOSSER (1971) reported that diazepam (0.5–1.5 mg/kg i.v.) did not significantly affect monosynaptic reflex activity but depressed polysynaptic reflexes in the unanesthetized spinal cat. He also noted that diazepam had no effect on post-tetanic potentiation of the spinal monosynaptic reflex and recurrent inhibition (which is glycine mediated) but markedly enhanced the dorsal root reflex and presynaptic inhibition (see also Sect. H.IV.2); he arrived at the conclusion that enhancement of presynaptic inhibition may play an important role in the muscle-relaxing action of the drug.

SCHMIDT et al. (1967) noted that i.v. diazepam (from 0.05 to 1 mg/kg) depressed, but never abolished, monosynaptic and polysynaptic reflexes in the spinal cat. HUDSON and WOLPERT (1970) obtained a depression of the patellar reflex and the linguomandibular reflex by injecting diazepam (0.125–16 mg/kg) into cats. Moreover, these latter authors found that facilitation of the patellar reflex produced in the spinal cat by stimulation of the contralateral sciatic nerve was reduced by diazepam (0.125 mg/kg), while inhibition of the reflex by ipsilateral sciatic nerve stimulation (which is predominantly of the glycine-mediated postsynaptic type) was highly resistant to diazepam and yielded only at a very high dose (16 mg/kg). The depression by diazepam of the facilitation of the patellar reflex produced by stimulation of the contralateral sciatic nerve is in agreement with the observation that diazepam (0.025–0.2 mg/kg i.v.) in the midcollicular decerebrate cat (TSENG and WANG 1971 a), and diazepam (0.003 mg/kg i.v.), nitrazepam (0.00125 mg/kg i.v.), medazepam (0.125 mg/kg i.v.), and chlordiazepoxide (0.25 mg/kg i.v.) in chloralose-anesthetized rats (KAWASAKI and MATSUSHITA 1981) depressed the crossed extensor reflex. KAWASAKI and MATSUSHITA (1981) were able to antagonize the depressant effects of the benzodiazepines with bicuculline and proposed that the effect of benzodiazepines is mediated by GABA.

2. Presynaptic Inhibition

In spinal cats, diazepam (0.05–1 mg/kg i.v.) increased and prolonged the presynaptic inhibition of a monosynaptic reflex response (SCHMIDT et al. 1967; SCHMIDT 1971). The changes in presynaptic inhibition were also reflected by an increase and prolongation of the dorsal root potentials (DRPs) (see also CHIN et al. 1974); diazepam had no effect on the intensity and duration of postsynaptic inhibition (SCHMIDT et al. 1967). STRATTEN and BARNES (1971) found that inhibitory influences exerted by diazepam (0.05–2.0 mg/kg) at the spinal level of cats were directly related to primary afferent depolarization (PAD), which is the expression of presynaptic inhibition, and that picrotoxin and diazepam seem to act as antagonists at the same site at which PAD is brought about. They conclude that the only effect of diazepam at the spinal level is enhancement of presynaptic inhibition.

POLC et al. (1974) described that diazepam (1 mg/kg i.v.) markedly depressed monosynaptic and polysynaptic reflexes in the spinal cat, increased DRPs in amplitude and duration, and enhanced presynaptic inhibition of a monosynaptic reflex. They also found that thiosemicarbazide (which inhibits GABA synthesis) and bicuculline reduced presynaptic inhibition, DRPs, and the effect of diazepam on both. When diazepam was administered after AOAA, its effect on presynaptic inhibition was considerably enhanced. POLC et al. (1974) conclude that normal levels of GABA are a prerequisite for the facilitation by benzodiazepines of presynaptic inhibition. In a study that was conducted at the same time, BANNA et al. (1974) observed that pretreatment of spinal unanesthetized cats with semicarbazide completely blocked the enhancement by diazepam (1–4 mg/kg) of segmental dorsal root reflexes (which are due to PAD), and that pyridoxine hydrochloride restored the effect of diazepam; they also proposed that a link exists between diazepam and GABA.

In cats anesthetized with pentobarbital, diazepam in cumulative doses enhanced DRPs but did not significantly diminish the strychnine-induced reduction of glycine-mediated postsynaptic inhibition (CURTIS et al. 1976); this latter result indicated that diazepam did not interfere with glycine receptors in the mammalian spinal cord.

In a recent investigation, POLC et al. (1981) observed that the benzodiazepine antagonist Ro 15-1788 did not produce any of the effects evoked by benzodiazepines in the cat spinal cord but antagonized all benzodiazepine effects; however, it failed to reduce the effects of phenobarbital which were similar to those produced by benzodiazepines.

In spinal neurons of the mouse grown in dissociate cell culture, microiontophoretic administration of diazepam and chlordiazepoxide enhanced GABA-mediated postsynaptic inhibition like phenobarbital (MACDONALD and BARKER 1979a). Unlike phenobarbital, the benzodiazepines did not antagonize glutamate-mediated postsynaptic excitation.

In cells dissociated from embryonic chick spinal cords, pressure microinjection of chlordiazepoxide enhanced the GABA-induced increase in membrane conductance and synaptic potentials which were probably mediated by GABA (CHOI et al. 1977). These results were interpreted in terms of an association of benzodiazepines with GABAergic inhibition.

3. Supraspinal Influences

Some authors favor the view that the benzodiazepines exert little or no effect at the spinal level, and that reflex depression produced by these drugs is due to a depressant effect on the facilitatory system of the brain stem reticular formation (NGAI et al. 1966; PRZYBYLA and WANG 1968; NAKANISHI and NORRIS 1971; TSENG and WANG 1971 b).

GHELARDUCCI et al. (1966) noted that nitrazepam did not affect monosynaptic reflexes in unanesthetized unrestrained cats, or in decerebrate and spinal cats; it reduced the rigidity resulting from hyperactivity of the γ-motor system while sparing the rigidity due to hyperactivity of the α-motor system. It was therefore concluded that nitrazepam acts only on that part of the brain stem reticular formation which facilitates γ-motor activity.

Depression by diazepam (0.125 mg/kg i.v.) of the γ-type of rigidity in the intercollicular decerebrate cat was also reported by HUDSON and WOLPERT (1970). In addition, these authors observed that diazepam reduced the facilitation and, somewhat less effectively, inhibition of the patellar reflex and the linguo-mandibular reflex produced by stimulation of the brain stem reticular formation. Depression of decerebrate rigidity in the cat was also produced by various other benzodiazepines, including chlordiazepoxide (SCHALLEK et al. 1964).

In the chloralose-anesthetized rat and cat, electrical stimulation of cutaneous afferents evoked an early segmental-spinal reflex, a later spinal reflex which is mediated by long loops via the brain stem (see Sect. C.IV.3), and in the preganglionic splanchnic nerve also a short-latency and long-latency reflex component. Diazepam (0.1–1.4 mg/kg i.v.) markedly depressed the late reflex responses while the purely spinal reflex activity was much less affected by the drug (SCHLOSSER et al. 1975 a, b).

MENÉTREY et al. (1973) observed that "spontaneous" dorsal root potentials (DRPs) evoked by supraspinal activity bursts were reduced by i.v. diazepam (0.5–1 mg/kg), while segmental-spinal DRPs were enhanced by the drug. The authors conclude that diazepam exerts an effect at the spinal level leading to an enhanced presynaptic inhibition and an effect at the supraspinal level which reduces presynaptic inhibition operated from the brain.

IV. Brain

1. Neuron Activity

When recording with microelectrodes from neurons in the rat brain stem, DRAY and STRAUGHAN (1976) observed that chlordiazepoxide and flurazepam applied by microiontophoresis reduced spontaneous impulse discharges in a dose-dependent manner. Both drugs acted like GABA or glycine but were only half as potent as the inhibitory amino acids. They observed no selective interaction between the benzodiazepines and the two amino acids. Since, however, the depressant effect of flurazepam was never selectively modified by strychnine but consistently reduced by bicuculline, the authors assume that benzodiazepines interfere with GABA rather than glycine-mediated processes.

In unanesthetized unrestrained rats, chlordiazepoxide (5–40 mg/kg) and diazepam (5–20 mg/kg) reduced spontaneous activity in neurons of the hippocampus, preoptic area, and midbrain tegmentum (OLDS and OLDS 1969). POLC et al. (1981) noted that the benzodiazepine antagonist Ro 15-1788 diminished the depression produced by benzodiazepines on the spontaneous activity of neurons in the substantia nigra pars compacta, nucleus raphé dorsalis, locus ceruleus, and hippocampus without exerting an effect of its own or reducing the depressant effect of pentobarbital on these neurons.

2. Cerebellar Inhibition

The cerebellum has been ascribed an important role in the control of seizure activity, and part of the anticonvulsant action of phenytoin may result from an activation of inhibitory influences from the cerebellum (see Sect. B.III.3). Since benzodiazepines apparently act by facilitating GABAergic inhibition, it was conceivable that these compounds might also turn on cerebellar inhibition and thus reduce convulsive activity.

JULIEN (1972) observed in awake, immobilized cats that diazepam (1 and 2 mg/kg i.v.) markedly increased the discharge of cerebellar Purkinje cells. In cats with a penicillin-induced epileptogenic focus in the sensorimotor cortex, diazepam depressed epileptiform activity with a concomitant increase of Purkinje-cell discharge. Thus, diazepam would exert effects similar to those of phenytoin. However, JULIEN'S observation has not remained unquestioned, because HAEFELY et al. (1975) and PIERI and HAEFELY (1976) found that diazepam and clonazepam reduced the impulse discharge of cerebellar Purkinje cells in cats and rats. Such an effect had to be expected if benzodiazepines facilitated GABAergic inhibition in all parts of the central nervous system, including that mediating inhibition of the cerebellar Purkinje cells (COSTA et al. 1975a). The reduced activity of cerebellar Purkinje cells will entail a decreased release of GABA from the terminals of their axons (OBATA et al. 1967, 1970; OBATA and TAKEDA 1969; TEN BRUGGENCATE and ENGBERG 1971), which in all likelihood cannot be compensated for by a facilitatory action of benzodiazepines at these inhibitory synapses in the brain stem. Thus, the cerebellum does not seem to be important for the depression by these drugs of seizure activity. RAINES and ANDERSON (1976) noted that pentylenetetrazol produces clonic convulsions after cerebellectomy in the rat (see also KOPELOFF and ALEXANDER 1972), and that diazepam suppressed the convulsions in the absence of the cerebellum.

3. Evoked Responses and Afterdischarges

a) Cortex

OSTROVSKAYA et al. (1975) observed that diazepam (1 mg/kg) slowed the recovery cycle of cortical neurons determined in rats by direct cortical stimulation with the double-shock technique. The effect of diazepam was enhanced by pretreatment with thiosemicarbazide and antagonized by bicuculline. These results were considered to indicate that diazepam enhanced an inhibitory process mediated by GABA. Also in the cat cerebral cortex, diazepam (1 mg/kg) prolonged the recovery cycle by increasing postexcitatory inhibition following direct cortical stimulation and stimulation of peripheral nerves (ZAKUSOV et al. 1975). Similarly, RAABE and GUMNIT (1977) found that diazepam increased the postsynaptic inhibition in cat pyramidal tract cells. SCHALLEK et al. (1965) depressed the spontaneous activity of cortical neurons as well as the activity evoked by stimulation of the sciatic nerve when nitrazepam, 10 mg/kg, was injected i.v. in to cats; diazepam (10 mg/kg) reduced the spontaneous but not the evoked activity. Chlordiazepoxide (10 and 40 mg/kg) was ineffective on the threshold of cortical afterdischarges (SCHALLEK et al. 1964), while diazepam (5–10 mg/kg) has been reported to depress or abolish afterdischarges from the precruciate motor cortex in cats (HERNÁNDEZ-PEÓN et al. 1964). Responses evoked in the sensorimotor cortex by delivering stimuli to the ventrolateral thalamus of the cat showed depression of excitability and slight elevation of the threshold after the administration of diazepam (ENGLANDER et al. 1977). Diazepam (1.4–15 mg/kg i.p.) also depressed the afterdischarges evoked in the rat hippocampus and recorded from the cortex (ALBERTSON et al. 1977). In the cat *cerveau isolé* preparation, diazepam (2 mg/kg) caused a strong inhibition of the responses in the hippocampus to single stimuli delivered to the ipsilateral amygdala (MORILLO 1962).

In functionally isolated slabs of the cat cerebral cortex, diazepam reduced the excitability of the neurons determined by electrical stimulation of the surface (FRANK and JHAMANDAS 1970).

b) Subcortical Areas

Chlordiazepoxide (10–40 mg i.v.; SCHALLEK and KUEHN 1963; SCHALLEK et al. 1964) and diazepam (0.25–2 mg/kg i.v.) raised the threshold for eliciting thalamic afterdischarges and decreased the duration and amplitude of the responses.

HERNÁNDEZ-PEÓN et al. (1964) reported that diazepam (5 and 10 mg/kg) depressed or abolished the behavioral and electrical manifestations of the afterdischarges elicited from the basolateral complex of the amygdala and hippocampus in awake unrestrained cats with chronically implanted electrodes. Auditory potentials recorded from the midbrain reticular formation were also reduced by the drug.

The threshold of afterdischarges of the cat amygdala was increased by diazepam and nitrazepam each in a dose of 10 mg/kg (SCHALLEK et al. 1965). Both drugs administered in the same dose had no effect on the afterdischarge threshold in the caudate nucleus and the septum (SCHALLEK and KUEHN 1965).

Visually evoked hippocampal responses were depressed by systemic administration of nitrazepam (STEINER and HUMMEL 1968). Diazepam (1.4–15 mg/kg i.p.) depressed the afterdischarges in the rat hippocampus evoked by electrical stimulation (ALBERTSON et al. 1977). MORILLO et al. (1962) stimulated the lateral nucleus of the cat amygdala and found that chlordiazepoxide (2.5 and 10 mg/kg i.v.) markedly depressed the response recorded from the basal hippocampus, while the drug showed no effect on the diffuse thalamocortical system.

Diazepam enhanced and prolonged the presynaptic inhibition elicited by conditioning stimulation of the median nerve and acting on the response evoked in the cuneate nucleus of the decerebrate cat by delivering at test stimulus to the ulnar nerve (HAEFELY et al. 1975). Moreover, it also enhanced GABA-mediated postsynaptic inhibition in the cuneate nucleus (POLC and HAEFELY 1976).

4. Focal Seizure Activity

Diazepam effectively depressed seizure activity evoked in the cat cortex after injection of penicillin into the amygdala, pyriform cortex, and ventral hippocampus

(GOGERTY and GUNN 1964). When focal seizure activity was evoked by injections of penicillin into the rat cortex, diazepam only transiently suppressed focal ictal activity and self-sustained afterdischarges, had a weak effect on interictal spikes, and had no effect on the interictal spiking in the mirror focus (CELESIA et al. 1973). EDMONDS et al. (1974) failed to observe any changes produced by diazepam (15 and 30 mg/kg orally) on the focal seizure activity appearing in freely moving rats after intracortical injections of penicillin. It is worth noting in this context that microiontophoretic administration of GABA to neurons in a penicillin-induced spiking focus in the rabbit cortex had no effect on the activity of the neuron when the amino acid was applied with currents which normally produced a block of neuron activity (CLARKE and HILL 1972). This would agree with the antagonism between penicillin and GABA in the mammalian brain (CURTIS et al. 1972) and amphibian afferent terminals [(DAVIDOFF 1972b), for interaction between penicillin and GABA in seizure disorders see Chap. 7 by MELDRUM)]. SHARER and KUTT (1971) noted that an i.v. infusion of diazepam in relatively large amounts to the lightly anesthetized cat reduced penicillin-induced cortical spike activity and afterdischarges, while small amounts suppressed the jerking of the limbs.

Focal seizure activity produced by local cortical administration of ouabain was reduced by clonazepam (PETSCHE 1972). Diazepam (0.25–0.5 mg/kg i.v.) suppressed the spiking activity following local freezing of the cat cortex (HORI et al. 1979). Focal seizure discharges produced by scarring lesions in the visual or motor cortex of cats could be depressed by diazepam but were slightly more resistant to the effect of the drug than the pentylenetetrazol-induced state of recurrent seizure activity in the electroencephalogram (SPEHLMANN and COLLEY 1968).

Chronic administration of diazepam (2 mg/kg i.p. daily for 2–3 months) suppressed epileptiform discharges in the mirror foci, but had little or no effect on seizure activity in the primary focus produced by implantation of aluminum oxide or penicillin into the olfactory bulb or hippocampus (GUERRERO-FIGUEROA et al. 1968). Diazepam and clonazepam decreased the amplitude of the potentials in the secondary cortical foci but had little or no effect on the primary (subcortical) epileptogenic foci evoked by irritative lesions and electrical stimulation in the septum, amygdala, and hippocampus (GUERRERO-FIGUEROA et al. 1969); when lesions were placed in the reticular formation, hypothalamus, and intralaminar nuclei of the thalamus, diazepam (but not clonazepam) also exerted a slight effect on the primary focus. Nitrazepam abolished local (hippocampal) and general seizure activity evoked by microinjection of acetylcholine into the amygdaloid complex (HERNÁNDEZ-PEÓN and ROJAS-RAMÍREZ 1966).

GUERRERO-FIGUEROA et al. (1967) noted that diazepam administered chronically at different daily doses to kittens abolished the spike-and-wave discharges in the electroencephalogram and the facial tic-like contractions and other signs resembling those of clinical petit mal which were induced by implantation of aluminum oxide or penicillin in the intralaminar thalamic nuclei or reticular formation.

Intraamygdaloid microinjections of diazepam (2 × 50 μg into the pars anterior) protected rabbits against convulsions and seizure activity in the electroencephalogram produced by i.v. infusions of pentylenetetrazol up to 40 mg/kg; seizures occurred after administration of pentylenetetrazol, 15 mg/kg, when the animals were not pretreated with intraamygdaloid diazepam (NAGY and DECSI 1979).

The clonus resulting from kindling in response to repeated stimulation of the frontal cortex of the rat was depressed by diazepam and the GABA-transaminase (GABA-T) inhibitor ethanolamine-*o*-sulfate (GOFF et al. 1978). Barbiturates and benzodiazepines were found to be the most effective drugs in attenuating kindled amygdaloid seizures in rats (ALBERTSON et al. 1980).

LOTHMAN and SOMJEN (1976) induced convulsions in the spinal cord of the functionally decapitate cat by topical or systemic administration of penicillin, recorded seizure activity from the cord surface as well as from ventral and dorsal roots, and observed tonic and clonic movements of the limbs. Since they found that diazepam administered by i.v. infusions in doses up to 7 mg/kg was ineffective in suppressing seizures, they concluded that diazepam exerts its anticonvulsant effect by acting at supraspinal sites.

V. Summary

There is strong evidence in favor of the view that benzodiazepines produce their various effects exclusively by facilitating GABA-mediated inhibition of neuron activity. They are very potent in models of primary generalized epilepsy and against most chemical convulsants. It seems likely that they exert not only their anxiolytic but also their anticonvulsant effect by acting on the limbic system, particularly at the amygdaloid complex.

J. Miscellaneous

I. Carboanhydrase Inhibition: Acetazolamide

SHANES (1958) found that carbonic anhydrase inhibitors such as acetazolamide and various sulfonamides act as "stabilizers" for a variety of depolarizing conditions in frog and rabbit nerves, which means that these drugs reduce or prevent any change of the membrane potential. He assumes that the "stabilizing" effect is independent of the specific effect of these drugs on carbonic anhydrase.

In the spinal cord of the cat carbon dioxide (5%–40%) and acetazolamide (25–200 mg/kg i.v.) depress the monosynaptic reflex to a larger extent than the polysynaptic reflex discharges. Despite the pronounced depression of the monosynaptic reflex, post-tetanic potentiation of the monosynaptic reflex is not affected. Neither the time of synaptic recovery nor the response of the spinal motoneurons to repetitive stimulation was influenced by carbon dioxide or acetazolamide (ESPLIN and ROSENSTEIN 1963).

Presynaptic inhibition in the spinal cord of unanesthetized cats was reduced by carbon dioxide, and the degree of this reduction was directly related to the degree of depression by carbon dioxide of the monosynaptic reflex (MIYAHARA et al. 1966).

II. Local Anesthetics

Local anesthetics prevent the generation of impulses and block their conduction in nerve fibers mainly by reducing the sodium conductance of the neuron membrane (STRAUB 1956; STRICHARTZ 1973; RITCHIE 1975, 1979). They are clinically used as antiarrhythmic agents, particularly in ventricular arrhythmias.

BERNHARD et al. (1955) found that lidocaine 0.6–3.0 mg/kg, administered by i.v. infusion was effective in controlling status epilepticus. MORRIS (1979) noted that bolus injection and infusion of lidocaine rapidly interrupted focal motor status epilepticus, when phenytoin, phenobarbital, or diazepam had been employed in vain. The bolus dose of 25 mg was given i.v. as a 2% solution over a period of 15 min. Simultaneously, a continuous i.v. infusion of a 2% lidocaine solution was begun at a rate of 27 μg/kg per minute. Although there was no effect on the patient's interictal electroencephalogram or electrocardiogram, there was a marked decrease in duration and frequency of the seizures.

The duration of afterdischarges following electroshock therapy was significantly shortened by pretreatment of the patients with i.v. lidocaine (OTTOSON 1955).

In electroseizures evoked in mice, local anesthetics such as lidocaine or tetracaine exerted an anticonvulsive effect of the same order of magnitude as phenobarbital or phenytoin, but their effect was much shorter in duration (FREY 1962); like phenytoin, local anesthetics were ineffective against pentylenetetrazol-induced clonic convulsions. The incidence of electrically induced convulsions in mice was reduced by lidocaine in a dose range of 12.5–100 mg/kg as a function of the dosage (ESSMAN 1965).

JULIEN (1973) administered lidocaine to cats with penicillin-induced epileptogenic foci and found that focal seizure activity was reduced at blood levels of 0.5–4.0 μg/ml, which were rapidly attained after i.m. or i.v. administration of the drug. Blood levels above 5 μg/ml were accompanied by an increased cortical excitability or even by convulsions. These high blood levels, however, were not observed after i.m. injection.

References

Albertson TE, Peterson SL, Stark LG, Rauschenberger JE (1977) The behavioural and electrical interactions of electrically induced hippocampal seizures and four anticonvulsants. Proc West Pharmacol Soc 20:165–172

Albertson TE, Peterson SL, Stark LG (1978) Effects of phenobarbital and SC-13504 on partially kindled hippocampal seizures in rats. Exp Neurol 61:270–280

Albertson TE, Peterson SL, Stark LG (1980) Anticonvulsant drugs and their antagonism of kindled amygdaloid seizures in rats. Neuropharmacology 19:643–652

Alderdice MT, Trommer BA (1980) Differential effects of the anticonvulsants phenobarbital, ethosuximide and carbamazepine on neuromuscular transmission. J. Pharmacol Exp Ther 215:92–96

Anderson RJ, Raines A (1974) Suppression by diphenylhydantoin of afferent discharges arising in muscle spindles of the triceps surae of the cat. J Pharmacol Exp Ther 191:290–299

Arushanyan EB, Zavyalov AV, Melnichuk PV (1967) Trimethadione effect upon the background activity of intercalary neurons of the spinal cord and their responses to an afferent and suprasegmental stimulation (in Russian). Farmakol Toksikol 30:655–658
Ayala GF, Johnston DJ (1977) The influences of phenytoin on the fundamental electrical properties of simple neural systems. Epilepsia 18:299–307
Ayala GF, Johnston D, Lin S, Dichter HN (1977a) The mechanism of action of diphenylhydantoin on invertebrate neurons. II. Effects on synaptic mechanisms. Brain Res 121:259–270
Ayala GF, Lin S, Johnston D (1977b) The mechanism of action of diphenylhydantoin on invertebrate neurons. I. Effects on basic membrane properties. Brain Res 121:245–258
Baldino F Jr, Geller HM (1981) Sodium valproate enhancement of γ-aminobutyric acid (GABA) inhibition: electrophysiological evidence for anticonvulsant activity. J Pharmacol Exp Ther 217:445–450
Banna NR, Jabbur SJ, Saadé NE (1974) Antagonism of the spinal action of diazepam by semicarbazide. Br J Pharmacol 51:101–103
Barker JL (1975a) CNS depressants: effects on post-synaptic pharmacology. Brain Res 92:35–56
Barker JL (1975b) Inhibitory and excitatory effects of CNS depressants on invertebrate synapses. Brain Res 93:77–90
Barker JL (1975c) Selective depression of postsynaptic excitation by general anesthetics. In: Fink BR (ed) Molecular mechanisms of anesthesia. Progress in anesthesiology, vol 1. Raven, New York, pp 135–153
Barker JL, Gainer H (1973) Pentobarbital: selective depression of excitation postsynaptic potentials. Science 182:720–722
Bazemore RP, Zuckermann EC (1974) On the problem of diphenyl-hydantoin-induced seizures. An experimental approach. Arch Neurol 31:243–249
Besson JM, LeBars D, Oliveras J-L (1978) L'analgésie morphinique: données neurobiologiques. Ann Anesthésiol Fr 19:343–369
Bernhard CG, Bohm E, Höjeberg S (1955) A new treatment of status epilepticus. Intravenous injections of a local anesthetic (lidocaine). Arch Neurol Psychiatr 74:208–214
Blaustein MP (1968) Barbiturates block sodium and potassium conductance increases in voltage-clamped lobster axons. J Gen Physiol 51:293–307
Blaustein MP (1976) Barbiturates block calcium uptake by stimulated and potassium-depolarized rat sympathetic ganglia. J Pharmacol Exp Ther 196:80–86
Blaustein MP, Ector AC (1975) Barbiturate inhibition of calcium uptake by depolarized nerve terminals in vitro. Mol Pharmacol 11:369–378
Blum B (1964) A differential action of diphenylhydantoin on the motor cortex of the cat. Arch Int Pharmacodyn Ther 149:45–55
Blume HW, Lamour Y, Arnauld E, Layton BS, Renaud LP (1979) Sodium di-*n*-propylacetate (valproate) action on single neurons in rat cerebral cortex and hippocampus. Brain Res 171:182–185
Bowery NG, Dray A (1976) Barbiturate reversal of amino acid antagonism produced by convulsant agents. Nature 264:276–278
Bowery NG, Dray A (1978) Reversal of the action of amino acid antagonists by barbiturates and other hypnotic drugs. Br J Pharmacol 63:197–215
Braestrup C, Squires RF (1977) Specific benzodiazepine receptors in rat brain characterized by high affinity ^{3}H-diazepam binding. Proc Natl Acad Sci USA 74:3805–3809
Braestrup C, Squires RF (1978) Pharmacological characterization of benzodiazepine receptors in the brain. Eur J Pharmacol 48:263–270
Brooks CMcC, Eccles JC (1947) A study of the effects of anaesthesia and asphyxia on the mono-synaptic pathway through the spinal cord. J Neurophysiol 10:349–360
Brooks CMcC, Koizumi K, Siebens AA (1956) Inhibitory action of bulbar and suprabulbar reticular formation on the spinal reflex pathway. Am J Physiol 184:497–504
Capek R, Esplin B (1973) Ethosuximide induced depression of repetitive transmission in the spinal monosynaptic pathway. Pharmacologist 15:161

Capek R, Esplin B (1977) Effects of ethosuximide on transmission of repetitive impulses and apparent rates of transmitter turnover in the spinal monosynaptic pathway. J Pharmacol Exp Ther 201:320–325

Carnay L, Grundfest S (1974) Excitable membrane stabilization by diphenylhydantoin and calcium. Neuropharmacology 13:1097–1108

Celesia GG, Booker HE, Sato S (1973) Effects of diazepam on experimentally induced cortical epilepsy and their correlation with drug concentration. EEG Clin Neurophysiol 34:727

Cheymol J, Van Den Driessche J, Allain P, Eben-Moussi E (1967) Diazépam et curarisation. Anesth Analg (Paris) 24:329–336

Chin JH, Smith CM (1962) Effects of some central nervous system depressants on the phasic and tonic stretch reflex. J Pharmacol Exp Ther 136:276–283

Chin JH, Crankshaw DP, Kendig JJ (1974) Changes in the dorsal root potential with diazepam and with analgesics aspirin, nitrous oxide, morphine and meperidine, Neuropharmacology 13:305–315

Chiu P, Olsen DM, Borys HK, Karler R, Turkanis SA (1979) The influence of cannabidiol and Δ^9-tetrahydrocannabinol on cobalt epilepsy in rats. Epilepsia 20:365–375

Choi DW, Farb DH, Fischbach GD (1977) Chlordiazepoxide selectively augments GABA action in spinal cord cell cultures. Nature 269:342–344

Clarke G, Hill RG (1972) Effects of a focal penicillin lesion on responses of rabbit cortical neurones to putative neurotransmitters. Br J Pharmacol 44:435–441

Costa E, Guidotti A (1979) Molecular mechanisms in the receptor action of benzodiazepines. Ann Rev Pharmacol Toxicol 19:531–545

Costa E, Guidotti A, Mao CC (1975a) Evidence for involvement of GABA in the action of benzodiazepines: studies on rat cerebellum. In: Costa E, Greengard P (eds) Mechanisms of action of benzodiazepines. Advances in biochemical psychopharmacology 14. Raven, New York, pp 113–130

Costa E, Guidotti A, Mao CC, Suria A (1975b) New concepts on the mechanism of action of benzodiazepines. Life Sci 17:167–185

Craig CR, Shideman FE (1971) Metabolism and anticonvulsant properties of mephobarbital and phenobarbital in rat brains. J Pharmacol Exp Ther 176:35–42

Crane P, Swanson PD (1970) Diphenylhydantoin and the cations and phosphates of electrically stimulated brain slices. Neurology (Minneap) 20:1119–1123

Crankshaw DP, Raper C (1970) Mephenesin, methocarbamol, chlordiazepoxide and diazepam: actions on spinal reflexes and ventral root potentials. Br J Pharmacol 38:148–156

Crawford JM (1970) Anaesthetic agents and the chemical sensitivity of corticol neurones. Neuropharmacology 9:31–46

Curtis DR, Game CJA, Johnston GAR, McCulloch RM, MacLachlan RM (1972) Convulsive action of penicillin. Brain Res 43:242–245

Curtis DR, Game CJA, Lodge D (1976) Benzodiazepines and central glycine receptors. Br J Pharmacol 56:307–311

Davenport J, Schwindt PC, Crill WG (1977) Penicillin-induced spinal seizures: selective effects on synaptic transmission. Exp Neurol 56:132–150

David J, Grewal RS (1976) Effect of carbamazepine (Tegretol®) on seizure and EEG patterns in monkeys with alumina-induced focal motor and hippocampal foci. Epilepsia 17:415–422

Davidoff RA (1972a) Diphenylhydantoin increases spinal presynaptic inhibition. Trans Am Neurol Assoc 97:193–196

Davidoff RA (1972b) Penicillin and presynaptic inhibition in the amphibian spinal cord. Brain Res 36:218–222

Davis HL, Johnson DD, Crawford RD (1978) Epileptiform seizures in domestic fowl. IX. Implications of the absence of anticonvulsant activity of ethosuximide in a pharmacological model of epilepsy. Can J Physiol Pharmacol 56:893–896

Deisz RA, Lux HD (1977) Diphenylhydantoin prolongs postsynaptic inhibition and iontophoretic GABA action in the crayfish stretch receptor. Neurosci Lett 5:199–203

Delgado-Escueta AV, Horan MP (1980) Phenytoin: biochemical membrane studies. In: Glaser GH, Penry JK, Woodbury DM (eds) Antiepileptic drugs: mechanisms of action. Advances in neurology 27. Raven, New York, pp 377–398

De Salva SJ, Oester YT (1960) The effect of central depressants on certain spinal reflexes in the acute high cervical cat. Arch Int Pharmacodyn Ther 124:255–262

De Sousa RC, Grosso A (1973) Effects of diphenylhydantoin on transport processes in frog skin (*Rana ridibunda*). Experientia 29:1097–1098

De Weer P (1980) Phenytoin: blockage of resting sodium channels. In: Glaser GH, Penry JK, Woodbury DM (eds) Antiepileptic drugs: mechanisms of action. Advances in neurology 27. Raven, New York, pp 353–361

Dolce G (1969) Über den antiepileptischen Aktionsmechanismus von 5-Carbamyl-5*H*-dibenzo (b,f) azepin. Neurophysiologische Untersuchungen an Katzen. Arzneimittelforsch 19:1257–1262

Dow RC, Forfar JC, McQueen JK (1973) The effects of some anticonvulsant drugs on cobalt-induced epilepsy. Epilepsia 14:203–212

Downes H, Williams JK (1969) Effects of a convulsant barbiturate on the spinal monosynaptic pathway. J Pharmacol Exp Ther 168:283–289

Dray A, Straughan DW (1976) Benzodiazepines: GABA and glycine receptors on single neurons in the rat medulla. J Pharm Pharmacol 28:314–315

Dretchen KL, Standaert FG, Raines A (1977) Effects of phenytoin on the cyclic nucleotide system in the motor nerve terminal. Epilepsia 18:337–348

Eccles JC (1946) Synaptic potentials of motoneurons. J Neurophysiol 9:87–120

Eccles JC (1965) Pharmacology of central inhibitory synapses. Br Med Bull 21:19–25

Eccles JC, Krnjević K (1959) Presynaptic changes associated with post-tetanic potentiation in the spinal cord. J Physiol (Lond) 149:274–287

Eccles JC, Schmidt R, Willis WD (1963) Pharmacological studies on presynaptic inhibition. J Physiol (Lond) 168:500–530

Edmonds HL, Stark LG, Hollinger MA (1974) The effects of diphenylhydantoin, phenobarbital, and diazepam on the penicillininduced epileptogenic focus in the rat. Exp Neurol 45:377–386

Elazar Z, Gottesfeld Z (1975) Effect of drug-induced increase of brain GABA levels on penicillin focus. Experientia 31:671–678

Englander RN, Johnson RN, Brickley JJ, Hanna GR (1977) Effects of antiepileptic drugs on thalamocortical excitability. Neurology (Minneap) 27:1134–1139

Esplin DW (1957) Effects of diphenylhydantoin on synaptic transmission in cat spinal cord and stellate ganglion. J Pharmacol Exp Ther 120:301–323

Esplin DW (1963) Criteria for assessing effects of depressant drugs on spinal cord synaptic transmission, with examples of drug selectivity. Arch Int Pharmacodyn Ther 143:479–497

Esplin DW, Curto EM (1975) Effects of trimethadione on synaptic transmission in the spinal cord; antagonism of trimethadione and pentylenetetrazol. J Pharmacol Exp Ther 121:457–467

Esplin DW, Freston JW (1960) Physiological and pharmacological analysis of spinal cord convulsions. J Pharmacol Exp Ther 130:68–80

Esplin DW, Rosenstein R (1963) Analysis of spinal depressant actions of carbon dioxide and acetazolamide. Arch Int Pharmacodyn Ther 143:498–513

Esplin DW, Zablocka B (1969) Effects of tetanization on transmitter dynamics. Epilepsia 10:193–210

Esplin DW, Zablocka-Esplin B (1969) Mechanisms of action of convulsants. In: Jasper HH, Ward AA, Pope A (eds) Basic mechanisms of the epilepsies. Little Brown, Boston, pp 167–183

Essman WB (1965) Xylocaine induced protection against electrically induced convulsions in mice. Arch Int Pharmacodyn Ther 157:166–173

Evans RH (1979) Potentiation of the effects of GABA by pentobarbitone. Brain Res 171:113–120

Fariello R, Mutani R (1970) Modificazioni dell'attività del focus epilettogeno cortico-motorio da allumina indotte dal sale di sodio dell'acido *n*-dipropilacetico (DPA). Acta Neurol (Napoli) 25:116–122

Faugier-Grimaud S (1978) Action of anticonvulsants on pentylenetetrazol-induced epileptiform activity on invertebrate neurones (*Helix apsersa*). Neuropharmacology 17:905–918

Fertziger AP, Liuzzi SE, Dunham PB (1971) Diphenylhydantoin (Dilantin): stimulation of potassium influx in lobster axons. Brain Res 33:592–596

Frank GB, Jhamandas K (1970) Effects of general depressant drugs on the electrical responses of isolated slabs of cat cerebral cortex. Br J Pharmacol 39:707–715

Franz DN, Esplin DW (1965) Prevention by diphenylhydantoin of posttetanic enhancement of action potentials in nonmyelinated nerve fibres. Pharmacologist 7:174

Frey H-H (1962) On the anticonvulsant activity of local anaesthetics. Acta Pharmacol Toxicol 19:205–211

Frey H-H (1969) Determination of the anticonvulsant potency of unmetabolized trimethadione. Acta Pharmacol Toxicol 27:295–300

Fromm GH (1969) Pharmacological consideration of anticonvulsants. Headache 9:35–41

Fromm GH, Landgren S (1963) Effect of diphenylhydantoin on single cells in the spinal trigeminal nucleus. Neurology (Minneap) 13:34–37

Fromm GH, Killian JM (1967) Effect of some anticonvulsant drugs on the spinal trigeminal nucleus. Neurology (Minneap) 17:275–280

Fromm GH, Kohli CM (1972) The role of inhibitory pathways in petit mal epilepsy. Neurology (Minneap) 22:1012–1020

Fromm GH, Chatta AS, Terrence CF, Glass JD (1981 a) Role of inhibitory mechanisms in trigeminal neuralogia. Neurology 31:683–687

Fromm GH, Glass JD, Chatta AS, Martinez AJ (1981 b) Effect of anticonvulsant drugs on inhibitory and excitatory pathways. Epilepsia 22:65–73

Gallagher BB, Baumel IP (1972) Primidone: biotransformation. In: Vida JA (ed) Anticonvulsants. Academic, New York, pp 11–55

Gallagher JP, Inokuchi H, Nakamura J, Shinnick-Gallagher P (1981) Effects of anticonvulsants on excitability and GABA sensitivity of cat dorsal root ganglion cells. Neuropharmacology 20:427–433

Gangloff H, Monnier M (1957) The action of anticonvulsant drugs tested by electrical stimulation of the cortex, diencephalon and rhinencephalon in the unanesthetized rabbit. EEG Clin Neurophysiol 9:43–58

Gent JP, Phillips NI (1980) Sodium di-*n*-propylacetate (valproate) potentiates responses to GABA and muscimol on single neurones. Brain Res 197:275–278

Ghelarducci B, Lenzi G, Pompeiano O (1966) A neurophysiological analysis of the postural effects of a benzodiazepine. Arch Int Pharmacodyn Ther 163:403–421

Goff D, Miller AA, Webster RA (1978) Anticonvulsant drugs and folic acid on the development of epileptic kindling in rats. Br J Pharmacol 64:406 P

Gogerty JH, Gunn CG (1964) Effects of various centrally acting agents on penicillin-induced temporal lobe seizures in cats. Fed Proc 23:349

Goldring JM, Blaustein MP (1980) Barbiturates: physiological effects II. In: Glaser GH, Penry JK, Woodbury DM (eds) Antiepileptic drugs: mechanisms of action. Advances in neurology 27. Raven, New York, pp 523–531

Goodman LS, Swinyard EA, Toman JEP (1946 a) Studies on the anticonvulsant properties of diphenylhydantoin. Fed Proc 5:180

Goodman LS, Swinyard EA, Toman JEP (1946 b) Further studies on the anticonvulsant properties of tridione (3,5,5-trimethyloxazollidinedione). Fed Proc 5:179–180

Goodman LS, Toman JEP, Swinyard EA (1946 c) The anticonvulsant properties of tridione. Laboratory and clinical investigations. Am J Med 1:213–228

Grossmann W, Jurna I, Nehles J (1974 a) Activation by diphenylthiohydantoin of inhibitory influences on spinal motor activity. Eur J Pharmacol 27:214–220

Grossmann W, Jurna I, Richter D (1974 b) Activating effect of diphenylhydantoin on spinal motoneurones. Neuropharmacology 13:803–811

Grossmann W, Jurna I, Theres C (1974c) The excitatory effect of diphenylthiohydantoin on spinal reflex activity. Neuropharmacology 13:813–817

Grossmann W, Jurna I, Theres C (1974d) The site of action of the optical isomers of 1-methyl-5-phenyl-5-propyl barbituric acid. Naunyn-Schmiedeberg's Arch Pharmacol 282:367–377

Guberman A, Gloor P, Sherwin AL (1975) Response of generalized penicillin epilepsy in the cat to ethosuximide and diphenylhydantoin. Neurology (Minneap) 25:758–764

Guerrero-Figueroa R, Rye MM, Gallant DM (1967) Effects of diazepam on three per second spike and wave discharges. Curr Ther Res 9:522–535

Guerrero-Figueroa R, Rye MM, Guerrero-Figueroa C (1968) Effects of diazepam on secondary subcortical epileptogenic tissues. Curr Ther Res 10:150–166

Guerrero-Figueroa R, Rye MM, Heath RG (1969) Effects of two benzodiazepine derivates on cortical and subcortical epileptogenic tissues in the cat and monkey. 1. Limbic system structures. Curr Ther Res 11:27–39

Haefely W, Kulcsár A, Möhler H, Pieri L, Polc P, Schaffner R (1975) Possible involvement of GABA in the central actions of benzodiazepines. In: Costa E, Greengard P (eds) Mechanisms of action of benzodiazepines. Advances in biochemical psychopharmacology 14. Raven, New York, pp 131–151

Haefely W, Polc P, Schaffner R, Keller HH, Pieri L, Möhler H (1979) Facilitation of GABA-ergic transmission by drugs. In: Krogsgaard-Larsen P, Scheel-Krüger J, Kofod H (eds) GABA-neurotransmitters. Munksgaard, Copenhagen, pp 357–375

Halpern LM, Julien RM (1972) Augmentation of cerebellar Purkinje discharge rate after diphenylhydantoin. Epilepsia 13:377–385

Hamilton JT (1967) Muscle relaxant activity of chlordiazepoxide and diazepam. Can J Physiol Pharmacol 45:191–199

Hartmann JF (1966) High sodium content of cortical astrocytes. Electron microscopic evidence. Arch Neurol 15:633–642

Hasbani M, Pincus JH, Lee SH (1974) Diphenylhydantoin and calcium movement in lobster nerves. Arch Neurol 31:250–254

Hauptmann A (1912) Luminal bei Epilepsie. MMW 59:1907–1909

Heinbecker P, Bartley SH (1940) Action of ether and nembutal on the nervous system. J Neurophysiol 3:219–236

Heinemann U, Lux HD (1973) Effects of diphenylhydantoin on extracellular (K+) in cat cortex. EEG Clin Neurophysiol 34:735

Hernández-Peón R (1964) Anticonvulsive action of G 32883. Neuropsychopharmacology 3:303–311

Hernández-Peón R (1965) Central action of G-32883 upon transmission of trigeminal pain impulses. Med Pharmacol Exp 12:73–80

Hernández-Peón R, Rojas-Ramírez JA (1966) Central mechanisms of tranquilizing, anticonvulsant and relaxant actions of Ro 4-5360. Neuropharmacology 5:263–267

Hernández-Peón, Rojas-Ramírez JA, O'Flaherty JJ, Mazzuchelli-O'Flaherty AL (1964) An experimental study of the anticonvulsive and relaxant actions of valium. Neuropharmacology 3:405–412

Hershkowitz N, Raines A (1978) Effects of carbamazepine on muscle spindle discharges. J Pharmacol Exp Ther 204:581–591

Hershkowitz N, Dretchen KL, Raines A (1978) Carbamazepine suppression of post-tetanic potentiation at the neuromuscular junction. J Pharmacol Exp Ther 207:810–816

Herz A, Fuster J (1964) Über die Wirkung von Barbituraten und Amphetamin auf die Entladungstätigkeit corticaler Neurone. Naunyn-Schmiedebergs Arch Pharmacol 249:146–161

Holm E, Kelleter, R, Heinemann H, Hamann K-F (1970) Elektrophysiologische Analyse der Wirkun von Carbamazepin auf das Gehirn der Katze. Pharmakopsychiat Neuro-Psychopharmakol 3:187–200

Honda H, Allen MB (1973) The effect of an iminostilbene derivative (G 32883) on peripheral nerves. J Med Ass Georgia 62:38–42

Hori M, Ito T, Yoshida K, Shimizu M (1979) Effect of anticonvulsants on spiking activity induced by cortical freezing in cats. Epilepsia 20:25–36

Huang L-YM, Barker JL (1980) Pentobarbital: stereospecific actions of (+) and (−) isomers revealed on cultured mammalian neurons. Science 207:195–197

Hudson RD, Wolpert MK (1970) Central muscle relaxant effects of diazepam. Neuropharmacology 9:481–488

Iadarola MJ, Gale K (1981) Cellular compartments of GABA in brain and their relationship to anticonvulsant activity. Mol Cell Biochem 39:305–330

Ito T, Hori M, Yoshida K, Shimizu M (1977) Effect of anticonvulsants on thalamic afterdischarge in rats and cats. Jpn J Pharmacol 27:823–831

Ito T, Hori M, Yoshida K, Shimizu M (1979) Effect of anticonvulsants on experimental cortical epilepsy induced by tungstic acid gel in rats. Arch Int Pharmacodyn Ther 241:287–299

Johnston D, Ayala GF (1975) Diphenylhydantoin: action of a common anticonvulsant on bursting pacemaker cells in *Aplysia*. Science 189:1009–1011

Julien RM (1972) Cerebellar involvement in the antiepileptic action of diazepam. Neuropharmacology 11:683–691

Julien RM (1973) Lidocaine in experimental epilepsy: correlation of anticonvulsant effect with blood concentrations. EEG Clin Neurophysiol 34:639–645

Julien RM (1974) Experimental epilepsy: cerebro-cerebellar interactions and antiepileptic drugs. In: Cooper IS, Riklan M, Snider RS (eds) The cerebellum, epilepsy and behaviour. Plenum, New York, pp 97–117

Julien RM, Halpern LM (1970) Stabilization of excitable membrane by chronic administration of diphenylhydantoin. J Pharmacol Exp Ther 175:206–211

Julien RM, Halpern LM (1971) Diphenylhydantoin: evidence for a central action. Life Sci 10:575–582

Julien RM, Hollister RP (1975) Carbamazepine: mechanisms of action. In: Penry JK, Daly DD (eds) Advances in neurology, vol II. Raven, New York, pp 263–276

Julien RM, Laxer KD (1974) Cerebellar responses to penicillin-induced cerebral cortical epileptiform discharge. EEG Clin Neurophysiol 37:123–132

Kästner I, Klingenberg F, Müller M (1968) Untersuchungen zur zentralnervösen Wirkung des Ethosuximids. Arch Psychiatr Nervenkr 211:365–376

Kästner I, Klingenberg F, Müller M (1970) Zur Wirkung des Ethosuximids auf die Kobalt-induzierte „Epilepsie“ der Ratte. Arch Int Pharmacodyn Ther 186:220–226

Kao LI, Crill WE (1972a) Penicillin-induced segmental myoclonus. I. Motor responses and intracellular recording from motoneurones. Arch Neurol 26:156–161

Kao LI, Crill WE (1972b) Penicillin-induced segmental myoclonus. II. Membrane properties of cat spinal motoneurones. Arch Neurol 26:162–168

Kawasaki K, Matsushita A (1981) Sensitive depressant effect of benzodiazepines on the crossed extensor reflex in chloralose-anesthetized rats. Life Sci 28:1391–1398

Kerwin RW, Olpe H-R, Schmutz M (1980) The effect of sodium-*n*-dipropyl acetate on γ-aminobutyric acid-dependent inhibition in the rat cortex and substantia nigra in relation to its anticonvulsant activity. Br J Pharmacol 71:545–551

Kobayashi K, Iwata Y, Mukawa J (1967) Preferential action of Tegretol (G-32883) to limbic seizure – clinical and experimental analyses. No To Shinkei 19:991–1005

Kopeloff LM, Alexander GJ (1972) Mechanism of *p*-chlorophenylalanine-mediated increase in seizure susceptibility: inhibition by cerebellar ablation. Proc Soc Exp Biol Med 139:647–651

Korey SR (1951) Effect of dilantin and mesantoin on the giant axon of the squid. Proc Soc Exp Biol Med 76:297–299

Krip G, Vazquez AJ (1971) Effects of diphenylhydantoin and cholinergic agents on the neuronally isolated cerebral cortex. EEG Clin Neurophysiol 30:391–398

Krupp P (1969) The effect of Tegretol® on some elementary neuronal mechanisms. Headache 9:42–46

Krupp P, Bianchi CP, Suarez-Kurtz G (1969) On the local anesthetic effect of barbiturates. J Pharm Pharmacol 21:763–768

LaManna J, Lothman E, Rosenthal M, Somjen G, Younts W (1977) Phenytoin, electric, ionic, and metabolic responses in cortex and spinal cord. Epilepsia 18:317–329

Larrabee MG, Posternak JM (1952) Selective action of anesthetics on synapses and axons in mammalian sympathetic ganglia. J Neurophysiol 15:91–114
Laxer KD, Robertson LT, Julien RM, Dow RS (1980) Phenytoin: relationship between cerebellar function and epileptic discharges. In: Glaser GH, Penry JK, Woodbury DM (eds) Antiepileptic drugs: mechanism of action. Advances in neurology 27. Raven, New York, pp 415–427
Leeb-Lundberg F, Snowman A, Olsen RW (1980) Barbiturate receptor sites are coupled to benzodiazepine receptors. Proc Natl Acad Sci USA 77:7468–7472
Lipicky RJ, Gilbert DL, Stillman IM (1972) Diphenylhydantoin inhibition of sodium conductance in squid giant axon. Proc Nat Acad Sci USA 69:1758–1760
Löscher W, Frey H-H (1977) Effect of convulsant and anticonvulsant agents on level and metabolism of γ-aminobutyric acid in mouse brain. Naunyn-Schmiedebergs Arch Pharmacol 296:263–269
Lothman EW, Somjen GG (1976) Motor and electrical signs of epileptiform activity induced by penicillin in the spinal cords of decapitate cats. EEG Clin Neurophysiol 41:237–252
Louis S, Kutt H, McDowell F (1968) Intravenous diphenylhydantoin in experimental seizures. II. Effect on penicillin-induced seizures in the cat. Arch Neurol 18:472–477
Louis S, Kutt H, McDowell F (1971) Modification of experimental seizures and anticonvulsant efficacy by peripheral stimulation. Neurology (Minneap) 21:329–336
Løyning Y, Oshima T, Yokota T (1964) Site of action of thiamylal sodium on the monosynaptic spinal reflex pathway in cats. Neurophysiol 27:408–428
MacDonald RL, Barker JL (1979a) Enhancement of GABA-mediated postsynaptic inhibition in cultured mammalian spinal cord neurons: a common mode of anticonvulsant action. Brain Res 167:323–336
MacDonald RL, Barker JL (1979b) Anticonvulsant and anesthetic barbiturates: different postsynaptic actions in cultured mammalian neurons. Neurology (Minneap) 29:432–447
MacDonald RL, Bergey GK (1979) Valproic acid augments GABA-mediated postsynaptic inhibition in cultured mammalian neurons. Brain Res 170:558–562
Mandell AJ, Bach LM (1957) Failure of the bulbar inhibitory reticular formation to affect somatic reflex activity in the unanesthetized cat. Am J Physiol 190:330–332
Mareš P, Kolínová M, Fischer J (1977) The influence of pentobarbital upon a cortical epileptogenic focus in rats. Arch Int Pharmacodyn Ther 226:313–323
Menétrey D, Decaud-Gasarabwe J, Besson JM (1973) Effects of diazepam on dorsal root potentials induced by cortical paroxysmal activity. Eur J Pharmacol 24:158–163
Merritt HH, Putnam TJ (1938) A new series of anticonvulsant drugs tested by experiments on animals. Arch Neurol Psychiatr 39:1003–1015
Merrit HH, Putnam TJ (1939) Sodium diphenylhydantoinate in treatment of convulsive seizures. Arch Neurol Psychiatr 42:1053–1058
Millichap JG, Woodbury DM, Goodman LS (1959) Mechanism of the anticonvulsant action of acetazoleamide, a carbonic anhydrase inhibitor. J Pharmacol Exp Ther 115:251–258
Miyahara JT, Esplin D, Zablocka B (1966) Differential effects of depressant drugs on presynaptic inhibition. J Pharmacol Exp Ther 154:119–127
Möhler H, Okada T (1977) Benzodiazepine receptor: demonstration in the central nervous system. Science 198:849–851
Möhler H, Okada T (1978) Biochemical identification of the site of action of benzodiazepines in human brain by ^{3}H-diazepam binding. Life Sci 22:985–996
Morillo A (1962) Effects of benzodiazepines upon amygdala and hippocampus of the cat. Neuropharmacology 1:353–359
Morillo A, Revzin AM, Knauss T (1962) Physiological mechanisms of action of chlordiazepoxide in cats. Psychopharmacologia (Berlin) 3:386–394
Morrell F, Bradley W, Ptashne M (1958) Effect of diphenylhydantion on peripheral nerve. Neurology (Minneap) 8:140–144

Morris HH (1979) Lidocaine: a neglected anticonvulsant? South Med J 72:1564–1566
Musgrave FS, Purpura DP (1963) Effects of dilantin on focal epileptogenic activity of cat neocortex. EEG Clin Neurophysiol 15:923
Mutani R, Fariello R (1969) Effetti dell'acido *n*-dipropilacetico (Depakine) sull'attività del focus epilettogeno corticale da cobalto. Riv Patol Nerv Ment 90:40–49
Mutani R, Doriguzzi T, Fariello R, Furlan PM (1968) Azione antiepilettica del sale di sodio dell'acido *N*-dipropilacetico. Studio sperimentale sul gatto. Riv Patol Nerv Ment 89:24–33
Nagy J, Decsi L (1979) Further studies on the site of action of diazepam: anticonvulsant effect in the rabbit. Neuropharmacology 18:39–45
Nakanishi T, Norris FH Jr (1971) Effect of diazepam on rat spinal reflexes. J Neurol Sci 13:189–195
Narahashi T, Moore JW, Poston RN (1969) Anesthetic blocking of nerve membrane conductances by internal and external applications. J Neurobiol 1:3–22
Narahashi T, Frazier DT, Deguchi T, Cleaves CA, Ernau MC (1971) The active form of pentobarbital in squid giant axons. J Pharmacol Exp Ther 177:25–34
Neuman RS, Frank GB (1977) Effects of diphenylhydantoin and phenobarbital on voltage-clamped myelinated nerve. Can J Physiol Pharmacol 55:42–47
Ngai SH, Tseng DTC, Wang SC (1966) Effect of diazepam and other central nervous system depressants on spinal reflexes in cats: a study of site of action. J Pharmacol Exp Ther 153:344–351
Nicoll RA (1972) The effects of anaesthetics on synaptic excitation and inhibition in the olfactory bulb. J Physiol (Lond) 223:803–814
Nicoll RA (1975a) Pentobarbital: action on frog motoneurons. Brain Res 96:119–123
Nicoll RA (1975b) Presynaptic action of barbiturates in the frog spinal cord. Proc Nat Acad Sci USA 72:1460–1463
Nicoll RA (1978) Pentobarbital: differential postsynaptic actions on sympathetic ganglion cells. Science 199:451–452
Nicoll RA, Iwamoto ET (1978) Action of pentobarbital on sympathetic ganglion cells. J Neurophysiol 41:977–986
Nicoll RA, Wojtowicz JM (1980) The effects of pentobarbital and related compounds on frog motoneurons. Brain Res 191:225–237
Nicoll RA, Eccles JC, Oshima T, Rubia I (1975) Prolongation of hippocampal inhibitory postsynaptic potentials by barbiturates. Nature 258:625–627
Obata K, Takeda K (1969) Release of γ-aminobutyric acid into the fourth ventricle induced by stimulation of the cat's cerebellum. J Neurochem 16:1043–1047
Obata K, Ito M, Ochi R, Sato N (1967) Pharmacological properties of the postsynaptic inhibition by Purkinje cell axons and the action of γ-aminobutyric acid on Deiters neurones. Exp Brain Res 4:43–57
Obata K, Takeda K, Shinozaki H (1970) Further study on pharmacological properties of the cerebellar-induced inhibition of Deiter's neurones. Exp Brain Res 11:327–342
Olds ME, Olds J (1969) Effects of anxiety-relieving drugs on unit discharges in hippocampus, reticular midbrain, and preoptic area in the freely moving rat. Neuropharmacology 8:87–103
Olsen RW (1981a) GABA-benzodiazepine-barbiturate receptor interactions. J Neurochem 37:1–13
Olsen RW (1981b) The GABA postsynaptic membrane receptor-ionophore complex. Site of action of convulsant and anticonvulsant drugs. Mol Cell Biochem 39:261–279
Olsen RW, Leeb-Lundberg F (1981) Convulsant and anticonvulsant drug binding sites related to GABA-regulated chloride ion channels. In: Costa E, Di Chiara G, Gessa GL (eds) GABA and benzodiazepine receptors. Advances in biochemical psychopharmacology 26. Raven, New York, pp 93–102
Olsen RW, Ticku MK, Van Ness PC, Greenlee D (1978) Effects of drugs on γ-aminobutyric acid receptors, uptake, release and synthesis in vitro. Brain Res 139:277–294
Olsen RW, Ticku MK, Greenlee D, Van Nees P (1979) GABA receptor and ionophore binding sites: interaction with various drugs. In: Krogsgaard-Larsen P, Scheel-Krüger J, Kofod H (eds) GABA-neurotransmitters. Munksgaard, Copenhagen, pp 165–178

Olsen RW, Leeb-Lundberg F, Napias C (1980) Pictrotoxin and convulsant binding site in mammalian brain. Brain Res Bull [Suppl 2] 5:217–221
Ostrovskaya RU, Molodavkin GM, Porfiryeva RP, Zubovskaya AM (1975) The mechanism of anticonvulsive action of diazepam (in Russian). Biull Eksp Biol Med 79:50–53
Ottoson JO (1955) The effect of xylocaine in electric convulsive treatment. Experientia 11:453–454
Peck EJ Jr, Miller AL, Lester BR (1976) Pentobarbital and synaptic high-affinity receptive sites for gamma-aminobutyric acid. Brain Res Bull 1:595–597
Perry JG, McKinney L, De Weer P (1978) The cellular mode of action of the anti-epileptic drug 5,5-diphenylhydantoin. Nature 272:271–273
Petsche H (1972) Zum Nachweis des kortikalen Angriffspunktes des antikonvulsiven Benzodiazepinderivats Clonazepam (Ro 5-4023) Z EEG EMG 3:145–153
Pieri L, Haefely W (1976) The effect of diphenylhydantoin, diazepam and clonazepam on the activity of Purkinje cells in the rat cerebellum. Naunyn-Schmiedebergs Arch Pharmacol 296:1–4
Pincus JH (1972) Diphenylhydantoin and ion flux in lobster nerve. Arch Neurol 26:4–10
Pincus JH (1977) Anticonvulsant actions at a neuromuscular synapse. Neurology (Minneap) 27:374–375
Pincus JH, Yaari Y, Argov Z (1980) Phenytoin: electrophysiological effects at the neuromuscular junction. In: Glaser GH, Penry JK, Woodbury DM (eds) Antiepileptic drugs: mechanisms of action. Advances in neurology 27. Raven, New York, pp 363–376
Polc P, Haefely W (1976) Effects of two benzodiazepines, phenobarbitone, and baclofen on synaptic transmission in the cat cuneate nucleus. Naunyn-Schmiedebergs Arch Pharmacol 294–121–131
Polc P, Möhler H, Haefely W (1974) The effect of diazepam on spinal cord activities: possible sites and mechanisms of action. Naunyn-Schmiedebergs Arch Pharmacol 284:319–337
Polc P, Laurent J-P, Scherschlicht R, Haefely W (1981) Electrophysiological studies on the specific benzodiazepine antagonist Ro 15-1788. Naunyn-Schmiedebergs Arch Pharmacol 316:317–325
Prince DA (1968) Inhibition in „epileptic" neurones. Exp Neurol 21:307–321
Prince DA, Wilder BJ (1967) Control mechanisms in cortical epileptogenic foci. „Surround" inhibition. Arch Neurol 16:194–202
Prince DA, Lux HD, Neher E (1973) Measurement of extracellular potassium activity in cat cortex. Brain Res 50:489–495
Przybyla AC, Wang SC (1968) Locus of central depressant action of idazepam. J Pharmacol Exp Ther 163:439–447
Puro DG, Woodward DJ (1973) Effects of diphenylhydantoin on activity of rat cerebellar Purkinje cells. Neuropharmacology 12:433–440
Raabe W, Gumnit RJ (1977) Anticonvulsant action of diazepam: increase of cortical postsynaptic inhibition. Epilepsia 18:117–120
Raines A, Anderson RJ (1976) Effects of acute cerebellectomy on maximal electroshock seizures and anticonvulsant efficacy of diazepam in the rat. Epilepsia 17:177–182
Raines A, Standaert FG (1966) Pre- and postjunctional effects of diphenylhydantoin at the cat soleus neuromuscular junction. J Pharmacol Exp Ther 153:361–366
Raines A, Standaert FG (1967) An effect of diphenylhydantoin on posttetanic hyperpolarization of intramedullary nerve terminals. J Pharmacol Exp Ther 156:591–597
Raines A, Standaert FG (1969) Effects of anticonvulsant drugs on nerve terminals. Epilepsia 10:211–227
Raines A, Sohn YJ, Levitt B (1971) Spinal excitatory and depressant effects of sodium diphenylthiohydantoinate. J Pharmacol Exp Ther 177:350–359
Ransom BR, Barker JL (1975) Pentobarbital modulates transmitter effects on mouse spinal neurones grown in tissue culture. Nature 254:703–705
Ransom BR, Barker JL (1976) Pentobarbital selectively enhances GABA-mediated postsynaptic inhibition in tissue cultured mouse spinal neurons. Brain Res 114:530–535
Richards CD (1972) On the mechanism of barbiturate anaesthesia. J Physiol (Lond) 227:749–767

Richards CD (1974) The action of general anaesthetics on synaptic transmission within the central nervous system. In: Halsey MJ, Miller RA, Sutton JA (eds) Molecular mechanisms in general anaesthesia. Churchill Livingstone, Edinburgh, pp 90–111

Ritchie JM (1975) Mechanism of action of local anesthetic agents and biotoxins. Br J Anaesthesiol 74:191–198

Ritchie JM (1979) A pharmacological approach to the structure of sodium channels in myelinated axons. Ann Rev Neurosci 2:341–362

Ritchie JM, Straub RW (1975) The hyperpolarization which follows activity in mammalian non-medullated fibres. J Physiol (Lond) 136:80–97

Roberts E (1980) Epilepsy and antiepileptic drugs: a speculative synthesis. In: Glaser GH, Penry KJ, Woodbury DM (eds) Antiepileptic drugs: mechanisms of action. Advances in neurology 27. Raven, New York, pp 667–713

Roldán E, Radil-Weiss T, Chocholová L (1971) The influence of barbiturates on paroxysmal EEG activity induced by hippocampal and/or thalamic cobalt foci. Psychopharmacologia (Berlin) 19:273–281

Rosenberg P, Bartels E (1967) Drug effects on the spontaneous electrical activity of the squid giant axon. J Pharmacol Exp Ther 155:532–544

Saad SF, El Masry AM, Scott PM (1972) Influence of certain anticonvulsants on the concentration of γ-aminobutyric acid in the cerebral hemispheres of mice. Eur J Pharmacol 17:386–392

Sabelli HC, Diamond BI, May J, Haudala HS (1977) Differential interactions of phenobarbital and pentobarbital with beta-adrenergic mechanisms in vitro and in vivo. Exp Neurol 54:453–466

Salt TE, Tulloch IF, Walter DS (1980) Anti-epileptic properties of sodium valproate in rat amygdaloid kindling. Br J Pharmacol 68:134P

Sato M, Austin GM, Yai H (1967) Increase in permeability of postsynaptic membrane to potassium produced by Nembutal. Nature 215:1506–1508

Schallek W, Kuehn A (1963) Effects of trimethadione, diphenylhydantoin and chlordiazepoxide on after-discharges in brain of cat. Proc Soc Exp Biol Med 112:813–817

Schallek W, Kuehn A (1965) An action of mogadon on the amygdala of the cat. Med Pharmacol Exp 12:204–208

Schallek W, Zabransky F, Kuehn A (1964) Effects of benzodiazepines on central nervous system of cat. Arch Int Pharmacodyn Ther 149:467–483

Schallek W, Thomas J, Kuehn A, Zabransky F (1965) Effects of mogadon on responses to stimulation of sciatic nerve, amygdala and hypothalamus of cat. Neuropharmacology 4:317–326

Schauf CL, Davis FA, Marder J (1974) Effects of carbamazepine on the ionic conductances of myxicola giant axons. J Pharmacol Exp Ther 189:538–543

Schlosser W (1971) Action of diazepam on the spinal cord. Arch Int Pharmacodyn Ther 194:93–102

Schlosser W, Franco S, Sigg EB (1975a) Differential attenuation of somatovisceral and viscerosomatic reflexes by diazepam, phenobarbital and diphenylhydantoin. Neuropharmacology 14:525–531

Schlosser W, Zavatsky E, Franco S, Sigg EB (1975b) Analysis of the action of CNS depressant drugs on somato-somatic reflexes in the cat. Neuropharmacology 14:517–523

Schmidt RF (1963) Pharmacological studies on the primary afferent depolarization of the toad spinal cord. Pflügers Arch 277:325–346

Schmidt RF (1964) The pharmacology of presynaptic inhibition. In: Progress in brain research vol 12, Elsevier, Amsterdam, pp 119–134

Schmidt RF (1971) Presynaptic inhibition in the vertebrate central nervous system. Ergeb Physiol 63:19–101

Schmidt RF, Vogel ME, Zimmermann M (1967) Die Wirkung von Diazepam auf präsynaptische Hemmung und andere Rückenmarksreflexe. Naunyn-Schmiedebergs Arch exp Path Pharmakol 258:69–82

Schmutz M, Olpe H-R, Koella WP (1979) Central actions of valproate sodium. J Pharm Pharmacol 31:413–414

Schoepfle GM (1957) Pentothal block of single nerve fibres and subsequent revival by means of anodal depolarization. Fed Proc 16:114
Scholfield CN (1977) Prolongation of post-synaptic inhibition by barbiturates. Br J Pharmacol 59:507P
Scholfield CN, Harvey JA (1975) Local anaesthetics and barbiturates: effects on evoked potentials in isolated mammalian cortex. J Pharmacol Exp Ther 195:522–531
Schwarz JR, Vogel W (1977) Diphenylhydantoin: excitability reducing action in single myelinated nerve fibres. Eur J Pharmacol 44:241–249
Seeman P, Chen S, Chau-Wong S, Staiman A (1974) Calcium reversal of nerve blockade by alcohols, anesthetics, tranquilizers and barbiturates. Can J Physiol Pharmacol 52:526–534
Seyama I, Narahashi T (1975) Mechanism of blockade of neuromuscular transmission by pentobarbital. J Pharmacol Exp Ther 192:95–104
Shanes AM (1958) Electrochemical aspects of physiological and pharmacological action in excitable cells. Part I. The resting cell and its alteration by extrinsic factors. Pharmacol Rev 10:59–164
Shapovalov AI (1964) Intracellular microelectrode investigation of effect of anesthetics on transmission of excitation in the spinal cord. Fed Proc 23:T113–T116
Sharer L, Kutt H (1971) Intravenous administration of diazepam. Effects on penicillin-induced focal seizures in the cat. Arch Neurol 24:169–175
Sherwin I (1973) Suppressant effects of diphenylhydantoin on the cortical epileptogenic focus. Neurology (Minneap) 23:274–281
Slater GE, Johnston GD (1978) Sodium valproate increases potassium conductance in *Aplysia* neurones. Epilepsia 19:379–384
Sohn RS, Ferrendelli JA (1976) Anticonvulsant drug mechanisms. Arch Neurol 33:626–629
Sohn YJ, Levitt B, Raines A (1970) Anticonvulsant properties of diphenylthiohydantoin. Arch Int Pharmacodyn Ther 188:284–289
Somjen G (1943) Effects of anesthetics of spinal cord of mammals. Anesthesiology 28:135–143
Somjen GG (1963) Effect of ether and thiopental on spinal presynaptic terminals. J Pharmacol Exp Ther 140:396–402
Somjen GG, Gill M (1963) The mechanism of the blockade of synaptic transmission in the mammalian spinal cord by diethyl ether and by thiopental. J Pharmacol Exp Ther 140:19–30
Spehlmann R, Colley B (1968) Effect of diazepam (Valium®) on experimental seizures in unanesthetized cat. Neurology (Minneap) 18:52–60
Staiman A, Seeman P (1964) The impulse-blocking concentrations of anesthetics, alcohol, anticonvulsants, barbiturates and narcotics on phrenic and sciatic nerves. Can J Physiol Pharmacol 52:535–557
Steiner FA, Hummel P (1968) Effects of nitrazepam und phenobarbital on hippocampal and lateral geniculate neurones in the cat. Neuropharmacology 7:61–69
Strasberg P, Krnjević K, Schwartz S, Elliott KAC (1967) Penetration of blood-brain barrier by γ-aminobutyric acid at sites of freezing. J Neurochem 14:755–760
Stratten WP, Barnes CD (1971) Diazepam and presynaptic inhibition. Neuropharmacology 10:685–696
Straub R (1956) Effects of local anaesthetics on resting potential of myelinated nerve fibres. Experientia 12:182–187
Straughan DW (1974) Convulsant drugs: amino acid antagonism and central inhibition. Neuropharmacology 13:494–508
Strichartz GR (1973) The inhibition of sodium currents in myelinated nerve by quaternary derivatives of lidocaine. J Gen Physiol 62:37–57
Strobos RRJ, Spudis EV (1960) Effects of anticonvulsant drugs on cortical and subcortical seizure discharges in cats. Arch Neurol 2:399–406
Suria A, Costa E (1973) Benzodiazepines and posttetanic potentiation in sympathetic ganglia of the bullfrog. Brain Res 50:235–239

Suria A, Costa E (1974) Diazepam inhibition of post-tetanic potentiation in bull frog sympathetic ganglia: possible role of prostaglandins. J Pharmacol Exp Ther 189:690–696
Suria A, Costa E (1975a) Action of diazepam, dibutyryl cGMP, and GABA on presynaptic nerve terminals in bull frog sympathetic ganglia. Brain Res 87:102–106
Suria A, Costa E (1975b) Diazepam depolarization of presynaptic terminals in bullfrog sympathetic ganglia: mediation through GABA? Psychopharmacol Bull 11:56–57
Swanson PD, Crane PO (1970) Diphenylhydantoin and the cations and phosphates of electrically stimulated brain slices. Neurology (Minneap) 20:1119–1123
Swanson PD, Crane PO (1972) Diphenylhydantoin and movement of radioactive sodium into electrically stimulated cerebral slices. Biochem Pharmacol 21:2829–2905
Takeuchi H (1969) Modifications par le phénobarbital des propriétés électriques du neurone à potentiel de membrane stable (neurone géant A d'*Aplysia*). CR Soc Biol (Paris) 162:488–490
Takeuchi H, Chalazonitis N (1968) Effects du phénobarbital sur les neurones autoactifs. CR Soc Biol (Paris) 162:491–493
Tappaz M, Pacheco H (1973) Effects de convulsivants et d'anticonvulsivants sur la capture de GABA^{14}C par les coupes de cerveau de rat. J Pharmacol (Paris) 4:295–306
Ten Bruggencate G, Engberg I (1971) Iontophoretic studies in Deiters nucleus of the inhibitory actions of GABA and related amino acids and the interactions of strychnine and pictrotoxin. Brain Res 25:431–448
Theobald W, Kunz HA (1963) Zur Pharmakologie des Antiepilepticums 5-carbamyl-5*H*-dibenzo [b.f.] azepin. Arzneimittelforsch 13:122–125
Theobald W, Krupp P, Levin P (1970) Neuropharmacologic aspects of the therapeutic action of carbamazepine in trigeminal neuralgia. In: Hassler R, Walker AE (eds) Trigeminal neuralgia: pathogenesis and pathophysiology. Thieme, Stuttgart, pp 107–114
Thesleff S (1956) The effect of anesthetic agents on skeletal muscle membrane. Acta Physiol Scand 37:335–349
Ticku MK (1980) Is the picrotoxinin binding site at the GABA synapse a site of action for barbiturates. Brain Res Bull [Suppl 2] 5:919–923
Ticku MK, Olsen RW (1977) Gamma-aminobutyric acid-stimulated chloride permeability in crayfish muscle. Biochim Biophys Acta 464:519–529
Ticku MK, Olsen RW (1978) Interaction of barbiturates with dihydropicrotoxinin binding sites related to the GABA receptor-ionophore system. Life Sci 22:1643–1652
Toman JEP (1949) The neuropharmacology of antiepileptics. EEG Clin Neurophysiol 1:33–44
Toman JEP (1952) Neuropharmacology of peripheral nerve. Pharmacol Rev 4:168–218
Toman JEP, Swinyard EA, Goodman LS (1946) Properties of maximal seizures, and their alteration by anticonvulsant drugs and other agents. J Neurophysiol 9:231–239
Tseng T-C, Wang SC (1971a) Locus of action of centrally acting muscle relaxants, diazepam and tybamate. J Pharmacol Exp Ther 178:350–360
Tseng T-C, Wang SC (1971b) Locus of central depressant action of some benzodiazepine analogues. Proc Soc Exp Biol Med 137:526–531
Van Dujn H, Beckmann MKF (1975) Dipropylacetic acid (Depakine®) in experimental epilepsy in the alert cat. Epilepsia 16:83–90
Vastola EF, Rosen A (1960) Suppression by anticonvulsants of focal electrical seizures in the neocortex. EEG Clin Neurophysiol 12:327–332
Vazquez AJ, Diamond BI, Sabelli HC (1975) Differential effects of phenobarbital and pentobarbital on isolated nervous tissue. Epilepsia 16:601–608
Vernadakis A, Parker KK (1980) Drugs and the developing central nervous system. Pharmacol Ther 11:593–647
Vernadakis A, Woodbury DM (1960) Effects of diphenylhydantoin and adrenocortical steroids on free glutamic acid, glutamine, and gamma-aminobutyric acid concentrations of rat cerebral cortex. In: Roberts E, Boxter CF, van Harreveld A, Wiersma CAG, Adey WR, Killam KF (eds) Inhibition in the nervous system and gamma-aminobutyric acid. Pergamon, New York, pp 242–248

Voskuyl RA, Ter Keurs HEDJ, Meinardi H (1975) Actions and interactions of dipropylacetate and penicillin on evoked potentials of excised prepiriform cortex of guinea pig. Epilepsia 16:583–592

Watson EL, Woodbury DM (1972) Effects of diphenylhydantoin on active sodium transport in frog skin. J Pharmacol Exp Ther 180:767–776

Weakly JN (1969) Effect of barbiturates on "quantal" synaptic transmission in spinal motoneurones. J Physiol (Lond) 204:63–77

Weinreich D (1971) Ionic mechanism of post-tetanic potentiation at the neuromuscular junction of the frog. J Physiol (Lond) 212:431–446

Wikler A (1945) Effects of morphine, nembutal, ether, and eserine on two-neuron and multineuron reflexes in the cat. Proc Soc Exp Biol Med 58:193–196

Wilson WA, Zbicz KL, Cote IW (1980) Barbiturates: inhibition of sustained firing in *Aplysia* neurons. In: Glaser GH, Penry JK, Woodbury DM (eds) Antiepileptic drugs: mechanisms of action. Advances in neurology 27. Raven, New York, pp 533–540

Withrow CD (1980) Oxazolidinediones. In: Glaser GH, Penry JK, Woodbury DM (eds) Antiepileptic drugs: mechanisms of action. Advances in neurology 27. Raven, New York, pp 577–586

Withrow CD, Stout RJ, Barton LJ, Beacham WS, Woodbury DM (1968) Anticonvulsant effects of 5,5-dimethyl-2,4-oxazolid-inedione (DMO). J Pharmacol Exp Ther 161:335–341

Woodbury DM (1955) Effect of diphenylhydantoin on electrolytes and radiosodium turnover in brain and other tissues of normal, hyponatremic and postictal rats. J Pharmacol Exp Ther 115:74–95

Woodbury DM (1980) Convulsant drugs: mechanisms of action. In: Glaser GH, Penry JK, Woodbury DM (eds) Antiepileptic drugs: mechanisms of action. Advances in neurology 27. Raven, New York, pp 249–303

Woodbury DM, Esplin DW (1959) Neuropharmacology and neurochemistry of anticonvulsant drugs. Proc Assoc Res Nerv Ment Dis 37:24–56

Woodbury DM, Kemp JW (1970) Some possible mechanisms of action of antiepileptic drugs. Pharmakopsychiat Neuro-Psychopharmakol 3:201–226

Zakusov VV, Ostrovskaya RV, Markovitch VV, Molodavkin GM, Bulayev VM (1975) Electrophysiological evidence for an inhibitory action of diazepam upon cat brain cortex. Arch Int Pharmacodyn Ther 214:188–205

Zukin SR, Young AB, Snyder SH (1974) Gamma-aminobutyric acid binding to receptor sites in the rat central nervous system. Proc Natl Acad Sci USA 71:4802–4807

Clinical Pharmacology of Antiepileptic Drugs

CHAPTER 24

Clinical Pharmacokinetics of Antiepileptic Drugs

E. PERUCCA and A. RICHENS

A. Hydantoin Drugs

I. Phenytoin

Among the various hydantoin compounds which have been tested for anticonvulsant activity in man, phenytoin is by far the most widely prescribed. Phenytoin is normally given orally, although parenteral administration may be occasionally used. Its pharmacokinetics has been studied extensively.

1. Pharmacokinetics in Adults

a) Absorption

Phenytoin, a weak acid with a pK_a of about 9, is poorly soluble in aqueous media. This poor solubility limits its rate of absorption from the gastrointestinal tract. Microcrystalline preparations, in which the crystal size has been substantially reduced, present a much greater area for dissolution to take place and therefore are better absorbed than phenytoin acid in the amorphous form. Absorption rate can also be enhanced by administering the sodium salt, which is more water soluble. In the acid medium of the stomach, phenytoin sodium precipitates rapidly as the acid, but the precipitate is finely divided and it is absorbed as well as the microcrystalline preparations. The most important determinant of phenytoin absorption is therefore particle size rather than whether it is given as an acid or as a salt (RICHENS 1979).

Due to the occurrence of saturation kinetics the quantitative determination of phenytoin bioavailability may require complex calculations (NEUVONEN 1979). Peak serum levels are usually attained between 2 and 12 h after oral dosing and the extent of absorption is high (80%–95% of the administered dose) (LUND et al. 1974; GUGLER et al. 1976; JUSKO et al. 1976). Some commercially available preparations, however, are absorbed to an extent much lower than this. In Scandinavia, one preparation containing phenytoin acid in amorphous form has been shown to be absorbed poorly as compared with other formulations containing the sodium salt (LUND 1974; TAMMISTO et al. 1976). Marked increases in serum phenytoin levels, sometimes associated with the development of clinical signs of intoxication, have been reported when patients stabilized on the former preparation were changed over to other formulations which were subsequently found to have greater bioavailability (LUND 1974). Problems with generic inequivalence between different formulations have been described in many other countries (for review, see NEUVONEN 1979). In an American study the innovator's preparation

(Parke-Davis) of phenytoin was found to have lower bioavailability than other preparations (Melikian et al. 1977). In Australia, clinically important changes in bioavailability have been reported as a result of a change in the excipient used during the manufacturing process (Tyrer et al. 1974).

The bioavailability of preparations containing phenytoin sodium is not necessarily greater than that of preparations containing the acid. In a British study a change from phenytoin sodium to phenytoin acid was found to cause a mean increase of 40% in serum phenytoin concentration (Stewart et al. 1975). The effect was most marked in patients with high serum phenytoin levels, as would be expected for a drug which shows saturation kinetics within the therapeutic concentration range. A rise in serum phenytoin levels after changing from one preparation containing the sodium salt to three preparations containing the acid has also been reported in a Finnish study (Tammisto et al. 1976). It should be emphasized, however, that in these two studies the molar dosage of phenytoin was approximately 10% higher for the acid than for the sodium salt (100 mg phenytoin sodium is equivalent to approximately 92 mg phenytoin acid). Because of the occurrence of saturation kinetics, this small difference in dose may be sufficient to cause appreciable and disproportionate changes in serum concentration.

There is suggestive evidence that the bioavailability of phenytoin is increased by intake of food and reduced in the presence of general malabsorption or concomitant administration of certain antacids (Melander 1978; Melander et al. 1979; Neuvonen 1979).

When phenytoin is administered intramuscularly, the drug precipitates within the tissues, and the absorption is slow and erratic (Wilensky and Lowden 1973; Kostenbauer et al. 1975; Wilder and Ramsey 1976). Changing to this route of administration for a few days (e.g. to cover an abdominal operation) may result in progressive fall in serum concentration with a swing to toxic levels on resumption of oral therapy, while absorption from the intramuscular sites continues. In order to maintain a constant serum phenytoin concentration, Wilder et al. (1974) recommend giving an intramuscular dose 50% higher than the patient's oral maintenance dose for the time necessary to cover the medical or surgical emergency. On resumption of oral therapy, a dose equivalent to half the original oral dose should then be given for the same period as that during which the intramuscular route was needed. Although this approach is pharmacokinetically sound, it does not avoid the problem of pain, tissue damage and haemorrhage after intramuscular injection of the drug. In the authors' opinion, intramuscular administration of phenytoin should be avoided altogether. If necessary, the drug may be given as an intravenous infusion.

b) Distribution and Plasma Protein Binding

The apparent volume of distribution of phenytoin is in the range of 0.5–0.8 litres/kg (Odar Cederlöf and Borgå 1974; Gugler et al. 1976). When the volume of distribution is calculated on the basis of the unbound concentration in serum values of 5–8 litres/kg are found: this indicates that phenytoin is highly bound to cellular structures, as would be expected from its high lipophilicity.

Following intravenous administration, phenytoin crosses the blood-brain barrier and enters the human brain rapidly (Wilder et al. 1977). In patients receiving chronic treatment, total brain concentrations are about 0.6–1.5 times the total serum concentration (HOUGHTON et al. 1975a; GOLDBERG and CRANDALL 1978; SIRONI et al. 1980). The existence of a positive correlation between the concentration in brain and in serum provides the rational basis for the usefulness of monitoring serum phenytoin levels.

In serum, phenytoin is reversibly bound (90% on average) to proteins, mainly albumin (PERUCCA 1980). The unbound fraction of the drug is virtually constant over the therapeutic serum concentration range. Early studies suggesting that the intersubject variation in the degree of binding is considerable have been criticized on methodological grounds (BARTH et al. 1976) and more recent results indicate that in normal subjects and otherwise healthy epileptic patients not receiving displacing agents, the interindividual variation in unbound fraction is relatively small (no more than twofold) (BARTH et al. 1976; YACOBI et al. 1977).

The factors affecting the binding of phenytoin to serum proteins have been reviewed by PERUCCA (1980). The unbound fraction of the drug correlates negatively with the plasma concentration of albumin (LUNDE et al. 1970; PORTER and LAYZER 1975), triglycerides and pre-β-lipoproteins (GUELEN and DEIMANN 1980) and positively with plasma bilirubin (HOOPER et al. 1974a) and α-lipoproteins (GUELEN and DEIMANN 1980). Binding is also dependent on temperature and plasma pH (LUNDE et al. 1970). The existence of a possible relationship between unbound phenytoin fraction and free fatty acid (FFA) concentration is controversial (FREDHOLM et al. 1975; BORGÅ et al. 1978; GIACOMINI et al. 1980). Conditions associated with reduced phenytoin binding include neonatal age (RANE et al. 1971; FREDHOLM et al. 1975), old age (HAYES et al. 1975), pregnancy (PERUCCA et al. 1981a), postoperative states (ELFSTROM 1977) and associated treatment with displacing agents (see Chap. 28).

The binding of phenytoin to plasma proteins is often reduced in patients with hepatic disease (HOOPER et al. 1974a; OLSEN et al. 1975; BLASHKE et al. 1975). This may be related to a combination of factors such as a decrease in plasma albumin concentration (BLASHKE et al. 1975), a displacing effect of bilirubin (HOOPER et al. 1974a) and possibly a change in conformational structure of the albumin molecule (WALLACE and BRODIE 1976). Because of the greater variability in unbound phenytoin fraction in these patients, the total plasma phenytoin levels are poorly correlated with either efficacy or toxicity (BLASHKE et al. 1975).

Reduced phenytoin binding also accompanies renal disease, and the degree of impairment of binding correlates inversely with the plasma albumin concentration and directly with the severity of renal failure as reflected by the serum creatinine level (REIDENBERG et al. 1971; EHRNEBO and ODAR-CEDERLÖF 1975; ODAR-CEDERLÖF and BORGÅ 1976). Plasma-binding capacity returns to near normal values within 10–15 days after renal transplantation (ODAR-CEDERLÖF 1977). The defect in binding capacity of uraemic plasma is only partially accounted for by a reduced albumin concentration, and a marked impairment can be demonstrated even in the presence of a normal albumin concentration (REIDENBERG et al. 1971). It is likely that endogenous inhibitors such as peptides which accumulate in uraemia may compete for binding sites on the albumin molecule (SJOHOLM et al. 1976; KINNIBURGH and BOYD 1981). As a result of this displacing effect, patients in renal failure have much lower serum phenytoin levels than non-uraemic controls (ODAR-CEDARLÖF and BORGÅ 1974). Since a greater proportion of the drug is in the free form, uraemic patients may have their seizures controlled at lower serum phenytoin levels than normal. REYNOLDS et al. (1976) suggested that a realistic optimal range of serum phenytoin levels in uraemia will probably be in the order of 5–10 μg/ml (20–40 μmol/litre).

Abnormally low degrees of phenytoin binding to plasma proteins have been reported by GUGLER and AZARNOFF (1976) in patients with nephrotic syndrome who showed no evidence of renal failure.

Phenytoin binds reversibly to the red cells (KURATA and WILKINSON 1974; EHRNEBO and ODAR-CEDERLÖF 1975). The amount of drug which penetrates the erythrocyte is proportional to the unbound concentration in plasma. Therefore, the blood/plasma concentration ratio (corrected for the haematocrit) can be used as an indirect index of the fraction of free drug in plasma (BORONDY et al. 1973; KURATA and WILKINSON 1974).

The unbound concentration of phenytoin has been shown to correlate well with the drug concentration in the CSF (TRIEDMAN et al. 1960; LUND et al. 1972; TROUPIN and FRIEL 1975). It has been suggested that a practical means of obtaining an estimate of the unbound phenytoin concentration is by determining the concentration of the drug in saliva, which correlates positively with both the unbound drug in plasma (BOCHNER et al. 1974; TROUPIN and FRIEDL 1975; REYNOLDS et al. 1976; MCAULIFFE et al. 1977; ANAVEKAR et al. 1979) and the drug concentration in the CSF (SCHMIDT and KUPFERBEG 1975; TROUPIN and FRIEL 1975; PAXTON et al. 1977a). The salivary/plasma ratio has been shown to be independent of changes in salivary flow (PAXTON et al. 1976, 1977a) and salivary pH (MUCKLOW et al. 1978). Although it has been suggested that phenytoin therapy can be more appropriately monitored by salivary rather than plasma concentrations, there are several problems. Salivary phenytoin levels are much lower than total plasma levels, and many laboratories cannot perform reliable measurements of such low concentrations (GRIFFITHS et al. 1980). Moreover, salivary phenytoin levels have generally been found to be more variable and erratic than plasma levels (BARTH et al. 1976; PAXTON et al. 1977b, PERUCCA et al. 1980a). Mixed salivary levels have been reported either to overestimate (BOCHNER et al. 1974; REYNOLDS et al. 1976) or underestimate (PAXTON et al. 1977a; ANAVEKAR et al. 1979) the free plasma concentration. With mixed saliva, differences in concentration may occur between the sediment and the supernatant, so that different results will be obtained depending on whether the homogenate or the clear supernatant is used for the analysis (ANAVEKAR et al. 1979). Other factors that may adversely affect the assay include the presence of sputum, food, food contaminants, protein-rich exudate (particularly in patients with gingivitis) and drug residues in the mouth (particularly with syrups and chewing tablets). The latter may be present for up to 3 h after dosing (AYERS and BURNETT 1977; PAXTON and FOOTE 1979). Some of these problems can be circumvented by measuring the concentration of the drug in parotid rather than mixed saliva. Even then, however, inconsistent results may be found, particularly at toxic concentrations (ANAVEKAR et al. 1979).

Phenytoin is excreted in tears at concentrations proportional to those found in plasma and in the CSF (MONACO et al. 1981).

Phenytoin is excreted in the breast milk of treated mothers. The milk/plasma ratio is in the range of 0.15–0.55 (MIRKIN 1971; RANE et al. 1974; KANEKO et al. 1979).

c) Metabolism and Urinary Excretion

Like other lipophilic drugs, phenytoin readily crosses biological membranes and therefore is extensively reabsorbed from the renal tubuli. Less than 5% of an administered dose of phenytoin is excreted unchanged in urine (GLAZKO et al. 1969; KARLEN et al. 1975; PERUCCA et al. 1980a). The proportion of the dose excreted unchanged increases with increasing serum concentration (HOUGHTON and RICHENS 1974a). The elimination of phenytoin from the body is dependent on the rate of metabolism, which takes place largely in the liver. The major catabolic pathway involves the para-hydroxylation of one of the phenol rings, leading to the formation of 5-*p*-hydroxyphenyl, 5-phenylhydantoin (p-HPPH) (BUTLER 1957). Other minor metabolites identified with variable degree of certainty in man include: 5,5-bis-(4-hydroxyphenyl)-hydantoin (THOMPSON et al. 1976), a dihydrodiol (ATKINSON et al. 1970; HORNING et al. 1971; GERBER et al. 1971), possibly formed by wave of an epoxide intermediate (GLAZKO 1973), a methylated catechol derivative (MIDHA et al. 1977) and an *N*-glucuronide of phenytoin (SMITH et al. 1977). A meta-hydroxylated derivative has also been found in human urine. This compound may be formed during the analytical procedure and therefore may not represent a true metabolite (ATKINSON et al. 1970; GERBER et al. 1971). Most of the hydroxylated metabolites are conjugated with glucuronic acid, excreted partly in the bile, and undergo enterohepatic circulation. These metabolites have little or no antiepileptic activity.

In epileptic patients, the serum concentration of conjugated p-HPPH is approximately $^1/_2$–$^1/_{20}$ that of the parent drug, but it may be increased as much as tenfold in the presence of impaired renal function. The serum concentration of unconjugated p-HPPH, on the other hand, is only 2%–6% of the phenytoin concentration and is increased only twofold in uraemia (HOPPEL et al. 1977; BORGÅ et al. 1979).

Small amounts of phenytoin and p-HPPH are excreted in the faeces (BOCHNER et al. 1972). Most of the administered dose can be recovered in urine as unchanged drug (<5%) or its biotransformation products. The percentage of the dose excreted as conjugated or unconjugated p-HPPH varies from about 20% to 90% (GLAZKO et al. 1969; BOROFSKY et al. 1973; KARLEN et al. 1975; PERUCCA et al. 1980a; SLOAN et al. 1981). The proportion of the drug excreted as the para-hydroxylated metabolite decreases with increasing dosage (HOUGHTON and RICHENS 1974; EADIE et al. 1976), in agreement with the evidence that this metabolic pathway is saturable (see below).

The metabolic oxidation of phenytoin is under genetic control, being probably influenced by the same D^H and D^L alleles that regulate the hydroxylation of debrisoquine (SLOAN et al. 1981). This suggests that impaired metabolism of phenytoin may occur in about 9% of the population, being transmitted as an autosomal recessive trait. Interethnic differences in rate of phenytoin metabolism occur (ANDOH et al. 1980; KROMANN et al. 1981).

The metabolism of phenytoin is dose dependent and hence better described by Michaelis-Menten than first-order kinetics (ARNOLD and GERBER 1970; ATKINSON and SHAW 1973; MAWER et al. 1974; RICHENS 1975; RICHENS and DUNLOP 1975; RAMBECK et al. 1979). The reason for this is that the para-hydroxylation pathway becomes easily saturated within the therapeutic serum concentration range. Individual estimates of K_m (the serum concentration at which 50% saturation occurs) and D_{max} (the maximum dose that can be metabolized) under in vivo conditions have been obtained (see below).

In animal experiments, p-HPPH (and the catechol metabolites) have been shown to inhibit phenytoin para-hydroxylation via a feedback mechanism (ASHLEY and LEVY 1972, 1973; GLAZKO 1973; LEVY 1976). However, no consistent changes in the clearance or half-life of phenytoin were found following prolonged infusion of p-HPPH in human volunteers (PERUCCA et al. 1978 a). These results, together with other lines of evidence from independent investigators (HOPPEL et al. 1977), suggest that the dose dependency of phenytoin metabolism in man is due to enzyme saturation rather than to feedback inhibition by metabolite formation.

d) Half-life and Clearance

Due to the occurrence of saturation kinetics, the decline in serum phenytoin concentration may not be log-linear and therefore a true half-life value cannot be calculated (RICHENS 1979). There are two ways of circumventing this problem. One is to administer a small dose of the drug, so that peak concentration is below the point at which saturation is important. Following intravenous administration of such doses to adult subjects, the decline in serum phenytoin concentration is usually biphasic, with a rapid distribution phase followed by a slower elimination phase (GUGLER et al. 1976; PERUCCA et al. 1980 a). The half-life of the distribution phase has been estimated to be about 0.6 ± 0.3 h (GUGLER et al. 1976). Irregularities with secondary peaks often complicate the interpretation of serum concentration data during the distributive phase (GATTI et al. 1977; PERUCCA et al. 1980 a): it is possible that these are related to an enterohepatic circulation of the drug (ALBERT et al. 1974). The elimination half-life of phenytoin after single-dose administration to normal volunteers or epileptic patients is usually in the range of 8–25 h and the plasma clearance 15–60 ml/h per kilogram (LUND et al. 1974; KOSTENBAUER et al. 1975; ROBINSON et al. 1975; GUGLER et al. 1976; GATTI et al. 1977; FRIGO et al. 1979; MAKKI et al. 1980; PERUCCA et al. 1980 a; KROMANN et al. 1981).

The drawback of determining phenytoin clearance and half-life after administration of single small doses is that the values obtained are not relevant to the therapeutic situation when, due to the occurrence of enzyme saturation, the elimination is much slower than this. The alternative approach used to circumvent this problem consists in administering a labelled tracer dose. The advantage of the latter technique is that the elimination of the tracer can be measured during steady state in a patient who is continued on a maintenance dose of the drug (HOUGHTON and RICHENS 1974). Provided that the serum phenytoin concentration remains constant throughout the sampling time, the disappearance of the tracer will not be accompanied by changes in the state of saturation of the enzyme and therefore a true half-life value can be calculated.

By using this technique, it can be shown that the half-life of phenytoin gradually lengthens as the serum concentration of unlabelled drug increases. Values of 20–60 h are frequently observed at therapeutic concentrations (Fig. 1), and a value of 140 h has been recorded in one intoxicated patient (HOUGHTON and RICHENS 1974; RICHENS 1979). The validity of this technique must be based on the assumption that the kinetics of the tracer are similar to the kinetics of unlabelled drug (i.e. that no "isotopic effect" is seen); however, BROWNE et al. (1981) have recently shown that 2[^{13}C]phenytoin and 1,3[^{15}N]phenytoin are handled in the same way as unlabelled drug.

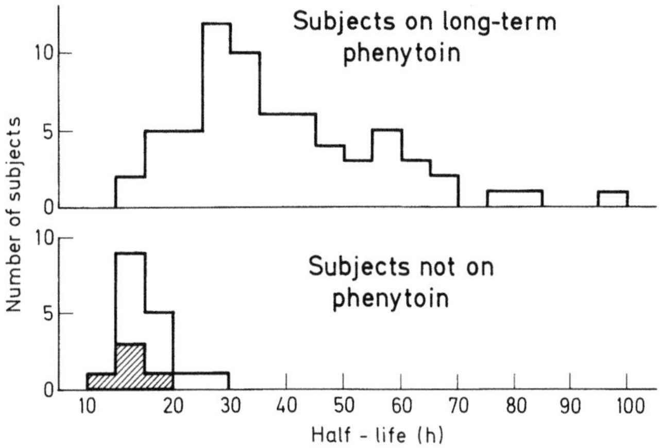

Fig. 1. Serum half-life of a tracer dose of phenytoin administered to 66 patients receiving maintenance therapy with the drug (*top*). Half-life values of the tracer in subjects not receiving unlabelled phenytoin are shown for comparison purposes. Five of the latter subjects were on phenobarbitone or primidone (*hatched*) while the remainder were drug-free healthy volunteers (RICHENS 1979)

Several factors are known to affect phenytoin elimination. Among these, genetic factors are particularly important (see above). Half-life values as long as 80 h have been occasionally described after single-dose administration in individuals with a deficient para-hydroxylating capacity (KUTT et al. 1964; PERUCCA et al. 1978a, 1980a; VASKO et al. 1980). Interethnic differences in phenytoin kinetics have been reported (ANDOH et al. 1980; KROMANN et al. 1981; LEE and CHAN 1981). KROMANN et al. (1981), for example, found that Eskimos have much shorter phenytoin half-lives and much higher clearance values than Danes.

Age is another important factor affecting phenytoin elimination. HOUGHTON et al. (1975) provided evidence that, in an adult population, the clearance of the drug decreases with increasing age. HAYES et al. (1975), on the other hand, found higher clearance values in elderly patients, but this observation must be interpreted in the light of the evidence that their patients had low albumin levels. Since phenytoin is subject to restrictive elimination, an increase in unbound fraction would be expected to result also in enhancement of the metabolic clearance.

There is some evidence that females show greater clearance values than males, but the difference is of little clinical importance (HOUGHTON et al. 1975). Kinetics in children are discussed below.

In pregnancy, serum phenytoin levels tend to fall (DAM et al. 1979), probably because of reduced binding to plasma proteins (PERUCCA et al. 1981 a) and increased clearance by both maternal and fetal livers.

In chronic hepatic disease the metabolism of phenytoin may be reduced and intoxication can occur (KUTT et al. 1964). Acute viral hepatitis was found not to affect phenytoin metabolism (BLASHKE et al. 1975) but infectious mononuclesis has been accompanied by an increase in phenytoin clearance (LEPPIK et al. 1979; BRAUN and GOLDSTONE 1980). Alcohol can both inhibit and induce phenytoin metabolism, the latter effect being unmasked on alcohol withdrawal (SANDOR et al. 1981).

e) Steady-State Serum Levels and Serum Level/Dose Relationship

In patients started on maintenance therapy, steady-state serum phenytoin levels are usually attained after 5–20 days. Since the half-life of phenytoin is longer at higher serum levels, the time to reach steady-state lengthens with increasing daily dose. If an immediate effect is required, a loading dose may be given (WILDER et al. 1973). The relatively long half-life of the drug implies that fluctuations in

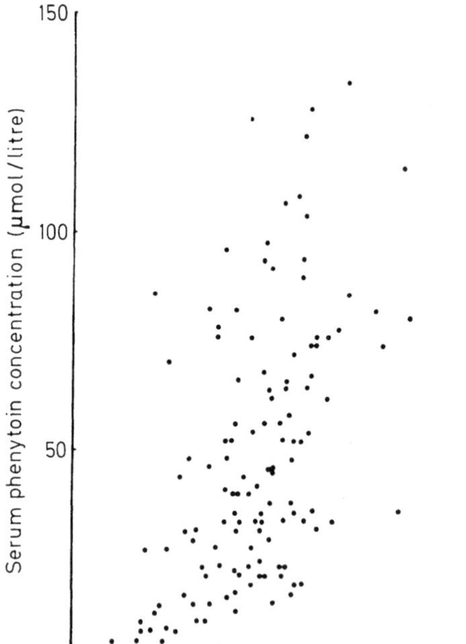

Fig. 2. Distribution of serum phenytoin concentrations in 131 epileptic patients on admission to a residential centre. Most were receiving other antiepileptic drugs in combination (RICHENS 1979)

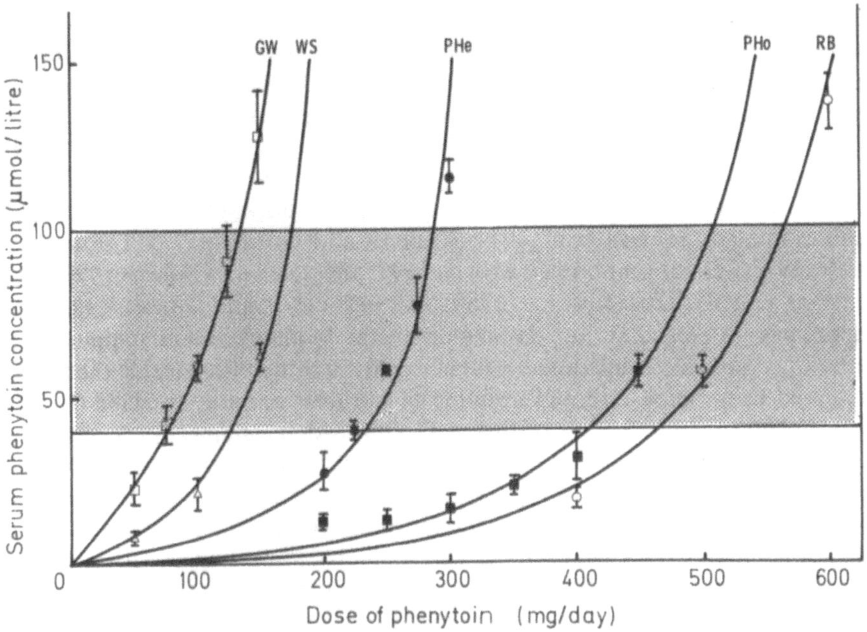

Fig. 3. Relationship between serum phenytoin concentration and daily dose in five epileptic patients. Each *point* represents the mean (±SD) of three to eight separate measurements of serum phenytoin at steady state. Curves were fitted by computer using the Michaelis-Menten equation. The *shaded area* corresponds to the therapeutic serum concentration range (the upper limit is slightly higher than that usually quoted) (RICHENS and DUNLOP 1975)

serum levels during the dose interval are not marked. Due to the dose-dependent elimination, the higher the steady-state serum concentration, the smaller (in percentage terms) is the degree of fluctuation. In most patients, once-daily dosing of the drug is adequate for clinical purposes (STRANDJORD and JOHANNESSEN 1974; COCKS et al. 1975).

There is a striking interindividual variability in steady-state serum phenytoin concentrations in patients receiving the same dose (Fig. 2). This is determined to a large extent by differences in rate of drug metabolism, the effect of which is exaggerated by the occurrence of saturation kinetics.

Within patients, the occurrence of saturation kinetics gives rise to a curvilinear relationship between steady-state concentration and dose (Fig. 3). The relationship is very steep within the therapeutic range of serum concentrations and even relatively minor adjustments in dosage can cause disproportionate changes in serum concentration. Due to the influence of genetic and environmental factors, the dose at which saturation is approached varies considerably from patient to patient. These findings are important in several ways: (1) dosage requirements need to be carefully individualized, ideally by monitoring the serum concentration; (2) if phenytoin therapy is regulated by monitoring the serum concentration, increments in dose should be no greater 50 mg when the concentration comes close to the therapeutic range (for the calculation of the desired dose adjustment see below); (3) serum concentrations within the therapeutic range are likely to be unstable because a few forgotten tablets or a small change in bioavailability will produce a disproportionate change in serum level; (4) the effects of drug interactions will be exaggerated; these interactions are considered in Chap. 28.

The non-linear relationship between dose and serum concentration makes phenytoin a difficult drug to use. Several methods for the calculation of the dosage increments necessary to produce a desired serum level have been proposed and evaluated (MAWER et al. 1974; RICHENS and DUNLOP 1975; LUDDEN et al. 1976, 1977; MARTIN et al. 1977; MULLEN 1978; MULLEN and FORSTER 1979; RAMBECK et al. 1979; DRIESSEN et al. 1980; VAN DER VELDE and DRIESSEN 1981). One approach is to calculate the parameters of the Michaelis-Menten equation (K_m and D_{max}) for each individual patient before treatment is started; the dosage required to produce a desired serum level can then be easily predicted (MAWER et al. 1974). A disadvantage of this method, however, is that several serum concentration measurements after administration of a single dose are required. Alternatively, individual K_m and D_{max} values can be derived from serum phenytoin levels at steady state provided that the serum concentration of the drug at at least two different daily dosages is known beforehand (LUDDEN et al. 1976, 1977; MULLEN 1978). An even more practical approach that requires the knowledge of only one serum concentration point is provided by the use of nomograms such as those proposed by RICHENS and DUNLOP (1975), MARTIN et al. (1977) and RAMBECK et al. (1979). The nomogram by RAMBECK et al. (1979) makes use of an average K_m value derived from a large population of patients. Its validity is based on the assumption that K_m does not vary among individuals and since this is clearly incorrect dosage predictions based on the nomogram will prove erroneous in some patients (VAN DER VELDE and DRIESSEN 1981). When only one serum concentration point is known, the accuracy of Richens and Dunlop's and Martin's nomograms is also limited. In a recent study, Richens and Dunlop's nomogram was reported to give the best predictions among various methods tested; even then, however, considerable inaccuracies were often found (DRIESSEN et al. 1980; VAN DER VELDE and DRIESSEN 1981).

2. Pharmacokinetics in Neonates, Infants and Children

Data on the gastrointestinal absorption of phenytoin in neonates and infants are controversial. While most authors agree on poor absorption of the drug during the 1st month of life (PAINTER et al. 1978), relatively high serum concentrations of phenytoin have been reported by LOUGHNAN et al. (1977) in some neonates of 1 week of age after oral administration of 8 mg/kg per day in suspension form (for a list of references on phenytoin absorption in the newborn see MORSELLI et al. 1980). In older infants and in children, phenytoin is well absorbed.

The serum unbound fraction of phenytoin is 1.5–2 times higher in normobilirubinaemic neonates than in adults and as a result serum levels of total drug provide a misleading underestimate of the concentration of pharmacologically active drug in these infants. The unbound fraction is increased even further in the presence of hyperbilirubinaemia (EHRNEBO et al. 1971; FREDHOLM et al. 1975). Values of protein binding close to those observed in adults are approached within the age of 3 months (LOUGHNAN et al. 1977). Reported values of apparent volume of distribution are in the order of 0.8 litres/kg (LOUGHNAN et al. 1977) or 1.2 ± 0.2 litres/kg (PAINTER et al. 1977) for neonates and 0.8 litres/kg for children (GARRETTSON and JUSKO 1975).

In neonates of epileptic mothers, the serum concentration of phenytoin at birth is comparable to that observed in the mother. Due to the occurrence of saturation kinetics, the decay of serum concentration is initially slow, but when the concentration has fallen to values below those at which saturation occurs, half-life values between 6 and 35 h are seen (RANE et al. 1974). This indicates that these neonates have a comparatively well-developed metabolizing capacity, probably due to transplacental autoinduction. Neonates not exposed to phenytoin in utero metabolize the drug much more slowly. The elimination may be particularly impaired in prematures. After 2–3 weeks of life, the phenytoin half-life in full-term neonates is in the range of 6–15 h, probably reflecting the maturation of the microsomal system. Infants older than 2 months have half-lives as short as 5–6 h (LOUGHNAN et al. 1977).

Throughout childhood, the elimination of phenytoin remains faster than that observed in adults. Like adults, however, children exhibit saturation kinetics within the clinically occurring serum concentration range (GARRETTSON and KIM 1970; DODSON 1980). Estimates of the Michaelis-Menten parameters have been determined in children by EADIE et al. (1976) and BLAIN et al. (1981). While K_m values were found to be similar in children and adults, D_{max} values were found to be markedly higher in children. After correction for differences in the ratio of liver weight to body weight in children and in adults, however, D_{max} values have been reported to be similar in the two groups. Important interethnic differences in phenytoin elimination in children occur (LEE and CHAN 1981).

One important implication of the faster elimination of phenytoin in infants and children is that paediatric patients require on average higher doses (in mg/kg body weight) than adults in order to achieve optimal serum levels (JALLING et al. 1970; HOOPER et al. 1973; BERMAN 1976). The optimal phenytoin dose (mg/kg body weight) increases with decreasing age. Body surface, however, may be a better guide to dosage than body weight in a paediatric population (RICHENS 1979).

Serum phenytoin levels usually show greater diurnal fluctuation in paediatric patients than in adults. Despite the suggestion that once daily dosing is adequate in children (BUCHANAN et al. 1973 b), more frequent administration may be necessary in some cases. As in adults, the attainment of steady-state serum levels may be accelerated by administering a loading dose at the onset of therapy; large initial doses have been associated with a high incidence of a concentration-dependent skin-rash (WILSON et al. 1976).

II. Mephenytoin (Methoin)

Mephenytoin (3-methyl-5-ethyl 5-phenylhydantoin) is rapidly absorbed from the gastrointestinal tract, peak serum levels occurring at 2–4 h after oral intake (PIPPENGER et al. 1978). In vivo, the drug is demethylated to 5-ethyl-5-phenylhydantoin (Nirvanol), which is itself an effective anticonvulsant (BUTLER and WADDELL 1958; KUPFERBERG and YONEKAWA 1975), known for its bone-marrow toxicity (JONES and JACOBS 1932). Nirvanol, in turn, is hydroxylated to 5-ethyl-5-(*p*-hydroxyphenyl)-hydantoin, which is excreted in urine (BUTLER 1956a). Direct parahydroxylation of mephenytoin also occurs (KÜPFER et al. 1980). Many other metabolites of mephenytoin have been described, including a dihydrodiol probably formed by way of an epoxide intermediate (GERBER et al. 1979). There is evidence that the elimination of Nirvanol is slower than that of mephenytoin. In two patients who had received mephenytoin, TROUPIN et al. (1976) reported Nirvanol half-lives of 74 an 144 h respectively. In one patient, the half-life of mephenytoin was 32 h. After starting chronic therapy, serum Nirvanol levels rise gradually over a period of a few weeks (BUTLER and WADDELL 1958). TROUPIN et al. (1976) found that during prolonged administration serum mephenytoin levels were only 8% of the combined mephenytoin-Nirvanol levels. Combined mephenytoin-Nirvanol levels in the saliva and in the cerebrospinal fluid were about 60% of the concentration in serum, suggesting a moderate degree of serum protein binding. It is likely that Nirvanol is responsible for a major part of the therapeutic and toxic effects seen in patients treated with mephenytoin.

III. Ethotoin

Ethotoin is rapidly absorbed from the gastrointestinal tract, peak serum levels being observed within 2–4 h after a single oral dose (SJÖ et al. 1975b). In epileptic patients the concentration of the drug in the cerebrospinal fluid is approximately 12% of the plasma concentration, suggesting extensive binding to plasma proteins (MIYAMOTO et al. 1975). Only a small amount of ethotoin is excreted unchanged in the urine of man. In dogs the major metabolic pathways involve the conversion to 5-phenylhydantoin, 3-ethyl-5-(*p*-hydroxyphenyl)-hydantoin and its glucuronide, and phenylhydantoic acid (DUDLEY et al. 1970). The dealkylated and para-hydroxylated metabolites have been identified in the urine of man (SJÖ et al. 1975).

SJÖ et al. (1975) provided evidence that ethotoin undergoes saturation kinetics. Following a single oral dose of 30 mg/kg the decline in serum concentration was not log-linear and showed an upward convexity. The elimination became first order at concentrations below 40 μmol/litre ($\sim$8 μg/ml). Half-life values calculated from this apparently terminal phase ranged from 3 to 6 h. SJÖ et al. (1975b) reported that in patients started on chronic treatment serum ethotoin levels tended to decrease in the 1st week in spite of a constant daily dose, possibly due to autoinduction. Within patients, the dose-level relationship is similar to that observed with phenytoin, increments in dose producing a disproportionately great rise in serum concentration (LUND et al. 1973; SJÖ et al. 1975b). A large interindividual variation is observed in the serum levels of patients receiving the same dose. Because of the relatively rapid elimination, serum levels fluctuate considerably even when the drug is given in three divided daily doses (LUND et al. 1973).

B. Barbiturates and Chemically Related Anticonvulsants

I. Phenobarbital (Phenobarbitone)

1. Pharmacokinetics in Adults

a) Absorption

Phenobarbital is well absorbed from the gastrointestinal tract (ALVIN et al. 1975). On the basis of available data, the oral bioavailability of conventional preparations of the drug is assumed to be high (80%–100%) (MORSELLI and FRANCO-MORSELLI 1980; POWELL et al. 1981). There are, however, commercially available formulations with low bioavailability (ALVARES et al. 1981). With most preparations, peak serum levels are usually attained 1–3 h after the intake of a single oral dose (VISWANATHAN et al. 1978; SANNITA et al. 1980), but may occur after as late as 12–18 h following ingestion of a large dose (LOUS 1954). MOOLENAAR et al. (1979) provided evidence that the free acid may be less rapidly and less reliably absorbed than the sodium salt.

Following intramuscular administration, the absorption profile of phenobarbital is similar to that observed after oral intake of a similar dose. The intramuscular bioavailability, however, may be slightly lower than the oral availability (VISWANATHAN et al. 1979).

The rectal absorption of phenobarbital in adults has been recently investigated (MOOLENAAR et al. 1979). Following rectal administration of the free acid or the sodium salt in aqueous dosage forms, peak serum phenobarbital levels were comparable with those observed after oral intake of a similar dose. The time required to achieve peak levels, however, was longer after rectal (3–4 h) than after oral administration (1–2 h). The rectal absorption of phenobarbital sodium from fatty suppositories was similar to that observed after rectal administration in aqueous form. A much slower absorption rate was observed if the free acid was used in the fatty suppository.

b) Distribution and Plasma Protein Binding

Phenobarbital has an apparent volume of distribution of about 0.6 litres/kg, which indicates a relatively extensive penetration into tissues (POWELL et al. 1981). The concentration of the drug in human brain is, at steady state, approximately 60%–110% of the serum level (SHERWIN et al. 1973; VAJDA et al. 1974; HOUGHTON et al. 1975a; SIRONI et al. 1980). Since phenobarbital is a weak acid with a pK_a of 7.2, its degree of ionization varies considerably within the physiological range of plasma and tissue pH. As un-ionized molecules have much greater lipid solubility and membrane permeability, a fall in plasma pH may result in an appreciable transfer of drug out of the circulation into the tissues. A transfer in the opposite direction is observed during alkalosis (WADDELL and BUTLER 1957a).

Phenobarbital is approximately 50% bound to serum proteins (LOUS 1954; WADDELL and BUTLER 1957; MCAULIFFE et al. 1977; CHEN et al. 1982). The concentration of the drug in the CSF is similar to the unbound concentration in plasma (JOHANNESSEN and STRANDJORD 1975a). The concentration of phenobarbital in saliva, on the other hand, is dependent not only on the unbound fraction in plasma but also on salivary pH. After correction for the difference in pH between plasma and saliva, salivary levels of phenobarbital can be used as an estimate of the free plasma concentration (MCAULIFFE et al. 1977; NISHIHARA et al. 1979).

In a mixed population of children and adults, MONACO et al. (1979) found a positive correlation between the concentration of phenobarbital in tears and that in plasma and CSF.

Phenobarbital is excreted in appreciable amounts in breast milk. The milk-plasma concentration ratio is in the range of 0.2–0.6 (KANEKO et al. 1979).

c) Metabolism and Urinary Excretion

Approximately 45%–65% of the administered dose of phenobarbital is metabolized (MORSELLI and FRANCO-MORSELLI 1980). A major metabolic pathway common to all species including man is the aromatic hydroxylation to para-hydroxyphenobarbital (BUTLER 1956b; WHYTE and DEKABAN 1977). This metabolite is pharmacologically inactive and is excreted in urine, partly in glucuronide form (KÅLLBERG et al. 1975). It has been suggested that another important metabolic pathway in man is the conversion to the *N*-glucoside (TANG et al. 1979). Other metabolites identified so far in man or other species include α-phenyl-γ-butyrolactone (ANDRESEN et al. 1976), a catechol derivative (HORNING et al. 1975), an hydroxyethyl derivative (HARVEY et al. 1972; GLAZKO 1975) and a dihydrodiol (HARVEY et al. 1972). The latter is probably formed by way of an epoxide intermediate.

The urinary excretion of unchanged phenobarbital is quantitatively important, since it accounts for about 20%–40% of the administered dose (MORSELLI and FRANCO-MORSELLI 1980). The renal excretion of the drug can be markedly increased by alkalinizing the urine or by increasing the rate of urinary flow (WADDELL and BUTLER 1957b; POWELL et al. 1981).

d) Half-life and Clearance

In adults the elimination half-life of phenobarbital ranges from 50 to 170 h and clearance values range from 2 to 13 ml/h per kilogram (LOUS 1954; BUTLER et al. 1954; ALVIN et al. 1975; MORSELLI and FRANCO-MORSELLI 1980; POWELL et al. 1981). Under most experimental conditions, the elimination of the drug has been found to follow a first-order process but there are a few reports suggestive of dose-dependent kinetics. VISWANATHAN et al. (1979) found that the half-life of phenobarbital following discontinuation of chronic treatment in three subjects was considerably longer than that observed in the same subjects following administration of a single dose. Further evidence that phenobarbital may show saturation kinetics has been presented by WILSON and WILKINSON (1973) and by EADIE et al. (1977a). If enzyme saturation occurs, however, its clinical implications are likely to be far less important than those seen in the case of phenytoin because a substantial amount of the administered dose of phenobarbital is excreted unchanged in urine. In the presence of reduced metabolizing capacity, the proportion of drug excreted unchanged in urine will rise and this will limit the extent to which accumulation can take place (ALVIN et al. 1975). Nevertheless, patients with cirrhosis or acute viral hepatitis have a longer plasma half-life than control subjects (ALVIN et al. 1975). Pregnancy is associated with an increased clearance of phenobarbital (MYGIND et al. 1976).

e) Steady-State Levels and Serum Level/Dose Relationship

The observation that phenobarbital has a long elimination half-life has two important therapeutic implications. First, serum phenobarbital levels fluctuate little during the dosing interval, and once daily administration is acceptable. Second, it may take up to 15–30 days for the serum levels to reach steady state following an adjustment in dosage. In patients being started on phenobarbital treatment, the time required to reach steady state can be reduced to less than 1 week by doubling the maintenance dose for the first 4 days (SVENSMARK and BUCHTHAL 1963). This practice, however, has the disadvantage of producing excessive sedation during the initial stages of treatment. When the maintenance dose is given from the beginning, the slow and gradual rise in serum levels is accompanied by the development of tolerance, and therefore central adverse effects are less common.

A considerable interindividual variation is observed in steady-state serum phenobarbital levels of patients receiving the same dose, although the scatter is not as great as that observed with phenytoin (EADIE et al. 1977; KAWASHIMA et al. 1980). The within-patient relationship between serum phenobarbital concentration and dosage has been little investigated. In one study, increments in phenobarbital dosage were found to produce, in some epileptic patients, a disproportionately great increase in serum concentration, but interpretation of these data was complicated by the observation that serum levels of phenobarbital metabolically derived from methylphenobarbital were linearly related to the dose of the latter compound (EADIE et al. 1977a). In a more recent study, PERUCCA et al. (1981b) found that doubling the phenobarbital dose from 15 to 30 mg/day in four subjects caused a consistent doubling of the steady-state serum concentration of the drug. These doses, however, are relatively low compared with those normally used in the treatment of epilepsy.

2. Pharmacokinetics in Neonates, Infants and Children

In the neonate, phenobarbital is absorbed relatively rapidly when given by the intramuscular route (WALLIN et al. 1974; BRACHET-LIERMAIN et al. 1975). The drug is absorbed from the gastrointestinal tract during the 1st few days of extrauterine life (WALLIN et al. 1974); relatively high serum phenobarbital levels were achieved giving 3 mg/kg intramuscularly on the day of birth followed by 5 mg/kg per day orally for the next 6 days. BOUTROY et al. (1980) found peak serum phenobarbital levels of 53 ± 16 µmol/litre (12.4 ± 3.8 µg/ml) following administration of a single dose of 12 mg/kg by nasogastric tube to premature and full-term neonates in the first 3 h of extrauterine life for the prophylaxis of hyperbilirubinaemia. The absorption of phenobarbital following oral administration in neonates is slower and less predictable than that following intramuscular administration (MORSELLI 1977b), but in older infants and in children, the absorption is more rapid and efficient (JALLING 1974).

The rectal absorption of phenobarbital in infants and children has been investigated by HEIMANN et al. (1978). The sodium salt was found to be relatively well absorbed from fatty suppositories. Average times required to achieve peak serum levels were 2.2, 3.3 and 4.2 h depending on the formulation used. The absorption of the free acid from the same suppository forms was considerably slower.

The binding of phenobarbital to plasma protein is reduced in the newborn, particularly in the presence of high bilirubin levels (EHRNEBO et al. 1971). This implies that, at any given serum level of total drug, the concentration of pharmacologically active drug is higher in newborns than in adults. The apparent volume of distribution is also increased during the first 2–3 months of life (HEIMANN and GLADTKE 1977).

The elimination half-life of phenobarbital may be prolonged in neonates, particularly those born prematurely. Half-life values of 60–200 h, with extremes up to 400 h, have been observed during the first few days of extrauterine life (JALLING et al. 1973; WALLIN et al. 1974; HEIMANN and GLADTKE 1977; BOREUS et al. 1978; PITLICK et al. 1978; BOUTROY et al. 1980). The slow elimination in these neonates is probably due to decreased renal excretion as well as to incomplete maturation of the drug-metabolizing enzymes. During the first few weeks of life the half-life of phenobarbital shortens progressively; values between 30 and 130 h are reported between the ages of 2 months and 5 years (GARRETTSON and DAYTON 1970; JALLING 1974; HEIMANN and GLADTKE 1977; PAINTER et al. 1978). In five children aged 5–10 years, MORSELLI (1977b) found half-life values ranging from 21 to 78 h. These data indicate that infants and children eliminate the drug more rapidly than adults and they require a higher dose (on a body weight basis) to produce a given serum level (SVENSMARK and BUCHTHAL 1964; ROSSI et al. 1979). Due to the long half-life of the drug, once daily dosing is acceptable also in children (WALSON et al. 1980).

II. Methylphenobarbital (Mephobarbital)

a) Absorption

Methylphenobarbital (mephobarbital) is rapidly absorbed from the gastrointestinal tract (EADIE et al. 1978; HOOPER et al. 1981). Following the ingestion of a single dose, peak serum levels are usually attained within 6–8 h. Although the oral availability of the drug has been little investigated, a critical evaluation of available data (BUTLER and WADDELL 1958) suggests that this is incomplete. In a recent study in which single doses of methylphenobarbital were given both orally and intravenously to two normal subjects, the oral bioavailability was estimated to be 70% and 75% respectively (HOOPER et al. 1981).

b) Distribution

The apparent volume of distribution of methylphenobarbital is very high (about 2 litres/kg), which is in accordance with the high lipid solubility of this drug (EADIE et al. 1978; HOOPER et al. 1981).

c) Metabolism and Urinary Excretion

Methylphenobarbital is extensively metabolized in the body. Only 1%–2% of the administered dose is excreted unchanged in urine (SVENDSEN and BROCHMAN-

HANSSEN 1962; EADIE et al. 1978). Two major metabolic pathways have been identified: demethylation to phenobarbital and para-hydroxylation to *p*-hydroxymethylphenobarbital (p-HMP).

After administration of a single oral dose of methylphenobarbital, phenobarbital appears in serum within a few hours and reaches peak levels in 3–8 days, at a time when the concentration of the parent drug has already declined to low values (EADIE et al. 1978; HOOPER et al. 1981). In patients treated with barbiturates or other enzyme-inducing antiepileptic drugs, the demethylation takes place at a faster rate so that peak serum phenobarbital levels occur earlier and are considerably higher (EADIE et al. 1978). The urinary excretion of the metabolites of methylphenobarbital is still incompletely known. In two normal subjects, HOOPER et al. (1981) found that about 30% of a single oral dose of methylphenobarbital was excreted in urine as p-HMP during the following 10 days; the fraction of the dose recovered in urine as phenobarbital and *p*-hydroxyphenobarbital over the same period was below 10%. Other metabolites of phenobarbital were not measured and therefore no reliable quantitation of the demethylation process could be obtained. There is evidence, however, that in patients receiving long-term treatment with methylphenobarbital or other enzyme-inducing drugs, the rate of conversion to phenobarbital is higher than that observed in normal subjects given a single dose. In these chronically treated patients, up to 50% of an administered dose of methylphenobarbital may in fact be converted to phenobarbital (EADIE et al. 1978).

d) Half-life

The elimination half-life of methylphenobarbital ranges from 30 to 70 h (HORNING et al. 1975; EADIE et al. 1978; HOOPER et al. 1981). Considerably shorter values (10–30 h), however, have been described in patients receiving concurrent treatment with enzyme-inducing drugs (EADIE et al. 1978). In two normal subjects given a single intravenous dose of the drug, clearance values were found to be 0.03 and 0.04 litres/kg per hour respectively (HOOPER et al. 1981). Higher values may be found in induced patients.

e) Steady-State Serum Levels and Serum Level/Dose Relationship

Steady-state serum levels of the parent drug are expected to be achieved in 3–15 days of starting therapy. The times necessary to achieve steady-state serum levels of phenobarbital are appreciable longer (up to 4–5 weeks) and give rise to concentrations that exceed those of methylphenobarbital by a factor of 3–10 (EADIE et al. 1978) or more (KUPFERBERG and LONGACRE-SHAW 1979). EADIE et al. (1977a, 1978) have shown that steady-state serum levels of both compounds are positively correlated with the methylphenobarbital dose, although the interindividual variation in the serum levels observed at any given dose is considerable. Within patients, the relationship between the dose of methylphenobarbital and the serum levels of both parent drug and metabolically derived phenobarbital is linear. Although methylphenobarbital itself has antiepileptic properties, it is likely that the pharmacological effects of the drug are largely mediated by phenobarbital.

III. Eterobarbital

Eterobarbital (dimethoxymethylphenobarbital) is a barbiturate derivative that has been claimed to be as effective as, but less sedating than, phenobarbital. The disposition of this compound in man has been investigated by GOLDBERG et al. (1979). They found that eterobarbital is entirely degraded in the gastrointestinal tract or, more likely, in the portal circulation during its first passage through the liver. Degradation occurs in two steps: first the monomethoxymethyl metabolite is formed; then this is metabolized to phenobarbital. Monomethoxy-methylphenobarbital has a very short half-life and is present in the circulation in very low concentrations during chronic therapy. Eterobarbital itself is not detectable in serum, whereas phenobarbital accumulates in substantial amounts. It appears therefore that the pharmacological effects of eterobarbital are largely, if not entirely, mediated by metabolically derived phenobarbital.

IV. Primidone

Primidone is a desoxybarbiturate that is partly converted to phenobarbital in vivo. The drug is invariably used by the oral route.

1. Pharmacokinetics in Adults

a) Absorption

Primidone is rapidly absorbed from the gastrointestinal tract, peak serum levels being attained between 0.5 and 7 h following a single oral dose (BOOKER et al. 1970; GALLAGHER et al. 1972; CLOYD et al. 1981). Studies based on the urinary recovery of unchanged drug and metabolites in children indicate that at least 90% of an orally administered dose is absorbed (KAUFFMAN et al. 1977). In one study, no important diffferences in oral biovailability between various formulations were found (BORST and LOOKWOOD 1975).

b) Distribution and Plasma Protein Binding

Primidone distributes evenly in all organs and tissues. The apparent volume of distribution of the drug is estimated to be approximately 0.6 litres/kg (MORSELLI and FRANCO-MORSELLI 1980). Brain concentrations have been found to be around 90% of the serum concentrations (HOUGHTON et al. 1975 a).

Information on the degree of binding of primidone to plasma proteins is conflicting. In an early study, BAUMEL et al. (1972) reported that neither primidone nor the metabolite phenylethylmalonamide (PEMA) bind to any significant extent to plasma proteins. MCAULIFFE et al. (1977), however, found that in 21 patients receiving chronic treatment with primidone the fraction of the drug bound to plasma proteins was about 35% (CHEN et al. 1982). The plasma protein binding of phenobarbital is about 50% (WADDELL and BUTLER 1957a).

The concentration of primidone in saliva and in cerebrospinal fluid has been shown to be positively correlated with the concentration in plasma. Salivary and cerebrospinal fluid/plasma ratios are in the range of 0.7–1 (HOUGHTON et al. 1975 a; TROUPIN and FRIEL 1975; SCHOTTELIUS and FINCHAM 1977; MCAULIFFE et al. 1977; MONACO et al. 1981). BARTELS et al. (1979) showed that the salivary/plasma ratio of primidone is dependent on the salivary flow, at variance with data previously reported by SCHMIDT and KUPFERBERG (1975). The discrepancy could be attributed to differences in the collection technique.

MONACO et al. (1981) reported a tears/plasma primidone concentration ratio of 0.45 ± 0.3 in 28 patients.

Primidone has been detected in the breast milk of nursing mothers treated with the drug. The milk/serum concentration ratio is in the order of 0.6–1.0 (KANEKO et al. 1979).

c) Metabolism and Urinary Excretion

In man, primidone is partly metabolized to PEMA and phenobarbital and partly excreted unchanged in urine. Crystalluria has been observed in cases associated with acute primidone intoxication (BAILEY and JATLOW 1972; BRILLMAN et al. 1974; CATE and TENSER 1975). Little information is available on the fraction of the administered dose which is metabolized in adults. Studies based on the urinary recovery of primidone and its metabolites in children receiving chronic therapy with the drug indicate that 15%–65% of the dose is excreted unchanged in urine, 16%–65% is converted to PEMA and only 1%–8% is converted to phenobarbital (KAUFFMAN et al. 1977). Induction of primidone metabolism has been demonstrated (see Chap. 28). The metabolism of the drug is faster after multiple doses than after a single dose, but this effect seems to be inconsistent (CLOYD et al. 1981).

After administration of a single oral dose of primidone to patients treated with other antiepileptic drugs, PEMA can be detected in the circulation within 24 h (CLOYD et al. 1981). Phenobarbital also appears within a few hours (EADIE and TYRER 1980). In patients not receiving other antiepileptic drugs, the appearance of detectable amounts of PEMA and phenobarbital in the circulation may be delayed more than 24 and 48 h respectively (CLOYD et al. 1981).

Both PEMA and phenobarbital have a longer half-life than primidone and therefore accumulate in serum during chronic administration. It is likely that a large proportion of the pharmacological activity in patients treated with primidone is due to metabolically derived phenobarbital. In animal studies, PEMA has been shown to have anticonvulsant activity of its own, which may be synergic with that of phenobarbital (BAUMEL et al. 1972). It is unclear, however, whether PEMA contributes significantly to the overall pharmacological activity of primidone in man.

d) Half-life and Clearance

Primidone is eliminated according to a first-order process with a half-life value ranging from 4 to 22 h (BOOKER et al. 1970; BAUMEL et al. 1972; BRILLMAN et al. 1974; SCHOTTELIUS and FINCHAM 1978; CLOYD et al. 1981). CLOYD et al. (1981) found that in patients receiving concurrent therapy with other antiepileptic drugs primidone half-lives (8 ± 3 h) were considerably shorter than in patients given a single primidone dose in the absence of associated therapy (15 ± 5 h). In the same study, clearance values determined after a single oral dose were reported to average 35 ml/kg per hour and 52 ml/kg per hour respectively. These values were calculated on the assumption that absorption was complete and therefore they may be overestimates. In patients started on single-drug therapy, there was a trend for clearance values to be higher after multiple- than after single-dose administration.

Following administration of primidone, the half-life of the metabolite PEMA ranges from 17 to 36 h (BAUMEL et al. 1972; GALLAGHER et al. 1972). These values are overestimates because PEMA was still being formed during the period of sampling. After administration of PEMA itself, half-life values are shorter and vary from 10 to 25 h (COTTRELL et al. 1982).

e) Steady-State Serum Levels and Serum Level/Dose Relationship

Steady-state serum primidone levels are usually attained within 2 days following initiation of treatment. Steady-state levels of PEMA are reached within about 1 week. In the case of metabolically derived phenobarbital, it may take 15–25 days before a stable concentration is obtained. This time factor needs to be taken into account in view of the evidence that the pharmacological action of primidone is largely, if not entirely, mediated by its conversion to phenobarbital.

Patients receiving the same primidone dose show large differences in the serum primidone levels achieved at steady state. These differences are related partly to the difficulty in standardizing precisely the sampling time in respect to the marked fluctuations during the dosing interval and partly to interpatient variability in the absorption and disposition of the drug (SCHOTTELIUS and FINCHAM 1978). GALLAGHER and BAUMEL (1972) suggested that increments in primidone dose can result in disproportionate changes in the serum concentration, possibly due to saturation of the enzyme system responsible for the conversion to phenobarbital. This suggestion, which was based on the comparison between different groups of patients, remains to be confirmed in a within-subject study.

There is statistically significant positive correlation between the administered dose of primidone and the serum concentration of metabolically derived phenobarbital, although the degree of interindividual variation is considerable (EADIE et al. 1977 a). At steady state the serum concentration of phenobarbital is always greater than that of primidone, but the precise ratio between the two varies greatly from one patient to another and also within the same patient, depending on the time of sampling and the influence of associated anticonvulsant therapy. REYNOLDS et al (1975) and SCHOTTELIUS and FINCHAM (1978) found that in patients receiving maintenance therapy with primidone alone serum phenobarbital levels were on average 35%–60% higher than those of the parent drug. In patients receiving phenytoin in combination, serum primidone levels were reduced and serum phenobarbital levels were increased. Serum phenobarbital levels in these patients were two to four times higher than those of the parent drug, suggesting an increased metabolic conversion of primidone into phenobarbitone. These results have recently been confirmed by HEIPERTZ et al. (1979). These authors, however, reported serum phenobarbital: primidone ratios considerably greater than those observed by the other groups. In addition to phenytoin, carbamazepine also appears to stimulate the conversion of primidone to phenobarbital. In most patients, a primidone dose ranging from 5 to 15 mg/kg per day appears to be required in order to produce a concentration of phenobarbital around 85 μmol/litre (~20 μg/ml) (EADIE et al. 1977; SCHOTTELIUS and FINCHAM 1978). The same level can also be achieved with a phenobarbital dose of 1–2 mg/kg.

Information on the steady-state serum concentration of PEMA in patients treated with primidone is relatively scarce. BAUMEL et al. (1972) and HAIDUKE-

WYCH and RODIN (1980) found that in large populations of patients PEMA levels were on average similar to primidone levels. Similar observations were made by HEIPERTZ et al. (1979) in patients receiving primidone in combination with phenytoin; in patients treated with primidone alone, PEMA levels were on average approximately one-half the primidone levels.

2. Pharmacokinetics in Neonates, Infants and Children

Neonates of mothers taking primidone have at birth serum levels of primidone, PEMA and phenobarbital comparable with those observed in the mother. The disposition of transplacentally acquired primidone and its metabolites has been investigated by NAU et al. (1980). In six neonates, primidone was excreted with a half-life of 23 ± 10 h, which is longer than that found in adults. The half-life of PEMA was 35 ± 6 h. Phenobarbital half-lives ranged from 70 to 160 h.

KAUFFMAN et al. (1977) studied the disposition of primidone in 12 children aged 7–14 years. Half-life values in these children were comparable with those described in adults. The urinary recovery of primidone and its metabolites in urine (see p. 679) suggested that the oral absorption of the drug was virtually complete. BATTINO et al. (1980) found that at steady state children had a lower primidone serum level/dose ratio than adults.

COTTRELL et al. (1982) reported a PEMA half-life value of 16 h in a 10-year-old child given a single oral dose of PEMA.

The kinetics of phenobarbital in neonates, infants and children is discussed in Sect. B.I.2.

C. Carbamazepine

Carbamazepine is a dibenzazepine derivative structurally related to the tricyclic antidepressants. The drug is always given by the oral route. Its pharmacokinetics have been extensively investigated.

1. Pharmacokinetics in Adults

a) Absorption

Due to lack of a preparation suitable for intravenous use, no information is available on the absolute bioavailability of carbamazepine in man. There is evidence, however, that the gastrointestinal absorption of the drug is slow, irregular and possibly incomplete (PALMER et al. 1973; LEVY et al. 1975; STRANDJORD and JOHANNESSEN 1975; BERTILSSON 1978). Following administration of a single oral dose in tablet form, peak serum levels are usually obtained after 4–18 h (KAUKO and TAMMISTO 1974; MORSELLI et al. 1975), sometimes after as late as 24–35 h (FAIGLE and FELDMAN; GERARDIN and HIRZ 1976; COTTER et al. 1977). Since carbamazepine is poorly soluble in aqueous media, it is likely that the delayed absorption is due to a slow dissolution rate which, in turn, is dependent on the particle size of the drug (RICHTER and TERHAAG 1978). Based on the recovery of radio-labelled drug in urine and faeces, FAIGLE and FELDMANN (1975) calculated that the fraction absorbed from gelatine capsules is at least 70%. However, considerable differences in rate and/or extent of absorption between different formulations have been described (LEVY et al. 1975; RICHTER and TERHAAG 1978; ANTTILA et al. 1979; DAN et al. 1981). LEVY et al. (1975) reported that the bioavailability of single doses of carbamazepine is enhanced by food but these findings could not be confirmed after repeated administration (TEDESCHI et al. 1981).

The possibility that carbamazepine shows dose-dependent absorption has been commented upon by several investigators. It is known that the time required to reach maximal concentrations increases considerably with increasing doses (GERARDIN et al. 1976; COTTER et al. 1977). In a patient who ingested an overdose of 20 g, peak serum carbamazepine levels were attained after as late as 3 days (GRUSKA et al. 1971). Although the fraction absorbed is likely to remain constant with single doses ranging from 50 to 400–600 mg (RAWLINS et al. 1975; LEVY et al. 1975; GERARDIN and HIRZ 1976), at higher doses bioavailability may be reduced (LEVY et al. 1975). Dose-dependent absorption during chronic administration would be consistent with the suggestion that the bioavailability of carbamazepine might be increased by increasing the frequency of administration whilst maintaining the total daily dose constant, but evidence in support of the latter hypothesis is conflicting. Perhaps the most convincing evidence of dose-dependent absorption during chronic therapy comes from the observation that the increase in serum carbamazepine levels is often lower than expected from the increment in dose (PERUCCA et al. 1980 b).

b) Distribution and Plasma Protein Binding

Carbamazepine is a neutral and fairly lipophilic compound that diffuses easily across biological membranes. The volume of distribution of the drug determined after oral administration ranges from 0.8 to 4 litres/kg (PALMER et al. 1973; EICHELBAUM et al. 1975; MORSELLI et al. 1975; RAWLINS et al. 1975; COTTER et al. 1977; WESTENBERG et al. 1978). These figures have been calculated on the assumption that absorption is complete and therefore may represent slight overestimates.

In rats, carbamazepine distributes uniformly in various organs, the highest concentration being found in the liver and the kidney (MORSELLI and FRIGERIO 1975). In brain tissue of epileptic patients the drug is found at concentrations which are approximately 50% higher than in plasma (FRIIS et al. 1978). In non-epileptic patients undergoing brain surgery for removal of cerebral tumour, MORSELLI et al. (1977) found higher carbamazepine brain: plasma ratios in the parieto-occipital area than in the temporal area. Brain: plasma concentration ratios of approximately 1–2 have been reported for the active metabolite carbamazepine-10,11-epoxide (MORSELLI et al. 1977; FRIIS et al. 1978).

Carbamazepine is about 65%–80% bound to plasma proteins (DI SALLE et al. 1974; HOOPER et al. 1975; RAWLINS et al. 1975; JOHANNESSEN et al. 1976; MCAULIFFE et al. 1977; MACKICHAN et al. 1981). Over the therapeutic plasma concentration range, the degree of binding is virtually constant (HOOPER et al. 1975; RAWLINS et al. 1975; JOHANNESSEN et al. 1976; MACKICHAN et al. 1981). The plasma protein binding of the epoxide metabolite is generally lower (30%–80%) (MORSELLI et al. 1975; JOHANNESSEN et al. 1976; MACKICHAN et al. 1981); in one study, the free fraction of the epoxide was shown to correlate positively with the free fraction of the parent compound (MACKICHAN et al. 1981). None of the currently used antiepileptic drugs appear to influence carbamazepine binding to a clinically significant extent (MORSELLI et al. 1975; HOOPER et al. 1975). The free fraction of the drug is normal in patients with renal disease and only marginally increased in patients with hepatic disease (HOOPER et al. 1975).

HOOPER et al. (1975) found that the concentration of carbamazepine in red cells was only 38% ± 18% of the plasma concentration. The 10,11-epoxide metabolite has been reported not to enter the red cell to any important extent (PYNNONEN and YRJANA 1977).

The relationship between the concentrations of carbamazepine in plasma and in saliva has been examined by several investigators. In general, salivary levels of both carbamazepine and carbamazepine-10,11-epoxide have been shown to correlate positively with the respective total and free concentrations in plasma (PYNNONEN 1977; MCAULIFFE et al. 1977; RYLANCE et al. 1977; WESTENBERG et al. 1978; MACKICHAN et al. 1981). On average, the concentration of carbamazepine in saliva is about 26%–27% of the total plasma concentration. For the epoxide, the average salivary : plasma ratio is about 0.40 (MACKICHAN et al. 1981). Since saliva can be considered as a natural ultrafiltrate of plasma, the suggestion has been made that salivary levels could provide a reliable indicator of the free concentration in plasma. Support for this hypothesis is provided by the observation that salivary levels of both carbamazepine and its 10,11-epoxide correlate better with the free than with the total plasma levels of these compounds (MACKICHAN et al. 1981). The concentrations of carbamazepine and the 10,11-epoxide metabolite in saliva, however, have often been found to be higher than their respective free plasma concentrations, possibly due to evaporation of saliva in the mouth during the collection procedure (TROUPIN and FRIEL 1975; MACKICHAN et al. 1981).

The concentration of carbamazepine and its 10,11-epoxide in CSF also provides an indication of their free concentration in plasma (TROUPIN and FRIEL 1975). Published figures for CSF: plasma concentration ratios are in the order of 0.2–0.3 for carbamazepine and 0.3–0.7 for the metabolite (JOHANNESSEN and STRANDJORD 1972; EICHELBAUM et al. 1976; JOHANNESSEN et al. 1976).

MONACO et al. (1979) found a positive correlation between the concentration of carbamazepine in tears and those in plasma and in the CSF.

The concentration of carbamazepine in breast milk is approximately 20%–60% of the total plasma concentration (PYNNONEN and SYLLANPAA 1975; PYNNONEN et al. 1977b; KANEKO et al. 1979; NIEBYL et al. 1979).

c) Metabolism and Urinary Excretion

Only 1%–2% of an orally administered dose of carbamazepine is excreted unchanged in urine (FAIGLE and FELDMAN 1975; MORSELLI et al. 1975). Most of the drug is converted to oxidized metabolites which are excreted in the urine and in the bile in glucuronide form. At least 12 different such metabolites have been identified in man (Fig. 4) (for details see BERTILSSON 1978 and LYNN et al. 1978). Direct *N*-glucuronidation without prior oxidation also occurs. It has been speculated that the carbamazepine *N*-glucuronide is excreted in the bile, hydrolysed in the gastrointestinal tract to the a glycone and reabsorbed. TERHAAG et al. (1978),

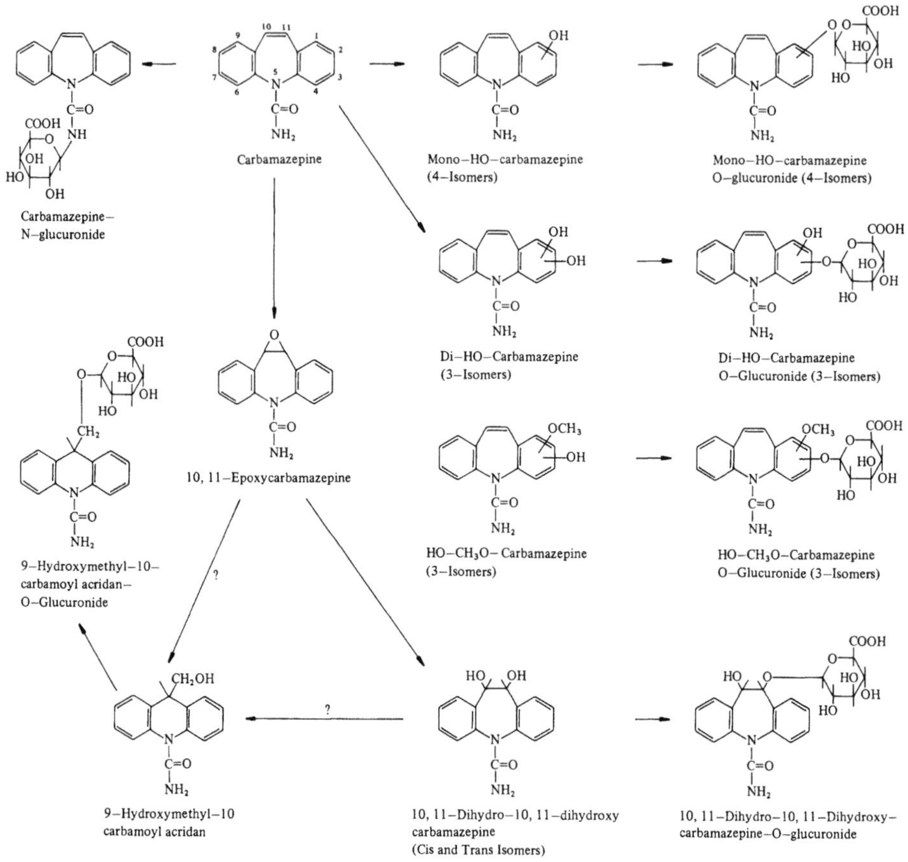

Fig. 4. Proposed pathways of carbamazepine metabolism (LYNN et al. 1978)

however, provided evidence that the extent to which carbamazepine undergoes enterohepatic circulation is probably negligible.

Considerable attention has been focused on carbamazepine-10,11-epoxide which, unlike other epoxides, is chemically stable. Although this metabolite accounts for only a small fraction of the urinary excretion (BERTILSSON 1978), it is found in patients' serum at concentrations which are between 15% and 55% (5% –81% in children) those of the parent drug. Since the plasma protein binding of the epoxide is lower than that of carbamazepine, the free concentrations of both compounds at steady state are sometimes found to be similar (BERTILSSON 1978). The main interest of these observations stems from the fact that in animals carbamazepine-epoxide has appreciable anticonvulsant activity (FRIGERIO and MORSELLI 1975). Whether the epoxide plays a significant role in the therapeutic action of carbamazepine in epileptic patients is unknown.

d) Half-life and Clearance

Following single-dose administration to normal volunteers the half-life of carbamazepine ranges from 20 to 65 h (PALMER et al. 1973; EICHELBAUM et al. 1975; LEVY et al. 1975; MORSELLI et al. 1975; RAWLINS et al. 1975; STRANDJORD and JOHANNESSEN 1975). After repeated administration, however, autoinduction occurs and the half-life is shortened. EICHELBAUM et al. (1975) administered 200 mg carbamazepine three times a day for 15–21 days and when treatment was discontinued, the half-lifes (20.9 ± 5.0 h) were considerably shorter than those previously observed in the same patients after a single dose (35.6 ± 15.3 h). Since carbamazepine has not been given intravenously to man, clearance data have been calculated after oral administration on the assumption that bioavailability is complete. Average values quoted in the literature are in the order of 10–20 ml/kg per hour after a single dose and 80–130 ml/kg per hour after multiple doses (for review, see EADIE and TYRER 1980).

The possibility that carbamazepine undergoes dose-dependent kinetics has been raised by COTTER et al. (1975) and GERARDIN et al. (1976), who found that the elimination half-life of the drug shortened with increasing drug dose. No evidence of this effect, however, was found by LEVY et al. (1975).

Apart from autoinduction and, possibly, dose-dependent kinetics, other factors affect carbamazepine elimination (for review, see PYNNONEN 1979). The effect of associated anticonvulsant therapy is probably the most important; treatment with phenytoin, phenobarbital or primidone leads to induction of carbamazepine metabolism, as indicated by a shortened half-life and a reduced carbamazepine to carbamazepine-10,11-epoxide ratio in the serum. WESTENBERG et al. (1978) found carbamazepine half-lives of 10.6±0.7 h in patients on combined anticonvulsant therapy as compared with half-lives of 18.3 ± 5 h in patients taking carbamazepine alone. EICHELBAUM et al. (1979) demonstrated that in some patients on combined antiepileptic drug therapy carbamazepine half-lives can be as short as 5–6 h.

The kinetics of the 10,11-epoxide metabolite have normally been studied under post-steady-state conditions in patients given carbamazepine (EICHELBAUM et al. 1975; MORSELLI et al. 1975). The reported half-life values of the epoxide in these patients (6–23 h) may be overestimates since the metabolite was still being formed during the time of sampling.

e) Steady-State Serum Levels and Serum Level/Dose Relationship

In patients started on chronic medication, maximal serum carbamazepine levels are usually observed after 3–4 days and thereafter decline gradually over a period of weeks due to the autoinduction effect (EICHELBAUM et al. 1975; PYNNONEN et al. 1980), eventually reaching serum levels much lower than those predicted from single-dose kinetics (RAWLINS et al. 1975; GERARDIN et al. 1976).

Steady-state serum carbamazepine levels are much lower in patients taking phenytoin, phenobarbital and primidone in addition as a result of enzyme induction by these drugs (CHRISTIANSEN and DAM 1973; CEREGHINO et al. 1975; JOHANNESSEN and STRANDJORD 1975 b; PERUCCA and RICHENS 1980).

At steady state, the serum concentration of carbamazepine is positively correlated with that of the epoxide, but the relationship is not sufficiently strong to enable a meaningful prediction to be made of the concentration of the epoxide from the level of parent drug (STRANDJORD and JOHANNESSEN 1980; TOMSON et al. 1980). In adults, the carbamazepine-10,11-epoxide: carbamazepine ratio in plasma ranges from 0.10 to 0.55 (BERTILSSON 1978; STRANDJORD and JOHANNESSEN 1980; TOMSON et al. 1980); the ratio is higher in patients treated with other enzyme-inducing antiepileptic drugs simultaneously (CHRISTIANSEN and DAM 1973; PYNNONEN et al. 1978; WESTENBERG et al. 1978; MACKICHAN et al. 1981).

Because of their relatively short half-lives, serum carbamazepine and carbamazepine epoxide levels fluctuate considerably during the dosing interval, particularly in patients receiving associated drug therapy. JOHANNESSEN et al. (1976) found that in patients receiving carbamazepine in two or three divided daily doses mean fluctuations in serum carbamazepine levels were similar (approximately 55%), whereas smaller fluctuations (36% on average) were seen with four daily doses. As expected, fluctuations are considerably less in patients receiving carbamazepine alone (HÖPPENER et al. 1980). These data suggest that once daily dosing of carbamazepine is inadequate. Two or, preferably, three divided doses are probably suitable for most patients, even though in some cases more frequent dosing may be required to prevent the occurrence of transient side effects associated with high serum levels (HÖPPENER et al. 1980).

Even if the time of sampling is carefully standardized, marked interindividual differences are observed in the serum concentration of carbamazepine and carbamazepine-10,11-epoxide in patients receiving the same maintenance dose (EICHELBAUM et al. 1976; JOHANNESSEN et al. 1976; LANDER et al. 1977; PYNNONEN et al. 1978; PERUCCA et al. 1978b) (Fig. 5). The poor correlation between serum level and dose in different patients underlines the usefulness of measuring the serum carbamazepine level as a means of optimizing therapy. The clinical usefulness of measuring the serum levels of the epoxide, on the other hand, has not been established, since it is still unclear whether this metabolite contributes to the overall pharmacological effect.

A rational approach to adjustments in dosage based on serum carbamazepine levels estimations is possible only if the within-patient relationship between serum level and dose is known. This relationship, however, is still unclear. HOOPER et al. (1974b) found that in ten patients receiving concurrent therapy with other antiepileptic drugs, increments in carbamazepine dose resulted in disproportionately large increases in the serum concentration at steady state. Although these results were interpreted as evidence of saturation of carbamazepine metabolism within the therapeutic dose range, the same authors were subsequently unable to reproduce a similar concentration-dose relationship in patients treated with carbamazepine alone. In the latter patients, the rate of rise in plasma drug level (relative to dose) was found to decrease as dosage was increased in the given individual (LANDER et al. 1977). Unfortunately, the interpretation of these results was limited by the fact that most of the patients could be studied at only two dose-serum concentration points.

No evidence of saturation kinetics of carbamazepine was found by TOMSON et al. (1980); the relationship between serum carbamazepine concentration and dose was linear, but in at least two of their patients the increase in serum concentration was much less than would have been expected from the increment in dose.

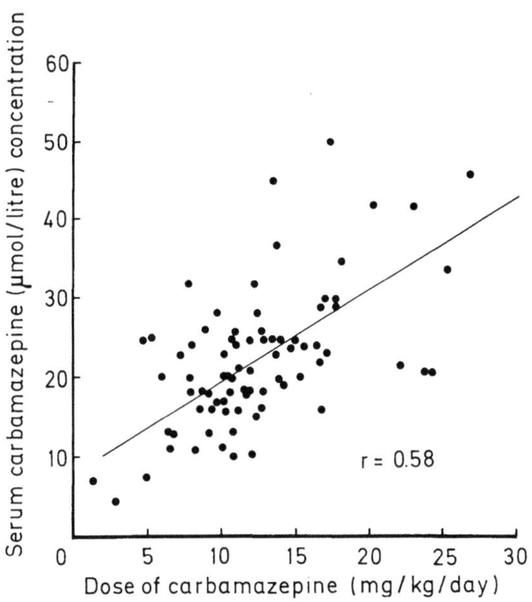

Fig. 5. Distribution of serum carbamazepine concentrations in 80 institutionalized epileptic patients. Most patients were receiving other antiepileptic drugs in combination (PERUCCA et al. 1978c)

PERUCCA et al. (1980b) have re-examined this question in patients receiving long-term therapy; information on the serum carbamazepine concentration at at least three separate dose levels was obtained. In all but one patient, a strong positive correlation between serum carbamazepine level and dose was found. In many patients, however, the increases in serum concentration produced by stepwise increases in dose were considerably smaller than expected from the magnitude of the dose increment (Fig. 6). These and the other findings discussed above suggest that at least in some patients there is a tendency for serum levels to plateau after an initial steep rise. These data are also consistent with the observation that in a treated population of patients carbamazepine level/dose ratios tend to decrease with increasing drug dosage (KUMPS 1981). Such a dose/level relationship could be explained by the occurrence of dose-dependent elimination (autoinduction) or, alternatively, dose-dependent absorption or plasma protein binding. It is not possible to decide which is responsible on current evidence.

2. Pharmacokinetics in Neonates, Infants and Children

REY et al. (1979) administered a single dose of carbamazepine (12–22 mg/kg) to seven neonates and five children. The drug was given as tablets, crushed and mixed with water or milk in eight cases. Peak serum carbamazepine levels (13–42 µmol/litre, i.e. 3–10 µg/ml) were achieved after between 2 and 7 h in the newborn and after 2 and 9 h in the children.

PYNNÖNEN and SILLANPÄA (1975) studied a neonate breast fed by a mother taking carbamazepine. After 30 days of breast-feeding the serum carbamazepine concentration in the infant was more than one-half the serum concentration in the mother.

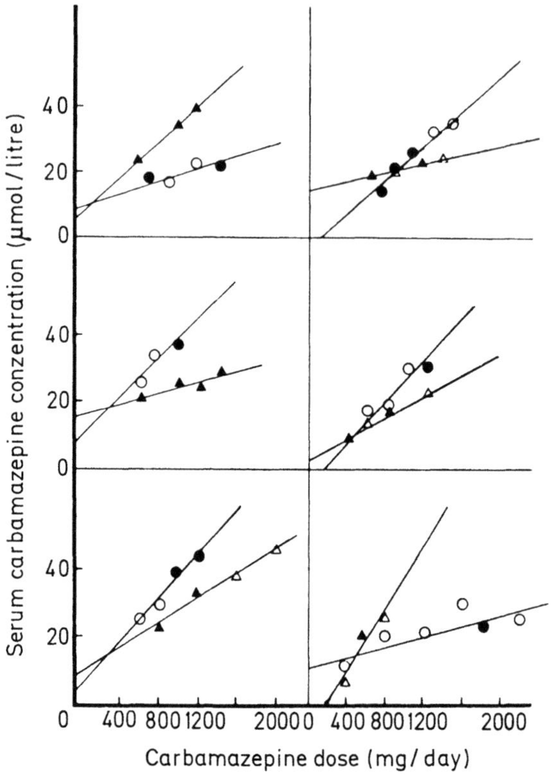

Fig. 6. Relationship between steady-state serum carbamazepine concentrations and dose in 12 institutionalized epileptic patients. *Open symbols* represent individual values and *closed symbols* the mean of two or more values. Most patients were receiving concurrent therapy with other antiepileptic drugs (PERUCCA et al. 1980 b)

Carbamazepine readily crosses the placenta. The concentration of the drug in the tissues of the human fetus and newborn has been studied by PYNNÖNEN et al. (1977 b). In fetuses carbamazepine is localized mainly in the liver and the kidney, whereas in neonates studied at autopsy the drug was localized mostly in the heart, liver and kidney and cerebral cortex.

PYNNÖNEN et al. (1977 a) found in children a CSF: plasma ratio of 0.33 ± 0.16 for carbamazepine.

The rate of disappearance of transplacentally transferred carbamazepine was studied by RANE et al. (1975). Half-life values (8.2, 10.5, 10.8, 27.7, and 28.1 h) were similar to those observed in adults after multiple doses but shorter than those observed after single doses. This indicates that these newborns have a well-developed metabolizing capacity, probably due to transplacental induction. In the patients studied by REY et al. (1979), the half-life of carbamazepine ranged from 4.7 to 12.6 h in the newborns and from 2.4 to 15.1 h in the children. These low values may partly reflect induction of carbamazepine metabolism by concurrently administered antiepileptic drugs.

The occurrence of autoinduction of carbamazepine metabolism in children has been demonstrated (BERTILSSON et al. 1980). Steady-state serum levels of carbamazepine in children tend to be lower than those observed in adults receiving equivalent doses (per unit of body weight). Children, however, have greater carbamazepine-10,11-epoxide ratios than adults (PYNNÖNEN et al. 1977a). Children on combined antiepileptic drug therapy have lower serum carbamazepine levels and higher carbamazepine-10,11-epoxide: carbamazepine ratios than children treated with carbamazepine alone, as in adults (RANE et al. 1976). Fluctuations in serum carbamazepine levels in children are comparable with those observed in adults. In many patients, three divided daily doses are required to minimize excessive fluctuations during the dosing intervals (RYLANCE et al. 1979).

D. Valproic Acid

Valproic acid is normally given orally but other routes of administration have been occasionally employed.

1. Pharmacokinetics in Adults

a) Absorption

Both valproic acid and its sodium salt are readily absorbed from the gastrointestinal tract. Following administration of conventional formulations or syrups, peak serum levels are usually attained within 1–3 h when the drug is taken on an empty stomach and within 3–8 h when it is taken after a meal (KLOTZ and ANTONIN 1977; PERUCCA et al. 1978c, d; CHUN et al. 1980). Since valproic acid may cause local gastric irritation, enteric-coated preparations have been developed which result in rapid liberation of the drug in the small intestine. Intake of an enteric-coated preparation under fasting conditions has been shown to result in a lag time of approximately 1–2 h, after which absorption occurs uninhibited (GUGLER et al. 1977). The lag time increases to 3–12 h when enteric-coated sodium valproate is taken together with a meal (LEVY et al. 1980). Slow-release formulations of valproic acid have been developed with the purpose of minimizing fluctuations in serum levels during the dosing interval (MEIJER and MEINARD 1976; OLDIGS et al. 1979). The amide derivative (depamide), which is marketed in some countries, can also be considered a delayed-release preparation of valproic acid (PINDER et al. 1977; PISANI et al. 1981).

A number of studies in which oral and intravenous preparations were used have demonstrated that the oral availability of conventional preparations of valproic acid (or its sodium salt) is complete (KLOTZ and ANTONIN 1977; PERUCCA et al. 1978c, d). The bioavailability of an enteric-coated formulation has also been shown to be complete irrespective of whether it was given on an empty stomach or together with a meal (LEVY et al. 1980). OLDIGS et al. (1979) found that a retard preparation was equivalent in its extent of absorption to an enteric-coated formulation.

The absorption profile of valproic acid after rectal administration has been investigated by MOOLENAAR et al. (1980). The absorption from an aqueous microenema of the sodium salt was found to be fast, the bioavailability being equivalent to that of a conventional oral preparation. When the drug was given in suppository form, the free acid was absorbed more rapidly than the sodium salt.

b) Distribution and Plasma Protein Binding

In man, valproic acid has a small apparent volume of distribution (0.14–0.20 litres/kg), suggesting that the penetration of the drug is mainly restricted to the circulation and rapidly exchangeable body water (KLOTZ and ANTONIN 1977; PERUCCA et al. 1978c, d). When the apparent volume of distribution is calculated on the basis of the unbound plasma concentration, however, values of about 1–2 litres/kg are found, which are comparable with those obtained in the case of other more lipophilic drugs (GUGLER et al. 1977). Patients receiving combination therapy with other antiepileptic drugs have larger volumes of distribution than drug-free normal volunteers (PERUCCA et al. 1978d).

Valproic acid is extensively (average 90%) bound to plasma proteins (JORDAN et al. 1976; KLOTZ and ANTONIN 1977; GUGLER and MULLER 1978; LÖSCHER 1978; PATEL and LEVY 1979; BREWSTER and MUIR 1980). The degree of binding is reduced in the presence of elevated levels of free fatty acids (FFA) (MONKS and RICHENS 1979; PATEL and LEVY 1979); diurnal variations in FFA concentration may therefore result in corresponding variations in free valproic acid fraction (PATEL et al. 1980). Free fatty acids released in plasma during equilibrium dialysis can lead to erroneously high values of estimated free drug fraction (ZIMMERMAN et al. 1981; RIVA et al. 1982), an observation that casts doubts on the interpretation of results obtained in some of the early studies on valproic acid binding. RIVA et al. (1982) have shown that the storage of samples for 8–24 h without freezing can also result in release of FFA with a corresponding elevation of the free fraction of the drug. Therapeutic concentrations of other antiepileptic drugs do not appear to alter valproic acid binding to a clinically important extent (PATEL and LEVY 1979).

The unbound fraction of valproic acid in plasma increases with increasing concentrations as a result of saturation of binding sites. In an in vivo study, CRAMER and MATTSON (1979) found that the percentage unbound of the drug is 5% at serum concentrations between 140 and 420 μmol/litre (20–60 μg/ml), 8% at 560 μmol/litre (80 μg/ml) and over 20% at 1,015 μmol/litre (145 μg/ml). Similar concentration-dependent changes in unbound fraction have been described in vivo (BOWDLE et al. 1980; RIVA et al. 1982). These findings have several implications. Due to the marked fluctuations in serum valproic acid levels, the fraction unbound changes during a dosage interval (LEVY et al. 1981). Also the dose-concentration relationship of the drug may be non-linear at higher concentrations, total serum levels increasing comparatively less than might be expected from the increment in dose (GRAM et al. 1979). Since only the unbound fraction is available to produce biological effects at the receptor sites, serum levels of total (free and bound) valproic acid would not be expected to reflect accurately the concentration of pharmacologically active drug, suggesting that optimal therapeutic monitoring should be based upon the measurement of free drug (LEVY 1980).

The plasma protein binding of valproic acid is reduced in conditions associated with hypoalbuminaemia, e.g. pregnancy (DAM et al. 1979), renal disease (GUGLER and MULLER 1978; BRUNI et al. 1979; BREWSTER and MUIR 1980) and hepatic disease (KLOTZ et al. 1978). The binding defect observed in many of these conditions, however, cannot be entirely explained by a reduction in concentration of the binding protein. The concentration of valproic acid in the CSF is similar to the unbound concentration of the drug in plasma (MEIJER and HESSING-BRANDT 1973; WULFF et al. 1977; GUGLER and VON UNRUH 1980). On the other hand, the concentration in saliva is strongly influenced by changes in salivary pH and does not show a consistent relationship with either free or total concentration in plasma (GUGLER et al. 1977; GUGLER and VON UNRUH 1980).

The concentration of valproic acid in breast milk of mothers treated with the drug is in the order of 1%–16% of the plasma concentration (ESPIR et al. 1976; ALEXANDER 1979; DICKINSON et al. 1979; PLASSE et al. 1979).

c) Metabolism and Urinary Excretion

Less than 5% of the administered dose of valproic acid is excreted unchanged in the urine of man (GUGLER and VON UNRUH 1980). Most of the drug is either directly conjugated with glucuronic acid (about 20% of the dose) or converted to oxidized metabolites. GUGLER and VON UNRUH (1980) listed more than 20 potential valproic acid metabolites. The main metabolic pathways involve glucuronidation (or other conjugation reactions) and β-, ω_1- and ω_2-oxidation. In addition to the list of putative metabolites GUGLER and VON UNRUH (1980) reported a number of compounds which have been detected in the body fluids of valproic acid-treated patients or experimental animals; some of these possible metabolites (e.g. methylmalonic acid) are excreted in relatively large amounts in the urine of some patients. Since valproic acid is a FFA of simple structure, it is possible that some of its metabolites are also normally occurring body constituents, perhaps accumulating in larger amounts as a result of the pharmacological action of the drug. This possibility causes major identification problems.

The hypothesis that metabolites may be wholly or partly responsible for the effects of valproic acid has been raised. LÖSCHER (1981) has demonstrated that the main plasma metabolites are three products of β-oxidation: 2-en-valproic acid, 3-hydroxy-valproic acid and 3-keto-valproic acid. The products of ω-oxidation, 4-hydroxy-valproic acid and 5-hydroxy-valproic acid, were quantitatively less important. When evidence on the anticonvulsant activity of these metabolites in experimental models was taken into account, it was considered unlikely that they make an important contribution to the pharmacological effect.

d) Half-life and Clearance

After intravenous administration of a single dose of valproic acid, the decline in the serum concentration of the drug is biphasic, with a rapid distributive phase followed after 4–6 h by a slower elimination phase (KLOTZ and ANTONIN 1977; PERUCCA et al. 1978c, d). After oral administration of a conventional preparation, the biphasic pattern may not be so evident and the log-linear part of the serum level curve (β-phase) may commence within 3–4 h after the attainment of the peak concentration (PERUCCA et al. 1978c, d). In some patients, however, the onset of the β-phase may be delayed for up to 12 h after oral dosing, so that a correct calculation of the elimination half-life can only be made by using serum concentration data obtained after that time (GUGLER et al. 1977). In subjects not taking other drugs, e.g. normal volunteers, the elimination half-life of valproic acid has been estimated at 8–10 h (LOISEAU et al. 1976), 9 ± 1 h (RICHENS et al. 1976), 13 ± 2 h (PERUCCA et al. 1978c), 14 ± 4 h (KLOTZ and ANTONIN 1977) and 16 ± 4 h (GUGLER et al. 1977). Half-life values determined after a single dose were found to be virtually identical to those determined in the same subject after multiple dosing (GUGLER et al. 1977).

In patients treated with other antiepileptic drugs such as phenytoin, phenobarbital and carbamazepine, the half-life of valproic acid is considerably shorter than that observed in normal volunteers. Values reported in these patients include 6 ± 0.6 h (RICHENS et al. 1976), 6–10 h (MATTSON et al. 1978) and 10 ± 1 h (PERUCCA et al. 1978d).

Since the apparent volume of distribution of valproic acid is larger in patients treated with other antiepileptic drugs (PERUCCA et al. 1978d; BOWDLE et al. 1979), the total body clearance of the drug in the presence of associated anticonvulsant therapy is much higher than that observed in normal volunteers. This suggests that valproic acid metabolism is induced by other antiepileptic drugs.

KLOTZ and ANTONIN (1977) drew attention to the fact that valproic acid is subject to restrictive, flow-independent elimination. This implies that its plasma clearance should be directly proportional to the free (unbound) fraction. Since the unbound fraction increases with increasing concentration, one would also expect the clearance to be concentration dependent (see also next section). BOWDLE et al. (1980) were unable to demonstrate this, however, and they concluded that the dose-dependent kinetics of valproic acid are more complex than predicted, being influenced by changes in free fraction as well as by autoinhibition or saturation of metabolism.

e) Steady-State Serum Levels and Serum Level/Dose Relationship

In most patients, steady-state serum valproic acid levels are reached within 2–3 days of starting maintenance therapy. A large variability is observed in steady-state serum valproic levels of patients receiving the same dose (GUGLER and VON UNRUH 1980). This is due partly to interindividual differences in clearance rate and partly to the difficulty in standardizing precisely the time of sampling in respect to the fluctuations in serum levels during the dosing interval. Due to the enhancement of valproic acid clearance by other antiepileptic drugs, patients receiving combination therapy have much lower steady-state valproic acid levels than patients receiving equivalent doses of valproate alone (MIHALY et al. 1979).

Information on the serum level/dose relationship within patients is inconclusive, especially in the light of the evidence that valproic acid may show complex dose-dependent kinetics. GUGLER et al. (1977) found that the steady-state concentration of valproic acid was lower than predicted from single-dose kinetics and suggested that the discrepancy was due to a reduction in the degree of plasma protein binding at higher concentrations. NUTT and KUPFERBERG (1979) reported that the relationship between serum valproic acid concentration and dose was linear but the *Y*-axis intercept of the regression line was positive in all patients, suggesting that the relationship might have been curvilinear over a lower dosage range. A definitely curvilinear relationship was observed by GRAM et al. (1979) in 11 patients who were studied at three separate dose levels. The rise in valproic acid serum levels was smaller than the increment in dose, probably due to decreased plasma protein binding at higher concentrations. A similar type of curvilinear relationship was observed by BOWDLE et al. (1980). In this study, evidence was presented that the disposition of the drug may be further complicated by the occurrence of inhibition of metabolism.

Because of the decrease in protein binding at higher concentrations the curvilinear relationship probably does not apply to the levels of free drug. Indeed available information suggests that increments in free drug levels may be even greater than the increment in dose. Under these circumstances total serum levels may underestimate the amount of pharmacologically active drug and lead to incorrect dose adjustments (LEVY 1979).

2. Pharmacokinetics in Neonates, Infants and Children

Valproic acid readily crosses the placental barrier and is found in the neonate's plasma at concentrations comparable with those observed in maternal plasma (BRACHET-LIERMAIN and DEMARQUEZ 1977).

The gastrointestinal absorption of the drug in the premature and full-term neonate has been reported to be relatively slow, peak serum levels being attained between 3 and 8 h. In infants, the absorption rate is faster and comparable with that observed in adults (BRACHET-LIERMAIN and DEMARQUEZ 1977).

The plasma protein binding of valproic acid is lower in the newborn than in adults. Elimination half-lives of 10–67 h have been reported during the first 10 days of life (BRACHET-LIERMAIN and DEMARQUEZ 1977; DICKINSON et al. 1979; IRVINE-MEEK et al. 1981). Half-life values range from 9 to 22 h in infants aged 0.5–2 months and from 7 to 13 h in older infants and children (SCHOBBEN et al. 1975; BRACHET-LIERMAIN and DEMARQUEZ 1977; IRVINE-MEEK et al. 1981). These findings suggest that the valproic acid metabolizing capacity is low during the first 2 months of extrauterine life but reaches normal values after this period. JOHANNESSEN and HENDRIKSEN (1977) found that in children under 12 years of age serum valproic acid levels were not significantly different from those observed in adults given equivalent doses per kilogram body weight.

E. Succinimides

I. Ethosuximide

Ethosuximide is the most widely prescribed of the succinimide drugs. The drug is always administered orally.

1. Pharmacokinetics in Adults

a) Absorption

Ethosuximide is well absorbed from the gastrointestinal tract. Peak serum levels normally occur within 4 h after a single oral dose but may be delayed for up to

7 h during chronic administration (HANSEN and FELDBERG 1964; CHANG et al. 1972; BUCHANAN et al. 1973; GOULET et al. 1976). No information is available on the absolute bioavailability of the drug in man.

b) Distribution and Plasma Protein Binding

The apparent volume of distribution of ethosuximide, calculated on the assumption that absorption is complete, is about 0.7 litres/kg (BUCHANAN et al. 1973; WARREN et al. 1980). Animal studies indicate that the drug is present in brain at concentrations similar to those found in plasma (PATEL et al. 1977). The plasma protein binding of the drug is negligible (CHANG et al. 1972; MCAULIFFE et al. 1977). The concentration of the drug in CSF and in saliva is similar to that in plasma (SHERWIN and ROBB 1972; BUCHANAN et al. 1973 a; MCAULIFFE et al. 1977).

Ethosuximide is excreted into breast milk. Average reported values of milk/plasma ratio are 0.94 (KOUP et al. 1978), 0.79 (KANEKO et al. 1979) and 0.80 (RANE and TUNELL 1981). A ratio of 1.03 has been reported for colostrum (RANE and TUNELL 1981).

c) Metabolism and Urinary Excretion

During chronic therapy, approximately 20% of the administered dose of ethosuximide is excreted unchanged in urine. Another 60% is excreted as the isomers of 2-(1-hydroxyethyl)-2-methylsuccinimide (GOULET et al. 1976). Other known metabolites of ethosuximide in man include: 2-ethyl-2-methyl-3-hydroxysuccinimide, 2-acetyl-2-methylsuccinimide, 2-(2-hydroxyethyl)-2-methylsuccinimide and 2-ethyl-2(hydroxymethyl)succinimide (for details see SHERWIN 1978 and EADIE and TYRER 1980). Some of these metabolites are excreted in urine in conjugated form.

d) Half-life and Clearance

In adults, the half-life of ethosuximide is approximately 55 h (GOULET et al. 1976; WARREN et al. 1980) or 52 ± 24 h (EADIE et al. 1977). Clearance values, calculated on the assumption that absorption is complete, are in the order of 10 ml/kg per hour. Higher clearance values and moderately shorter half-lives have been reported in subjects receiving concurrent treatment with enzyme-inducing drugs (WARREN et al. 1980).

e) Steady-State Serum Levels and Serum Level/Dose Relationship

Steady-state serum ethosuximide values are usually reached within 7–12 days after initiation of treatment. Because of the long half-life, once daily administration is probably satisfactory for clinical purposes, at least in adults (GOULET et al. 1976).

SMITH et al. (1979) found that, in patients mostly treated with other antiepileptic drugs, average daily doses around 30 mg/kg were required to achieve steady-state serum ethosuximide levels between 280 and 700 µmol/litre (~40–100 µg/ml). There is, however, a large interindividual variation in the serum levels of patients receiving the same dose (BROWNE et al. 1975). GOULET et al. (1976) found that steady-state serum ethosuximide levels were directly proportional to dosage;

the pattern of metabolite excretion did not suggest dose-dependent kinetics. SMITH et al. (1979), however, reported that in some patients increments in ethosuximide dose resulted in a disproportionate increase in serum concentration. This seems to be the only report in which evidence of dose-dependent kinetics has been given.

2. Pharmacokinetics in Neonates, Infants and Children

KOUP et al. (1979) found that in one full-term neonate the serum concentration of transplacentally transferred ethosuximide was similar to that observed in the mother and declined with a half-life of 41 h.

Ethosuximide may also be transferred from the mother to the baby through breast milk. RANE and TUNELL (1981) found that the plasma concentration of the drug during the first 5 months of age in a suckling infant was about 30% of the maternal plasma concentration. There was a tendency for the infant's plasma/milk concentration to decrease over the 1st month, possibly due to an increase in drug clearance.

In children, ethosuximide is readily absorbed from the gastrointestinal tract. BUCHANAN et al. (1969) found that the absorption profile when the drug is given as a syrup is similar to when it is given as capsules.

The apparent volume of distribution (calculated on the assumption that bioavailability is complete) in children is about 0.7 litres/kg, which is similar to that found in adults (BUCHANAN et al. 1969). The half-life of ethosuximide in children is about 30 h on average and once daily dosing is probably acceptable in a paediatric population (BUCHANAN et al. 1969, 1976). Children require relatively larger doses than adults in order to achieve comparable serum levels (for review, see MORSELLI 1977b and SHERWIN 1978).

II. Methsuximide

Methsuximide is rapidly absorbed from the gastrointestinal tract, peak serum levels being usually attained within 2 h after a single oral dose (GLAZKO and DILL 1972). The elimination half-life of methsuximide is about 1–5 h (GLAZKO and DILL 1972; PORTER et al. 1979) but is shorter after repeated administration than after a single dose, suggesting the occurrence of autoinduction (GLAZKO and DILL 1972).

Only negligible amounts of unchanged drug are excreted unchanged in urine. Methsuximide is extensively metabolized; the most important biotransformation product is *N*-desmethylmethsuximide, which is pharmacologically active and has a half-life of 23–57 h (PORTER et al. 1979). Several other metabolites have been described, some of which are probably formed by way of an epoxide intermediate (HORNING et al. 1973). *N*-Desmethylmethsuximide accumulates in serum at concentrations which are on average about 700 times higher than those of the parent drug (STRONG et al. 1974; PORTER et al. 1979). It is likely that during chronic treatment the metabolite is largely responsible for the pharmacological effect (BARRON et al. 1974; STRONG et al. 1974; PORTER et al. 1979). In patients receiving long-term therapy, serum levels of the desmethylated derivative are positively correlated with the dose of the parent drug. RAMBECK (1979) has clearly shown that within patients the serum *N*-desmethylmethsuximide concentration is linearly related to the methsuximide dose.

III. Phensuximide

Phensuximide is rapidly absorbed from the gastrointestinal tract (GLAZKO et al. 1954). Animal studies indicate that the drug has a relatively uniform distribution in most tissues. In man, the half-life of phensuximide ranges from 4 to 12 h (GLAZKO and DILL 1972; PORTER et al. 1979). The drug is partly converted to *N*-desmethylphensuximide. This metabolite (unlike *N*-desmethylmethsuximide) is rapidly eliminated (probably by further biodegradation) and therefore its concentration in serum at steady state is much lower than that of the parent drug (PORTER et al. 1979). The failure of phensuximide and its desmethyl metabolite to accumulate during prolonged treatment could provide an explanation for the relatively weak antiepileptic effect of phensuximide compared with methsuximide.

F. Benzodiazepines

Benzodiazepine drugs are frequently used intravenously for status epilepticus and orally in certain types of epilepsy, particularly myoclonic epilepsy. Discussion here will be confined to diazepam and clonazepam.

I. Diazepam

Most of the available information on the pharmacokinetics of the drug has been obtained in non-epileptic patients.

1. Pharmacokinetics in Adults

a) Absorption

Diazepam is rapidly absorbed from the gastrointestinal tract, peak serum levels being usually attained within 30–90 min after an oral dose (MANDELLI et al. 1978). The rate of absorption of the drug is age dependent, being particularly faster in children and delayed in the elderly. The bioavailability of many of the commercially available pharmaceutical preparations is considered to be high, probably around 75%–90% or even greater (KLOTZ et al. 1975; MANDELLI et al. 1978; DIVOLL-ALLEN and GREENBLATT 1981). There may be, however, considerable differences in bioavailability between separate formulations (BERLIN et al. 1975). Concomitant intake of food has been reported to delay the absorption of the drug, but to enhance its bioavailability (GREENBLATT et al. 1978a). Compared with the findings obtained after oral intake, intramuscular administration of diazepam has been reported to result in lower peak serum levels and in slower and less predictable absorption (HILLESTAD et al. 1974b; KANTO 1975). Other authors, however, have described a relatively rapid intramuscular absorption (DIVOLL-ALLEN and GREENBLATT 1981). The site and the technique of injection may be important in this respect. GAMBLE et al. (1975) found that serum diazepam levels after injection into the thigh were higher than those observed after injection into the buttock. When the injection was given by doctors, serum diazepam levels were twice as high as those observed when the injection was given by nurses.

Considerable interest has focused on the absorption of diazepam following rectal administration, particularly in children. When diazepam is given as a rectal solution, the absorption is rapid and efficient (AGURELL et al. 1975; MEBERG et al. 1978; DHILLON and RICHENS 1981 a). The absorption of the drug from suppository forms is dependent on the pharmaceutical preparation used. With certain suppositories peak serum levels can be achieved as rapidly as after oral administration, whereas with other formulations the absorption may be incomplete, erratic and delayed (KANTO 1975; DHILLON and RICHENS 1981 a).

Diazepam is frequently used intravenously. Since the drug is poorly soluble in water, precipitation may occur when it is added to normal saline or dextrose solutions (MORRIS 1978). It has been suggested that for prolonged infusions a dilution factor of at least 1:20 should be adhered to. An additional problem is that diazepam adsorbs to plastic. When stored in plastic intravenous fluid bags, about 95% of the drug may be lost in 24 h. With slow intravenous infusion in diluted form, more than 50% of the dose may become adsorbed to the infusing set (MACKICHAN et al. 1979). The problem can be avoided by using for infusion a glass syringe connected to high-density polyethylene tubing (COSSUM and ROBERTS 1981). In most clinical situations, however, the desired therapeutic effect can be achieved by direct slow injection of the commercially available preparation and no dilution is required.

b) Distribution and Plasma Protein Binding

Diazepam is a highly lipophilic substance which distributes rapidly to all body tissues. In animal studies, brain concentrations higher than the plasma concentrations have been found within a few minutes after intravenous injection (MORSELLI et al. 1973 a).

The apparent volume of distribution of the drug in adults has been reported to range from 0.6 to 2 litres/kg (KLOTZ et al. 1975; MANDELLI et al. 1978; GREENBLATT et al. 1980; DHILLON and RICHENS 1981 b; OCHS et al. 1981). The volume of distribution increases with increasing age (KLOTZ et al. 1975; OCHS et al. 1981). Females have greater volumes of distribution than age-matched male controls (OCHS et al. 1981).

In serum, diazepam is extensively (98%–99%) bound to proteins; the degree of binding is virtually constant over the therapeutic concentration range. In normal subjects, the interindividual variation in unbound fraction is about twofold (ABEL et al. 1979). ROUTLEDGE et al. (1980 b) have demonstrated that there is a positive relationship between the extent of binding and the serum concentration of both albumin and α_1-acid glycoprotein. The unbound fraction of diazepam is greater in women on oral contraceptives than in women not taking these drugs. The latter, in turn, have higher free fraction values than males (ROUTLEDGE et al. 1981). Other studies, however, have failed to provide evidence for these sex-related differences (DIVOLL-ALLEN and GREENBLATT 1981). Conditions associated with decreased protein binding of diazepam include pregnancy (PERUCCA et al. 1981 c), old age (GREENBLATT et al. 1980), hypoalbuminaemic states in general (THIESSEN et al. 1976), renal failure (KANGAS et al. 1976), elevated levels of free fatty acids (GUGLER et al. 1974; ROUTLEDGE et al. 1980) and concurrent treatment with displacing agents such as valproic acid. Binding can also change depending on whether the sample is drawn in the fasting or postprandial state (ABEL et al. 1979).

The salivary concentration of diazepam has been shown to correlate positively with the unbound concentration in serum (GILES et al. 1977; DI GREGORIO et al. 1978; DIXON and CREWS 1978). The levels of diazepam in the CSF have been shown to be of the same order of magnitude as the free concentration in plasma (KANTO et al. 1975).

The major plasma metabolite, *N*-desmethyldiazepam, is also extensively bound to serum proteins (MANDELLI et al. 1978). The unbound fraction of this metabolite, however, is about twice as high as that of the parent drug (ABEL et al. 1979; GREENBLATT et al. 1980; HALLSTROM et al. 1980; DIVOLL-ALLEN and GREENBLATT 1981). The concentration of the *N*-desmethyldiazepam in saliva and CSF is comparable with the unbound concentration in serum (KANTO et al. 1975; HALLSTROM et al. 1980). HENDEL (1975), however, reported that long-term treatment with diazepam can lead to a substantial increase in the CSF/plasma ratio of the *N*-desmethylated metabolite.

Both diazepam and *N*-desmethyldiazepam are excreted in appreciable amounts in breast milk (BRANDT 1976; WILSON et al. 1980). For diazepam, the milk/plasma ratio is about 0.1 (ERKKOLA and KANTO 1972).

c) Metabolism and Urinary Excretion

Only negligible amounts of diazepam are excreted unchanged in urine (KAPLAN et al. 1973). The main route of elimination of the drug involves biotransformation to a number of metabolites. Among these metabolites, *N*-desmethyldiazepam (nordiazepam) is probably the most important from the clinical point of view. *N*-Desmethyldiazepam, which is pharmacologically active, appears in serum within 1 h of diazepam administration and due to its half-life being longer than that of the parent drug accumulates in considerable amounts during chronic medication (MANDELLI et al. 1978; GREENBLATT et al. 1981). Other metabolites include 3-hydroxy-diazepam (temazepam), oxazepam, *p*-hydroxy-phenyl-oxazepam and *p*-hydroxy-phenyl-*N*-desmethyldiazepam (MANDELLI et al. 1978; EADIE and TYRER 1980). Some of these compounds are pharmacologically active but they are rapidly eliminated or found in insufficient amounts to be of marked clinical relevance. Conjugated metabolites recovered in urine account for at least 60%–80% of the administered dose of diazepam (MORSELLI and FRANCO-MORSELLI 1980).

d) Half-life and Clearance

Following administration of a single intravenous dose, the decline in serum diazepam concentration is biphasic, with a short distributive phase followed by a slower elimination phase. In young normal subjects the elimination half-life ranges from 20 to 65 h (GREENBLATT et al. 1980), with average values around 30 h. Clearance values in adults are in the order of 15–30 ml/h per kilogram (KLOTZ et al. 1976a, b, 1977; DHILLON and RICHENS 1981 b). KLOTZ et al. (1975) found that in adults the half-life of diazepam increases linearly with age, from average values of 20 h at 20 years to 90 h at 80 years. Since the plasma clearance showed no significant age dependence, the prolongation of the half-life in the elderly must be related to an increase in the volume of distribution. A moderate decrease in diazepam clearance has been reported in elderly male patients (GREENBLATT et al. 1980).

There is suggestive evidence that after multiple dosing the half-life of diazepam may be longer and its clearance values lower than those determined after administration of a single dose (KLOTZ et al. 1976b). This may be due to accumulation of *N*-desmethyldiazepam having an inhibitory effect on diazepam metabolism. Two recent studies aimed at investigating this possibility, however, have yielded conflicting results (ABERNETHY and GREENBLATT 1981; KLOTZ and REIMANN 1981).

The metabolism of diazepam is induced in patients taking other antiepileptic drugs such as carbamazepine and primidone. DHILLON and RICHENS (1981b) reported half-life values of 13 ± 4 h in these patients compared with 34 ± 12 h in age-matched controls. Serum *N*-desmethyldiazepam levels were higher and their peak serum concentration occurred earlier in the patients than in the controls. In contrast, diazepam elimination is reduced in patients with liver disease (KLOTZ et al. 1975, 1977; BRANCH et al. 1976; ANDREASEN et al. 1976).

The elimination half-life of the main active metabolite, *N*-desmethyldiazepam, is longer than that of the parent drug. In patients dosed with desmethyldiazepam or its pro-drug clorazepate, the half-life of *N*-desmethyldiazepam ranges from 50 to 120 h (MANDELLI et al. 1978), with slightly shorter values in patients taking concurrent therapy with other antiepileptic drugs (WILENSKY et al. 1978). The possibility that the metabolite follows dose-dependent kinetics has been raised. In three out of six patients treated with *N*-desmethyldiazepam and nortriptyline in combination, TOGNONI et al. (1975) found that the elimination of the former compound from the circulation was biphasic. A slow initial component corresponding to half-lives of 96–349 h was followed, at plasma levels below 2,000 nmol/litre (~550 ng/ml), by a faster elimination, with half-life values ranging from 26 to 33 h.

e) Steady-State Serum Levels and Serum Level/Dose Relationship

With multiple dosing, steady-state serum diazepam levels are usually reached after approximately 7–8 days. This period may be shortened in patients receiving enzyme-inducing drugs in combination, but may be prolonged to 12–15 days in the elderly. In one study, serum diazepam levels after 2–5 years of treatment were found to be much lower than those observed after 15 days (KANTO et al. 1974). Reduced patients' compliance during long-term therapy may be an explanation for these findings, which are in contrast with the observation that diazepam clearance may be reduced after multiple- compared with single-dose administration (KLOTZ et al. 1976b). GREENBLATT et al. (1981) found that the steady-state levels of the drug were not influenced by the duration of therapy.

When trying to relate serum levels to clinical effect, it is necessary to take into account the presence of the active metabolite *N*-desmethyldiazepam. Since this metabolite has a relatively long half-life, it accumulates progressively during chronic treatment and its steady-state concentrations may not be reached until at least 10–25 days have elapsed following initiation of treatment.

A large variation is observed in serum diazepam levels of patients receiving the same dose. In patients receiving single-drug therapy, doses of 15–20 mg/day are generally associated with serum levels between 350–2,100 nmol/litre (100–600 ng/ml) (BERLIN et al. 1975; DÅSBERG et al. 1974; HILLESTAD et al. 1974a; GREENBLATT et al. 1981).

GREENBLATT et al. (1981) found that the plasma levels of the parent drug in patients on chronic therapy were significantly correlated with those of the *N*-desmethyl metabolite. The mean desmethyldiazepam/diazepam plasma ratio was 1.26. Other authors reported ratios between 0.6 and 5 (MANDELLI et al. 1978); if the lower degree of plasma protein binding of *N*-desmethyldiazepam is taken into account (DIVOLL-ALLEN and GREENBLATT 1981) it is evident that in patients receiving chronic therapy the unbound concentration of the metabolite usually exceeds that of the parent drug. Particularly high metabolite/parent drug ratios are likely to be found in patients receiving other enzyme-inducing antiepileptic drugs.

During chronic treatment, oxazepam and 3-hydroxy-diazepam (temazepam) levels are about 5%–10% of the diazepam level.

2. Pharmacokinetics in Neonates, Infants and Children

Diazepam and *N*-desmethyldiazepam readily cross the placental barrier, reach to fetus (ERKKOLA et al. 1974) and are found at birth in neonatal plasma at concentrations comparable with those present in maternal plasma (MANDELLI et al. 1975).

Relatively large doses of diazepam given to the nursing mother can result in appreciable transfer of the drug and its active metabolites to the baby through the milk (WILSON et al. 1980). This can result in sedation, weight loss and EEG changes in the newborn (PATRICK et al. 1972). A daily dose of 10 mg given to the mother, however, is probably insufficient to produce adverse effects in the suckling newborn (MANDELLI et al. 1978).

Following oral administration to premature and full-term neonates, diazepam is rapidly absorbed. In infants and children peak serum levels are usually attained within 30–60 min, suggesting that the rate of absorption is faster than that observed in adults (MANDELLI et al. 1978). Rectal absorption is also rapid when the drug is given as a suspension or a solution (AGURELL et al. 1975; KNUDSEN 1977). With suppositories, both the rate and extent of absorption are largely influenced by the pharmaceutical preparation used. Intramuscular diazepam results in somewhat delayed peak serum levels and is not recommended when a rapid effect is required, e.g. in a convulsing child.

The apparent volume of distribution of diazepam in infants and children has been reported to be about 1.1 and 2.0 litres/kg respectively (MORSELLI et al. 1973 b), which is within the range observed in adults. Higher values of volume of distribution have been reported in another study (MORSELLI et al. 1974). The plasma protein binding of diazepam is lower in neonates than in adults. Due to the markedly reduced diazepam binding in late pregnancy, however, the free fraction of the drug is lower in the neonate than in the mother.

Human fetal liver microsomes can metabolize diazepam as early as the 13th week of gestation (ACKERMANN and RICHTER 1977). The elimination half-life in the newborn is dependent on the gestation age. Apparent serum half-lives of 40–100 h (with clearance values of about 27 ml/kg per hour) have been observed in premature neonates, whereas in full-term neonates half-lives vary from 20 to 50 h

(MORSELLI et al. 1974; MORSELLI 1977 a). The slow elimination in the premature neonate is probably due to incomplete maturation of the enzyme system responsible for the hydroxylation of both diazepam and its *N*-desmethyl derivative (MANDELLI et al. 1978). A much faster elimination rate, associated with an increased formation of hydroxylated and conjugated metabolites, has been observed in premature and full-term newborns exposed to enzyme-inducing agents in utero or during the first days of extrauterine life.

MORSELLI (1977 a) reported in infants half-life values ranging from 8 to 14 h, which are considerably shorter than those observed in adults. Half-lives of 15–21 h (with clearance values of about 107 ml/kg per hour) have been described in children (MORSELLI et al. 1974; MORSELLI 1974 a).

II. Clonazepam

a) Absorption

Clonazepam is rapidly and completely absorbed from the gastrointestinal tract. Peak serum levels are usually achieved within 1–4 h after an oral dose both in adults and in children (KAPLAN et al. 1974; BERLIN and DAHLSTRÖM 1975; DREIFUSS et al. 1975; SJÖ et al. 1975 a; PINDER et al. 1976; EADIE et al. 1977 b).

b) Distribution and Plasma Protein Binding

Clonazepam distributes rapidly to the various organs, with a preferential uptake by the brain structures (KNOP et al. 1975). Reported values of apparent volumes of distribution are usually in the range of 1.5–4.4 litres/kg (BERLIN and DAHLSTRÖM 1975; EADIE et al. 1977). The degree of binding to plasma proteins is about 85%–90% (KHOO et al. 1980).

c) Metabolism and Urinary Excretion

Less than 5% of an administered dose of clonazepam is excreted unchanged in urine (KAPLAN et al. 1974; SJÖ et al. 1975 a).

Clonazepam is extensively metabolized in the body. A major metabolic pathway involves the reduction of the nitro group to generate an amino derivative which is subsequently acetylated (KNOP et al. 1974; SJÖ et al. 1975). The rate of acetylation is determined by the acetylator phenotype (MILLER et al. 1981). Hydroxylation in position-3 of clonazepam and of its 7-amino and 7-acetamido derivatives is also possible (ESCHENOF 1973). Apparently all the metabolites are biologically inactive (MORSELLI and FRANCO-MORSELLI 1978).

Both 7-amino- and 7-acetamido-clonazepam have been detected in human plasma. The concentration of the former of these metabolites has been found to range between 30% and 300% of those of the parent drug (SJÖ et al. 1975 a), but further studies are required to confirm this.

The metabolites of clonazepam are excreted in urine partly in conjugated (glucuronide and sulphate) form (PINDER et al. 1976). SJÖ et al. (1975) found that, at steady state, 5%–20% of a clonazepam dose appears in urine as the 7-amino and 7-acetamido metabolites.

d) Half-life and Clearance

Following intravenous administration, serum clonazepam levels decline bi-exponentially, with a short distributive phase followed by a slower elimination phase.

In most studies, elimination half-lives have been found to be in the range of 20–60 h (NAESTOFT et al. 1973; KAPLAN et al. 1974; BERLIN and DAHLSTRÖM 1975; KNOP et al. 1975; PINDER et al. 1976). Somewhat shorter half-lives are observed in patients receiving combined treatment with barbiturates, phenytoin or carbamazepine (LAI et al. 1978; KHOO et al. 1980). Clonazepam clearance values of 92 ± 51 ml/kg per hour have been reported (EADIE et al. 1977). DREIFUSS et al. (1975) found that in ten epileptic children the half-life of clonazepam ranged from 22 to 33 h. These values are comparable with those observed in adults.

The rate of elimination of the drug following discontinuation of subchronic treatment has been found to be similar to that observed after a single dose (BERLIN and DAHLSTRÖM 1975). Despite the relatively long half-life, divided daily dosing may be preferred in order to avoid adverse effects associated with high peak serum levels.

e) Steady-State Serum Levels and Serum Level/Dose Relationship

Steady-state serum clonazepam levels are usually achieved 4–10 days after the initiation of treatment. There are wide interindividual variations in the levels achieved at the same dose. In patients receiving daily doses of 6 mg for up to 12 months SJÖ et al. (1975) found plasma clonazepam levels ranging from 100 to 250 nmol/litre (30–80 ng/ml). Lower levels are observed in patients treated with barbiturates, phenytoin and carbamazepine in combination (HUANG et al. 1974; SJÖ et al. 1975). Within patients, the relationship between serum clonazepam concentration and dosage appears to be linear (SJÖ et al. 1975; EADIE 1976). At steady state, the ratio between the plasma concentration of clonazepam and that of the 7-amino metabolite ranges from 1 : 3 to 3 : 1 (SJÖ et al. 1975).

G. Oxazolidinediones

I. Trimethadione (Troxidone)

Trimethadione is rapidly absorbed from the gastrointestinal tract, peak serum levels occurring within 30 min after a single oral dose (BOOKER 1972).

Assuming complete absorption, BOOKER (1972) calculated that the apparent volume of distribution of unchanged drug is about 0.6 litres/kg. The volume of distribution of the metabolite dimethadione is probably somewhat smaller (WITHROW and WOODBURY 1972). Dimethadione is a weak acid ($pK_a = 6.1$) and changes in tissue pH, by altering its degree of ionization, could have an important influence on the distribution of this compound.

Only a small fraction of the administered dose of trimethadione is excreted unchanged in urine. The drug is converted almost entirely to dimethadione, which is pharmacologically active (CHAMBERLIN et al. 1965; FREY 1969). The metabolite does not appear to undergo further degradation and is excreted in urine (WADDELL and BUTLER 1957 b).

The half-life of unchanged trimethadione is about 16 h (BOOKER 1972). The active metabolite dimethadione is very extensively reabsorbed from the renal tubuli and has a very slow rate of elimination; JENSEN (1962) and CHAMBERLIN et al. (1965) reported dimethadione half-life values of approximately 10 days.

Alkalinization of urine reduces the amount of dimethadione reabsorbed from the renal tubuli and hastens its elimination (WADDELL and BUTLER 1957b; JENSEN 1962).

In patients started on trimethadione treatment, serum levels of unchanged drug reach a plateau after about 4–5 days. It may take a much longer period (30 days or more) before a steady-state concentration of dimethadione is achieved (JENSEN 1962). At steady state, serum dimethadione levels are approximately 20 times higher than the trimethadione levels. Serum levels of both parent drug and metabolite are positively correlated with the administered dose (BOOKER 1972). Since the concentration of dimethadione is so greatly in excess of that of the parent compound, it is likely that the metabolite plays a major part in the pharmacological effect seen in patients stabilized on trimethadione therapy. CHAMBERLIN et al. (1965) found that dimethadione alone controls petit mal when given in doses sufficient to produce serum levels equivalent to those observed during trimethadione treatment. The long period required to reach steady-state dimethadione levels may explain why in some patients there is a delay between the onset of trimethadione therapy and the attainment of a full therapeutic response (CHAMBERLIN et al. 1965).

II. Paramethadione

Paramethadione is rapidly absorbed from the gastrointestinal tract (HOFFMAN and CHUN 1975). In man, the drug is rapidly converted into the *N*-demethylated metabolite, 5-ethyl-5-methyl-2,4-oxazolidinedione. The half-life of the parent drug is about 16 h (HOFFMAN and CHUN 1975), whereas that of the metabolite is extremely long. In two subjects started on treatment with paramethadione (900 mg daily) serum levels of the metabolite were found to be steadily rising after 2 weeks (BUTLER 1955). Following discontinuation of treatment, serum metabolite levels declined very slowly with half-life values of 11 and 19 days respectively. These data suggest that it may take more than 2 months for the serum level of the metabolite to reach steady state after an adjustment in paramethadione dose. At steady state, serum levels of the demethylated derivative are expected to exceed greatly those of the parent drug. The possible contribution of the metabolite to the pharmacological effect is unclear. This should be kept in mind, especially in view of the analogy with the situation described above in respect to trimethadione and dimethadione (BUTLER and WADDELL 1958).

H. Acetazolamide

Acetazolamide, in doses up to 5–10 mg/kg, is rapidly and completely absorbed from the gastrointestinal tract. Larger doses may be erratically absorbed. In man, the apparent volume of distribution is said to be about 0.2 litres/kg (WOODBURY 1972). Acetazolamide is a weak acid with a pK_a of 7.4, and therefore its degree of tissue penetration is markedly influenced by pH changes within the physiological range. In rodents, the drug accumulates in tissues with high carbonic anhydrase content, e.g. the erythrocytes, salivary glands, liver and thyroid. The brain concentration is lower than the serum concentration. Acetazolamide is 90%–95%

bound to plasma proteins. The degree of binding is inversely related to the plasma concentration (WOODBURY 1972).

In patients receiving effective antiepileptic doses (about 10 mg/kg per day) serum acetazolamide levels are 10–14 μg/ml. In man, acetazolamide is excreted entirely unchanged in urine, partly through an active secretory process. After administration of a single dose the decline of the serum levels is characterized by fast and slow components (WOODBURY 1972). The initial (rapid) phase reflects largely a redistribution process and is characterized by a half-life of about 1.5 h. The elimination half-life should also be relatively short if virtually 100% of a single oral dose is excreted in urine within 24 h. WOODBURY (1972) discussed the evidence for a tissue compartment represented by the drug-carbonic anhydrase complex. Elimination of the drug from this complex is a slow process with a half-life of several days.

J. Sulthiame

Sulthiame is a sulphonamide drug with weak carbonic anhydrase-inhibiting properties, mainly known for its ability to elevate serum phenytoin levels in epileptic patients (HOUGHTON and RICHENS 1976b). When given orally, the drug is absorbed fairly rapidly with peak serum levels occurring after 1–5 h (OLESEN 1968). From a study in which radio-labelled sulthiame was given to six subjects, DIAMOND and LEVY (1963) concluded that the absorption is almost complete. The recovery of radioactivity in urine and faeces, however, was grossly incomplete and therefore definitive proof of a high oral availability is lacking.

In animals, sulthiame penetrates readily into tissues and is found in the brain at concentrations similar to those observed in serum (GREEN and KUPFERBERG 1972). OLESEN (1968) found that in epileptic patients 17%–69% of the administered dose is excreted unchanged in urine. An additional fraction of the urinary excretion is in the form of a metabolite, probably a hydroxylated derivative (DIAMOND and LEVY 1963; GREEN and KUPFERBERG 1972).

The elimination half-life of sulthiame is short, as indicated by considerable fluctuations in the serum levels at steady state (GREEN et al. 1974). OLESEN (1968) found sulthiame levels of 0.5–12 μg/ml in fasting samples collected from patients receiving daily doses between 3 and 14.5 mg/kg. In patients receiving doses between 400 and 3,600 mg (mean 1,993 mg) daily, TROUPIN et al. (1974) reported sulthiame levels of 29 μg/ml on average, with most patients in the 10–50 μg/ml range. In the latter study, serum sulthiame levels were found to be linearly related to dose.

K. Pheneturide

No information is available on the absolute bioavailability of pheneturide. Apparent volumes of distribution calculated after a single oral dose on the assumption that absorption is complete are about 3.3 litres/kg on average (GALEAZZI et al. 1979). It is likely that the drug is partly bound to plasma proteins, since the cerebrospinal fluid/serum concentration ratio is about 40% (MIYAMOTO et al.

1975). Half-lives calculated following a single oral dose in normal volunteers range from 32 to 90 h. GALEAZZI et al. (1979) found that following discontinuation of subchronic treatment with pheneturide (1 g daily for 10 days) in four subjects, half-life values were shorter and apparent volumes of distribution were smaller than those determined in a separate group of subjects after a single dose. Pheneturide is probably extensively metabolized. Only a small fraction of the orally administered dose is excreted unchanged in urine.

References

Abel JG, Sellers EM, Naranjo CA, Shaw J, Kadar D, Romach MK (1979) Inter- and intrasubject variation in diazepam free fraction. Clin Pharmacol Ther 26:247–255
Abernethy DR, Greenblatt DJ (1981) Metabolite-parent drug interaction study: desmethyldiazepam effect in diazepam kinetics. Clin Pharmacol Ther 29:230–231
Ackermann E, Richter K (1977) Diazepam metabolism in human foetal and adult liver. Eur J Clin Pharmacol 11:43–49
Agurell S, Berlin A, Ferngren H, Hellstrom B (1975) Plasma levels of diazepam after parenteral and rectal administration in children. Epilepsia 16:277–283
Albert KS, Sakmar E, Hallmark MR, Weidler DJ, Wagner JG (1974) Bioavailability of diphenylhydantoin. Clin Pharmacol Ther 16:727–735
Alexander FW (1979) Sodium valproate and pregnancy. Arch Dis Child 54:240
Alvarez N, Hartford E, Cavalleri E (1981) Low blood levels of phenobarbital due to poor gastrointestinal solubility of phenobarbital tablets. Ann Neurol 9:305–310
Alvin J, McHorse TS, Hoyumpa A, Bush MT, Schenker S (1975) The effect of liver disease in man on the disposition of phenobarbital. J Pharmacol Exp Ther 192:224–235
Anavekar SN, Saunders RH, Wardell WM, Shoulson I, Emmings FG, Cook CE, Gringeri AJ (1979) Parotid and whole saliva in the prediction of serum total and free phenytoin concentrations. Clin Pharmacol Ther 24:629–637
Andoh B, Idle JR, Sloan TP, Smith RL, Woolhouse N (1980) Inter-ethnic and inter-phenotype differences among Ghanaians and Caucasians in the metabolic hydroxylation of phenytoin. Br J Clin Pharmacol 9:282–283P
Andresen BD, Davis FT, Templeton JL (1976) Synthesis and characterization of alpha-phenyl gamma butyrolactone, a metabolite of glutethimide, phenobarbital and primidone, in human urine. Res Commun Chem Pathol Pharmacol 15:21–30
Andreasen PB, Hendel J, Greisen G, Hvidberg EF (1976) Pharmacokinetics of diazepam in disordered liver function. Eur J Clin Pharmacol 10:115–120
Anttila M, Kahela P, Panelius M, Yriänä T, Tikkanen R, Aaltonen R (1979) Comparative bioavailability of two commercial preparations of carbamazepine tablets. Eur J Clin Pharmacol 15:421–425
Arnold K, Gerber N (1970) The rate of decline of diphenylhydantoin in human plasma. Clin Pharmacol Ther 11:121–134
Ashley JJ, Levy G (1972) Inhibition of diphenylhydantoin elimination by its major metabolite. Res Commun Chem Pathol Pharmacol 4:297–306
Ashley JJ, Levy G (1973) Kinetics of diphenylhydantoin elimination in rats. J Pharmacokinet Biopharm 1:99–102
Atkinson AJ Jr, Mac Gee J, Strong J, Garteiz D, Gaffney TE (1970) Identification of 5-toxicity. Clin Pharmacol Ther 14:521–528
Atinson AJ Jr, Mac Gee J, Strong J, Garteiz D, Gaffney TE (1970) Identification of 5-meta-hydroxyphenyl-5-phenylhydantoin as a metabolite of diphenylhydantoin. Biochem Pharmacol 19:2483–2491
Ayers GI, Burnett D (1977) Drug formulations and salivary phenytoin measurements. Lancet I:656–657
Bailey DN, Jatlow PI (1972) Clinical analysis of massive crystalluria following primidone overdose. Am J Clin Pathol 58:583–589

Barron SJ, Darcey BA , Booker HE (1974) Metabolism and kinetics of methsuximide in man. Neurology 24:386

Bartels H, Günther E, Wallis S (1979) Flow-dependent salivary primidone levels in epileptic children. Epilepsia 20:431–436

Barth N, Alvan G, Borgå O, Sjöqvist F (1976) Two-fold interindividual variation in plasma protein binding of phenytoin in patients with epilepsy. Clin Pharmacokinet 1:444–452

Battino D, Bossi L, Croci D, Cusi C, Gomeni C, Moise A, Spina S (1980) Plasma levels of primidone and phenobarbital in children and adults: influence of age and associated therapy. Acta Neurol Scan [Suppl] 62:101

Baumel IP, Gallagher BB, Mattson RH (1972) Phenylethylmalonamide (PEMA) An important metabolite of primidone. Arch Neurol 27:34–41

Berlin A, Dahlström H (1975) Pharmacokinetics of the anticonvulsant drug clonazepam evaluated from single oral dose and intravenous doses and by repeated oral administration. Eur J Clin Pharmacol 9:155–159

Berlin A, Siwers B, Agurell S, Hiort A, Sjöqvist F, Ström S (1975) Determination of bioavailability of diazepam in various formulations from steady-state plasma concentration data. Clin Pharmacol Ther 13:733–744

Berman PH (1976) Management of seizure disorders with anticonvulsant drugs: current concepts. Pediatr Clin North Am 23:443–459

Bertilsson L (1978) Clinical pharmacokinetics of carbamazepine. Clin Pharmacokinet 3:128–143

Bertilsson L, Höjer B, Tybring G, Osterloh J, Rane A (1980) Autoinduction of carbamazepine metabolism in children examined by a stable isotope technique. Clin Pharmacol Ther 27:83–88

Blain PG, Mucklow JC, Bacon CJ, Rawlins MD (1981) Pharmacokinetics of phenytoin in children. Br J Clin Pharmacol 12:659–662

Blashke TF, Meffin PJ, Melmon KL, Rowland M (1975) Influence of acute viral hepatitis on phenytoin kinetics and protein binding. Clin Pharmacol Ther 17:685–691

Bochner F, Hooper WD, Tyrer JH, Eadie MJ (1972) Factors involved in an outbreak of phenytoin intoxication. J Neurol Sci 16:481–487

Bochner F, Hooper WD, Sutherland JM, Eadie MJ, Tyrer JH (1974) Diphenylhydantoin concentrations in saliva. Arch Neurol 3:57–59

Booker HE (1972) Trimethadione and other oxazolidinediones. Relation of plasma levels to clinical control. In: Woodbury DM, Penry JK, Schmidt RP (eds) Antiepileptic drugs. Raven, New York, pp 403–407

Booker HE, Hosokowa K, Burdette RD, Darcey B (1970) A clinical study of serum primidone levels. Epilepsia 11:395–402

Boreus LO, Jalling B, Wallin A (1978) Plasma concentrations of phenobarbital in mother and child after combined prenatal and postnatal administration for prophylaxis of hyperbilirubinemia. J Pediatr 93:695–698

Borgå O, Juhlin-Dannfeldt A, Dahlqvist R (1978) Plasma levels and protein binding of phenytoin during exercise in man. The effect of elevated free fatty acids. Pharmacology 16:37–43

Borgå O, Hoppel C, Odar-Cederlöf I, Garle M (1979) Plasma levels and renal excretion of phenytoin and its metabolites in patients with renal failure. Clin Pharmacol Ther 26:306–314

Borofsky LG, Louis S, Kutt H (1973) Diphenylhydantoin in children. Pharmacology and efficacy. Neurology 23:967–972

Borondy P, Dill WA, Chang T, Buchanan R, Glazko A (1973) Effect of protein binding on the distribution of 5,5-diphenylhydantoin between plasma and red cells. Ann NY Acad Sci 222:82–87

Borst SI, Lookwood CH (1975) Plasma level studies on different brands of sodium diphenylhydantoin (DPH) and primidone. Int J Clin Pharmacol Biopharm 12:309–314

Boutroy MJ, Royer-Morrot MJ, Legras B, Royer RJ, Vert P, Moreau RM (1980) Pharmacocinétique du phénobarbital chez le nouveau-né. In: Mathieu H, Pantonnier G, Olive G (eds) Pharmacologie de developpement, INSERM Seminar vol 89 pp 329–338

Bowdle TA, Levy RH, Cutler RE (1979) Effect of carbamazepine on valproic acid kinetics in normal subjects. Clin Pharmacol Ther 26:629–634
Bowdle TA, Patel IH, Levy RH, Wilensky AJ (1980) Valproic acid dosage and plasma protein binding and clearance. Clin Pharmacol Ther 28:486–492
Brachet-Liermain A, Demarquez JL (1977) Pharmacokinetics of dipropyl acetate in infants and young children. Pharm Weekbl [Sci] 112:293–297
Brachet-Liermain A, Goutieres F, Aicardi J (1975) Absorption of phenobarbital after the intramuscular administration of single doses in infants. J Pediatr 87:624–626
Branch RA, Morgan MH, James J, Read AE (1976) Intravenous administration of diazepam in patients with chronic liver disease. Gut 17:975–983
Brandt R (1976) Passage of diazepam and desmethyldiazepam in breast milk, Arzneimittelforsch 26:454–457
Braun CW, Goldstone JM (1980) Increased clearance of phenytoin as the presenting feature of infectious mononucleosis. Ther Drug Monit 2:355–357
Brewster D, Muir NC (1980) Valproate plasma protein binding in the uremic condition. Clin Pharmacol Ther 27:76–82
Brillman J, Gallagher BB, Mattson RH (1974) Acute primidone intoxication. Arch Neurol 30:255–258
Browne TR, Dreifuss FE, Dynen PR, Goode DJ, Penry JK, Porter RJ, White BG, White PT (1975) Ethosuximide in the treatment of absence (*petit mal*) seizures. Neurology 25:515–524
Browne TR, Van Langenhove A, Costello CE, Biemann K, Greenblatt DJ (1981) Kinetic equivalence of stable-isotope-labelled and unlabelled phenytoin. Clin Pharmacol Ther 29:511–515
Bruni J, Wang LH, Marbury TC, Lee CS, Wilder BJ (1979) Protein binding of valproic acid in uremic patients. Neurology 30:557–559
Buchanan RA, Fernandez L, Kinkel AW (1969) Absorption and elimination of ethosuximide in children. J Clin Pharmacol 9:393–398
Buchanan RA, Kinkel AW, Smith TC (1973a) The absorption and excretion of ethosuximide. Int Clin Pharmacol Ther Toxicol 7:213–218
Buchanan RA, Turner JL, Moyer CF, Heffelfinger JC (1973b) Single daily dose of diphenylhydantoin in children. J Pediatr 83:479–483
Buchanan RA, Kinkel AW, Turner J, Heffelfinger JC (1976) Ethosuximide dosage regimens. Clin Pharmacol Ther 19:142–147
Butler TC (1955) Metabolic demethylation of 3,5-dimethyl-5-ethyl 2,4-oxazolidinedione (paramethadione, paradione) J Pharmacol Exp Ther 113:178–185
Butler TC (1956a) The metabolic conversion of 3-methyl-5-ethyl-5-phenylhydantoin (mesantoin) and of 5-ethyl-5-phenylhydantoin (nirvanol) to 5-ethyl-5-(*p*-hydroxyphenyl)-hydantoin. J Pharmacol Exp Ther 117:160–165
Butler TC (1956a) The metabolic hydroxylation of phenobarbital. J Pharmacol Exp Ther 116:326–336
Butler TC (1957) The metabolic conversion of 5-5-diphenylhydantoin to 5-(*p*-hydroxyphenyl)-5-phenylhydantoin. J Pharmacol Exp Ther 119:1–11
Butler TC, Waddell WJ (1958) *N*-Methylated derivatives of barbituric acids, hydantoin and oxazolidinedione used in the treatment of epilepsy. Neurology [Suppl 1] 8:106–112
Butler TC, Mahaffee C, Waddell WJ (1954) Phenobarbital: studies of elimination, accumulation, tolerance and dosage schedule. J Pharmacol Exp Ther 111:425–435
Cate JC, Tenser R (1975) Acute primidone overdosage with massive crystalluria. Clin Toxicol 8:385–389
Cereghino JJ, Brock JT, Van Meter JC, Penry JK, Smith LD, White BG (1975) The efficacy of carbamazepine combinations in epilepsy. Clin Pharmacol Ther 18:733–741
Chamberlin HR, Waddell WJ, Butler TC (1965) A study of the product of demethylation of trimethadione in the control of petit mal epilepsy. Neurology 15:449–454
Chang T, Dill WA, Glazko AJ (1972) Ethosuximide. Absorption, distribution and excretion. In: Woodbury DM, Penry JK, Schmidt RP (eds) Antiepileptic drugs. Raven, New York, pp 417–423

Chen SS, Perucca E, Lee J-N, Richens A (1982) Serum protein binding and free concentration of phenytoin and phenobarbitone in pregnancy. Br J Clin Pharmacol 4:551–554

Christiansen J, Dam M (1973) Influence of phenobarbital and diphenylhydantoin on plasma carbamazepine levels in patients with epilepsy. Acta Neurol Scand 49:543–546

Chun AHC, Hoffman DJ, Friedmann N, Carrigan PJ (1980) Bioavailability of valproic acid under fasting/nonfasting regimens. J Clin Pharmacol 20:30–36

Cloyd JC, Miller KW, Leppik IE (1981) Primidone kinetics: effects of concurrent drugs and duration of therapy. Clin Pharmacol Ther 29:402–407

Cocks DA, Critchley EMR, Hayward HW, Owen V, Mawer GE, Woodcock BG (1975) Control of epilepsy with a single daily dose of phenytoin sodium. Br J Clin Pharmacol 2:449–553

Cossum PA, Roberts MS (1981) Availability of isosorbide dinitrate, diazepam and chlormethiazole from i.v. delivery systems. Eur J Clin Pharmacol 19:181–185

Cotter LM, Eadie MJ, Hooper WD, Lander CM, Smith GA, Tyrer JH (1977) The pharmacokinetics of carbamazepine. Eur J Clin Pharmacol 12:451–456

Cottrell PR, Street JM, Berry DJ, Schäfer H, Pisani F, Perucca E, Richens A (1982) Pharmacokinetics of phenylethylmalonamide (PEMA) in normal subjects and in patients treated with antiepileptic drugs. Epilepsia 23:307–313

Cramer JA, Mattson RH (1979) Valproic acid: *in vitro* plasma protein binding and interaction with phenytoin. Ther Drug Monit 1:105–116

Dam M, Christiansen J, Munck O, Mygind KI (1979) Antiepileptic drugs: metabolism in pregnancy. Clin Pharmacokinet 4:53

Dam M, Christiansen J, Christiansen CB, Helles A, Jaegerskou A, Schmiegelow M (1981) Carbamazepine: a clinical biopharmaceutical study. Eur J Clin Pharmacol 20:59–64

Dasberg HH, Van Der Kleijn E, Guelen PJR, Van Praag HM (1974) Plasma concentrations of diazepam and its metabolite *N*-desmethyldiazepam in relation to anxiolytic effect. Clin Pharmacol Ther 15:473–483

Dhillon S, Richens A (1981 a) Bioavailability of rectally administered diazepam in adult epileptic patients. Br J Clin Pharmacol 11:437–438P

Dhillon S, Richens A (1981 b) Pharmacokinetics of diazepam in epileptic patients and normal volunteers following intravenous administration. Br J Clin Pharmacol 12:841–844

Diamond S, Levy L (1963) Metabolic studies on a new anti-epileptic drug: Riker 594. Curr Ther Res 5:325–330

Dickinson RG, Harland RC, Lynn RK, Smith WB, Gerber N (1979) Transmission of valproic acid (Depakene) across the placenta: half-life of the drug in mother and baby. J Pediatr 94:832–835

Di Gregorio GJ, Peraino AJ, Ruch E (1978) Diazepam concentrations in parotid saliva, mixed saliva and plasma. Clin Pharmacol Ther 24:720–725

Di Salle E, Pacifici GM, Morselli PL (1974) Studies on plasma protein binding of carbamazepine. Pharmacol Res Commun 6:193–202

Divoll-Allen MRN, Greenblatt DJ (1981) Absolute bioavailability of oral and intramuscular diazepam. Clin Pharmacol Ther 29:240–241

Dixon R, Crews T (1978) Diazepam: determination in micro samples of blood, plasma, and saliva by radioimmunoassay. J Anal Toxicol 2:210–213

Dodson EW (1980) Phenytoin elimination in childhood: effect of concentration-dependent kinetics. Neurology 30:196–199

Dreifuss FE, Penry JK, Rose SW, Kupferberg HJ, Dyken P, Sato S (1975) Serum clonazepam concentrations in children with absence seizures. Neurology, 25:255–258

Driessen O, Van Der Velde E, Höppener R (1980) Practical and theoretical aspects of phenytoin administration. II Prediction of plasma concentration. Eur Neurol 19:103–114

Dudley KH, Bius DL, Butler TC (1970) Metabolic fates of 3-ethyl-5-phenylhydantoin (ethotoin, Peganone®), 3-methyl-5-phenyl-hydantoin and 5-phenylhydantoin. J Pharmacol Exp Ther 175:27–37

Eadie MJ (1976) Plasma level monitoring of anticonvulsants. Clin Pharmacokinet 1:52–66

Eadie MJ, Tyrer JH (1980) Anticonvulsant therapy, Churchill-Livingstone, Edinburgh

Eadie MJ, Tyrer JH, Bochner F, Hooper WD (1976) The elimination of phenytoin in man. Clin Exp Pharmacol Physiol 3:217–224
Eadie MJ, Lander CM, Hooper WD, Tyrer JH (1977a) Factors influencing plasma phenobarbitone levels in epileptic patients. Br J Clin Pharmacol 4:541–547
Eadie MJ, Tyrer JH, Smith GA, McKauge L (1977b) Pharmacokinetics of drugs used for petit mal absence epilepsy. Clin Exp Neurol 14:172–183
Eadie MJ, Bochner F, Hooper WD, Tyrer JH (1978) Preliminary observations on the pharmacokinetics of methylphenobarbitone. Clin Exp Neurol 15:131–144
Ehrnebo M, Odar-Cederlöf I (1975) The binding of amobarbital, pentobarbital and diphenylhydantoin to blood cells and plasma proteins in healthy volunteers and uremic patients. Eur J Clin Pharmacol 8:445–453
Ehrnebo M, Agurell S, Jalling B, Boreus LO (1971) Age differences in drug binding by plasma proteins: studies on human foetuses, neonates and adults. Eur J Clin Pharmacol 3:189–193
Eichelbaum M, Ekbom K, Bertilsson L, Ringberger VA, Rane A (1975) Plasma kinetics of carbamazepine and its epoxide in man during single and multiple dosing. Eur J Clin Pharmacol 8:337–341
Eichelbaum M, Bertilsson L, Lund L, Palmer L, Sjöqvist F (1976) Plasma levels of carbamazepine and carbamazepine-10,11-epoxide during carbamazepine therapy in epileptic patients. Eur J Clin Pharmacol 9:417–421
Eichelbaum M, Köthe KW, Hoffmann F, Von Unruh GE (1979) Kinetics and metabolism of carbamazepine during combined antiepileptic therapy. Clin Pharmacol Ther 26:366–371
Elfström J (1977) Plasma protein binding of phenytoin after cholecystectomy and neurosurgical operations. Acta Neurol Scand 55:455–464
Erkkola R, Kanto J (1972) Diazepam and breast feeding. Lancet I:1235–1236
Erkkola R, Kanto J, Sellman R (1974) Diazepam in early human pregnancy. Acta Obstet Gynaecol, Scand 53:135–138
Eschenof VE (1973) Untersuchungen über das Schicksal des Antikonvulsivums Clonazepam im Organismus der Ratte, des Hundes und des Menschen. Arzneimittelforsch 23:390–400
Espir MLE, Benton P, Will E, Hayes MJ, Walker G (1976) Sodium valproate (Epilim)–some clinical and pharmacological aspects. In: Legg NJ (ed) Clinical and pharmacological aspects of sodium valproate (Epilim) in the treatment of epilepsy. MCS Consultants, Tunbridge Wells, pp 145–151
Faigle JW, Feldmann KF (1975) Pharmacokinetic data of carbamazepine and its major metabolites in man. In: Schneider H, Janz D, Gardner-Thorpe C, Meinardi M, Sherwin AS (eds) Clinical pharmacology of anti-epileptic drugs. Springer, Berlin Heidelberg New York, pp 159–165
Fredholm BB, Rane A, Persson B (1975) Diphenylhydantoin binding to proteins in plasma and its dependence on free fatty acids and bilirubin concentration in dogs and newborn infants. Pediatr Res 9:26–30
Frey HH (1969) Determination of the anticonvulsant potency of unmetabolized trimethadione. Acta Pharmacol Toxicol 27:295–300
Frigerio A, Morselli PL (1975) Carbamazepine: biotransformation. In: Penry JK, Daly DD (eds) Advances in neurology, vol II. Raven, New York pp 275–280
Frigo GM, Lecchini S, Gatti G, Perucca E, Crema A (1979) Modification of phenytoin clearance by valproic acid in normal subjects. Br J Clin Pharmacol 8:553–556
Friis ML, Christiansen J, Hvidberg EF (1978) Brain concentrations of carbamazepine and carbamazepine-10,11-epoxide in epileptic patients. Eur J Clin Pharmacol 14:47–51
Galeazzi RL, Egli M, Wad N (1979) Pharmacokinetics of phenylethylacetylurea (pheneturide) an old antiepileptic drug. J Pharmacokinet Biopharm 7:453–462
Gallagher BB, Baumel IP (1972) Primidone. Biotransformation. In: Woodbury DM, Penry JK, Schmidt RP (eds). Antiepileptic drugs, Raven, New York, pp 361–366
Gallagher BB, Baumel IP, Mattson RH (1972) Metabolic disposition of primidone and its metabolites in epileptic subjects after single and repeated administration. Neurology 22:1186–1192

Gamble JAS, Dundee JW, Assaf RAE (1975) Plasma diazepam levels after single oral and intramuscular administration. Anaesthesia 30:164–169

Garrettson LK, Dayton PG (1970) Disappearance of phenobarbital and diphenylhydantoin from serum of children. Clin Pharmacol Ther 11:674–679

Garrettson LK, Jusko WJ (1975) Diphenylhydantoin elimination kinetics in overdosed children. Clin Pharmacol Ther 17:481–491

Garrettson LK, Kim OK (1970) Apparent saturation of diphenylhydantoin metabolism in children. Pediat Res 4:455

Gatti G, Perucca E, Caravaggi M, Poloni M, Frigo GM, Crema A (1977) Pharmacokinetics of phenytoin following intravenous administration in epileptic patients. Farmaco (Prat) 32:470–474

Gerardin A, Hirz J (1976) The quantitative assay of carbamazepine in biological material and its application to basic pharmacokinetic studies. In: Birkmayer H (ed) Epileptic seizures, behaviour, pain. Huber, Berne, pp 151–164

Gerardin AP, Abadie FV, Campestrini JA, Theobald W (1976) Pharmacokinetics of carbamazepine in normal humans after single and repeated oral doses. J Pharmacokinet Biopharm 4:521–535

Gerber N, Weller WL, Lynn R, Rangno RE, Sweetman BJ, Bush MT (1971) Study of dose-dependent metabolism of 5,5-diphenylhydantoin in the rat using new methodology for isolation and quantitation of metabolites *in vivo* and *in vitro*. J Pharmacol Exp Ther 178:567–579

Gerber N, Thompson RM, Smith RG, Lynn RK (1979) Evidence for the epoxide-diol pathway in the biotransformation of mephenytoin. Epilepsia 20:287–294

Giacomini K, Giacomini J, Blaschke T (1980) Heparin decreases plasma protein binding of drugs. Clin Pharmacol Ther 27:256

Giles HH, Zilm DH, Frecker RC, Macleod SM, Sellers EM (1977) Saliva and plasma concentrations of diazepam after a single oral dose. Br J Clin Pharmacol 4:711–712

Glazko AJ (1973) Diphenylhydantoin metabolism. A prospective review. Drug Metab Dispos 1:711–714

Glazko AJ (1975) Antiepileptic drugs: biotransformation, metabolism and serum half-life. Epilepsia 16:367–391

Glazko AJ, Dill WA (1972) Other succinimides. Methsuximide and phensuximide. In: Woodbury DM, Penry JK, Schmidt RP (eds) Antiepileptic drugs. Raven, New York, pp 455–464

Glazko AJ, Dill WA, Wolf LM, Miller CA (1954) The determination and physiological disposition of Milontin (*N*-methyl-α-phenylsuccinimide). J Pharmacol Exp Ther 111:413–424

Glazko AJ, Chang T, Baukema J, Dill WA, Goulet JR, Buchanan RA (1969) Metabolic disposition of diphenylhydantoin in normal human subjects following intravenous administration. Clin Pharmacol Ther 10:498–504

Goldberg MA, Crandall PH (1978) Human brain binding of phenytoin. Neurology 28:881–885

Goldberg MA, Gal J, Cho AK, Jenden DJ (1979) Metabolism of dimethoxymethylphenobarbital (Eterobarb) in patients with epilepsy. Ann Neurol 5:121–126

Goulet JR, Kinkel AW, Smith TC (1976) Metabolism of ethosuximide. Clin Pharmacol Ther 20:213–218

Gram L, Flachs H, Wurtz-Jorgensen A, Parnas J, Andersen B (1979) Sodium valproate, serum level and clinical effect in epilepsy: a controlled study. Epilepsia 20:303–312

Green JR, Kupferberg HJ (1972) Sulfonamides and derivatives Sulthiame. In: Woodbury DM, Penry JK, Schmidt RP (eds) Antiepileptic drugs. Raven, New York, pp 477–485

Green JR, Troupin AS, Halpern LM, Friel P, Kanarek P (1974) Sulthiame: evaluation as an anticonvulsant. Epilepsia 15:329–349

Greenblatt DJ, Allen MD, Maclaughlin DS, Harmatz JS, Shader RI (1978a) Diazepam absorption: effects of antacids and food. Clin Pharmacol Ther 24:600–609

Greenblatt DJ, Divoll-Allen M, Harmatz JS, Shader RI (1980) Diazepam disposition determinants. Clin Pharmacol Ther 27:301–312

Greenblatt DJ, Laughren TP, Allen MD, Harmatz JS, Shader RI (1981) Plasma diazepam and desmethyl-diazepam concentrations during long-term diazepam therapy. Br J Clin Pharmacol 11:35–40

Griffiths A, Hebdige S, Perucca E, Richens A (1980) Quality control in drug measurements. Ther Drug Monit 2:51–60

Gruska H, Beyer KH, Kubicki S, Schneider H (1971) Klinik, Toxikologie und Therapie eine schweren Carbamazepine-Vergiftung. Arch Toxicol 27:193–203

Guelen PJM, Deimann LGJ (1980) Influence of plasma lipids on the protein binding of diphenylhydantoin and its clinical significance. In: Johannessen SI, Morselli PL, Pippenger CE, Richens A, Schmidt D, Meinardi H (eds) Antiepileptic therapy: advances in drug monitoring. Raven, New York, pp 185–192

Gugler R, Azarnoff DL (1976) Drug protein binding and the nephrotic syndrome. Clin Pharmacokinet 1:25–35

Gugler R, Muller G (1978) Plasma protein binding of valproic acid in healthy subjects and in patients with renal disease. Br J Clin Pharmacol 5:441–446

Gugler R, Von Unruh GE (1981) Clinical pharmacokinetics of valproic acid. Clin Pharmacokinet 5:67–83

Gugler R, Shoeman DW, Azarnoff DL (1974) Effect of *in vivo* elevation of free fatty acids on protein binding of drugs. Pharmacology 12:160

Gugler R, Manion CV, Azarnoff DL (1976) Phenytoin: pharmacokinetics and bioavailability. Clin Pharmacol Ther 19:135–142

Gugler R, Schell A, Eichelbaum M, Fröscher W, Schultz HV (1977) Disposition of valproic acid in man. Eur J Clin Pharmacol 12:125–132

Haidukewych D, Rodin EA (1980) Monitoring 2-ethyl-3-phenylmalonamide in serum by gas-liquid chromatography: application to retrospective study in epilepsy patients dosed with primidone. Clin Chem 26:1537–1539

Hallstrom C, Lader MH, Curry SH (1980) Diazepam and its *N*-desmethyldiazepam concentrations in saliva, plasma and CSF. Br J Clin Pharmacol 9:333–339

Hansen SE, Feldberg L (1964) Absorption and elimination of Zarontin. Dan Med Bull 11:54–55

Harvey DJ, Glazener L, Stratton C, Nowlin J, Hill RM, Horning MG (1972) Detection of a 5-(3,4-dihydroxy-1,5-cyclo-hexadiene-1-yl)-metabolite of phenobarbital and mephobarbital in rat, guinea pig and human. Res Commun Chem Pathol Pharmacol 3:557–566

Hayes MJ, Langman MJS, Short AH (1975) Changes in drug metabolism with increasing age. II. Phenytoin clearance and protein binding. Br J Clin Pharmacol 2:73–79

Heimann G, Gladtke E (1977) Parmacokinetics of phenobarbital in childhood. Eur J Clin Pharmacol 12:305–310

Heimann G, Neuwald F, Gladtke E (1978) Die rektale Absorption von Phenobarbital bei Kindern unter dem Einfluß verschiedener Vehikel. Arzneimittelforsch 28:1023–1027

Heipertz R, Guthoff A, Bernhardt W (1979) Primidone metabolism in renal insufficiency and acute intoxication. J Neurol 221:101–104

Hendel J (1975) Cumulation in the cerebrospinal fluid of the *N*-desmethyl metabolite after long-term treatment with diazepam in man. Acta Pharmacol Toxicol 37:17–22

Hillestad L, Hansen T, Melsom H (1974a) Diazepam metabolism in normal man. II. Serum concentration and clinical effect after oral administration and cumulation. Clin Pharmacol Ther 16:485–489

Hillestad L, Hansen T, Melsom H, Driveness A (1974b) Diazepam metabolism in normal man. I. Serum concentrations and clinical effects after intravenous, intramuscular and oral administration. Clin Pharmacol Ther 16:479–484

Hoffman DJ, Chun AHC (1975) Paramethadione and metabolite serum levels in humans after a single oral paramethadione dose. J Pharm Sci 64:1702–1703

Hooper WD, Eadie MJ, Tyrer JH (1973) Plasma diphenylhydantoin levels in Australian children. Aust NZ J Med 4:456–461

Hooper W, Bochner F, Eadie MJ, Tyrer JH (1974a) Plasma protein binding of diphenylhydantoin. Effects of sex hormones, renal and hepatic disease. Clin Pharmacol Ther 15:276–282

Hooper WD, Dubetz DK, Eadie MJ, Tyrer JH (1974b) Preliminary observations on the clinical pharmacology of carbamazepine (Tegretol). Proc Aust Ass Neurol 11:189–198

Hooper WD, Dubetz DK, Bochner F, Cother LM, Smith GA, Eadie MJ, Tyrer JH (1975) Plasma protein binding of carbamazepine. Clin Pharmacol Ther 17:433–440

Hooper WD, Kunze HE, Eadie MJ (1981) Pharmacokinetics and bioavailability of methylphenobarbital in man. Ther Drug Monitor 3:39–44

Hoppel C, Garle M, Rane A, Sjöqvist F (1977) Plasma concentrations of 5-(4-hydroxyphenyl)-5-phenylhydantoin in phenytoin treated patients. Clin Pharmacol Ther 21:294–300

Höppener RJ, Kuyer A, Meijer JWA, Hulsman J (1980) Correlation between daily fluctuations of carbamazepine serum levels and intermittent side effects. Epilepsia 21:341–350

Horning MG, Stratton C, Wilson A, Horning EC, Hill RM (1971) Detection of 5-(3,4-dihydroxy-1,5-cyclohexadiene-1-yl)-5-phenylhydantoin (Dilantin) in the newborn human. Anal Lett 4:537–545

Horning MG, Butler C, Harvey DJ, Hill RM, Zion TE (1973) Metabolism of *N*,2-dimethyl-2-phenylsuccinimide (methsuximide) by the epoxide diol pathway in rat, guinea pig and human. Res Commun Chem Pathol Pharmacol 6:565–578

Horning MG, Nowlin J, Butler CM, Letratanangkoon K, Sommer K, Hill RM (1975) Clinical applications of gas-chromatograph/mass spectrometer/computer systems. Clin Chem 21:1282–1287

Houghton GW, Richens A (1974a) Rate of elimination of tracer doses of phenytoin at different steady-state serum concentrations in epileptic patients. Br J Clin Pharmacol 1:155–161

Houghton GW, Richens A (1974b) Phenytoin intoxication induced by sulthiame in epileptic patients. J Neurol Neurosurg Psych 37:275–281

Houghton GW, Richens A, Toseland PA, Davidson S, Falconer MA (1975a) Brain concentrations of phenytoin, phenobarbitone and primidone in epileptic patients. Eur J Clin Pharmacol 9:73–78

Houghton GW, Richens A, Leighton M (1975b) Effect of age, height, weight and sex on serum phenytoin concentration in epileptic patients. Br J Clin Pharmacol 2:251–256

Huang CY, McLeod JG, Sampson D, Hensley WJ (1974) Clonazepam in the treatment of epilepsy. Med J Aust 2:5–8

Irvine-Meek JM, Hall KW, Otten NH, Leroux M, Budnik M, Seshia SS (1981) Pharmacokinetic study of valproic acid in a neonate. Clin Pharmacol Ther 29:253–254

Jalling B (1974) Plasma and cerebrospinal fluid concentrations of phenobarbital in infants given single doses. Dev Med Child Neurol 16:785–793

Jalling B, Boreus LO, Rane A, Sjöqvist F (1970) Plasma concentrations of diphenylhydantoin in young infants. Pharmacologia Clinica 2:200–202

Jalling B, Boreus LO, Kallberg N, Agurell S (1973) Disappearance of circulating prenatally administered phenobarbital. Eur J Clin Pharmacol 6:234–238

Jensen BN (1962) Trimethadione in serum of patients with petit mal epilepsy. Dan Med Bull 9:74–79

Johannessen SI, Strandjord RE (1972) The concentration of carbamazepine (Tegretol®) in serum and in cerebrospinal fluid in patients with epilepsy. Acta Neurol Scand [Suppl 51] 48:445–446

Johannessen SI, Strandjord RE (1975a) Absorption and protein binding in serum of several antiepileptic drugs. In: Schneider H, Janz D, Gardner-Thorpe C, Meinardi H, Sherwin AL (eds) Clinical pharmacology of antiepileptic drugs. Springer, Berlin Heidelberg New York, pp 262–273

Johannessen SI, Strandjord RE (1975b) The influence of phenobarbitone and phenytoin on carbamazepine serum levels. In: Schneider H, Janz D, Gardner-Thorpe C, Meinardi H, Sherwin AL (eds) Clinical pharmacology of antiepileptic drugs. Springer, Berlin Heidelberg New York, pp 201–205

Johannessen SI, Gerna M, Bakke J, Strandjord RE, Morselli PL (1976) CSF concentrations and serum protein binding of carbamazepine and carbamazepine 10,11-epoxide in epileptic patients. Br J Clin Pharmacol 3:575–582

Johannessen SI, Hendriksen O (1977) Serum levels of di-*n*-propyl-acetate in epileptic patients. Pharm Weekbl [Sci] 112:287–289

Jones TD, Jacobs JL (1932) The treatment of obstinate chorea with Nirvanol with notes on its mode of action. JAMA 99:18–21

Jordan BJ, Shillingford JS, Steed KP (1976) Preliminary observations on the protein-binding and enzyme-inducing properties of sodium valproate (Epilim). In: Legg, N (ed) Clinical and pharmacological aspects of sodium valproate (Epilim) in the treatment of epilepsy. MCS Consultants, Tunbridge Wells, pp 112–116

Jusko WJ, Koup JR, Alvan G (1976) Nonlinear assessment of phenytoin bioavailability. J Pharmacokinet Biopharm 4:327–336

Kållberg N, Agurell S, Ericsson Ö, Bucht E, Jalling B, Boréus LO (1975) Quantitation of phenobarbital and its main metabolites in human urine. Eur J Clin Pharmacol 9:161–168

Kaneko S, Sato T, Suzuki K (1979) The levels of anticonvulsants in breast milk. Br J Clin Pharmacol 7:624–627

Kangas L, Kanto J, Forsstrom J, Iisalo E (1976) Protein binding of diazepam and *N*-demethyldiazepam in patients with poor renal function. Clin Nephrol 5:114–118

Kanto J (1975) Plasma concentrations of diazepam and its metabolites after peroral, intramuscular, and rectal administration. Int J Clin Pharmacol Biopharm 12:427–432

Kanto J, Iisalo E, Lehtinen V, Salminen J (1974) The concentration of diazepam and its metabolites in the plasma after an acute and chronic administration. Psychopharmacologia 36:123–131

Kanto J, Kangas L, Surtola T (1975) Cerebrospinal fluid concentrations of diazepam and its metabolites in man. Acta Pharmacol Toxicol 36:328–334

Kaplan SA, Jack ML, Alexander K, Weinfeld RE (1973) Pharmacokinetic profile of diazepam in man following single intravenous and oral chronic oral administration. J Pharm Sci 62:1789–1796

Kaplan SA, Alexander K, Jack ML, Puglisi CV, De Silva JAF, Lee TL, Weinfeld RE (1974) Pharmacokinetic profiles of clonazepam in dog and humans and of flunitrazepam in dog. J Pharm Sci 63:527–537

Karlen B, Garle M, Rane A, Gutova M, Lindeborg B (1975) Assay of diphenylhydantoin (phenytoin) metabolites in urine by gas-chromatography. Metabolite pattern in humans. Eur J Clin Pharmacol 8:359–363

Kaufman RE, Habersang R, Lansky L (1977) Kinetics of primidone metabolism and excretion in children. Clin Pharmacol Ther 22:200–205

Kauko K, Tammisto P (1974) Comparison of two generically equivalent carbamazepine preparations. Ann Clin Res [Suppl II] 6:21–25

Kawashima K, Ishijima B, Yoshimizu N, Sato F (1980) Determination of dose-plasma concentration relationship of phenobarbital in epileptic patients by a new specific radioimmunoassay. Arch Int Pharmacodyn Ther 244:166–176

Khoo K-C, Mendels J, Rothbart M, Garland WA, Colburn WA, Min BH, Lucek R, Carbone JJ, Boxenbaum HG, Kaplan SA (1980) Influence of phenytoin and phenobarbital on the disposition of single oral dose of clonazepam. Clin Pharmacol Ther 28:368–375

Kinniburgh DW, Boyd ND (1981) Isolation of peptides from uremic plasma that inhibit phenytoin binding to normal plasma proteins. Clin Pharmacol Ther 30:276–280

Klotz U, Antonin KH (1977) Pharmacokinetics and bioavailability of sodium valproate. Clin Pharmacol Ther 21:736–743

Klotz U, Reimann I (1981) Clearance of diazepam can be impaired by its major metabolite desmethyldiazepam. Eur J Clin Pharmacol 21:161–163

Klotz U, Avant GR, Hoyumpa A, Schenker S, Wilkinson GR (1975) The effect of age and liver disease on the disposition and elimination of diazepam in adult man. J Clin Invest 55:347–359

Klotz U, Antonin KH, Bieck PR (1976a) Pharmacokinetics and plasma binding of diazepam in man, dog, rabbit, guinea pig and rat. J Pharmacol Exp Ther 199:67–73

Klotz U, Antonin KH, Bieck PR (1976b) Comparison of the pharmacokinetics of diazepam after single and subchronic doses. Eur J Clin Pharmacol 10:121–126

Klotz U, Antonin KH, Brüger H, Bieck PR (1977) Disposition of diazepam and its major metabolite desmethyldiazepam in patients with liver disease. Clin Pharmacol Ther 21:430–436

Klotz U, Rapp T, Muller WA (1978) Disposition of valproic acid in patients with liver disease. Eur J Clin Pharmacol 13:55–60

Knop HJ, Van Der Kleijn E, Edmunds LC (1975) Pharmacokinetics of clonazepam in man and laboratory animals. In: Schneider M, Janz D, Gardner-Thorpe C, Meinardi H, Sherwin AL (eds) Clinical pharmacology of antiepileptic drugs. Springer, Berlin, pp 247–259

Knudsen FO (1977) Plasma diazepam in infants after rectal administration in solution and by suppository. Acta Paediatr Scand 66:563–567

Kostenbauer HB, Rapp RP, McGovern JP, Foster TS, Perrier DG, Blacker HM, Hulon WC, Kinkel AW (1975) Biovailability and single-dose pharmacokinetics of intramuscular phenytoin. Clin Pharmacol Ther 18:449–456

Koup JR, Rose JQ, Cohen ME (1978) Ethosuximide pharmacokinetics in a pregnant patient and her newborn. Epilepsia 19:535–539

Kromann N, Christiansen J, Flachs H, Dam M, Hvidberg EF (1981) Differences in single dose phenytoin kinetics between Greenland Eskimos and Danes. Ther Drug Monit 3:239–246

Kumps AH (1981) Dose-dependency of the ratio between carbamazepine serum level and dosage in patients with epilepsy. Ther Drug Monit 3:271–274

Küpfer A, Brilis GM, Watson JT, Harris TM (1980) A major pathway of mephenytoin metabolism in man. Aromatic hydroxylation to *p*-hydroxymephenytoin. Drug Metab Dispos 8:1–4

Kupferberg HJ, Longacre-Shaw J (1979) Mephobarbital and phenobarbital plasma concentrations in epileptic patients treated with mephorbital. Ther Drug Monit 1:117–122

Kupferberg HJ, Yonekawa W (1975) The metabolism of 3-methyl-5-ethyl-5-phenylhydantoin (mephenytoin) to 5-ethyl-5-phenylhydantoin (Nirvanol) in mice in relation to anticonvulsant activity. Drug Metab Dispos 3:26–29

Kurata D, Wilkinson GR (1974) Erythrocyte uptake and plasma binding of diphenylhydantoin. Clin Pharmacol Ther 16:677–684

Kutt H, Winters W, Scherman R, McDowell F (1964) Diphenylhydantoin and phenobarbital toxicity. The role of liver disease. Arch Neurol 11:649–656

Kutt H, Wolk M, Scherman R, McDowell F (1964) Insufficient para-hydroxylation as a cause of diphenylhydantoin toxicity. Neurology 14:542–548

Lai AA, Levy RH, Cutler RE (1978) Time course of interaction between carbamazepine and clonazepam in normal man. Clin Pharmacol Ther 24:316–323

Lander CM, Eadie MJ, Tyrer JH (1977) Factors influencing plasma carbamazepine concentrations. Proc Aust Assoc Neurol 14:184–193

Lee HS, Chan KY (1981) Phenytoin and phenobarbitone plasma level-dose relationships in Chinese epileptic children in Singapore. Ther Drug Monit 3:247–252

Leppik IE, Ramani V, Sawchuk R, Gumnit R (1979) Increased clearance of phenytoin during infectious mononucleosis. N Engl J Med 300:481–482

Levy G (1976) Pharmacokinetic approaches to the study of drug interactions. Ann NY Acad Sci 281:24–39

Levy RH (1980) Monitoring of free valproic acid levels? Ther Drug Monit 2:199–201

Levy RH, Pitlick WH, Troupin AS, Green JR, Neal JM (1975) Pharmacokinetics of carbamazepine in normal man. Clin Pharmacol Ther 17:657–668

Levy RH, Cenraud B, Loiseau P, Akbaraly R, Brachet-Liermain A, Guyot M, Gomeni R, Morselli PL (1980) Meal-dependent absorption of enteric-coated sodium valproate. Epilepsia 21:273–280

Levy RH, Bowdle TA, Patel IH, Wilensky AJ (1981) Variability in valproate binding and clearance: implications in therapeutic monitoring. Epilepsia 22:240–241

Loiseau P, Brachet A, Henry P (1975) Concentration of dipropylacetate in plasma. Epilepsia 16:609–615

Löscher W (1978) Serum protein binding and pharmacokinetics of valproate in man, dog, rat and mouse. J Pharmacol Exp Ther 204:255–261

Löscher W (1981) Concentration of metabolites of valproic acid in plasma of epileptic patients. Epilepsia 22:169–178

Loughnan PM, Greenwald A, Purton WW, Aranda JV, Watters G, Neims AH (1977) Pharmacokinetic observations of phenytoin disposition in the newborn and young infant. Arch Dis Child 52:302–309

Lous P (1954) Plasma levels and urinary excretion of three barbituric acids after oral administration to man. Acta Pharmacol Toxicol

Ludden TM, Hawkins DW, Allen JP, Hoffman SF (1976) Optimum phenytoin-dosage regimens. Lancet I:307–308

Ludden TM, Allen JP, Valutsky WA, Vicuna AV, Nappi JM, Hoffman SF, Wallace JE, Lalka D, McNay JL (1977) Individualization of phenytoin dosage regimens. Clin Pharmacol Ther 21:287–293

Lund L (1974) Clinical significance of generic inequivalence of three different pharmaceutical preparations of phenytoin. Eur J Clin Pharmacol 7:119–124

Lund L, Berlin A, Lunde PKM (1972) Plasma protein binding of diphenylhydantoin in patients with epilepsy. Clin Pharmacol Ther 13:196–200

Lund L, Alvan G, Berlin A, Alexanderson B (1974) Pharmacokinetics of single and multiple doses of phenytoin in man. Eur J Clin Pharmacol 7:81–86

Lund M, Sjö O, Hvidberg E (1973) Plasma concentrations of ethotoin in epileptic patients. In: Schneider H, Janz D, Gardner-Thorpe C, Meinardi H, Sherwin AL (eds) Clinical pharmacology of antiepileptic drugs. Springer, Berlin Heidelberg New York, pp 111–114

Lunde PKM, Rane A, Yaffe SJ, Lund L, Sjöqvist F (1970) Plasma protein binding of diphenylhydantoin in man. Interactions with other drugs and the effect of temperature and plasma dilution. Clin Pharmacol Ther 13:196–200

Lynn RK, Smith RG, Thompson RM, Deinzer ML, Griffin D, Gerber N (1978) Characterization of glucuronide metabolites of carbamazepine in human urine by gas-chromatography and mass-spectrometry. Drug Metab Dispos 6:494–501

Mackichan J, Duffner PK, Cohen ME (1979) Adsorption of diazepam to plastic tubing. N Engl J Med 301:332–333

Mackichan J, Duffner PK, Cohen ME (1981) Salivary concentrations and plasma protein binding of carbamazepine and carbamazepine 10,11-epoxide in epileptic patients. Br J Clin Pharmacol 12:31–37

Makki KA, Perucca E, Richens A (1980) Metabolic effects of folic acid in folate-deficient epileptic patients. In: Johannessen SI et al. (eds) Antiepileptic therapy: advances in drug monitoring. Raven, New York, pp 391–398

Mandelli M, Morselli PL, Nordio S, Pardi G, Sereni F, Tognoni G (1975) Placental transfer of diazepam and its disposition in the newborn infant. Clin Pharmacol Ther 17:564–572

Mandelli M, Tognoni G, Garattini S (1978) Clinical pharmacokinetics of diazepam. Clin Pharmacokinet 3:72–91

Martin E, Tozer TN, Sheiner LB, Riegelman S (1977) The clinical pharmacokinetics of phenytoin. J Pharmacokinet Biopharm 5:579–596

Mattson RH, Cramer JA, Williamson PD, Novelly R (1978) Valproic acid in epilepsy: clinical and pharmacological effects. Ann Neurol 3:20–25

Mawer GE, Mullen PW, Rodgers R, Robins AJ, Lucas SB (1974) Phenytoin dose adjustment in epileptic patients. Br J Clin Pharmacol 1:163–168

McAuliffe JJ, Sherwin AL, Leppik IE, Fayle SA, Pippenger CE (1977) Salivary levels of anticonvulsants: a practical approach to drug monitoring. Neurology 27:409–413

Meberg A, Langslet A, Bredesen JE, Lunde PKM (1978) Plasma concentration of diazepam and *N*-desmethyldiazepam in children after a single rectal or intramuscular dose of diazepam. Eur J Clin Pharmacol 14:273–276

Meijer JWA, Hessing-Brandt L (1973) Determination of lower fatty acids, particularly the antiepileptic drug dipropylacetic acid, in biological material by means of microdiffusion and gas-chromatography. Clin Chim Acta 43:215–222

Meijer JWA, Meinardi H (1976) Pharmacokinetic studies on sodium valproate. In: Legg NJ (ed) Clinical and pharmacological aspects of sodium valproate (Epilim) in the treatment of epilepsy. MCS Consultants, Tunbridge Wills pp 70–74

Melander A (1978) Influence of food on the bioavailability of drugs. Clin Pharmacokinet 3:337–351

Melander A, Brante G, Johansson Ö, Lindberg T, Wåhlin-Boll E (1979) Influence of food on the absorption of phenytoin in man. Eur J Clin Pharmacol 15:269–274

Melikian AP, Straughn AB, Slywka GWA, Whyatt PL, Meyer MC (1977) Bioavailability of 11 phenytoin products. J Pharmacokinet Biopharm 5:133–146

Midha KK, Hindmarsh KW, McGilveray JJ, Cooper JK (1977) Identification of urinary catechol metabolites of phenytoin in humans, monkeys and dogs by GLC and GLC-mass spectrometry. J Pharm Sci 66:1596–1602

Mihaly GW, Vajda FJ, Miles JL, Louis WJ (1979) Single and chronic dose pharmacokinetic studies of sodium valproate in epileptic patients. Eur J Clin Pharmacol 16:23–29

Miller ME, Garland WA, Min BH, Ludwick BT, Ballard RH, Levy RH, (1981) Clonazepam acetylation in fast and slow acetylators. Clin Pharmacol Ther 30:343–347

Mirkin BL (1971) Diphenylhydantoin: placental transport, fetal localization, neonatal metabolism, and possible teratogenic effects. J Pediatr 78:329–337

Miyamoto K, Seino M, Ikeda Y (1975) Consecutive determination of the levels of twelve antiepileptic drugs in blood and cerebrospinal fluid. In: Schneider H, Janz D, Gardner-Thorpe C, Meinardi H, Sherwin AL (eds) Clinical pharmacology of antiepileptic drugs. Springer, Berlin Heidelberg New York, pp 323–330

Molenaar F, Korning B, Huizinga T (1979) Biopharmaceutics of rectal administration of drugs in man. 7. Absorption rate and bioavailability of phenobarbital and its sodium salt from rectal dosage forms. Int J Pharmaceutics 4:99–110

Molenaar F, Grunig WJ, Huizinga T (1980) Absorption rate and bioavailability of valproic acid and its sodium salt from rectal dosage form. Eur J Clin Pharmacol 17:309–315

Monaco F, Mutani R, Mastropaolo C, Tondi M (1979) Tears as the best practical indicator of the unbound fraction of an anticonvulsant drug. Epilepsia 20:705–710

Monaco F, Piredda S, Mastropaolo G, Tondi M, Mutani R (1981) Diphenylhydantoin and primidone in tears. Epilepsia 22:185–188

Monks A, Richens A (1979) Serum protein binding of valproic acid and its displacement by palmitic acid *in vitro*. Br J Clin Pharmacol 8:187–189

Morris ME (1978) Compatibility of diazepam injection following dilution with intravenous fluids. Am J Hosp Pharm 35:669–672

Morselli PL (1977 a) Psychotropic drugs. In: Morselli PL (ed) Drug disposition during development. Spectrum, New York, pp 431–476

Morselli PL (1977 b) Antiepileptic drugs. In: Morselli PL (ed) Drug disposition during development. Spectrum, New York, pp 311–360

Morselli PL, Franco-Morselli R (1980) Clinical pharmacokinetics of antiepileptic drugs in adults. Pharmacol Ther 10:65–101

Morselli PL, Frigerio A (1975) Metabolism and pharmacokinetics of carbamazepine. Drug Metab Rev 4: 97–113

Morselli PL, Cassano GB, Placidi GF, Muscettola GB, Rizzo M (1973 a) Kinetics of the distribution of ^{14}C-diazepam and its metabolites in various areas of cat brain. In: Garattini S, Mussini E, Randall O (eds) The benzodiazepines. Raven, New York, pp 129–143

Morselli PL, Principi N, Tognoni G, Reali E, Belvedere G, Standen SM, Sereni F (1973 b) Diazepam elimination in premature and full-term infants and children. J Perinat Med 1:133–141

Morselli PL, Mandelli M, Tognoni G, Principi N, Pardi G, Sereni F (1974) Drug interaction in the human fetus and in the newborn infant. In: Morselli PL, Garattini S, Cohen SN (eds) Drug interactions. Raven, New York, pp 259–270

Morselli PL, Monaco F, Gerna M, Recchia M, Riccio A (1975) Bioavailability of two carbamazepine preparations during chronic administration to epileptic patients. Epilepsia 16:759–764

Morselli PL, Baruzzi A, Gerna M, Bossi L, Porta M (1977) Carbamazepine and carbamazepine-10,11-epoxide concentrations in human brain. Brit J Clin Pharmacol 4:535–540

Morselli PL, Franco-Morselli R, Bossi L (1980) Clinical pharmacokinetics in newborns and infants. Age-related differences and therapeutic implications. Clin Pharmacokinet 5:485–527

Mucklow JC, Bending MR, Kahn GC, Dollery CT (1978) Drug concentration in saliva. Clin Pharmacol Ther 24:563–570

Mullen PW (1978) Optimal phenytoin therapy: a new technique for individualizing dosage. Clin Pharmacol Ther 23:228–232

Mullen PW, Foster PW (1979) Comparative evaluation of six techniques for determining the Michaelis-Menten parameters relating phenytoin dose and steady-state serum concentrations. J Pharm Pharmacol 31:100–104

Mygind KJ, Dam M, Christiansen J (1976) Phenytoin and phenobarbital plasma clearance during pregnancy. Acta Neurol Scand 54:160–166

Naestoft J, Lund M, Larsen NE, Hvidberg E (1973) Assay and pharmacokinetics of clonazepam in humans. Acta Neurol, Scand 49:103–108

Nau H, Rating D, Häuser I, Jäger E, Koch S, Helge H (1980) Placental transfer and pharmacokinetics of primidone and its metabolites phenobarbital, PEMA and hydroxyphenobarbital in neonates and infants of epileptic mothers. Eur J Clin Pharmacol 18:31–41

Neuvonen PJ (1979) Bioavailability of phenytoin: clinical pharmacokinetic and therapeutic implications. Clin Pharmacokinet 4:91–103

Niebyl JR, Blake DA, Freeman JM, Luff RP (1979) Carbamazepine levels in pregnancy and lactation. Obstet Gyneaecol 53:139–140

Nishihara K, Uchino K, Saitoh Y, Honda Y, Makagawa F, Tamura Z (1979) Estimation of plasma unbound phenobarbital concentration by using mixed saliva. Epilepsia 20:37–45

Nutt JG, Kupferberg HJ (1979) Linear relationship between plasma concentration and dosage of sodium valproate. Epilepsia 20:589–592

Ochs H, Greenblatt DJ, Divoll M, Abernethy DR, Feyerabend H, Dengler HJ (1981) Diazepam kinetics in relation to age and sex. Pharmacology 23:24–40

Odar-Cederlöf I (1977) Plasma protein binding of phenytoin and warfarin in patients undergoing renal transplantation. Clin Pharmacokinet 2:147

Odar-Cederlöf I, Borgå O (1974) Kinetics of diphenylhydantoin in uraemic patients: consequences of decreased plasma protein binding. Eur J Clin Pharmacol 7:31–37

Odar-Cederlöf I, Borgå O (1976) Impaired plasma protein binding of phenytoin in uremia and displacement effect of salicylic acid. Clin Pharmacol Ther 20:36–47

Oldigs HD, Bartels H, Wallis S, Warecka A, Grob-Selbeck G (1979) The effect of galenics on the blood level fluctuations of dipropylacetate – comparative investigation of small intestine-soluble coated pills and a retard form in children. Epilepsia 20:85–90

Olesen OV (1968) Determination of sulthiame (Ospolot®) in serum and urine by thin-layer chromatography: serum levels and urinary output in patients under long-term treatment. Acta Pharmacol Toxicol 26:22–28

Olsen GD, Bennett WM, Porter GA (1975) Morphine and phenytoin binding to plasma proteins in renal and hepatic disease. Clin Pharmacol Ther 17:677–684

Painter MJ, Pippenger C, Carter G, Pitlick W (1977) Metabolism of phenobarbital and phenytoin by neonates with seizures. Neurology 27:370

Painter MJ, Pippenger C, Macdonald H, Pitlick W (1978) Phenobarbital and diphenylhydantoin levels in neonates with seizures. J Pediatr 92:315–319

Palmer L, Bertilsson L, Collste P, Rawlins M (1973) Quantitative determination of carbamazepine in plasma by mass fragmentography. Clin Pharmacol Ther 14:827–832

Patel IH, Levy RH (1979) Valproic acid binding to human serum albumin and determination of free fraction in the presence of anticonvulsants and free fatty acids. Epilepsia 20:85–90
Patel IH, Levy RH, Rapport RL (1977) Distribution characteristics of ethosuximide in discrete areas of rat brain. Epilepsia 18:533–541
Patel IH, Levy RH, Venkataramanan R, Viswanathan CT, Moretti-Ojemann L (1980) Diurnal variation in protein binding of valproic acid and phenytoin and the role of free fatty acids. Clin Pharmacol Ther 22:277
Patrick MJ, Tilstone WJ, Reavey P (1972) Diazepam and breast feeding. Lancet I:542–543
Paxton JW, Foote S (1979) Aberrantly high phenytoin concentrations in saliva. Precaution in monitoring phenytoin concentration. Br J Clin Pharmacol 8:508–509
Paxton JW, Whiting B, Rowell F, Ratcliffe JG, Stephen KW (1976) Salivary concentrations of antiepileptic drugs. Lancet 2:639–640
Paxton JW, Rowell FJ, Ratcliffe JG, Lambie DG, Nanda R, Melville ID, Johnson RH (1977a) Salivary phenytoin radioimmunoassay: a single method for the assessment of non protein bound drug concentrations. Eur J Clin Pharmacol 11:71–74
Paxton JW, Whiting B, Stephen KW (1977b) Phenytoin concentrations in mixed parotid and submandibular saliva and serum measured by radioimmunoassay. Br J Clin Pharmacol 4:185–192
Perucca E (1980) Plasma protein binding of phenytoin in health and disease: relevance to therapeutic drug monitoring. Ther Drug Monit 2:331–344
Perucca E, Richens A (1980) Reversal of carbamazepine-induced water intoxication by phenytoin: a pharmacokinetic interaction. J Neurol Neurosurg Psych 43:540–545
Perucca E, Makki K, Richens A (1978a) Is phenytoin metabolism dose-dependent by enzyme-saturation or by feedback inhibition? Clin Pharmacol Ther 24:46–51
Perucca E, Garratt A, Hebdige S, Richens A (1978b) Water intoxication in epileptic patients receiving carbamazepine. J Neurol Neurosurg Psych 41:713–718
Perucca E, Gatti G, Frigo GM, Crema A (1978c) Pharmacokinetics of valproic acid after oral and intravenous administration. Br J Clin Pharmacol 5:313–318
Perucca E, Gatti G, Frigo GM, Crema A, Calzetti S, Visintini D (1978d) Disposition of sodium valproate in epileptic patients. Br J Clin Pharmacol 5:495–499
Perucca E, Hebdige S, Gatti S, Lecchini S, Frigo GM, Crema A (1980a) Interaction between phenytoin and valproic acid: plasma protein binding and metabolic effects. Clin Pharmacol Ther 28:779–789
Perucca E, Bittencourt P, Richens A (1980b) Effect of dose increments on serum carbamazepine concentration in epileptic patients. Clin Pharmacokinet 6:576–582
Perucca E, Ruprah M, Richens A (1981a) Altered drug binding to serum proteins in pregnant women: relevance to therapeutic drug monitoring. JR Soc Med 74:422–426
Perucca E, Ruprah M, Richens A, Park BK, Betteridge DJ, Hedges A (1981b) Effect of low-dose phenobarbitone on five indirect indices of hepatic microsomal enzyme-induction and plasma lipoproteins in normal subjects. Br J Clin Pharmacol 12:592–596
Perucca E, Ruprah M, Richens A (1981c) Decreased serum protein binding of diazepam and valproic acid in pregnant women. Br J Clin Pharmacol 12:276P
Pinder RM, Brogden RN, Speight TM, Avery GS (1976) Clonazepam: a review of its pharmacological properties and therapeutic efficacy in epilepsy. Drugs 12:321–361
Pinder RM, Brogden RN, Speight TM, Avery GS (1977) Sodium valproate: a review of its pharmacological properties and therapeutic efficacy in epilepsy. Drugs 13:81–123
Pippenger CE, Penry JK, Kutt H (1978) Antiepileptic drugs. Quantitative analysis and interpretation. Raven, New York, pp 326
Pisani F, Fazio A, Oteri G, Di Perri R (1981) Dipropylacetic acid plasma levels; diurnal fluctuations during chronic treatment with dipropylacetamide. Ther Drug Monit 3:297–301
Pitlick W, Painter M, Pippenger C (1978) Phenobarbital pharmacokinetics in neonates. Clin Pharmacol Ther 23:346–350
Plasse JC, Revol M, Chabert G, Ducerf F (1979) Neonatal pharmacokinetics of valproic acid. In: Schaaf H, Van Der Kleijn E (eds) Progress in clinical pharmacy. Biomedical, Elsevier/North Holland, pp 247–252

Porter RJ, Layzer RB (1975 Plasma albumin concentration and diphenylhydantoin binding in man. Arch Neurol 32:298–303

Porter RJ, Penry JK, Lacy JR, Newmark ME, Kupferberg HJ (1979) Plasma concentrations of phensuximide, methsuximide, and their metabolites in relation to clinical efficacy. Neurology 29:1509–1513

Powell JR, Nelson E, Conrad KA, Likes K, Byers J, Perrier D (1983) Phenobarbital clearance, elimination with alkaline diuresis, and bioavailability in adults. Clin Pharmacol Ther 29:273–274

Pynnönen S (1977) The pharmacokinetics of carbamazepine in plasma and saliva of man. Acta Pharmacol Toxicol 41:465–471

Pynnönen S (1979) Pharmacokinetics of carbamazepine in man: a review. Ther Drug Monit 1:409–431

Pynnönen S, Sillanpäa M (1975) Carbamazepine and mother's milk. Lancet II:563

Pynnönen S, Yrjana T (1977) The significance of the simultaneous determination of carbamazepine and its 10,11-epoxide from plasma and human erythrocytes. Int J Clin Pharmacol Biopharm 15:222–226

Pynnönen S, Sillanpäa M, Frey H, Iisalo E (1977 a) Carbamazepine and its 10,11-epoxide in children and adults with epilepsy. Eur J Clin Pharmacol 11:129–133

Pynnönen S, Kanto J, Sillanpäa M, Erkkola R (1977 b) Carbamazepine: placental transport, tissue concentrations in foetus and newborn, and level in milk. Acta Pharmacol Toxicol 41:244–253

Pynnönen S, Sillanpäa M, Frey H, Iisalo E (1978) Carbamazepine and its 10,11-epoxide in children and adults with epilepsy. Eur J Clin Pharmacol 11:129–133

Pynnönen S, Frey H, Syllanpäa M (1980) The autoinduction of carbamazepine during long-term therapy. Int J Clin Pharmacol Ther Toxicol 18:247–252

Rambeck B (1979) Pharmacological interactions of mesuximide with phenobarbital and phenytoin in hospitalized epileptic patients. Epilepsia 20:147–156

Rambeck B, Boenigk HE, Dunlop A, Mullen PW, Wadsworth J, Richens A (1979) Predicting phenytoin dose: a revised nomogram. Ther Drug Monit 2:325–333

Rane A, Tunell R (1981) Ethosuximide in human milk and in plasma of a mother and her nursed infant. Br J Clin Pharmacol 12:855–858

Rane A, Lunde PKM, Jalling B, Yaffe SJ, Sjöqvist F (1971) Plasma protein binding of diphenylhydantoin in normal and hyperbilirubinaemic infants. J Pediatr 78:877–882

Rane A, Garle M, Borgå O, Sjöqvist F (1974) Plasma disappearance of transplacentally transferred diphenylhydantoin in the newborn studied by mass fragmentography. Clin Pharmacol Ther 13:39–45

Rane A, Bertilsson L, Palmer L (1975) Disposition of placentally transferred carbamazepine (Tegretol®) in the newborn. Eur J Clin Pharmacol 8:283–284

Rane A, Hojer B, Wilson JT (1976) Kinetics of carbamazepine and its 10,11-epoxide metabolite in children. Clin Pharmacol Ther 19:276–283

Rawlins MD, Collste P, Bertilsson L, Palmer L (1975) Distribution and elimination kinetics of carbamazepine in man. Eur J Clin Pharmacol 8:91–96

Reidenberg MM, Odar-Cederlöf I, Von Bahr C, Borgå O, Sjöqvist F (1971) Protein binding of diphenylhydantoin and desmethylimipramine in plasma from patients with poor renal function. N Engl J Med 285:264–267

Rey E, D'Athis P, De Lauture D, Dulac O, Aicardi J, Olive G (1979) Pharmacokinetics of carbamazepine in the neonate and the child. Int J Clin Pharmacol Biopharm 17:90–96

Reynolds EH, Fenton G, Fenwick P, Johnson AL, Laundy M (1975) Interaction of phenytoin and primidone. Br Med J 2:594–595

Reynolds F, Ziroyanis P, Jones N Smith SE (1976) Salivary phenytoin concentrations in epilepsy and in chronic renal failure. Lancet II:384–386

Richens A (1975) A study of the pharmacokinetics of phenytoin (diphenylhydantoin) in epileptic patients and the development of a nomogram for making dose increments. Epilepsia 16:627–646

Richens A (1979) Clinical pharmacokinetics of phenytoin. Clin Pharmacokinet 4:153–169

Richens A, Dunlop A (1975) Serum phenytoin levels in the management of epilepsy. Lancet II:247–248

Richens A, Scoular IT, Ahmad S, Jordan BJ (1976) Pharmacokinetics and efficacy of Epilim in patients receiving long-term therapy with other antiepileptic drugs. In: Legg NJ (ed) Clinical and pharmacological aspects of sodium valproate (Epilim) in the treatment of epilepsy. MCS Consultants, Tunbridge Wells, pp 78–88

Richter K, Terhaag B (1978) The relative bioavailability and pharmacokinetics of carbamazepine. Int J Clin Pharmacol 16:377–379

Riva R, Albani F, Baruzzi A, Galvani I, Perucca E (1982) Determination of unbound valproic acid concentration in plasma by equilibrium dialysis and gas-liquid chromatography. Methodological aspects and observations in epileptic patients. Ther Drug Monit 4:341–352

Robinson JD, Morris BA, Aherne GW, Marks V (1975) Pharmacokinetics of a single dose of phenytoin in man measured by radioimmunoassay. Br J Clin Pharmacol 2:345–350

Rossi LN, Nino LM, Principi N (1979) Correlation between age and plasma level/dosage ratio for phenobarbital in infants and children. Acta Paediatr Scand 68:431–434

Routledge PA, Kitchell BB, Bjornsson TD, Skinner, BS, Linnoila M, Shand DG (1980a) Diazepam and *N*-desmethyldiazepam redistribution after heparin. Clin Pharmacol Ther 27:528–532

Routledge PA, Stargel WW, Kitchell BB, Shand DG (1980b) Determinants of plasma protein binding of diazepam. Clin Pharmacol Ther 27:282

Routledge PA, Stargel WW, Kitchell BB, Barchowsky A, Shand DG (1981) Sex related differences in the plasma protein binding of lignocaine and diazepam. Br J Clin Pharmacol 11:245–250

Rylance GW, Butcher GM, Moreland T (1977) Saliva carbamazepine levels in children. Br Med J 2:1481

Rylance GW, Moreland TA, Butcher GM (1979) Carbamazepine dose-frequency requirements in children. Arch Dis Child 54:454–458

Sandor P, Sellers EM, Dumbrell RM, Khouw V (1981) Effect of short- and long-term alcohol use on phenytoin kinetics in chronic alcoholics. Clin Pharmacol Ther 30:390–397

Sannita WG, Rapallino MV, Rodriguez G, Rosadini G (1980) EEG effects and plasma concentrations of phenobarbital in volunteers. Neuropharmacology 19:927–930

Schmidt D, Kupferberg H (1975) Diphenylhydantoin, phenobarbital and primidone in saliva, plasma and CSF, Epilepsia 16:735–741

Schobben F, Van Der Kleijn E, Gabreëls FJM (1975) Pharmacokinetics of di-*n*-propylacetate in epileptic patients. Eur J Clin Pharmacol 8:97–105

Schottelius DD, Fincham RW (1978) Clinical application of serum primidone levels. In: Pippenger CE, Penry JK, Kutt H (eds) Antiepileptic drugs, quantitative analysis and interpretation. Raven, New York, pp 273–282

Sherwin AL (1978) Clinical pharmacology of ethosuximide. In: Pippenger CE, Penry JK, Kutt H (eds) Antiepileptic drugs: quantitative analysis and interpretation. Raven, New York, pp 283–295

Sherwin AL, Robb JP (1972) Ethosuximide: relation of plasma level to clinical control. In: Woodbury DM, Penry JK, Schmidt RP (eds) Antiepileptic drugs. Raven, New York, pp 443–448

Sherwin AL, Eisen AA, Sokolowsky CD (1973) Anticonvulsant drugs in human epileptogenic brain. Correlation of phenobarbital and diphenylhydantoin levels with plasma. Arch Neurol 29:73–77

Sironi VA, Cabrini G, Porro MG, Ravagnati L, Marossero F (1980) Antiepileptic drug distribution in cerebral cortex, Ammons's horn, and amygdala of man. J Neurosurg 52:686–692

Sjö O, Hvidberg EF, Naestoft J, Lund M (1975a) Pharmacokinetics and side effects of clonazepam and its 7-amino metabolite in man. Eur J Clin Pharmacol 8:249–254

Sjö O, Hvidberg EF, Larsen N-E, Lund M, Naestoft J (1975b) Dose-dependent kinetics of ethotoin in man. Exp Pharmacol Physiol 2:185–192

Sjoholm I, Kober A, Odar-Cederlöf I, Borgå O (1976) Protein binding of drugs in uremic and normal serum. The role of endogenous binding inhibitors. Biochem Pharmacol 25:1205–1213

Sloan TP, Idle JR, Smith RL (1981) Influence of D^H/D^L alleles regulating debrisoquine oxidation on phenytoin metabolism. Clin Pharmacol Ther 29:493–497

Smith RG, Davies GD, Lynn RK, Gerber N (1977) Hydantoin ring glucuronidation: characterization of a new metabolite of 5,5-diphenylhydantoin in man and the rat. Biomed Mass Spectrom 4:275–279

Smith GA, McKauge L, Dubetz D, Tyrer JH, Eadie MJ (1979) Factors influencing plasma concentrations of ethosuximide. Clin Pharmacokinet 4:38–52

Stewart MJ, Ballinger BR, Devlin EJ, Miller AY, Ramsay AC (1975) Bioavailability of phenytoin. A comparison of two preparations. Eur J Clin Pharmacol 9:209–212

Strandjord RE, Johannessen SI (1974) One daily dose of diphenylhydantoin for patients with epilepsy. Epilepsia 15:317–327

Strandjord RE, Johannessen SI (1975) A preliminary study of serum carbamazepine levels in healthy subjects and in patients with epilepsy. In: Schneider H, Janz D, Gardner-Thorpe C, Meinardi H, Sherwin A (eds) Clinical pharmacology of antiepileptic drugs. Springer, Berlin Heidelberg New York, pp 181–188

Strandjord RE, Johannessen SI (1980) Single drug therapy with carbamazepine in patients with epilepsy: serum levels and clinical effect. Epilepsia 21:655–662

Strong JM, Abe T, Gibbs EL, Atkinson AJ Jr (1974) Plasma levels of methsuximide and *N*-desmethyl-methsuximide during methsuximide therapy. Neurology 24:250–255

Svendsen A, Brochmann-Hanssen E (1962) Gas chromatography of barbiturates: application to the study of their metabolism and excretion in humans. J Pharm Sci 51:494–495

Svensmark O, Buchthal F (1963) Accumulation of phenobarbital in man. Epilepsia 4:199–206

Svensmark O, Buchthal F (1964) Diphenylhydantoin and phenobarbital. Serum levels in children. Am J Dis Child 108:82–87

Tammisto P, Kauko K, Viukari M (1976) Bioavailability of phenytoin. Lancet I:254–255

Tang BK, Kalow W, Grey AA (1979) Metabolic fate of phenobarbital in man. *N*-Glucoside formation. Drug Metab Dispos 7:315–318

Tedeschi G, Cenraud B, Guyot M, Gomeni R, Morselli PL, Levy RH, Loiseau P (1981) Influence of food on carbamazepine absorption. In : Dam M, Gram L, Penry JK (eds) Advances in epileptology: XIIth epilepsy international symposium. Raven, New York, pp 563–567

Terhaag B, Richter K, Diettrich H (1978) Concentration behaviour of carbamazepine in bile and plasma of man. Int J Clin Pharmacol 16:607–609

Thiessen JJ, Sellers EM, Denbeigh P, Dolman L (1976) Plasma protein binding of diazepam and tolbutamide in chronic alcoholics. J Clin Pharmacol 16:345–351

Thompson RM, Beghin J, Fife WK, Gerber N (1976) 5,5-bis (4-hydroxyphenyl)hydantoin, a minor metabolite of diphenylhydantoin (Dilantin) in the rat and human. Drug Metab Dispos 4:349–356

Tognoni G, Gomeni R, De Maio D, Alberti GG, Franciosi P, Sireghi G (1975) Pharmacokinetics of *N*-demethyldiazepam in patients suffering from insomnia and treated with nortriptyline. Br J Clin Pharmacol 2:227–232

Tomson T, Tybring G, Bertilsson L, Ekbom C, Rane A (1980) Carbamazepine therapy in trigeminal neuralgia. Clinical effects in relation to plasma concentration. Arch Neurol 37:699–703

Triedman HM, Fishman RA, Yahr MD (1960) Determination of plasma and cerebrospinal fluid levels of Dilantin in the human. Trans Am Neurol Assoc 85:166–169

Troupin AS, Friel (1975) Anticonvulsant levels in saliva, serum and cerebrospinal fluid. Epilepsia 16:223–227

Troupin AS, Moretti-Ojemann L, Dodrill CB (1976) Mephenytoin: a reappraisal. Epilepsia 17:403–414

Troupin AS, Green JR, Levy RH (1974) Carbamazepine as an anticonvulsant: a pilot study. Neurology 24:863–869

Tyrer JH, Eadie MJ, Sutherland JM, Hooper WD (1974) Outbreak of anticonvulsant intoxication of an Australian city. Br Med J 4:271–273

Vajda F, Williams FM, Davidson S, Falconer MA, Breckenridge A (1974) Human brain, cerebrospinal fluid and plasma concentrations of diphenylhydantoin and phenobarbital. Clin Pharmacol Ther 15:597–603

Van Der Velde, EA, Driessen O (1981) Prediction of phenytoin dosage in relation to the variability of phenytoin plasma concentration. Br J Clin Pharmacol 1:41–52

Vasko MR, Bell RD, Daly DD, Pippenger CEJ (1980) Inheritance of phenytoin hypometabolism: a kinetic study of one family. Clin Pharmacol Ther 27:96–103

Viswanathan CT, Booker HE, Welling PG (1978) Bioavailability of oral and intramuscular phenobarbital. J Clin Pharmacol 18:100–105

Viswanathan CT, Booker HE, Welling PG (1979) Pharmacokinetics of phenobarbital following single and repeated doses. J Clin Pharmacol 19:282–289

Waddell WJ, Butler TC (1957a) The distribution and excretion of phenobarbital. J Clin Invest 36:1217–1226

Waddell WJ, Butler TC (1957b) Renal excretion of 5,5-dimethyl-2,4-oxazolidinedione (product of demethylation of trimethiadione). Proc Soc Exp Biol Med 96:563–565

Wallace S, Brodie MJ (1976) Decreased drug binding in serum from patients with chronic hepatic disease. Eur J Clin Pharmacol 9:429–432

Wallin A, Jalling B, Boréus LO (1974) Plasma concentrations of phenobarbital in the neonate during prophylaxis for neonatal hyperbilirubinemia. J Pediatr 85:392–397

Walson PD, Mimaki T, Curless R, Mayersohn M, Perrier D (1980) Once daily doses of phenobarbital in children. J Pediatr 97:303–305

Warren JW, Benmaman JD, Braxton B, Wannamaker BB, Levy RH (1980) Kinetics of a carbamazepine-ethosuximide interaction. Clin Pharmacol Ther 28:646–651

Westenberg HGM, Van Der Kleijn E, Oei TT, De Zeeuw RA (1978) Kinetics of carbamazepine and carbamazepine-epoxide, determined by use of plasma and saliva. Clin Pharmacol Ther 23:320–328

Whyte MP, Dekaban AS (1977) Metabolic fate of phenobarbital. A quantitative study of *p*-hydroxyphenobarbital elimination in man. Drug Metab Dispos 5:63–70

Wilder BJ, Ramsay RE (1976) Oral and intramuscular phenytoin. Clin Pharmacol Ther 19:360–364

Wilder BJ, Serrano EE, Ramsay E (1973) Plasma diphenylhydantoin levels after loading and maintenance doses. Clin Pharmacol Ther 14:797–801

Wilder BJ, Serrano EE, Ramsey E, Buchanan RA (1974) A method for shifting from oral to intramuscular diphenylhydantoin administration. Clin Pharmacol Ther 16:507–513

Wilder BJ, Ramsay RE, Willmore LJ, Feussner GF, Perchalski RJ, Shumate JB (1977) Efficacy of intravenous phenytoin in the treatment of status epilepticus: kinetics of central nervous system penetration. Ann Neurol 1:511–518

Wilensky AJ, Levy RH, Troupin AS, Moretti-Ojemann L, Friel P (1978) Clorazepate kinetics in treated epileptics. Clin Pharmacol Ther 24:22–30

Wilensky AJ, Lowden JA (1973) Inadequate serum levels after intramuscular administration of diphenylhydantoin. Neurology 23:318–324

Wilson JT, Wilkinson GR (1973) Chronic and severe phenobarbital intoxication in a child treated with primidone and diphenylhydantoin. J Pediatr 83:484–489

Wilson JT, Hojer B, Rane A (1976) Loading and conventional dose therapy with phenytoin in children; kinetic profile of parent drug and main metabolite in plasma. Clin Pharmacol Ther 20:48–58

Wilson JT, Brown RD, Cherek DR, Dail JW, Hilman B, Jobe PC, Manno BR, Manno JE, Redetzki HM, Stewart JJ (1980) Drug excretion in human breast milk: principles, pharmacokinetics and projected consequences. Clin Pharmacokinet 5:1–66

Withrow CD, Woodbury DM (1972) Trimethadione and other oxazolidinediones. Absorption, distribution and excretion. In: Woodbury DM, Penry JK, Schmidt RP (eds) Antiepileptic drugs. Raven, New York, pp 389–392

Woodbury DM (1972) Sulfonamides and derivatives Acetazolamide. In: Woodbury DM, Penry JK, Schmidt RP (eds) Antiepileptic drugs. Raven, New York, pp 465–475

Wulff K, Flachs H, Wurtz-Jorgensen A, Gram L (1977) Clinical pharmacological aspects of valproate sodium. Epilepsia 18:149–157

Yacobi A, Lampmann T, Levy G (1977) Frequency of distribution of free warfarin and free phenytoin fraction values in serum of healthy human adults. Clin Pharmacol Ther 21:283–286

Zimmermann CL, Patel IH, Levy RH, Edwards D, Nelson SD, Hutchinson M (1981) Protein binding of valproic acid in the presence of elevated free fatty acids in patient and normal human serum. Epilepsia 22:11–17

CHAPTER 25

Monitoring Antiepileptic Drug Levels

E. F. HVIDBERG

A. Introduction

Numerous studies and years of clinical experience support the assumption that the care of epileptic patients can often be improved by monitoring the plasma (serum) levels of the antiepileptic drug(s) used. The purpose of this chapter is to describe and analyze the background for the use of antiepileptic drug level monitoring and to evaluate the documentation for the possible benefit of this activity.

Epilepsy was, in fact, the first disease in which a rational approach to therapeutic drug monitoring was applied. The pioneering work was predominantly carried out by a Danish research team with phenytoin and phenobarbital in the late 1950s and through the 1960s (e.g., BUCHTHAL and SVENSMARK 1960; BUCHTHAL et al. 1960; SVENSMARK et al. 1960; SVENSMARK and BUCHTHAL 1963). These studies are now considered "classical" not only for antiepileptic drugs, but also for the concept of therapeutic drug monitoring in general. The subsequent decades of progress created and modeled this important tool for the epileptologist, and numerous experimental and review articles, as well as clinical communications, have dealt with this area of clinical neuropharmacology.

Two factors in particular have been responsible for this development: first, the pharmacology, escpecially the pharmacokinetics, of several antiepileptic drugs, has been investigated intensively during the past years, revealing that knowledge of the interindividual differences in kinetic parameters, particularly in the dose/plasma concentration ratio, is of great significance for rational drug therapy, not least for antiepileptic drugs. Second, chemical and biochemical technology has provided the medical community with a wide range of analytical procedures capable of determining drug plasma levels for routine purposes with great specificity and accuracy. Indeed, the development of analytical techniques, being the prerequisite for both advances in pharmacokinetics and routine drug determinations, long ago outpaced developments in therapeutics. Consequently, whole new sets of problems are emerging, because "plasma-level services" are becoming available in such an abundance that only financial cost will limit their use. To this concern may be added another one, discussed in particular by LATINI et al. (1980). They emphasized the existing gap between (experimental) clinical pharmacokinetics and routine therapy, partly resulting in very little attention being paid to the problem of evaluating the clinical relevance of drug monitoring programs through, e.g., controlled studies. Although these authors did not exemplify their considerations with antiepileptics, their point of view is extremely relevant also for these drugs. It may, therefore, be fair to state that, even if monitoring (at our present stage of knowledge) is considered advantageous, both its wise use and correct utilization may be harmed or impeded by uncontrolled development.

The *theoretical background* for therapeutic drug monitoring is based on the concept that the concentration of a given drug measured in the plasma is reversibly correlated to the concentration of the drug at the receptor site, and thus correlated to the clinical effect. Expressed in more practical pharmacological terms: the primary prerequisite for plasma drug monitoring is that a plasma concentration/response relationship is established in a dose/response-like fashion, based on controlled trials and other prospective studies.

The *clinical background* for therapeutic monitoring of anticonvulsant drugs is based on numerous studies demonstrating that seizure control improves as the plasma level of antiepileptic drugs increases, both in groups of patients (for review see KUTT and PENRY 1974) and in individual patients (ROWAN et al. 1975). Furthermore, high concentrations are often associated with increasing toxicity. This is, however, not the same as a proof for the value of drug level monitoring.

B. Justification for Monitoring Plasma Concentration Levels of Antiepileptic Drugs

Although conclusive documentation for improved quality in patient care due to therapeutic drug monnitoring is still lacking, it is extremely important that the arguments put forward for its justification are fully understood and accepted. Thus therapeutic drug monitoring in general should be considered (cf. EADIE 1976)

1. If great interindividual variations in the kinetics – and therefore large differences in the concentration/dose ratio – call for an individual tailoring of the drug dosage
2. If the drug exhibits a narrow therapeutic margin
3. If the drug has a "difficult" kinetic profile, e.g., gives rise to relatively large fluctuations in plasma concentrations, evinces saturation kinetics at therapeutic levels, shows a tendency to (auto)-induction, fills up deep compartments very slowly, etc.
4. In special risk groups, e.g., neonates, elderly patients, pregnant women, patients with impaired capacity of the elimination organs (liver, kidneys), etc.
5. If other drugs are added to a therapeutic regime and kinetic drug interactions are a possibility
6. To ensure adherence to the treatment schedule, i.e., control of compliance

As an elaboration of, and in addition to, these more general principles many epileptologists would ascribe to the following points (JOHANNESSEN 1981), suggesting that antiepileptic drug level monitoring – apart from routine monitoring to ensure drug compliance – should be used:

1. When antiepileptic drugs therapy is initiated and after dosage adjustments
2. In the case of therapeutic failure or when clinical signs of side effects or intoxication occur
3. After the addition of a drug which may interact with the first, or if any change occurs in a patient's normal physiological state, e.g., pregnancy or intercurrent illness

Based on these principles, monitoring of antiepileptic drugs has been regarded by some authors as being the most important advance in the treatment of epilepsy during the past decades (BARTELS 1980). However, a more critical attitude may also be adopted, e.g., that the only clear indication for measuring antiepileptic drug levels is to affirm suspected toxic signs in patients whose clinical picture is difficult to interpret. Also, much more solid evidence may be demanded for the correlation between effect and plasma concentrations before embarking on a large monitoring program. In this context it should be emphasized that great differences do exist in the justification for monitoring plasma levels of the various antiepileptic drugs (RICHENS 1981), e.g., between phenytoin and valproate.

As a consequence of these and other uncertainties interest in drug-level monitoring is not equally enthusiastic at all centers. Nevertheless, it cannot be disregarded that the general experience over the past decade has supported the idea that therapeutic drug monitoring in epileptic patients does improve the therapy, although certain provisions must be taken.

Whatever attitude is taken, the definition of an optimal (or therapeutic) plasma concentration range is essential for the use of drug-level monitoring.

C. The Concept of the Therapeutic Level

Many factors will influence the patients' ability to keep the plasma concentration of an antiepileptic drug within the so-called therapeutic level. Most of these factors will be discussed in detail in other chapters of this volume, including, e.g., the kinetics of the drugs, interindividual variability in kinetic parameters, diseases in the elimination organs, age, pregnancy, drug interactions, and patient compliance.

Just as important for the concept of the therapeutic level, as are the kinetic aspects, are, however, the individual pharmacodynamic factors, which may determine the optimal therapeutic concentration in the single patient, e.g., severity of disease, physiological conditions, and comedication. Likewise toxicity will appear at quite different levels in different patients. Details will be discussed in Sect. I. Consequently, the individual level at which seizure control is effected (sometimes at the expense of acceptable side effects) will vary from patient to patient. Group studies will only result in a useful initial goal. It is therefore clinically important to emphasize this distinction between the concepts of the "individual" level and the "average" (or "statistical") range. This problem has repeatedly been discussed over the years (e.g., EADIE 1976), but may have been put most clearly by KUTT (1972) who, writing about phenytoin, stated that: ".... the therapeutic level range of 10–20 mg/l is an empirical compromise and was arrived at by observations of frequent intoxication with levels over 20 mg/l, and generally poor seizure control with levels below 10 mg/l .... Yet, the range is a useful initial goal, later to be adjusted to the individual patient's need." This concept is undoubtedly still valid, and its principles can be used for most antiepileptic drugs with respect to drug-level monitoring.

However, it cannot be concealed that quite negative views are sometimes also expressed about the clinical value of therapeutic ranges (cf. discussion after CHADWICK et al. 1977). Such pessimism may originate from the fact that too much emphasis on a therapeutic level increases the chances of misinformation, which could lead to erroneous antiepileptic therapy. Furthermore, it could also be argued that as long as the monitoring system is based on total plasma concentrations and not on the free fraction, which is supposed to be in equilibrium with the tissue concentration (see later), the basis of the whole system may be unreliable.

D. Clinical Evaluation of Therapeutic Levels

In order to provide reasonable evidence for the existence of a therapeutic plasma level it is not sufficient to perform retrospective studies, e.g., merely recording the effect and plasma levels in a group of already treated patients. This may be a good starting point for further investigations, but not adequate as to the final design. Furthermore, research in this area must go hand in hand with both good human kinetic studies and solid clinical competence.

Determination of a therapeutic plasma range is no different from any other clinical evaluation process: after some preliminary investigations it is necessary to prove or disprove a given hypothesis by means of prospective clinical trials. However, to perform theoretically correct investigations is a difficult and especially very elaborate task, as it demands several controlled trials to prove or disprove both an upper and a lower limit. In principle, the trial must be designed in such a way that the null hypothesis (i.e., no difference in the outcome between two groups presenting levels over and under the tested limit) can be rejected or verified. Double-blind techniques (possibly with open therapeutic steering) may be required, and it is essential to have a sufficient number of patients in each trial to avoid type II errors. As such investigations may also involve considerable ethical problems, it is no wonder that only few studies of this kind have been published. This state of affairs leaves the justification for therapeutic drug monitoring in a difficult situation. On the other hand, even controlled studies will only define a more "general" therapeutic range, i.e., in groups of patients, not fully taking into account the possibility of individual aberrations. Prospective studies which attempt to substantiate individual tailoring in antiepileptic drug therapy within – or beyond – the accepted ranges in a few patients are therefore also of great value.

Although not only applicable to trials concerned with the evaluation of therapeutic levels, the following questions should also be considered in connection with such trials (cf. BERTILSSON 1978):

1. Were the included patients resistant to other entiepileptics? Were they currently on other drugs? Did they have adequate plasma levels of these? Were they diagnosed, observed, and explained adequately?
2. Was the actual treatment monitored with plasma levels frequently enough to establish that the patients were in steady state? Was good compliance ensured?
3. Were active metabolites measured?
4. Was the analytical method adequately specific and sensitive?
5. When were the blood samples taken and was the timing consistent?
6. Was the therapeutic effect investigated at more than one plasma level in the individual patients?

7. What were the control measures, and did they include bias-reducing techniques such as blinding and proper effect measuring?

Against this background it would be reasonable to ask what has been done in general to establish sufficient evidence for the so-called therapeutic levels of antiepileptic drugs. Seen from a critical point of view, the answer is not encouraging. Prospective studies are few and the number of patients included are often limited. Even uncontrolled or retrospective studies are infrequent. Clinical experiences and single-case studies seem to fill the gap to some extent, and good and quite convincing examples have also been published recently (e.g., BOOKER 1980, RICHENS 1981). However, this may be acceptable for antiepileptic drugs that have been in use for several years, but in order to establish a basis for rational therapy with newer or future drugs it is necessary to develop a procedure for the evaluation of therapeutic drug monitoring with a much firmer structure. This could be done along with the normal drug evaluation scheme ("the phase system"), as proposed by HVIDBERG (1980). General principles for the use of plasma-level monitoring in clinical trials of new antiepileptic drugs have been given by MILLIGAN and RICHENS (1981).

E. Therapeutic Plasma Concentration Ranges for the Individual Antiepileptic Drugs

The following section will primarily be concerned with the evidence (or lack of) for the correlation between plasma levels and effects, and not with the general pharmacokinetic problems or other factors influencing the plasma level.

I. Phenytoin

Generally recommended therapeutic range: 10–20 mg/liter (40–80 μmol/liter). Generally accepted toxic limit: 25 mg/liter (100 μmol/liter).

It is noteworthy that the plasma concentration range originally suggested as being "therapeutic" in the earliest papers (BUCHTHAL and SVENSMARK 1960, BUCHTHAL et al. 1960, SVENSMARK et al. 1960) is the same as that used today, although this range is based on data from very few patients. A limited number of patients were arbitrarily divided into two small groups, one with above and one with below 10 mg/liter, and compared with respect to seizure frequency. The toxic level was determined in a similar way. Nevertheless, almost all later investigations, supplied by the many years of clinical experience, have pointed to the very same figures. This seems to be valid for all age groups, e.g., also neonates (PAINTER et al. 1978).

It serves no purpose to analyze all these studies, and only a few will be discussed. One of the more significant prospective studies was carried out by LUND (1974), who related seizure frequency to average plasma level over a 3-year span of treatment in 34 patients with grand mal epilepsy. The strength of this investigation is the dose/response-like fashion in which the results have been calculated. The inherited and unavoidable problems are the lack of contemporary controls and the possible influence of the time factor. Similar results have been reported by others, e.g., LOISEAU et al. (1977), although these results are less distinct because of comedication with phenobarbital. Their optimal phenytoin plasma level was 7–15 mg/liter. In a prospective study of 117 Latin American adults of whom 110 were on phenytoin monotherapy, GALDAMES et al. (1980) found satisfactory seizure control in a range of 10.2–25.8 mg/liter.

KUTT et al. (1964) specifically looked at the toxic level. From this and other studies (see KUTT 1972) several of the dose-related CNS signs of intoxication (nystagmus, ataxia, mental side effects) can be correlated to increasing plasma concentrations, and the diagram in Kutt's article is now a classical one. It refers, however, to a general pattern for a number of patients, and for the individual patient the toxic signs may start at quite different levels, although very rarely below 15 mg/liter. GANNAWAY and MAWER (1981) found that in a group of patients in whom the phenytoin dose was slowly increased, tolerance varied quite considerably, the threshold for symptomatic intoxication (ataxia) ranging form 35 to 60 mg/liter. The intraindividual toxic limit, on the other hand, does not show major variations, as the clinical symptoms can be correlated quite well to phenytoin levels in the single patient (BEIER et al. 1978).

Some prospective studies suggest that the concept of a therapeutic range for phenytoin is of no use (e.g., FEELEY et al. 1979), as excellent control is obtained in too many patients at concentrations outside (particularly below) the stated limits. Out of 20 patients taking phenytoin and phenobarbital, 19 were seizure free with phenytoin levels below 10 mg/liter (FELDMAN and PIPPENGER 1976), but many such patients, who suffer seizures again upon stopping the therapy, are on multiple-drug treatment. It is therefore not easy to evaluate the situation for phenytoin alone, and a substantial number of studies (most of them retrospective) have confirmed that the best therapeutic results are obtained in the originally suggested plasma concentration range (cf. SCHMIDT 1977a; RICHENS 1979).

However, the previously mentioned dependency on seizure type is important and among others an interesting study of GANNAWAY and MAWER (1981) is relevant to these problems. They transferred 18 poorly seizure controlled patients from multiple-drug therapy to monotherapy with phenytoin and 17 of these showed no deterioration. Eleven of these patients suffering from partial seizures did not improve during a (slow) increase in dose and plasma level (from 15 mg/liter to individual threshold for intoxication). However, four patients with generalized seizures did improve at higher concentrations.

At present the main problem about monitoring phenytoin plasma levels seems to be how to keep the patients's plasma concentration within the accepted range. Several studies indicate that up to half of outpatients have a phenytoin concentration below the accepted lower limit, and in many of these patients seizures are poorly controlled (cf. GUELEN and VAN DER KLEIJN 1978; KOCH-WESER 1981). It is evident, therefore, that the concentration range usually administered for phenytoin is a useful factor in the clinical control of epilepsy, and will continue to be so.

II. Carbamazepine

Generally recommended therapeutic range: 5–10 mg/liter (21–42 μmol/liter). Generally accepted toxic limit: 11 mg/liter (45 μmol/liter).

Only few controlled clinical trials have been performed with the specific aim of relating plasma levels to the therapeutic or toxic activity of carbamazepine.

However, studies including clinical observation, retrospective analysis, and prospective comparisons with other antiepileptic drugs have correlated the levels obtained with the clinical outcome. Such studies have suggested ranges anywhere between <4 and 16 mg/liter in adults, although the majority of studies recommend 5–10 mg/liter.

Early studies (FREY and YRJÄNÄ 1970; MØLLER 1971; PARSONAGE 1972; MEINARDI 1972; CEREGHINO et al. 1973, 1974, 1975), of which some are prospective, do not explicitly titrate a lower and an upper limit. However, it can be deduced from the results that levels below 1.5 mg/liter are definitely ineffective, while the first trace of toxic effects might be seen at the same level in some patients (MEINARDI 1972). On the other hand, some patients seem to tolerate concentrations above 11 mg/liter. Several of the early studies may not be comparable with recent ones as, e.g., the time at which the blood samples are taken by be different and the analytical methods not sufficiently specific.

SCHNEIDER (1975a) demonstrated a positive correlation of plasma concentration to clinical effect, with complete control of psychomotor seizures at an average level of 5.9 ($\pm$2.7) mg/liter. The patient material covered both institutionalized patients and patients in whom therapy was recently initiated. Side effects were observed from a level of about 8 mg/liter, and for both therapeutic effect and toxicity considerable variations were noted. The significance for drug-level monitoring of the suggested therapeutic range (5–11 mg/liter) in this study is clouded by the fact that the "therapeutic concentrations" are based on fasting morning samples, while the "side effect concentrations" are based on samples taken 3 h after the morning dose.

In a study by STRANDJORD and JOHANNESSEN (1975), it was reported that 21 of 28 patients on a constant carbamazepine dose had serum levels between 5.5 and 13.3 mg/liter without side effects. MONACO et al. (1976) likewise found a decrease in seizure frequency, when plasma levels of carbamazepine were kept between 4 and 10 mg/liter. Carbamazepine was compared with phenytoin in a controlled study using patients with psychomotor seizures (SIMONSEN et al. 1976). The two drugs were found equally effective when carbamazepine plasma concentrations ranged from 6 to 10 mg/liter. It is noteworthy that it was not necessarily the same patients who responded to the two drugs in this crossover trial. In a long-term follow-up study by STRANDJORD and JOHANNESSEN (1980) in patients with simple and complex partial seizures, the mean plasma level for patients was about 5.5 mg/liter (epoxide 0.6 mg/liter) and for patients previously treated with other antiepileptic drugs about 6.8 mg/liter (epoxide 0.7 mg/liter). Seizure control was good in both groups. However, in a group of poorly controlled patients the plasma carbamazepine (as well as the epoxide) was within the range giving seizure control in the rest of the patients. The authors emphasize the considerable interindividual differences in optimal carbamazepine levels.

By adding carbamazepine to patients suffering from partial seizures with complex symptomatology, but adequately controlled on phenytoin, 14–20 mg/liter, EICHELBAUM et al. (1976) were not able to demonstrate any further reduction in seizure frequency at an average carbamazepine level of 5 mg/liter. Increased levels in some of the patients to about 8 mg/liter resulted in side effects, but no improvements in seizure control. Similar results are reported by KUTT et al. (1975). The seizure type as well as the active carbamazepine metabolite (see later) may account for these negative results, whose general value could be questioned. However, it does not seem convincing that phenytoin was tried at sufficiently high levels.

TROUPIN et al. (1977) demonstrated in a comparative trial with phenytoin in patients with focal and major generalized seizures that for carbamazepine the "clinical range" of the plasma concentration was 8–12 mg/liter, with a total range of 2–18 mg/liter. However, an appreciable difference in plasma level in terms of effectiveness could not be revealed and this was also the case for toxicity. Studies of this kind therefore seem to describe the individual variations in plasma levels rather than presenting evidence for an optimal concentration range. However, such information is also of value and sometimes lost in later investigations. In similar patients, DAM et al. (1975) found that a level above 4 mg/liter was necessary to obtain seizure control. Rearranged, these results demonstrate an excellent dose/response relationship. In contrast to some other studies psychomotor seizures could not be controlled with carbamazepine alone.

TESTA et al. (1980) found in a heterogenic group of epileptic patients, who also took other drugs, that carbamazepine concentrations averaged 4.2 ($\pm$1.4) mg/liter in those patients who showed a substantial decrease in seizure frequency after carbamazepine had been administered. FORSYTHE et al. (1979) demonstrated that 6 mg/liter was the lowest carbamazepine level associated with complete control of seizures in a study on epileptic children. The observations of the last-mentioned studies contribute to a definition of the lower limit of the therapeutic concentration range, but they do not explain the relation between effect and plasma levels. In a study in patients with intermittent side effects from carbamazepine, HÖPPENER et al. (1980) found these side effects correlated to fluctuations in plasma concentrations over the day, particularly when they exceeded 8 mg/liter. After changing the scheme of intake in such a way that the plasma levels did not exceed this concentration, the side effects disappeared, but not at the expense of adequate seizure control. Such types of study design contribute greatly to the definition of an upper limit of the therapeutic range.

In spite of shortcomings in methods and design, the studies cited seem to indicate a lower limit for effectiveness of about 4–5 mg/liter for grand mal, but higher and more doubtful levels for psychomotor seizures. Several review articles also agree with this (e.g., HVIDBERG and DAM 1976; SCHMIDT 1977a; BERTILSSON 1978). Somewhat more problematical is the upper limit, as the intensity of side effects does not always seem to follow the plasma level (LEVY et al. 1975). As previously mentioned, discrete side effects (nystagmus) were observed by MEINARDI (1972) at very low levels, but analytical problems may have influenced these early results. The majority of patients in other studies did not experience side effects until they were above 8–11 mg/liter (cf. KUTT 1978a).

Although a therapeutic plasma range is not based on solid scientific grounds, monitoring carbamazepine can be considered useful based on the information obtained so far. Monitoring carbamazepine levels is consequently often recommended as a routine in epileptic patients (BATTINO et al. 1980).

Some of the difficulties in defining a therapeutic plasma range for carbamazepine might be caused by the active metabolite, CBZ-10,11-epoxide (see p. 748).

III. Phenobarbital

Generally recommended therapeutic range 10–30 (40) mg/liter [45–140(180)μmol/liter].

Generally accepted toxic limit: 40 mg/liter (180 μmol/liter).

It is puzzling that phenobarbital, in spite of being the oldest antiepileptic drug still in clinical use, has been investigated so sparsely with respect to both human pharmacokinetics and plasma level/effect relationship. Although a therapeutic level of 10–25 mg/liter was suggested by SVENSMARK and BUCHTHAL (1963), the first prospective studies were only published several years later (BUCHTHAL et al. 1968; BUCHTHAL and SVENSMARK 1971; BUCHTHAL and LENNOX-BUCHTHAL 1972). The original evidence rests on close observation of both EEG and clinical manifestations in 11 adults with grand mal seizures and in 60 children with febrile convulsions. An effect of phenobarbital was not seen unless the concentration was above 10–15 mg/liter. The same authors found the toxic limit to be about 30 mg/liter, but with large individual variations as also observed earlier (PLAA and HINE 1960). In another prospective investigation in 15 patients (SCHMIDT and JANZ 1977) the therapeutic level ranged from 14 to 76 mg/liter, with an average of 39.5 mg/liter, while the subtherapeutic concentration of phenobarbital had a mean of 25.6 mg/liter in the same patients. All but one of these were, however, treated with primidone, a precursor of phenobarbital (see below). Another group of 17 patients , who had been free of seizures for years, showed an average phenobarbital concentration of 25.2 mg/liter. These findings – although from a small number of patients – point to the already proposed therapeutic range, but they also emphasize the considerable interindividual variation. SCHMIDT and JANZ (1977) ascribe these variations mostly to the difference in severity of disease, but other explanations such as different degree of tolerance development may also be likely (BOOKER 1972a).

Few pharmacokinetic studies with phenobarbital have been carried out during the past years, and certainly only very few relating effect to plasma levels. KUPFERBERG and LONGACRE-SHAW (1979) found phenobarbital concentrations of 4–32 mg/liter in 11 patients adequately treated with mephobarbital, which is metabolized to phenobarbital. Only minute concentrations of mephobarbital were detected. In a complicated study by LOISEAU et al. (1977), the therapeutic level for phenobarbital was found to be 15–25 mg/liter, but also in this study the design was not aimed at a real evaluation of the level/effect relationship. Other studies with phenobarbital determination have been carried out with primidone (see below). In neonates a level of 12–30 mg/liter (JALLING 1975) or about 20 mg/liter (PAINTER et al. 1978) was found to be effective. It should be mentioned that effects on the EEG in normal volunteers correlated very well with the plasma levels of phenobarbital injected i.v., although these (2–8 mg/liter) were below the usually accepted lower limit for anticonvulsant activity (SANNITA et al. 1980).

The plasma levels originally suggested as the therapeutic range for phenobarbital now seem to be accepted to such a degree that new investigations about their validity hardly appear, although the original studies are about 15 years old and based on only a few patients. Particularly the upper limit is not very well defined, and individual differences here seem more pronounced for phenobarbital than for other antiepileptic drugs, although this has not been evaluated.

IV. Primidone

Generally accepted therapeutic range:

Parent compound	3–12 mg/liter	(13–55 μmol/liter)
Phenobarbital	10–30 mg/liter	(45–140 μmol/liter)
Phenylethylmalonamide	?	

Suggested toxic limit:

Parent compound	15 mg/liter	(75 μmol/liter)
Phenobarbital	40 mg/liter	(180 μmol/liter)
Phenylethylmalonamide	?	

The major problem for primidone with respect to therapeutic plasma ranges lies in the fact that we are dealing with a complex system of active compounds.

BUTLER and WADDELL (1956) and later OLESEN and DAM (1967) demonstrated that therapeutic doses of primidone resulted in plasma levels of phenobarbital with a definite anticonvulsant effect. The other metabolite phenylethylmalonamide (PEMA), as well as primidone itself, also exerts antiepileptic activity, and it is this triangle of substances which is probably responsible for the effect of primidone (SCHOTTELIUS and FINCHAM 1978). The problem is, however, their mutual strength of anticonvulsant activity. This has not been evaluated in man, and may be impossible to do. However, about 85% of the effect in the steady state must be ascribed to phenobarbital, and it has still to be shown whether or not the two other components really contribute clinically to the antiepileptic activity during primidone treatments (FREY and LÖSCHER 1980).

No controlled or other prospective studies have been published relating levels of primidone itself to effect. The lower limit for primidone was suggested by KUTT and PENRY (1974) to about 5 mg/liter and the upper limit to 10 mg/liter (KUTT 1974), while others (BOOKER 1972b; SCHMIDT 1977b) refer to a toxic level of 20 mg/liter. Retrospectively, SCHOTTELIUS and FINCHAM (1978) considered a therapeutic range of 3–12 mg/liter to be correct, and found that toxicity is not seen below 15 mg/liter. These authors used plasma samples obtained 2–4 h after the drug was ingested. The cited values may, however, be considered as more or less speculative, because the simultaneously generated concentration of phenobarbital can be crucial. Interestingly, BOOKER (1972b) reported that substitution of primidone with phenobarbital in some patients resulted in the same therapeutic effect, but they recovered from certain side effects, suggesting a different profile of adverse reactions in the two therapeutic situations, of which both include phenobarbital. In a recent review (JOHANNESSEN 1981), no final solution for the monitoring problem in primidone-treated patients could be offered, except that monitoring of phenobarbital was considered essential, while additional monitoring of primidone may be beneficial. Determination of PEMA was not considered justified.

The individual variation in the metabolism of primidone, whether genetic in origin or influenced by xenobiotics (e.g., other drugs), magnifies the problems, but serves also – in theory – as reasonable justification for monitoring of primidone and phenobarbital during primidone treatment. The prerequisite for doing so, well-founded documentation for the therapeutic levels, has not, however, been established. Phenobarbital monitoring can help to avoid phenobarbital intoxication during primidone therapy, but on logical grounds it is all that can be advocated until more studies have been performed.

V. Ethosuximide

Generally accepted therapeutic range: 40–100 mg/liter (285–710 μmol/liter).

Assumed toxic limit: 130 mg/liter (1,000 μmol/liter).

The control of petit mal seizures with ethosuximide seems to be fairly well correlated to plasma concentration (SHERWIN and ROBB 1972; SHERWIN 1978), but only few prospective investigations have been performed to define a therapeutic plasma range. HAERER et al. (1970) reported a range of 11–55 mg/liter in a group of patients with absence seizures (with or without other kinds of seizures) and for the majority showing improvements during the treatment. However, this finding can hardly be taken as a documentation for a therapeutic range. PENRY et al. (1972) found maximum clinical control with plasma ethosuximide between 40 and 80 mg/liter in patients who responded to the treatment. Similar results, although with greater variation, were reported by SHERWIN and ROBB (1972). PENRY (1975) and BROWNE et al. (1975) reported essentially the same outcome, i.e., excellent seizure control in responsive patients at plasma levels of about 60 mg/liter. In a prospective study, SHERWIN (1978) pointed to some important features: Significant reduction in seizure frequency was seen in a number of patients with frequent attacks of absence seizures after 2½ years of treatment with ethosuximide, and during this period the mean plasma levels increased from 57 to 76 mg/liter (due to dose increments). Such an increase was not observed in patients who continued to have frequent attacks. Although an age-related improvement is known in this disease, the author finds the reported improvement as a result of the dose adjustments made on the basis of the plasma level determinations. Another finding by SHERWIN (1978) is that individual treatment schedules with plasma concentrations as high as 150 mg/liter may sometimes prove useful, although he recommends an average therapeutic range of 40–100 mg/liter.

The toxic limit has been very poorly investigated, probably because side effects of ethosuximide are quite rare. Some very high concentrations, e.g., 135 and 168 mg/liter (SOLOW and GREEN 1971) and up to 153 mg/liter were reported not to be associated with side effects. Similarly, in a pharmacokinetic study covering up to 3 years' observation at different steady-state levels, several of 46 patients had plasma levels above 120 mg/liter, some even 180 mg/liter, but with no reports of toxicity (SMITH et al. 1979).

The correlation between plasma concentration of ethosuximide and the control of absence seizures is well established in patients in which the drug shows an effect at all, but documentation for a therapeutic plasma range is very scanty. The average level to be aimed at may be 60–70 mg/liter, although some patients may show a benefit up to 150 mg/liter without toxicity. A toxic limit has not really been defined. The basis for monitoring ethosuximide levels may consequently be considered quite weak.

VI. Benzodiazepines

1. Diazepam

Therapeutic plasma range: not known
Toxic level: not known
The relation between diazepam plasma concentration and the various clinical effects in man has been investigated very little. In nonepileptic patients correlations have been looked for between various effects of diazepam and diazepam plasma levels. The antianxiety activity showed no correlation (MANDELLI et al. 1978), while the effective plasma levels after i.v. injection seemed to be 400–500 µg/liter for changes in, e.g., reaction times (HILLESTAD et al. 1974; HARDER et al. 1976). Effects on spasticity in normal volunteers were seen at concentrations of between 300 and 2,200 µg/liter (LOSSIUS et al. 1980). For anticonvulsant activity only few results are available which relate effect to plasma levels. MORSELLI and FRANCO-MORSELLI (1980) refer to statements that plasma concentrations of at least 1,000–1,200 µg/liter are necessary to suppress ictal discharges, and BOOKER and CELESIA (1973) found that a peak level of 500–600 µg/liter could suppress interictal discharges in photosensitive subjects. After rectal administration of diazepam, FERNGREN (1974) noted convulsions in one child at a concentration of 130 µg/liter, while AGURELL et al. (1975) found the anticonvulsant level in two children to be 150 and 200 µg/liter, respectively. However, KNUDSEN (1977) observed febrile convulsions in a child with a concentration of about 1,200 µg/liter. After i.v. injections or rectal application, with the doses usually applied in status epilepticus, it seems reasonable to believe that the lower anticonvulsant concentration of diazepam may be 300–500 µg/liter. The lack of documentation may, however, be of little direct clinical significance, as plasma concentration monitoring in status epilepticus is not feasible.

Anticonvulsant treatment with orally given diazepam is only rarely effective, except in minor motor seizures. Plasma concentrations of 100–300 µg/liter have been suggested as effective (KUTT 1978b), but no investigation seems to have been performed to substantiate this claim. Acute side effects have been noted at concentrations above 400 µg/liter (MORSELLI and FRANCO-MORSELLI 1980), but for chronic treatment there is no reliable information. Furthermore, it does not seem to have been investigated whether the rare respiratory depression seen after i.v. injection of diazepam coincides with extraordinarily high plasma levels, although levels exceeding 2,500 µg/liter have been suggested (MORSELLI and FRANCO-MORSELLI 1980).

In chronic diazepam treatment two conditions must be remembered. First, that the active metabolite *N*-desmethyl-diazepam is present in plasma concentrations higher than the parent compound (see later), and secondly that tolerance may develop. To which degree these conditions are of significance is apparently not known in the rarely applied chronic antiepileptic treatment with diazepam. Monitoring of plasma diazepam is therefore not to be advocated except, perhaps, for the control of patient compliance.

2. Clonazepam

Suggested therapeutic plasma range: 20–70 μg/liter (65–225 nmol/liter)
Assumed toxic levels: 100 μg/liter (320 nmol/liter)
For clonazepam very sparse documentation is available concerning the relation between plasma levels and antiepileptic effect (PINDER et al. 1976). DREIFUSS et al. (1975) and MORSELLI (1978) found levels between 20 and 70 μg/liter effective in absence seizures. Other retrospective studies (SJÖ et al. 1975, VAN DER KLEIJN 1975) suggest the therapeutic range to be 30–60 μg/liter. No firm correlation between plasma clonazepam and toxic effects have been reported, but MORSELLI (1978) found an increasing number of patients with severe toxicity above 100 μg/liter, and even an increased frequency of seizures at levels exceeding 180 μg/liter.

The indications for the use of clonazepam in epilepsy is more restricted than originally thought, as infantile spasms and absences seem to be the main indications (BROWNE 1978) Clonazepam is a difficult drug to handle in clinical practice. If, for example, dosage is increased too fast at the beginning of the treatment, severe side effects may occur (PINDER et al. 1976), but monitoring plasma levels is not useful in this situation. Furthermore, a diminished effect is often seen after 2–3 months of treatment, probably mostly at higher dosages (MORSELLI and FRANCO-MORSELLI 1980), but plasma-level monitoring has not given the explanation. Clonazepam seems to gain a place in the treatment of status epilepticus, but so far no investigation has been published concerning the effective plasma level in this situation.

Based on the above considerations routine monitoring of plasma levels can hardly be recommended.

VII. Valproic Acid

Suggested therapeutic plasma concentration range: 50–100 mg/liter (350–700 μmol/liter)
Suspected toxic level: 100 mg/liter (700 μmol/liter)
Considerable confusion seems to exist about therapeutic monitoring and optimal plasma levels of valproic acid. Some authors find no correlation between plasma levels and antiepileptic effect, while others seem to agree on an optimal plasma-concentration range of somewhere between 34 and 105 mg/liter (MEIJER and HESSING-BRAND 1973; MEINARDI et al. 1974; BARNES and BOWER 1975; SCHOBBEN et al. 1975; LOISEAU et al. 1975; CHARD 1976; RICHENS et al. 1976; VAJDA et al. 1976; BRUNI et al. 1978; GRAM et al. 1979; SCHULZ et al. 1979; HENRIKSEN and JOHANNESSEN 1980; KLOTZ and SCHNEIDER 1980). Furthermore, ROWAN et al. (1979) found a correlation between changes in plasma levels and changes in the EEG (serial monitoring). The majority of these investigations find a level above 50 (60) mg/liter necessary to obtain seizure control (cf. FRÖSCHER et al. 1978), but the impression prevails that considerable individual differences exist in the plas-

ma level/effect ratio. There are some indications that plasma levels exceeding 100 mg/liter are associated with increasing frequency of side effects (drowsiness, sedation, and perhaps also weight gain and hair loss), but observations are often made in patients undergoing polytherapy (HASSAN et al. 1976; GRAM et al. 1979; HENRIKSEN and JOHANNESSEN 1980; MORSELLI and FRANCO-MORSELLI 1980).

However, acute valproic acid toxicity is not a major therapeutic problem, and it is therefore difficult to determine an upper therapeutic level.

In spite of the many studies, the documentation supporting a therapeutic level for valproic acid is not very strong. A major reason for the difficulties in correlating the total plasma concentration levels of valproic acid to the clinical effects may be found in the variation in the plasma protein binding of valproic acid. In addition, the protein binding is dependent on total concentration. At lower concentrations the free fraction is average 10% (review: GUGLER and VON UNRUH 1980), while it increases more than 50% at concentrations of around 100 mg/liter (GRAM et al. 1979). Furthermore, considerable fluctuations of the plasma level are seen during the day because of rapid absorption and a relatively fast elimination rate. The small volume of distribution (cf. GUGLER and VON UNRUH 1980) makes these fluctuations more significant for the variations in the tissue concentrations. The use of the primary amide of dipropylacetic acid, dipropylacetamide, as a prodrug, greatly reduces the diurnal fluctuations of valproic acid (PISANI et al. 1981), but this is probably not sufficient to eliminate the problems. Thus it has also been shown that the free fraction of valproic acid may increase under influence of concomitant therapy and other factors (HAIDUKEWYCH and RODIN 1981). As a result of these problems the timing of blood sampling becomes critical, and consequently measuring the total plasma level of valproic acid does not result in a reliable parameter to be compared with clinical benefit or toxicity. Other kinetic factors may add to this problem, as valproic acid is metabolized and at least some of the metabolites are biologically active (LÖSCHER 1981) (see later).

The kinetic variability may explain the poor plasma level/effect correlation, but it may not be the whole explanation. An indication of the influence of pharmacodynamic factors is that the considerable daily fluctuation in plasma levels (and even greater in the levels of the unbound fraction) seen with a once-a-day dosage schedule do not make the clinical outcome inferior to the normal t.i.d. schedule with much less fluctuation (CENRAUD et al. 1981); rather the opposite (COVANIS et al. 1981; ROWAN et al. 1981). In this connection it is of note that clinical recovery from intoxication (peak plasma level 2,120 mg/liter) was not correlated to the eventual occurrence of "normal" plasma levels (i.e., <150 mg/liter). The slow recovery from coma was delayed for several days (PEDERSEN 1982).

At the present time there is no indication that monitoring total plasma concentration of valproic acid may be of benefit for the therapy (SCHOBBEN et al. 1980). One exception however, may be the control of patient compliance, and as most studies find a concentration of 50 mg/liter necessary for effective treatment, control may be justified if nonresponders are above this limit. Monitoring in the sense of, e.g., that given to phenytoin treatment would hardly be defensible until many more studies have been carried out and level/effect correlations have been verified. However, as suggested by LEVY (1980), monitoring the unbound plasma levels may seem benificial (cf. Sect. F).

VIII. Other Antiepileptic Drugs

Very little information is available on optimal plasma concentration ranges or therapeutic monitoring concerning antiepileptic drugs other than the ones dealt with in the previous sections.

Human kinetics have been studied to some extent for other hydantoin derivatives, but therapeutic ranges have not been substantiated (TROUPIN et al. 1979). Plasma levels usually obtained for mephenytoin are 5–16 mg/liter, and 25–40 mg/liter for its active metabolite 5-ethyl-5-phenyl-hydantoin (Nirvanol) (MILLICHAP 1972; SCHMIDT 1981). For ethotoin, concentrations of about 4–15 mg/liter have been observed (LUND et al. 1975). No information is available for phenytoin-3-norvalin (Neo-Citrullamon). Methylphenobarbital is metabolized quickly to phenobarbital, and plasma levels of the latter will determine the antiepileptic effect (cf. KUPFERBERG and LONGACRE-SHAW 1979). Trimethadione is metabolized to dimethadione and "therapeutic levels" of 20 mg/liter and 700 mg/liter, respectively, are suggested (EADIE 1976; SCHMIDT 1981). With an average dose of 5 mg/day nitrazepam plasma levels of 30–150 µg/liter were seen (BOSSI and MORSELLI 1977). Information on therapeutic plasma levels for carboanhydrase inhibitors is also scanty. For sulthiame a range of 6–10 mg/liter has been suggested (EGLI 1977). Levels of about 10–14 mg/liter are obtained for acetazolamide after doses of 10 mg/kg (SCHMIDT 1981).

No studies have been carried out in order to correlate plasma levels with effects for the above-mentioned drugs. The information on plasma levels cannot therefore be used as a basis for therapeutic drug monitoring, possibly not even as initial guidance. However, the use of these drugs is quite rare and the problems therefore very limited.

F. Protein Binding and Monitoring Antiepileptic Drug Levels

The kinetic details of the plasma protein binding of antiepileptic drugs are given elsewhere in this volume (Chap. 24), and only the implications for therapeutic drug monitoring will be discussed here. An excellent general review of this topic has recently been presented by ROWLAND (1980).

Measurement of the free fraction seems important, as this can diffuse across membranes into the biophase. The free fraction is therefore thought to interact with the receptors. Direct measurements of the free fraction in plasma require often much more sensitive analytical assays because of the lower concentration to be measured. For this reason and because of the more elaborate procedure to be applied (dialysis, ultracentrifugation, or the like), routine monitoring is at present almost exclusively based on the determination of the total concentration of the antiepileptic drug in plasma. Free fraction measurements are still predominantly considered experimental, devoted to clinical pharmacological investigations, and used as a routine in only few laboratories.

Other methods are available for the determination of the free fraction, such as measurements of CSF concentrations (not relevant for monitoring purposes), salivary concentration, and concentration in tears (see later). Finally, the determination of erythrocyte-binding can be used; thus binding to red blood cells of phenytoin and phenobarbital has been found to be fairly constant, e.g., unaffected by uremia. It has therefore been suggested that the erythrocyte/plasma ratio may serve as a screening method for abnormal plasma binding in the individual patient (GLAZKO 1973; BORONDY et al. 1973; KURATA and WILKINSON 1974; SHERWIN et al. 1976; EHRNEBO and ODAR-CEDERLÖF 1975, 1977). This approach does not seem to have gained much clinical interest and it has not been evaluated for its significance in larger patient materials. One important reason could be pitfalls in the interpretation of concentration data because of methodological problems. Thus, washed erythrocytes have a greater binding than whole blood erythrocytes (EHRNEBO and ODAR-CEDERLÖF 1977).

It should be noted that although the free fraction (as a *percentage* of the total concentration) is increased, e.g., during renal insufficiency, this parameter does not serve as a useful guideline for adjustments of the plasma level. The absolute concentration of unbound drug may be unchanged due to a compensatory increase in the apparent volume of distribution and plasma clearance (ODAR-CEDERLÖF and BORGÅ 1974; GUGLER et al. 1975). A decrease in plasma protein binding thus leads to a lower total plasma level, but should not trigger off an increased dose (REIDENBERG 1977).

Data on protein binding of antiepileptic drugs of special interest for drug level monitoring are:

1. The magnitude of the interindividual variation in protein binding
2. The degree of change (if any) in the binding imposed by, e.g., renal disease and drug interactions
3. The occurrence of concentration-dependent binding within the therapeutic range

If these problems are applied to the individual antiepileptic drugs, only few answers can be extracted. For phenytoin the interindividual variation in protein binding is somewhat controversial. BOOKER and DARCEY (1973) observed large variations, which might have been due to technical problems, while BARTH et al. (1976), YACOBI et al. (1977), and MONKS (1978) all found a mere twofold variation in the free fraction in adults with normal liver and kidney function. The protein binding of phenytoin is, however, influenced by several factors (for review see PERUCCA 1980), as renal and liver disease have a great impact on the binding. Likewise, the extremes of age (newborns, old age), pregnancy, burns, surgery, and a number of drugs have a considerable influence on the protein binding of phenytoin. On the whole, therefore, measuring the free fraction of phenytoin would seem advantageous in clinical practice, because a false impression of the active part may be obtained in certain situations (such as in renal disease), leading to wrong clinical decisions. However, as stated above the methodology is not yet geared to direct routine determinations, and salivary concentrations may also be problematical (see later). Protein binding of phenytoin does not seem to be concentration dependent.

Half of the amount of phenobarbital in plasma is bound to proteins (BUCHANAN and VAN DER WALT 1977), which is reflected in the CSF concentration. Interindividual differences do not seem to be of greater importance. Renal and hepatic disease have not been reported to influence the protein binding of phenobarbital, and concentration-dependent binding is not likely.

The free fraction of carbamazepine has been reported in different studies to be 20%–44% (mean values) (for reviews see BERTILSSON 1978; PYNNÖNEN 1979; SILLANPÄÄ 1981). Methodological differences may account for at least part of this variability, but the twofold difference covers an even greater intersubject variability in the individual studies (RAWLINS et al. 1975). There is no hint of a dose-dependent protein binding. Comedication with phenobarbital or phenytoin does not result in displacement of carbamazepine from its binding sites (RAWLINS et al. 1975), and hepatic disorders seem to have no clinically relevant influence, although a minor reduction in protein binding was observed (HOOPER et al. 1975). The main impression is that monitoring the free drug level of carbamazepine in theory would be advantageous, e.g., by salivary concentration measurements, but that a lot of practical problems prevail.

Primidone and ethosuximide are both bound to plasma proteins to a very low degree. The benzodiazepines are highly bound, 82%–90% (HVIDBERG and DAM 1976) but as plasma-level monitoring of these drugs in epileptic patients plays no role, the problems concerned with variability in protein binding are of no clinical relevance in this connection.

For valproic acid it is quite different. Considerable variations in protein binding have been demonstrated, and the binding seems sensitive to a number of influences (KLOTZ et al. 1978; BREWSTER and MUIR 1980; BRUNI et al. 1980; HAIDUKEWYCH and RODIN 1981; RODIN and HAIDUKEWYCH 1981). Relating the free fraction to antiepileptic effect of valproic acid may reveal a much better correlation than total valproic acid concentration and it may be possible to explain some cases of nonresponders and other irregularities. At the present time monitoring free fraction levels of valproic acid, however, may be regarded as a tool of investigation rather than as a routine, although LEVY (1980) suggested that monitoring the free fraction would be an advantage.

G. Monitoring Antiepileptic Drug Therapy by Measurements in Biological Fluids Other than Plasma

I. General Considerations

For several reasons it would seem logical to use body fluids other than blood for monitoring antiepileptic drug levels. The noninvasive way of obtaining saliva, tears, and urine is an advantage to the patient, particularly children. The possibility of direct determination of the free fraction in low-protein fluids such as saliva, tears, and cerebrospinal fluid (CSF) may further appear to be a more correct approach (see above). Although such considerations are based on sound theories, practical application does not always seem very attractive. Measurements of urinary concentrations may only serve as a semiquantitative control of compliance and are of no use in monitoring drug levels in the body. CSF levels cannot, of course, be measured as a routine procedure, but they are of great value for the investigation of the passage of a drug into the central nervous system. This leaves two possibilities in clinical practice: saliva and tears. The former has attracted considerable interest and a great number of investigations have therefore appeared during recent years.

II. Monitoring Salivary Levels of Antiepileptic Drugs

The kinetics of antiepileptic drugs in saliva will be treated thoroughly elsewhere. It suffices here to state that the following factors will determine the concentration in saliva (cf. MUCKLOW et al. 1978; STEPHEN et al. 1980).

1. The protein binding of the drug in plasma
2. The protein binding of the drug in saliva, often considered nil (protein in saliva is about 3 g/liter)
3. The pH of plasma (approximately 7.4)
4. The pH of saliva (varying)
5. The physicochemical properties of the drug, including the pK_a value and partition coefficient
6. Transport mechanisms: active secretion or passive diffusion into saliva

Using the Henderson-Hasselbalch equation, the concentration of the drug in saliva can be estimated as follows, providing only passive diffusion is the driving force:

$$C_s = C_p \frac{1+10(pK_a - pH_s)}{1+10(pK_a - pH_p)} \frac{f_p}{f_s}.$$

C_s and C_p are the drug concentrations in saliva and plasma, respectively. pH_s and pH_p are the pH values in saliva and plasma. The fractions of unbound drug in saliva and plasma are designated f_s and f_p, respectively.

A prerequisite for the utilization of salivary concentrations in therapeutic drug monitoring is that a direct correlation exists between the levels of drug in saliva and plasma over a wide range of concentrations. Acceptable correlations have been reported particularly for drugs, which are largely un-ionized at normal plasma pH (HORNING et al. 1977; MUCKLOW et al. 1978). For substances with a high degree of ionization the salivary concentration is highly dependent on the actual pH in saliva and fluctuations can be considerable due to pH changes in saliva. Monitoring salivary concentrations in such cases may, therefore, be problematical or even meaningless.

By applying the above-mentioned principles it can be predicted for a number of antiepileptic drugs that salivary concentrations would be a reliable reflection of the free fraction of the drug in plasma. In fact, it has been shown that for phenytoin, carbamazepine, primidone, ethosuximide, and diazepam a good correlation does exist between salivary drug levels and levels of the free fraction of the drug in plasma. For phenobarbital, which has a more critical pK_a value, the reports have not been consistent, and for valproic acid no correlation has been found.

Although in theory it seems better to monitor salivary drug levels instead of plasma levels, and also in practice it has been shown to be so (cf., e.g., KRISTENSEN and LARSEN 1980), many authors have pointed out the problems and limitations involved (RICHENS 1979; MORSELLI and FRANCO-MORSELLI 1980; STEPHEN et al. 1980; JOHANNESSEN 1981). The problems can be summarized as follows:

1. The practical problems of obtaining saliva (preferably serous saliva from the parotid gland) in sufficient amounts and uncontaminated by food, etc. should not

be disregarded. The measured drug concentration may have been influenced by the sampling conditions.

2. By examining the original data from many studies an appreciable variation in the saliva/plasma ratio can be noted between the patients included, although the correlations are acceptable on average.

3. The lower drug concentrations in saliva require analytical methods of much higher sensitivity than needed for measuring total drug concentrations in plasma. The likelihood of increased analytical variability is consequently great.

4. The saliva/plasma relationship for drug concentrations may only be valid for steady-state conditions.

5. Salivary drug concentrations can only be used for monitoring certain drugs (see above), and, although some studies find that comedication with, e.g., other antiepileptic drugs has no influence on the saliva/plasma ratio, the possibility of drug interaction does not seem to have been investigated in depth.

6. At the present state of knowledge it seems reasonable to believe that the unbound fraction of a drug is a better and more pharmacologically correct determinant for the observed action of the drug than the total concentration. However, it still has to be proven that it is *clinically* advantageous to measure the free fraction.

In practice measuring salivary drug concentrations does not seem to play the role that could be expected from the theoretical considerations. A critical attitude has been expressed by several authors (MORSELLI and FRANCO-MORSELLI 1980; PERUCCA 1980; JOHANNESSEN 1981), and the above-stated difficulties and hesitations are the main reasons. However, being aware of these problems, determinations of salivary concentrations will be – under well-standardized conditions of saliva collection and by the use of sensitive analytical procedures – a convenient way of determining the free concentration of some drugs, e.g., in situations where alterations in protein binding may be suspected. Furthermore, the non-invasive sampling technique is especially suitable for monitoring antiepileptic drugs in children. Finally, it may be a convenient way of controlling patients compliance.

It is, however, fair to state that at the present time much more research, as well as cost-benefit calculations, is needed before measuring salivary drug concentrations finds its place in the clinical control of epileptic patients. Just as for monitoring plasma levels it is a prerequisite to establish a relationship between salivary drug levels and antiepileptic effect in order to create a firm basis for its clinical use. Such investigations are rather few, as almost all studies have focused on the correlation between salivary and plasma levels.

1. Phenytoin

Several studies indicate a good to excellent correlation between salivary and plasma leves for phenytoin over a wide range, in both children and adults and independent of comedication (BOCHNER et al. 1974; TROUPIN and FRIEL 1975; SCHMIDT and KUPFERBERG 1975; COOK ET AL. 1975; REYNOLDS ET AL 1976; HORNING et al. 1977; BLOM and GUELEN 1977; PAXTON et al. 1977; ANAVEKAR et al. 1978; MUCKLOW et al. 1978; ZYSSET et al. 1981; KNOTT et al. 1982). The majority of investigators find a salivary/plasma ratio of about 0.1 corresponding to the commonly observed free fraction in plasma of about 10%. These results indicate that phenytoin is dialyzed into saliva ((RICHENS 1979), i.e., transported by simple diffusion to an equilibrium with the nonprotein bound fraction in plasma. However, it has been suggested that other, more complex mechanisms are involved, e.g., ultrafiltration or active transport (STEPHEN et al. 1980). Thus, some data (ANAVEKAR et al. 1978) may be consistent with a saturated active transport, but there has been no confirmation of this probability. The problem of which kind of saliva (parotid, submaxillar, mixed) should be preferred has been investigated in some studies. The general conclusion seems to be that parotid saliva is preferable (ANAVEKAR et al. 1978; STEPHEN et al 1980), although the differences are not great.

Based on the studies cited above (including several review articles), a therapeutic salivary concentration range of 1.0–2.0 mg/liter can be suggested. Insofar as this range is a reliable expression of the free fraction of phenytoin, salivary concentration monitoring would be justified (i.e., preferred to plasma-level monitoring) in several diseased states in which the protein binding of phenytoin is known to be altered (for review see PERUCCA 1980) or in the case of comedication with displacing agents as valproic acid (KNOTT et al. 1982).

Together with carbamazepine, phenytoin is the most extensively investigated antiepileptic drug with respect to salivary concentrations, but several of the previously stated difficulties in the use of plasma concentration ranges certainly also apply to saliva. The enthusiasm may also be lowered by the finding of BRUGMANN et al. (1979) that, although a very good correlation was demonstrated between the free fraction in plasma and salivary concentrations, the latter were (apparently for unknown reasons) in some cases extremely high in comparison with plasma. The authors state that precautions are advisable before therapeutic decisions are taken on the basis of saliva determinations.

2. Carbamazepine

Carbamazepine fulfils the criteria for a drug whose concentration in saliva should correlate over a wide concentration range with the unbound fraction of the drug in plasma, and several studies have confirmed this experimentally (CHAMBERS et al. 1977; MCAULIFFE et al. 1977; TROUPIN et al. 1977; GUELEN and VAN DER KLEIJN 1978; WESTENBERG et al. 1978; PAXTON and DONALD 1980; KRISTENSEN and LARSEN 1980; MACKICHAN et al. 1981). In fact, the free fraction shows a much better correlation with the salivary concentration than the total plasma concentration, which seems to indicate that the protein binding of carbamazepine can be predicted by determination of salivary concentrations in the individual patient. The (probably) active metabolite CBZ-10-11-epoxide could not be detected in saliva by WESTENBERG et al. (1978), but this was possible for MACKICHAN et al. (1981), although the sensitivity of the methods (both of them liquid chromatography) were apparently similar. MACKICHAN et al. (1981) were also able to demonstrate a very high degree of correlation between the free fraction of this metabolite and its salivary concentration. For both carbamazepine and its epoxide metabolite the average concentrations in saliva were found to be higher than the free fraction in plasma. For carbamazepine this was not significant, but for the metabolite it amounted to a difference of almost one-third. Similar findings have been reported by TROUPIN and FRIEL (1975) and CHRISTIANSEN and

DAM (1977). For carbamazepine, technical explanations (e.g., evaporation of saliva during sampling) could be possible, but if these findings are confirmed for the epoxide, other reasons should be examined, e.g., active transport mechanisms.

The therapeutic salivary concentration level for carbamazepine has definitely not been demonstrated, but based on the published studies (see above) it might be suggested to range from 1.5 to 2.5 mg/liter. Because of the lack of evidence for any therapeutic or toxic effect of the epoxide metabolite, it serves no purpose to suggest a "therapeutic" level for this substance in saliva.

3. Phenobarbital

The physicochemical conditions for phenobarbital are not favorable for monitoring drug levels by measuring salivary concentrations. Its pK_a value of 7.3 is close to the physiological pH, and its concentration in saliva is therefore very sensitive to variations in pH (see above).

In a study by SCHMIDT and KUPFERBERG (1975) the pH of the saliva samples was not stated, the average saliva/plasma ratio was lower than would be expected from its degree of plasma protein binding, and the variation was considerable (mean 0.33, range 0.2–0.6). HORNING et al. (1977) obtained similar results (0.31–0.37). These results are possibly a reflection of the pH variations in saliva and/or variations in protein binding. MCAULIFFE et al. (1977) found that phenobarbital was clearly influenced by the pH of the salvia, and several authors have recommended that phenobarbital levels in saliva should be corrected for pH (GUELEN and VAN DER KLEIJN 1978; NISHIHARA et al. 1979; MORSELLI and FRANCO-MORSELLI 1980; JOHANNESSEN 1981). Monitoring phenobarbital by salivary concentrations is therefore more problematical than for, e.g., phenytoin and carbamazepine and should only be recommended for general use if the results are corrected for salivary pH.

4. Primidone

On the basis of the low protein binding in plasma (<10%) the concentration of primidone should be almost equal in saliva and plasma, which in fact has also been found experimentally (SCHMIDT and KUPFERBERG 1975; BLOM and Guelen 1977; HORNING et al. 1977). Its metabolite phenobarbital behaves as described above, which means that the salivary concentrations of phenobarbital have to be corrected for salivary pH. There are no reports of the other metabolite, PEMA, in saliva.

If primidone levels are to be monitored in saliva the therapeutic range for plasma can be applied for the parent compound. For phenobarbital the same reservations as stated above must be taken.

5. Ethosuximide

Ethosuximide is virtually unbound to plasma proteins and is undissociated at physiological pH. Salivary concentrations should therefore equal plasma concentrations. Experimentally the saliva/plasma ratio has been found to be from 0.9 to 1.0 (SCHMIDT 1976; BLOM and GUELEN 1977; MCAULIFFE et al. 1977; HORNING et al. 1977; GUELEN and VAN DER KLEIJN 1978; PIREDDA and MONACO 1981). Often used in children, monitoring salivary concentrations of ethosuximide should be of special advantage, but no investigations seem to have been published as to the therapeutic benefit of salivary level monitoring in this situation.

6. Benzodiazepines

Concentrations of diazepam in saliva show excellent correlation with the plasma concentration of the non-protein bound fraction (DIGREGORIO et al. 1978). Similar results have been demonstrated for nitrazepam (KANGAS et al. 1979). No information is apparently available about clonazepam. For diazepam the salivary concentration is about 3% of the total plasma concentration. It remains to be shown that monitoring diazepam levels in saliva would be of any benefit for the acute use of diazepam in status epilepticus, but it seems quite doubtful.

7. Valproic Acid

Investigations of valproic acid in saliva have almost unanimously demonstrated a very low degree of correlation between plasma and salivary concentrations (GUGLER et al. 1977; PINDER et al. 1977; BLOM and GUELEN 1977; GUELEN and VAN DER KLEIJN 1978). This is predictable as the pK_a is about 5, which means a high degree of ionization. The plasma protein binding of valproic acid is variable and saturable (see previously, and for this reason is would be desirable to have access to a clinical estimate of the free fraction (cf. e.g., HAIDUKEWYCH and RODIN 1981). However, no clinical experimental study has tried to correlate salivary concentrations (corrected for salivary pH) to the clinical effect of valproic acid, with the specific aim of monitoring valproic acid levels in patients. This possibility has – possibly for good reasons – been rejected due to the lack of correlation between saliva and plasma concentrations, but it should be borne in mind that total valproic acid levels in plasma are not well correlated to the antiepileptic effect.

III. Monitoring Antiepileptic Drugs in Tears

Only few investigations have been carried out with the purpose of monitoring drug levels in tears, and such studies have mainly focused on pharmacokinetic conditions, e.g. the correlation between the free fraction in plasma and levels of CSF, saliva, and tears. However, for a number of antiepileptic drugs a good correlation could be demonstrated between drug concentration in saliva, tears and other biological fluids (MONACO et al. 1979, 1981; PIREDDA and MONACO 1981).

Phenytoin is distributed rapidly to all extracellular fluids and found in tears in a concentration similar to the non-protein fraction of plasma (MORSELLI and FRANCO-MORSELLI 1980; MONACO et al. 1979, 1981). For carbamazepine, with a protein binding of between 60% and 73%, the tear/plasma ratio was found to be 44% (MONACO et al. 1979), which is rather high compared with saliva or CSF in other studies (SILLANPÄÄ 1981). This may partly be due to a cross-reaction between carbamazepine and its epoxide metabolite in the enzyme multiplied immunoassay technique (EMIT) assay. A closer connection was observed between tear/plasma and tear/CSF ratios for carbamazepine. For phenobarbital, tears also seem to be a good indicator of the unbound fraction, but not necessarily for primidone (MONACO et al. 1979, 1981). For ethosuximide the concentration in tears seems to correlate well with those in CSF plasma, and saliva (PIREDDA and MONACO 1981), but the number of observations are still few. Valproic acid has apparently been measured in tears, but results have not yet been published (cf. PIREDDA and MONACO 1981).Until now mainly a single research team (MONACO et al.) has been engaged in studying antiepileptic drugs in tears. The number of patients investigated are relatively few and the methodology not fully tested. It is therefore too early to judge this approach, which could be particularly acceptable in the treatment of epileptic children.

H. Active Metabolites and Monitoring Antiepileptic Drug Levels

Several antiepileptic drugs form biologically active substances in the body. Such metabolites may have a considerable influence on the use and interpretation of results obtained for therapeutic drug monitoring (EADIE 1976). The problem has been reviewed for drugs in general by ATKINSON and STRONG (1977) and ATKINSON et al. (1980), but the examples given by these authors do not include antiepileptics. Such examples have, however, been given by DRAYER (1976) and LANE and LEVY (1980).

In general the problems imposed by active metabolites can be summarized as follows:

1. The effects of a drug may, partly or totally, rely on active metabolites. Conventional dose/response curves may not disclose this, but by substituting dose with plasma concentration it is essential to correlate the active principles to the effect, if such concentrations are to be used for monitoring purposes. Recent investigations using modern analytical technology have revealed that active metabolites contribute to the antiepileptic effect for several drugs, and that these metabolites may behave differently than the parent compound, both concerning pharmacokinetics and pharmacodynamics. The therapeutic situation is no different in principle from that encountered in combination therapy.
2. Because of interindividual differences in drug metabolism, the amount of active metabolites produced may vary between patients. The quantitative and qualitative impact of active metabolites may consequently be of an individually different nature, and this will only be realized if the metabolites are measured separately and both their effect profile and concentration/response curves are determined independently.
3. Active metabolites may be accumulated in the body during renal failure, changing the normal ratio between metabolite(s) and parent compound.
4. Hepatic insufficiency may also alter the ratio between metabolite(s) and parent compound.
5. Interactions between an active metabolite and its parent compound have been described (ELSASS et al. 1980; KLOTZ and REIMANN 1981). Just as for other drug interactions, precise kinetic mapping is essential for the subsequent understanding of the clinical relevance.

In principle, therefore, therapeutic drug monitoring of antiepileptic drugs should be based on measurements of all active substances as well as on knowledge of the pharmacology of these, including concentration/effect curves.

I. Phenytoin

All phenytoin metabolites are biologically inactive or their activity is of no clinical relevance (GLAZKO and CHANG (1972). The main metabolite 5-(*p*-hydroxyphenyl)-5-phenylhydantoin (HPPH) is largely conjugated before excretion. Small amounts of other metabolites have also been identified (HORNING et al. 1971; BORGÅ et al. 1972; GLAZKO 1973, 1975; MIDHA et al. 1977; MAGUIRE et al. 1979), HPPH may accumulate in patients with renal insufficiency (BOCHNER et al. 1973), but the clinical significance thereof has not been verified, and a feedback inhibition of HPPH on the metabolism of phenytoin has been excluded (PERUCCA et al. 1978). An intermediate epoxide metabolite has been supposed to be formed, but the evidence is not convincing (MORSELLI and FRANCO-MORSELLI 1980). HPPH is 60%–65% bound to plasma albumin, and there is no indication of an interaction between phenytoin and HPPH at the level of protein binding.

At the present time there is no reason to believe that any of the phenytoin metabolites interferes kinetically or dynamically with the treatment of phenytoin, for which reason they will have no influence on monitoring plasma levels if they do not interfere with the analysis of phenytoin.

II. Carbamazepine

The main pathway for carbamazepine metabolism in man is through a stable epoxide, CBZ-10,11-epoxide, to a diol, trans-10,11-dihydro-10,11-hydroxy-CBZ (for reviews see PYNNÖNEN 1979; SILLANPÄÄ 1981). The epoxide has anticonvulsant properties in experimental animals (FAIGLE et al. 1977) probably equal to those of carbamazepine (FRIGERIO and MORSELLI 1975). The epoxide metabolite has, however, not yet been subjected separately to clinical testing and there is at present no real knowledge about its possible contribution of the antiepileptic effect during carbamazepine treatment. It has been suggested that the epoxide is reponsible for certain side effects, but no substantial evidence is available (FRIGERIO et al. 1976).

Carbamazepineepoxide levels in plasma are about 10%–20% of that of carbamazepine (STRANDJORD and JOHANNESSEN 1980), but the protein binding is lower, about 50% (SILLANPÄÄ 1981). This means that the ratio between the free (and active) fraction of the two substances is higher (closer to 1) than the total levels indicate. Several of the previously mentioned investigations of carbamazepine effects have included separate determinations of the metabolite in plasma, but so far no investigators have been able to titrate its pharmacodynamic contribution. The plasma level of the metabolite tends to increase relatively if phenytoin, phenobarbital, or primidone is added to the treatment (DAM et al. 1975; SCHNEIDER 1975b: MORSELLI et al. 1976). The fluctuations in plasma levels seem considerable. Comedication with other antiepileptic drugs seems to change the brain/plasma ratio for carbamazepine epoxide but not for carbamazepine itself

(FRIIS et al. 1978; FRIIS and CHRISTIANSEN 1978). If this is true the plasma level of carbamazepine at which a therapeutic effect is obtained may be different in patients treated with other drugs compared with patients in carbamazepine monotherapy, provided the carbamazepine epoxide is active. This has not been investigated.

As it can be understood from the above-cited studies and reviews, a relationship between the carbamazepine epoxide metabolite and an antiepileptic or toxic effects has not been established. Therapeutic monitoring of the metabolite is therefore problematical. Further evidence is needed if routine monitoring of the epoxide metabolite is to be advocated, but for kinetic investigations measuring this metabolite is important.

III. Phenobarbital

Parahydroxylation of phenobarbital, the main metabolic pathway, results in an inactive metabolite of which about half is excreted unconjugated (KÅLLBERG et al. 1975; BOREUS et al. 1978). A dihydrodiol metabolite is formed through an epoxide intermediate (HILL et al. 1977), but no indication of biological action seems to have been observed. Thus, the problems of active metabolites are not relevant for the treatment with phenobarbital.

IV. Primidone

The monitoring problems with primidone treatment are partly due to its two metabolites PEMA and phenobarbital. Of the metabolites only phenobarbital has been reasonably well investigated, although its therapeutic level in the presence of the two other active substances may be different from phenobarbital levels obtained by phenobarbital treatment alone. This question has not yet been settled. The problems have been discussed on p. 734.

V. Ethosuximide

At least 80% of ethosuximide is metabolized in man (CHANG et al. 1972b; SHERWIN 1978), but none of the metabolites have been shown to exert anticonvulsant properties (CHANG et al. 1972a). So far no studies have been published about the plasma levels of these metabolites, and it is therefore not known whether they may influence the concentration/response curve of the parent drug. The likelihood of this is, however, minimal.

VI. Benzodiazepines

Diazepam has been the subject of several studies concerning the influence of its active metabolites. These are *N*-desmethyl diazepam (NDDZ) and methyloxazepam, which may both be transformed into oxazepam or directly conjugated with glucuronic acid (GARATTINI et al. 1973; MORSELLI and FRANCO-MORSELLI 1980). Interest tends to concentrate on NDDZ, because both the dynamics and kinetics of this metabolite are similar to those of diazepam. It appears in plasma only about 15 min after diazepam administration, and after repeated doses it accumulates to a higher plasma level than the parent compound because of its longer half-life (DASBERG et al. 1974). As diazepam is almost only used in epileptics for acute intravenous or rectal treatment of status epilepticus, the metabolite problem does not seem relevant in this respect. However, it has been shown that the presence of NDDZ (from a previous treatment) may affect the cerebral effects of an acutely given dose of diazepam (ELSASS et al. 1980), but whether this also holds true for the anticonvulsant effect is not known. Monitoring NDDZ cannot be recommended on these grounds.

For clonazepam very few studies have been carried out, but its metabolites are all claimed to be inactive (MORSELLI and FRANCO-MORSELLI 1980).

VII. Valproic Acid

Several different metabolites are known in man, but their quantification and kinetic and dynamic profiles have not been evaluated to a degree that can be utilized in clinical situations. LÖSCHER (1981) studied five metabolites in plasma from a number of patients treated with valproic acid. From this study it appears that on average 90% of the antiepileptic effect of valproic acid in man can be accounted for by the parent compound itself, if the anticonvulsant activity of the metabolites in animals is taken into consideration. In Löscher's (1981) work, however, there is a considerable individual variation in the ratios between valproic acid and its metabolites. It cannot, therefore, be excluded that this could cause a different concentration/effect relationship in some patients. However, bearing in mind the monitoring problems already stated (see p. 738), it is premature to have any idea of the influence of active metabolites on plasma level monitoring of valproic acid.

J. Pharmacodynamic Aspects of Monitoring Antiepileptic Drug Levels

Much discussion on therapeutic ranges is concerned with the many factors which may influence the concentrations as such, e.g., differences in bioavailability and metabolic rates, drug interactions, age, pregnancy, compliance, etc., in fact, all the factors and situations which constitute justifications for drug-level monitoring (EADIE 1976; JOHANNESSEN 1981). However, not only the plasma levels can vary, but also the pharmacodynamics of the treatment may change or be different between patients (EADIE 1976); however, very little is known about this important problem from experimental investigations. The amount of an antiepileptic drug at the (theoretical) receptor site needed to control seizure activity may be influenced by many factors, such as the severity and type of disease, and comedication.

The strength of an epileptic focus seems to be an important determinant of the actual plasma level at which seizure control is exerted in the individual patient. Thus, it is a common observation that the severity of the epileptic disorder to a certain degree governs the level at which the antiepileptic drugs exert seizure control. The strength of the seizure focus is therefore of importance when the therapeutic level is investigated, as pointed out by many authors (e.g., KUTT 1972; EADIE 1976; SCHMIDT 1977a; SCHMIDT and MACHUS 1980). Thus, patients treated with phenytoin alone require higher therapeutic plasma levels for complex partial seizures than for grand mal (SCHMIDT 1977a). In patients where computed tomography scanning revealed organic lesions of the brain (CAZZULLO et al. 1981), significantly higher drug levels were required to achieve clinical effectiveness than in patients without detectable structural lesions. GANNAWAY and MAWER (1981) found that patients with poorly controlled epilepsy responded to levels of phenytoin well above the usual therapeutic range after they had been transferred from multiple-drug therapy.

The problem of how comedication influences the seizure control level is a different question. It has not been fully elucidated whether the therapeutic range for a given drug is the same with or without the presence of one or more other antiepileptic drugs in plasma. In other words, can the level of one drug be reduced in the presence of another drug, and if so, are we dealing with a synergistic effect. In a symposium discussion, MORSELLI (1977) stated "that the therapeutic range for multiple therapy is perhaps a little lower than for each drug alone. Potentiation does not seem to occur therefore." SCHMIDT (1977a) cites unpublished results showing that with treatment of phenytoin alone a higher phenytoin level is necessary to control grand mal seizures than with comedication of primidone. Others may have different experiences, but the question does not seem to have been subjected to experimental evaluation. Often kinetic interactions between two antiepileptic drugs will result in a change in plasma level of one or both of the involved drugs (for details see Chap. 28). However, if such changes in levels are not extreme, little is known about the significance of such shifts in levels in relation to the individual therapeutic concentration for the single drug. The study of this problem is very difficult, but the answer is of clinical importance, because multiple-drug treatment is still predominant in antiepileptic therapy (REYNOLDS and SHORVON 1981).

K. Practical Problems of Monitoring Antiepileptic Drug Levels

I. Timing of Sampling

A major prerequisite for obtaining plasma concentration results that are meaningful for drug-level monitoring is that the blood sample is taken at a time when reproducible results can be anticipated (EADIE 1976). The more fluctuation in plasma levels during a dose interval, the more problems can be expected. The pre-dose level, particularly the absolute trough level (before the morning dose), has often been suggested as superior from a kinetic point of view. This level can be reproduced with the greatest certainty (JOHANNESSEN 1981), but for practical reasons it may not always be possible to postpone the morning dose too long, especially in outpatients. The long half-life and often extended absorption time for phenytoin, phenobarbital, and ethosuximide tend to reduce fluctuation, rendering the sampling time less critical for these drugs, but for the majority of other antiepileptic drugs the pre-dose level should be preferred. Few investigations have, however, been published with the specific aim of evaluating the timing problems.

Whatever practical arrangement is preferred for blood sampling, it is necessary to standardize the procedure for the individual patient in terms of sampling time so that evaluations are performed under comparable conditions in each patient. Sampling for drug monitoring should therefore be a well-structured part of the therapeutic strategy for the individual patient.

Another timing problem relates to the steady-state conditions. It is essential to make sure when such conditions in fact have been reached, but for long-term treatment this is of course not a real problem. In theory about 90% of the steady-state level is reached after four to five half-lives, and the average half-life of the drugs in question should, therefore, be known. However, this kinetic parameter is subject to considerable individual variation and furthermore (auto)-induction may occur during the first weeks of treatment, particularly for carbamazepine (Sillanpää 1981). The time at which a true steady state will be reached (if no loading dose is given) can vary considerably and is sometimes very long. Control of the plasma level is therefore necessary at least two to three times after an appropriate length of time after initiation of the treatment.

II. Handling of Blood Samples and Results

The analytical methods used for the determination of antiepileptic drugs are discussed in the respective drug chapters. However, a few practical items will be emphasized here. For all practical purposes and for the majority of analytical procedures there is no reason to make a distinction between serum and plasma samples. Nevertheless, it is advisable in each case to make sure which kind of sample the laboratory prefers for the individual analytical assay.

It is important to separate serum/plasma from the blood cells as fast as possible, but thereafter the sample can be stored at 4 °C for several days, except for clonazepam, which will be destructed fairly rapidly (Knop et al. 1975). If a sample must be kept for a longer period (e.g., >2 weeks), it should be stored frozen (−20 °C). For routine monitoring it is, however, of great importance to obtain the result as quickly as possible, and the long-term storing problems have therefore more relevance for research purposes. It does not seem to have been evaluated to what degree freezing and thawing may influence the protein binding of antiepileptics. Analytical assays of antiepileptic drugs must be carried out in skilled laboratories, whether these are labeled clinical chemistry, clinical pharmacology, or what else. Trained chemists and inter- and intralaboratory quality control of drug assays (Gerson 1980; Ayers et al. 1981) are essential. With respect to interpretation of the plasma concentration results, no universal and standardized solution can be given. However, it has been repeatedly emphasized (e.g., Milano Collaborative Group for Studies on Epilepsy 1977) that a dialogue must be established between the treating epileptologist and the clinical pharmacologist. Plasma-level monitoring cannot be used out of context with clinical pharmacokinetics, and only a combination can improve the results of any monitoring system. It is therefore of great importance that each blood sample is accompanied by a series of items of relevant information (name, age, sex, weight, diagnosis, all drugs and doses, time of sampling, time for last dose, length of treatment, etc.).

L. Utilization of the Monitoring of Antiepileptic Drug Levels

Criticism has been voiced, not only against the use of "therapeutic ranges" (see previously), but in general also against the use of monitoring plasma levels at all. These critics find that a well-executed antiepileptic therapy should rest solely on sound clinical judgments, although such viewpoints are rarely documented and published. In practical clinical circumstances, it has, however, repeatedly been shown that seizures are poorly controlled in a substantial number of outpatients and that a large number of these show low ("subtherapeutic") concentrations (GUELEN and VAN DER KLEIJN 1978). Likewise, clinical experience finds that toxic symptoms are better interpreted if it is revealed that the plasma level is above the usually accepted therapeutic range. Nevertheless, it is a fact that the documentation presented in support of the benefit obtained by monitoring antiepileptic drug levels is almost entirely anecdotal and retrospective. Only few attempts have been made to examine in depth the cost/benefit problem in a controlled way, i.e., by prospective randomized, blind studies on patients in monotherapy. It has virtually not been evaluated whether routine drug concentrations are worthwhile determining, and whether this time and money-consuming activity augments the quality of life for the epileptic patients in the long run, considering all aspects. However, in addition to the many individual reports and personal statements in favor of monitoring, there is also a logical reasoning based on pharmacological and clinical grounds which cannot be neglected. Essentially this reasoning is expressed in the reasons for monitoring given in Sect. B.

Much emphasis has been put on kinetic investigations and very little on prospective evaluations of the clinical significance of the practical use of plasma-level monitoring (cf. LATINI et al. 1980), but a few studies have been undertaken to determine whether plasma concentration monitoring has had a beneficial effect on the therapeutic outcome. THE MILANO COLLABORATIVE GROUP FOR STUDIES ON EPILEPSY (1977) made an integrated monitored approach in so-called difficult patients for 16 months and concluded that "... the knowledge of antiepileptic drug plasma levels does seem to have a noticeable impact on both therapeutic decision and the therapeutic efficacy ... provided that an adequate dialogue is established between the attending neurologist and the clinical pharmacologist." Although this statement is encouraging, only scanty clinical data on the seizure pattern were given. CHADWICK et al. (1977) found that serum-level monitoring was of particular value in 31 newly diagnosed, prospectively followed patients, of which only 3 needed addition of a second drug in the course of approximately 15 months of treatment. Such studies, although interesting, suffer from lack of controls and appropriate design, and cannot, therefore, substitute for real documentation in this respect.

A similar aspect of the drug-level monitoring question was studied by SHORVON et al. (1978) and further commented upon by REYNOLDS (1980). In a long-term prospective study of phenytoin and carbamazepine in previously untreated new referrals with grand mal and/or partial epilepsy, it became clear that seizures were well controlled in about one-third of the patients at a plasma drug level below the usually accepted therapeutic range. However, the clinical value of the therapeutic plasma concentration range was illustrated by the fact that continuing seizures at low levels in up to one-fourth of the patients could subsequently be controlled, if their plasma levels were adjusted to the therapeutic range. Similar observations have been made by many others (cf. GUELEN and VAN DER KLEIJN 1978; KOCH-WESER 1981) and also in prospective trials other than those discussed above (BROEKER et al. 1981). The advantage of prospective studies of this kind is that they substantiate the value of an "optimal" plasma range for the treatment schedules. It appears that the same clinical benefit may not have been obtained without the use of plasma-level monitoring, although the scientific proof is weak as such. However, particularly in the light of the possibility of avoiding a subsequent multiple-drug therapy that otherwise most probably would have been the result, the outcome of these studies is of great interest, but the application of carefully practiced clinical skill might have resulted in the same benefit.

A more controlled way of clarifying the problems about the possible advantage of drug-level monitoring is to follow two groups, which only differ with respect to the use of plasma concentrations in monitoring the patients. Using this approach TATZER and GROH (1980) compared 41 pediatric patients undergoing carbamazepine treatment whose blood levels were regularly measured with 77 patients who were not monitored in this way. In 71% of the first group good seizure control was obtained, in contrast to 61% in the second group, and other advantages were also noted. The differences are not striking, although significant, and the design not satisfactory (no random allocation), but the data support the benefit of drug-level monitoring. However, FRÖSCHER et al. (1981) designed their study as a randomized trial, lasting for 1 year. In total, data from 105 epileptic patients were available for assessment (out of 127 at the start of the trial). The patients were randomly allocated into two groups, one in which an attempt was made to keep plasma levels within the therapeutic range of the actual drug, and the other in which the physician giving the treatment was not informed of the results of the plasma level, so that he was unable to adjust the therapy on this basis. The therapeutic results were not statistically different in the two groups, but the results revealed that a reduction in seizure frequency was associated with an increase in the plasma level for both groups. The authors conclude that under the conditions of the study, information on plasma levels did not further improve the antiepileptic therapy. This study is open to criticism, as, e.g., the quality of the treatment may have been increased in both groups because of the trial conditions. However, it does dispute the general benefit of drug-level monitoring, not necessarily in the single cases, but in groups comparisons. The cited studies reveal the fact that correlation between concentration and effect/side effects does not necessarily or automatically mean benefit from drug-level monitoring.

Another approach was made by BERGMANN et al. (1981), in a prospective utilization study. It was observed that 63% of the first-time analyses of phenytoin were below the usual therapeutic range on a prescribed mean daily dose of 300 mg. High plasma concentrations of phenytoin were seen more frequently in older patients. For the patients in whom consecutive analyses were made, the subsequent concentrations showed a tendency toward the therapeutic range. The authors themselves point to the shortcomings of this study, these being the lack of attempts to relate the phenytoin concentrations to effect, the lack of control material, and the lack of compliance control. Nevertheless, this type of study can (besides describing the actual clinical situation) serve as an indication in favor of utilizing the analytical drug service and of cooperating with the clinical pharmacologists.

No study yet seems to have included an evaluation of the financial costs spent in connection with a drug-level monitoring system. Both cost/benefit analyses and "production control" investigations should have a high priority, also in the light of the growing interest for evaluating medical technology. Investigations of this kind within the area of antiepileptic drug treatment are highly desirable, as technological developments are moving fast. Abuse of drug-level monitoring with replacement of clinical judgment by laboratory data (instead of supporting the former) is a real risk, which can only be combated by scientific investigations of the utilization of drug-level monitoring.

References

Agurell S, Berlin A, Ferngren H, Hellström B (1975) Plasma levels of diazepam after parenteral and rectal administration in children. Epilepsia 16:277–283

Anavekar SN, Saunders RH, Wardell WM, Shalson I, Emmings FG, Cook CE, Gringeri AJ (1978) Parotid and whole saliva in the prediction of serum total and free phenytoin concentrations. Clin Pharmacol Ther 24:629–637

Atkinson AJ Jr, Strong JM (1977) Effect of active drug metabolites on plasma level-response correlations. J Pharmacokinet Biopharm 5:95–109

Atkinson AJ Jr, Stec GP, Lertora JJL, Ruo TI, Thenot JP (1980) Impact of active metabolites on monitoring plasma concentrations of therapeutic drugs. Ther Drug Monit 2:19–27

Ayers G, Burnett D, Griffiths A, Richens A (1981) Quality control of drug assay. Clin Pharmacokinet 6:106–117

Barnes SE, Bower BD (1975) Sodium valproate in the treatment of intractable childhood epilepsy. Dev Med Child Neurol 17:175–181

Bartels H (1980) Rational usage of therapeutic drug monitoring in antiepileptic treatment. Eur J Pediatr 133:193–199

Barth N, Alvan G, Borgå O, Sjöqvist F (1976) Two-fold interindividual variation in plasma protein binding of diphenylhydantoin and warfarin in patients with epilepsy. Clin Pharmacokinet 1:444–452

Battino D, Bossi L, Croci D, Franceschetti S, Gomeni C, Moise A, Vitali A (1980) Carbamazepine plasma levels in children and adults: influence of age, dose, and associated therapy. Ther Drug Monit 2:331–344

Beier R, Zschiesche M, Cammann R (1978) Phenytoinintoxikation und Serumspiegel. Psychiatr Neurol Med Psychol 30:414–423

Bergman U, Rane A, Sjöqvist F, Wiholm B-E (1981) Digoxin and phenytoin analyses as part of consultations in clinical pharmacology: a study on the use of drugs. Ther Drug Monit 3:259–269

Bertilsson L (1978) Clinical pharmacokinetics of carbamazepine. Clin Pharmacokinet 3:128–143

Blom GF, Guelen PJM (1977) The distribution of anti-epileptic drugs between serum, saliva and cerebrospinal fluid. In: Gardner-Thorpe C, Janz D, Meinardi H, Pippenger CE (eds) Antiepileptic drug monitoring. Pitman Medical, Tunbridge Wells, pp 287–297

Bochner F, Hooper WD, Tyrer JH, Eadie MJ (1973) The renal handling of diphenylhydantoin and 5-(*p*-hydroxyphenyl)-5-phenylhydantoin. Clin Pharmacol Ther 14:791–796

Bochner F, Hooper WD, Sutherland JM, Eadie MJ, Tyrer JH (1974) Diphenylhydantoin concentrations in saliva. Arch Neurol 31:57–59

Booker HE (1972a) Phenobarbital, mephobarbital, and metharbital. Relation and plasma levels to clinical control. In: Woodbury DM, Penry JK, Schmidt RP (eds) Antiepileptic drugs. Raven, New York, pp 329–334

Booker HE (1972b) Primidone. Toxicity. In: Woodbury DM, Penry JK, Schmidt RP (eds) Antiepileptic drugs. Raven, New York, pp 377–383

Booker HE, (1980) Intensive monitoring of antiepileptic drug serum levels. In: Wada JA, Penry JK (eds) Advances in epileptology: the Xth epilepsy international symposium. Raven, New York, pp 53–58

Booker HE, Celesia GG (1973) Serum concentrations of diazepam in subjects with epilepsy. Arch Neurol 29:191–194

Booker HE, Darcey B (1973) Serum concentrations of free diphenylhydantoin and their relationship to clinical intoxication. Epilepsia 14:177–184

Boreus LO, Jalling B, Kållberg N (1978) Phenobarbital metabolism in adults and in newborn infants. Acta Paediatr Scand 67:193–200

Borgå O, Garle M, Gutova M (1972) Identification of 5-(3.4-dihydroxyphenyl)-5-phenylhydantoin as a metabolite of 5.5-diphenylhydantoin (phenytoin) in rats and man. Pharmacology 7:129–137

Borondy P, Dill WA, Chang T, Buchanan RA, Glazko AJ (1973) Effect of protein binding on the distribution of 5,5-diphenylhydantoin between plasma and red cells. In: Anton, Solomon (eds) Drug-protein binding. New York Academy of Sciences, pp 82–87

Bossi L, Morselli PL (1977) Hypnotics. In: Morselli PL (ed) Drug disposition during development. Spectrum, New York, p 361

Brewster D, Muir NC (1980) Valproate plasma protein binding in the uremic condition. Clin Pharmacol Ther 27:76–82

Broeker H, Müller D, Müller J, Walther H (1980) Zum Antikonvulsivablutspiegelverhalten therapieresistenter Epilepsiepatienten. Psychiatr Neurol Med Psychol (Leipz) 32:541–549

Browne TR (1978) Drug therapy reviews: clinical pharmacology of antiepileptic drugs. Am J Hosp Pharm 35:1048–1056

Browne TR, Dreifuss FE, Dryken PR, Goode DJ, Penry JK, Porter RJ, White BG, White PT (1975) Ethosuximide in the treatment of absence (petit mal) seizures. Neurology 25:515–524

Brugmann G, Kleinau E, Nolte R, Petruch F (1979) Comparison of phenytoin determinations in plasma, plasma dialysate and saliva for control of antiepileptic therapy in children. Klin Wochenschr 57:93–94

Bruni J, Wilder BJ, Willmore LJ, Pershalski RJ, Villareal HJ (1978) Steady state kinetics of valproic acid in epileptic patients. Clin Pharmacol Ther 24:324–332

Bruni J, Wang LH, Marbury TC, Lee CS, Wilder BJ (1980) Protein binding of valproic in uremic patients. Neurology 30:557–559

Buchanan N, Van der Walt LA (1977) The binding of phenobarbitone and phenytoin to kwashiorkor serum. S Afr Med J 52:518–521

Buchthal F, Lennox-Buchthal MA (1972) Phenobarbital. Relation of serum concentration to control of seizures. In: Woodbury DM, Penry JK, Schmidt RP (eds) Antiepileptic drugs. Raven, New York, pp 335–343

Buchthal F, Svensmark O (1960) Aspects of the pharmacology of phenytoin (Dilantin®) and phenobarbital relevant to their dosage in the treatment of epilepsy. Epilepsia 1:373–384

Buchthal F, Svensmark O (1971) Serum concentration of diphenylhydantoin (phenytoin) and phenobarbital and their relation to therapeutic and toxic effects. Psychiatr Neurol Neurochir 74:7–36

Buchthal F, Svensmark O, Schiller PJ (1960) Clinical and electroencephalographic correlations with serum levels of diphenylhydantoin. Arch Neurol 2:624–630

Buchthal F, Svensmark O, Simonsen H (1968) Relation of EEG and seizures to phenobarbital in serum. Arch Neurol 19:567–572

Butler TC, Waddell WJ (1956) Metabolic conversion of primidone (Mysoline) to phenobarbital. Proc Soc Exp Biol Med 93:544–546

Cazzullo CL, Altamura AC, Cornaggia CM, Canger R, Pruneri C (1981) Therapeutic plasma levels of some anticonvulsants in focal epilepsy in relation to computerized axial tomography. Encephale 7:191–197

Cenraud B, Guyot M, Levy RH, Brachet-Liermain A, Morselli PL, Loiseau P (1981) Effect of dosage regimen on valproic acid plasma levels. In: Dam M, Gram L, Penry JK (eds) Advances in epileptology. The XIIth epilepsy international symposium. Raven, New York, pp 549–553

Cereghino JJ, Van Meter JC, Brock JT, Penry JK, Smith LD, White BG (1973) Preliminary observations of serum carbamazepine in epileptic patients. Neurology 23:357–366

Cereghino JL, Brock JT, Van Meter JC, Penry JK, Smith LD, White BG (1974) Carbamazepine for epilepsy – a controlled prospective evaluation. Neurology 24:401–410

Cereghino JJ, Brock JT, Van Meter JC, Penry JK, Smith LD, White BG (1975) The efficacy of carbamazepine combinations in epilepsy. Clin Pharmacol Ther 18:733–741

Chadwick D, Vydelingum L, Galbraith A, Reynolds EH (1977) The value of serum phenytoin levels in new referrals with epilepsy. One drug in the treatment of epilepsy. In: Gardner-Thorpe C, Janz D, Meinardi H, Pippenger CE (eds) Antiepileptic drug monitoring. Pitman Medical, Tunbridge Wells, pp 187–196

Chambers RE, Homeida M, Hunter KR, Teague RH (1977) Salivary carbamazepine concentrations. Lancet 1:656–657

Chang T, Burkett AR, Glazko AJ (1972a) Ethosuximide. Biotransformation. In: Woodbury DM, Penry JK, Schmidt RP (eds) Antiepileptic drugs. Raven, New York pp 425–429

Chang T, Wesley AD, Glazko AJ (1972a) Ethosuximide. Absorption, distribution, and excretion. In: Woodbury DM, Penry JK, Schmidt RP (eds) Antiepileptic drugs. Raven, New York, pp 417–423

Chard CR (1976) A simple method for the determination of Epilim in serum. In: Legg (ed) Clinical and pharmacological aspects of sodium valproate (Epilim) in the treatment of epilepsy. MCS Consultants, Tunbridge Wells, pp 89–91

Christiansen J, Dam M (1977) Plasma and salivary levels of carbamazepine and carbamazepine-10,11,epoxide during pregnancy. In: Gardner-Thorpe C, Janz D, Meinardi H, Pippenger CE (eds) Antiepileptic drug monitoring. Pitman Medical, Tunbridge Wells, pp 128–135

Cook CE, Arnerson E, Poole WK, Lesser P, O'Tuama L (1975) Phenytoin and phenobarbital concentrations in saliva and plasma measured by radioimmunoassay. Clin Pharmacol Ther 18:742–747

Covanis A, Jeavons PM, Gupta AK (1981) Monotherapy with once daily sodium valproate (epilim). In: Dam M, Gram L, Penry JK (eds) Advances in epileptology. The XIIth epilepsy international symposium. Raven, New York, pp 527–532

Dam M, Jensen A, Christiansen J (1975) Plasma level and effect of carbamazepine in grand mal and psychomotor epilepsy. Acta Neurol Scand [Suppl] 60:33–38

Dasberg HH, Van der Kleijn E, Guelen PJR, Van Praag HM (1974) Plasma concentrations of diazepam and of its metabolite *N*-desmethyl-diazepam in relation to anxiolytic effect. Clin Pharmacol Ther 15:473–483

Di Gregorio GJ, Piraino AJ, Ruch E (1978) Diazepam concentrations in parotid saliva, mixed saliva and plasma. Clin Pharmacol Ther 24:720–725

Drayer DE (1976) Pharmacologically active drug metabolites: therapeutic and toxic activities, plasma urine data in man, accumulation in renal failure. Clin Pharmacokinet 1:426–443

Dreifuss FE, Penry JK, Rose SW, Kupferberg HJ, Dyken P, Sato S (1975) Serum clonazepam concentrations in children with absence seizures. Neurology 25:255–258

Eadie MJ (1976) Plasma level monitoring of anticonvulsants. Clin Pharmacokinet 1:52–66

Egli M (1977) Pharmacokinetik der Antiepileptika: ihre Bedeutung für die praktische Epilepsietherapie. Schweiz Med Wochenschr 107:1513–1518

Ehrnebo M, Odar-Cederlöf I (1975) Binding of amobarbital, pentobarbital and diphenylhydantoin to blood cells and plasma proteins in healthy volunteers and uraemic patients. Eur J Clin Pharmacol 8:445–453

Ehrnebo M, Odar-Cederlöf I (1977) Distribution of pentobarbital and diphenylhydantoin between plasma and cells in blood: effect of salicylic acid, temperature and total drug concentration. Eur J Clin Pharmacol 11:37–43

Eichelbaum M, Bertilsson L, Lund L, Palmër L, Sjöqvist F (1976) Plasma levels of carbamazepine and carbamazepine-10,11-epoxide, during treatment of epilepsy. Eur J Clin Pharmacol 9:417–421

Elsass P, Hendel J, Hvidberg EF, Hansen T, Gymoese E, Rathje J (1980) Kinetics and neuropsychologic effects of IV diazepam in the presence and absence of its active *N*-desmethyl metabolite in humans. Psychopharmacology 70:307–312

Faigle JW, Feldmann KF, Baltzer V (1977) Anticonvulsant effect of carbamazepine. An attempt to distinguish between potency of the parent drug and its epoxide metabolite. In Gardner-Thorpe C, Janz D, Meinardi H, Pippenger CE (eds) Antiepileptic drug monitoring. Pitman Medical, Tunbridge Wells, pp 104–108

Feeley M, Duggan B, O'Callagan M, Callaghan N (1979) The therapeutic range for phenytoin – a reappraisal. Ir J Med Sci 148:44–49

Feldman RG, Pippenger CE (1976) The relation of anticonvulsant drug levels to complete seizure control. J Clin Pharmacol 16:51–59

Ferngren HG (1974) Diazepam treatment for acute convulsions in children. Epilepsia 15:27–37

Forsythe WI, Prendergast MP, Toothill C, Broughton PM (1979) Carbamazepine serum levels in children with epilepsy: a micro immuno-assay technique. Dev Med Child Neurol 21:441–447

Frey H-H, Löscher W (1980) Kann Primidone mehr als Phenobarbital? Versuch einer pharmakologischen Analyse. Nervenarzt 51:359–362

Frey H, Yrjänä T (1970) Carbamazepine titer of epileptic patients. Scand J Clin Lab Invest [Suppl] 25, 113:90

Frigerio A, Morselli PL (1975) Carbamazepine: biotransformation. In: Penry JK, Daly DD (eds) Advances in neurology, vol 11. Raven, New York, pp 295–308

Frigerio A, Cavo-Briones M, Belvedere G (1976) Formation of stable epoxides in the metabolism of tricyclic drugs. Drug Metabol Rev 5:197–218

Friis ML, Christiansen J (1978) Carbamazepine, carbamazepine-10,11-epoxide and phenytoin concentrations in brain tissue of epileptic children. Acta Neurol Scand 58:104–108

Friis ML, Christiansen J, Hvidberg EF (1978) Brain concentrations of carbamazepine and carbamazepine-10,11-epoxide in epileptic patients. Eur J Clin Pharmacol 14:47–51

Fröscher W, Schultz H-U, Gugler R (1978) Valproinsäure in der Behandlung der Epilepsien unter besonderer Berücksichtigung des Serumspiegels. Fortschr Neurol Psychiat 46:327–341

Fröscher W, Eichelbaum M, Gugler R, Hildenbrand G, Penin H (1981) A prospective randomized trial on the effect of monitoring plasma anticonvulsant levels in epilepsy. J Neurol 224:193–201

Galdames DG, Saavedra IN, Ortiz MA, Aguilera LI, Valenzuela AL, Concha GL, Droguest PA, Morales ER (1980) Plasma levels of diphenylhydantoin and the control of adult epileptic seizures: a Chilean experience. Epilepsia 21:467–474

Gannaway DJ, Mawer GE (1981) Serum phenytoin concentration and clinical response in patients with epilepsy. Br J Clin Pharmacol 12:833–839

Garattini S, Marcucco F, Morselli PL, Mussini E (1973) The significance of measuring blood levels of benzodiazepines. In: Davies DS, Pritchard BNC (eds) Biological effects of drugs in relation to their plasma concentration. MacMillan, London, pp 211–225

Gerson B (1980) Quality control in therapeutic drug monitoring: intra-laboratory precision and medical requirements. Ther Drug Monit 2:225–232

Glazko AJ (1973) Diphenylhydantoin metabolism – a prospective review. Drug Metabol Dispos 1:711–714

Glazko AJ (1975) Antiepileptic drugs: biotransformation, metabolism and serum half-life. Epilepsia 16:367

Glazko AJ, Chang T (1972) Diphenylhydantoin. Absorption, distribution and excretion. In: Woodbury, Penry, Schmidt (eds) Antiepileptic drugs. Raven, New York, pp 127–136
Gram L, Flachs H, Würtz-Jørgensen A, Parnas J, Andersen B (1979) Sodium valproate, serum level and clinical effect in epilepsy: a controlled study. Epilepsia 20:303–312
Guelen, PJM, Van Der Kleijn E (1978) Rational anti-epileptic drug therapy. Elsevier/North-Holland, Amsterdam
Gugler R, Von Unruh GE (1980) Clinical pharmacokinetics of valproic acid. Clin Pharmacokinet 5:67–83
Gugler R, Shoeman DW, Huffmann DH, Cohlmia JB, Azarnoff DL (1975) Pharmacokinetics of drugs in patients with the nephrotic syndrome. J Clin Invest 55:1182–1189
Gugler R, Schell A, Eichelbaum M, Fröscher W, Schultz H-U (1977) Disposition of valproic acid in man. Eur J Clin Pharmacol 12:125–132
Haerer AF, Buchanan RA, Wiygul FM (1970) Ethosuximide blood levels in epileptics. J Clin Pharmacol 10:370–374
Haidukewych EA, Rodin E (1981) Free (unbound) valproic acid in epilepsy patients medicated with coanticonvulsants: in vivo variable concentration and explanation for "nontherapeutic" plasma levels. In: Dam M, Gram L, Penry JK (eds) Advances in epileptology. The XIIth epilepsy international symposium. Raven, New York, pp 555–562
Harder F, Elsass P, Hendel J, Hvidberg EF, Hjørting-Hansen E (1976) Clinical and psychological effects of intra-venous diazepam related to plasma levels. Int J Oral Surg 5:226–239
Hassan MN, Laljee HVK, Parsonage MJ (1976) Sodium valproate in the treatment of resistant epilepsy. Acta Neurol Scand 54:209–218
Henriksen O, Johannessen SI (1980) Clinical observations of sodium valproate in children: an evaluation of therapeutic serum levels. In: Johannessen SI, Morselli PL, Pippenger CE, Richens A, Schmidt D, Meinardi H (eds) Antiepileptic therapy: advances in drug monitoring. New York, Raven, pp 253–261
Hill RM, Verniaud WM, Morgan NF, Nowlin J, Glazener L, Horning MG (1977) Urinary excretion of phenobarbital in a neonate having withdrawal symptoms. Am J Dis Child 131:546–550
Hillestad L, Hansen T, Melsom H, Drivenes A (1974) Diazepam metabolism in normal man. I. Serum concentrations and clinical effects after intravenous, intramuscular, and oral administration. Clin Pharmacol Ther 16:479–484
Hooper WD, Dubetz DK, Bochner F, Cotter LM, Smith GA, Eadie MJ, Tyrer JH (1975) Plasma protein binding of carbamazepine. Clin Pharmacol Ther 17:433–440
Höppener RJ, Kuyer A, Meijer JWA, Hulsman J (1980) Correlation between daily fluctuations of carbamazepine serum levels and intermittent side effects. Epilepsia 21:341–350
Horning MG, Stratton C, Wilson A, Horning EC, Hill RM (1971) Detection of 5(3,4-dihydroxy-1,5-cyclohexadien-1-yl)-5 phenylhydantoin as a major metabolite of 5,5, diphenylhydantoin (Dilantin) in the newborn human. Anal Lett 4:537–545
Horning MG, Brown L, Nowlin J, Lertratanangkoon K, Kellaway P, Zion TE (1977) Use of saliva in therapeutic drug monitoring. Clin Chem 23:157–164
Hvidberg EF (1980) Monitoring drug plasma levels in clinical practice. A procedure for evaluation is needed. Eur J Clin Pharmacol 17:317–319
Hvidberg EF, Dam M (1976) Clinical pharmacokinetics of anticonvulsants. Clin Pharmacokinet 1:161–188
Jalling B (1975) Plasma concentrations of phenobarbital in the treatment of seizures in newborns. Acta Paediatr Scand 64:514–525
Johannessen SI (1981) Antiepileptic drugs: pharmacokinetic and clinical aspects. Ther Drug Monit 3:17–37
Kållberg N, Agurell S, Ericsson O, Bucht E, Jalling B, Borëus LO (1975) Quantitation of phenobarbital and its main metabolites in human urine. Eur J Clin Pharmacol 9:161–168
Kangas L, Allonen H, Lammintausta R, Salonen M, Pekkarinen A (1979) Pharmacokinetics of nitrazepam in saliva and serum after a single oral dose. Acta Pharmacol Toxicol (Copenh) 45:20–24

Klotz U, Reiman I (1981) Clearance of diazepam can be impaired by its major metabolite desmethyldiazepam. Eur J Clin Pharmacol 21:161–163
Klotz U, Schneider C (1980) Valproic acid in childhood epilepsy: anticonvulsive efficacy in relation to its plasma levels. Int J Clin Pharmacol Ther Toxicol 18:461–465
Klotz U, Rapp T, Müller WA (1978) Disposition of valproic acid in patients with liver disease. Eur J Clin Pharmacol 13:55–60
Knop HJ, Van Der Kleijn E, Edmunds LC (1975) The determination of clonazepam in plasma by gas-liquid chromatography. Pharm Weekblad [Sci] 110:297–309
Knott C, Hamshaw-Thomas A, Reynolds F (1982) Phenytoin-valproate interaction of saliva monitoring in epilepsy. Br Med J 284:13–16
Knudsen FU (1977) Plasma diazepam in infants after rectal administration in solution and by suppositories. Acta Paediatr Scand 66:563–567
Koch-Weser J (1981) Serum drug concentrations in clinical perspectives. Ther Drug Monit 3:3–16
Kristensen O, Larsen HF (1980) Value of saliva samples in monitoring carbamazepine concentrations in epileptic patients. Acta Neurol Scand 61:344–350
Kupferberg HJ, Longacre-Shaw J (1979) Mephobarbital and phenobarbital plasma concentrations in epileptic patients treated with mephobarbital. Ther Drug Monit 1:117–122
Kurata D, Wilkinson GR (1974) Erythrocte uptake and plasma binding of diphenylhydantoin. Clin Pharmacol Ther 16:355–362
Kutt H (1972) Diphenylhydantoin: interactions with other drugs in man. In: Woodbury DM, Penry JK, Schmidt RP (eds) Antiepileptic drugs. Raven, New York, pp 169–180
Kutt H (1974) Pharmacodynamic and pharmacokinetic measurements of antiepileptic drugs. Clin Pharmacol Ther 16:243–250
Kutt H (1978a) Clinical pharmacology of carbamazepine. In: Pippenger CE, Penry JK, Kutt H (eds) Antiepileptic drugs: quantitative analysis and interpretation. Raven, New York, pp 297–305
Kutt H (1978b) Evaluation of Unusual antiepileptic drug concentrations. In: Pippenger CE, Penry JK, Kutt H (eds) Antiepileptic drugs: quantitative analysis and interpretation. Raven, New York, pp 307–314
Kutt H, Penry JK (1974) Usefulness of blood levels of antiepileptic drugs. Arch Neurol 31:283–288
Kutt H, Winters W, Sherman R (1964) Diphenylhydantoin and phenobarbital toxicity. The role of liver disease. Arch Neurol 11:649–656
Kutt H, Solomon G, Wasterlain C, Peterson H, Louis S, Carruthers R (1975) Carbamazepine in difficult to control epileptic out-patients. Acta Neurol Scand Suppl 60:27–32
Lane EA, Levy RH (1980) Prediction of steady-state behavior of metabolite from dosing of parent drug. J Pharm Sci 69:610–612
Latini R, Bonati M, Tognoni G (1980) Clinical role of blood levels. Ther Drug Monit 2:3–9
Levy RH (1980) Monitoring of free valproic acid levels? Ther Drug Monit 2:199–201
Levy RH, Pitlick WH, Troupin AS, Green JR, Neal JM (1975) Pharmacokinetics of carbamazepine in normal man. Clin Pharmacol Ther 17:657–668
Loiseau P, Brachet-Liermain A, Henry P (1975) Concentrations of dipropylacetate in plasma. Epilepsia 16:609–615
Loiseau P, Brachet-Liermain A, Legroux M, Jogeix M (1977) Value of anticonvulsant level determination in the treatment of epilepsies. Nouv Presse Med 6:813–817
Lossius R, Dietrichson P, Lunde PKM (1980) Effect of diazepam and desmethyldiazepam in spasticity and rigidity. Acta Neurol Scand 61:378–383
Löscher W (1981) Concentration of metabolites of valproic acid in plasma of epileptic patients. Epilepsia 22:169–178
Lund L (1974) Anticonvulsant effect of diphenylhydantoin relative to plasma levels. Arch Neurol 31:289–294
Lund M, Sjö O, Hvidberg E (1975) Plasma concentrations of ethotoin in epileptic patients. In: Schneider H, Janz D, Gardner-Thorpe C, Meinardi H, Sherwin AL (eds) Clinical pharmacology of anti-epileptic drugs. Springer, Berlin Heidelberg New York, pp 111–114

MacKichan JJ, Duffner PK, Cohen ME (1981) Salivary concentrations and plasma protein binding of carbamazepine and carbamazepine 10,11-epoxide in epileptic patients. Br J Clin Pharmacol 12:31–37

Maguire J, Kraus BL, Butler TC, Dudley KH (1979) Determination of 5-(3,4-dihydroxy-1,5-cyclohexadien-1-yl)-5-phenylhydantoin (dihydrodiol) and quantitative studies of phenytoin metabolism in man. Ther Drug Monit 1:359–370

Mandelli M, Tognoni G, Garattini S (1978) Clinical pharmacokinetics of diazepam. Clin Pharmacokinet 3:72–91

McAuliffe JJ, Sherwin Al, Leppik LE, Pippenger CE (1977) Salivary levels of anticonvulsants: a practical approach to drug monitoring. Neurology 27:409–413

Meijer JWA, Hessing-Brand L (1973) Determination of lower fatty acid, particularly the antiepileptic dipropylacetic acid, in biological material by means of microdiffusion and gas chromatography. Clin Chim Acta 43:215–222

Meinardi H (1972) Other antiepileptic drugs. Carbamazepine. In: Woodbury DM, Penry JK, Schmidt RP (eds) Antiepileptic drugs. Raven, New York, pp 487–496

Meinardi H, Hanke NFJ, Van Beveren J (1974) Sodium di-*n*-propylacetate: estimation of effective serum levels. Pharm Weekblad 109:47–47

Midha KK, Hindmarsh KW, McGilveray IJ, Cooper JK (1977) Identification of urinary catechol and methylated catechol metabolites of phenytoin in humans, monkeys and dogs by GLC and GLC-mass-spectrometry. J Pharm Sci 66:1596–1602

Milano Collaborative Group for studies on Epilepsy (1977) Long-term intensive monitoring in the difficult patient. Preliminary results of 16 months of observations – usefulness and limitations. In: Gardner-Thorpe C, Janz D, Meinardi H, Pippenger CE (eds) Antiepileptic drug monitoring. Pitman Medical, Tunbridge Well, pp 197–213

Millichap JG (1972) Other hydantoins. Mephenytoin, ethotoin, and albutoin. In: Woodbury DM, Penry JK, Schmidt RP (eds) Antiepileptic drugs. Raven, New York, pp 275–281

Milligan N, Richens A (1981) Methods of assessment of antiepileptic drugs. Br J Clin Pharmacol 11:443–456

Møller J (1971) Determination of serum concentration of carbamazepine in child neurology. In: Lund L (ed) Measurements of plasma concentrations of antiepileptic drugs. Methodological and clinical aspects (in Swedish). Konferens Lidingö 1971, pp 72–79

Monaco F, Riccio A, Benna P, Covacich A, Durelli L, Fantini M, Furlan PM, Gilli M, Mutani R, Troni W, Gerna M, Morselli PL (1976) Further observation on carbamazepine plasma levels in epileptic patients – relationship with therapeutic and side effects. Neurology 26:936–943

Monaco F, Mutani R, Mastropaolo C, Tondi M (1979) Tears as the best practical indicator of the unbound fraction of an anticonvulsant drug. Epilepsia 20:705–710

Monaco F, Piredda S, Mastropaolo C, Tondi F, Mutani R (1981) Diphenylhydantoin and primidone in tears. Epilepsia 22:185–188

Monks A (1978) Binding of phenytoin and valproic acid by human serum proteins. PhD Thesis, University of London

Morselli PL (1977) Antiepileptic drugs. In: Morselli PL (ed) Drug disposition during development. Spectrum Publishers, New York, pp 311–360

Morselli PL (1978) Clinical significance of monitoring plasma levels of benzodiazepine tranquillizers and antiepileptic drugs: In: Deniker P, Radouco-Thomas C, Villeneuve A (eds) Neuropsychopharmacology. Pergamon, Oxford, pp 877–888

Morselli PL, Franco-Morselli R (1980) Clinical pharmacokinetics of antiepileptic drugs in adults. Pharmacol Ther 10:65–102

Morselli PL, Bossi L, Gerna M (1976) Pharmacokinetic studies with carbamazepine in epileptic patients. In: Birkmayer (ed) Epileptic seizures – behavior – pain. Huber, Bern, pp 141–150

Mucklow JC, Binding MR, Kahn GC, Dollery CT (1978) Drug concentration in saliva. Clin Pharmacol Ther 24:563–570

Nishihara K, Uchino K, Saitoh Y, Honda Y, Nakagawa F, Tamura Z (1979) Estimation of plasma unbound phenobarbital concentration by using mixed saliva. Epilepsia 20:37–45

Odar-Cederlöf I, Borgå O (1974) Kinetics of diphenylhydantoin in uraemic patients: consequences of decreased plasma protein binding. Eur J Clin Pharmacol 7:31–37

Olesen OV, Dam M (1967) The metabolic conversion of primidone (mysoline®) to phenobarbitone in patients under long-term treatment. Acta Neurol Scand 43:348–356

Painter MJ, Pippenger C, MacDonald H, Pitlick W (1978) Phenobarbital and diphenylhydantoin levels in neonates with seizures. J Pediatr 92:315–319

Parsonage M (1972) Clinical experience with carbamazepine (Tegretol) as an anticonvulsant. In: Wink CAS (ed) Tegretol in epilepsy. Proceeding of an international meeting. Nicholls, Manchester, pp 69–76

Paxton JW, Donald RA (1980) Concentrations and kinetics of carbamazepine in whole saliva, parotid saliva, serum ultrafiltrate, and serum. Clin Pharmacol Ther 28:695–702

Paxton JW, Whiting B, Stephen KW (1977) Phenytoin concentrations in mixed, parotid and submandibular saliva and serum measured by radioimmunoassay. Br J Clin Pharmacol 4:185–191

Pedersen B (1982) Intoxication after large overdose of sodium valproate. Br J Clin Pract Symp 18 [Suppl] 152–153

Penry JK (1975) Correlation of serum ethosuximide levels with clinical effects. In: Schneider H, Janz D, Gardner-Thorpe C, Meinardi H, Sherwin AL (eds) Clinical pharmacology of antiepileptic drugs. Springer, Berlin, Heidelberg New York, pp 217–220

Penry JK, Porter RJ, Dreifuss FE (1972) Ethosuximide. Relation of plasma levels to clinical control. In: Woodbury DM, Penry JK, Schmidt RP (eds) Antiepileptic drugs. Raven, New York, pp 431–441

Perucca E (1980) Plasma protein binding of phenytoin in health and disease: relevance to therapeutic drug monitoring. Ther Drug Monit 2:315–322

Perucca E, Makki K, Richens A (1978) Is phenytoin metabolism dose-dependent by enzyme saturation or by feedback inhibition? Clin Pharmacol Ther 24:46–51

Pinder RM, Brogden RN, Speight TM, Avery GS (1976) Clonazepam: a review of its pharmacological properties and therapeutic efficacy in epilepsy. Drugs 12:321–361

Pinder RM, Brogden RN, Speight TM, Avery GS (1977) Sodium valproate: a review of its pharmacological properties and therapeutic efficacy in epilepsy. Drugs 13:81–123

Piredda S, Monaco F (1981) Ethosuximide in tears, saliva, and cerebrospinal fluid. Ther Drug Monit 3:321–323

Pisani F, Fazio A, Giancarla O, Perri RD (1981) Dipropylacetic acid plasma levels: diurnal fluctuations during chronic treatment with dipropylacetamide. Ther Drug Monit 3:297–301

Plaa GL, Hine CH (1960) Hydantoin and barbiturate blood levels observed in epileptics. Arch Int Pharmacodyn Ther 78:375

Pynnönen S (1979) Pharmacokinetics of carbamazepine in man: a review. Ther Drug Monit 1:409–431

Rawlins MD, Collste P, Bertilsson L, Palmér L (1975) Distribution and elimination kinetics of carbamazepine in man. Eur J Clin Pharmacol 8:91–96

Reidenberg MM (1977) The binding of drugs to plasma proteins and the interpretation of measurements of plasma concentrations of drugs in patients with poor renal function. Am J Med 62:466–470

Reynolds EH (1980) Clinical application of the monitoring of anticonvulsant drug levels. In: Drug concentrations in neuropsychiatry. Ciba Foundation Symposium 74 (new series). Excerpta Medica, Elsevier, New York, pp 199–214

Reynolds EH, Shorvon S (1981) Monotherapy or polytherapy for epilepsy? Epilepsia 22:1–10

Reynolds F, Zyroyanis PN, Jones NF, Smith SE (1976) Salivary phenytoin concentrations in epilepsy and in chronica renal failure. Lancet II:384–386

Richens A (1979) Clinical pharmacokinetics of phenytoin. Clin Pharmacol 4:153–169

Richens A (1981) Monitoring antiepileptic drug therapy. Editorial. Ther Drug Monit 3:1–2

Richens A, Scoular IT, Ahmed S, Jordan BJ (1976) Pharmacokinetics and efficacy of Epilim in patients receiving long term therapy with other antiepileptic drugs. In: Legg (ed) Clinical and pharmacological aspects of sodium valproate (Epilim) in the treatment of epilepsy. MCS Consultants, Tunbridge Wells, pp 78–88

Rodin EA, Haidukewych D (1981) Fluctuations in free valproic acid (VPA) levels of epileptic patients. In: Dam M, Gram L, Penry JK (eds) Advances in epileptology. The XIIth epilepsy international symposium. Raven, New York, pp 541–548

Rowan AJ, Pippenger CE, McGregor PA, French JH (1975) Seizure activity and anticonvulsant drug concentration. 24-hour sleep-waking studies. Arch Neurol 32:281–288

Rowan AJ, Binnie CD, de Beer-Pawlikowski NKB, Goedhart DM, Gutter T, Van Der Geest P, Meinardi H, Meijer JWA (1979) Sodium valproate: serial monitoring of EEG and serum levels. Neurology 29:1450–1459

Rowan AJ, Overweg J, Meijer JWA (1981) Monodose therapy with valproic acid: 24-hours telemetric EEG and serum level studies. In: Dam M, Gram L, Penry JK (eds) Advances in epileptology. The XIIth epilepsy international symposium. Raven, New York, pp 533–539

Rowland M (1980) Plasma protein binding and therapeutic drug monitoring. Ther Drug Monit 2:29–37

Sannita WG, Rapallino MV, Rodriguez G, Rosadini G (1980) EEG effects and plasma concentrations of phenobarbital in volunteers. Neuropharmacology 19:927–930

Schmidt D (1976) Salivary concentrations of antiepileptic drugs. Lancet II:639

Schmidt D (1977 a) The value of antiepileptic drug determinations for the treatment of epilepsy. In: Majkowski J (ed) Posttraumatic epilepsy and pharmacological prophylaxis. Polish chapter of the International League against Epilepsy, Warsaw

Schmidt D (1977 b) Die Behandlung der Epilepsien mit Hilfe der Blutspiegelbestimmung. Nervenarzt 48:183–196

Schmidt D (1981) Behandlung der Epilepsien. Georg Thieme, Stuttgart New York

Schmidt D, Janz D (1977) Therapeutic plasma concentrations of phenytoin and phenobarbitone. In: Gardner-Thorpe C, Janz D, Meinardi H, Pippenger CE (eds) Antiepileptic drug monitoring. Pitman Medical, Kent, pp 214–225

Schmidt D, Kupferberg HJ (1975) Diphenylhydantoin, phenobarbital and primidone in saliva, plasma and cerebrospinal fluid. Epilepsia 16:735–741

Schmidt D, Machus B (1980) The use of blood levels in the treatment of patients with Lennox syndrome. In: Johannessen SI, Morselli PL, Pippenger CE, Richens A, Schmidt D, Meinardi H (eds) Antiepileptic therapy: advances in drug monitoring. Raven, New York, pp 279–285

Schneider H (1975 a) Carbamazepine: an attempt to correlate serum levels with antiepileptic and side effects. In: Schneider H, Janz D, Gardner-Thorpe C, Meinardi H, Sherwin AL (eds) Clinical pharmacology of anti-epileptic drugs. Springer, Berlin Heidelberg New York, pp 151–158

Schneider H (1975 b) Carbamazepine: the influence of other antiepileptic drugs on its serum level. In: Schneider H, Janz D, Gardner-Thorpe C, Meinardi H, Sherwin AL (eds) Clinical pharmacology of anti-epileptic drugs. Springer, Berlin Heidelberg New York, pp 189–196

Schobben, F, Van Der Kleijn E, Gabreëls FJM (1975) Pharmacokinetics of di-*n*-propylacetate in epileptic patients. Eur J Clin Pharmacol 8:97–105

Schobben F, Vree TB, Van Der Kleijn E, Claessens R, Renier WO (1980) Metabolism of valproic acid in monkey and man. In: Johannessen SI, Morselli PL, Pippenger CE, Richens A, Schmidt D, Meinardi H (eds) Antiepileptic therapy: advances in drug monitoring. Raven, New York, pp 93–100

Schottelius DD, Fincham RW (1978) Clinical application of serum primidone levels. In: Pippenger CE, Penry JK, Kutt H (eds) Antiepileptic drugs: quantitative analysis and interpretation. Raven, New York, pp 273–282

Schulz H-U, Fröscher W, Gugler R, Eichelbaum M (1979) Untersuchungen zum therapeutischen Bereich der Valproinsäure. Med Welt 30:59–61

Sherwin AL (1978) Clinical pharmacology of ethosuximide. In: Pippenger CE, Penry JK, Kutt H (eds) Antiepileptic drugs: quantitative analysis and interpretation. Raven, New York, pp 283–295

Sherwin AL, Robb JP (1972) Ethosuximide. Relation of plasma levels to clinical control. In: Woodbury DM, Penry JK, Schmidt RP (eds) Antiepileptic drugs. Raven, New York, pp 443–448

Sherwin AL, Harvey C, Leppik I, Gonda A (1976) Correlation between red cells and free plasma phenytoin levels in renal disease. Neurology 26:874–878

Shorvon SD, Chadwick D, Galbraith AW, Reynolds EH (1978) One drug for epilepsy. Br Med J 1:474–476

Sillanpää M (1981) Carbamazepine. Pharmacology and clinical uses. Acta Neurol Scand [Suppl 88] 64

Simonsen N, Zander-Olsen P, Kühl V, Lund M, Wendelboe J (1976) A comparative controlled study between carbamazepine and diphenylhydantoin in psychomotor epilepsy. Epilepsia 17:169–176

Sjö O, Hvidberg EF, Naestoft J, Lund M (1975) Pharmacokinetics and side-effects of clonazepam and its 7-amino-metabolite in man. Eur J Clin Pharmacol 8:249–254

Smith GA, McKauge L, Dubetz D, Tyrer JH, Eadie MJ (1979) Factors influencing plasma concentrations of ethosuximide. Clin Pharmacokinet 4:38–52

Solow EN, Green JB (1971) The determination of ethosuximide in serum by chromatography. Preliminary results of clinical application. Clin Chim Acta 33:87–90

Stephen KW, MacFarlance CB, Speirs CF (1980) Factors determining the passage of drugs from blood into saliva. Br J Clin Pharmacol 9:51–55

Strandjord RE, Johannessen SI (1975) A preliminary study of serum carbamazepine levels in healthy subjects and in patients with epilepsy. In: Schneider H, Janz D, Gardner-Thorpe C, Meinardi H, Sherwin AL (eds) Clinical pharmacology of anti-epileptic drugs. Springer, Berlin Heidelberg New York, pp 181–188

Strandjord RE, Johannessen SI (1980) Single-drug therapy with carbamazepine in patients with epilepsy: Serum levels and clinical effect. Epilepsia 21:655–662

Svensmark O, Buchthal F (1963) Accumulation of phenobarbital in man. Epilepsia 4:199–206

Svensmark O, Schiller PJ, Buchthal F (1960) 5,5-Diphenylhydantoin (Dilantin®) blood levels after oral or intravenous dosage in man. Acta Pharmacol Toxicol (Copenh) 16:331–346

Tatzer E, Groh C (1980) Is the therapy with carbamazepine more effective when measuring blood levels? Paediatr Paedol 15:293–296

Testa G, Ermani M, Giaretta D, Pellegrini A, Paleari C (1980) Clinicopharmacologic study of blood carbamazepine levels in a group of epileptic patients. Riv Neurol 50:241–252

Troupin AS, Friel P (1975) Anticonvulsant level in saliva, serum and cerebrospinal fluid. Epilepsia 16:223–227

Troupin A, Ojemann LM, Halpern L, Dodrill C, Wilkus R, Friel P, Feigl P (1977) Carbamazepine – a double-blind comparison with phenytoin. Neurology 27:511–519

Troupin AS, Friel P, Lovely MP, Wilensky AJ (1979) Clinical pharmacology of mephenytoin and ethotoin. Ann Neurol 6:410–414

Vajda F, Morris P, Drummer O, Bladin P (1976) Studies on sodium valproate – a new anticonvulsant. In: Legg (ed) Clinical and pharmacological aspects of sodium valproate (Epilim) in the treatment of epilepsy. MCS Consultants, Tunbridge Wells, pp 92–100

Van Der Kleijn E, Guelen PJM, Van Wijk C, Baars I (1975) Clinical pharmacokinetics in monitoring chronic medication with anti-epileptic drugs. In: Schneider H, Janz D, Gardner-Thorpe C, Meinardi H, Sherwin AL (eds) Clinical pharmacology of anti-epileptic drugs. Springer, Berlin, pp 11–33

Westenberg HGM, Van Der Kleijn E, Oei TT, De Zeuw RA (1978) Kinetics of carbamazepine and carbamazepine-epoxide, determined by use of plasma and saliva. Clin Pharmacol Ther 23:320–328

Yacobi A, Lampman T, Levy G (1977) Frequency of distribution of free warfarin and free phenytoin fraction values in serum of healthy human adults. Clin Pharmacol Ther 21:283–286

Zysset T, Rüdeberg A, Vassella F, Küpfer A, Bircher J (1981) Phenytoin therapy for epileptic children: evaluation of salivary and plasma concentrations and of methods of assessing compliance. Dev Med Child Neurol 23:66–75

CHAPTER 26

Clinical Use of Antiepileptic Drugs

M. J. EADIE

A. Introduction

Although the main use of antiepileptic drugs in contemporary clinical practice is in the treatment of epilepsy, these drugs are occasionally employed for other purposes. The present chapter will deal mainly with the use of antiepileptic drugs for epilepsy, but their other uses will be considered briefly towards the end of the chapter.

B. Use of Antiepileptic Drugs in Epilepsy

I. Indications for the Use of Antiepileptic Drugs

The decision to prescribe an antiepileptic drug for epilepsy in an individual patient depends on four main considerations.

1. The risk of the patient having further epileptic seizures
2. The disadvantages that further attacks would constitute for the patient
3. The risks that the treatment may hold for the patient
4. The likely effectiveness of the therapy that can be offered

Often the natural history of a patient's seizure disorder will not be known at the time when a decision must be taken about the need for treatment with antiepileptic drugs. If there have already been recurrent seizures, even very minor ones, it is likely that further attacks will occur unless treatment is given. However, if the patient is seen after a solitary epileptic episode, the prognosis is less clear. Often such patients will prove to have subsequent seizures, but sometimes a solitary seizure can be due to a set of circumstances which is unlikely to recur, e.g. an attack of meningitis. Therefore, the patient may never experience another epileptic event. Further, if benign febrile convulsions of infancy are considered a form of epilepsy (and there is good reason why they should be) the risk of a solitary febrile convulsion going on to subsequent recurrent seizures is so low that many would feel antiepileptic drug therapy is not indicated. In the past it was often felt that it was usually unnecessary to prescribe antiepileptic drugs until at least two epileptic episodes had occurred in a given patient. Present-day thinking often tends to favour earlier therapy, but the need to treat the patient after a solitary seizure is still rather controversial.

The second consideration concerning the need for treatment is the disadvantage that a further attack would hold for the patient. This disadvantage is determined by individual circumstances. Thus for an ophthalmic surgeon or a television announcer, any further epileptic attack would have serious implications for the subject's subsequent career; a single attack at a critical moment could be professionally disastrous. Yet for a severely mentally retarded, institutionalized child, or for a middle-aged housewife living alone with her husband, with convenient access to shopping, an occasional epileptic attack may have little consequence.

If the risk of subsequent epilepsy, and its disadvantages for the patient, appear sufficient to justify treatment, there remain to be considered the questions of the effectiveness of the treatment that can be offered and the disadvantages that treatment may have for the patient. There is an increasing realization that skilful, vigorously pursued antiepileptic drug therapy, making use of the best contemporary knowledge and technology, can control a substantial percentage of cases of recent onset epilepsy not due to active brain disease. If full control can be maintained for long enough there is often permanent cure. Further, modern knowledge permits adverse effects of treatment to be kept to an acceptably low level in most instances.

Over recent years, the indications for using antiepileptic drugs in epilepsy have gradually changed. Treatment with these drugs has become more effective and safer at the same time as it has been increasingly realized that the longer epilepsy is left inadequately treated, or untreated, the less is the chance that the epilepsy can ever be cured. All these factors have combined to produce an increasingly vigorous contemporary attitude to the drug therapy of epilepsy. Nevertheless, the decision to treat should always be taken after considering the individual patient's circumstances carefully.

II. Aim of Antiepileptic Drug Therapy

In the past there seems to have been a general, though largely implicit, expectation that the most that antiepileptic therapy could achieve was the suppression of the clinical manifestations of epilepsy. If seizures failed to recur after therapy was ceased, that was an added benefit but not one that could reasonably be anticipated in most cases. The reason for any apparent cure of epilepsy that happened to occur was often not formally defined. Gradually a number of items of evidence have accumulated which make it probable that prolonged total suppression of epilepsy can, in a significant proportion of instances, lead to disappearance of the epileptic process. The aim of treating epilepsy has become increasingly seen as achieving a cure of epilepsy, rather than simply suppressing a symptom.

In general the longer epilepsy has been present before it is brought under complete control the less the chances that therapy can ever be withdrawn without relapse of seizures. Complete control of epilepsy means more than the prevention of all major overt expressions of epilepsy – it means the total suppression of all clinical manifestations of epilepsy, however minor these manifestations may be. Further, one is moving towards the view that such complete control should also lead to the disappearance of all paroxysmal activity from the EEG. Such paroxysmal activity, if originally present, often will not disappear as soon as clinical epileptic seizures cease. However, if paroxysmal activity does not ultimately disappear from the EEG the writer's experience has been that the epilepsy will usually recur after antiepileptic drug therapy is ceased. Further, if epilepsy is due to a progressive disease, e.g. a tumour, even if clinical seizures can be prevented by anticonvulsant treatment, it is very likely that they will recur after treatment is withdrawn. The cause of a patient's epilepsy is thus a significant factor in determining any realistic aim of the treatment of the epilepsy. The possibility of curing epilepsy is also related to the duration of complete suppression of epilepsy that is achieved. The available figures suggest that cure rate increases with length of total control of epilepsy. Thus JUUL-JENSEN (1964) found two chances in three of cure after 2 years of control, HOLOWACH et al. (1972) three chances in four after 4 years of control, and OLLER-DAURELA et al. (1976) four chances in five after 5 years of control.

With the increasing realization that careful, prolonged antiepileptic drug therapy offers a reasonable prospect of achieving the lasting cure of epilepsy in many patients, it becomes important for the clinician to define his aim in treating epilepsy in each individual patient. In most circumstances, the initial aim should be the enduring cure of epilepsy. Sometimes, even from the outset, this aim may be unrealistic, or its attainment not worthwhile, as when epilepsy is only a minor component of the patient's overall disability, e.g. in a person who is mentally retarded enough to be quite unable to lead an independent existence. Sometimes, during the course of antiepileptic drug therapy, it may become apparent that complete suppression of a patient's seizures cannot be obtained without an unacceptable degree of adverse effects of treatment, or without undue disruption of the individual's or the individual's family's social or emotional life. In such circumstances the clinician must settle for the best degree of control of epilepsy compatible with the patient's and the patient's family's wellbeing. Thus the clinician may need to redefine the goal of the therapy he has prescribed. Not to define a reasonable aim of therapy is likely to lead to less than optimum treatment.

III. Selection of an Antiepileptic Drug

The choice of an antiepileptic drug to treat a patient's epilepsy depends on the interplay of four considerations:

1. The specificity of the drug for the patient's type(s) of seizures
2. The effectiveness of the drug for the patient's type(s) of seizures
3. The safety of the drug relative to the alternative drugs
4. The ease of use of the drug

1. Specificity of Antiepileptic Drugs for Particular Types of Seizure

Experience in humans has shown that certain forms of epilepsy respond best to particular antiepileptic drugs, while other antiepileptic drugs are comparatively ineffective for the same forms of epilepsy. It is not so much a case of absolute as of relative specificity of antiepileptic drugs for each type of epileptic seizure. A correlation between the major varieties of seizures, classified on the basis proposed by the International League Against Epilepsy (GASTAUT 1969) and the types of antiepileptic drugs effective for these forms of epilepsy is shown in Fig. 1.

Most of the antiepileptic drugs have overlapping specificities for different types of seizure and there are drugs available which may be effective to a useful

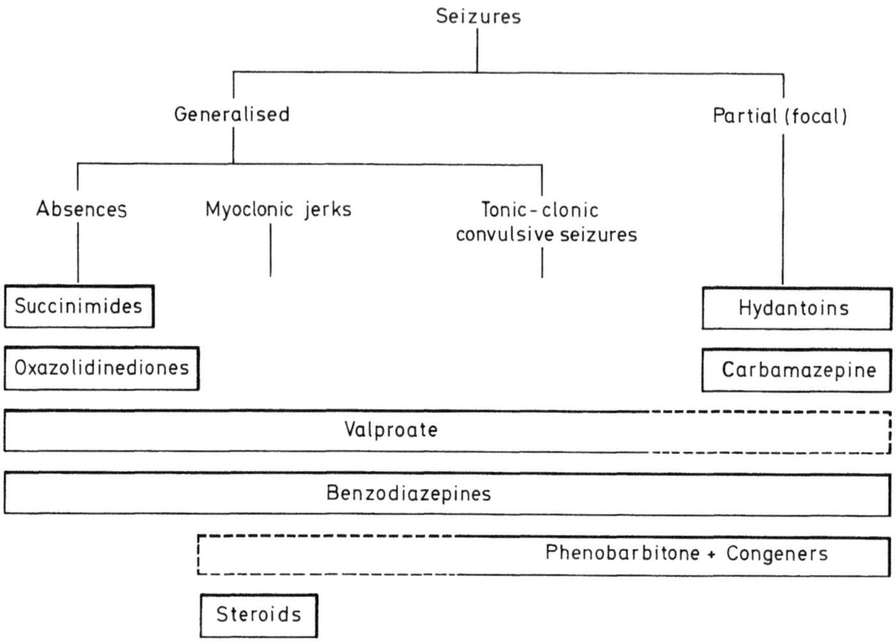

Fig. 1. Correlation between type of seizure and potentially effective antiepileptic drugs (EADIE 1981). *Broken lines* indicate that the response of the type of epilepsy to the drug is inconsistent

extent for practically all types of epileptic seizure. The simple correlation shown in Fig. 1 does not bring out several points of practical importance. Within the group of myoclonic seizures there are certain age-related subgroups of epilepsies which have relatively specific therapeutic requirements. Infantile spasms with hypsarrhythmia (the West syndrome), if they respond to any agent, respond best to adrenal corticosteroids, which may be provided directly, or indirectly, via corticotrophin or cosyntropin (tetracosactrin). Childhood myoclonic-astatic seizures (the Lennox-Gastaut syndrome) do not respond to steroids, but may respond to valproate or certain benzodiazepines (clonazepam, nitrazepam). Adolescence or adult life onset myoclonic seizures respond to the latter drugs, but also to phenobarbital or its congeners (methylphenobarbital and primidone). The conventional view is that phenytoin and methoin (another hydantoin), carbamazepine, and phenobarbital and its congeners, are each effective therapies for both partial (focal) seizures, in all their variety of clinical expressions and whether or not they become secondarily generalized, and also for generalized epilepsy causing convulsive seizures. The correlations shown in Fig. 1 also do not bring out the quantitative aspect of antiepileptic drug use. Some two-thirds of patients with epilepsy have partial (focal) seizures, while simple absences and myoclonic seizures together probably take in only about 10% of all cases of epilepsy. Consequently drugs used for partial epilepsy are the most frequently prescribed antiepileptic drugs in the community despite the relatively small space partial epilepsy occupies in Fig. 1.

A patient may have more than one type of seizure. Persons with absences, or myoclonic jerks, may at other times have tonic-clonic seizures of generalized epilepsy. Agents such as the oxazolidinediones and succinimides are often reasonably effective for absences, but not for convulsive seizures. Hence a second antiepileptic drug may be needed if these drugs are used for absence seizures. However, valproate or clonazepam will usually cover adequately against both types of seizure in the one patient.

2. Comparative Efficacy of Antiepileptic Drugs Specific for Particular Types of Seizure

Antiepileptic efficacy and antiepileptic specificity are closely related and in the foregoing discussion of specificity questions of relative efficacy have sometimes arisen.

a) Absences

Among the succinimides – phensuximide, methsuximide and ethosuximide – the latter appears the most effective agent for absences. Ethosuximide, the benzodiazepine clonazepam and valproate are all very effective drugs for this type of epilepsy. The choice between these drugs would need to be made on grounds other than comparative efficacy. The oxazolidinediones (mainly trimethadione and paramethadione) are not little used. One's impression is that they were not as effective as ethosuximide, but this impression may not be valid because the oxazolidinediones were never the subject of any large-scale use guided by pharmacokinetic principles, as the other three more recently introduced drugs have been. However, when there are a number of effective alternatives available for a relatively uncommon form of epilepsy, it seems unlikely that there would be much purpose in re-evaluating the efficacy of trimethadione.

b) Myoclonic Seizures

As indicated above, in infantile spasms adrenal corticosteroids are the only agents capable of stopping the attacks and also of reversing the associated mental retardation. However, they are effective in only about 50% of cases. The benzodiazepines clonazepam and nitrazepam have some effect in stopping the myoclonic jerks, but do not halt the mental deterioration. In the Lennox-Gastaut type of myoclonic epilepsy of childhood valproate appears the most effective drug, though it is far from efficacious. Clonazepam or nitrazepam is sometimes of benefit, and rarely ethosuximide, carbamazepine, phenobarbital (or its congeners) or sulthiame may be of use. For adolescent or adult life onset myoclonic epilepsy, valproate, clonazepam and phenobarbital, methylphenobarbital or primidone are all effective. There is probably not a great deal to choose between these drugs purely on grounds of efficacy.

c) Convulsive Generalized Epilepsy

For convulsive generalized epilepsy, valproate, phenobarbital or the latter's congeners appear effective drugs, while carbamazepine and phenytoin will suppress clinical seizures though apparently not the fundamental epileptic process.

d) Partial (Focal) Seizures (With or Without Secondary Generalization and Convulsions)

For partial (focal) seizures, experience suggests that the hydantoins, phenytoin, and methoin, carbamazepine, and phenobarbital, methylphenobarbital and primidone are probably virtually equipotent. Clonazepam is sometimes of benefit in cases that have not been fully controlled by the drugs mentioned immediately above. However, seizure control may not develop until some weeks after clonazepam has been introduced. Clonazepam monotherapy has not been extensively studied in this type of epilepsy. Valproate has not proved as effective in partial seizures as in generalized seizures. In partial seizures it has nearly always been used combined with other antiepileptic drugs. Valproate interacts pharmacokinetically with phenobarbital (or drugs biotransformed to phenobarbital, viz. methylphenobarbital or primidone) to produce raised plasma phenobarbital levels (SCHOBBEN et al. 1975). Therefore at least some of the apparent benefit from valproate in partial seizures may not have been due to the anticonvulsant actions of the drug itself but to the interaction increasing the effects of phenobarbital simultaneously present. Similarly, the effectiveness of sulthiame as an independent antiepileptic drug in partial seizures is uncertain. The drug has often been studied in combination with other agents, and in some patients sulthiame causes phenytoin accumulation (RICHENS and HOUGHTON 1973). In one well-designed study sulthiame monotherapy was clearly shown to be inferior to phenytoin monotherapy in the same population with partial seizures (GREEN et al. 1974). The succinimide methsuximide is reputedly useful in partial seizures, but the writer has found it of little value for this indication.

3. Comparative Safety of Antiepileptic Drugs

The question of comparative safety may be considered in relation to two viewpoints. Firstly, there is safety relative to the safety of the alternative effective drugs. Secondly, safety may be assessed relative to the disadvantages of the types of seizure for which the drug is used. To some extent the latter is an individual matter, depending on each patient's life circumstances, but there are also general hazards that apply for each major seizure type.

a) Absences

Of the effective drugs for this form of epilepsy, ethosuximide appears to be comparatively safe, causing very occasional idiosyncratic reactions (skin rashes, bone marrow function alterations) and mild alimentary tract dysfunction, and in overdosage produces drowsiness and ataxia.

Valproate has the advantage that it produces less drowsiness than any other antiepileptic drug. It can cause mild alimentary tract disturbance and occasional behaviour disorder. There are reports of its causing thrombocytopenia (WINFIELD et al. 1976), a bleeding tendency (SUTOR and JESDINSKY-BUSCHER 1976) and pancreatitis (BATALDEN et al. 1979). Recently there have been reports of a series of cases of relatively sudden onset hepatotoxicity associated with the use of the drug, often with clinical and biochemical features resembling the Reye syndrome (GERBER et al. 1979). The mortality has been substantial in these cases. Evidence is beginning to appear that use of the drug in pregnancy may be associated with an increased risk of lumbosacral neural tube defects in the offspring (ROBERT and GUIBARD 1982).

Clonazepam has the typical overall safety of a benzodiazepine, with very few idiosyncratic reactions. Not infrequently it produces some drowsiness, irritability and aggression, particularly if too high a dose is used too early in the course of treatment. Tolerance to the drug varies rather considerably from patient to patient, and adverse effects do not appear to correlate closely with plasma clonazepam concentrations. Very gradual introduction of the drug does reduce the adverse effects of therapy and increases patient acceptance of the drug.

Trimethadione is a relatively toxic drug which can cause agranulocytosis (WELLS 1957) and nephrotic syndromes (BARNETT et al. 1948). Occasionally it has produced a myasthenia-like condition (BOOKER et al. 1970). It commonly causes troublesome glare phenomena (SLOAN and GILGER 1947) and carries a substantial risk of dysmorphogenesis in man if taken in pregnancy (GERMAN et al. 1970).

With its lesser efficacy and greater level of toxicity, trimethadione would rarely be acceptable as therapy for absence epilepsy. Of the more effective drugs, ethosuximide and clonazepam are safe from the point of view of the patient's life, though clonazepam causes more minor but annoying problems unless its dose is handled carefully. It does, however, protect against any type of associated convulsive seizure, while ethosuximide probably does not. The rare but dangerous hepatotoxicity that is now being reported with the use of valproate is a relative contraindication to the use of this drug for a form of epilepsy which is comparatively benign, and for which there are two effective, safer alternatives.

b) Myoclonic Seizures

For infantile spasms there is no adequate alternative to adrenal glucocorticoids. The use of cosyntropin or corticotrophin may reduce the risks adrenal suppression from glucocorticoid therapy at the price of causing more mineralocorticoid-type unwanted effects. In relation to childhood Lennox-Gastaut myoclonic epilepsy, valproate is so much more effective than any alternative therapy in a disorder which is nearly always severely disruptive for the patient's quality of life that the drug's benefits outweigh its apparently rare but grave hazards. However, some might argue that the safer, but less effective, clonazepam should be tried first. In adolescent and adult onset myoclonic epilepsy there are several effective alternatives to valproate, and the epilepsy in its own right is usually much less disruptive to the patient's way of life than earlier onset myoclonic seizures. These alternative drugs (clonazepam, nitrazepam, and phenobarbital and its congeners) all produce sedative-type unwanted effects, but life-threatening adverse effects must be exceedingly rare. Clonazepam has one disadvantage over the barbiturates. If clonazepam therapy is ceased abruptly, there is a greater danger of withdrawal fits.

c) Generalized Tonic-Clonic Seizures

Here the argument about anticonvulsant safety is similar to that for later onset myoclonic epilepsy. The risk of serious valproate hepatotoxicity, small though it may be, tends to rank this drug behind the barbiturates, carbamazepine and phenytoin as the preferred drugs for this type of epilepsy.

d) Partial (Focal) Seizures

Of the hydantoins, phenytoin and methoin are effective drugs, but the use of methoin carries a significant risk of aplastic anaemia (TROUPIN et al. 1976). This grave hazard makes the drug virtually unacceptable in contemporary therapy. Of the three barbiturates, primidone has one particular disadvantage over phenobarbital and methylphenobarbital. In a few patients the first primidone dose can produce such extreme drowsiness for 24 h (or longer) that the patient will be reluctant to take the drug again. On the whole, the barbiturates produce more sedation than carbamazepine, and that drug causes more sedation than phenytoin for a similar anticonvulsant effect. Conversely, in overdosage, all these drugs cause cerebellar ataxia, but the risks appear greatest for phenytoin. The barbiturates produce fewer idiosyncratic adverse effects than phenytoin or carbamazepine. Skin rashes are not infrequent in the first weeks of therapy with phenytoin and carbamazepine, and can contraindicate the further use of these drugs. There were early reports of significant haematological toxicity from carbamazepine, but these effects no longer appear to occur with any significant frequency (LIVINGSTONE et al. 1978). Carbamazepine has a dose-related antidiuretic effect (WALES 1975), though this rarely causes clinical problems. Phenytoin has two further characteristic, frequent and troublesome adverse effects which are disadvantages in long-term therapy, viz. hirsuties and gum hypertrophy. All the drugs being considered in this section can cause folate deficiency and osteomalacia, all are probably occasional dysmorphogens and phenytoin is a rare cause of hepatitis and of a strange pseudolymphoma syndrome (EADIE and TYRER 1980a).

From the point of view of relative freedom from serious adverse effects, carbamazepine on the whole would seem preferable to its alternatives. Most clinicians would probably prefer phenytoin to the barbiturates, considering that the advantage it offered of less sedation outweighed its increased incidence of idiosyncratic unwanted effects. One wonders whether this attitude is necessarily valid if the use of the barbiturates is based on a careful application of pharmacokinetic principles. Among the barbiturates there may be grounds for preferring phenobarbital or methylphenobarbital to primidone.

4. Relative Ease of Use of the Various Antiepileptic Drugs

The last factor helping determine the choice of an antiepileptic drug for a particular patient's epilepsy is the relative ease of use of the available drugs suitable for the type of seizure which the patient has. Ease of use of a drug depends on its pharmacokinetic parameters and on the available dosage forms, and needs to be considered in relation to both long-term oral and short-term parenteral use. At first sight, ease and convenience of use might seem a rather trivial factor in determining choice of a drug, compared with considerations such as specificity of action, efficacy and safety. However, in practice convenience of use is of major importance in relation to long-term administration. Probably the main cause of therapeutic failure in contemporary long-term antiepileptic drug treatment is imperfect patient compliance. Ease and convenience of drug administration is a major factor in promoting compliance. In general, if a drug can be taken orally in one or two dosage units once or twice daily, the prospect of full compliance over long periods of time is enhanced. However, ease of use involves considerations other than achieving full compliance. These other issues include ease of making dosage adjustments and delay in achieving maximum effect after dosage changes.

The antiepileptic drugs are considered from the viewpoint of ease of use, in the order in which they have been discussed throughout this section:

a) Ethosuximide

Ethosuximide has a half-life of the order of 2–2½ days in adults and 1½ days in children. This comparatively slow elimination rate means that the drug is suitable for once daily administration, since its steady state plasma levels are not likely to fluctuate excessively over a 24-h dosage interval. However, the same slow elimination rate means that it will take up to 2 weeks for a steady state to apply after a dosage change. Therefore dosage alterations at shorter intervals than this run the risk of not allowing time for a maximum pharmacological effect from one dosage to appear before a new dosage is perscribed. Despite the drug's suitability for once daily administration because of its pharmacokinetic properties, the size of the usual ethosuximide dosage (often some 20–30 mg/kg per day), relative to the size of the usual individual dosage unit (250 mg), poses a problem. For older children and adolescents, the single daily dose may involve swallowing four to six or more individual dosage units, a situation which does not promote compliance.

b) Clonazepam and Nitrazepam

Both drugs have half-lives of the order of 24–36 hours. They are therefore suitable for once or twice daily administration, and achieve steady-state conditions about 1 week after a dosage change. The oral dosage units (0.5 and 2 mg in the case of clonazepam; 5 mg for nitrazepam) are reasonably sized for the average patient given the drug once or twice daily, though relatively high doses are sometimes required. Clonazepam is available for parenteral use, which offers the convenience of being able to use the same drug parenterally, or orally, as necessary.

c) Valproate

Valproate is marketed as the free acid, or as the sodium salt, in tablet or capsule form. The drug is hygroscopic so that in humid climates the tablets need to be kept foil wrapped until shortly before use. The short half-life of valproate, of the order of 8 h, means that steady state conditions are achieved quickly, within 2 days of a dosage change. Conversely, the short half-life and the drug's rapid absorption mean that interdosage plasma-level fluctuation is likely to be substantial and may allow the plasma level to fall to subtherapeutic values at stages over the dosage interval if the drug is taken less often than three times a day. The range of size of dosage units (200, 300, 500, and 600 mg) is reasonably suitable for such frequency of administration in most patients.

d) Phenobarbital

With its long half-life (3–4 days), phenobarbital is well suited to once daily administration from the point of view of small interdosage plasma-level fluctuations. However, the time to achieve a steady state after a dosage change (2–3 weeks) is annoyingly long. One wonders if some of phenobarbital's reputation for producing mental dulling may not be related to an excessive dosage being used because of failure to wait for steady state conditions to apply before the dosage is adjusted upwards. Phenobarbital also has the relative disadvantage that its steady state plasma levels in the individual tend to rise disproportionately relative to sequential dosage increments of equal size (EADIE et al. 1977). This is a further factor which may lead the unwary into prescribing excessive dosage of the drug. The drug is marketed as the acid, or the sodium salt, in a reasonable variety of dosage units (15, 30, 60, 100 mg) in tablet form, and as a 20% solution in a dosage unit of 1 ml for parenteral use.

e) Methylphenobarbital

Though almost certainly an anticonvulsant in its own right, in man methylphenobarbital is biotransformed to phenobarbital. This metabolite has a lower clearance and smaller apparent volume of distribution than the parent substance (EADIE et al. 1978). Phenobarbital therefore comes to exert the major antiepileptic effect when methylphenobarbital is used and is the determinant of the optimal dosage interval and time to achieve a maximum overall antiepileptic effect. The elimination half-life of methylphenobarbital (18–36 h) is reasonably long. Its own plasma levels are unlikely to fluctuate excessively if the drug is given once daily. A reasonable range of dosage unit sizes (30-, 60- and 200-mg tablets) is available but there is no commercially marketed parenteral form. The ease of use of oral methylphenobarbital is reasonably similar to that of phenobarbital, with two qualifications, one disadvantageous, one beneficial. The disadvantage arises from there being a second antiepileptic drug in the system to be accounted for when methylphenobarbital is used. The advantage is that, when methylphenobarbital is used, steady state plasma phenobarbital levels in the individual rise in direct proportion to drug dose, at least until levels reach the upper part of the therapeutic range (EADIE et al. 1977). The latter fact confers on methylphenobarbital a distinct advantage over phenobarbital.

f) Primidone

Because of its biotransformation, when primidone is used three different antiepileptic drugs are simultaneously present in the body (primidone itself, phenobarbital and phenylethylmalonamide). Primidone (half-life 6–10 h) and phenylethylmalonamide are fairly rapidly eliminated. Therefore the derived phenobarbital becomes the chief determinant of optimal dosage interval and of time to achieve maximum antiepileptic effects. The situation is like that which applies for methylphenobarbital except that (a) there is a third variable (a second metabolite) to be accounted for, (b) the rapid absorption and short half-life of primidone may allow unacceptably high peak levels of the drug to occur (with drowsiness) if primidone is given in full dosage once daily at any time other than bedtime, and (c) the quantitative effect of primidone dosage increase on steady-state plasma phenobarbital level in the individual does not appear to be adequately documented. The dosage unit (250 mg, divisible) is a reasonably convenient one, but no parenteral preparation is available

g) Carbamazepine

The 20- to 40-h half-life of the drug, with a possible anticonvulsant metabolite (carbamazepine-10,11-epoxide) that is more rapidly eliminated than the parent substance, make once daily administration of carbamazepine a practicable proposition, particularly since the drug's absorption after oral administration is slow. The delay in achieving steady state conditions after a dosage change (some 5–7 days) is not onerous is most circumstances. Steady state plasma levels of the drug in the individual tend to increase less than would be expected in response to a series of dose increments of equal size (COTTER et al. 1977), though the situation is different if phenytoin is used concurrently (HOOPER et al. 1974). Phenytoin undergoes a very consistent pharmacokinetic interaction with carbamazepine, resulting in lowered plasma carbamazepine concentrations (CHRISTIANSEN and DAM 1973). This interaction makes the phenytoin-carbamazepine combination difficult to handle. Carbamazepine, probably because of its poor aqueous solubility, is not available for parenteral use. The oral tablets, 100 mg and 200 mg, are reasonably sized for convenient use.

h) Phenytoin

The dominant elimination pathway for phenytoin is one which is better described by Michaelis-Menten than by exponential elimination kinetics. Therefore in a strict sense one should not speak of the elimination half-life of phenytoin. However, when first-order kinetics have been applied to phenytoin plasma-level data, half-lives of the order of 22 ± 9 h (ARNOLD and GERBER 1970) have been calculated. These values would suggest that the drug is suitable for twice daily, and perhaps for once daily, administration. For practical purposes steady state conditions should apply 4–6 days after a dosage change. Actually, phenytoin is slowly absorbed from the alimentary tract and proves quite suitable for once daily oral use. The main inconvenience in using phenytoin results from its Michaelis-Menten elimination kinetics. These are reflected in disproportionate rises in steady state plasma phenytoin levels relative to dosage increments in individual patients. This phenomenon was documented in man nearly a decade ago (BOCHNER et al. 1972) and has been amply confirmed since (RICHENS and DUNLOP 1975; LUDDEN et al. 1976; MULLEN 1978). Despite this, and the publication of nomograms (RICHENS and DUNLOP 1975) and other mathematical aids to phenytoin dosage adjustment, phenytoin overdosage still occurs with considerable frequency because of clinicians' lack of awareness of the non-linear relation between plasma level and dose in the individual.

Phenytoin (as the free acid or the sodium salt) is available in 30-, 50- and 100-mg strengths for oral use in tablets, capsules or suspension. A parenteral preparation is marketed. This solution is inconvenient to use intravenously because the low aqueous solubility of the drug at physiological pH leads to precipitation problems and because the solvent, if the solution is administered rapidly, may cause hypotension. For intramuscular administration, the preparation is so inefficient (WILDER and RAMSAY 1976) that its use can scarcely be justified.

5. The Actual Choice of an Antiepileptic Drug

The foregoing discussion should have set the background for the logical choice, or hierarchal ranking of choices, of an antiepileptic drug for all the more important types of epilepsy. Clearly some will place greater weights of preference on one factor rather than another. The writer's own ranking of choices of antiepileptic drugs is set out in Table 1. There is, in reality, a further factor which may determine each clinician's choice of an antiepileptic drug when he deals with his patient. Despite any amount of compelling logic favouring one drug, if a clinician knows another drug well, and is satisfied with it, he may rightly prefer it to the drug which has the theoretically stronger case.

Table 1. Choice of antiepileptic drug, ranked in order of preference for different seizure type

Seizures

Generalized			Partial (focal)
Absences	Myoclonic seizures	Convulsive	
1. Clonazepam 2. Ethosuximide 3. Valproate	(a) Infantile spasms 1. Corticosteroids 2. Clonazepam 3. Valproate (b) Childhood 1. Valproate 2. Clonazepam 3. Nitrazepam 4. Ethosuximide 5. Phenobarbital or congener 6. Carbamazepine (c) Adolescence and later 1. Phenobarbital or congener 2. Valproate 3. Clonazepam	1. Phenobarbital or congener 2. Carbamazepine 3. Phenytoin 4. Valproate 5. Clonazepam	1. Carbamazepine 2. Phenytoin 3. Phenobarbital or congener 4. Clonazepam 5. Sulthiame

Despite the ranking of drugs shown in Table 1, the writer must confess that in practice he does not follow his own logic in all instances. Thus, even though a major antiepileptic drug (e.g. carbamazepine, phenytoin) must usually be taken in addition, he prefers ethosuximide to clonazepam in absence epilepsy; whenever possible he tends to use other agents in preference to valproate, because he is concerned about the occasional, unpredictable and often life-threatening hepatotoxicity of this drug; he has no strong preference between carbamazepine and phenytoin in partial (focal) seizures, except for favouring phenytoin with its lesser degree of sedation when a rapid anticonvulsant effect is needed; and among the barbiturates he prefers methylphenobarbital, because of its greater ease of dose adjustments.

IV. Use of Antiepileptic Drugs in Practice

1. Principles

The following principles apply in antiepileptic drug therapy:

1. The most appropriate single drug for the patient's seizure type should be used from the outset.

2. Unless the patient's seizures occur so frequently that clinical response provides a convenient guide to therapy, the initial dose of the antiepileptic drug should be calculated to provide a plasma drug level within the therapeutic range for that drug (Table 2). The attaining of such a plasma level should be confirmed by plasma drug measurement once time has elapsed for a steady state to apply. To allow the patient to develop tolerance to sedative adverse effects of an antiepileptic drug it may be better to increase the dose of the drug over several weeks, rather than to provide the full expected therapeutic dose from the outset.

Table 2. Therapeutic ranges of plasma level for the antiepileptic drugs in common use, together with typical daily drug doses likely to be required to produce plasma drug levels in the therapeutic ranges

Drug	Therapeutic range		Typical dose (mg/kg/day)
	(mg/litre)	(μmol/litre)	
Ethosuximide	40–100	300–700	30
Clonazepam	0.025–0.075	0.08–0.24	0.15
Valproate (sodium)	50–100	300–600	15–30
Phenobarbital	10–30	45–130	2–3
Methylphenobarbital	As for phenobarbital		4–5
Primidone	As for phenobarbital		10
Carbamazepine	6–12	25–50	10–20
Phenytoin	10–20	40–80	6 (adults) 11 (children)

3. If unacceptable adverse effects occur, or if the plasma drug level is unsatisfactory, or if the patient's epilepsy is not controlled, the dose should be adjusted. As far as possible, doses should be changed only after the steady state clinical effects of the dose are known. Dosage adjustments should be made in knowledge of the non-linearities that may occur in the individual patient between steady state plasma drug level and drug dose for several of the anticonvulsants.

4. The aim of treatment should be seen as the total suppression of all manifestations of epilepsy without the production of an unacceptable level of adverse effects. The primary aim is not the production of a plasma drug level within a particular "therapeutic" concentration range. So long as the aim of treatment is achieved the plasma drug level (whatever it may be) is appropriate for the patient and serves as a guide for his or her future management.

5. If the aim of therapy is met, drug treatment in full dosage is continued for so long a time (3–5 years) that the epileptic process has a good chance of dying out. The decision to withdraw therapy is then taken in the light of all the patient's circumstances. During this prolonged course of therapy, plasma levels should be monitored at intervals to help ensure compliance. Levels should also be measured after any change in any concurrent therapy and if altered physiological circumstances develop, e.g. pregnancy. In such circumstances dose alteration may be required to maintain satisfactory plasma concentrations.

6. If the aim of therapy cannot be met by any non-toxic dose of a single antiepileptic drug, the dose of that drug should be reduced slightly to a non-toxic

one. A second appropriate antiepileptic drug should then be added and its dose adjusted as was the dose of the first drug. The situation is now made more complex by the possibility of pharmacokinetic interactions between the two drugs. This complexity would be obviated if the first drug were withdrawn. However, to do this would run the risk of making the patient's epilepsy worse if the second drug happened to be less effective than the first. Therefore it usually proves better to monitor the plasma levels of both drugs and to be prepared to adjust the dose of the first drug, if necessary, while trying to find the optimal dose of the second drug. As far as possible, the dose of only one drug should be changed at one time. This simplifies interpretation of the consequences of any dosage change. Dosage alterations are better not made until steady state plasma levels of the drugs have had time to apply.

7. If the aim of therapy cannot be met by maximum tolerated doses of two drugs in combination, a third appropriate drug may be added following the guidelines set down above (6).

8. If the aim of therapy cannot be met by maximum tolerated doses of all available appropriate antiepileptic drugs, the best accommodation between control of epilepsy and toxicity that can be obtained for the individual must be sought. In these circumstances it may be anticipated that antiepileptic therapy will have to be continued indefinitely, with little prospect of ultimate cure of the epilepsy.

The above principles are based largely on common sense and simple pharmacokinetic considerations. However, the argument for using a single drug from the outset may be worth examination. Certainly such a therapeutic policy produces a pharmacokinetically "cleaner" situation, and empirically a single appropriate drug has been shown to produce a very good chance of full sustained control of recent onset epilepsy (SHORVON et al. 1978). Nevertheless, if it could be shown that different antiepileptic drugs interrupted the epileptic process at different biochemical stages there would be an argument for the use of drug combinations from the outset, to suppress epilepsy as well as possible. The available antiepileptic drugs do have multiple known biochemical effects and do not share all these effects in common. Unfortunately though, the biochemical actions which produce the antiepileptic effects of the drugs are not known. Therefore the essential background knowledge is not available to enable a valid case to be made for the use of multiple drugs at the outset of therapy.

2. Use of Individual Antiepileptic Drugs

a) Ethosuximide

Ethosuximide provides efficient therapy for only one type of seizure – absences. Here there is rarely need for haste in obtaining full control of attacks. It is therefore possible to introduce ethosuximide gradually. Since absences nearly always occur frequently, it is usually possible to use the clinical response to find the minimum effective dose of the drug. If ethosuximide is used as sole antiepileptic agent for absence attacks, convulsive seizures may develop soon after (SCHMIDT and WILDER 1968). To avoid this contingency, phenytoin, carbamazepine or phenobarbital (or one of its congeners) is commonly prescribed with ethosuximide. In this case it is sensible to prescribe the major antiepileptic drug (e.g. carbamazepine) first, to establish the patient on a satisfactory dose and to see that there is no early toxicity which might preclude further use of the drug. Ethosuximide may then be commenced in a dose of 10–15 mg/kg per day, which for the age group in which absences occur often proves to be 250 mg twice or three times daily. Although once daily ethosuximide dosage is practicable, most patients find twice daily therapy completely acceptable. Dosage of this frequency does not appear to produce compliance problems. Every 2 weeks (to allow time for a steady state to develop after the previous dosage change) the daily dose of ethosuximide may be increased by 250 mg, until all absences cease, or unacceptable adverse effects develop. Plasma ethosuximide levels are used largely as reference values against which to check subsequent patient compliance. The plasma level of the major antiepileptic drug being taken concurrently with ethosuximide should be measured in the steady state after each ethosuximide dosage change, to ensure that pharmacokinetic interactions have not occurred. Such interactions could decrease protection against convulsive generalized seizures or else cause the major drug to accumulate and produce toxic effects which might be incorrectly attributed to ethosuximide. The upper limit of ethosuximide dose is determined by the occurrence of unacceptable adverse effects. Such effects often comprise mental dullness, drowsiness and ataxia and may not occur until plasma ethosuximide levels exceed 150 mg/litre.

Once a satisfactory dose of ethosuximide is found, full dosage is continued for several years. If the patient remains free of all absences for this time, and paroxysmal activity disappears from the EEG, there is a good chance that the absence epilepsy is cured. The ethosuximide may then be gradually withdrawn over several months. The author's practice is to have the patient continue taking the major antiepileptic drug for another year or two, until late adolescence, though there is no hard evidence that such a cautious attitude is necessary.

b) Benzodiazepines (Clonazepam and Nitrazepam)

Although the benzodiazepines, and in particular clonazepam, have a wide spectrum of action against different types of seizures there does not seem to be an extensive body of experience with these drugs except in myoclonic seizures. To some extent this may reflect the availability of older, well-established and reasonably satisfactory alternative drugs for many of the forms of epilepsy for which clonazepam may also be effective. Clonazepam in fact is probably often used only after alternative therapy has failed. Therefore its true effectiveness as a primary drug in previously untreated epilepsy is probably not yet known.

When clonazepam or nitrazepam is used, it seems best to introduce the drug in low dosage, administering it orally once or twice daily. Dosage is increased not more often than every 5–7 days to allow time for the full clinical effect of one steady state plasma level of the drug to appear before another drug level is produced. The benzodiazepines may cause drowsiness, irritability and, in the case of clonazepam, aggression. The incidence and severity of these problems can be reduced if low doses of the drugs are used initially, and increased gradually. Thus while the effective daily clonazepam dose for an older child, or adult, will often be in the range 4–10 mg, and the nitrazepam dose in the range 5–20 mg, it may be best to commence clonazepam with 0.5 mg twice daily and nitrazepam with 2.5 mg at night and to increase the dose no more than once a week, depending on the clinical response. Plasma benzodiazepine concentrations seem to prove a poor guide to the prospective therapeutic efficacy of benzodiazepines. However, the levels serve as a useful point of reference for assessing subsequent correctness of compliance with the therapeutic regimen. If benzodiazepine doses are increased gradually, some patients tolerate surprisingly large doses of the drugs and obtain benefit from these.

Some authors have stated that, with time, the initial benefits of clonazepam therapy may be lost. The explanation of this phenomenon is uncertain. Perhaps at times it is simply a consequence of compliance failure for a drug which, if ceased abruptly, tends to produce withdrawal fits (EDWARDS 1974).

Assuming a satisfactory clonazepam (or nitrazepam) dose is found (and the upper limit of dosage is set by the patient's ability to tolerate sedation from the drug), that dosage should be continued until the patient has been totally free from seizures for 3–5 years, and until all paroxysmal activity has disappeared from the EEG. Then withdrawal of therapy may be considered, with drug doses being reduced gradually, over several months.

Clonazepam, or diazepam, may be used parenterally to treat all varieties of status epilepticus. Nitrazepam is not widely available in a form suitable for injection. Diazepam, at least, is not efficiently absorbed after intramuscular injection (HILLESTAD et al. 1974) and both benzodiazepines are better given intravenously, either directly into a vein or into the tubing of a running infusion. If benzodiazepines are injected into reservoirs of solutions for parenteral infusion there is substantial risk of the drugs precipitating out, leading to the risk of incorrect dosage. Intravenously, diazepam is given at a rate of 2 mg/min and clonazepam at a rate of 0.5 mg/min, with frequent monitoring of heart rate, blood pressure and respiration. Administration continues until seizures cease or vegetative function begins to become imperiled. If clonazepam is given too rapidly, there is a danger of respiratory arrest.

c) Valproate

Oral sodium valproate, or valproic acid, therapy may commence with a dose of 200 mg t.d. three times daily in the older child or adult, and perhaps half that amount (or 200 mg twice daily if the available dosage forms are indivisible) in the younger child. If the patient's type of epilepsy is one in which seizures occur frequently (e.g. childhood myoclonic seizures), dosage increments may be made as often as every second day to obtain seizure control. If it is decided to use valproate in types of epilepsy where seizures are infrequent, it may be reasonable to build up the dose to obtain minimum (i.e. trough or immediately predose) plasma valproate levels of 50–100 mg/litre and to then make further dose increments only as indicated by clinical considerations. Apart from some upper alimentary tract irritation, which can be reduced by giving the drug with meals or with antacids, valproate causes little immediate toxicity. In particular, when given as the sole antiepileptic drug, it usually causes little drowsiness. There are recommendations that liver function should be monitored every 1–2 months for the first 6–12 months of valproate therapy to detect incipient hepatotoxicity from the drug. One doubts whether this policy will prove reliable. The literature suggests that liver function tests may not become seriously abnormal in valproate hepatotoxicity until the Reye type of syndrome produced by the drug has already appeared (JACOBI et al. 1980). In view of recent suggestions that there may be an increased risk of teratogenesis if the drug is taken during pregnancy (ROBERT and GUIBARD 1982), the decision to use the drug in women of child-bearing age should be taken very carefully.

When a satisfactory valproate dose is found, this dose should be continued for 3–5 years, with monitoring of predose plasma valproate levels often enough to help ensure compliance with the dosage regime. It may be possible to simplify the therapeutic regime by using 500 or 600 mg dosage units instead of 200 or 300 mg units. Bleeding and coagulation profiles and platelet counts should be checked at intervals since the drug can effect these. If the appropriate symptoms arise, it should be remembered that valproate may cause pancreatitis (COULTER and ALLEN 1980) and may also cause sudden clouding of consciousness in the presence of conventionally non-toxic plasma drug levels (SACKELLARES et al. 1979). If the epilepsy for which valproate has been given is considered cured on clinical and EEG grounds, the drug may be withdrawn in stages, over several weeks or longer.

Valproate may be used rectally for status epilepticus (VAJDA et al. 1978), and there seems no reason a priori why it could not be given intravenously for this purpose. However, no adequate information regarding its use by the latter route is available.

d) Adrenal Corticosteroids, Cosyntropin or Corticotrophin

Adrenal corticosteroids, provided directly or indirectly via the relevant trophic hormone, are useful for only one type of epilepsy, infantile spasms (hypsarrhythmia, West's syndrome). At an earlier time there was a belief that the trophic hormones were more effective than the steroids themselves (FINNE 1963 cited by JEAVONS and BOWER 1964),but this view no longer seems to be held. Hypsarrhythmia may be treated with intramuscular corticotrophin gel 20 IU daily or cosyntropin 0.5 mg daily. If, after 10 days, the attacks continue, the dose should be doubled. If that dose fails, a trial of a directly acting corticosteroid may be carried out. However, in that circumstance one should not be sanguine about the outcome. The initial glucocorticoid dose might be 5 mg four times a day for prednisone or prednisolone, or 0.5 mg four times a day for dexamethasone. The dose should be doubled if attacks persist after 10 days. Once steroids have fully controlled infantile spasms for about 2 weeks and the hypsarrhythmic appearance is no longer seen in the EEG, treatment can usually be ceased with little risk of relapse. If the initial and the doubled dose of steroids fail, the use of steroids may be abandoned. The infantile spasms in that patient are refractory to steroid therapy and only symptomatic treatment with valproate or benzodiazepines is then likely to be of any use.

e) Phenobarbital

In most circumstances where phenobarbital is used, the patient's seizures are unlikely to occur frequently enough for the clinical response to provide a convenient guide to the likely effectiveness of the therapy. The initial phenobarbital dose should therefore be set to achieve a steady state plasma phenobarbital level a little above the lower therapeutic limit (15 mg/litre). For adolescent or adult myoclonic seizures the lower therapeutic limit is probably around 7 mg/litre, so that here an initial plasma phenobarbital level of 10 mg/litre will often prove satisfactory. Some patients will experience unacceptable drowsiness if the initial phenobarbital dose is sufficient to yield a plasma level as high as 15 mg/litre (the required dose usually being in the range 1–2 mg/kg per day, the higher figure applying for children, the lower for the aged). It may be better to use about half the calculated effective daily phenobarbital dose initially, giving the drug once or twice daily, and after 3 weeks to measure the plasma phenobarbital level. Unless the plasma level is already satisfactory, the phenobarbital dose may then be increased to bring the plasma drug level to around 15 mg/litre. It should be remembered that each phenobarbital dose increment will tend to produce a disproportionately large increase in plasma level compared with the increase produced by the previous dose increment of the same size. Unless unacceptable adverse effects have occurred, in which case the phenobarbital dose must be reduced, the drug dose sufficient to keep the plasma level around 15 mg/litre is continued until the clinical response establishes whether this dose is sufficient. If not, and further seizures occur, the plasma phenobarbital level should be measured immediately in case the reason for the therapeutic failure is imperfect compliance (or, rarely, increased clearance of the drug with time). If the plasma level has not fallen, an increased dose is required. The increase in dose should be made bearing in mind the nonlinearity between plasma phenobarbital level and dose in the individual. The steady state plasma level may be remeasured 3 weeks (or longer) after the dose increase to provide a reference value for later therapeutic decisions. The clinical response is used to determine the need for subsequent dosage changes. Whenever possible, decisions about dosage should be taken only when steady state conditions apply (in general, at least 3 weeks after the most recent phenobarbital dosage change). If necessary, phenobarbital dose may be increased to the patient's limit of tolerance. It should be remembered that the drug may cause insidious mental dulling, particularly in children, whose school performance should therefore be kept under review. Deteriorating school performance in the presence of full seizure control and absence of paroxysmal activity in the EEG suggests a need for a reduced phenobarbital dose and possibly for the introduction of a second appropriate antiepileptic drug. During long-term phenobarbital therapy it may be wise to check at intervals for evidence of clinically significant folate deficiency or osteomalacia.

If phenobarbital therapy produces full clinical and EEG control of seizures without unacceptable adverse effects, full dosage of the drug may be continued for 3–5 years, with periodic monitoring of plasma levels to help ensure compliance. At the end of that period, a decision about whether to withdraw therapy may be taken. If the drug is to be ceased its dosage is usually reduced in stages over 2 or 3 months.

Phenobarbital may be given by intravenous or intramuscular injection. For an adult, the dose to achieve a plasma level of 10 mg/litre in a previously untreated patient is usually about 400 mg, which can be given in an acceptably small volume by intramuscular injection. Intravenously, half such a dose should be given over 5–10 min, with the remainder of the dose perhaps being given more gradually afterwards.

f) Methylphenobarbital

Methylphenobarbital is used similarly to phenobarbital. However, the dosages required tend to be about 75% greater than phenobarbital doses. Plasma phenobarbital levels provide an adequate guide to therapy except in very occasional patients who seem to have disproportionately high plasma levels of methylphenobarbital relative to phenobarbital (normally the two are in a 1:7 to 1:10 ratio (EADIE et al. 1978). Plasma methylphenobarbital levels above 3 mg/litre seem to be associated with drowsiness in patients, even if simultaneous plasma phenobarbital levels are not particularly high. It is necessary to use assay methods which distinguish between methylphenobarbital and its congener to be in a position to detect this phenomenon. Some commonly used assays, e.g. enzyme multiplied immune test (EMIT) assays, may not differentiate between drug and metabolite in plasma. It should be mentioned that methylphenobarbital doses are easier to adjust than phenobarbital doses, when using plasma phenobarbital levels for guidance, because of the wider range of linearity between plasma phenobarbital level and methylphenobarbital dose.

g) Primidone

The method of use of primidone, and its indications, are reasonably similar to those which apply for phenobarbital. It is wise to give an initial single low oral test dose of primidone (e.g. 62.5 mg) to detect the occasional patient who cannot tolerate the drug because of extreme drowsiness. The average primidone dose to produce a steady state plasma phenobarbital level of 15 mg/litre is around 10 mg/kg per day. To allow time for a degree of tolerance to the sedative effects of the drug to develop, about half this dose might be prescribed initially and the dose increased after 3 or 4 weeks.

Although therapeutic ranges of plasma primidone levels are quoted, one wonders how useful these often are in their own right when a second anticonvulsant (phenobarbital) is present simultaneously. Further, to obtain reproducible values, minimum primidone levels need to be measured (i.e. predose or trough levels). In practice, plasma phenobarbital levels provide a satisfactory and convenient guide to primidone therapy. These levels vary so little in the steady state that they can be measured at any stage over a 12- or even a 24-h dosage interval.

h) Carbamazepine

A carbamazepine dose of 8–10 mg/kg per day is likely to yield a plasma carbamazepine level of 6–12 mg/litre, which is often satisfactory for therapeutic purposes. The drug induces its own metabolism over a period of about 3 weeks after therapy is begun. To allow time for this effect, it may be reasonable to use about half the expected daily carbamazepine dose for the 1st week or two, and then the full dose. The drug may be given twice daily. This staged introduction of the full dose of carbamazepine seems to avoid the early drowsiness which may otherwise occur. Some 3 weeks after carbamazepine therapy is begun the plasma carbamazepine level may be measured. If the level is below 6 mg/litre the dose should be increased unless the clinical response indicates that the dose is already appropriate, or unless adverse effects have developed which make a dose reduction or change of drug imperative. Plasma carbamazepine levels in the individual tend to increase less than would be expected with serial dose increments of equal size, so long as phenytoin is not taken concurrently. Once plasma carbamazepine levels are in the therapeutic range, further dosage adjustments are made on clinical grounds. Doses should be increased no more often than at weekly intervals (to allow steady state conditions to develop after each change) until adverse effects (mainly drowsiness or its consequences, or ataxia) preclude further dosage increase. This may not occur until plasma carbamazepine levels are well above 12 mg/litre, a figure often quoted as the upper limit of the therapeutic range.

If carbamazepine alone in maximum tolerated dosage will not control a patient's epilepsy, a second appropriate antiepileptic drug may be added to the therapy. If carbamazepine therapy is successful it is continued in full dosage, with periodic monitoring of plasma carbamazepine levels and checking for late manifestations of toxicity, until so many years' freedom from epilepsy have elapsed that withdrawal of therapy can be considered. The withdrawal is often carried out in stages over 2 or 4 months or longer.

i) Phenytoin

Phenytoin is usually used for types of epilepsy in which seizures are relatively infrequent. Therefore clinical response is usually not a practicable guide to the potential adequacy of the initial phenytoin dose. Consequently, the initial aim of oral phenytoin therapy becomes the achieving of a steady state plasma phenytoin level of between 10 and 20 mg/litre. In the majority of patients levels in this range can be attained by prescribing 5 mg/kg per day for adults, or 10 mg/kg per day for children under 10 years (Eadie and Tyrer 1980 a). Since phenytoin causes relatively little drowsiness, the full dose can be taken from the outset. The plasma phenytoin level should be checked 5–7 days after the outset of therapy and the dose then adjusted upwards or downwards to bring the plasma level into the desired range. Due to the dominantly Michaelis-Menten type of elimination kinetics of the drug, once plasma phenytoin levels are above 5 or 6 mg/litre relatively small dose changes can produce major changes in plasma drug level. Various mathematical methods for adjusting the drug dose to achieve a desired plasma level are available (e.g. Richens and Dunlop 1975; Ludden et al. 1976). However, for practical purposes, if the plasma phenytoin level in an adult is between 5 and 8 mg/litre the patient will probably tolerate a 100-mg/day dose increment without overdosage, and if the level is between 8 and 10 mg/litre a 30-mg or 50-mg increment.

Once steady state plasma phenytoin levels are in the therapeutic range, providing no unacceptable adverse effects have developed, the clinical response of the seizures may be used as a guide to any further dosage change. If necessary, phenytoin dose can be increased to take the plasma phenytoin level into the range 20–25 mg/litre to try to control epilepsy. Levels above 25 mg/litre are almost always associated with troublesome toxic manifestations. Levels in the range 20–25 mg/litre represent a pharmacokinetically brittle and sometimes clinically toxic situation in which the body has little additional capacity to eliminate the drug. Therefore with levels in this range any slight reduction in hepatic mixed oxidase function, or the temporary presence of any other substance which competes for the metabolic pathway utilized by phenytoin, may lead to phenytoin accumulation, and overt toxicity.

If a satisfactory phenytoin dose is found, this dose should be continued for several years. Because of the rather critically poised clearance capacity of the drug when its plasma levels are in the therapeutic range, every effort should be made to obtain full compliance so that hard-won control of epilepsy is not lost. The plasma phenytoin level should be checked whenever intercurrent illness is treated, to reduce the risk of overdosage type toxicity or of therapeutic failure. Throughout the course of phenytoin therapy the patient's general health should be supervised carefully, though most of the serious idiosyncratic adverse effects of the drug occur early in the course of therapy. If withdrawal of phenytoin is decided upon, dosage of the drug may be reduced in stages over 2 or 3 months. Phenytoin doses up to 250 mg can be given over 5–10 min by direct intravenous injection. Because of toxic effects from the solvent in intravenous phenytoin solutions, larger single doses of the drug are more safely given in 100- to 200-mg quantities, each introduced over several minutes into the tubing of an intravenous saline or glucose infusion. The whole course of intravenous phenytoin administration may then take many minutes to a few hours, and frequent monitoring of cardiac and respiratory function and blood pressure is desirable. Intramuscular phenytoin is too inefficient for satisfactory use.

V. Combinations of Antiepileptic Drugs

Not infrequently, two antiepileptic drugs must be used in combination because maximum tolerated doses of the first drug have failed to control a patient's epilepsy. The principles involved in the management of such combination therapy have already been set out. In practice some combinations are more commonly encountered than others and may be worth separate comments because of the pharmacokinetic interactions that may occur.

1. Ethosuximide with Phenytoin

This combination, used in patients with generalized epilepsy with absence seizures, often presents no particular problems. Ethosuximide dosage increase may cause phenytoin accumulation (FRANTZEN et al. 1967) and toxicity, but this eventuality can be avoided if plasma phenytoin levels are monitored after ethosuximide dosage changes.

2. Valproate with Phenobarbital (or Methylphenobarbital or Primidone)

When valproate is added to the therapy of a patient already taking phenobarbital, or a drug metabolized to phenobarbital, the plasma phenobarbital level is likely to rise substantially over a period of several weeks (SCHOBBEN et al. 1975; VAKIL et al. 1976; ADAMS et al. 1978). If plasma phenobarbital levels are not monitored, adverse effects due to phenobarbital accumulation are likely to be regarded as direct consequences of the valproate dose. This dose may then be reduced, rather than the dose of phenobarbital being reduced.

3. Valproate with Phenytoin

Valproate therapy poduces somewhat unpredictable effects on whole plasma phenytoin levels (RICHENS et al. 1976). These levels may rise in the short term (WINDORFER and SAUER 1977; ADAMS et al. 1978) but fall in the longer term (ADAMS et al. 1976). In addition valproate decreases the plasma protein binding of phenytoin (PATSALOS and LASCELLES 1977), so that measurement of plasma water (or salivary) phenytoin is desirable for adequate assessment of the situation.

4. Phenytoin with Phenobarbital (or Methylphenobarbital or Primidone)

Phenytoin intake may cause raised plasma phenobarbital levels in patients taking primidone (FINCHAM et al. 1974; REYNOLDS et al. 1975; WINDORFER and SAUER 1977). With this exception, combinations of phenytoin and barbiturates in man produce little in the way of pharmacokinetic interactions which significantly alter the plasma levels of the drugs concerned. Such combinations are therefore advantageous for clinicians who do not have ready access to plasma drug level measurements.

5. Phenytoin with Carbamazepine

This is a very troublesome combination from the viewpoint of interactions. Increase in carbamazepine dose may raise (LANDER et al. 1975) or lower (HOOPER et al. 1974) plasma phenytoin level. Increase in phenytoin dose will consistently, and significantly, lower plasma carbamazepine levels (CHRISTIANSEN and DAM 1973; LANDER et al. 1975, 1977). Plasma-level monitoring of both substances will clarify the situation. However, the combination of the drugs may be difficult, and at times frustrating, to handle. The unwary clinician may become bewildered or irritated at what he interprets as the patient's chaotically inconsistent compliance with the prescribed therapy.

6. Carbamazepine with Phenobarbital

Although concurrent phenobarbital intake is reported as causing a fall in plasma carbamazepine level (CHRISTIANSEN and DAM 1973; CEREGHINO et al. 1975), the writer has not seen this interaction cause plasma-level changes of any great magnitude, or sufficient to produce therapeutic difficulty.

7. Phenytoin with Sulthiame

A number of authors have reported that sulthiame intake may cause a major rise in plasma phenytoin levels (HANSEN et al. 1968; OLESEN and JENSEN 1969; RICHENS and HOUGHTON 1973). The present writer has rarely seen this interaction, but judged from the literature his experience is unusual.

VI. Indications for Cessation of Antiepileptic Drug Therapy

Unless the patient insists on ceasing treatment, the only indication for withdrawing antiepileptic drugs should be the occurrence of unacceptable adverse effects or the belief that the patient's epilepsy is cured. The best contemporary evidence suggests that a belief that epilepsy is cured might reasonably be held in the following circumstances:

1. The epilepsy is not due to active brain disease
2. There has been no clinical trace of epilepsy, however minor, for at least 3 years, and preferably for 4 or 5 years
3. All paroxysmal activity has disappeared from the EEG

In these circumstances, the decision to cease therapy can be considered, weighing the disadvantage that further seizures would hold for the patient against his reluctance to take unnecessary therapy. Drug withdrawal is best carried out gradually, at a time when the patient's life situation is comparatively unstressful and his health good.

If attacks recur, they generally do so within the 1st year after treatment is ceased.

C. Use of Antiepileptic Drugs for Indications Other than Epilepsy

I. Migraine

Phenytoin has proved useful in the prophylaxis of childhood migraine and in adult migraine when the aura comprises dysphasia or disturbance of brain stem function, commonly manifested as vertigo, i.e. basilar artery migraine (EADIE and TYRER 1980 b).

II. Tic Douloureux

Since 1962 carbamazepine has been accepted as the most effective available prophylactic agent for tic douloureux (BLOM 1962). Phenytoin is less useful, though certainly not without benefit (PENNYBACKER 1961). There are recent reports that clonazepam is also effective (CHANDRA 1976; COURT and KASE 1976).

III. Other Varieties of Pain

Other varieties of neurogenic pain, e.g. glossopharyngeal neuralgia (EKBOM and WESTERBERG 1966) and tabetic lightening pains (EKBOM 1972), sometimes respond to carbamazepine. Pain due to damage to central pain pathways in the medulla or thalamus is sometimes treated with carbamazepine or phenytoin, on occasions with some apparent benefit. The pain of Fabry's disease (ceramide trihexoside lipidosis) is said to respond to phenytoin (LOCKMAN et al. 1973) and carbamazepine (SHIBASAKI et al. 1973).

IV. Hyperinsulinism

Phenytoin causes decreased insulin secretion (MALHERBE et al. 1972), which may produce some relief from the manifestations of insulinoma (KNOPP et al. 1972). This relief may mislead diagnostically if the manifestations of insulinoma mimic those of epilepsy, as they often do.

V. Dyskinesia

Clonazepam has been reported useful in postanoxic action myoclonus (GOLDBERG and DORMAN 1976) and chorea (PIERIS et al. 1976).

VI. Cardiac Arrhythmia

Phenytoin is sometimes used to treat supraventricular cardiac arrhythmias (Bigger et al. 1968)

VII. Myotonia

Phenytoin has been reported useful in treating myotonia (Munsat 1967).

VIII. Miscellaneous

A miscellany of sometimes ill-defined conditions have been reported to benefit from the administration of phenytoin (Bogoch and Dreyfus 1970). The evidence often appears rather dubious.

References

Adams DJ, Luders H, Pippenger C (1978) Sodium valproate in the treatment of intractable seizure disorders: a clinical and electroencephalographic study. Neurology 28:152–157

Arnold K, Gerber N (1970) The rate of decline of diphenylhydantoin in human plasma. Clin Pharmacol Ther 11:121–134

Barnett, HL, Simons DJ, Wells RE Jr (1948) Nephrotic syndrome during Tridione therapy. Am J Med 4:760–764

Batalden, PB, Van Dyne BJ, Cloyd J (1979) Pancreatitis associated with valproic acid therapy. Pediatrics 64:520–522

Bigger JT Jr, Schmidt DH, Kutt H (1968) Relationship between the plasma level of diphenylhydantoin sodium and its cardiac antiarrhythmic effect. Circulation 38:363–374

Blom S (1962) Trigeminal neuralgia: its treatment with a new anticonvulsant drug (G-32883) Lancet I:839–840

Bochner F, Hooper WD, Tyrer JH, Eadie MJ (1972) The effect of dosage increments on blood phenytoin concentrations. J Neurol Neurosurg Psychiatr 35:873–876

Bogoch S, Dreyfus J (1970) The broad range of use of diphenylhydantoin. Dreyfus Medical Foundation.

Booker HE, Chun RWM, Sanguino M (1970) Myasthenia gravis syndrome associated with trimethadione. J Am Med Assoc 212:2262–2263

Cereghino JJ, Brock JT, Van Meter JC, Penry JK, Smith LD, White BG (1975) The efficacy of carbamazepine combinations in epilepsy. Clin Pharmacol Ther 18:733–741

Chandra B (1976) The use of clonazepam in the treatment of tic douloureux (a preliminary report). Proc Aust Assoc Neurol 13:119–122

Christiansen J, Dam M (1973) Influence of phenobarbital and diphenylhydantoin on plasma carbamazepine levels in patients with epilepsy. Acta Neurol Scand 49:543–546

Cotter LM, Eadie MJ, Hooper WD, Lander CM, Smith GA, Tyrer JR (1977) The pharmacokinetics of carbamazepine. Eur J Clin Pharmacol 12:451–456

Coulter DL, Allen RJ (1980) Pancreatitis associated with valproic acid therapy for epilepsy. Ann Neurol 7:92

Court JE, Kase CS (1976) Treatment of tic douloureux with a new anticonvulsant (clonazepam). J Neurol Neurosurg Psychiatr 39:297–299

Eadie MJ (1981) Anticonvulsant therapy – present and future. Trends Pharmacol Sci 2:37–39

Eadie MJ, Tyrer JR (1980a) Anticonvulsant therapy. Pharmacological basis and practice 2nd edn. Churchill-Livingstone, Edinburgh

Eadie MJ, Tyrer JH (1980b) Neurological clinical pharmacology. Adis, New York

Eadie MJ, Lander CM, Hooper WD, Tyrer JH (1977) Factors influencing plasma phenobarbitone levels in epileptic patients. Br J Clin Pharmacol 4:541–547

Eadie MJ, Bochner F, Hooper WD, Tyrer JH (1978) Preliminary observations on the pharmacokinetics of methylphenobarbitone. Clin Exp Neurol 15:131–144

Edwards VE (1974) Side effects of clonazepam therapy. Proc Aust Assoc Neurol 11:199–202
Ekbom K (1972) Carbamazepine in the treatment of tabetic lightning pains. Arch Neurol 26:374–378
Ekbom, KA, Westerberg CE (1966) Carbamazepine in glossopharyngeal neuralgia. Arch Neurol 14:595–596
Fincham RW, Schottelius DD, Sahs AL (1974) The influence of diphenylhydantoin on primidone metabolism. Arch Neurol 30:259–262
Finne PH (1963) Nord Med 69:197 cited by Jeavons PM, Bower BD (1964) Infantile spasma. Clinics in developmental medicine 15 Heinemann, London
Frantzen E, Hansen JM, Hansen OE, Kristensen M (1967) Phenytoin (Dilantin®) intoxication. Acta Neurol Scand 43:440–446
Gastaut H (1969) Clinical and electroencephalographical classification of epileptic seizures. Epilepsia [Suppl] 10:2
Gerber N, Dickinson RG, Harland RC, Lynn RK, Houghton D, Antonias JI, Schimschock JC (1979) Reye-like syndrome associated with valproic acid therapy. J Pediatr 95:142–144
German J, Kowal A, Ehlers KH (1970) Trimethadione and human teratogenesis. Teratology 3:349–362
Goldberg MA, Dorman JD (1976) Intention myoclonus: successful treatment with clonazepam. Neurology 26:24–26
Green JR, Troupin AS, Halpern LM, Friel P, Kanarek P (1974) Sulthiame: evaluation as an anticonvulsant. Epilepsia 15:329–349
Hansen JM, Kristensen M, Skovsted L (1968) Sulthiame (Ospolot) as inhibitor of diphenylhydantoin metabolism. Epilepsia 9:17–22
Hillestad L, Hansen T, Melsom H, Drivenes A (1974) Diazepam metabolism in normal man. Serum concentrations and clinical effects after intravenous, intramuscular, and oral administration. Clin Pharmacol Ther 16:479–484
Holowach J, Thurston DL, O'Leary J (1972) Prognosis in childhood epilepsy. Follow-up study of 148 cases in which therapy had been suspended after prolonged anticonvulsant control. N Engl J Med 286:169–174
Hooper WD, Du Betz DK, Eadie MJ, Tyrer JH (1974) Preliminary observation on the clinical pharmacology of carbamazepine ("Tegretol"). Proc Aust Assoc Neurol 11:189–198
Jacobi G, Thorbeck R, Ritz A, Janssen W, Schmidts HL (1980) Fatal hepatotoxicity in child on phenobarbitone and sodium valproate. Lancet I: 712–713
Jeavons PM, Bower BD (1964) Infantile spasms. Clinics in Developmental Medicine, vol 15. Heinemann, London
Juul-Jensen P (1964) Frequency of recurrence after discontinuance of anticonvulsant therapy in patients with epileptic seizures. Epilepsia 5:352–363
Knopp RH, Sheinin JC, Freinkel N (1972) Diphenylhydantoin and an insulin secreting islet adenoma. Arch Int Med 130:904–908
Lander CM, Eadie MJ, Tyrer JH (1975) Interactions between anticonvulsants. Proc Aust Assoc Neurol 12:111–116
Lander CM, Eadie MJ, Tyrer JH (1977) Factors influencing plasma carbamazepine concentrations. Clin exp Neurol 14:184–193
Livingstone S, Pauli LL, Pruce I (1978) No proven relationship of carbamazepine therapy to blood dyscrasias. Neurology 28:101
Lockman LA, Hunninghake DB, Krivit W, Desnick RJ (1973) Relief of pain of Fabry's disease by diphenylhydantoin. Neurology 23:871–875
Ludden TM, Hawkins DW, Allen JP, Hoffmann SF (1976) Optimum phenytoin dosage regimens. Lancet I:307–308
Malherbe C, Burrill KC, Levin SR, Karam JH, Forsham PH (1972) Effect of diphenylhydantoin on insulin secretion in man. N Engl J Med 286:339–342
Mullen PW (1978) Optimal phenytoin therapy: a new technique for individualizing dosage. Clin Pharmacol Ther 23:228–232

Munsat TL (1967) Therapy of myotonia. A double-blind evaluation of diphenylhydantoin, procainamide, and placebo. Neurology 17:359–367
Olesen OV, Jensen ON (1969) Drug-interaction between sulthiame (Ospolot (R)) and phenytoin in the treatment of epilepsy. Dan Med Bull 16:154–158
Oller-Daurella L, Pamies R, Oller L (1976) Reduction or discontinuance of antiepileptic drugs in patients seizure free for more than 5 years. In: Janz D (ed) Epileptology. Thieme, Stuttgart, pp 218–227
Patsalos PN, Lascelles PT (1977) Effect of sodium valproate on plasma protein binding of diphenylhydantoin. J Neurol Neurosurg Psychiatr 40:570–574
Pennybacker J (1961) Some observations on trigeminal neuralgia. In: Garland H (ed) Scientific aspects of neurology. Livingstone, Edinburgh, pp 153–167
Pieris JB, Boralessa H, Lionel NDW (1976) Clonazepam in the treatment of choreiform activity. Med J Aust I:225–227
Reynolds EH, Fenton G, Fenwick P, Johnson AL, Laundy M (1975) Interaction of phenytoin and primidone. Br Med J 2:594–595
Richens A, Dunlop A (1975) Serum-phenytoin levels in management of epilepsy. Lancet II:247–248, 1305–1306
Richens A, Houghton GW (1973) Phenytoin intoxication caused by sulthiame. Lancet II:1442–1443
Richens A, Scoular IT, Ahmad S, Jordan BJ (1976) Pharmacokinetics and efficacy of Epilim in patients receiving long-term therapy with other anticonvulsants. In: Legge NJ (ed) Clinical and pharmacological aspects of sodium valproate (Epilim) in the treatment of epilepsy. MCS Consultants, Tunbridge Wells, pp 78–88
Robert E, Guibard P (1982) Maternal valproic acid and congenital neural tube defects. Lancet II:937
Sackellares JC, Lee SI, Dreifuss FE (1979) Stupor following administration of valproic acid to patients receiving other antiepileptic drugs. Epilepsia 20:697–703
Schmidt RP, Wilder BJ (1968) Epilepsy. Davis, Philadelphia
Schobben E, Van Der Kleijn E, Gabreels FJM (1975) Pharmacokinetics of di-*N*-propylacetate in epileptic patients. Eur J Clin Pharmacol 8:97–105
Shibasaki H, Tabira T, Inoue N, Goto I, Kuroiwa Y (1973) Carbamazepine for painful crises in Fabry's disease. J Neurol Sci 18:47–51
Shorvon SD, Chadwick D, Galbraith AW, Reynolds EH (1978) One drug for epilepsy. Br Med J I:474–476
Sloan LL, Gilger AP (1947) Visual effects of Tridione®. Am J Ophthalmol 30:1387–1405
Sutor AH, Jesdinsky-Buscher C (1976) The effect of dipropylacetate (Ergenyl) upon haemostasis during anticonvulsant therapy. Fortschr Med 94:411–414
Troupin AS, Ojemann LM, Dodrill CB (1976) Mephenytoin: a reappraisal. Epilepsia 17:403–414
Vajda FJE, Mihaly GW, Miles JL, Donnan GA, Bladin PF (1978) Rectal administration of sodium valproate in status epilepticus. Neurology 28:897–899
Vakil SD, Critchley EMR, Philips JC, Fahim V, Haydock C, Cocks A, Dyer T (1976) The effect of sodium valproate (Epilim) on phenytoin and phenobarbitone blood levels. In: Legge NJ (ed) Clinical and pharmacological aspects of sodium valproate (Epilim) in the treatment of epilepsy. MCS Consultants, Tunbridge Wells, pp 75–77
Wales JK (1975) Treatment of diabetes insipidus with carbamazepine. Lancet IV:948–956
Wells CE (1957) Trimethadione: its dosage and toxicity: Arch Neurol Psychiatr 77:140–155
Wilder BJ, Ramsay RE (1976) Oral and intramuscular phenytoin. Clin Pharmacol Ther 19:360–364
Windorfer A, Sauer W (1977) Drug interactions during anticonvulsant therapy in childhood. Diphenylhydantoin, primidone, phenobarbitone, clonazepam, nitrazepam, carbamazepine and dipropylacetate. Neuropediatrie 8:29–41
Winfield DA, Benton P, Espir, MLE, Arthur LJH (1976) Sodium valproate and thrombocytopenia. Br Med J II:981

CHAPTER 27

Adverse Effects

D. SCHMIDT

A. Introduction

Although any review devoted to adverse effects alone without reference to therapeutic benefits is in danger of exaggerating the side effects of antiepileptic drug therapy – and many side effects are less disabling than uncontrolled seizures – it is reasonable to expect that many of the changes in the neurological, psychological, and medical status of a patient may in fact not be due to epilepsy itself but are rather due to the adverse effects of drugs. A growing concern about the adverse effects of antiepileptic drugs has led to many reports on their unintended reactions. In these studies adverse effects ranged from rather rare and mostly unpredictable drug-induced diseases to more frequent, transient, and mostly mild, dose-dependent side effects. In this review adverse effects are classified from a clinical point of view. Section C.I covers the more common side effects encountered during treatment with each individual antiepileptic drug, and in Sect. C.II each organ or organ system is reviewed separately as it is adversely affected by antiepileptic drug treatment. Furthermore, this overview is primarily based on the more recent literature, since earlier reviews on acute or chronic toxicity (PLAA 1975; REYNOLDS 1975) have covered the data published up to 1975. In addition, the interested reader is referred to a more detailed recent monograph on adverse effects of antiepileptic drugs (SCHMIDT and SELDON 1982).

B. Mechanism of Adverse Effects

As outlined in the "Introduction", adverse effects may be classified into more frequent side effects, which are mostly mild and reversible due to their dose dependency, and rather rare and frequently unpredictable drug-induced diseases. The pathophysiological basis of adverse drug reactions has recently been reviewed in detail (REYNOLDS 1975; PERUCCA and RICHENS 1980; SCHMIDT and SELDON 1982).

I. Dose-Dependent Side Effects

In recent years the plasma concentrations of antiepileptic drugs have been monitored in patients with clinical signs of dose-dependent drug toxicity. This has led to the definition of toxic plasma concentrations of individual antiepileptic drugs above which a majority of patients can be expected to develop side effects. In order to put these statistical data in a proper clinical perspective it is useful to be aware of the great variability in toxic concentrations from patient to patient. Furthermore, intraindividual variation may be seen in clinical toxicity with rising plasma concentration of the drug. Therefore, it seems useful to consider separately (a) the pharmacokinetic mechanism of the increase in plasma concentration and (b) the pathophysiological basis of clinical drug toxicity.

The pathogenetic mechanisms leading to an increase in plasma concentration of antiepileptic drugs include an increase in daily dose, drug interactions, and changes in physiological conditions or additional disease, as reviewed in other chapters in the section on "Clinical Pharmacology" in this volume.

The factors regulating the clinical response to an increase in the plasma concentration are less known. A number of clinical variables have been shown to influence the clinical toxicity in relation to the plasma concentration. These include the development of tolerance, i.e., clinical drug toxicity is diminished or disappears during continued drug treatment as reviewed in Chap. 11. In addition, the abrupt termination of antiepileptic drug treatment may lead to withdrawal reactions as outlined in Chap. 11. The age of the patient may influence the clinical toxicity of a drug, e.g., the sedative effects of plasma concentrations of diazepam are stronger in older patients (REIDENBERG et al. 1978). Hypoalbuminemic patients carry a higher risk of developing side effects during phenytoin treatment (*Boston Collaborative Drug Surveillance Program* 1973), probably due to an increased unbound fraction of the plasma phenytoin concentration.

II. Drug-Induced Diseases

For most of the drug-induced diseases we are only beginning to understand the pathogenetic mechanisms involved. Nevertheless, it has become increasingly apparent that antiepileptic drug-induced diseases do develop in high-risk subgroups of epileptic patients. The nature of these risk factors differs with the respective disease. Antiepileptic drugs may therefore act by precipitation of clinical disease in predisposed patients. An example is the increased incidence of anticonvulsant osteomalacia, which mainly occurs in patients with insufficient nutrition, lack of sun exposure, and poor physical exercise. These factors alone induce osteomalacia even without antiepileptic drug treatment.

There are only a few examples where we know that disease is caused or aggravated by an altered target organ response of the individual. The precipitation of acute porphyria with enzyme-inducing antiepileptic drugs is such an example (MAGNUSSEN et al. 1975). Myasthenia gravis may be worsened by the intake of antiepileptic drugs, especially hydantoins (BRUMLIK and JACOBS 1974).

The increased knowledge of risk factors for each of the antiepileptic drug-induced diseases will help to define high-risk groups for specific complications of antiepileptic drug treatment. This will improve our ability for risk-counseling prior to the introduction of new drug treatment and will alert the patient and the physician to the detection of early diagnostic features. This in turn will improve the management of drug-induced diseases.

Finally, the most common antiepileptic drug-induced diseases are due to hypersensitivity reactions. The pathophysiological basis for hypersensitivity reactions has been reviewed by PERUCCA and RICHENS (1980).

C. Adverse Effects

The following section reviews the clinical drug toxicity observed in studies on the therapeutic and toxic effects of individual antiepileptic drugs. The toxic effects noted in these studies are mostly dose related and usually subside after dose reduction or withdrawal of the drug. Antiepileptic drug-induced or chronic toxicity is reviewed separately for each organ system (Sect. C.II) and will therefore not be referred to in the following section on each individual drug.

I. Adverse Effects of Individual Antiepileptic Drugs

1. Hydantoins

Phenytoin is by far the most commonly used hydantoin and a primary antiepileptic drug. Mephenytoin is used less often due to its side effects. Methetoin, ethotoin, and albutoin are tertiary antiepileptic drugs.

a) Phenytoin

The majority of patients develop only mild and transient side effects during treatment with phenytoin, mostly at plasma concentrations above 20 μg/ml (Kutt et al. 1964; Plaa 1975). Buchthal et al. (1960) reported as early as 1960 that none of their 86 patients with plasma levels below 14 μg/ml showed signs of toxicity, while above a plasma concentration of 30 μg/ml nearly 75% of the patients complained of side effects. Despite considerable individual variability, a certain sequence of clinical symptoms of drug toxicity can be observed in the individual patient with increasing plasma levels. Phenytoin intoxication may begin at plasma levels of 20 μg/ml with anxiety and increasing irritability, followed by a fine resting-tremor, diplopia, and fatigue. Nystagmus may appear on extreme lateral gaze. With plasma concentrations above 30 μg/ml ataxia and bulbar speech appear (Kutt et al. 1964). At plasma concentrations above 40 μg/ml impaired memory and reduced intellectual performance may set in (Kutt et al. 1964).

Marked bulbar speech, nystagmus on straight forward gaze, loss of appetite, vomiting, and weight loss may occur, frequently together with increasing apathy and sedation. Neurological and psychiatric syndromes are discussed in Sect. C.II.1. At plasma concentrations above 60 μg/ml the patient may develop somnolence and coma (Kutt et al. 1964).

Hypersensitivity reactions with exanthema have also been recorded (Haruda 1979). No significant hemodynamic side effects are seen in otherwise healthy epileptic patients, as reviewed in Sect. C.II.8.c. Gingival hyperplasia and hirsutism may develop (Sect. C.II.8.b). Fatal intoxications with phenytoin have been reported with a plasma concentration of 94 μg/ml 24 h after ingestion (Laubscher 1966). On the other hand, patients have survived the ingestion of 3.9–21.5 g phenytoin and plasma concentrations of 112 μg/ml with subsequent peritoneal dialysis (Theil et al. 1961; Tenckhoff et al. 1968). Children have tolerated doses of up to 300 mg/kg and plasma concentrations of 108–112 μg/ml (Wilder et al. 1973; Pruitt et al. 1975). It is therefore difficult to give a reasonable estimate of the mean lethal dose of phenytoin.

The most common cause for phenytoin intoxications is a dose increment of more than 50 mg, which disregards the nonlinear pharmacokinetics of phenytoin at plasma concentrations of above 15–20 μg/ml, where a small dose increment results in a steep rise in the plasma concentration. Another common factor is the interaction with other drugs, either antiepileptic drugs or other medications.

Hemodialysis, forced diuresis, peritoneal dialysis, or complete substitution transfusion and charcoal hemoperfusion have had little clinical effect in patients with phenytoin intoxication. Intensive care treatment with control of the plasma concentration is most successful.

b) Mephenytoin

The side effects of mephenytoin range from harmless eosinophilia, lymphadenopathy, sedation, and allergic exanthemas in about 5% of the patients (LOSCALZO 1952) up to occasionally fatal aplastic anemias (ABBOTT and SCHWAB 1954). Altogether, about 3% of the patients treated with mephenytoin develop serious aplastic anemia (see Sect. C.II.2).

c) Miscellaneous Hydantoins

Methetoin, 1-methyl-5,5-phenylethylhydantoin, is as effective as phenytoin but has more severe side effects, including exanthema (10%), drowsiness (18%), and leukopenia (3%) (LOGOTHETIS 1967). Side effects of ethotoin are thought to occur less frequently than with phenytoin. They include exanthema (2%), anorexia and vomiting (3%), lymphadenopathy, drowsiness, nystagmus, and ataxia. Gingival hyperplasia and hirsutism are not reported (MILLICHAP 1972).

Reports on the clinical toxicity of albutoin include exanthema, nausea, vomiting and abdominal discomfort and weight loss (CEREGHINO et al. 1972; MILLICHAP 1972).

2. Phenobarbital

In spite of a number of reports on the antiepileptic effects of phenobarbital, which is the oldest of the modern antiepileptic drugs, specific studies on its side effects in adult patients are scarce. PATEISKY and PRESSLICH (1970) reported drowsiness, vertigo, impaired sexual potency, leukopenia, tachycardia, and bulbar speech as side effects in 15 out of 40 adult patients receiving Barbexaclone (*N*-benzoyl-phenobarbital). Unfortunately the corresponding plasma concentrations were not available. Most studies on adverse effects were conducted on children with febrile convulsions, and it was discovered that over half of the patients showed adverse effects at plasma concentrations of 10–12 μg/ml (THORN 1975). A recent report summarized the potential risk of phenobarbital treatment for febrile convulsions (*Consensus Statement* 1980). Side effects or toxic reactions were reported in up to 40% of infants or children receiving phenobarbital. These reactions included: (1) behavioral changes with hyperactivity up to extreme irritability, and only rarely somnolence, (2) disturbances in sleep rhythms with prolonged nocturnal waking periods, and (3) interference with higher cortical or cognitive functions, e.g., inattentiveness, impaired short-term memory, or reduced general comprehension. The therapy was discontinued in up to one-third of the patients (12% – 32%) (THORN 1975; HECKMATT et al. 1976; WOLF et al. 1977) due to hyperactivity behavioral disturbances, loss of sleep, drowsiness, exanthema, and ataxia. Drowsiness is undoubtedly the most frequent complaint of patients receiving phenobarbital. It usually begins at the onset of treatment and mostly subsides in a few weeks, probably due to the development of tolerance to the sedative action. During long-term treatment adult patients show sedation and ataxia (sometimes without nystagmus) at plasma levels of 50–60 μg/ml and above. Impaired concentration, lack of appetite, and loss of initiative may be due to phenobarbital intoxication.

At plasma levels of 80 μg/ml, patients who are under long-term treatment show ataxia of the trunk, nausea, vomiting, and nystagmus. If the plasma values rise above 100 μg/ml phenobarbital, the patient becomes soporous. A coarse, continuous nystagmus becomes apparent as well as the inability to sit upright in bed due to severe dizziness and ataxia of the trunk. At plasma levels above 120 μg/ml, the patient becomes comatose (HANCOCK 1974). Such high plasma levels are tolerated only in chronically treated epileptic patients who have developed a tolerance for the sedative effect of phenobarbital.

The sudden withdrawal of phenobarbital from epileptic patients may lead to withdrawal symptoms, including exacerbation of seizures that sometimes proceeds to a status epilepticus (BUCHTHAL et al. 1968). Even neonatal infants of epileptic mothers who took phenobarbital during pregnancy suffer from withdrawal symptoms like irritability, hypotonia, and vomiting (ERITH 1975).

The lethal dose varies from 4 to 6 g for previously untreated patients (MOESCHLIN 1972). On the other hand, a dose of 25 g was survived (PUKA and SZAJEWSKI 1975). Forced diuresis and alkalinization may improve the rate of survival. Activated charcoal impairs the absorption of phenobarbital and may be given in severe intoxications.

3. Primidone

In spite of its early introduction in 1952, only a few studies have investigated the adverse effects of primidone. During treatment with primidone, sedative side effects and ataxia occur in about 20% of the patients, usually at plasma levels of more than 8 μg/ml primidone. At a daily dose of more than 2,000 mg, lethargy, dysarthria, ataxia, and difficulties in getting up in the morning are reported in one-third of patients (RODIN et al. 1976). Primidone treatment has had to be discontinued in 10%–20% of all patients due to adverse effects (e.g., TROLLE 1961).

Most of the side effects occur during the onset of primidone treatment. Vertigo, nausea, vomiting, drowsiness, and ataxia are usually caused by a high initial dose and can be avoided by a gradual increase in total dose. Among previously untreated patients, the initial adverse effects are in large part due to primidone rather than its metabolites phenobarbital or phenylethylmalonamide (PEMA) (BRILLMAN et al. 1974). Phenobarbital, one of the major metabolites of primidone, usually appears in the serum of patients 24–96 h after initiation of therapy (FINCHAM et al. 1974). If the patient has already received antiepileptic drugs such as phenobarbital, phenytoin, or carbamazepine, the primidone dose can be increased more rapidly because the patient has developed a tolerance (GALLAGHER et al. 1973). This tolerance is due to pharmacokinetic changes, with an increased metabolism of primidone, and to the development of a functional adaptation in the brain (GALLAGHER et al. 1973). At serum primidone levels in excess of 100 μg/

ml, dysarthric speech, ataxia, and somnolence or sopor are usually present. Nystagmus may not be seen in all patients.

Despite a dose reduction or withdrawal the phenobarbital levels may continue to rise in the next 24 h. The plasma concentration of primidone falls rapidly with a biological half-life of 15 h (BRILLMAN et al. 1974). At less than 80 μg/ml primidone, the patients are tired and nystagmus becomes evident; vertigo, nausea, nystagmus, ataxia, and dysarthria recede within the next 2 days. After 5 days the patients are generally neurologically normal.

The abrupt discontinuation of primidone can lead to withdrawal symptoms such als sleeplessness, irritability, tremor, and grand mal. The symptoms do not appear during the rapid drop in primidone plasma levels but rather between the 5th and 11th day after discontinuing primidone, when phenobarbital seems to fall below a critical level (personal observation).

Fatal intoxications have very rarely been reported with primidone alone (MORLEY and WYNNE 1957), primidone and phenobarbital (FAZEKAS and RENGEL 1960), and primidone and methsuximide (JOHNSON et al. 1976). During the first 24 h of an intoxication with plasma concentrations of more than 100 μg/ml primidone, white shimmering primidone crystals can be observed in the urine as sediment (MORLEY and WYNNE 1957). Treatment of primidone intoxication consists of forced diuresis or dialysis.

4. Carbamazepine

Side effects occur in approximately one of three patients during treatment with carbamazepine. The list of adverse effects is long, with drowsiness, diplopia, ataxia, exanthema, vertigo, leukopenia, nystagmus, headaches, tremor, dry mouth, and behavioral disturbances appearing in order of decreasing frequency (SCHMIDT and SELDON 1982). Most of the side effects are mild, transient, and dose dependent. A correlation between serum carbamazepine levels and side effects has been reported (TOMSON et al. 1980). During multiple-drug therapy side effects are seen more often due to drug interactions.

Exanthema occurs in about 3.7% of patients and is usually treated by the withdrawal of carbamazepine (GAYFORD and REDPATH 1969). Bone marrow depression, leukopenia, or aplastic anemia may be dose-dependent side effects or hypersensitivity reactions. In one case, carbamazepine caused a double quotidian fever in a patient with no other adverse reactions or evidence of hypersensitivity (STEWART et al. 1980). Ingestion of 20 g (100 tablets) (GRUSKA et al. 1971) and plasma concentrations of 35 μg/ml registered 5 h after ingestion were not fatal. Recently two fatal intoxications were reported by KRARUP and MOGENSEN (1981). Overdosage with carbamazepine results in tremor, agitation, and changes in reflexes, followed by reduced levels of consciousness, hypertension, and coma. Treatment should be supportive.

5. Valproic Acid

Side effects are seen in about a fourth of the patients treated with valproic acid only. These include increased appetite, hair loss, sleepiness, tremor, paresthesias, increased weight, and drowsiness. The sedative side effects often seem to be due to a rise in the phenobarbital plasma concentration when valproic acid is added to phenobarbital (SIMON and PENRY 1975; PINDER et al. 1977; RUUSKANEN et al. 1979). Gastrointestinal discomfort, nausea, and vomiting are noticeably rarer when enteric-coated preparations are taken (JOHANNESSEN and HENRIKSEN 1980; SHERARD et al. 1980). Hematological side effects of valproic acid are reviewed in Sect. C.II.2. Acute liver failure or pancreatitis have recently raised doubts about the choice of valproic acid as the preferred drug for primary generalized epilepsies (see Sect. C.II.5). However, a mild increase in transaminase levels in asymptomatic patients has little clinical significance and is reversible upon dose reduction (see Sect. C.II.5). Exposure to valproic acid during early pregnancy has been associated with an increased presumptive risk for neural tube defects in the offspring as reviewed in Sect. C.II.4. WILDER et al. (1978) report a rare case of a hypersensitivity reaction with exanthema due to valproic acid. BOWDLE et al. (1979) reported an acute intoxication with drowsiness, reduced ability to concentrate, malaise, stammering or slurred speech, and frequent bad dreams in six volunteers given 1–1.5 g valproic acid daily. CHADWICK et al. (1978) described two epileptic patients who developed an acute toxic encephalopathy. STEIMAN et al. (1979) described a coma in a 19-month-old boy (11 kg) who accidentally ingested about 2,250 mg valproic acid. Naxolone (0.01 mg/kg) was given intravenously, and within 3 minutes the infant awoke and was able to sit up. There have been rare cases of coma during valproic acid therapy, but whether they are caused by valproic acid alone or are due to a phenobarbital intoxication is unclear since few patients received valproic acid alone, and since the plasma concentrations were not determined in all patients receiving additional antiepileptic drugs. TIFT (1980) reported one case of valproic acid-induced fatal coma after a high initial dose. An autopsy revealed massive pulmonary edema.

6. Trimethadione

LIVINGSTON and BOKS (1955) reported photophobia in 20% of 1,200 children treated with trimethadione. In addition, they reported diplopia, vertigo, increased irritability, drowsiness, headaches, insomnia, and personality and behavioral changes in their patients. In 3% of the patients exanthemas were seen. Exanthema was associated with pancytopenia, fever, arthralgia, and hepatitis in isolated cases (LIVINGSTON and BOKS 1955). In 4% of the cases hiccups occurred during early treatment and subsided spontaneously. Fatal cases due to hematological disorders have been reported (DREYER 1959). Furthermore, trimethadione was held responsible for the development of nephrotic syndromes in several cases (CHAMBERLIN et al. 1965).

7. Succinimides

a) Ethosuximide

Ethosuximide produced adverse effects in 112 out of 694 patients (16%). These were either gastrointestinal complaints including hiccups or rare psychiatric complications. The medication was discontinued in 5% (33 out of 694) of the cases due to insomnia, psychotic episodes, dyspepsia, aplastic anemia, or vomiting

(SCHMIDT 1981 a). Occasionally the patients complain of agonizing headaches. One case of a fatal aplastic anemia occurring during ethosuximide treatment is worth mentioning (FISCHER et al. 1965); however, the patient also received acetazolamide and mephobarbital. Despite anecdotal reports there is no good clinical evidence that ethosuximide contributes to the exacerbation of generalized tonic-clonic seizures (LORENTZ DE HAAS and KUILMAN 1964).

b) Methsuximide

Methsuximide led to adverse effects in every third patient (STRONG et al. 1974). Furthermore, the incidence of side effects is higher with multiple-drug therapy due to a methsuximide-induced increase in the plasma concentrations of phenytoin or phenobarbital. Gastrointestinal symptoms like nausea and hiccups are secondary to the sedative side effects (SCHMIDT 1981 a).

In two patients with an overdose of methsuximide, coma developed which was fatal in one case (KARCH 1973; BAEHLER et al. 1980). In both cases, *N*-desmethylmethsuximide, a metabolite of methsuximide, was primarily responsible for the CNS depression.

8. Benzodiazepines

a) Clonazepam

Clonazepam often causes side effects as demonstrated by 334 out of 674 patients (50%) in uncontrolled studies (SCHMIDT and SELDON 1982). In controlled studies the incidence rose to 72% (60%–74%). In most cases, however, they were mild and reversible (PINDER et al. 1976; BROWNE 1978). Nonetheless, in 6%–10% of all cases clonazepam had to be discontinued, i.e., several times more often than reported for either ethosuximide or valproic acid treatment.

The most common side effect is sedation, followed by muscular hypotonia and ataxia. Hypersalivation also occurs, accompanied by increased bronchial secretion, which can create respiratory insufficiency. Finally, it has been suggested that clonazepam induces tonic seizures (BITTENCOURT and RICHENS 1981).

Behavioral disturbances may be associated with clonazepam treatment, especially in children. The affected children are variously described as irritable, aggressive, and excitable (BROWNE 1976; see Sect. C.II.1). An additional difficulty is the incidence of ictal withdrawal symptoms (BROWNE 1978) and the development of tolerance to the anticonvulsant effect. WELCH et al. (1977) described cyclic coma in a case of clonazepam overdose in which agitated alertness alternated with unresponsive coma with pinpoint pupils.

b) Diazepam

The most serious but fortunately rare side effects after intravenous injection of diazepam are apnea, hypotension, cardiac arrest, and obtundation. After intravenous administration for status epilepticus mild to severe hypotension or respiratory depression occurred in 5.2% of 246 patients, including one fatal case with additional sedative medication (SCHMIDT 1982a). In otherwise apparently healthy patients with epilepsy slow intravenous administration usually produces no clinically significant hypotension or hypoventilation (NIEDERMEYER 1970). The pathogenesis of the hypotensive and respiratory depressant action of diazepam may involve the solvent propylene glycol (MATTSON 1972). Risk factors for increased incidence of side effects include additional intake of drugs such as barbiturates, lidocaine/epinephrine, methaqualone, chlordiazepoxide, and even a rapid (bolus) injection of as little as 2.5 or 5 mg. Dose-dependent side effects such as drowsiness, ataxia, and dizziness are seen in up to 10%–40% of patients at the onset of oral treatment (BROWNE and PENRY 1973).

Diazepam and *N*-desmethyldiazepam are transferred through the placenta and will remain in neonatal plasma for several days, causing mostly sedative effects and muscular hypotonia (ANDRE et al. 1973), especially in premature babies with sligthly lower Apgar scores (ROSANELLI 1970), and possibly neonatal withdrawal symptoms (REMENTERIA and BHATT 1977). Usually mild thrombophlebitis occurs in about 3%–7% of all patients after intravenous administration (LANGDON et al. 1973). There are reported cases of accidental intra-arterial injection leading to extensive tissue necrosis and amputation (GOULD and LINGAM 1977).

c) Nitrazepam

Nitrazepam is primarily utilized as an adjunct to standard anticonvulsant drugs and causes mostly mild side effects in the majority of patients. In 15% of patients the drug had to be discontinued due to drowsiness, ataxia, bulbar speech, and an increase in the seizure frequency (PETERSON 1967; SNYDER 1968). Increased salivation, drooling, and bronchial secretion increase the risk of pneumonia (MILLICHAP and ORTIZ 1966). HIRSCH (1968) reported that a 15-year-old girl survived ingestion of 130 mg nitrazepam.

9. Miscellaneous Antiepileptic Drugs

a) Acetazolamide

The toxicity of acetazolamide was extensively reviewd by WOODBURY (1972), who considers it as one of the least toxic of the antiepileptic drugs. Apart from hypersensitivity reactions, all adverse effects appear to be related to the inhibition of carbonic anhydrase. Acetazolamide may impair the absorption of primidone (SYVERSEN et al. 1977).

b) Adrenocorticotrophic Hormone, Corticoids

Treatment of infantile spasms with adrenocorticotrophic hormone (ACTH) or corticoids leads to side effects in up to one-third of the treated children (with a mortality of 4.9%) (RIIKONEN and DONNER 1980). The authors describe oliguria and hyperkalemia leading to tubular necrosis, and infections, which were more common with large doses of ACTH (120 units) than with small ones (40 units). Other adverse effects include arterial hypertension; Cushing syndrome; osteoporosis; electrolyte disturbances; stomach, intestinal, and intracerebral hemorrhages; heart failure secondary to excessive fluid retention; sometimes fatal septic infections; pneumonias; and urinary and gastrointestinal infections (LACY and PENRY 1976). During ACTH treatment a transient increase of the internal and external subarachnoid space was detected by cranial computed tomography (MAEKAWA et al. 1980).

c) Beclamide

Several patients complained about nausea and anorexia (WILSON et al. 1959).

d) Bromides

Nowadays bromides are used only rarely in patients who do not tolerate barbiturates or hydantoins due to a porphyria (MAGNUSSEN et al. 1975) or as a last resort in drug treatment of intractable epilepsy or in patients with anticonvulsant-induced aplastic anemia. MOSES and KLAWANS (1979) accumulated a comprehensive list of symptoms of bromide intoxication.

e) Sulthiame

The acute toxic effects of sulthiame have recently been reviewed by GREEN and KUPFERBERG (1972) and PLAA (1975). Over one-third of the patients receiving sulthiame demonstrate side effects. Tachypnoea, paresthesia, and weight loss are peculiar side effects of sulthiame. Gastrointestinal disturbances, weight loss, dizziness, and ataxia are among the frequent adverse effects (SCHMIDT and SELDON 1982). In one patient a polyneuropathy was observed during sulthiame treatment (FILIPIDIS and SUCHENWIRTH 1968). An overdose of sulthiame (LAUBENTHAL and RAFFAUF 1963; ROCKLEY 1965), which ended fatally in one case (AHREND et al. 1969), and acute renal failure during sulthiame treatment (AVIRAM et al. 1965) have been reported.

II. Antiepileptic Drug-Induced Diseases

1. Neurological and Psychiatric Disorders Including Neuropsychological Disturbances

a) Neurological Disorders

A vestibular-cerebellar syndrome with gaze nystagmus, ataxia, and dysarthria may develop at high plasma concentrations of individual antiepileptic drugs (PLAA 1975). Cerebellar atrophy or degeneration (MCLAIN et al. 1980), a diffuse loss of Purkinje cells (GHATAK et al. 1976), and lamellar inclusions in the cerebellar cortex (DEL CERRO and SNIDER 1970) were reported in epileptic patients treated with phenytoin. The available equivocal evidence suggests that phenytoin may contribute to cerebellar degeneration in high-risk patients (see SCHMIDT and SELDON 1982). In some patients a so-called anticonvulsant encephalopathy has been observed with progressive mental deterioration, brain stem and cerebellar signs, electroencephalographic changes, and an increased seizure frequency during treatment with phenytoin (LEVY and FENICHEL 1965; MEISTRUP-LARSEN et al. 1979), carbamazepine (SALCMAN and PIPPENGER 1975), and valproic acid (CHADWICK et al. 1978; COULTER and ALLEN 1980 b). Furthermore, diazepam or nitrazepam may induce tonic seizures or even status epilepticus (TASSINARI et al. 1972; BITTENCOURT and RICHENS 1981). Tremor may develop during treatment with valproic acid (HYMAN et al. 1979), phenytoin (GITLIN and MORRIS 1976), and primidone (FORMAN et al. 1979). A transient, total external ophthalmoplegia and a loss of oculovestibular and oculocephalic reflexes may develop in comatose patients with phenytoin or primidone intoxication (ORTH et al. 1967; SPECTOR et al. 1976). Transient hemiplegia and pathological grasp reflexes have been reported in single cases and in doubtful relation to drug treatment. Increased CSF protein, cell count, and meningeal irritation have been associated with phenytoin treatment (see REYNOLDS 1975). Facial hyperkinesia, choreoathetosis, bradykinesia, dyskinesia, and asterixis have been observed quite often without other signs of CNS drug toxicity. Phenytoin may also intensify phenothiazine-induced tardive dyskinesia. A mild, mostly sensory polyneuropathy has been noted in 8.5%–18% of epileptic patients receiving long-term treatment with phenytoin, often together with other anticonvulsants (SO and PENRY 1981). Anticonvulsant-induced EEG changes are dependent on the type of drug and its plasma concentration and on as yet less well-defined individual factors (SCHMIDT 1982b).

b) Psychiatric Disorders

Somnolence, stupor, and finally a comatose state may develop with toxic plasma concentrations (ROSEMAN 1961; WILDER and RAMSAY 1974). In some patients confusion or "hysterical" behavior may be the leading psychopathological manifestations of antiepileptic drug toxicity (NIEDERMEYER et al. 1970). SHERARD et al. (1980) reported on five patients who were treated with barbiturates and showed emotional upset, aggression, or hyperactivity when valproic acid was added. But the symptoms remitted when the barbiturate dosage alone was reduced. At plasma levels above 100 μg/ml valproic acid alone may lead to altered behavior and confusion (CHADWICK et al. 1978). A high plasma concentration or clinical drug toxicity is, however, not necessarily present in patients developing anticonvulsant-induced psychotic episodes. MCDANAL and BOLMAN (1975) described a delayed, phenytoin-induced psychotic episode at phenytoin plasma concentrations of as low as 3.2 μg/ml. ROSEMAN (1961) described a case of delirium following phenytoin withdrawal. Finally, a so-called "alternative psychosis" may develop when seizures have been controlled and epileptic discharges have disappeared from the EEG (LANDOLT 1956). Ethosuximide seems to be more often involved than other antiepileptic drugs in the development of alternative psychoses. Valproic acid, in contrast, does not seem to precipitate alternative psychoses. The clinical features of these acute psychotic episodes include paranoid thoughts and sometimes hallucinations heralded by insomnia, withdrawal, and anxiety.

c) Neuropsychological Disturbances

The correlation between antiepileptic drug treatment and impairment of cognitive function or behavior is difficult to evaluate (TRIMBLE and REYNOLDS 1976; STORES 1975; TRIMBLE 1983). There are only a few prospective neuropsychological studies of epileptic patients before and during treatment with antiepileptic drugs. Thus there are often methodological difficulties in defining the psychological status prior to the epilepsy and the influence of antiepileptic drugs or the effect of seizures on the neuropsychological status. We will therefore shortly summarize the relatively few studies on specific neuropsychological side effects of the individual drugs.

The neuropsychological effects of 1–30 months of treatment with ethosuximide and phenobarbital have been tested by GUEY et al. (1967). The

Wechsler IQ test for children indicated decreasing IQs. The score of the Bender test of visual retention dropped in 60% of the patients. The Rorschach test indicated an increase in stereotyping and aggressivity in eight out of one nine patients. BROWNE et al. (1975) tested language, perception, motor performance, intelligence, and cognition in 37 children with previously untreated absences. Out of the 37 patients 17 improved their performance; only one achieved a lower score.

Several studies have compared the neuropsychological effects of carbamazepine with those of other anticonvulsants. Patients treated with carbamazepine showed fewer psychopathic changes on the Minnesota Multifactorial Personality Inventory and fewer depressive tendencies than those treated with primidone (RODIN et al. 1974) or phenytoin (DODRILL and TROUPIN 1977). SCHAIN et al. (1977) replaced primidone, phenobarbital, or phenytoin by carbamazepine and found an increased attentiveness in 37 out of 45 epileptic children. In a double-blind study of 22 patients who were difficult to treat, DODRILL (1975) found consistently worse neuropsychological test results and more frequent seizures during therapy with sulthiame compared with treatment with phenytoin alone. Negative effects of phenytoin on learning were shown by ROWLEY and GAURON (1977). THOMPSON (1983), in a recent review suggested that there is little evidence that phenytoin has any adverse effects on behavior; on the other hand, it may have a detrimental effect on cognitive functions, especially at high plasma concentrations. Valproic acid would seem to be the compound with the least influence on cognitive and behavioral impairment when compared with phenytoin or phenobarbital (TRIMBLE 1982).

Phenobarbital and primidone are usually thought to have sedative side effects. Surprisingly, few controlled studies have been performed. HUTT et al. (1968) and IDESTRÖM et al. (1972) found a decrease in attentiveness related to the plasma concentration of phenobarbital and phenytoin. WAPNER et al. (1962), in a study of 36 epileptic children, noted no change in learning abilities after 6 weeks of treatment with phenobarbital. The exacerbation of hyperkinetic syndromes among children treated with phenobarbital was recognized early (OUNSTED 1955). In a careful prospective study on the influence of phenobarbital on the psychomotor development and behavior in preschool children with convulsions, a transient deterioration of fine motor functions and behavioral disturbances was found in most children during the first weeks and months. The problems subsided thereafter and at a 1-year follow-up, the drug-induced changes had disappeared (HELLSTRÖM and BARLACH-CHRISTOFFERSEN 1980). This report underlines the need for further studies on the correlation of adverse behavioral effects and impairment of cognitive function of phenobarbital to its plasma concentrations.

It is quite possible that antiepileptic drugs contribute to or exacerbate underlying behavioral or neuropsychological disturbances of the individual patient. If that is the case, it may be possible to define subgroups of epileptic patients who are especially vulnerable to neuropsychological side effects of antiepileptic drugs.

2. Blood Disorders Including Lymphoma

a) Aplastic Anemia (Panmyelopathy, Pancytopenia)

Mephenytoin is most frequently incriminated in the development of anticonvulsant-induced aplastic anemia (DREYER 1959; HEIMPEL 1974). Rare case reports include phenytoin, primidone, trimethadione, ethosuximide, phenacemide, methsuximide, and 3-methyl-5-phenylhydantoin and carbamazepine (PISCIOTTA 1975; REYNOLDS 1975; SCHMIDT and SELDON 1982). Aplastic anemia may appear from 2 weeks to 2 years after the onset of treatment (DREYER 1959; ROBINS 1962; PISCIOTTA 1975) and usually includes anemia, thrombocytopenia, and leukopenia accompanied by neutropenia. Phenytoin has been implicated in the development of reversible erythroid aplasia and a dose-related panmyeloid hypoplasia (PARKER and GUMNIT 1974). Early diagnosis of aplastic anemia is essential. Any fever of unknown etiology accompanied by general weakness and anemia is suggestive of aplastic anemia. Even frequent differential blood counts have no good predictive value for the usually rapid development of aplastic anemia. The mortality may be as high as 77% (ISAACSON et al. 1956; ROBINS 1962).

b) Megaloblastic Anemia

Megaloblastic anemia develops in about 0.15%–0.75% of patients receiving anticonvulsants (see REYNOLDS 1975). In the great majority of cases, it has been associated with phenytoin alone or in combination with phenobarbital, primidone alone or in combination with phenobarbital, mephenytoin, or the combination of phensuximide and phenobarbital (see SCHMIDT and SELDON 1982). Megaloblastic anemia may appear 1 month to 21 years after starting anticonvulsant treatment. The patients often have additional psychiatric symptoms. Macrocytosis (in the absence of anemia) has been observed in 30%–40% of all patients being treated with phenytoin or phenobarbital. Macrocytosis is thus much more frequent but apparently of little clinical relevance.

The pathogenesis of megaloblastic anemia has not been conclusively determined, but folate deficiency is primarily implicated (see SCHMIDT and SELDON 1982). CHASSAGNON et al. (1967) suggest folic acid substitution with 5–25 mg daily; however, as little as 500 μg daily has produced remission (FLEXNER and HARTMANN 1960). Withdrawal of the anticonvulsant is usually not necessary.

c) Folate Deficiency

Low serum folate levels without anemia have been noted in 10%–91% of epileptic patients (NORRIS and PRATT 1974; see REYNOLDS 1975). The pathogenetic mechanism is controversial (see REYNOLDS 1975). Uncontrolled studies and individual case histories led to the fear that the substitution of folate could precipitate seizures or psychiatric complications (REYNOLDS 1975). This was not confirmed in controlled studies (NORRIS and PRATT 1974). At present no definite disorder can be attributed to lowered folate levels in nonanemic patients. Therefore, substitution therapy is not recommended. In addition, administration of folate lowers the plasma concentrations of phenytoin or phenobarbital.

No vitamin B_{12} deficiency has yet been discovered among patients treated with antiepileptic drugs (CARNEY 1969). Hypochromic anemia has been observed in individual cases during treatment with ethosuximide and phensuximide (WEINSTEIN and ALLEN 1966).

Acquired hemolytic anemia secondary to autoantibodies has been diagnosed during treatment with phenytoin and mephenytoin in some patients (SNAPPER et al. 1953). Some patients develop a syndrome resembling infectious mononucleosis during the first weeks of phenytoin therapy (KLECKNER et al. 1975).

d) Agranulocytosis and Leukopenia

Agranulocytosis has been observed usually during the first 3 months of treatment with phenytoin alone, phenobarbital, ethosuximide, carbamazepine, trimethadione, and mephenytoin, as well as with a multiple-drug therapy with carbamazepine (PISCIOTTA 1975; REYNOLDS 1975; SCHMIDT and SELDON 1982). Agranulocytosis is usually associated with other signs of hypersensitivity, e.g., fever, rash, splenomegaly, eosinophilia, lymphadenopathy and increased serum glutamic oxaloacetic transferase or serum glutamic pyruvic transferase values. Antibody-mediated suppression of granulopoiesis has been suggested to be a major mechanism in the induction of agranulocytosis (TAETLE et al. 1979).

Leukopenia and a slight thrombocytopenia may develop during the first 3 weeks of treatment with phenytoin or carbamazepine, even at low plasma levels, and disappear during the treatment without a reduction in the dose of the drug. Unfortunately long-term studies on this effect of carbamazepine or phenytoin are lacking. Lymphocytopenia has been reported with phenytoin therapy by MACKINNEY and BOOKER (1972). This was not confirmed by SEAGER (1976).

e) Lymphadenopathy

Patients receiving anticonvulsant therapy may develop significant lymphadenopathy as part of a hypersensitivity reaction usually 1 week to 4 months after the onset of treatment. The diagnosis may be difficult and lymph node biopsy may be misleading (SALTZSTEIN and ACKERMAN 1959; SPARBERG 1963). A number of drugs have been implicated. These include phenytoin alone (LAPES et al. 1976b; SEYFEDDINIPUR 1976), phenobarbital (MCGEACHY and BLOOMER 1953), trimethadione, mephenytoin, phensuximide, and ethotoin (SALTZSTEIN and ACKERMAN 1959; HYMAN and SOMMERS 1966). Withdrawal of the offending drug is followed by regression of the lymphadenopathy within 1–2 weeks, but it can recur after reexposure (SEYFEDDINIPUR 1976). Very rarely a malignant lymphoma may develop from benign lymphadenopathy (LAPES et al. 1976a).

f) Malignant Lymphoma

Malignant lymphoma has been observed among patients after 2–28 years of treatment with phenytoin (BICHEL 1975) and a combination of phenobarbital with mephobarbital or primidone and ethosuximide (SALTZSTEIN and ACKERMAN 1959; ANTHONY 1970; LI et al. 1975). In contrast to the benign lymphadenopathies, the histologically and clinically malignant lymphomas usually appear after year-long therapy and without signs of hypersensitivity. If discontinuation or substitution of the drug brings no remission, a malignant lymphoma may be suspected (ALBERTO et al. 1971). Hodgkin's disease (LEDERLIN et al. 1976) and a lymphosarcoma and immunoblastic lymphadenopathy (LAPES et al. 1976b) were associated with phenytoin treatment (THIBAUT et al. 1976).

g) Thrombocytopenia

Isolated thrombocytopenia without megaloblastic anemia has been rarely observed during treatment with phenytoin (FINCHAM et al. 1979), acetazolamide

(BERTINO et al. 1957), primidone (PARKER 1974), phenobarbital, valproic acid (STOLZIS and SCHEFFNER 1975; SMITH 1976), clonazepam (VEALL and HOGARTH 1975), and carbamazepine (CEREGHINO et al. 1975). Thrombocytopenia is usually accompanied by other hypersensitivity reactions like lymphadenopathy, exanthema, fever, and eosinophilia. JOIST et al. (1973) found that phenobarbital impairs platelet function as measured by in vitro tests.

RICHARDSON et al. (1976) noticed a decrease in the number of thrombocytes in asymptomatic children under treatment with valproic acid. They believed the reduction to be caused by an inhibition of the thrombocyte aggregation. Studies by VOSS et al. (1976). SUTOR and JESDINSKY-BUSCHER (1976), WINFIELD et al. (1976), and BRAUN and HELWIG (1977) on a total of nine children found hematomas, nose-bleeding, and increased bleeding after operations, partly associated with high doses of valproic acid alone and plasma concentrations up to 244 µg/ml. Stopping the valproic acid treatment improved the clinical and laboratory findings (BRAUN and HELWIG 1977).

TARGAN et al. (1975) described a case of purpura fulminans with disseminated intravascular clotting occurring 4 weeks after the beginning of phenytoin therapy.

h) Coagulation Defects

Cases of neonatal hemorrhage after maternal anticonvulsant therapy have been reported (see Sect. C.II.4.c).

3. Immunological Disorders

a) Immunoglobulins

Low serum immunoglobulin A levels of less than 0.6 mg/ml are found in about 12% of epileptic patients treated with phenytoin (AARLI 1980). An IgA deficiency with less than 0.05 mg/ml appears in 2%–15% of phenytoin-treated patients. On the other hand, in some patients phenytoin may even lead to an increase in serum IgA concentrations (AARLI 1980). In contrast to phenytoin, carbamazepine seems to raise IgA serum levels, at least in patients not previously exposed to phenytoin (STRANDJORD et al. 1980).

A number of reports indicated a relationship between IgA deficiency and primary generalized epilepsies of hereditary origin (FONTANA et al. 1976), histocompatibility antigen HLA 2 (AARLI 1980), and a history of febrile convulsions.

Patients with symptomatic or acquired epilepsies develop no IgA deficiency if left untreated or when treated with phenytoin (FONTANA et al. 1976). It is not known whether the observed IgA deficiency has any clinical relevance (AARLI 1980).

Phenytoin may also have an effect on lymphoid tissue in the gut. The number of IgA-containing plasma cells is reduced in biopsies of intestinal mucosa of epileptic children treated with phenytoin (see AARLI 1980).

Immunoglobulins G and M have repeatedly been found to be normal or only slightly altered among untreated and treated epileptic patients (FONTANA et al. 1978; AARLI 1980).

b) Antinuclear Antibodies

Data concerning the occurrence of antinuclear antibodies is still preliminary and controversial. SINGSEN et al. (1976) found antinuclear antibodies in 14 out of 70 children receiving ethosuximide and/or phenytoin. Such children should receive careful observation, but their treatment need not be changed.

c) Cellular Immune Response

In addition to the impairment of the humoral immune reaction, deficiencies of the cellular immune reaction have been reported (SEAGER et al. 1975). Whether the number of lymphocytes remains normal during phenytoin therapy is controversial (SEAGER 1976). SORRELL and FORBES (1975) found low lymphocyte counts in carbamazepine-treated patients. NEILAN and LEPPIK (1980) report that phenytoin treatment does not acutely inhibit the formation of T-lymphocyte rosettes. Some patients who were treated with phenytoin or carbamazepine demonstrated delayed hypersensitivity reactions to common antigens less often than healthy persons (SORRELL and FORBES 1975). It remains uncertain if or to what extent the deficiencies described can be attributed to the effects of medication or to specific characteristics of epileptic patients. The complement system is apparently not impaired in treated or untreated epileptic patients (SORRELL and FORBES 1975).

d) Lupus Erythematosus

Lupus erythematosus may appear within 9 days to several years after the onset of treatment with phenytoin (BONARD 1964), mephenytoin (RUPPLI and VOSSEN 1957), trimethadione (BENTON et al. 1962), primidone (ALARCON-SEGOVIA 1969), ethosuximide (SINGSEN et al. 1976), carbamazepine (SIMPSON 1966), or a combination of drugs (SINGSEN et al. 1976).

The pathogenesis of the lupus erythematosus syndrome has not yet been defined. Epilepsy may be the initial symptom of idiopathic systemic lupus erythematosus and may antedate other manifestations by years (FEINGLASS et al. 1976), so that the drugs which were given to treat the seizures could mistakenly be considered the cause of the syndrome. Epileptic patients who develop the syndrome while under anticonvulsant therapy have a higher antinuclear antibody titer than other patients. However, the positive titer is frequent among epileptic patients and should not be considered suggestive of the lupus erythematosus sydrome (BEERNINK and MILLER 1973).

Discontinuation of the antiepileptic drug and the administration of corticoids led to remission in 84% of cases, but 10% of patients died. If continuing anticonvulsant therapy is necessary, emergency treatment with diazepam injections or chronic administration of less often involved drugs such as phenobarbital may be useful. Dermatomyositis and a scleroderma-like syndrome have been rarely described in patients taking antiepileptic drugs (SCHMIDT and SELDON 1982).

4. Adverse Effects During Pregnancy

Antiepileptic drug treatment of a pregnant woman could have adverse effects on (a) the pregnancy and the delivery, (b) the prenatal development of the child, and (c) the postnatal development of the child. A recent workshop dealt with the problems of parental epilepsy, pregnancy, and the child (JANZ et al. 1982) and includes a detailed bibliography, so here we shall review only a few pertinent points.

a) Pregnancy and Delivery

In a recent study of 7,652 deliveries in Norway, bleeding appeared to be the only significantly increased complication during pregnancy, labor and delivery in epileptic women (EGENAES 1982). HIILESMAA et al. (1982) found no correlation between epilepsy, drugs, and pregnancy complications.

b) Prenatal Development of the Child

Antiepileptic drugs could possibly adversely affect the prenatal development in three ways: (1) antiepileptic drug exposure could lead to a higher incidence of major malformations; this aspect deals with the teratogenicity of antiepileptic drugs; (2) antiepileptic drugs could possibly lead to minor anomalies in infants exposed to them in utero, which have been lumped together in the so-called fetal antiepileptic drug syndrome; (3) postnatal development could be influenced by exposure to antiepileptic drugs during pregnancy or through breast feeding of the infant.

α) Teratogenicity. Children of epileptic mothers show malformations in about 0,5%. i.e., about twice as often as the general population. An attempt was made to investigate the influence of antiepileptic drugs on the increased malformation rate by comparing the incidence of malformations in children of treated (0,78%) and untreated (0.34%) epileptic mothers, and children of epileptic fathers (0.8%) (JANZ 1982). The most frequent malformations involve the cardiovascular system, cheilo- and/or palatoschisis, skeletal abnormalities, central nervous system, and gastrointestinal and urogenital tract (JANZ 1982). A number of difficult to control variables confound our insight into the role of antiepileptic drugs in the development of malformations. These include the difficulty of comparing treated and untreated patients, who may differ in the clinical properties of their epilepsies, age, seizure frequency, and psychosocial data. In addition, there may be a genetic association of epilepsy and certain malformations. Several but not all studies have demonstrated an increased frequency of malformations among the relatives of malformed children (JANZ 1982). Also, children of epileptic fathers show a malformation incidence only slightly lower than that for epileptic mothers. Based on retrospective surveys exposure to valproic acid during early pregnancy may possibly increase the risk of neural tube defects in the offspring (US Public Health Service 1982). Until further clarification through prospective studies, treatment with valproic acid at the lowest effective plasma concentrations should be initiated only after careful consideration in women liable to become pregnant. It seems entirely possible that subsequent studies will succeed in establishing high-risk subgroups of epileptic women in whom antiepileptic drugs in fact contribute but are not solely responsible for a higher incidence of malformations.

β) Fetal Antiepileptic Drug Syndrome. Apart from the major malformations of children of epileptic parents exposed to antiepileptic drugs during pregnancy a number of so-called minor anomalies have recently been observed in these children and been called fetal antiepileptic drug syndrome (Table 1). The terminology "fetal hydantoin syndrome" or "fetal phenobarbital syndrome" is a specific but inadequately supported incrimination of these drugs. The features of these syndromes overlap considerably, and many of the infants were exposed to several drugs. Therefore, the term "fetal antiepileptic drug syndrome" is preferable.

The number of individual minor anomalies is higher in children of antiepileptic drug-treated mothers than in untreated epileptic mothers. Children of untreated epileptic mothers have more minor anomalies than children of healthy mothers (RATING et al. 1982). Infants who were exposed to antiepileptic drugs during gestation and who have a malformation or more than a total of nine anomalies also have a poorer prognosis for normal mental development than others (HILL and TENNYSON 1982). The pathogenetic mechanism of the development of minor anomalies is not fully clarified. Although antiepileptic drugs are frequently incriminated, additional pathogenetic factors may exist.

c) Postnatal Development of the Child

There has been growing interest in the influence that antiepileptic drugs could have on the immediate and long-term postnatal development of the child exposed

Table 1. Anomalies in the fetal antiepileptic drug syndrome. (HANSON and SMITH 1975)

Growth and performance
Motor or mental deficiency
Microcephaly
Prenatal growth deficiency
Postnatal growth deficiency
Craniofacial
Short nose with low nasal bridge
Hypertelorism
Epicanthic folds
Ptosis of eyelid
Strabismus
Low-set and/or abnormal ears
Wide mouth
Prominent lips
Cleft palate
Metopic sutural ridging
Wide fontanelles
Limb
Hypoplasia of nails and distal phalanges
Fingerlike thumb
Abnormal palmar creases
Five or more digital arches
Other
Short or webbed neck, low hairline
Coarse hair
Widely spaced, hypoplastic nipples
Rib, sternal, or spinal anomalies
Hernias
Undescended testes

to the drugs in utero. BATTINO et al. (1982) associated intrauterine exposure to phenytoin, barbiturates, and trimethadione with clinical and subclinical coagulopathies, usually on the first postnatal day. The abnormalities are similar to the ones resulting from vitamin K deficiency and are reversed by vitamin K_1 administration. BATTINO et al. (1982) also found that prothrombin time, partial prothrombin time, and prothrombin activity were lower in newborns of epileptic mothers, but were still in the normal range. One case of bleeding occurred in 49 neonates. Fatal neonatal hemorrhage has been reported after maternal antiepileptic drug therapy despite phytonadione prophylaxis at birth and additional doses at the onset of bleeding (BLEYER and SKINNER 1976). A review of 21 cases of neonatal hemorrhage was given recently by BLEYER and SKINNER (1976). Neonatal hypocalcemia was reported after intrauterine exposure to antiepileptic drugs (FRIIS and SARDEMANN 1977).

BOSSI et al. (1982) studied the adverse effects of antiepileptic drugs in newborn babies of epileptic women. The plasma half-lives of phenobarbital, primidone, carbamazepine, and valproic acid were equal to or greater than in adults and definitely greater than in older infants. Possible drug-related problems included withdrawal symptoms (6% of the cases, plus another 14% with a few signs of withdrawal), CNS depression (4%), and cephalohematoma (2%). Neonates exposed to barbiturates in late pregnancy may develop restlessness, tremor, hyperreflexia, and vasomotor instability 6–7 days after birth. Antiepileptic drugs are also transferred to the breast-fed infant. Respiratory depression, hypothermia, and hypotonia may develop in infants of women taking more than 30 mg diazepam daily. The milk and serum concentrations of ethosuximide are roughly equal due to the minimal plasma protein binding, while the ratio is less than one for phenytoin, valproic acid, and carbamazepine. The drug transfer to the infant may result in poor sucking, perhaps due to the infant's becoming drowsy during feeding (KANEKO et al. 1982; GRANSTRÖM et al. 1982). However, opinions are still divided. Certainly the concentrations of medications in the breast-fed child can reach several micrograms per milliliter or up to 100% of the maternal plasma levels. Socioeconomic factors and substandard motherly care may also contribute adversely to the postnatal development of children of epileptic parents, but the role of these factors has not been adequately established.

The long-term physical, mental, and social development of the child exposed in utero to antiepileptic drugs has been studied very little. The possible influence of antiepileptic drugs is thus difficult to estimate. In a recent Finnish study, antiepileptic drug treatment or epilepsy seemed to have no great effect on the development of the child during the 1st years of life (GRANSTRÖM 1982). In an Italian neuropediatric follow-up of infants born to epileptic mothers, no relationship between maternal drug treatment and neurological features in the offspring was found (LATIS et al. 1982). At school age there was no difference in psychomotor and mental development in children of epileptic mothers or fathers (BECK-MANNAGETTA and JANZ 1982). The possibility that antiepileptic drugs used during pregnancy may lead to unexpected, late manifestations is suggested by the reports of BLATTNER et al. (1977) on malignant mesenchymoma 18 years after prenatal exposure to phenytoin, and of PENDERGRASS and HANSON (1976) and SHERMAN and ROIZEN (1976) on neuroblastoma also in children exposed in utero to phenytoin. In addition, HOYT and BILLSON (1978) found optic nerve hypoplasia in children of epileptic women treated with antiepileptic drugs during pregnancy.

Recommendations on pregnancy counseling were recently reviewed (SCHMIDT and SELDON 1982). Pregnancy need not be discouraged, and abortions need not be routinely advised if pregnancy has occurred. Discontinuation or a dose reduction of antiepileptic drugs during pregnancy is unwarranted in view of the possible serious side effects of repeated seizures on maternal and fetal health. Frequent therapeutic drug monitoring is useful as plasma concentrations may decrease during pregnancy. Neonates exposed in utero to antiepileptic drugs should be examined for evidence of bleeding. Breast feeding an infant should not be discouraged. If signs of poor sucking or sedation are found, early weaning must be considered.

5. Disorders of the Digestive System

a) Gastrointestinal System

Nausea, epigastric discomfort, and loss of appetite have developed after administration of valproic acid and ethosuximide. Hiccups and attacks of epigastric pain were described in patients taking ethosuximide (BURKE 1964). ACTH or corticoids may induce peptic ulcers.

b) Hepatic Injury

Antiepileptic drugs may influence hepatic function in three different ways. Accordingly, it seems useful to deal separately with the acute and chronic hepatic injury and increased liver enzymes in clinically asymptomatic patients.

α) Acute Hepatic Injury. This type of hepatic disease usually begins with signs of a hypersensitivity reaction within the first 10 weeks of treatment with phenytoin alone or in combination with phenobarbital, with trimethadione as a single drug or in combination with mephenytoin, thiohydantoin, 5-phenyl-5-thienyl-hydantoin, or phenobarbital (ZIMMERMAN 1979). The changes are usually reversible following withdrawal of the medication. The hepatic lesion is cytotoxic, and the clinical manifestations of hepatic disease resemble those of severe viral hepatitis (ZIMMERMAN 1979). The mechanism of hepatotoxicity of the antiepileptic drugs has not been elucidated. The evidence for a delayed hypersensitivity or an idiosyncratic reaction seems to be the most convincing (ZIMMERMAN 1979). The prognosis is guarded. Approximately one-third of the patients have a fatal outcome in hepatic failure. In the remaining patients complete remission sets in within a few weeks after withdrawal of the medication. In recent years a number of fatal cases of acute liver failure have been described mainly in patients who were under 10 years old, had additional psychomotor retardation or neurological handicaps, and had taken valproic acid for 3–6 months (DONAT et al. 1979; SUCHY et al. 1979; ADDISON and GORDON 1980; JACOBI et al. 1980; LE BIHAN et al. 1980; WARE and MILLWARD-SADLER 1980; SPATZ et al. 1981; STENZEL et al. 1981). The acute liver failure leads to somnolence, stupor, or coma. Petechiae, prolonged bleeding from injection sites, and gastrointestinal blood loss have been described. Initial symptoms and signs included jaundice, vomiting, lethargy, general malaise, weight loss, edema, ataxia, facial swelling, vertigo, and tremor. Pathological findings indicate centrilobular necroses with microvesicular fat deposits in the hepatocytes (WARE and MILLWARD-SADLER 1980), signs of toxic hepatitis (ADDISON and GORDON 1980), fat uptake in small and medium vacuoles (LE BIHAN et al. 1980), and severe hepatocyte destruction leading to extensive fibrosis, pseudoductular proliferation, mononuclear cell infiltration, and the disappearance of the normal lobular structure (DONAT et al. 1979). Despite a number of proposals the mechanism of valproic acid-induced acute liver failure has not yet been elucidated. GERBER et al. (1979) drew attention to the similarity to the Reye syndrome and Jamaican vomiting sickness due to methylene-cyclopropylacetic acid. A fatal Reye-like syndrome has been described in a 8-year-old epileptic boy following the administration of valproic acid (YOUNG et al. 1980). Since the valproic acid plasma levels in these patients are mostly not very high, an idiosyncratic or hypersensitivity reaction is usually assumed. Recently TRIPP et al. (1981) described a child with ornithine carbamyl transferase deficiency, which died upon treatment with valproic acid. This mechanism cannot, however, be implicated in all cases of liver failure accompanying valproic acid therapy.

β) Chronic Hepatic Injury. The most comprehensive study on chronic hepatic injury in epileptic patients has been carried out in an epilepsy institution by ZIEGLER and SINAZADEH (1975). In only three of the 540 cases (0.6%) was a causal relationship with antiepileptic drug intake considered likely. These included a fatal acute liver failure in one patient receiving phenytoin and phenobarbital. The other two patients were shown to have fatty infiltration of the liver at autopsy. They had received primidone or phenytoin. Acute fatal liver failure was seen in 2.4% of the epileptic patients and in 2.6% of the control group of nonepileptic, institutionalized patients. Two careful additional studies found no evidence for hepatotoxicity in clinically asymptomatic epileptic patients receiving long-term anticonvulsant treatment (KOCH et al. 1975; JACOBSEN et al. 1976).

ZUCKER et al. (1977) recorded the only fatal case of acute hepatitis with extensive parenchymal necrosis during multiple-drug therapy with carbamazepine and phenobarbital. POPPER et al. (1965) observed unspecific hepatitis without accompanying cholestasis and granulomatous hepatitis which appeared with phenytoin treatment. Chronic hepatitis with slightly increased SGOT and SGPT activity developed only in one case of the extremely rare, progressive myoclonus epilepsy (Lafora's disease) (HUCHZERMEYER and GERHARD 1974).

It is interesting that tuberculosis, treated or untreated, as well as tuberculostatic therapy, even when given to patients without tuberculosis, carries an as yet unexplained increased risk of developing antiepileptic drug-induced liver disease (DOLD and REICHENMILLER 1969).

γ) Increased Liver Enzyme Activity. Untreated, otherwise healthy patients with epilepsy have normal liver enzyme values (BARTELS et al. 1974). Following a generalized tonic-clonic seizure, lactate dehydrogenase (LDH), SGOT, SGPT, and creatine kinase levels in the serum can be temporarily elevated for a few days, the latter probably due to destruction of skeletal muscle cells during the seizure (MATZ et al. 1977). In contrast, liver enzyme levels may be elevated in anticonvulsant-treated epileptic patients. In one study, in 93% of 642 patients gamma-glutamyl transferase (gamma-GT) was increased (SCHMIDT 1981 a). The interpretation of an isolated raised gamma-GT level is still controversial. It seems most likely that an isolated gamma-GT increase is a biochemical feature of a drug-induced adaptive phenomenon of liver without clinical relevance. Histologically, long-term antiepileptic drug treatment leads to a hypertrophy of the smooth endoplasmic reticulum. More specifically, agranuloreticular hypertrophy has been observed during anticonvulsant treatment (ALTMANN 1980). It does not justify a reduction of the dosage or even a withdrawal of the drug in an asymptomatic patient without convincing biochemical evidence for hepatotoxicity. Alkaline phosphatase is increased in about 28% of antiepileptic drug-treated epileptic patients. KRUSE (1968) reported that an elevated alkaline phosphatase level among children and youth is the most reliable biochemical marker for early osteomalacia or rickets. Among adults the bone and liver fractions of the isoenzymes are usually equal (ROSALKI 1976), whereas among 16- to 20-year-olds the liver fraction is usually larger than the bone fraction (ROWE 1974).

If SGOT and SGPT levels are elevated, as they may be in 13% and 4% respectively of patients, hepatic damage should be excluded by clinical and additional biochemical investigations, even though the incidence of liver disease among epileptic patients is below 1%. Increases in SGOT and SGPT levels appeared in 8% and 6%, respectively, of patients treated with valproic acid. The concentrations did not usually rise above twice the normal values, and they returned to normal after a dosage reduction (WILLMORE et al. 1978).

Raised leucine amino peptidase levels suggest additional hepatic disease (RUNDLE and SUDELL 1973). Increased amylase is suggestive of pancreatitis, which has been seen rarely with valproic acid treatment.

c) Porphyria

In patients affected by acute intermittent porphyria severe attacks are known to be precipitated by some antiepileptic drugs, such as barbiturates, hydantoins, clonazepam, and valproic acid (MAGNUSSEN et al. 1975). In these patients bromide has been recommended (BONKOWSKY et al. 1980).

d) Biliary Tract

ZIEGLER (1970 a) found that gallstones appear more than twice as often among institutionalized epileptic patients than among institutionalized nonepileptic patients.

e) Pancreas

Recently cases of pancreatitis associated with valproic acid treatment have been reported (BATALDEN et al. 1979; CAMFIELD et al. 1979; SASAKI et al. 1980; COULTER and ALLEN 1980 a; MURPHY et al. 1981).

6. Hormonal and Metabolic Disorders

a) Thyroid Hormones

It has long been known that protein-bound iodine (PBI) (REYNOLDS 1975), total thyroxine (T_4) (HEYMA et al. 1977), free thyroxine (FT_4) (CAPLAN et al. 1977), and free thyroxine index (FTI) (STJERNHOLM et al. 1975; HEYMA et al. 1977) may be reduced in patients receiving antiepileptic drugs. In addition, a slightly elevated tri-iodothyronine uptake (T_3U) has been found (CAPLAN et al. 1977). Phenytoin (HEYMA et al. 1977; CAPLAN et al. 1977) and carbamazepine (ROOTWELT et al. 1978; AANDERUD and STRANDJORD 1980; STRANDJORD et al. 1981), valproic acid, phenytoin, primidone, and carbamazepine (FICHSEL and KNÖPFLE 1978) have been implicated. The thyrotropin (TSH) levels remain unchanged even after stimulation with thyrotropin-releasing factor (TRF) in adults and children following the administration of phenytoin or carbamazepine (HEYMA et al. 1977; FICHSEL and KNÖPFLE 1978).

Enhanced degradation of T_4 and T_3 due to enzyme induction and displacement of T_4 from its binding sites on thyroxine-binding globulin (TBG) has been discussed (see FICHSEL and KNÖPFLE 1978). The clinical significance of these laboratory findings remains small, unless clinical dysfunction of the thyroid gland is seen, and they do not justify hormone substitution therapy (HEYMA et al. 1977). In patients treated with antiepileptic drugs, hypothyroidism should only be assumed in the presence of pituitary insufficiency or an abnormally high thyrotropin concentration (CAPLAN et al. 1977; STJERNHOLM et al. 1975). AANDERUD and STRANDJORD (1980) described two cases of hypothyroidism following therapy with carbamazepine and phenytoin. Both patients became euthyroid after withdrawal of the antiepileptic drugs. Substitution with L-thyroxine may decrease the plasma concentration of anticonvulsants.

b) Adrenal Hormones

GALLAGHER (1976) demonstrated that phenytoin leads to increased cortisol production and raises the 24-h cortisol secretion rate. There is some evidence that endogenous corticoadrenal or exogenous steroids are more readily cartabolized due to enzyme induction.

c) Sexual Hormones

In a prospective study, morphologically abnormal spermatozoa and decreased numbers of spermatozoa were found more frequently than expected in antiepileptic drug-treated epileptic patients (CHRISTIANSEN and LUND 1976). The secretion of androsterone, ethiocolanolone, and dehydroepiandrosterone was reduced in some patients, and the secretion of estrogen was increased. However, it is unjustified to relate any change in sexual hormones or complaints of sexual dysfunction directly to the effects of anticonvulsants before other somatic and psychological factors have been evaluated.

Many antiepileptic drugs induce the metabolism of oral contraceptives and may therefore considerably impair the contraceptive effect (JANZ and SCHMIDT 1974). The interaction leads to a tenfold increase of spotting and breakthrough bleeding and to a higher failure rate of the contraceptives. The onset of bleeding disturbances under oral contraceptives frequently indicates a deficient contraceptive action (SCHMIDT 1981 b). When irregular bleedings occur, an oral contraceptive with a higher estrogen content should be given immediately. If the bleedings persist, other contraceptive methods should be considered.

d) Miscellaneous Hormones

Phenytoin therapy appears to promote increased secretion of follicle-stimulating hormone (FSH) and luteinizing hormone (LH) (SCHMITZ et al. 1975). No definite change in the basic TSH serum concentration has been observed among epileptic patients under treatment (FICHSEL and KNÖPFLE 1978). Both carbamazepine and phenytoin diminished the growth hormone response secondary to insulin hypoglycemia (LONDON et al. 1980). Elevated growth hormone levels were found in female epileptic patients receiving phenytoin and carbamazepine while male patients and controls had normal values (LUOMA et al. 1980b). LONDON et al. (1980) found a rise in prolactin levels after 7-day administration of carbamazepine or phenytoin.

e) Metabolic Disturbances

High concentrations of phenytoin have occasionally led to temporary hyperglycemia and an abnormal glucose tolerance test (see REYNOLDS 1975). A side effect may even occasionally be advantageous. NIKKILÄ et al. (1978) and LUOMA et al. (1980a) reported that phenytoin and phenobarbital may increase serum high-density lipoprotein (HDL). Since HDL appears to be inversely related to the risk of coronary heart disease, these authors suggest that the observed increase may actually be a beneficial side effect of antiepileptic drug treatment.

Carbamazepine can lead to hyponatremia (PERUCCA et al. 1978) and water intoxication (ASHTON et al. 1977). In patients with diabetes insipidus, carbamazepine leads to a notable decrease in diuresis (PERLEMUTER et al. 1975). Phenytoin is reported to inhibit the release of antidiuretic hormone (ADH) in syndromes with increased ADH secretion (see REYNOLDS 1975). Aside from the effects antiepileptic drugs have on folic acid, vitamin B_{12}, vitamin K or vitamin D, hydantoins, and succinimides may reduce the activity of erythrocyte glutamic oxalacetic transaminase and the level of pyridoxalphosphate in serum (REINKEN 1975). Interestingly, HAGBERG et al. (1966) reported an antiepileptic effect of vitamin B_6 substitution among epileptic children.

Altered serum levels of copper, manganese, and zinc have been reported among epileptic patients, but the etiology (epilepsy, seizures, antiepileptic drugs) has not been determined (REYNOLDS 1975). The concentration of magnesium in patients' serum is generally normal (KATZ et al. 1976).

7. Disorders of Bones and Mineral Metabolism

The association between long-term antiepileptic drug treatment and impairment of the calcium and vitamin D metabolism and clinical osteomalacia was recognized as recently as 1968 by KRUSE, even though phenytoin and phenobarbital had been in therapeutic use for 30 and 40 years. Among the biochemical features, decreased early-morning calcium, decreased phosphate, increased alkaline phosphatase, low 25-hydroxy-cholecalciferol in serum, and increased calcium elimination in 24-h urine samples are most frequently found (KRUSE 1975; HAHN et al. 1975; REYNOLDS 1975). The optimal screening is done at the end of winter. Radiological findings have been reported in 6%–15% of patients with biochemical abnormalities (PRAGER et al. 1977). Finally, a bone biopsy may be considered.

Overt clinical osteomalacia occurs in about 5% of children and adolescents treated with antiepileptic drugs and in about 1%–5% of adult epileptic patients (KRUSE 1975) and has mostly been reported in series with a small number of patients. There is general agreement that overt osteomalacia usually occurs in a specific, high-risk subgroup of epileptic patients. It is more frequent in institutionalized children and adolescents with severe epilepsy treated with several antiepileptic drugs in high doses. Patients with deficient sun exposure, inadequate nutrition, and muscular inactivity have an increased relative risk of developing antiepileptic drug-associated osteomalacia. Malabsorption, partial gastrectomy, kidney disease, and consumptive diseases are additional risk factors (HAHN 1976).

The most commonly assumed pathogenetic mechanism of antiepileptic drug-associated osteomalacia is vitamin D deficiency through the antiepileptic drug-induced increased production of inactive or less active vitamin D metabolites (HAHN et al. 1975) and a decrease in 1,25-hydroxycholecalciferol (25-OHCC), which is the most potent vitamin D metabolite (SHAFER and NUTTALL 1975). In fact, reduced 25-OHCC levels were reported by Hahn et al. (1975), but the 1,25-dihydroxymetabolite, which is physiologically produced from 25-OHCC in the kidneys, was not depressed (JUBIZ et al. 1977), and, furthermore, 25-OHCC is not therapeutically effective in all patients (CHRISTIANSEN et al. 1975). It seems therefore possible that other mechanisms may be involved. The absorption of calcium but not of vitamin D is impaired by antiepileptic drugs (SHAFER and NUTTALL 1975). Calcium absorption can be improved by the intake of 25-OHCC (CASPARY et al. 1975).

Among the antiepileptic drugs, phenytoin, phenobarbital, and, in only one case, carbamazepine have been incriminated in the development of clinical osteomalacia. Acetazolamide may precipitate the development of osteomalacia (MALLETTE 1977). Other antiepileptic drugs like pheneturide, exazolidinediones, and ethosuximide have not been documented to be involved.

Even though there is no doubt that antiepileptic drugs do indeed lead to hypocalcemia, elevated alkaline phosphatase, reduced bone density, and depressed anorganic phosphate – for example, REUNANEN et al. (1976) reported that 10%–40% of the antiepileptic drug-treated patients had abnormalities in one or more of these parameters – it is apparent that additional risk factors are necessary for the development of overt clinical osteomalacia. Furthermore, the incidence of bone disease depends very much on the sensitivity of the screening procedure involved. Clinical examination or radiography will detect the small number of patients with overt and severe disease, but a much higher incidence of laboratory abnormalities (many of them in asymptomatic patients) will be detected by surveys based on the serum concentration of alkaline phosphatase or 25-OHCC, or by using the photon absorption measurement of bone density.

There is general agreement that clinically overt osteomalacia is treated with high doses of vitamin D_3 until the clinical symptoms and signs disappear (HAHN and AVIOLI 1975). Whether the asymptomatic patient with one or more laboratory abnormalities should receive prophylactic treatment with vitamin D is controversial (OFFERMANN et al. 1979). Any prophylactic program in which vitamin D is prescribed should be administered with caution, and appropriate measures should be taken to avoid vitamin D toxicity (ANAST 1975).

8. Miscellaneous Disorders

a) Skin Disorders

Antiepileptic drugs may induce various dermatological diseases (Table 2). In most cases a hypersensitivity reaction will develop within the initial 4–10 weeks of treatment. Discontinuation of the implicated drug is necessary, and re-exposure is dangerous. For a detailed discussion the reader is referred to a recent review (SCHMIDT and SELDON 1982).

b) Connective Tissue and Myopathies

α) Gingival Hyperplasia. Gingival hyperplasia is observed in approximately one-third of all epileptic patients who are treated with phenytoin. It appears 2–4 months after the start of treatment and is more frequent with high salivary concentrations of phenytoin (BABCOCK and NELSON 1964) and poor oral hygiene. It disappears within 2–5 months after reduction or discontinuation of phenytoin.

β) Facial Changes. Two-thirds of all institutionalized patients with severe epilepsies develop coarsened facial features during drug therapy, usually with a combination of several drugs (FALCONER and DAVIDSON 1973). Gingival hyperplasia and calvarial thickening (KATTAN 1970) are more common among epileptic patients with facial changes than among those without.

γ) Dupuytren's Contracture, Wound Repair. Dupuytren's contracture is found in one-third to one-half of all male patients and among one-fourth of all female patients under treatment for epilepsy (LUND 1941). Among the general population the incidence of Dupuytren's contracture is 1%–18% for men and 0.5%–9% for women; it rises with increasing age (CRITCHLEY et al. 1976). Dupuytren's contracture is often bilateral and can be accompanied by knuckle pads, i.e., subcutaneous fibromas on the middle joints of the fingers (CRITCHLEY et al. 1976). In addition to Dupuytren's contracture fibromas of the mucous membrane of the mouth and of the plantar fascia of the foot may develop (*Ledderhose* syndrome).

Table 2. Adverse dermatological effects of individual antiepileptic drugs. (SCHMIDT and SELDON 1982)

	Phenytoin	Mephenytoin	Pheno-barbital	Primidone	Carbama-zepine	Valproic acid	Ethosuxi-mide	Trimetha-dione
Exanthemas	+		+		+	+	+	+
Exfoliative dermatitis	+		+	+	+		+	
Stevens-Johnson syndrome	+	+	+	+	+		+	+
Lyell syndrome	+	+	+	+	+			
Dermatomyositis	+		+	+	+		+	+
Erythema nodosum			+					
Pigmentation	+	+						
Hair alteration	+	+				+		+
Acne	+		+	+				

Among the factors leading to an increased incidence of Dupuytren's contracture, phenobarbital treatment has been incriminated most often (SCHMIDT and SÖRENSEN 1981). French authors were the first to become aware of a painful stiffness in the shoulder among epileptic patients, and they named it *rhumatisme gardénalique* after phenobarbital (BLANQUART et al. 1974). The syndrome appears in about 7% of epileptic patients treated with phenobarbital or, as recently shown, with primidone but not other antiepileptic agents (JANZ, personal communication). Both shoulders and other joints may be affected. Even with continued phenobarbital therapy the syndrome recedes within a few months. Faster gingival wound healing and faster repair of leg ulcers were reported in patients who were given phenytoin (see REYNOLDS 1975).

δ) Myopathy. A myasthenic syndrome has been reported in a total of five patients during treatment with phenytoin, mephenytoin, and trimethadione. Withdrawal of the antiepileptic drug led to remission after a few weeks. In one case a relapse occurred upon re-exposure. In some cases other myopathies have been reported together with biochemical features of hypothyroidism and osteomalacia and have been associated with phenytoin treatment or multiple-drug therapy (see SCHMIDT and SELDON 1982).

c) Heart and Vascular System

Bradycardia and a reversible complete heart block occurred in elderly patients with cardiovascular disorders after administration of more than 600 mg carbamazepine daily for trigeminal neuralgia (HERZBERG 1978; HAMILTON 1978). In addition, BEERMANN et al. (1975) reported a patient in whom carbamazepine suppressed the conduction of an already defective Purkinje fiber system, thus inducing ventricular arrest with subsequent Adams-Stokes attacks.

Intravenous infusion of phenytoin causes no significant hemodynamic change in blood pressure or pulse rate among epileptic patients who are otherwise healthy (a normal ECG and no clinical signs of cardiac disease) (SCHMIDT and VOGEL 1977). Patients over 65 years of age with low blood pressure and coronary disease clearly have a higher risk of hemodynamic and respiratory depression when receiving intravenous phenytoin treatment (WALLIS et al. 1968). The injection rate for phenytoin should not be more than 25 mg/min (SCHMIDT and VOGEL 1977). The intravenous administration of phenytoin is contraindicated in the presence of sinoatrial and severe atrioventricular blocks (HANSEN et al. 1974).

d) Respiratory System

Lung diseases have not been convincingly associated with antiepileptic drug therapy except for rare cases of pulmonary reactions with antiepileptic drug-induced lupus erythematosus, lymphoma of the mediastinum, or hypersensitivity reactions (BAYER et al. 1976).

e) Kidney Disorders

Nephrotic syndromes may be induced by 4 months to 2 years of treatment with oxazolidinediones (trimethadione, paramethadione), and mortalities have been reported (BRIGGS and EMERY 1949). A reversible nephrotic syndrome has also been seen with mephenytoin, phenytoin, sulthiame, and carbamazepine (see SCHMIDT and SELDON 1982).

f) Oncogenic and Mutagenic Effects

Careful Danish and English studies (CLEMMESEN et al. 1974; WHITE et al. 1979) in over 10,000 epileptic patients found no evidence for an oncogenic effect of antiepileptic drugs. This is interesting because antiepileptic drugs, which have an enzyme-inducing effect, stimulate tumor growth in animal experiments (PERAINO et al. 1975). The cancer ratio among epileptic patients was considerably lower than that of the control group, perhaps because of the higher mortality rate of institutionalized epileptic patients (ZIEGLER 1970b). In contrast, SCHNEIDERMAN (1974) found a higher incidence of liver tumors. In addition, carcinomas of the gallbladder seemed to occur more frequently when compared with nonepileptic cancer patients. COHNEN and HEREDIA (1977) described one case of a plasmocytoma which developed during phenytoin therapy. ENDTZ et al. (1973) mentioned a case of leukemia which developed during phenytoin therapy. The existing studies do not yet enable any reliable conclusions to be drawn about a causal relationship between antiepileptic drug treatment and the development of neoplasms. The available data provide no convincing evidence for mutagenic effects of antiepileptic drugs (OBE et al. 1980).

References

Aanderud S, Strandjord RE (1980) Hypothyroidism induced by anti-epileptic therapy. Acta Neurol Scand 61:330–332

Aarli JA (1980) Effect of phenytoin on the immune system. In: Hassell TM, Johnston M, Dudley KH (eds) Phenytoin-induced teratology and gingival pathology. Raven, New York, pp 25–34

Abbott JA, Schwab RS (1954) Mesantoin in the treatment of epilepsy. N Engl J Med 250:197–205

Addison GM, Gordon NS (1980) Sodium valproate and acute hepatic failure. Dev Med Child Neurol 22:248–249

Ahrend K-F, Nagy L, Tiess D (1969) Zur Morphologie und Analytik der Sultiamum-Intoxikation. Arch Toxikol 25:229–237

Alarcón-Segovia D (1969) Drug-induced lupus syndromes. Mayo Clin Proc 44:664–681

Alberto P, Cougn R, Maurice P, Weber J (1971) Trois cas de lymphome malin ou pseudolymphome chez des épileptiques traités par la diphenylhydantoine. Schweiz Med Wochenschr 101:1773–1774

Altmann H-W (1980) Drug-induced liver reactions: a morphological approach. In: Grundmann E (ed) Drug-induced pathology. Springer, New York, pp 69–142

Anast CS (1975) Anticonvulsant drugs and calcium metabolism. N Engl J Med 292:587-588

André M, Sibout M, Petry J-M, Vert P (1973) Dépression respiratoire et neurologique chez le prématuré nouveau-né de mère traitée par Diazépam. J Gynecol Obstet Biol Reprod 2:357–366

Anthony JJ (1970) Malignant lymphoma associated with hydantoin drugs. Arch Neurol 22:450–454

Ashton MG, Ball SG, Thomas TH, Lee MR (1977) Water intoxication associated with carbamazepine treatment. Br Med J 1:1134–1135

Aviram A, Czaczkes JW, Rosenmann E (1965) Acute renal failure associated with sulthiame. Lancet I:818

Babock JR, Nelson GH (1964) Gingival hyperplasia and dilantin content of saliva: a pilot study. J Am Dent Assoc 68:195–198
Baehler RW, Work J, Smith W, Dominic JA (1980) Charcoal hemoperfusion in the therapy for methsuximide and phenytoin overdose. Arch Intern Med 140:1466–1468
Bartels H, Petersen C, Schulze W (1974) Der Einfluß von antikonvulsiver Langzeitbehandlung auf die Aktivitäten einiger in der Diagnostik hepatobiliärer Erkrankung gebräuchlicher Serumenzyme. Monatsschr Kinderheilkd 122:674–675
Batalden PB, Van Dyne BJ, Cloyd J (1979) Pancreatitis associated with valproic acid therapy. Pediatrics 64:520–522
Battino D, Bossi L, Canger R, Margstkler E, Molteni B, Rossi E, Spina S (1982) Coagulation function in newborns treated in utero with antiepileptic drugs. In: Janz D, Dam M, Richens A, Bossi L, Helge H, Schmidt D (eds) Epilepsy, pregnancy, and the child. Raven, New York, pp 383–385
Bayer AS, Targan SR, Pitchon HE, Guze LB (1976) Dilantin® toxicity: miliary pulmonary infiltrates and hypoxemia. Ann Intern Med 85:475–476
Beck-Mannagetta G, Janz D (1982) Data on psychomotor and mental development in children of epileptic parents: a retrospective study. In: Janz D, Dam M, Richens A, Bossi L, Helge H, Schmidt D (eds) Epilepsy, pregnancy, and the child. Raven, New York, pp 443–445
Beermann B, Edhag O, Vallin H (1975) Advanced heart block aggravated by carbamazepine. Br Heart J 37:668–671
Beernink DH, Miller JJ (1973) Anticonvulsant-induced antinuclear antibodies and lupus-like disease in children. J Pediatr 82:113–117
Benton JW, Tynes B, Register HB, Alford C, Holley HL (1962) Systemic lupus erythematosus occurring during anticonvulsive drug therapy. J Am Med Assoc 180:115–118
Bertino JR, Rodman T, Myerson RM (1957) Thrombocytopenia and renal lesions associated with acetazolamide (Diamox) therapy. Arch Intern Med 99:1006–1008
Bichel J (1975) Hydantoin derivatives and malignancies of the haemopoietic system. Acta Med Scand 198:327–382
Bittencourt PRM, Richens A (1981) Anticonvulsant-induced status epilepticus in Lennox-Gastaut syndrome. Epilepsia 22:129–134
Blanquart F, Houdent G, Deshayes P (1964) L'algo dystrophie iatrogène gardénalique. Sem Hop Paris 50:499–503
Blattner WA, Henson DE, Young RC, Fraumeni JF Jr (1977) Malignant mesenchymoma and birth defects. J Am Med Assoc 238:334–335
Bleyer WA, Skinner AL (1976) Fatal neonatal hemorrhage after maternal anticonvulsant therapy. J Am Med Assoc 235:626–627
Bonard EC (1964) Pseudocollagenose ou pseudolymphome malin? Effet fâcheux d'un dérive de l'hydantoine. Schweiz Med Wochenschr 94:57–59
Bonkowsky HL, Sinclair PR, Emery S, Sinclair JF (1980) Seizure management in acute hepatic porphyria: risks of valproate and clonazepam. Neurology 30:588–592
Bossi L, Battino D, Caccamo ML, Giambattista M, Latis GO, Oldrini A, Spina S (1982) Pharmacokinetics and clinical effects of antiepileptic drugs in newborns of chronically treated epileptic mothers. In: Janz D, Dam M, Richens A, Bossi L, Helge H, Schmidt D (eds) Epilepsy, pregnancy, and the child. Raven, New York, pp 373–381
Boston Collaborative Drug Surveillance Program (1973) Diphenylhydantoin side effects and serum albumin levels. Clin Pharmacol Ther 14:529–532
Bowdle TA, Patel IH, Wilensky AJ, Comfort C (1979) Hepatic failure from valproic acid. N Engl J Med 301:435–436
Braun W, Helwig H (1977) Unerwünschte Wirkungen von Valproinat (Ergenyl). Gynaekol Praxis 1:349–352
Briggs JN, Emery JL (1949) Toxic effects of tridione. Lancet I:59–62
Brillman J, Gallagher BB, Mattson RH (1974) Acute primidone intoxication. Arch Neurol 30:255–258
Browne TR (1976) Clonazepam: a review of a new anticonvulsant drug. Arch Neurol 33:326–332
Browne TR (1978) Clonazepam. N Engl J Med 299:812–816

Browne TR, Penry JK (1973) Benzodiazepines in the treatment of epilepsy. Epilepsia 14:277–310

Browne RT, Dreifuss FE, Dyken PR, Goode DJ, Penry JK, Porter RJ, White BG, White PT (1975) Ethosuximide in the treatment of absence (petit mal) seizures. Neurology 25:515–524

Brumlik J, Jacobs RS (1974) Myasthenia gravis associated with diphenylhydantoin therapy for epilepsy. Can J Neurol Sci 1:127–129

Buchthal F, Svensmark O, Schiller PJ (1960) Clinical and electroencephalographic correlations with serum levels of diphenylhydantoin. Arch Neurol 2:624–630

Buchthal F, Svensmark O, Simonsen H (1968) Relation of EEG and seizures to phenobarbital in serum. Arch Neurol 19:567–572

Burke CW (1964) Gastrointestinal side-effects of ethosuximide. Lancet II:966

Camfield PR, Bagnell P, Camfield CS, Tibbles JAR (1979) Pancreatitis due to valproic acid. Lancet I:1198–1199

Caplan RH, Mordon R, Kristoff K, Wickus G (1977) Diphenylhydantoin effects on thyroid function tests. Ann Neurol 1:603–604

Carney MWP (1969) Serum vitamin B_{12} values in 374 psychiatric patients. Behav Neuropsychiatry 1:19–23

Caspary WF, Hesch RD, Matte R, Ritter H, Kattermann R, Emrich D (1975) Effect of vitamin D and 25-hydroxycholecalciferol on intestinal calcium absorption in epileptics under anticonvulsant therapy. Horm Metab Res 7:271–272

Cereghino JJ, Brock JT, Penry JK (1972) Albutoin. In: Woodbury DM, Penry JK, Schmidt RP (eds) Antiepileptic drugs. Raven, New York, pp 283–291

Cereghino JJ, Brock JT, Van Meter JC, Penry JK, Smith LD, White BG (1975) The efficacy of carbamazepine combinations in epilepsy. Clin Pharmacol Ther 18:733–741

Chadwick DW, Cumming WJK, Livingstone I, Cartlidge NEF (1978) Acute intoxication with sodium valproate. Ann Neurol 6:552–553

Chamberlin HR, Waddell WJ, Butler TC (1965) A study of the product of demethylation of trimethadione in the control of petit mal epilepsy. Neurology 15:449–454

Chassagnon C, Eysette M, Gibert M, Fournis Y (1976) Anemie megaloblastique au cours d'un traitement par la mysoline. J Med (Lyon) 48:1163–1167

Christiansen P, Lund M (1976) Sexual potency, testicular function and excretion of sexual hormones in male epileptics. In: Janz D (ed) Epileptology, proceedings of the seventh international symposium on epilepsy. Thieme, Stuttgart, pp 190–191

Christiansen C, Rødbro P, Munck O, Munck O (1975) Actions of vitamins D_2 and D_3 and 25-OHD_3 in anticonvulsant osteomalacia. Br Med J 2:363–365

Clemmesen J, Fuglsang-Frederiksen V, Plum CM (1974) Are antivonvulsants oncogenic? Lancet I:705–707

Cohnen G, Heredia D-M (1977) Plasmozytom nach Phenytoin-Therapie? Münch Med Wochenschr 119:309–310

Consensus Statement (1980) Febrile seizures: long-term management of children with fever-associated seizures. Pediatrics 66:1009–1012

Coulter DL, Allen RJ (1980 a) Pancreatitis associated with valproic acid therapy for epilepsy. Ann Neurol 7:92

Coulter DL, Allen RJ (1980 b) Secondary hyperammonaemia: a possible mechanism for valproate encephalopathy. Lancet I:1310–1311

Critchley EMR, Vakil SD, Hayward HW, Owen VMH (1976) Dupuytren's disease in epilepsy: result of prolonged administration of anticonvulsants. J Neurol Neurosurg Psychiatry 39:498–503

Del Cerro PM, Snider RS (1970) Cerebellar alterations resulting from Dilantin intoxication: an ultrastructural study. In: Fields WS, Willis WD (eds) The cerebellum in health and disease. Green, St. Louis, pp 380–409

Dodrill CB (1975) Effects of sulthiame upon intellectual, neuropsychological, and social functioning abilities among adult epileptics: comparison with diphenylhydantoin. Epilepsia 16:617–625

Dodrill CB, Troupin AS (1977) Psychotropic effects of carbamazepine in epilepsy: a double-blind comparison with phenytoin: Neurology 27:1023–1028

Dold U, Reichenmiller HE (1969) Akute Leberzellschädigung beim Menschen durch gleichzeitige Gabe von Isonikotinsäurehydrazid und Antiepileptika (Diphenylhydantoin oder Carbamazepin). Med Welt 1:48–54
Donat JF, Bocchini JA, Gonzalez E, Schwendimann RN (1979) Valproic acid and fatal hepatitis. Neurology 29:273–274
Dreyer R (1959) Therapieschäden durch antiepileptische Mittel unter besonderer Berücksichtigung schwerer Nebenwirkungen an Hand der Literatur und einiger Fälle. Fortschr Neurol Psychiatr 27:401–423
Egenaes J (1982) Outcome of pregnancy in women with epilepsy – Norway, 1967 to 1978: complications during pregnancy and delivery. In: Janz D, Dam M, Richens A, Bossi L, Helge H, Schmidt D (eds) Epilepsy, pregnancy, and the child. Raven, New York, pp 81–85
Endtz LJ, Leeksma, CHW, Kerkhofs H, Mulder OG, Mosmans FA, Meinardi H (1973) Leucémia aiguë causée par la Diphénylhydantoïne? Rev Neurol (Paris) 129:296–300
Erith MJ (1975) Withdrawal symptoms in newborn infants of epileptic mothers. Br Med J 3:40
Falconer MA, Davidson S (1973) Coarse features in epilepsy as a consequence of anticonvulsant therapy. Lancet II:1112–1114
Fazekas IG, Rengel B (1960) Tödliche Vergiftung (Selbstmord) mit Mysoline und Phenobarbiturat. Arch Toxikol 18:213–223
Feinglass EJ, Arnett FC, Dorsch CA, Zizic TM, Stevens MB (1976) Neuropsychiatric manifestations of systemic lupus erythematosus: diagnosis, clinical spectrum, and relationship to other features of the disease. Medicine 55:323–339
Fichsel H, Knöpfle G (1978) Effects of anticonvulsant drugs on thyroid hormones in epileptic children. Epilepsia 19:323–336
Filipidis V, Suchenwirth R (1968) Polyneuritis nach Sulfaphenylbutansultam (Ospolot). Med Monatschr 22:129–130
Fincham RW, Schottelius DD, Sahs AL (1974) The influence of diphenylhydantoin on primidone metabolism. Arch Neurol 30:259–262
Fincham RW, Hamilton HE, Schottelius DD (1979) Late onset thrombocytopenia with phenytoin therapy. Ann Neurol 6:370
Fischer M, Korskjaer G, Pedersen E (1965) Psychotic episodes in Zarondan treatment. Epilepsia 6:325–334
Flexner JM, Hartmann RC (1960) Megaloblastic anemia associated with anticonvulsant drugs. Am J Med 28:386–396
Fontana A, Grob PJ, Sauter R, Joller H (1976) IgA deficiency, epilepsy, and hydantoin medication. Lancet II:228–231
Fontana A, Grob PJ, Sauter R (1978) Immunoglobulin abnormalities in relatives of IgA deficient epileptics. J Neurol 217:207–212
Forman MB, Chouler C, Milne FJ (1979) Primidone-induced "uraemic flap". Lancet II:1250–1251
Friis B, Sardemann, H (1977) Neonatal hypocalcaemia after intrauterine exposure to anticonvulsant drugs. Arch Dis Child 52:239–241
Gallagher BB (1976) Adrenal hyperplasia in epileptic patients. In: Kellaway P, Petersen I (eds) Quantitative analytic studies in epilepsy. Raven, New York, pp 165–169
Gallagher BB, Baumel IP, Mattson RH, Woodbury SG (1973) Primidone, diphenylhydantoin and phenobarbital – aspects of acute and chronic toxicity. Neurology 23:145–149
Gayford JJ, Redpath TH (1969) The side-effects of carbamazepine. Proc Roy Soc Med 62:615–616
Gerber N, Dickinson RG, Harland RC, Lynn RK, Houghton D, Antonias JI, Schimschock JC (1979) Reye-like syndrome associated with valproic acid therapy. J Pediatr 95:142–144
Ghatak NR, Santoso RA, McKinney WM (1976) Cerebellar degeneration following long-term phenytoin therapy. Neurology 26:818–820
Gitlin N, Morris HB (1976) Flapping tremor associated with administration of diphenylhydantoin sodium. S Afr Med J 50:1427
Gould JDM, Lingam S (1977) Hazards of intra-arterial diazepam. Br Med J 2:298–299

Granström M-L (1982) Development of the children of epileptic mothers: preliminary results from the prospective Helsinki study. In: Janz D, Dam M, Richens A, Bossi L, Helge H, Schmidt D (eds) Epilepsy, pregnancy, and the child. Raven, New York, pp 403–408

Granström M-L, Bardy AH, Hiilesmaa VK (1982) Prolonged feeding difficulties of infants of primidone mothers during neonatal period: preliminary results from the prospective Helsinki study. In: Janz D, Dam M, Richens A, Bossi L, Helge H, Schmidt D (eds) Epilepsy, pregnancy, and the child. Raven, New York, pp 357–358

Green JR, Kupferberg HJ (1972) Sulthiame. In: Woodbury DM, Penry JK, Schmidt RP (eds) Antiepileptic drugs. Raven, New York, pp 477–485

Gruska H, Beyer K-H, Kubicki S, Schneider H (1971) Course, toxicology and therapy of a case of severe carbamazepine poisoning. Arch Toxikol 27:193–203

Guey J, Charle C, Coquery C, Roger J, Soulayrol R (1967) Study of psychological effects of ethosuximide (Zarontin) on 25 children suffering from petit mal epilepsy. Epilepsia 8:129–141

Hagberg B, Hamfelt A, Hansson O (1966) Tryptophan load tests and pyridoxal-5-phosphate levels in epileptic children. Acta Paediatr Scand 55:371–384

Hahn TJ (1976) Bone complications of anticonvulsants. Drugs 12:201–211

Hahn TJ, Avioli LV (1975) Anticonvulsant osteomalacia. Arch Intern Med 135:997–1000

Hahn TJ, Hendin BA, Scharp CR, Boisseau VC, Haddad JG Jr (1975) Serum 25-hydroxycalciferol levels and bone mass in children on chronic anticonvulsant therapy. N Engl J Med 292:550–554

Hamilton DV (1978) Carbamazepine and heart block. Lancet I:1365

Hancock BW (1974) Acute barbiturate poisoning in young epileptics. Postgrad Med J 50:244–246

Hansen H-W, Marquort B, Pelz W (1974) Anwendungstechnik und Therapieergebnisse mit einem Phenytoin-Infusionskonzentrat. Dtsch Med Wochenschr 99:1961–1964

Hanson JW, Smith DW (1975) The fetal hydantoin syndrome. J Pediatr 87:285–290

Haruda F (1979) Phenytoin hypersensitivity: 38 cases. Neurology 29:1480–1485

Heckmatt JZ, Houston AB, Clow DJ, Stephenson JBP, Dodd KL, Lealman GT, Logan RW (1976) Failure of phenobarbitone to prevent febrile convulsions. Br Med J 1:559–561

Heimpel H (1974) Die Panmyelopathie und andere Formen der Pancytopenie. Springer, Berlin Heidelberg New York, pp 83–134 (Handbuch der Inneren Medizin, vol 2, part 4)

Hellström B, Barlach-Christoffersen M (1980) Influence of phenobarbital on the psychomotor development and behaviour in preschool children with convulsions. Neuropädiatrie 11:151–160

Herzberg L (1978) Carbamazepine and bradycardia. Lancet I:1097–1098

Heyma P, Larkins RG, Perry-Keene D, Peter CT, Ross D, Sloman JG (1977) Thyroid hormone levels and protein binding in patients on long-term diphenylhydantoin treatment. Clin Endocrinol 6:369–376

Hiilesmaa VK, Teramo K, Bardy AH (1982) Social class, complications, and perinatal deaths in pregnancies of epileptic women: preliminary results of the prospective Helsinki study. In: Janz D, Dam M, Richens A, Bossi L, Helge H, Schmidt D (eds) Epilepsy, pregnancy, and the child. Raven, New York, pp 87–90

Hill RM, Tennyson LM (1982) Significant anomalies in the antiepileptic drug syndrome: comment. In: Janz D, Dam M, Richens A, Bossi L, Helge H, Schmidt D (eds) Epilepsy, pregnancy, and the child. Raven, New York, pp 309–311

Hirsch W (1968) Mogadan „Roche" bei chronischer Hepatitis. Ther Ggw 107:686–695

Hoyt GS, Billson FA (1978) Maternal anticonvulsants and optic nerve hypoplasia. Br J Ophthalmol 62:3–6

Huchzermeyer H, Gerhard L (1974) Die Leber bei der progressiven Myoklonusepilepsie (Lafora's disease). Klin Wochenschr 52:559–567

Hutt SJ, Jackson PM, Belsham A, Higgins G (1968) Perceptual motor behaviour in relation to blood phenobarbitone level: a preliminary report. Dev Med Child Neurol 10:626–632

Hyman GA, Sommers SC (1966) The development of Hodgkin's disease and lymphoma during anticonvulsant therapy. Blood 28:416–427
Hyman NM, Dennis PD, Sinclair KGA (1979) Tremor due to sodium valproate. Neurology 29:1177–1180
Ideström C-M, Schalling D, Carlquist U, Sjöqvist F (1972) Acute effects of diphenylhydantoin in relation to plasma levels. Psychol Med 2:111–120
Isaacson S, Gold JA, Ginsberg V (1956) Fatal aplastic anemia after therapy with Nuvarone (3-methyl-5-phenylhydantoin). J Am Med Assoc 160:1311–1312
Jacobi G, Thorbeck R, Ritz A, Janssen W, Schmidts H-L (1980) Fatal hepatoxicity in child on phenobarbitone and sodium valproate. Lancet I:712–713
Jacobsen NO, Mosekilde L, Myhre-Jensen O, Pedersen E, Wildenhoff KE (1976) Liver biopsies in epileptics during anticonvulsant therapy. Acta Med Scand 199:345–348
Janz D (1982) On major malformations and minor anomalies in the offspring of parents with epilepsy: review of the literature: In: Janz D, Dam M, Richens A, Bossi L, Helge H, Schmidt D (eds) Epilepsy, pregnancy, and the child. Raven, New York, pp 211–222
Janz D, Schmidt D (1974) Anti-epileptic drugs and failure of oral contraceptives. Lancet I:1113
Janz D, Dam M, Richens A, Bossi L, Helge H, Schmidt D (1982) Epilepsy, pregnancy, and the child. Raven, New York
Johannessen SI, Henriksen O (1980) Pharmacokinetic observations of sodium valproate in healthy subjects and in patients with epilepsy. In: Johannessen SI, Morselli PL, Pippenger CE, Richens A, Schmidt D, Meinardi H (eds) Antiepileptic therapy: advances in drug monitoring. Raven, New York, pp 131–140
Johnson GF, Least CJ Jr, Serum JW, Solow EB, Solomon HM (1976) Monitoring drug concentrations in a case of combined overdosage with primidone and methsuximide. Clin Chem 22:915–921
Joist JH, Cazenave JP, Mustard JF (1973) The effect of barbituric acid derivatives on platelet function in vitro and in vivo. Thromb Diath Haemorrh 30:315–326
Jubiz W, Haussler MR, McCain TA, Tolman KG (1977) Plasma 1,25-dihydroxyvitamin D levels in patients receiving anticonvulsant drugs. J Clin Endocrinol Metab 44:617–621
Kaneko S, Suzuki K, Sato T, Ogawa Y, Nomura Y (1982) The problems of antiepileptic medication in the neonatal period: is breast-feeding advisable? In: Janz D, Dam M, Richens A, Bossi L, Helge H, Schmidt D (eds) Epilepsy, pregnancy, and the child. Raven, New York, pp 343–348
Karch SB (1973) Methsuximide overdose – delayed onset of profound coma. J Am Med Assoc 223:1463–1465
Kattan KR (1970) Calvarial thickening after Dilantin medication. Am J Roentgenol Radium Ther Nucl Med 110:102–105
Katz SH, Gerstman I, Lautenbacher HW, Hediger ML (1976) Failure to confirm anticonvulsant hypomagnesaemia. Br Med J 1:341
Kleckner HB, Yakulis V, Heller P (1975) Severe hypersensitivity to diphenylhydantoin with circulating antibodies to the drug. Ann Intern Med 83:522–523
Koch M, Quattrini A, Lorenzini I, Capurso L, Jezequel AM, Orlandi F (1975) Changes of the liver cell endoplasmic reticulum in patients treated with diphenylhydantoin and phenobarbital. Gastroenterology 7:219
Krarup G, Mogensen AM (1981) Carbamazepine intoxication (in Danish). Ugeskr Laeger 143:603–606
Kruse R (1968) Osteopathien bei antiepileptischer Langzeittherapie. Monatsschr Kinderheilkd 116:378–380
Kruse R (1975) Osteopathien, Kalzium- und Vitamin-D-Stoffwechsel-Störungen unter antiepileptischer Langzeittherapie. Bibl Psychiatr 151:114–143
Kutt H, Winters W, Kokenge R, McDowell F (1964) Diphenylhydantoin metabolism, blood levels, and toxicity. Arch Neurol 11:642–648
Lacy JR, Penry JK (1976) Infantile spasms. Raven, New York
Landolt H (1956) L'electroencéphalographie dans les psychoses épileptiques et les épisodes schizophréniques. Rev Neurol (Paris) 95:597–599

Langdon DE, Harlan JR, Bailey RL (1973) Thrombophlebitis with diazepam used intravenously. J Am Med Assoc 223:184–185
Lapes M, Antoniades K, Gartner W Jr, Vivacqua R (1976a) Conversion of a binding lymphoepithelial salivary gland lesion to a lymphocytic lymphoma during Dilantin therapy. Cancer 38:1318–1322
Lapes MJ, Vivacqua RJ, Antoniades K (1976b) Immunoblastic lymphadenopathy associated with phenytoin (diphenylhydantoin). Lancet I:198
Latis GO, Battino D, Boldi B, Breschi F, Ferraris G, Moise A, Molteni B, Simionata L (1982) Preliminary data of a neuropediatric follow-up of infants born to epileptic mothers. In: Janz D, Dam M, Richens A, Bossi L, Helge H, Schmidt D (eds) Epilepsy, pregnancy, and the child. Raven, New York, pp 419–423
Laubenthal F, Raffauf JH (1963) Begleit- und Nebenerscheinungen bei Ospolot-Anwendung. In: Selbach H (ed) Internationales Kolloquium über das Antikonvulsium Ospolot. Staufen, Kamp Lintfort, pp 124–133
Laubscher FA (1966) Fatal diphenylhydantoin poisoning. J Am Med Assoc 198:1120–1121
Le Bihan G, Bourreille J, Sampson M, Leroy J, Szekely AM, Coquerel A (1980) Fatal hepatic failure and sodium valproate. Lancet II:1298–1299
Lederlin P, Mangin Cheval MC, Macinot C, Thibaut G (1976) Les adenopathies au cours des traitements par hydantoines. Problemes histopathologiques. Ann Med Nancy 15:33–37
Levy LL, Fenichel GM (1965) Diphenylhydantoin activated seizures. Neurology 15:716–722
Li FP, Willard DR, Goodman R, Vawter G (1975) Malignant lymphoma after diphenylhydantoin (Dilantin) therapy. Cancer 36:1359–1362
Livingston S, Boks LL (1955) Use of the dione drugs (Propazone, Tridione, Paradione, Dimedione and Malidone) in treatment of epilepsy of children. N Engl J Med 253:138–142
Logothetis J (1967) Methetoin (N-3) treatment in epilepsy. Dis Nerv Syst 28:515–518
London DR, Loizou LA, Butt WR, Rovei V, Bianchetti G, Morselli PL (1980) The effect of anti-convulsant drugs (AED) on hormonal responses in normal volunteers. In: Johannessen SI, Morselli PL, Pippenger CE, Richens A, Schmidt D, Meinardi H (eds) Antiepileptic therapy: advances in drug monitoring. Raven, New York, pp 405–411
Lorentz de Haas AM, Kuilman M (1964) Ethosuximide (alpha-ethyl-alpha-methyl-succinimide) and grand mal. Epilepsia 5:90–96
Loscalzo AE (1952) Mesantoin in the control of epilepsy. Neurology 2:403–441
Lund M (1941) Dupuytren's contracture and epilepsy. Acta Psychol Neurol 16:465–492
Luoma PV, Myllylä VV, Sotaniemi EA, Lehtinen IA, Hokkanen EJ (1980a) Plasma high-density lipoprotein cholesterol in epileptics treated with various anticonvulsants. Eur Neurol 19:67–72
Luoma PV, Myllylä VV, Hokkanen E (1980b) Elevated serum growth hormone levels in patients treated with anticonvulsants. In: Canger R, Angeleri F, Penry JK (eds) Advances in epileptology: XIth epilepsy international symposium. Raven, New York, pp 431–433
MacKinney AA, Booker HE (1972) Diphenylhydantoin effects on human lymphocytes in vitro and in vivo. Arch Intern Med 129:988–992
Maekawa K, Ohta H, Tamai I (1980) Transient brain shrinkage in infantile spasms after ACTH treatment. Report of two cases. Neuropädiatrie 11:80–84
Magnussen CR, Doherthy JM, Hess RA, Tschudy DP (1975) Grand mal seizures and acute intermittent porphyria: the problem of differential diagnosis and treatment. Neurology 25:1121–1125
Mallette LE (1977) Acetazolamide-accelerated anticonvulsant osteomalacia. Arch Intern Med 137:1013–1017
Mattson RH (1972) The benzodiazepines. In: Woodbury DM, Penry JK, Schmidt RP (eds) Antiepileptic drugs. Raven, New York, pp 497–516
Matz DR, Rolf LH, Brune GG (1977) Serumenzymmuster bei cerebralen Krampfanfällen. Nervenarzt 48:632–635

McDanal CE Jr, Bolman WM (1975) Delayed idiosyncratic psychosis with diphenylhydantoin. J Am Med Assoc 231:1063
McGeachy TE, Bloomer WE (1953) The phenobarbital sensitivity syndrome. Am J Med 14:600–604
McLain LW, Martin JT, Allen JH (1980) Cerebellar degeneration due to chronic phenytoin therapy. Ann Neurol 7:18–23
Meistrup-Larsen K-I, Hermann S, Permin H (1979) Chronic diphenylhydantoin encephalopathy in mentally retarded children and adolescents with severe epilepsy. Acta Neurol Scand 60:50–55
Millichap JG (1972) Mephenytoin, ethotoin, and albutoin. In Woodbury DM, Penry JK, Schmidt RP (eds) Antiepileptic drugs. Raven, New York, pp 275–281
Millichap JG, Ortiz WR (1966) Nitrazepam in myoclonic epilepsies. Am J Dis Child 112:242–248
Moeschlin S (1972) Klinik und Therapie der Vergiftungen, 5th ed. Thieme, Stuttgart
Morley D, Wynne NA (1957) Actue primidone poisoning in a child. Br Med J 1:90
Moses H, Klawans HL (1979) Bromide intoxication. In: Vinken PJ, Bruyn GW (eds) Handbook of clinical neurology. North-Holland, Amsterdam, pp 295–300
Murphy MJ, Lyon LW, Taylor JW, Mitts G (1981) Valproic acid associated pancreatitis in an adult. Lancet I:41–42
Neilan BA, Leppik IE (1980) Phenytoin and formation of T lymphocyte rosettes. Arch Neurol 37:580–581
Niedermeyer E (1970) Intravenous diazepam and its anticonvulsive action. Johns Hopkins Med J 127:79–96
Niedermeyer E, Blumer D, Holscher E, Walker BA (1970) Classical hysterical seizures facilitated by anticonvulsant toxicity. Psychiatr Clin (Basel) 3:71–84
Nikkilä EA, Kaste M, Ehnholm C, Viikari J (1978) Elevation of high-density lipoprotein in epileptic patients treated with phenytoin. Acta Med Scand 204:517–520
Norris JW, Pratt RF (1974) Folic acid deficiency and epilepsy. Drugs 8:366–385
Obe G, Riedl L, Herha J (1980) Mutagenität von Antiepileptika. In: Doose H, Dam M, Gross-Selbeck G, Meinardi H (eds) Epilepsie 1979. Thieme, Stuttgart, pp 58–69
Offermann G, Pinto V, Kruse R (1979) Anticonvulsant drugs and vitamin D supplementation. Epilepsia 20:3–10
Orth DN, Almeida H, Walsh FB, Honda M (1967) Ophthalmoplegia resulting from diphenylhydantoin and primidone intoxication. J Am Med Assoc 201:225–227
Ounsted C (1955) The hyperkinetic syndrome in epileptic children. Lancet II:303–311
Parker WA (1974) Primidone thrombocytopenia. Ann Intern Med 81:559–560
Parker WA, Gumnit RJ (1974) Diphenylhydantoin toxicity: dose-dependent blood dyscrasia. Neurology 24:1178–1180
Pateisky K, Presslich O (1970) Wirkungen von Maliasin bei Epilepsie mit häufiger Anfallsfrequenz. In: Pateisky K, Lechner H (eds) Sozialmedizinische und therapeutische Aspekte der psychischen Veränderungen bei Epilepsie. Geigy, Basel, pp 108–113
Pendergrass TW, Hanson JW (1976) Fetal hydantoin syndrome and neuroblastoma. Lancet II:150
Peraino C, Fry RJM, Staffeldt E, Christopher JP (1975) Comparative enhancing effects of phenobarbital, amobarbital, diphenylhydantoin, and dichlorodiphenyltrichloroethane on 2-acetylaminofluorene-induced hepatic tumorigenesis in the rat. Cancer Res 35:2884–2890
Perlemuter L, Hazard J, Kazatchkine M, Guilhaume B, Bernheim R (1975) Action comparée de la carbamazepine et du clofibrate dans le diabete insipide, Etude de 7 cas. Nouv Presse Méd 4:2307–2319
Perucca E, Richens A (1980) The pathophysiological basis of drug toxicity. In: Grundmann E (ed) Current topics in pathology, vol 69, drug induced pathology. Springer, Berlin Heidelberg New York, pp 17–68
Perucca E, Garratt A, Hebdige S, Richens A (1978) Water intoxication in epileptic patients receiving carbamazepine. J Neurol Neurosurg Psychiatr 41:713–718
Peterson WG (1967) Clinical study of Mogadan. A new anticonvulsant. Neurology 17:878–880

Pinder RM, Brogden RN, Speight TM, Avery GS (1976) Clonazepam: a review of its pharmacological properties and therapeutic efficacy in epilepsy. Drugs 12:321–361
Pinder RM, Brogden RN, Speight TM, Avery GS (1977) Sodium valproate: a review of its pharmacological properties and therapeutic efficacy in epilepsy. Drugs 13:81–123
Pisciotta AV (1975) Hematologic toxicity of carbamazepine. In: Penry JK, Daly DD (eds) Advances in neurology, vol 11. Raven, New York, pp 355–368
Plaa GL (1975) Acute toxicity of antiepileptic drugs. Epilepsia 16:183–191
Popper H, Rubin E, Gardiol D, Schaffner F, Paronetto F (1965) Drug-induced liver disease. Arch Intern Med 115:128–136
Prager PJ, Krause K.-H, Ritz E, Schmidt-Gayk H (1977) Handskelettaufnahmen in Mammographietechnik bei Patienten unter antiepileptischer Medikation. Fortschr Röntgenstr 126:371–375
Pruitt AW, Zwiren GT, Patterson JH, Dayton PG, Cook CE, Wall ME (1975) A complex pattern of disposition of phenytoin in severe intoxication. Clin Pharmacol Ther 18:112–120
Puka J, Szajewski JM (1975) Case of exceptionally severe luminal poisoning (over 25 g) successfully treated with hemodialysis and forced diuresis. Pol Tyg Lek 30:1583–1585
Rating D, Jäger-Roman E, Koch S, Göpfert-Geyer I, Helge H (1982) Minor anomalies in the offspring of epileptic parents. In: Janz D, Dam M, Richens A, Bossi L, Helge H, Schmidt D (eds) Epilepsy, pregnancy, and the child. Raven, New York, pp 283–288
Reidenberg MM, Levy M, Warner H, Coutinho CB, Schwartz MA, Yu G, Cheripko J (1978) Relationship between diazepam dose, plasma level, age, and central nervous system depression. Clin Pharmacol Ther 23:371–374
Reinken L (1975) The influence of antiepileptic drugs on vitamin B_6 metabolism. Acta Vitaminol Enzymol 29:252–254
Rementeria JL, Bhatt K (1977) Withdrawal symptoms in neonates from intrauterine exposure to diazepam. J Pediatr 90:123–126
Reunanen MI, Sotaniemi EA, Hakkarainen HK (1976) Serum calcium balance during early phase of diphenylhydantoin therapy. Int J Clin Pharmacol 14:15–19
Reynolds EH (1975) Chronic antiepileptic toxicity: a review. Epilepsia 16:319–352
Richardson SGN, Fletcher DJ, Jeavons PM, Stuart J (1976) Sodium valproate and platelet function. Br Med J 1:221–222
Riikonen R, Donner M (1980) ACTH therapy in infantile spasms: side effects. Arch Dis Child 55:664–672
Robins MM (1962) Aplastic anemia secondary to anticonvulsants. Am J Dis Child 104:614–624
Rockley GJ (1965): Attempted suicide with sulthiame. Br Med J 2:632
Rodin EA, Rim CS, Rennick PM (1974) The effects of carbamazepine on patients with psychomotor epilepsy: results of a double-blind study. Epilepsia 15:574–561
Rodin EA, Rim CS, Kitano H, Lewis R, Rennick PM (1976) A comparison of the effectiveness of primidone versus carbamazepine in epileptic out-patients. J Nerv Ment Dis 163:41–46
Rootwelt K, Ganes T, Johannessen SI (1978) Effect of carbamazepine, phenytoin and phenobarbitone on serum levels of thyroid hormones and thyrotropin in humans. Scand J Clin Lab Invest 38:731–736
Rosalki SB (1976) Plasma enzyme changes and their interpretation in patients receiving anticonvulsant and enzyme-inducing drugs. In: Richens A, Woodford FP (eds) Anticonvulsant drugs and enzyme induction. Elsevier, Amsterdam, pp 27–35
Rosanelli K (1970) Über die Wirkung von pränatal verabreichtem Diazepam auf das Frühgeborene. Geburtshilfe Frauenheilk 30:713–724
Roseman E (1961) Dilantin toxicity. Neurology 11:912–921
Rowe DJF (1974) Alkaline phosphatase levels in epileptic subjects. Br Med J 3:686
Rowley VN, Gauron EF (1977) Effects of chronic administration of diphenylhydantoin on learning and offspring behavior. Psychopharmacology 53:259–262
Rundle AT, Sudell B (1973) Leucine aminopeptidase isoenzyme changes after treatment with anticonvulsant drugs. Clin Chim Acta 44:377–384

Ruppli H, Vossen R (1957) Nebenwirkung der Hydantoinkörpertherapie unter dem Bilde eines visceralen Lupus erythematosus. Schweiz Med Wochenschr 87:1555–1558
Ruuskanen I, Kilpeläinen HO, Riekkinen PJ (1979) Side effects of sodium valproate during long-term treatment in epilepsy. Acta Neurol Scand 60:125–128
Salcman M, Pippenger CE (1975) Acute carbamazepine encephalopathy. JAMA 231:915
Saltzstein SL, Ackerman LV (1959) Lymphoadenopathy induced by anticonvulsant drugs and mimicking clinically and pathologically malignant lymphomas. Cancer 12:164–182
Sasaki M, Tonoda S, Aoki Y, Katsumi M (1980) Pancreatitis due to valproic acid. Lancet I:1196
Schain RJ, Ward JW, Guthrie D (1977) Carbamazepine as an anticonvulsant in children. Neurology 27:476–480
Schmidt D (1981 a) Behandlung der Epilepsien. Thieme, Stuttgart
Schmidt D (1981 b) Effect of antiepileptic drugs on estrogen and progesterone metabolism and on oral contraception. In: Dam M, Gram L, Penry JK (eds) Advances in epileptology: XIIth epilepsy international symposium. Raven, New York, pp 423–431
Schmidt D (1982 a) Diazepam. In: Woodbury DM, Penry JK, Pippenger CE (eds) Antiepileptic drugs, 2nd ed. Raven, New York
Schmidt D (1982 b) The influence of antiepileptic drugs on the electroencephalogram. A review of controlled studies. Electroencephalogr Clin Neurophysiol [Suppl] 36:453–466
Schmidt D, Seldon L (1982) Adverse effects of antiepileptic drugs. Raven, New York
Schmidt D, Sörensen H (1981) Polyfibromatose durch Phenobarbital. In: Remschmidt HH, Rentz R, Jungmann R (eds) Epilepsie 1980. Thieme, Stuttgart, pp 198–201
Schmidt D, Vogel A (1977) Plasmakonzentrationen nach Injektion und Infusion von Phenytoin. Klin Wochenschr 55:219–223
Schmitz I, Janzik HH, Mayer K (1975) Persönlichkeitsstruktur und Sexualverhalten Anfallskranker unter Langzeitbehandlung mit DPH. Bibl Psychiatr 151:176–181
Schneiderman MA (1974) Phenobarbitone and liver tumors. Lancet II:1085
Seager J (1976) Lymphocytes in children treated with phenytoin. Lancet II:1205
Seager J, Wilson J, Jamison DL, Hayward AR, Soothill JF (1975) IgA deficiency, epilepsy, and phenytoin treatment. Lancet II:632–635
Seyfeddinipur N (1976) Lymphadenopathie bei Phenytoin-Behandlung. Dtsch Med Wochenschr 101:1454–1456
Shafer RB, Nuttall FQ (1975) Calcium and folic acid absorption in patients taking anticonvulsant drugs. J Clin Endocrinol Metab 41:1125–1129
Sherard ES Jr, Steiman GS, Couri D (1980) Treatment of childhood epilepsy with valproic acid: results of the first 100 patients in a 6-month trial. Neurology 30:31–35
Sherman S, Roizen N (1976) Fetal hydantoin syndrome and neuroblastoma. Lancet II:517
Simon D, Penry JK (1975) Sodium di-*n*-propylacetate (DPA) in the treatment of epilepsy. Epilepsia 16:549–573
Simpson JR (1966) "Collagen disease" due to carbamazepine (Tegretol). Br Med J 2:1434
Singsen BH, Fishman L, Hanson V (1976) Antinuclear antibodies and lupus-like syndromes in children receiving anticonvulsants. Pediatrics 57:529–534
Smith RB (1976) Sodium valproate: dosage for children. Mr Med J 2:1507
Snapper I, Marks D, Schwartz L, Hollander L (1953) Hemolytic anemia secondary to Mesantoin. Ann Intern Med 39:619–623
Snyder CH (1968) Myoclonic epilepsy in children: short-term comparative study of two benzodiazepine derivatives in treatment. South. Med J 61:17–20
So EL, Penry JK (1981) Adverse effects of phenytoin on peripheral nerves and neromuscular junction: a review. Epilesia 22:467–473
Sorrell TC, Forbes IJ (1975) Depression of immune competence by phenytoin and carbamazepine. Clin Exp Immunol 20:273–285
Sparberg M (1963) Diagnostically confusing complications of diphenylhydantoin therapy. Ann Inter Med 59:914–930
Spatz R, Kugler J, Pongratz D (1981) Neuronale Ceroidlipofuszinose. Akute Leberdystrophie mit letalem Ausgang unter antikonvulsiver Therapie mit Luminal, Rivotril und Ergenyl. In: Rundbrief der Deutschen Sektion der Internationalen Liga gegen Epilepsie, no 69, pp 42–43. Obtainable from: Liga gegen Epilepsie, Landstraße, Kehl-Kork

Spector RH, Davidoff RA, Schwartzman RJ (1976) Phenytoin-induced ophthalmoplegia. Neurology 26:1031–1034

Steiman, GS, Woerpel RW, Sherard ES Jr (1979) Treatment of accidental sodium valproate overdose with an opiate antagonist. Ann Neurol 6:274

Stenzel E, Panteli C, Schnabel R (1981) Leberkoma bei drei anfallskranken Geschwistern nach Valproat-Behandlung in zwei Fällen: In: Rundbrief der Deutschen Sektion der Internationalen Liga gegen Epilepsie, no 69, p 42. Obtainable from: Liga gegen Epilepsie, Landstraße, Kehl-Kork

Stewart CR, Vengrow MI, Riley TI (1980) Double quotidien fever caused by carbamazepine. N Engl J Med 302:1262

Stjernholm MR, Alsever RN, Rudolph MC (1975) Thyroid-function tests in diphenylhydantoin-treated patients. Clin Chem 21:1388–1392

Stolzis L, Scheffner D (1975) Thrombozytenwerte unter Ergenyl. Bibl Psychiat 151:161–165

Stores G (1975) Behavioural effects of anti-epileptic drugs. Dev Med Child Neurol 17:647–658

Strandjord RE, Aanderud S, Myking OL, Johannessen SI (1981) Influence of carbamazepine on serum thyroxine and triiodothyronine in patients with epilepsy. Acta Neurol Scand 63:111–121

Strandjord RE, Johannessen SI, Aarli JA (1980) Serum levels of immunglobulins in epileptic patients on carbamazepine treatment. In: Johannessen SI, Morselli PL, Pippenger CE, Richens A, Schmidt D, Meinardi H (eds) Antiepileptic therapy: advances in drug monitoring. Raven, New York, pp 399–403

Strong JM, Abe T, Gibbs EL, Atkinson AJ Jr (1974) Plasma levels of methsuximide and *N*-desmethyl methsuximide during methsuximide therapy. Neurology 24:250–255

Suchy FJ, Balisteri WF, Buchino JJ, Sondheimer JM, Bates SR, Kearns GL, Stull JD, Bove KE (1979) Acute hepatic failure associated with the use of sodium valproate. N Engl J Med 300:962–966

Sutor AH, Jesdinsky-Buscher C (1976) Veränderungen der Hämostase bei Epilepsie-Behandlung mit Dipropylessigsäure – Erweiterte Untersuchung. Fortschr Med 94:411–414

Syversen GB, Morgan JP, Weintraub M, Myers GJ (1977) Acetazolamide induced interference with primidone absorption. Case reports and metabolic studies. Arch Neurol 34:80–84

Taetle R, Lane TA, Mendelsohn J (1979) Drug-induced agranulocytosis: in vitro evidence for immune suppression of granulopoiesis and cross-reacting lymphocyte antibody. Blood 54:501–512

Targan SR, Chassin MRG, Guze LB (1975) Dilantin®-induced disseminated intravascular coagulation with purpura fulminans. Ann Intern Med 33:227–230

Tassinari CA, Dravet C, Roger J, Cano JP, Gastaut H (1972) Tonic status epilepticus precipitated by intravenous benzodiazepine in five patients with Lennox-Gastaut syndrome. Epilepsia 13:421–435

Tenckhoff H, Sherrard DJ, Hickman RO, Ladda RL (1968) Acute diphenylhydantoin intoxication. Am J Dis Child 116:422–425

Theil GB, Richter RW, Powell MR, Doolan PD (1961) Acute Dilantin poisoning. Neurology 11:138–142

Thibaut G, Guerci O, Puchelle JC (1976) Maladie de Hodgkin et hydantoines. Ann Med Nancy 15:29–32

Thompson PJ (1983): Phenytoin and psychosocial development. In: Morselli PL, Pippenger CE, Penry JK (eds) Antiepileptic drug therapy in pediatrics. Raven, New York, pp 193–198

Thorn I (1975) A controlled study of prophylactic long-term treatment of febrile convulsions with phenobarbital. Acta Neurol Scand [Suppl] 60:67–73

Tift JP (1980) Valproic acid. N Engl J Med 303:394

Tomson T, Tybring G, Bertilsson L, Ekbom K, Rane A (1980) Carbamazepine therapy in trigeminal neuralgia. Arch Neurol 37:699–703

Trimble MR (1983) Anticonvulsant drugs and psychosocial development: phenobarbitone, sodium valproate, and benzodiazepines. In: Morselli PL, Pippenger CE, Penry JK (eds) Antiepileptic drug therapy in pediatrics. Raven, New York, pp 201–212

Trimble MR, Reynolds EH (1976) Anticonvulsant drugs and mental symptoms: a review. Psychol Med 6:169–178

Tripp JH, Hargreaves T, Anthony PP, Searle JF, Miller P, Leonard JV, Patrick AD, Oberholzer VG (1981) Sodium valproate and ornithine carbamyl transferase deficiency. Lancet I:1165–1166

Trolle E (1961) Drug therapy of epilepsy. Acta Psychiatr Neurol Scand 36:187–199

US Public Health Service (1982) Valproic acid and spina bifida: a preliminary report – France. Morbidity and Mortality Weekly Report 31:565–566

Veall RM, Hogarth HC (1975) Thrombocytopenia during treatment with clonazepam. Br Med J 4:462

Voss H v, Petrich C, Karch D, Schulz H-U, Göbel U (1976) Sodium valproate and platelet function. Br Med J 2:179

Wallis W, Kutt H, McDowell F (1968) Intravenous diphenylhydantoin in treatment of acute repetitive seizures. Neurology 18:513–525

Wapner I, Thurston DL, Holowach J (1962) Phenobarbital, its effect on learning in epileptic children. J Am Med Assoc 182–937

Ware S, Millward-Sadler GH (1980) Acute liver disease associated with sodium valproate. Lancet II:1110–1113

Weinstein AW, Allen RJ (1966) Ethoxuximide treatment of petit mal seizures: a study of 87 pediatric patients. Am J Dis Child 111:63–67

Welch TR, Rumack BH, Hammond K (1977) Clonazepam overdose resulting in cyclic coma. Clin Toxicol 10:433–436

White SJ, McLean AEM, Howland C (1979) Anticonvulsant drugs and cancer: a cohort study in patients with severe epilepsy. Lancet II:458–460

Wilder BJ, Ramsay RE (1974) Psychological aberrations associated with antiepileptic drugs. Clin Electroencephogr 5:199–200

Wilder BJ, Buchanan RA, Serrano EE (1973) Correlation of acute diphenylhydantoin intoxication with plasma levels and metabolite excretion. Neurology 23:1329–1332

Wilder BJ, Willmore LJ, Villarreal HJ, Bruni J, Perchalski RJ (1978) Valproic acid: clinical, EEG and pharmacological studies in patients with absence seizures. Acute and long-term studies. Epilepsy Research Foundation of Florida. Gainesville, Florida

Willmore LJ, Wilder BJ, Bruni J, Villarreal HJ (1978) Effect of valproic acid on hepatic function. Neurology 28:961–964

Wilson J, Walton JN, Newell DJ (1959) Beclamide in intractable epilepsy: a controlled trial. Br Med J 1:1275–1278

Winfield DA, Benton P, Espir MLE, Arthur LJH (1976) Sodium valproate and thrombocytopenia. Br Med J 2:981

Wolf SM, Carr A, Davis DC, Davidson S, Dale EP, Forsythe A, Goldenberg ED, Hanson R, Lulejian GA, Nelson MA, Treitman P, Weinstein A (1977) The value of phenobarbital in the child who has a single febrile seizure: a controlled prospective study. Pediatrics 59:378–385

Woodbury DM (1972) Acetazolamide. In: Woodbury DM, Penry JK, Schmidt RP (eds) Antiepileptic drugs. Raven, New York, pp 465–475

Young RSK, Bergman I, Gang DL, Richardson EP Jr (1980) Fatal Reye-like syndrome associated with valproic acid. Ann Neurol 7:389

Ziegler H-K (1970 a) Epilepsie und Cholelithiasis. Z Neurol 198:305–308

Ziegler H-K (1970 b) Maligne Tumoren bei Epileptikern. Z Neurol 198:309–314

Ziegler H-K, Sinazadeh M (1975) Antiepileptika und Leberschaden. J Neurol 208:207–220

Zimmerman HJ (1979) Hepatotoxicity. The adverse effects of drugs and other chemicals on the liver. Appleton-Century-Crofts, New York, pp 395–417

Zucker P, Daum F, Cohen MI (1977) Fatal carbamazepine hepatitis. J Pediatr 91:667–668

CHAPTER 28

Antiepileptic Drug Interactions

E. PERUCCA and A. RICHENS

Antiepileptic drug interactions may be either pharmacokinetic or pharmacodynamic; this chapter discusses only the former. Due to the difficulties of extrapolating animal data to the clinical situation, this review will be restricted to studies which have been performed in normal human volunteers or in patients. Reference to animal experiments, however, will be made occasionally when these are considered to be particularly relevant to the interpretation of clinical findings.

A. Interactions Affecting the Kinetics of Antiepileptic Drugs

I. Drugs Which May Affect the Gastrointestinal Absorption of Antiepileptic Drugs

Drug interactions at the site of absorption in the gastrointestinal tract usually result in decreased bioavailability of antiepileptic drugs. A considerable number of such interactions have been reported.

1. Antacids

The absorption of phenytoin may be reduced by antacids containing calcium carbonate (GARRATT et al. 1979). Mixtures of aluminium hydroxide with magnesium hydroxide or magnesium trisilicate have also been reported to reduce phenytoin bioavailability (KULSHRESTHA et al. 1978; GARRATT et al. 1979), but this effect has not been consistently found (CHAPRON et al. 1979a; O'BRIEN et al. 1978). The absorption of barbiturates (HURWITZ 1977) and benzodiazepines (GREENBLATT et al. 1976; SHADER et al. 1978) may also be reduced by antacids.

2. Activated Charcoal

NEUVONEN et al. (1978, 1983) and NEUVONEN and ELONEN (1980) have shown that the gastrointestinal absorption of carbamazepine, phenobarbital, valproate, and phenytoin is decreased by activated charcoal. The greatest inhibitory effect on absorption was observed when charcoal was ingested within 5 min of administration of the antiepileptic drug.

Oral ingestion of activated charcoal during the postabsorptive phase markedly accelerates the elimination of phenobarbital and carbamazepine (NEUVONEN and ELONEN 1980), probably due to inhibition of reabsorption of enterally secreted drug by activated charcoal. For phenobarbital, this interaction has been exploited therapeutically in cases of intoxication in overdose patients (GOLDBERG and BERLINGER 1982).

3. Calcium Salts

Calcium sulphate used as an excipient in phenytoin capsules has been shown to cause a reduction in phenytoin bioavailability (BOCHNER et al. 1972). Gastric antacids containing calcium carbonate also reduce the bioavailability of phenytoin (GARRATT et al. 1979) but calcium gluconate does not appear to have an important influence (CHAPRON et al. 1979 a; HERISHANU et al. 1976).

4. Antineoplastic Drugs

FINCHAM and SCHOTTELIUS (1979) provided evidence that combination therapy with vinblastine, cisplatin and bleomycin may increase the dosage requirements of phenytoin, possibly by interfering with the absorption of the drug. Similar observations have recently been made by BOLLINI et al. (1983) with vinblastine, methotrexate, and 1,3 bis 2-chlorethylnitrosourea.

5. Ethanol

Serum levels of benzodiazepine drugs are increased by acute administration of ethanol. There are several possible mechanisms. Ethanol enhances the rate and possibly the extent of absorption of some benzodiazepines (HAYES et al. 1977; LAIZI et al. 1979; TAAEUBER et al. 1979) but some studies have failed to confirm this (SELLERS and HOLLOWAY 1978). Ethanol may modify the tissue distribution of benzodiazepines (TAAEUBER et al. 1979) but, more importantly, it can inhibit benzodiazepine metabolism (SELLERS et al. 1980) and potentiate benzodiazepine effects through a pharmacodynamic interaction (LAIZI et al. 1979).

6. Nasogastric Feeding

Nasogastric feeding formulas can inhibit dramatically the absorption of phenytoin, resulting in low serum levels during continuous nasogastric feeding and in signs of toxicity when feeding is discontinued (BAUER 1982).

7. Other Drugs

Oxacillin (FINCHAM et al. 1976) and theophylline (HENDELES 1979) may decrease the absorption of phenytoin and acetazolamide may decrease the absorption of primidone (SYVERSEN et al. 1977).

II. Drugs Which May Affect the Plasma Protein Binding of Antiepileptic Drugs

Phenytoin, valproic acid and diazepam bind extensively to plasma proteins. When agents that are highly bound are used in combination, interactions may occur which result in increased free fraction in the plasma. Since most antiepileptic drugs have a relatively large volume of distribution and are subject to restrictive clearance, the increase in free drug concentration and magnitude of pharmacological effect resulting from these interactions is likely to be short-lived and to be rapidly counteracted by enhanced elimination and redistribution into tissues. At steady state, the overall result of the interaction should be a decrease in the plasma concentration of total (free and protein-bound) drug, whereas the concentration of free drug should remain substantially unchanged (KOCH-WESER and SELLERS 1976; PERUCCA and RICHENS 1980b). Under these circumstances, the most important consequence of this interaction will be a change in the relationship between serum total drug concentration and pharmacological effect, with a corresponding shift of the therapeutic range of (total) serum levels towards lower values. In practice, the situation may be more complex in that the displacing agent may interfere not only with the plasma protein binding, but also with the tissue binding and metabolic inactivation of the affected drug. When this is the case, a clinically important modification of pharmacological effect is likely to be seen.

1. Valproic Acid

Valproic acid displaces phenytoin from plasma protein binding sites both in vitro (CRAMER and MATTSON 1979; MONKS et al. 1978; PATSALOS and LASCELLES 1977) and in vivo (DAHLQVIST et al. 1979; MATTSON et al. 1978; FRIEL et al. 1979; MONKS and RICHENS 1980; PERUCCA et al. 1980; RODIN et al. 1981; KNOTT et al. 1982). Although evidence is incomplete, a number of studies indicate that the interaction may be complex. A pharmacokinetic analysis of the work of MATTSON et al. (1978) and PERUCCA et al. (1980) suggests that valproic acid has a dual effect on phenytoin disposition: (a) it displaces phenytoin from plasma protein binding sites, thereby decreasing the concentration of total drug in serum and (b) it inhibits phenytoin metabolism, thereby increasing the concentration of free drug. The occurrence of a third effect, i.e. displacement of phenytoin from tissue binding sites, was also suggested on the basis of the data presented. A rise in free phenytoin *concentration* (suggestive of inhibition of phenytoin metabolism) in patients started on valproic acid has also been documented by BRUNI et al. (1980 a), RODIN et al. (1981), and KOCH et al. (1981).

JORDAN et al. (1976) have shown that valproic acid increases the unbound fraction of phenobarbital in vitro, but the effect is small and probably of little clinical significance. Carbamazepine is also displaced from protein binding sites by valproic acid (MATTSON et al. 1982). DHILLON and RICHENS (1981b, 1982) found that valproic acid displaces diazepam from plasma protein binding sites and increases the free concentration of diazepam in serum. The interaction may provide an explanation for the observation that the CNS-depressant effects of benzodiazepine drugs are potentiated by concurrent intake of sodium valproate.

2. Phenylbutazone

Phenylbutazone caused a moderate initial decrease, followed by a slight but significant elevation, in total serum phenytoin level (NEUVONEN et al. 1979). Because of a concomitant reduction in the degree of plasma protein binding, the free phenytoin concentration increased markedly during phenylbutazone treatment. These results suggest that phenylbutazone can both displace phenytoin from plasma protein binding sites and inhibit phenytoin metabolism.

FLEITMAN et al. (1980) showed that phenylbutazone displaces valproic acid from plasma proteins.

3. Aspirin and Salicylic Acid

Both aspirin and salicylic acid have been shown to displace phenytoin from plasma protein binding sites in vitro (ODAR-CEDERLÖF and BORGÅ 1976; PORTER and LAYZER 1975) and in vivo (FRASER et al. 1980; LEONARD et al. 1981; OLANOW et al. 1981; PAXTON 1980) causing a fall in total serum phenytoin level, with little or no change in free phenytoin concentration. FLEITMAN et al. (1980) and ORR et al. (1982) showed that salicylic acid displaces valproic acid from plasma proteins.

4. Heparin and Free Fatty Acids

Administration of heparin has been shown to decrease the plasma protein binding of phenytoin (GIACOMINI et al. 1980), diazepam (DESMOND et al. 1979) and *N*-desmethyldiazepam (ROUTLEDGE et al. 1980).

However, the change in plasma protein binding produced by in vivo administration of heparin seems to be at least in part artefactual, being mediated by in vitro accumulation of free fatty acids under the catalytic action of lipoprotein lipase released by heparin (BROWN et al. 1981).

5. Other Drugs

Diazoxide (ROE et al. 1975), halofenate (KARCH et al. 1977), sulphafurazole (LUNDE et al. 1970), sulphamethoxypyridazine (KURATA and WILKINSON 1974), tolbutamide (WESSELING and MOLS-THURKOW 1975) and azapropazone (GEANEY et al. 1983) have all been shown to displace phenytoin from plasma proteins in vivo or in vitro. HOOPER et al. (1971) reported that sulthiame may also increase the free fraction of phenytoin in plasma, but LUNDE et al. (1970) found no evidence of this effect. Intralipid increases the free fraction of valproic acid, probably through elevation of free fatty acids (ZIMMERMAN et al. 1981).

III. Drugs Which May Inhibit the Metabolism of Antiepileptic Drugs

Most antiepileptic drugs have a narrow therapeutic ratio, and an increase in steady-state serum levels as a result of inhibition of their metabolism can result in a clinically important potentiation of pharmacological response. Phenytoin metabolism appears to be particularly vulnerable to inhibition by other drugs since its para-hydroxylation is a saturable process.

Table 1. Other interactions (not mentioned in the text) which increase serum concentrations of antiepileptic drugs

Affected drug	Interfering drug	Reference
Phenytoin	Allopurinol	YOKOCHI et al. (1982)
	Azapropazone	GEANEY et al. (1983)
	Calcium carbide	OLESEN (1976)
	Chlorpheniramine	PUGH et al. (1975)
	Chlorpromazine	BIELMANN et al. (1978)
	Dicoumarol	HANSEN et al. (1966)
	Disulfiram	OLESEN (1967); SVENDSEN et al. (1976); VESELL et al. (1971)
	Ethanol	SANDOR et al. (1980)
	Imipramine	PERUCCA and RICHENS (1977)
	Methylphenidate	GARRETTSON et al. (1969); KUTT and LOUIS (1972)
	Phencoupromon	SKOVSTED et al. (1976)
	Phenyramidol	SOLOMON and SCHROGIE (1967)
	Sulphinpyrazone	HANSEN et al. (1980b)
	Thioridazine	VINCENT (1980)
	Tolbutamide	WESSELING and MOLS-THÜRKOW (1975)
	Viloxazine	ICI (unpublished data, 1974)
Carbamazepine	Nicotinamide	BOURGEOIS et al. (1982)
	Viloxazine	PISANI F et al. (1984)
Diazepam	Disulfiram	McLEOD et al. (1978)
	Ethanol (acute)	SELLERS et al. (1980)
	Steroid oral contraceptives	ABERNETHY et al. (1982)
N-Desmethylsuximide (active metabolite of methsuximide)	Phenytoin	RAMBECK (1979)
Phenobarbital	Dicoumarol	HANSEN et al. (1966)
	Frusemide	AHMAD et al. (1976)
	Methylphenidate	GARRETTSON et al. (1969)
Primidone	Nicotinamide	BOURGEOIS et al. (1982)
	Valproic acid[a]	WINDORFER et al. (1965)
Trimethadion	Valproic acid	FLACHS et al. (1979)
Valproic acid	Aspirin	ORR et al. (1982)

[a] Conflicting evidence

1. Sulthiame

Sulthiame, a sulphonamide with carbonic anhydrase inhibitory properties, is a powerful inhibitor of phenytoin metabolism (HANSEN et al. 1968; HOUGHTON and RICHENS 1974a, b; OLESEN and JENSEN 1969; RICHENS and HOUGHTON 1975). The interaction is illustrated by a prolongation of the half-life and by a marked rise in the steady-state serum concentration of phenytoin. Prospective studies have shown that the rise in serum phenytoin concentration following the addition of sulthiame may be delayed for up to 10–20 days, suggesting that the inhibition of metabolism is of a non-competive type. It is likely that at least part of both the therapeutic and toxic effects of sulthiame are mediated by this elevating effect on serum phenytoin levels.

RICHENS (1976) reported that sulthiame may also elevate serum levels of phenobarbital and primidone, possibly by inhibiting the metabolism of the latter drugs.

2. Valproic Acid

Serum phenobarbital levels may rise markedly following the administration of sodium valproate to patients receiving chronic barbiturate therapy (GUGLER and VON UNRUH 1980), leading to sedation and in some cases to serious phenobarbital intoxication. Valproic acid can prolong the half-life, reduce the plasma clearance and increase the urinary excretion of unchanged phenobarbital, indicating that inhibition of metabolism is the mechanism responsible for the interaction (BRUNI et al. 1980 b; KAPETANOVIC et al. 1981; PATEL et al. 1980).

Valproic acid may also inhibit phenytoin metabolism (PERUCCA et al. 1980; BRUNI et al. 1980 a). Because of the simultaneous displacement of phenytoin from plasma protein binding sites, a rise in total serum phenytoin concentration may not be consistently seen. Preliminary data suggest that valproic acid may also inhibit the metabolism of diazepam, in addition to displacing it from binding sites (DHILLON and RICHENS 1982).

3. Succinimides

FRANTZEN et al. (1967) reported that ethosuximide can raise serum phenytoin levels but RICHENS and HOUGHTON (1975) could find no evidence of the effect. Treatment with methsuximide has been reported to cause an elevation in the serum levels of both phenytoin (RAMBECK 1979) and phenobarbital (RAMBECK 1979; STENZEL et al. 1978).

4. Benzodiazepines

Both increases and decreases in serum phenytoin concentration have been described in patients given diazepam (PERUCCA and RICHENS 1980 c). Clonazepam does not appear to produce a consistent change in serum phenytoin, phenobarbital, and carbamazepine levels (JOHANNESSEN et al. 1977).

WINDORFER and SAUER (1977) claimed that clonazepam may cause a rise in serum primidone concentration but no evidence of this effect could be found by NANDA et al. (1977).

5. Pheneturide

When pheneturide is added to the treatment of patients on phenytoin, serum phenytoin levels may show an initial rise that is followed by a slow decline to steady-state values slightly above baseline (RICHENS and HOUGHTON 1975). The time course of the interaction is suggestive of initial enzyme-inhibition followed by progressive induction of phenytoin metabolism. HUISMAN et al. (1970) reported that pheneturide increases serum phenobarbital levels, probably by inhibiting its metabolism.

6. Other Antiepileptic Drugs

Phenobarbital may stimulate and inhibit the metabolism of phenytoin at the same time and the overall result of the interaction is unpredictable (KUTT 1972).

Phenytoin treatment usually tends to cause a rise in serum phenobarbital concentration (LAMBIE and JOHNSON 1981; MORSELLI et al. 1971; WINDORFER and SAUER 1977).

7. Antibiotics and Chemotherapeutic Agents

Isoniazid is a potent inhibitor of the metabolism of phenytoin (Fig. 1) (BRENNAN et al. 1970; KUTT et al. 1966, 1970). A rise in serum phenytoin levels and the development of clinical signs of phenytoin toxicity occur in a considerable proportion (10%–27%) of epileptic patients given this drug for the prophylaxis or the treatment of tuberculosis (MILLER et al. 1979; MURRAY 1962; KUTT et al. 1970). The interaction occurs mainly in slow acetylators and is potentiated in vitro by *p*-aminosalicylic acid, which is frequently used in combination with isoniazid.

The metabolism of primidone (SUTTON and KUPFERBERG 1975) and carbamazepine (BLOCK 1982; WRIGHT et al. 1982) can also be inhibited by isoniazid. OCHS et al. (1981) provided evidence that the metabolism of diazepam is also inhibited by isoniazid and that this effect can be reversed by the concurrent administration of rifampicin, a potent enzyme-inducer.

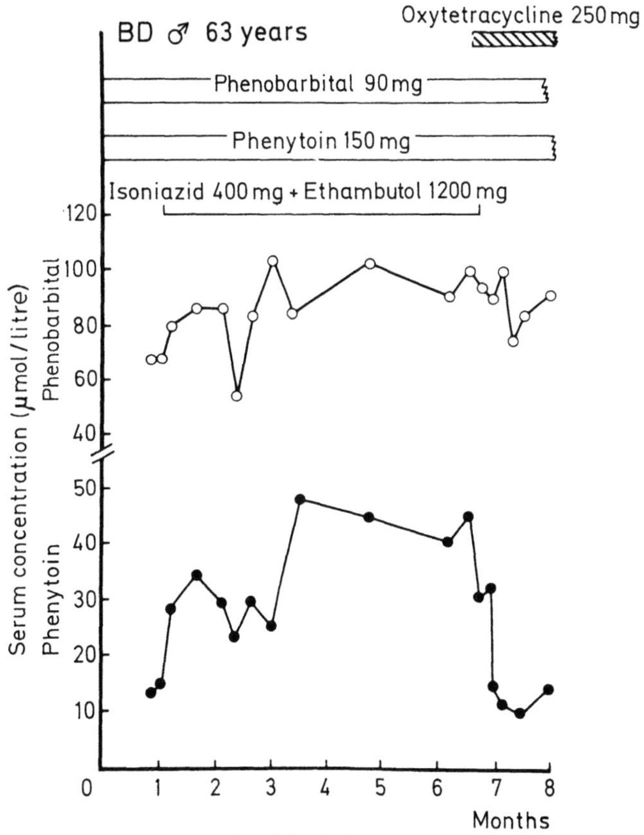

Fig. 1. Effect of treatment with isoniazid and ethambutol on the serum phenytoin and phenobarbital concentration in a 63-year-old epileptic patient (PERUCCA and RICHENS 1980c)

Sulphaphenazole, sulphadiazine, sulphamethizole, and sulphamethoxazole + trimethoprim (co-trimoxazole) and trimethoprim have all been shown to prolong the half-life and to decrease the metabolic clearance of phenytoin, while sulphamethoxypyridazine, sulphadimethoxine, and sulphamethoxydiazine appear to be devoid of this effect (LUMHOLTZ et al. 1975; HANSEN et al. 1979).

Chloramphenicol inhibits the metabolism of phenytoin and precipitates clinical signs of phenytoin intoxication (BALLEK et al. 1973; CHRISTENSEN and SKOVSTED 1969; KOUP et al. 1978; ROSE et al. 1977). Miconazole may also inhibit phenytoin metabolism (ROLAN et al. 1983). KOUP et al. (1978) showed that serum phenobarbital levels may also be elevated by chloramphenicol. DRAVET et al. (1977) and HEDRICK et al. (1983) showed that triacetyloleandomycin and erythromycin can inhibit carbamazepine metabolism.

8. Phenylbutazone

Phenylbutazone prolongs the half-life of phenytoin (ANDREASEN et al. 1973) and increases its serum concentration at steady state, precipitating clinical signs of phenytoin intoxication (NEUVONEN et al. 1979). Since the free fraction of phenytoin is increased in the presence of phenylbutazone, total serum phenytoin levels may underestimate the rise in the concentration of free, pharmacologically active drug.

9. Cimetidine

Cimetidine decreases the plasma clearance of diazepam, presumably by inhibiting its metabolism (KLOTZ and REIMANN 1980). Cimetidine can also increase the serum levels of carbamazepine (TELLERMAN-TOPPET et al. 1981) and phenytoin (HETZEL et al. 1981; see also FRIGO et al. 1983 for review), precipitating clinical signs of toxicity.

10. Propoxyphene

Propoxyphene may inhibit the metabolism of phenytoin (KUTT 1971), phenobarbital (HANSEN et al. 1980 a) and carbamazepine (DAM et al. 1977).

11. Other Drugs

Many other agents have been shown to increase the serum concentration of antiepileptic drugs (Table 1, p. 835).

IV. Drugs Which Stimulate the Metabolism of Antiepileptic Drugs

A number of interactions resulting in stimulation of metabolism of antiepileptic drugs have been described. Generally the stimulating agent is another antiepileptic drug. When this is the case, the clinical implications of the interaction are limited by the fact that the therapeutic efficacy of the added drug may compensate for the potentially adverse consequences of the fall in serum levels of the affected drug.

1. Phenytoin, Phenobarbital, and Primidone

Chronic treatment with phenytoin, phenobarbital, and primidone, alone or in combination, has been shown to increase the metabolic clearance and/or reduce the steady-state serum concentration of diazepam (DHILLON and RICHENS 1981 a), desmethyldiazepam (WILENSKY et al. 1978), clonazepam (KHOO et al. 1980; NANDA et al. 1977; SJÖ et al. 1975), carbamazepine (Fig. 2) (DAM et al. 1975; EICHELBAUM et al. 1979; PERUCCA and RICHENS 1980 a) and valproic acid (Fig. 3) (MIHALY et al. 1979; PERUCCA et al. 1978).

Stimulation of metabolism of primidone occurs in patients treated with phenytoin, phenobarbital and, possibly, carbamazepine (CLOYD et al. 1981; FINCHAM et al. 1974; REYNOLDS et al. 1975; SCHMIDT 1975). Since primidone is partly converted to phenobarbital, which has a long half-life and accumulates in serum, this interaction may result in potentiation rather than reduction of pharmacological effect.

As discussed above, phenobarbital may both stimulate and inhibit the metabolism of phenytoin.

2. Carbamazepine

Carbamazepine is a potent enzyme-inducing drug and may stimulate its own metabolism (RAWLINS et al. 1975) and also that of diazepam and clonazepam (LAI et al. 1978), primidone (see above), ethosuximide (WARREN et al. 1980) and phenytoin (HANSEN et al. 1971 b). BOWDLE et al. (1979) suggested carbamazepine may cause an increase in the plasma clearance and volume of distribution of valproic acid. The mechanisms underlying the latter effect is unclear.

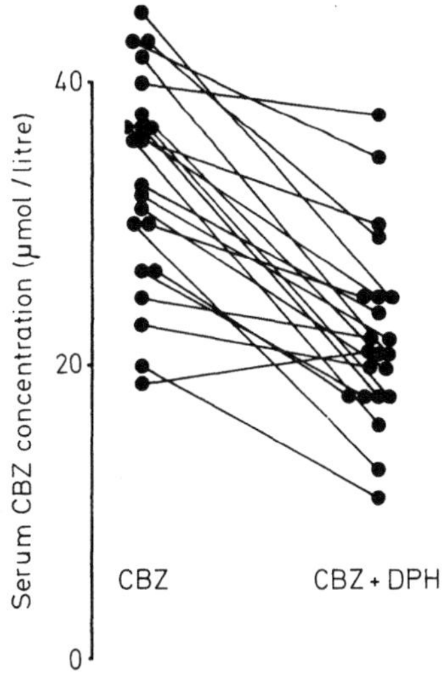

Fig. 2. Serum carbamazepine concentration in epileptic patients treated with carbamazepine alone (*CBZ*) or in combination with phenytoin (*CBZ+DPH*). Patients were matched according to carbamazepine dose (PERUCCA and RICHENS 1980 a)

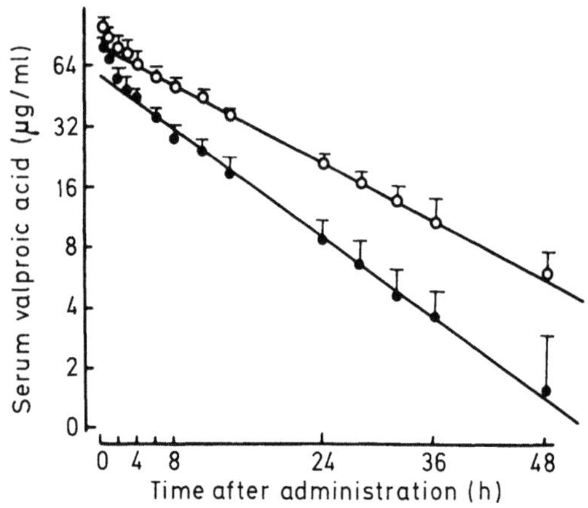

Fig. 3. Serum valproic acid concentration (mean ± SD) after intravenous administration of sodium valproate (800 mg) in six normal subjects (o–o) and in six epileptic patients receiving chronic drug therapy (●–●) (PERUCCA et al. 1978)

3. Folic Acid

Administration of folic acid to folate-depleted patients causes a reduction in serum concentration of phenytoin (BAYLIS et al. 1971; FURLANUT et al. 1978; MAKKI et al. 1980; MATTSON et al. 1973) and phenobarbital (MAKKI et al. 1980). These effects are probably mediated by stimulation of drug metabolism and may provide an explanation for the clinical observation that the control of seizures may be worsened following administration of folate.

4. Ethanol

Chronic intake of ethanol may result in acceleration of phenytoin elimination (KATER et al. 1969). SANDOR et al. (1980), however, found that ethanol also has enzyme-inhibiting properties; an increase in phenytoin clearance 1 week after cessation of drinking in 11 alcoholics was found.

5. Other Drugs

The metabolic clearance of diazepam is enhanced by concurrent treatment with antipyrine (OHNHAUS et al. 1979) and rifampicin (OCHS et al. 1981). It is possible that clozapine (RYAN and MATTHEWS 1970) and nitrofurantoin (HEIJERTZ and PILZ 1978) may also accelerate the elimination of phenytoin.

V. Drugs Which May Affect the Renal Excretion of Antiepileptic Drugs

1. Urine-Alkalinizing Agents

Alkalinization of urine enhances the elimination of phenobarbital by reducing the reabsorption of this acidic drug from the renal tubules (POWELL et al. 1981; WADDELL and BUTLER 1957). The effect can be exploited therapeutically in severe cases of phenobarbital intoxication.

B. Interactions Affecting the Kinetics of Other Drugs

I. Drugs Whose Gastrointestinal Absorption May Be Affected by Antiepileptic Drugs

There is evidence that antiepileptic drugs, phenytoin and barbiturates in particular, may have an inhibitory influence on the gastrointestinal absorption of other drugs. In spite of this, potential interactions at the absorption site have been little investigated. It is likely that some of the interactions resulting in reduced serum drug levels at steady state and presently considered to be due to enzyme induction (Sect. B.IV) are in fact mediated by inhibition of absorption.

Phenobarbital reduces the rate and extent of absorption of griseofulvin from the gastrointestinal tract (BUSFIELD et al. 1963; RIEGELMAN et al. 1970) and can cause therapeutic failure when griseofulvin is administered in conventional doses to epileptic patients. FINE et al. (1977) found that the oral availability of frusemide was reduced by phenytoin, providing an explanation for the observation that the diuretic response to frusemide is considerably reduced in drug-treated patients (AHMAD 1974).

There is suggestive evidence that phenytoin in combination with phenobarbital or carbamazepine can decrease the gastrointestinal absorption of nomifensine (NAWISHI and HATHAWAY 1982; NAWISHI et al. 1981). Certain barbiturates may decrease the absorption of dicoumarol (LEWIS 1966).

II. Drugs Whose Plasma Protein Binding May Be Affected by Antiepileptic Drugs

There is increasing evidence that treatment with certain antiepileptic drugs may result in significant alterations in plasma drug-binding capacity.

1. Methotrexate

Phenytoin can displace methotrexate from plasma protein binding sites and possibly potentiate methotrexate toxicity (REILLY 1973).

2. Hormones

Drug-treated epileptic patients have elevated levels of sex-hormone binding globulin (SHBG) (BARRAGRY et al. 1978; VICTOR et al. 1977); this abnormality may be related to enzyme induction (BACK et al. 1980). The change in the concentration of SHBG may complicate the interpretation of data on total serum sex hormone levels in epileptic patients (DANA-HAERI and RICHENS 1981). An increase in SHBG leading to decreased free concentration of steroid hormones has been implicated as a contributing factor to reduced efficacy of the contraceptive pill in patients treated with anticonvulsants (Editorial 1980). Phenytoin may compete with thyroxine for binding sites on the thyroxine-binding globulin (OPPENHEIMER 1968).

3. Lidocaine

ROUTLEDGE et al. (1981) found that patients treated with phenytoin in combination with other antiepileptic drugs had a reduced free fraction of lidocaine in plasma. The effect was mediated by an increase in the concentration of α_1-acid glycoprotein, probably as a result of the drug treatment. The change in lidocaine binding may alter the disposition kinetics of this drug (PERUCCA and RICHENS 1979 b; ROUTLEDGE et al. 1981).

4. Other Drugs

Phenytoin has been shown to displace some tricyclic antidepressants from plasma protein binding sites in vitro (BORGÅ et al. 1969).

III. Drugs Whose Metabolism May Be Inhibited by Antiepileptic Drugs

Interactions resulting in inhibition of metabolism of other drugs have rarely been described. NAPPI (1979) reported prolongation of the prothrombin time in two warfarin-treated patients given phenytoin in combination. It is possible that this effect was mediated by inhibition of warfarin metabolism.

FURLANUT and RIZZONI (1980) reported that valproic acid can prolong the half-life of antipyrine. However, no evidence of this effect was found by OXLEY et al. (1979) and PERUCCA et al. (1979).

IV. Drugs Whose Metabolism May Be Stimulated by Antiepileptic Drugs

Phenytoin, carbamazepine, phenobarbital, and primidone, when administered in therapeutic doses to patients with epilepsy, are potent inducers of the hepatic drug-metabolizing enzymes (PERUCCA and RICHENS 1981; PERUCCA et al. 1979; SOTANIEMI et al. 1978). A number of clinically important drug interactions are considered to be mediated by this effect.

1. Oral Anticoagulants

Patients treated with barbiturates eliminate dicoumarol and warfarin at an increased rate and therefore may require unusually large doses of these drugs for a satisfactory degree of anticoagulation to be achieved. A danger of this phenomenon is a rebound prolongation in prothrombin time when the enzyme-inducing agent is withdrawn without careful readjustment of the anticoagulant dose. Serious haemorrhagic reactions have been described as a result of this phenomenon (MACDONALD and ROBINSON 1968).

Both phenytoin and carbamazepine have also been shown to enhance the elimination of dicoumarol in man (HANSEN et al. 1971 a, b). ROSS and BEELEY (1980) reported a marked prolongation in prothrombin time following withdrawal of carbamazepine treatment but NAPPI (1979) found that phenytoin potentiated the anticoagulant effect of warfarin.

2. Antibiotics and Chemotherapeutic Agents

Patients treated with phenytoin, phenobarbital, and carbamazepine eliminate doxycycline at an abnormally fast rate (NEUVONEN and PENTTILA 1974; PENTTILA et al. 1974); this can result in reduced clinical effectiveness of the antibiotic. The elimination of chloramphenicol (BLOXHAM et al. 1979) may also be enhanced by concurrent antiepileptic drug therapy. DE RAUTLIN DE LA ROY et al. (1971) found a decrease in serum rifampicin levels in patients receiving phenobarbital but ACOCELLA et al. (1974) failed to detect any measurable effect of this drug treatment on rifampicin half-life. Phenobarbital stimulates the metabolism of metronidazole, thereby reducing its effect (GUPTA 1982; MEAD et al. 1982).

3. Corticosteroids and Metyrapone

Phenobarbital has been shown to cause deterioration in the therapeutic response to prednisolone in patients with rheumatoid arthritis (BROOKS et al. 1976) and to precipitate attacks of asthma in prednisone-dependent patients (BROOKS et al. 1972). Phenytoin and primidone have been shown to reduce the therapeutic efficacy of dexamethasone (BOYLAN et al. 1976; HANCOCK and LEVELL 1978; MCLELLAND and JACK 1978). Toxic reactions on stopping the enzyme-inducing drugs without an adequate adjustment in steroid dosage have also been reported (JUBIZ and MEIKLE 1979).

Induction of dexamethasone metabolism in phenytoin-treated patients is responsible for the failure of the low-dose dexamethasone suppression test, but the response to the high-dose test is unaffected (JUBIZ et al. 1970). Another test of adrenal function, the inhibition of cortisol biosynthesis by oral metyrapone, fails in phenytoin-treated patients due to induction of first-pass metabolism of metyrapone (FUJI et al. 1975; MEIKLE et al. 1969).

For more information on the interaction between antiepileptic drugs and corticosteroids the reader is referred to JUBIZ and MEIKLE (1979).

4. Oral Steroid Contraceptives

The efficacy of the contraceptive pill is reduced in patients treated with phenytoin, phenobarbital, primidone or carbamazepine. The effect is responsible for the high incidence of spotting and breakthrough bleeding and for the occasional occurrence of pregnancy in epileptic patients taking the contraceptive pill (HEMPEL and KLINGER 1976; Editorial 1980). The contraceptive failure is due to induction of progestagen and oestrogen metabolism, particularly the latter (BACK et al. 1981 b). The interaction is likely to take place largely in the gut wall, where ethinyloestradiol is extensively metabolized (BACK et al. 1981 a). Women taking antiepileptic drugs should be given a contraceptive preparation containing at least 50 μg ethinyloestradiol, but pregnancies have occurred even with this dose of oestrogen (COULAM and ANNEGERS 1979).

Phenytoin also decreases the activity of oestrogens when they are used therapeutically in the management of menopausal symptoms (NOTELOVITZ et al. 1981).

5. Cardioactive Drugs

Phenobarbital and phenytoin have been shown to shorten the half-life of quinidine and to produce a marked reduction in serum quinidine levels at steady state (DATA et al. 1976). Should antiepileptic drugs be discontinued, the dose of quinidine may need to be reduced to avoid toxicity (CHAPRON et al. 1979 b).

AITIO et al. (1981) showed that administration of enzyme-inducing drugs such as rifampicin and phenytoin accelerates the conversion of disopyramide to its *N*-dealkylated metabolite. This metabolite has some antiarrhythmic activity and therefore the suggestion that the interaction may lead to decreased effectiveness of disopyramide (AITIO and VUORENMAA 1980) must be taken with caution. Measurements of the serum level of the metabolite may prove valuable in these patients.

Pentobarbital (used as a model enzyme-inducing drug) has been shown to enhance the first-pass metabolism of metroprolol (HAGLUND et al. 1979) and alprenolol (ALVAN et al. 1977; COLLSTE et al. 1979), thereby reducing the oral availability of these β-blockers. Propranolol metabolism may also be induced by anticonvulsants (SOTANIEMI et al. 1979). Phenobarbital and phenytoin increase the rate of conversion of digitoxin to digoxin and/or other metabolites (JELLIFFE and BLANKENHORN 1966; SOLOMON et al. 1971; SOLOMON and ABRAMS 1972). KALDOR et al. (1975), however, failed to detect any change in digitoxin clearance following the administration of phenobarbital in ten patients. BOGAERT et al. (1971) found that phenobarbital stimulates the metabolism of nitroglycerin in man, and BEGG et al. (1982) found a marked acceleration of mexiletine metabolism in phenytoin-treated patients.

6. Antineoplastic Drugs

Phenytoin stimulates the metabolism of the radio-sensitizing drug misonidazole (GANGJI et al. 1980; WORKMAN et al. 1980), thereby reducing the incidence of toxic reactions (WASSERMAN et al. 1980). Barbiturates stimulate the metabolism of cyclophosphamide (JAO et al. 1972; MELLETT 1971). The implications of this interaction are unclear, also because cyclophosphamide has active metabolites.

KORANYI and GERO (1979) have provided evidence that phenytoin protects the beta-cells of the pancreas from the cytotoxic effects of streptozotocin; whether this is due to enhanced metabolism of streptozotocin or to a pharmacodynamic effect is unclear.

7. Non-Opiate Analgesics

Treatment with enzyme-inducing agents has been shown to decrease the oral availability of paracetamol (acetaminophen), probably by stimulating its first-pass metabolism in the liver (PERUCCA and RICHENS 1979 a). The half-life of paracetamol and the serum paracetamol concentration at steady state are also reduced in these patients (CUNNINGHAM and PRICE-EVANS 1981; PRESCOTT et al. 1981). The speculation has been made that induction of paracetamol metabolism by antiepileptic drugs can enhance the hepatotoxic potential by increasing the rate of formation of toxic metabolites, but recent studies do not support this hypothesis (PRESCOTT et al. 1981).

The metabolism of acetanilide, antipyrine, fenoprofen, and phenylbutazone has also been found to be increased in patients taking antiepileptic drugs. SHAHIDI (1968) showed that phenobarbital can increase the rate of conversion of phenacetin into the methaemoglobin-forming *ortho*-hydroxy metabolite and precipitate serious methaemoglobinaemic reactions in genetically predisposed patients.

8. Pethidine (Meperidine)

Phenytoin has been shown to increase both the systemic clearance and the first-pass metabolism of pethidine, thereby reducing its oral availability. The biotransformation of the metabolite nor-pethidine may also be stimulated by phenytoin (POND and KRETZSCHMAR 1981) or phenobarbital (STAMBAUGH et al. 1977, 1978). Increased conversion of pethidine to nor-pethidine may result in enhanced central nervous system toxicity (STAMBAUGH et al. 1977). The metabolism of methadone may also be stimulated (FINELLI 1976).

9. Vitamins

Antiepileptic drugs can cause rickets and osteomalacia by stimulating the metabolic inactivation of vitamin D (see HAHN 1976 and PERUCCA 1978 for review).

LABADARIOS et al. (1978) suggested that phenytoin and other enzyme-inducing agents cause folate deficiency by increasing the utilization of folic acid in synthetic metabolic reactions.

10. Theophylline

Phenytoin (MARQUIS et al. 1982; REED and SCHWARTZ 1982) and carbamazepine (ROSENBERRY et al. 1983) have been shown to accelerate the elimination of theophylline. Evidence on the effect of phenobarbital on theophylline metabolism is, however, conflicting (LANDAY et al. 1978; PFIASKY et al. 1977).

11. Neuroleptics

Serum levels of haloperidol and mesoridazine (active metabolite of thioridazine) are reduced by concurrent treatment with phenytoin and phenobarbital (LINNOILA et al. 1980). Chlorpromazine levels are also reduced by anticonvulsants (PERUCCA 1982).

12. Antidepressants

There is evidence that the metabolism of several antidepressant drugs is stimulated by enzyme-inducing antiepileptic drugs: desmethylchlorimipramine (TRAKSMAN et al. 1980), desmethylimipramine (HAMMER et al. 1967), imipramine (BALLINGER et al. 1974; HEWICK et al. 1977), mianserin (NAWISHI et al. 1981), nomifensine (NAWISHI and HATHAWAY 1982), nortriptyline (ALEXANDERSON et al. 1969; BRAITHWAITE et al. 1975) and protriptyline (MOODY et al. 1977).

13. Other Drugs

The metabolism of several other drugs may be induced by anticonvulsants. For a more complete list, the reader is referred to PERUCCA (1982).

V. Interactions Resulting in Altered Drug Excretion in Urine

Acetazolamide may alkalinize the urine and may therefore modify the renal excretion of a number of ionic compounds (see HANSTEN 1973 for review).

References

Abernethy DR, Greenblatt DJ, Divoll M, Arendt R, Ochs HR, Shader RI (1982) Impairment of diazepam metabolism by low-dose estrogen-containing oral contraceptive steroids. N Engl J Med 306:791–792

Acocella G, Bonollo L, Mainardi M, Margardoli P (1974) Kinetic studies on rifampicin. III. Effect of phenobarbital on the half-life of the antibiotic. Tijdschr Gastroenterol 17:151–158

Ahmad S (1974) Renal insensitivity to frusemide caused by chronic anticonvulsant therapy. Br Med J 3:657–659

Ahmad S, Clarke L, Hewett AJ, Richens A (1976) Controlled trial of frusemide as an antiepileptic drug in focal epilepsy. Clin Pharmacokinet 3:621–625

Aitio ML, Vuorenmaa T (1980) Enhanced metabolism and diminished efficacy of disopyramide by enzyme-induction. Br J Clin Pharmacol 9:149–152

Aitio ML, Mansbury L, Tala E, Haataja M, Aitio A (1981) The effect of enzyme induction on the metabolism of disopyramide in man. Br J Clin Pharmacol 11:279–286

Alexanderson B, Price-Evans DA, Sjöqvist F (1969) Steady-state levels of nortriptyline in twins: influence of genetic factors and drug therapy. Br Med J 4:764–768

Alvan G, Piafsky K, Lind N, Von Bahr C (1977) Effect of pentobarbital on the disposition of alprenolol. Clin Pharmacol Ther 22:316–321

Andreasen PB, Frøland A, Skovsted L, Andersen SA, Hauge M (1973) Diphenylhydantoin half-life in man and its inhibition by phenylbutazone: the role of genetic factors. Acta Med Scand 193:561–564

Back DJ, Breckenridge AM, Crawford FE, MacIver O, Orme MI'E, Perucca E, Richens A, Rowe PH, Smith E (1980) The effect of oral contraceptive steroids and enzyme-inducing drugs on sex hormone binding globulin capacity in women. Br J Clin Pharmacol 9:115P

Back DJ, Bates M, Breckenridge AM, Ellis A, Hall JM, MacIver M, Orme MI'E, Rowe PH (1981 a) The in vitro metabolism of ethinyloestradiol, mestranol and levonorgestrel by human jejunal mucosa. Br J Clin Pharmacol 11:275–278

Back DJ, Bates M, Bowden A, Breckenridge AM, Hall MJ, Jones H, MacIver M, Orme MI'E, Perucca E, Richens A, Rowe PH, Smith E (1981 b) The interaction of phenobarbital and other anticonvulsants with oral contraceptive steroid therapy. Contraception 22:495–503

Ballek RE, Reidenberg MM, Orr L (1973) Inhibition of diphenylhydantoin metabolism by chloramphenicol. Lancet I:150

Ballinger BR, Prealy A, Reid AH, Stevenson IH (1974) The effects of hypnotics on imipramine treatment. Psychopharmacology 39:267–274

Barragry JM, Makin HLJ, Trafford DJH, Scott DF (1978) Effect of anticonvulsants on plasma testosterone and sex hormone binding globulin levels. J Neurol Neurosurg Psychiatry 41:913–914

Bauer LA (1982) Interference of oral phenytoin absorption by continuous nasogastric feedings. Neurology 32:570–572

Baylis EM, Croley JM, Preece JM, Sylvester PE, Marks V (1971) Influence of folic acid on blood phenytoin levels. Lancet I:62–64

Begg EJ, Chinwah PM, Webb C, Day RO, Wade DN (1982) Enhanced metabolism of mexiletine after phenytoin administration. Br J Clin Pharmacol 14:219–223

Bielmann I, Luac T, Gagnon MA (1978) Clonazepam: its efficacy in association with phenytoin and phenobarbital in mental patients in generalized major motor seizures. Int J Clin Pharmacol 16:268–273

Block SH (1982) Carbamazepine-isoniazid interaction. Pediatrics 69:494–495

Bloxham RA, Durbin GM, Johnson T, Winterborn MH (1979) Chloramphenicol and phenobarbitone – a drug interaction. Arch Dis Child 54:76

Bochner F, Hooper WD, Tyrer JH, Eadie MJ (1972) Factors involved in an outbreak of phenytoin intoxication. J Neurol Scand 16:481–487

Bogaert MG, Rosseel MT, Belpaine FM (1971) Metabolism of nitroglycerine in man: influence of phenobarbital. Arch Int Pharmacodyn Ther 24:1303–1311

Bollini P, Riva R, Albani F, Ida N, Cacciari L, Bollini C, Baruzzi A (1983) Decreased phenytoin level during antineoplastic therapy: a case report. Epilepsia 24:75–78

Borgå O, Azarnoff DL, Forshell GP, Sjöqvist F (1969) Plasma protein binding of tricyclic antidepressants in man. Biochem Pharmacol 18:2135–2143

Bourgeois BFD, Dodson WE, Ferrendelli JA (1982) Interactions between primidone, carbamazepine and nicotinamide. Neurology 32:1122–1126

Bowdle TA, Levy RH, Cutler RE (1979) Effect of carbamazepine on valproic acid kinetics in normal subjects. Clin Pharmacol Ther 26:629–634

Boylan JJ, Owen DS, Chin JB (1976) Phenytoin interference with dexamethasone. JAMA 235:803–804

Braithwaite RA, Flanagan RA, Richens A (1975) Steady-state plasma nortriptyline concentrations in epileptic patients. Br J Clin Pharmacol 2:469–471

Brennan RW, Dehejia H, Kutt H, Verebely K, McDowell F (1970) Diphenylhydantoin intoxication attendant to slow inactivation of isoniazid. Neurology 20:687–693

Brooks SM, Werk EE, Ackerman SJ, Sullivan I, Thrasher K (1972) Adverse effects of phenobarbital on corticosteroid metabolism in patients with bronchial asthma. N Engl J Med 286:1125–1128

Brooks PM, Buchanan WW, Grove M, Downie NW (1976) Effects of enzyme-induction on metabolism of prednisolone. Clinical and laboratory study. Ann Rheum Dis 35:339–343

Brown JE, Kitchell BB, Bjornsson TD, Shand DG (1981) The artifactual nature of heparin-induced drug binding alteration. Clin Pharmacol Ther 30:636–643

Bruni J, Gallo JM, Lee CS, Perchalski RJ, Wilder BJ (1980a) Interactions of valproic acid with phenytoin. Neurology 30:1233–1236

Bruni J, Wilder BJ, Perchalski RJ, Hammond EJ, Villareal HJ (1980b) Valproic acid and plasma levels of phenobarbital. Neurology 30:94–97

Busfield D, Child KJ, Atkinson RM, Tomich EG (1963) An effect of phenobarbitone on blood levels of griseofulvin in man. Lancet II:1042

Chapron DJ, Kramer PA, Mariano SL, Hohnadel DC (1979a) Effect of calcium and antacids on phenytoin bioavailability. Arch Neurol 36:436–438

Chapron DJ, Numford D, Pitegoff GI (1979b) Apparent quinidine-induced digoxin toxicity after withdrawal of pentobarbital. Case of sequential drug interactions. Arch Intern Med 139:363–364

Christensen LK, Skovsted L (1969) Inhibition of drug metabolism by chloramphenicol. Lancet II:1397–1399

Cloyd JC, Miller KW, Leppik IE (1981) Primidone kinetics: effects of concurrent drugs and duration of therapy. Clin Pharmacol Ther 29:402–407

Collste P, Seideman P, Borg KO, Haglund K, Von Bahr C (1979) Influence of pentobarbital on effect and plasma levels of alprenolol and 4-hydroxy-alprenolol. Clin Pharmacol Ther 25:423–427

Coulam CB, Annegers JF (1979) Do anticonvulsants reduce the efficacy of oral contraceptives? Epilepsia 20:519–526

Cramer JA, Mattson RH (1979) Valproic acid: in vitro plasma protein binding and interaction with phenytoin. Ther Drug Monit 1:105–116

Cunningham JL, Price-Evans DA (1981) Acetanilide and paracetamol pharmacokinetics before and after phenytoin administration: genetic control of induction. Br J Clin Pharmacol 11:591–596

Dahlqvist R, Borgå O, Rane A, Walsh Z, Sjöqvist F (1979) Decreased plasma protein binding of phenytoin in patients on valproic acid. Br J Clin Pharmacol 8:547–552

Dam M, Jensen A, Christiansen J (1975) Plasma level and effect of carbamazepine in grand mal and psychomotor epilepsy. Acta Neurol Scand [Suppl] 60:33–38

Dam M, Kristensen CB, Hansen BS, Christiansen J (1977) Interaction between carbamazepine and propoxyphene in man. Acta Neurol Scand 56:603–607

Dana-Haeri J, Richens A (1981) Effect of antiepileptic drugs on the hypothalamic pituitary axis. Br Med J 282:902

Data JL, Wilkinson GR, Nies AS (1976) Interaction of quinidine with anticonvulsant drugs. N Engl J Med 294:699–702

De Rautlin de La Roy Y, Beauchant G, Breuil K, Patte F (1971) Diminution du taux sérique de rifampicine par le phenobarbital. Presse Med 79:350
Desmond PV, Roberts RK, Wilkinson GR, Wood AJJ, Dunn D, Schenker S (1979) The effect of heparin on benzodiazepine binding. Fed Proc 38:743
Dhillon S, Richens A (1981 a) Pharmacokinetics of diazepam in epileptic patients and normal volunteers following intravenous administration. Br J Clin Pharmacol 12:841–844
Dhillon S, Richens A (1981 b) Serum protein binding of diazepam and its displacement by valproic acid in vitro. Br J Clin Pharmacol 12:591–592
Dhillon S, Richens A (1982) Valproic acid and diazepam interaction in vivo. Br J Clin Pharmacol 13:553–560
Dravet C, Mesdjan E, Cenraud B, Roger J (1977) Interaction between carbamazepine and triacetyloleandomycin. Lancet I:810–811
Editorial (1980) Drug interactions with oral contraceptive steroids. Br Med J 281:93–94
Eichelbaum M, Kothe KW, Hoffmann F, Von Unruh GE (1979) Kinetics and metabolism of carbamazepine during combined antiepileptic therapy. Clin Pharmacol Ther 26:367–371
Fincham RW, Schottelius DD (1979) Decreased phenytoin levels in antineoplastic therapy. Ther Drug Monit 1:277–283
Fincham RW, Schottelius DD, Sahs AL (1974) The influence of diphenylhydantoin on primidone metabolism. Arch Neurol 30:259–262
Fincham RW, Wiley DE, Schottelius DD (1976) Use of phenytoin serum levels in a case of status epilepticus. Neurology 26:879–881
Fine A, Henderson IS, Morgan DR, Tilstone WJ (1977) Malabsorption of frusemide caused by phenytoin. Br Med J 2:1061–1062
Finelli PF (1976) Phenytoin and methadone tolerance. N Engl Med 294:110
Flachs H, Gram L, Würtz-Jørgensen A, Parnas J (1979) Drug levels of other antiepileptic drugs during concomitant treatment with sodium valproate. Epilepsia 20:187
Fleitman JS, Bruni J, Perrin JH, Wilder BJ (1980) Albumin-binding interactions of sodium valproate. J Clin Pharmacol 20:514–517
Frantzen E, Hansen JM, Hansen OE, Kristensen M (1967) Phenytoin (Dilantin®) intoxication. Acta Neurol Scand 43:440–446
Fraser DG, Ludden TM, Evens RP, Sutherland EW III (1980): Displacement of phenytoin from plasma binding sites by salicylate. Clin Pharmacol Ther 27:165–169
Friel PN, Leal KW, Wilensky AJ (1979) Valproic acid-phenytoin interaction. Ther Drug Monit 1:243–248
Frigo GM, Lecchini S, Caravaggi M, Gatti G, Tonini M, D'Angelo L, Perucca E, Crema A (1983) Reduction in phenytoin clearance caused by cimetidine. Eur J Clin Pharmacol 25:135–137
Fuji K, Hayashi M, Murata R (1975) Effect of diphenylhydantoin therapy on plasma 11-OHCS: interference in the effects of dexamethasone and metapirone. Brain Dev 7:354–360
Furlanut M, Rizzoni G (1980) Effetti del dipropilacetato sulla cinetica della antipirina (Abstr). Proceedings 20th Meeting of the Italian Pharmacological Society (SIF), Verona
Furlanut M, Benetello P, Avogaro A, Dainese R (1978) Effects of folic acid on phenytoin kinetics in healthy subjects. Clin Pharmacol Ther 24:294–297
Gangji D, Schwade JG, Strong JM (1980) Phenytoin-misonidazole: a possible metabolic interaction. Cancer Treat Rep 64:155–156
Garratt WR, Carter BL, Pellock JM (1979) Bioavailability of phenytoin administered with antacids. Ther Drug Monit 1:435–437
Garrettson LK, Perel JM, Dayton PG (1969) Methylphenidate interaction with both anticonvulsants and ethyl-biscoumacetate. JAMA 207:2053–2056
Geaney DP, Carver JG, Davies CL, Aronson JK (1983) Pharmacokinetic investigation of the interaction of azapropazone with phenytoin. Brit J Clin Pharmacol 15:727–734
Giacomini K, Giacomini J, Blaschke T (1980) Heparin decreases plasma protein binding of drugs. Clin Pharmacol Ther 27:256
Goldberg MJ, Berlinger WG (1982) Treatment of phenobarbital overdose with activated charcoal. JAMA 247:2400–2401

Greenblatt DJ, Shader RI, Harmatz JS, Franke K, Koch-Weser J (1976) Influences of magnesium and aluminium hydroxide mixture on chlordiazepoxide absorption. Clin Pharmacol Ther 19:234–239
Gugler R, Von Unrhuh GE (1980) Clinical pharmacokinetics of valproic acid. Clin Pharmacokinet 5:67–83
Gupta S (1982) Phenobarbital and metabolism of metronidazole. N Engl J Med 308:529
Haglund K, Seideman P, Collste B, Borg KO, Von Bahr C (1979) Influence of pentobarbital on metroprolol plasma levels. Clin Pharmacol Ther 26:326–329
Hahn TJ (1976) Bone complications of anticonvulsants. Drugs 12:210–211
Hammer W, Ideström CM, Sjöqvist F (1967) Chemical control of antidepressant drug therapy. Minerva Med Int Congr Ser 122:301–310
Hancock KW, Levell MJ (1978) Primidone/dexamethasone interaction. Lancet II:97–98
Hansen JM, Kristensen M, Skovsted L, Christensen LK (1966) Dicoumarol-induced diphenylhydantoin intoxication. Lancet II:265–266
Hansen JM, Kristensen M, Skovsted L (1968) Sulthiame (Ospolot®) as inhibitor of diphenylhydantoin metabolism. Epilepsia 9:17–22
Hansen JM, Siersbaek-Nielsen K, Kristensen M, Skovsted L, Christensen LK (1971 a) Effect of diphenylhydantoin on the metabolism of dicoumarol in man. Acta Med Scand 189:15–19
Hansen JM, Siersbaek-Nielsen K, Skovsted L (1971 b) Carbamazepine-induced acceleration of diphenylhydantoin and warfarin metabolism in man. Clin Pharmacol Ther 12:539–543
Hansen JM, Kampmann JP, Siersbaek-Nielsen K, Lumholtz IB, Arrøe M, Abilgaard V, Skovsted L (1979) The effect of different sulfonamides on phenytoin metabolism in man. Acta Med Scand [Suppl] 624:106–110
Hansen BS, Dam M, Brandt J, Hvidberg EF, Angelo H, Christensen JM, Lous P (1980 a) Influence of dextropropoxyphene on steady-state serum levels and protein binding of three antiepileptic drugs. Acta Neurol Scand 61:357–367
Hansen JM, Busk G, Niemi G, Haase NJ, Lumholtz B, Skovsted L, Kampmann JP (1980 b) Inhibition of phenytoin metabolism by sulfinpyrazone (Abstr 0584). In: Turner P, Padgham C (eds) Abstracts of the world conference on clinical pharmacology and therapeutics, London. MacMillan, London
Hansten PD (1973) Drug interactions. Lea and Febiger, Philadelphia
Hayes SL, Pablo G, Radomski T, Palmer RF (1977) Ethanol and oral diazepam absorption. N Engl J Med 296:186–189
Hedrick R, Williams F, Morin R, Lamb WA, Cate JCIV (1983) Carbamazepine-erythromycin interaction leading to carbamazepine toxicity in four epileptic children. Ther Drug Monit 5:405–407
Heijertz R, Pilz H (1978) Interaction of nitrofurantoin with diphenylhydantoin. J Neurol 218:297–301
Hempel E, Klinger W (1976) Drug stimulated biotransformation of hormonal steroid contraceptives: clinical implications. Drugs 12:442–448
Hendeles L (1979) Decreased oral phenytoin absorption following concurrent theophylline administration. J Allergy Clin Immunol 63:156
Herishanu Y, Eylath U, Ilan R (1976) Effect of calcium content of diet on absorption of diphenylhydantoin. Israel J Med Sci 12:1453–1456
Hetzel DJ, Bochner F, Hallpike JF, Sherman DJC, Hann CS (1981) Cimetidine interaction with phenytoin. Br Med J 282:1512
Hewick DS, Sparks RG, Stevenson IH, Watson ID (1977) Induction of imipramine metabolism following barbiturate administration. Br J Clin Pharmacol 4:399
Hooper WO, Sutherland JM, Bochner F, Tyrer JG, Eadie MJ (1971) The effect of certain drugs on the plasma protein binding of diphenylhydantoin. Aust NZ J Med 3:377–381
Houghton GW, Richens A (1974 a) Phenytoin intoxication induced by sulthiame in epileptic patients. J Neurol Psychiatry 37:275–281
Houghton GW, Richens A (1974 b) Inhibition of phenytoin metabolism by sulthiame in epileptic patients. Br J Clin Pharmacol 1:59–66

Huisman JW, van Heycop Ten Ham MW, van Zijl CHW (1970) Influence of ethylphenacemide on serum levels of other antiepileptic drugs. Epilepsia 11:207–215
Hurwitz A (1977) Antacid therapy and drug kinetics. Clin Pharmacol 2:269–280
Jao JY, Jusko WJ, Cohen JL (1972) Phenobarbital effects on cyclophosphamide pharmacokinetics. Cancer Res 32:2761–2764
Jelliffe RW, Blankenhorn DH (1966) Effect of phenobarbital on digitoxin metabolism. Clin Res 14:160
Johannessen SI, Strandjord RE, Munthe-Kaas AW (1977) Lack of effect of clonazepam on serum levels of diphenylhydantoin, phenobarbital and carbamazepine. Acta Neurol Scand 55:506–512
Jordan BJ, Shillingford JS, Steed KP (1976) Preliminary observations on the protein binding and enzyme-inducing properties of sodium valproate (Epilim). In: Legg NJ (ed) Clinical and pharmacological aspects of sodium valproate (Epilim) in the treatment of epilepsy, MCS consultants, Tunbridge Wells, pp 112–116
Jubiz W, Meikle AW (1979) Alterations of glucocorticoid actions by other drugs and disease states. Clin Pharmacokinet 18:113–121
Jubiz W, Meikle AW, Levinson RA, Mizutani S, West CD, Tyler FH (1970) Effect of diphenylhydantoin on the metabolism of dexamethasone. N Engl J Med 283:11–14
Kaldor A, Somogyi G, Debreczen LA (1975) Interaction of heart glycosides and pentobarbital. Int J Clin Pharmacol 12:403
Kapetenanovic IM, Kupferberg HJ, Porter RJ, Theodore W, Schulman E, Penry JK (1981) Mechanism of valproate-phenobarbital interaction in epileptic patients. Clin Pharmacol Ther 29:480–486
Karch FE, Wardell WM, Dambly M, Gringeri A (1977) Effect of halofenate on the serum binding of phenytoin. Br J Clin Pharmacol 4:625–626
Kater RMH, Roggin G, Tobon F, Zieve P, Iber FL (1969) Increased rate of clearance of drugs from the circulation of alcoholics. Am J Med Sci 258:35–39
Khoo KL, Mendels J, Rothbart M, Garland WA, Colburn WA, Min BH, Lucek R, Carbone JJ, Boxenbaum HG, Kaplan SA (1980) Influence of phenytoin and phenobarbital on the disposition of a single oral dose of diazepam. Clin Pharmacol Ther 28:368–375
Klotz V, Reimann I (1980) Delayed clearance of diazepam due to cimetidine. N Engl J Med 302:1012–1014
Knott C, Hamshaw-Thomas A, Reynolds F (1982) Phenytoin-valproate interaction: importance of saliva monitoring in epilepsy. Br Med J 284:13–16
Koch KM, Ludwick BT, Levy RH (1981) Phenytoin-valproic acid interaction in rhesus monkey. Epilepsia 22:19–25
Koch-Weser J, Sellers ES (1976) Binding of drugs to serum albumin. N Engl J Med 292:311–316
Koranyi L, Gero L (1979) Influence of diphenylhydantoin on the effect of streptozotocin. Br Med J 1:127
Koup JR, Gibaldi M, McNamara P, Hilligoss DM, Colburn WA, Bruck E (1978) Interaction of chloramphenicol with phenytoin and phenobarbital. Clin Pharmacol Ther 24:571–575
Kulshrestha VK, Thomas M, Wadsworth J, Richens A (1978) Interaction between phenytoin and antacids. Br J Clin Pharmacol 6:177–179
Kurata D, Wilkinson GR (1974) Erythrocyte uptake and plasma binding of diphenylhydantoin. Clin Pharmacol Ther 16:355–362
Kutt H (1971) Biochemical and genetical factors regulating Dilantin® metabolism in man. Ann NY Acad Sci 179:704–722
Kutt H (1972) Diphenylhydantoin. Interactions with other drugs in man. In: Woodbury DM, Penry IK, Schmid RP (eds) Antiepileptic drugs. Raven, New York, pp 169–180
Kutt H, Louis S (1972) Anticonvulsant drugs. II. Clinical pharmacological therapeutic aspects. Curr Ther (Phila) 13:58–82
Kutt H, Winters W, McDowell FH (1966) Depression of parahydroxylation of diphenylhydantoin by antituberculosis chemotherapy. Neurology 16:594–602
Kutt H, Brennan R, Dehejia H, Verebely K (1970) Diphenylhydantoin intoxication. A complication of isoniazid therapy. Am Rev Respir Dis 101:377–384

Labadarios D, Dickerson JWT, Parke DV, Lucas EG, Obuwa GH (1978) The effects of chronic drug administration on hepatic enzyme-induction and folate metabolism. Br J Clin Pharmacol 5:167–173
Lai AA, Levy RH, Cutler RE (1978) Time course of interaction between carbamazepine and clonazepam in normal man. Clin Pharmacol Ther 24:316–323
Laizi V, Linnoila M, Seppala T, Himberg JJ, Mattila MJ (1979) Pharmacokinetic and pharmacodynamic interactions of diazepam with different alcoholic beverages. Eur J Clin Pharmacol 16:262–270
Lambie DG, Johnson R (1981) The effects of phenytoin on phenobarbitone and primidone metabolism. J Neurol Neurosurg Psychiatry 44:148–151
Landay RA, Gonzalez MA, Taylor JC (1978) Effect of phenobarbital on theophylline disposition. J Allergy Clin Immunol 62:27–29
Leonard RF, Knott PJ, Rankin GO, Robinson DS, Melnick DE (1981) Phenytoin-salicylate interaction. Clin Pharmacol Ther 29:56–60
Lewis R (1966) Effect of barbiturates on anticoagulant therapy. N Engl J Med 274:110
Linnoila M, Viukari M, Vaisanen K, Auvinen J (1980) Effect of anticonvulsants on plasma haloperidol and thioridazine levels. Am J Psych 137:819–821
Lumholtz B, Siersbaek-Nielsen K, Skovsted L, Kampmann J, Hansen JM (1975) Sulfamethizole-induced inhibition of diphenylhydantoin, tolbutamide, and warfarin metabolism. Clin Pharmacol Ther 17:731–734
Lunde PKM, Rane A, Yaffe SJ, Lund L, Sjöqvist F (1970) Plasma protein bindings of diphenylhydantoin in man. Clin Pharmacol Ther 11:846–855
MacDonald MG, Robinson DS (1968) Clinical observations of possible barbiturate interference with anticoagulation. JAMA 204:97–99
MacLeod SM, Sellers EM, Giles HG, Billings BJ, Martin PR, Greenblatt DJ, Marshman JA (1978) Interaction of disulfiram with benzodiazepines. Clin Pharmacol Ther 24:583–589
Makki KA, Perucca E, Richens A (1980) Metabolic effects of folic acid replacement therapy in folate-deficient epileptic patients. In: Johannessen SI, Morselli PL, Pippenger CE; Richens A, Schmidt D, Meinardi H (eds) Antiepileptic therapy. Advances in drug monitoring. Raven, New York, pp 391–396
Marquis JF, Carruthers SG, Spence JD, Brownstone YS, Toogood JH (1982) Phenytoin-theophylline interaction. N Engl J Med 307:1189–1190
Mattson RH, Gallagher BB, Reynolds EH, Glass D (1973) Folate therapy in epilepsy. A controlled study. Arch Neurol 29:78–81
Mattson RH, Cramer JA, Williamson PC, Novelly RA (1978) Valproic acid in epilepsy: clinical and pharmacological effects. Ann Neurol 3:20–25
Mattson GF, Mattson RH, Cramer JA (1982) Interaction between valproic acid and carbamazepine: an in vitro study of protein binding. Ther Drug Monit 4:181–184
McLelland J, Jack W (1978) Phenytoin/dexamethasone interactions: a clinical problem. Lancet I:1096–1097
Mead PB, Gibson M, Schentag JJ, Ziemniak JA (1982) Possible alteration of metronidazole metabolism by phenobarbital. N Engl J Med 306:1490
Meikle AW, Jubiz W, Matsukura S, West CD, Tyler FH (1969) Effect of diphenylhydantoin on the metabolism of metyrapone and release of ACTH in man. J clin Endocrinol Metab 29:1553–1558
Mellett LB (1971) Chemistry and metabolism of cyclophosphamide. In: Vancil (ed) Immunosuppressive properties of cyclophosphamide. Mead and Johnson, Evansville, pp 6–34
Mihaly GW, Vajda FJ, Miles JL, Louis WJ (1979) Single and chronic dose pharmacokinetic studies of sodium valproate in epileptic patients. Eur J Clin Pharmacol 16:23–29
Miller RR, Porter J, Greenblatt DJ (1979) Clinical importance of the interaction of phenytoin and isoniazid. A report from the Boston collaborative drug surveillance program. Chest 75:356–358
Monks A, Richens A (1980) Effect of a single dose of sodium valproate on serum phenytoin concentration and protein binding in epileptic patients. Clin Pharmacol Ther 27:89–95

Monks A, Boobis S, Wadsworth J, Richens A (1978) Plasma protein binding interaction between phenytoin and valproic acid in vitro. Br J Clin Pharmacol 6:487–492
Moody JP, Whyte SF, McDonald AJ, Naylor GJ (1977) Pharmacokinetic aspects of protriptyline plasma levels. Eur J Clin Pharmacol 11:51–56
Morselli P, Rizzo M, Garattini S (1971) Interaction between phenobarbital and diphenylhydantoin in animals and in epileptic patients. Ann NY Acad Sci 179:88–107
Murray FJ (1962) Outbreak of unexpected reactions among epileptics taking isoniazid. Am Rev Respir Dis 86:729–732
Nanda RN, Johnson RH, Keogh HJ, Lambie DG, Melville ID (1977) Treatment of epilepsy with clonazepam and its effect on other anticonvulsants. J Neurol Neurosurg Psychiatry 40:538–543
Nappi J (1979) Warfarin and phenytoin interaction. Ann Intern Med 90:852
Nawishi S, Hathaway N (1982) Nomifensine pharmacokinetics in patients with epilepsy. Br J Clin Pharmacol 13:295
Nawishi S, Hathaway N, Turner P (1981) Interactions of anticonvulsant drugs with mianserin and nomifensine. Lancet II:870–871
Neuvonen PJ, Elonen E (1980) Effect of activated charcoal on absorption and elimination of phenobarbitone, carbamazepine and phenylbutazone in man. Eur J Clin Pharmacol 15:51–57
Neuvonen PJ, Penttila O (1974) Interaction between doxycycline and barbiturates. Br Med J 1:535–536
Neuvonen PJ, Elfving SM, Elonen E (1978) Reduction of absorption of digoxin, phenytoin and aspirin by activated charcoal in man. Eur J Clin Pharmacol 13:213–218
Neuvonen PJ, Lehtovaara R, Bardy A, Elonen E (1979) Antipyrine analgesics in patients on antiepileptic drug therapy. Eur J Clin Pharmacol 15:263–268
Neuvonen PJ, Kannisto H, Hirvisalo EL (1983) Effect of activated charcoal on absorption of tolbutamide and valproate in man. Eur J clin Pharmacol 24:243–246
Notelovitz M, Tjapkes J, Ware M (1981) Interaction between oestrogen and Dilantin in a menopausal woman. N Engl J Med 304:788–789
O'Brien LS, Orme MI'E, Breckenridge AM (1978) Failure of antacids to alter the pharmacokinetics of phenytoin. Br J Clin Pharmacol 6:176–177
Ochs HR, Greenblatt DJ, Roberts GM, Dengler HJ (1981) Interaction of diazepam with antituberculosis drugs. Clin Pharmacol Ther 29:270
Odar-Cederlöf I, Borgå O (1976) Impaired plasma protein binding of phenytoin in uremia and displacement effect of salicylic acid. Clin Pharmacol Ther 20:36–47
Ohnhaus EE, Park BK, Colombo JP, Heizmann P (1979) The effect of enzyme-induction on diazepam metabolism in man. Br J Clin Pharmacol 8:557–563
Olanow CW, Finn AL, Prussak C (1981) The effects of salicylate on the pharmacokinetics of phenytoin. Neurology 31:341–342
Olesen OV (1967) The influence of disulfiram and calcium carbide on the serum diphenylhydantoin. Excretion of HPPH in the urine. Arch Neurol 16:642–644
Olesen OV, Jensen ON (1969) Drug interaction between sulthiame (Ospolot®) and phenytoin in the treatment of epilepsy. Dan Med Bull 16:154–158
Oppenheimer JH (1968) Role of plasma proteins in the binding, distribution and metabolism of the thyroid hormones. N Engl J Med 278:1153
Orr JM, Abbott FS, Farrell K, Ferguson S, Sheppard I, Godolphin W (1982) Interaction between valproic acid and aspirin in epileptic children: serum protein binding and metabolic effects. Clin Pharmacol Ther 31:642–649
Oxley J, Hedges A, Makki KA, Monks A, Richens A (1979) Lack of hepatic enzyme-inducing effect of sodium valproate. Br J Clin Pharmacol 8:189–190
Patel JH, Levy RH, Cutler RE (1980) Phenobarbital-valproic acid interaction in normal man. Clin Pharmacol Ther 27:515–521
Patsalos PN, Lascelles PT (1977) Effect of sodium valproate on plasma protein binding of diphenylhydantoin. J Neurol Neurosurg Psychiatry 40:570–574
Paxton JW (1980) Effects of aspirin on salivary and serum phenytoin kinetics in healthy subjects. Clin Pharmacol Ther 27:170–178

Penttila O, Neuvonen PJ, Aho K, Lehtovaara R (1974) Interaction between doxycycline and some antiepileptic drugs. Br Med J 2:470–472
Perucca E (1978) Clinical consequences of microsomal enzyme-induction by antiepileptic drugs. Pharmacol Ther 2:285–314
Perucca E (1982) Pharmacokinetic interactions with antiepileptic drugs. Clin Pharmacokinet 7:57–84
Perucca E, Richens A (1977) Interaction between phenytoin and imipramine. Br J Clin Pharmacol 4:484–486
Perucca E, Richens A (1979a) Paracetamol disposition in normal subjects and in patients treated with antiepileptic drugs. Br J Clin Pharmacol 7:201–206
Perucca E, Richens A (1979b) Reduction of the oral availability of lignocaine by induction of first-pass metabolism in epileptic patients. Br J Clin Pharmacol 8:21–31
Perucca E, Richens A (1980a) Water intoxication produced by carbamazepine and its reversal by phenytoin. J Neurol Neurosurg Psychiatry 43:540–545
Perucca E, Richens A (1980b) Interpretation of drug levels: Relevance of plasma protein binding. Ciba Found Symp 74:51–68
Perucca E, Richens A (1980c) Anticonvulsant drug interactions, In: Tyrer J (ed) The treatment of epilepsy. MTP, Lancaster, pp 95–128
Perucca E, Richens A (1981) Drug interactions with phenytoin. Drugs 21:120–137
Perucca E, Gatti G, Frigo GM, Crema A, Calzetti S, Visintini D (1978) Disposition of sodium valproate in epileptic patients. Br J Clin Pharmacol 5:495–499
Perucca E, Hedges A, Makki K, Hebdige S, Wadsworth J, Richens A (1979) The comparative enzyme-inducing properties of antiepileptic drugs. Br J Clin Pharmacol 7:414–415P
Perucca E, Hebdige S, Gatti G, Lecchini S, Frigo GM, Crema A (1980) Interaction between phenytoin and valproic acid: plasma protein binding and metabolic effects. Clin Pharmacol Ther 28:779–789
Pfiasky KM, Sitar DS, Ogilvie RI (1977) Effect of phenobarbital on the disposition of intravenous theophylline. Clin Pharmacol Ther 22:336–339
Pisani F, Narbone MC, Fazio A, Crisafulli P, Primerano G, Amendola D'Agostino A, Oteri G, Di Perri R (1984) Effect of viloxazine on serum carbamazepine levels in epileptic patients. Epilepsia 25:482–485
Pond SM, Kretzschmar KM (1981) Decreased bioavailability and increased clearance of meperidine during phenytoin administration. Clin Pharmacol Ther 29:273
Porter RJ, Layzer RP (1975) Plasma albumin concentration and diphenylhydantoin binding in man. Arch Neurol 32:298–303
Powell JR, Nelson E, Conrad KA, Likes K, Byers J III, Perrier D (1981) Phenobarbital clearance, elimination with alkaline diuresis and bioavailability in adults. Clin Pharmacol Ther 29:273
Prescott LF, Critchley JAJH, Balali-Mood M, Pentland B (1981) Effect of microsomal enzyme-induction on paracetamol metabolism in man. Br J Clin Pharmacol 12:149–154
Pugh RNH, Geddes AM, Yeoman WB (1975) Interaction of phenytoin and chlorpheniramine. Br J Clin Pharmacol 2:173–174
Rambeck B (1979) Pharmacological interactions of methsuximide with phenobarbital and phenytoin in hospitalized epileptic patients. Epilepsia 20:147–156
Rawlins MD, Collste P, Bertilsson L, Palmer L (1975) Distribution and elimination kinetics of carbamazepine in man. Eur J Clin Pharmacol 8:91–96
Reed RC, Schwartz HJ (1982) Phenytoin-theophylline-quinidine interaction. N Engl J Med 308:724–725
Reilly MJ (1973) Drug information digest: methotrexate USP (amethopterin) and methotrexate sodium. Am J Hosp Pharm 30:543–548
Reynolds EH, Fenton G, Fenwick P, Johnson Al, Laundy M (1975) Interaction of phenytoin and primidone. Br Med J 2:594–595
Richens A (1976) Drug treatment of epilepsy. Kimpton, London, pp 108–109
Richens A, Houghton GW (1975) Effect of drug therapy on the metabolism of phenytoin. In: Schneider H, Janz D, Gardner-Thorpe C, Meinardi H, Sherwin AL (eds) Clinical pharmacology of antiepileptic drugs. Springer, Berlin Heidelberg New York

Riegelman S, Rowland M, Epstein WL (1970) Griseofulvin-phenobarbital interaction in man. JAMA 213:426–431
Rodin EA, De Sousa G, Haidukewych D, Lodhi R, Berchou RC (1981) Dissociation between free and bound phenytoin levels in presence of valproate sodium. Arch Neurol 38:240–242
Roe TF, Podosin RL, Blaskovics ME (1975) Drug interaction: diazoxide and diphenylhydantoin. J Pediatr 9:285
Rolan PA, Somogyi AW, Drew MJR, Cobain WG, South D, Bochner F (1983) Phenytoin intoxication during treatment with parenteral miconazole. Brit Med J 287:1760
Rose JQ, Choi HK, Schentag JJ, Kimbel WR, Jusko WJ (1971) Intoxication caused by interaction of chloramphenicol and phenytoin. JAMA 237:2630–2631
Rosenberry KR, Defusco CJ, Mansmann HC Jr, McGeady SJ (1983) Reduced theophylline half-life induced by carbamazepine therapy. J Pediat 102:472–474
Ross JRY, Buley L (1980) Interaction between carbamazepine and warfarin. Br Med J 280:1415–1416
Routledge PA, Kitchell BB, Bjornsson TD, Skinner T, Linnoila M, Shand DG (1980) Diazepam and *N*-desmethyldiazepam redistribution after heparin. Clin Pharmacol Ther 27:528–532
Routledge PA, Stargel WW, Finn AL, Barchowsky A, Shand DG (1981) Lignocaine disposition in blood in epilepsy. Br J clin Pharmacol 12:663–666
Ryan GM, Matthews PA (1970) Phenytoin metabolism stimulated by loxapine. Drug Intell clin Pharm 11:428
Sandor P, Sellers EM, Khouw V, Fan T (1980) Phenytoin disposition during alcohol ingestion and withdrawal. Clin Pharmacol Ther 27:283
Schmidt D (1975) The effect of phenytoin and ethosuximide on primidone metabolism in patients with epilepsy. J Neurol 209:115–123
Sellers EM, Holloway MR (1978) Drug kinetics and alcohol ingestion. Clin Pharmacokinet 3:440–452
Sellers EM, Naranjo CA, Giles HG, Frecker RL, Beeching RN (1980) Intravenous diazepam and oral ethanol interaction. Clin Pharmacol Ther 28:638–645
Shader RI, Anastasios G, Greenblatt DJ, Harmatz JS, Divoll Allen M (1978) Impaired absorption of desmethyldazepam from chlorazepate by magnesium-aluminium hydroxide. Clin Pharmacol Ther 24:308–315
Shahidi NT (1968) Acetophenetidin-induced methemoglobinemia. Ann NY Acad Sci 151:822–831
Skovsted L, Kristensen M, Hansen JM, Siersbaek-Nielsen K (1976) The effect of different oral anticoagulants on diphenylhydantoin and tolbutamide metabolism. Acta Med Scand 199:513–515
Sjö O, Hvidberg EF, Naestoft J, Lund M (1975) Pharmacokinetics and side effects of clonazepam and its 7-amino metabolite in man. Eur J clin Pharmacol 8:249–254
Solomon H, Abrams WB (1972) Interaction between digitoxin and other drugs in man. Am Heart J 83:277–280
Solomon HM, Schrogie JJ (1967) The effect of phenyramidol on the metabolism of diphenylhydantoin. Clin Pharmacol Ther 8:554–556
Solomon HM, Reich S, Spirt N, Abrams WB (1971) Interaction between digitoxin and other drugs in vitro and in vivo. Ann NY Acad Sci 179:362–369
Sotaniemi EA, Pelkonen RO, Ahokas J, Pirttiaho HI, Ahlqvist J (1978) Drug metabolism in epileptics: in vivo and in vitro correlations. Br J clin Pharmacol 5:71–76
Sotaniemi EA, Anttila M, Pelkonen RO, Järvensivu P, Sundquist H (1979) Plasma clearance of propranolol and sotalol and hepatic drug metabolizing enzyme activity. Clin Pharmacol Ther 26:153–161
Stambaugh JE, Wainer IW, Hemphill DM, Schwartz I (1977) A potentially toxic drug interaction between pethidine (meperidine) and phenobarbitone. Lancet I:398–399
Stambaugh JE, Wainer IW, Schwartz I (1978) The effect of phenobarbital on the metabolism of meperidine in normal volunteers. J Clin Pharmacol 18:482–490

Stenzel E, Boenigk HE, Rambeck B (1978) Methsuximide in the treatment of epilepsy. Epilepsia 19:114

Sutton G, Kupferberg HJ (1975) Isoniazid as an inhibitor of primidone metabolism. Neurology 25:1179–1181

Svendsen TL, Kristensen MB, Hansen JM, Skovsted L (1976) The influence of disulfiram on the half-life and clearance rate of diphenylhydantoin and tolbutamide in man. Eur J clin Pharmacol 9:439–441

Syversen GB, Morgan JP, Weintraub M, Myers GJ (1977) Acetazolamide-induced interference with primidone absorption: case reports and metabolic studies. Arch Neurol 34:80–84

Taeuber K, Badian M, Brittel HF, Toyen T, Rypp W, Sitting W, Wihlein M (1979) Kinetic and dynamic interaction of clobazam and alcohol. Br J clin Pharmacol 7:91–97S

Telerman-Toppet N, Duret ME, Coers C (1981) Cimetidine interaction with carbamazepine. Ann Int Med 94:544

Träskman L, Åsberg M, Bertilsson L, Cronholm B, Mellström B, Neckers LM, Sjöqvist F, Thoren P, Tybring G (1980) Plasma levels of chlorimipramine and its desmethyl-metabolite during treatment of depression. Clin Pharmacol Ther 6:600–610

Vesell ES, Passananti GT, Lee CH (1971) Impairment of drug metabolism by disulfiram in man. Clin Pharmacol Ther 21:785–792

Victor A, Lundbeg PO, Johansson EDB (1977) Induction of sex hormone binding globulin by phenytoin. Br Med J 2:934–935

Vincent FM (1980) Phenothiazine-induced phenytoin intoxication. Ann Intern Med 93:56–57

Waddel WJ, Butler TC (1957) The distribution and excretion of phenobarbital. J Clin Invest 36:1217–1226

Warren JW, Benmaman JD, Braxton B, Wannamaker BB, Levy RH (1980) Kinetics of a carbamazepine-ethosuximide interaction. Clin Pharmacol Ther 28:646–651

Wasserman TH, Phillips TI, Vauraalte G, Urtasun R, Partington J, Kozid D, Schwade JG, Gangji D, Strong JM (1980) Neurotoxicity of misonidazole. Potential modifying role of phenytoin sodium and dexamethasone. Br J Radiol 53:172–173

Wesseling H, Mols-Thürkow I (1975) Interaction of diphenylhydantoin (DPH) and tolbutamide in man. Eur J Clin Pharmacol 8:75–78

Wilenski AJ, Levy RH, Troupin AS, Moretti-Ojemann L, Friel P (1978) Clorazepate kinetics in treated epileptics. Clin Pharmacol Ther 24:22–30

Windorfer A, Sauer W (1977) Drug interactions during anticonvulsant therapy in childhood: diphenylhydantoin, primidone, phenobarbitone, clonazepam, nitrazepam, carbamazepine and dipropylacetate. Neuropediatrie 8:29–41

Windorfer A, Sauer W, Gaedeke R (1975) Elevation of diphenylhydantoin and primidone serum concentration by addition of dipropylacetate, a new anticonvulsant drug. Acta Pediatr Scand 64:771–772

Workman P, Bleehen NM, Wiltshire CR (1980) Phenytoin shortens the half-life of the hypoxic cell radiosensitizer misonidazole in man; implications for possible reduced toxicity. Br J Cancer 41:302–304

Wright JM, Stokes EF, Sweeney VP (1982) Isoniazid-induced carbamazepine toxicity and vice versa. A double drug interaction. N Engl J Med 307:1225–1227

Yokochi K, Yokochi A, Chiba K, Ishizaki T (1982) Phenytoin-allopurinol interaction: Michaelis-Menten kinetic parameters of phenytoin with and without allopurinol in a child with Lesch-Nyhan syndrome. Ther Drug Monit 4:353–358

Zimmerman CL, Patel IH, Levy RH, Edwards D, Nelson SD, Hutchinson M (1981) Protein binding of valproic acid in the presence of elevated free fatty acids in patient and normal human serum. Epilepsia 22:11–17

Subject Index

Absences
  comparative efficacy of drugs for 769
  drug treatment of 210, 770
Acetazolamide
  adverse effects 799
  electrophysiological effects 644
  metabolic tolerance to 268
  pharmacokinetics 703–704
  therapeutic level range 739
  tolerance to 273
Acetylcholine (ACh) 139, 153, 190, 300
Acetylcholinesterase 70
Acetylureas
  anticonvulsant activity 602–603
  chemistry 601
  drug interactions 605
  pharmacokinetics 604
  structure-activity relations 601
  toxicity 605–608
Acidosis, lactic 84, 85, 90, 91, 92
ACTH adverse effects 799
ADDP = Antiepileptic Drug Development Program 204
Agranulocytosis, drug-induced 804
Aicardi syndrome 15
Albutoin 200
  adverse effects 794
  in animal models 207
Alcohol 9,19
  excess 18
  withdrawal of 3, 5
Allobarbital, effects on brain 627
Alprazolam 229, 230
Alumina cream 304 f., 313
Amantadine 115
Amino acids, inhibitory ionic mechanism 155
Aminoacidurias 176
Amobarbital 219
  effects on membrane excitability 621
Amphetamine 102, 110, 112, 115, 119, 190
Anemia
  drug-induced aplastic 802
  megaloblastic 803
Anesthetics, local electrophysiological effects 645
Anoxemia 91
Anoxia 93,95
Anticonvulsant drugs, new 234 f.
  presynaptic action 167
Antiepileptic Drug Development (ADD) Program 341 ff.
Antiepileptic drugs 9, 13, 101, 142, 147
  action 5
    on neurotransmission 176
  activity and stereochemistry 199 ff.
  actual choice 775–776
  adverse effects 791–818
    in pregnancy 806–810
  affection of plasma protein binding 832–834
  clinical use 765–788
  comparative efficacy 769–770
  comparative safety 770–772
  combinations 785–786
  electrophysiological effects 611–645
  indications for cessation 786
  indications for the use of 765–766
  inhibition of metabolism 834–838
  interactions 831–845
    with analgesics 844
    with antidepressants 845
    with antineoplastic drugs 844
    with cardioactive drugs 843
    with oral contraceptives 843
    with vitamins 845
  metabolism stimulation 838–840
  monitoring 725–755
    active metabolites 747–750
    and protein binding 739–741
    in tears 746–747
    justifications for 726
    pharmakodynamic aspects 750–751
    salivary levels 742–746
    timing problems 751
    utilization of 753–755
  mutagenic effects 818
  oncogenic effects 818
  principles for the use 776–785

Antiepileptic drugs
  screening 69, 71
  selection of 767–776
  specifity 767–769
  teratogenicity 807
Antiepileptic drug therapy, aim of 766–767
Arrest-reaction model 292, 293
Atropine 139, 140, 143, 145, 147
Aura 10, 17
  dysphasic 20
  EEG patterns 38, 41
Aura continua 20, 23
  EEG 39
Autoreceptors 156

Baclofen 156, 163
Barbiturates 3, 160, 161, 165, 167, 169, 175, 177, 217 ff.
  anticonvulsant activity 153, 426 ff.
  clinical pharmacology 673–681
  CNS activity 423–425, 429–431
  drug interactions 438
  effects 155
    on brain 625–627
    on membrane excitability 620–621
    on spinal cord 623
    on synaptic transmission 621–622
  electrophysiological effects 620–645
  electroshock test in 218
  excretion 438
  influence on GABA synthesis 168
  interaction with
    antacids 831
    GABA 622–623
  metabolism 433–438
  neurotoxicity of 218
  pharmacodynamic effects 431
  pharmacokinetics 432
  structure-activity-relationships 422 ff.
  toxicology 439–441
Beclamide, adverse effects 800
Benzodiazepines 146, 160, 164, 165, 167, 169, 177, 199, 208
  adverse effects 798–799
  anticonvulsant activity 153, 581–583
  brain concentrations 583–585
  chemical structure 575
  clinical pharmacology 696–702
  dependence on 277
  distribution 577
  effects 155
    on brain 640–644
    on GABA sites 636
    on spinal cord 638
    on synaptic transmission 637
  electrophysiological effects 636–644
  high-affinity drug-binding sites 585–588
  influence on GABA synthesis 168
  interaction with
    antacids 831
    ethanol 832
  metabolic tolerance to 267, 270
  metabolism 577–581
  methods of determination 576
  monitoring of metabolites 749
  pharmacokinetics 577–581
  pharmacological effects 227 ff.
  protein binding 741
  salivary/plasma ratio 746
  seizure specifity 768
  therapeutic level ranges 736–737
  tolerance to 272
  use 779
Benzodiazepine sites 257 f., 270
Bicuculline (BCC) 81, 90, 140, 141, 156, 161, 164, 169, 256, 257, 297, 300, 321
Blood-brain barrier 92, 94, 102, 204, 236, 256, 421, 662
Boundary lipid 250
Bradycardia, drug-induced 817
Brain damage 90, 91, 93
Brain glucose 94
Bromides 251, 351
  adverse effects 800
Burst index (BI) 306

Calmoduline 253
Carbachol 143, 145
Carbamazepine 160, 167, 177, 223 ff., 250, 253, 257, 328
  acute toxicity 497
  adverse effects 796
  antiaggressive effects 489
  antiarrhythmic effects 490
  anticonvulsant activity 481–484
  antidiuretic effects 490
  antineuralgic effects 489
  bioavailability in adults 681
  carcinogenicity 498
  chemistry 479–481
  chronic toxicity 497
  combination with
    phenobarbital 786
    phenytion 786
  comparison with phenytoin 731, 732
  distribution 492
    in adults 682
  dose/response relationship 732
  drug interactions 496
  effects on
    alcohol-withdrawal symptoms 490
    brain 629

nerve fibers 627
sodium permeability 248
synaptic transmission 628
electrophysiological effects 627–630
elimination 495
elimination half-life 267
excretion 683
half-life and clearance 685
indications for 479
interaction with
activated charcoal 831
antibiotics 837
cimetidine 838
clonazepam 839
diazepam 839
dicoumarol 842
doxycycline 842
ethosuximide 839
phenobarbital 839
phenytoin 839
primidone 839
propoxyphene 838
theophylline 845
mechanisms of action 488
metabolic tolerance to 267
metabolism 493–495, 683
monitoring of metabolites 748
mutagenicity 498
neurobiochemical effects 485–488
overdosage 796
pharmacological effects 484
pharmacokinetics 492–496
in adults 681–687
in children 687
in infants 687
in neonates 687
plasma protein binding 682, 741
psychotropic effect 479
salivary/plasma ratio 744
seizure specifity 768
side effects 732, 772
steady state serum levels 685
suitability 774
tear/plasma ratio 746
teratology 497
therapeutic level range 730–731, 737
treatment of partial seizures .772
unwanted effects 492
use 783
for Tic Douloureux 787
in neurogenic pain 787
Carbamylcholine 145
Carbonic anhydrase inhibitors 595–598
anticonvulsant effects 595–597
clinical use 597
toxicity 598
Cardiazol *see* Pentylenetetrazol
Catecholaminergic system 102
Catecholamines 101, 103, 105, 108, 109, 110, 112, 113, 115, 116, 118, 119, 120, 121, 127, 128, 192
action on prostaglandins 189
cerveau isolé preparation 625, 642
Chlorpromazine 58
Cholineacetyltransferase 70
Cinromide 235
Clobazam 230, 231
Clomethiazol, tolerance to 273
Clonazepam 224, 227
adverse effects 798
elimination half-life 267
interaction with
carbamazepine 839
phenobarbital 839
phenytoin 839
primidone 839
pharmacokinetics 701–702
seizure specifity 768
side effects 771
suitability 773
tolerance to 273
treatment of
absences 771
myoclonic seizures 771
use 779
for Tic Douloureux 787
for dyskinesia 787
Clonidine 115, 116
Coagulation defects, drug-induced 805
Cobalt 306ff.
Cocaine 116
status epilepticus after 317
Coma 69
Comazepam 228
Comedication, influence of 751
Compliance 781
control of 726, 738, 741
Consciousness
disturbance of 20
impairment of 6, 7, 10, 11, 15, 22, 26
loss of 41, 293
Corticosteroids
seizure specifity 768
use 781
CSF 62
Cyheptamide 225, 226

Delirium, epileptic 21
Desmethyldiazepam, interaction with
phenobarbital 839
phenytoin 839
primidone 839

Diazepam 175, 199, 224, 227, 230, 250, 251, 254
adverse effects 798
bioavailability in adults 696
distribution in adults 697
dose-dependent side effects 792
effects
on brain 641–644
on spinal cord 638
on synaptic transmission 637
excretion 698
half-life and clearance 698
interaction with
antipyrine 840
carbamazepine 839
cimetidine 838
heparin 834
phenobarbital 839
phenytoin 836, 839
primidone 839
rifampicin 840
metabolic tolerance to 268, 273
metabolism 698
pharmacokinetics in
adults 696–700
children 700
infants 700
neonates 700
plasma protein binding 697
side effects 736
steady-state serum levels 699
therapeutic level range 736
Diisopropyl fluorophosphate (DFP) 144
Diphenylhydantoin *see* Phenytoin
Dipropylacetamide 738
Diseases, drug-induced 792, 800–818
Disorders, drug-induced
digestive 810–812
hormonal 812–814
immunological 805
metabolic 812–814
neurological 800
psychiatric 801
skin 816
Disturbances, drug-induced
neuropsychological 801–802
DOPA 70, 101, 102, 104, 105, 108, 109, 112, 113, 116, 118, 120, 153, 156
Doxenitoine 201
Drug monitoring
active metabolites 747–750
general 725
in cerebrospinal fluid 741
in saliva 741
in tears 741, 746–747
justifications for 726
pharmacodynamic aspects 750–751
salivary levels 742–746
timing problems 752
utilization of 753–755
Dupuytren's contracture, drug-induced 816
Dyskinesia 787
Dysmnesic symptoms 10
Dysphasia 9, 10

Eclampsia 3
EEG
clinical value 39
in hypsarrhythmia 13, 14, 15
spikes 36
Electroconvulsive shock (ECS) 79, 80, 81, 85, 90
Electroshock 87, 89, 121, 123, 141, 177, 190, 191, 199 ff.
Electroshock seizure threshold (EST) 103, 104, 120
Emprosthobonus 63
encéphale isolé preparation 292
Energy charge potential (ECP) 81
Enkephalin 298
Epilepsia partialis continua 22, 23
EEG 39
Epilepsy
active 3
alumina 144
audiogenic 25
awakening 5, 17, 18, 21
chronic 12, 13
cobalt 144
convulsive generalized comparative efficacy of drugs for 769
focal 5, 19, 24, 142, 143, 147, 307
EEG 47
induced by cobalt 162, 170
generalized 24, 174
EEG 42, 45
grand-mal 329
idiopathic 5, 17, 19, 24, 62, 64
juvenile absence 17
limbic 147
EEG 40
musicogenic 25
myoclonus 273
EEG 44
partial 177
amygdalar 292
pattern-sensitive 25
photogenic 25
photomyoclonic 59
photosensitive 26, 159, 163, 176
progressive 5
random 18, 19, 21

reflex 5, 24, 57, 66
refractory 352
residual 5
sleep 5, 18, 19, 21
spontaneous 147
startle 26
stationary 5
symptomatic 5, 19
temporal 20
vestibulogenic 25
Epilepsy, genetic models of 318
Epileptic palilalia 9
Epileptogenesis 109, 139, 147, 285, 301, 302
focal 142
GABA in 156
models on 311 ff.
secondary 312, 313
Estazolam 229
Eterobarb, pharmacology 421 ff.
Ethadione 208
Ethosuximide 160, 208, 250, 251, 254, 328
anticonvulsant effects 558–561
bioavailability 565
in adults 693
chemistry 557
combination with phenytoin 785
distribution 565
in adults 694
drug interactions 568
effects on
brain 636
neurochemical processes 563–564
synaptic transmission 635
elimination 567
elimination half-life 267
excretion 694
half-life and clearance 694
influence on behavior 562
influence on EEG 562
interaction with carbamazepine 839
metabolism 566–567, 694
monitoring in tears 747
pharmacokinetics 565–567
in adults 693–694
in children 695
in infants 695
in neonates 695
plasma protein binding 694
protein binding 741
salivary/plasma ratio 745
side effects 735, 770
steady-state serum levels 694
suitability 773
therapeutic level range 735, 739
toxicity 568
treatment of absences 770
use 778
Ethotoin 200
adverse effects 794, 797
clinical pharmocology 672, 678

Fabry's disease 787
Febrile convulsions 5
Fetal Antiepileptic Drug Syndrome 807–808
Flurazepam 228
Flurothyl 81, 85, 89
Folate deficiency, drug-induced 803
Folic acid interaction with
phenobarbital 840
phenytoin 840
Freezing, local 309
Friedmann syndrome 16, 17

GABA 89, 139, 143, 145, 153 ff., 176, 191, 303, 307
metabolism 159 f.
Schiff bases of 236
synthesis 157 f.
Gallstones, drug-induced 812
Glucocorticoids
side effects 771
treatment of myoclonic seizures 771
Glucose utilization 85, 92
Glutamate 145, 156, 176
as neurotransmitter 173
Glutamine 308
Glycine 168 ff., 308
as neurotransmitter 153, 155
Grand mal 4, 5, 11, 14, 16, 19, 20, 21, 22, 23, 24, 63, 65, 147, 207
awakening 18
EEG 44
nonfocal 18
solitary 17

Hallucinations 6, 10
Haloperidol 102
Hepatic injury, drug-induced 810
Hereditary epilepsy with complex focal 21
Herpin-Janz-Syndrome 18
Hexokinase 86, 87
Histamine 101, 128
Histidinaemia 176
Homocystinuria 158, 175, 176
Hydantoins 160, 167, 177, 200 ff.
acute toxicity 401
adverse effects 793–794
anticonvulsant potency in
animals 361
man 369
chemistry 352 f.

Hydantoins
chronic toxicity 403
clinical pharmacology 661–672
effects on
calcium 372
cardiac muscle 376
neurotransmitters 373
skeletal muscle 378
smooth muscle 376
sodium 371
excretion 400
influence on glycine 168
neuropharmacology 370
seizure specifity 768
structure-activity relationships 200, 353 ff.
teratogenic effects 404
therapeutic index of 203
5-Hydroxytryptamine (5-HT) 70, 101, 102, 104, 105, 116, 121, 125, 126, 127, 128, 130, 192
Hyperexcitability, withdrawal 276
Hyperglycinaemia 168
Hyperlysinaemia 176
Hyperplasia, drug-induced gingival 816
Hyperprolinaemia 176
Hypersalivation 19
Hypersynchrony
cholinergic 147
focal 144
Hyperthermia 91
Hyperventilation 58
Hypotonia, muscular 168
Hypoxemia 85, 90
Hypoxia and brain GABA 160
Hypsarrhythmia 45

Indometacin 192
Inheritance 19, 58, 59, 61, 64, 65, 68
Interactions in antiepileptic drugs 831–845
Intermittent light stimulation (ILS) 57, 58, 60, 69, 70
Iron 309
Ischaemia
and brain GABA 160
focal in infant monkeys 162

Jacksonian seizure 9

Kidney disorders, drug-induced 817
Kindling 109, 110, 123, 130, 139, 142, 145, 146, 290, 294, 314 ff., 330, 627, 632
anatomical specifity 315

Lafora bodies (LB) 61, 62
Lafora's disease 62
L-dopa *see* DOPA
Ledderhose syndrome, drug-induced 816
Lennox syndrome 4, 12, 15, 16, 768, 771
Leukopenia, drug-induced 804
Lidocaine 250, 317, 318
Lorazepam 229
Lupus erythematosus, drug-induced 806
Lymphadenopathy, drug-induced 804
Lymphoma, drug-induced malignant 804

MAO inhibitors 113, 116, 118, 127
Medazepam 229
Meningoencephalitis 3, 189
Mephenytoin 200, 203
adverse effects 794
biotransformation 396
clinical pharmacology 671
seizure specifity 768
side effects 772
therapeutic level range 739
treatment of partial seizures 772
Mephobarbital *see* Methylphenobarbital
Metergoline 125
Methetoin, adverse effects 794
Methohexital 61
Methoin *see* Mephenytoin
Methsuximide 216, 328
adverse effects 798
bioavailability 565
chemistry 557
clinical pharmacology 695
influence on behavoir 562
interaction with
phenobarbital 836
phenytoin 836
Methylphenobarbital 620, 739
clinical pharmacology 676–677
combination with
phenytoin 786
valproic acid 785
pharmacology 421 ff.
seizure specifity 768
suitability 774
therapeutic level range 733
use 783
Metrazol *see* pentylenetetrazol
Migraine, treatment with phenytoin 787
Monoamines 70, 101, 103, 108, 113, 129, 139
Monoepilepsy 5
Muscimol 156, 161, 163, 164, 256, 631
Myasthenia gravis, drug-induced 792
Myoclonus 67, 163
Myopathy, drug-induced 817

Neo-Citrullamon 739
Neuroleptics 102, 105

Neuromediators 101, 102
Neurotransmission 101, 102, 103
Nirvanol 671–672
Nitrazepam
  adverse effects 799
  seizure specifity 768
  side effects 771
  suitability 773
  therapeutic levels range 739
  tolerance to 273
  use 779
Nonpyknoleptic 4
Noradrenaline 70, 101, 153, 156, 190
Norepinephrine, *see* Noradrenaline

Oestrogens 158
Oligoepilepsy 5
Opisthotonus 60, 63, 64, 67, 69
Osteomalacia, drug-induced 792, 814
Ouabain 170
  competition with phenytoin 247
Oxazepam 228, 229
Oxazolidinediones 208 ff.
  clinical pharmacology 702–703
  electrophysiological effects 632–635
  seizure specifity 768
Oxotremorine 142

Pancreatitis, drug-induced 812
Paracetamol 192
Paralysis 85
Paramethadione 208
  anticonvulsant effects 537 ff.
  biochemical effects 543
  distribution 545
  drug interactions 547
  excretion 546–547
  influence on behavior 542
  influence on EEG 542
  metabolism 546
  pharmacokinetics 544–547, 703
  toxicity 547–548
Paroxysmal depolarization shift (PDS) 143
Penicillin 142, 143, 146, 170, 301, 328
Pentamethylenetetrazol, *see* Pentylenetetrazol
Pentetrazole *see* Pentylenetetrazol
Pentobarbital 165, 169, 175
  effects on membrane excitability 621
Pentylenetetrazol (PTZ) 58, 60, 61, 81, 89, 90, 101, 110, 112, 113, 115, 124, 125, 129, 130, 140, 141, 146, 170, 177, 191, 192, 286, 295 ff., 300, 307, 318, 321, 326
  action on prostaglandins 189
  death by 190
Pentylenetetrazol convulsion test 199 ff., 296, 327
Petit mal 4, 17, 147, 160
  EEG 44
  impulsive 17, 18
  retropulsive 17
Petit mal triad 5
Phenacemide
  anticonvulsant activity 602–604
  chemistry 601
  drug interactions 605
  metabolic tolerance to 270
  pharmacokinetics 604
  pharmacological profile 223
  toxicity 605–608
Phenelzine 70
Pheneturide
  pharmacokinetics 704
  interaction with
    phenobarbital 836
    phenytoin 836
Phenobarbital 160, 165, 175, 217, 218, 219, 221 ff., 224, 250, 251, 254, 328, 351
  adverse effects 782, 794–795
  bioavailability in adults 673
  combination with
    carbamazepine 786
    phenytoin 786
    valproic acid 785
  distribution in adults 673
  effect on sodium uptake 247
  excretion 674
  half-life and clearance 674
  interaction with
    activated charcoal 831
    carbamazepine 839
    clonazepam 839
    desmethyldiazepam 839
    diazepam 839
    doxycycline 842
    folic acid 840
    griseofulvin 841
    methsuximide 836
    metronidazole 843
    pheneturide 836
    phenytoin 836, 839
    prednisolon 843
    primidone 839
    propoxyphene 838
    urine-alkalinizing agents 840
    valproic acid 836, 839
  lethal dose 795
  metabolic tolerance to 269
  metabolism 674
  monitoring 725
    in tears 746, 747

Phenobarbital
pharmacokinetics
in adults 673–675
in children 675
in infants 675
in neonates 675
plasma protein binding 673
salivary/plasma ratio 745
seizure specifity 768
side effects 771
steady-state serum levels 675
suitability 773
therapeutic level range 733
tolerance to 271 f.
use 781
Phenobarbitone, *see* Phenobarbital
Phenoxybenzamine 70
Phensuximide 216
chemistry 557
clinical pharmacology 696
derivates 212
effects on neurochemical processes 563–564
influence on EEG 562 Phentolamine 70, 105, 108, 115, 117
Phenylacetyl ureas, structure-activity relationships 223
Phenylbutazone, interaction with
phenytoin 838
valproic acid 834
Phenylketonuria 176
Phenytoin 200, 201, 203, 223, 224, 257, 351 ff.
action on neuronal membranes 612–615
adverse effects 793
bioavailability
in adults 661
in animals 380
biotransformation 391
clinical effects 619
combination with
Carbamazepine 786
Ethosuximide 785
Methylphenobarbital 786
Phenobarbital 786
Primidone 786
Sulthiame 786
Valproic acid 786
concentrations in brain and cerebrospinal fluid 386
distribution in adults 662
diurnal fluctuation in serum levels 671
dosage calculation 670
dose-dependent side effects 792
effect on
brain 617–619
GABA 253
neurotransmitter metabolism 252
sodium conductance 245 f.
spinal cord 615
synaptic transmission 251, 615
thyrotropin release 251
elimination half-life 266
excitatory effects on spinal cord 616
excretion 665
extravascular distribution 384
half-life and clearance 666
inhibition by
sulthiamine 835
valproic acid 836, 839
in pregnancy 668
interaction with
activated charcoal 831
antacids 831
antibiotics 837
antineoplastic drugs 832
aspirin 834
azapropazone 834
calcium salts 832
carbamazepine 839
cimetidine 838
clonazepam 839
desmethyldiazepam 839
dexamethasone 843
diazepam 836, 839
diazoxide 834
diconmarol 842
doxycycline 842
folic acid 840
frusemide 841
halofenate 834
haloperidol 845
heparin 834
lidocaine 841
mesoridazine 845
methotrexate 841
methsuximide 836
nasogastric feeding 832
oxacillin 832
pethidine 845
pheneturide 836
phenobarbital 836, 839
phenylbutazone 838
primidone 839
propoxyphene 838
sulphafurazole 834
sulphamethoxypyridazine 834
sulthiame 834
theophylline 832, 845
tolbutamide 834
warfarin 842
interethnic differences
in kinetics 667
in metabolism 665
intoxication 793

maintenance therapy 668
metabolic tolerance to 268
metabolism in adults 665
metabolization of 206
monitoring 725, 727
in tears 746
of metabolites 748
pharmacokinetics
in adults 661–670
in animals 380
in children 671
in infants 670
in neonates 670
interethnic differences in children 671
plasma protein binding 383, 662, 740
salivary/plasma ratio 743
seizure specifity 768
side effects 772
steady-state serum levels 668
suitability 775
therapeutic level range 727, 729
tolerance to 272
toxicity 249
toxic level 729, 730
transport of 247
treatment of partial seizures 772
use 784
for migraine 787
for Tic Douloureux 787
in cardiac arrhythmia 788
in Fabry's disease 787
in hyperinsulinism 787
in myotonia 788
Phosphofructokinase (PFK) 85, 86
Photomyoclonic syndrome 56
Photosensitivity 19, 25, 57
Photostimulation 26
Physostigmine 140, 143, 144, 145, 147
Picrotoxin 140, 155, 156, 161, 169, 190, 225, 256, 257, 286, 297, 321, 326
Pimozide 102
Porphyria, drug-induced 792, 812
Pregnancy, antiepileptic drugs in 806–810
Premarin 299
Primidone
acute toxicology 468
adverse effects 795–796
antiarrhythmic effect 459
anticonvulsant activity in standard models 451–454
anticonvulsant potency in man 454–455
binding to serum proteins 460
bioavailability in adults 678
biochemical mechanism of action 457
chemistry 449–451
chronic toxicology 469
combination with
phenytoin 786
valproic acid 785
distribution in adults 678
drug interactions 466–468
effect on brain enzymes 458
efficiency 222
elimination 465
excretion 679
half-life and clearance 679
interaction with
acetazolamide 832
antibiotics 837
carbamazepine 839
clonazepam 839
desmethyldiazepam 839
dexamethasone 843
diazepam 839
phenobarbital 839
phenytoin 839
valproic acid 839
intoxications 470, 796
mechanism of anticonvulsant action 455 ff.
metabolism 462–465, 679
mutagenic effect 469
pharmacokinetics
in adults 678–681
in animals 459–466
in children 681
in infants 681
in neonates 681
physical dependence 458
plasma protein binding 678
protein binding 741
salivary/plasma ratio 745
sedative effect 458
seizure specifity 768
side effects 772
steady-state serum levels 680
suitability 774
teratogenic effect 469
therapeutic level range 734–735
treatment of partial seizures 772
use 783
withdrawal symptoms 796
L-Proline 156
Pronethalol 103, 113
Propanolol 70, 103, 109, 110, 113, 117
Pyknolepsy 4, 5, 17, 19
Pyridoxine 158
deficiency 161
dependency 158
Pyrogallol 116
Pyruvate kinase 87

Quinuclidyl-benzylate (QNB) 143, 146

Receptors, multiple 156
Relationships, structure-activity 199 ff.
Reserpine 101, 104, 105, 108, 109, 110, 112, 113, 115, 118, 119, 120, 121, 127
Rodent models 159, 163

Salaam convulsions 13, 14
Saliva/plasma ratio 743
Salivation 60, 63, 64, 67, 291
Schizophrenia 163
Schizophrenic behavior in cats 292
Scopolamine 145, 147
Seizure classification 9
Seizure monitoring 9
Seizures
  generalized tonic-clonic
    drug treatment of 771
  myoclonic
    comparative efficacy of drugs for 769
  partial (focal)
    comparative efficacy of drugs for 769
    drug treatment of 772
Serotonin (5-hydroxytryptamine) 101, 120, 153, 156
Side effects, dose-dependent 791
Spanioleptic 5, 17
Spikes
  monophasic 37
  multiphasic 37
Status epilepticus 9, 14, 15, 22, 23, 24, 61, 80, 82, 85, 90, 91, 92, 274
  after withdrawal of phenobarbital 277
  EEG 39
  in baboons 297
  in newborns 96
Stress convulsions 3, 5
Strychnine 116, 140, 141, 156, 168, 169, 170, 190, 206, 225, 286, 298, 300, 321, 326
Stun reaction 286
Succinimides 160, 209 ff.
  adverse effects 797–798
  anticonvulsant effects 558–561
  chemistry 557
  clinical pharmacology 693–696
  electrophysiological effects 635–636
  enzyme induction by 267
  seizure specifity 768
  structure-activity relationships 210
Sulfonamides 234
Sulthiame
  adverse effects 800
  combination with phenytoin 786
  inhibition of phenytoin metabolism 835
  pharmacokinetics 704
  therapeutic level range 739
Synaptosomes (synaptic vesicles) 155, 169, 247, 250, 253, 254, 311

Tachyphylaxis, after diazepam 274
Taurine 155, 169, 176
Tear/plasma ratio 746
Tetanus toxin 299
Tetrabenazine 108, 113, 127
Tetrodotoxin 249
Thiopental 61
  effects
    on brain 627
    on membrane excitability 621
THIP 156, 164
Therapeutic level, clinical evaluation 728
Therapeutic level, the concept of the 727
Thrombocytopenia, drug-induced 804
Tic Douloureux, treatment with carbamazepine 787
Tofizopam 227
Tremor, oxotremorine-induced 214
Triazolam 229
Trimethadione 160, 208, 209, 328
  adverse effects 797
  anticonvulsant effects 537 ff.
  biochemical effects 543
  distribution 545
  drug interactions 547
  effects
    on brain 634
    on spinal cord 633
    on synaptic transmission 633
  electrophysiological effects 632–635
  excretion 546–547
  influence
    on behavior 542
    on EEG 542
  metabolism 546
  pharmacokinetics 544–547, 702–703
  side effects 771
  therapeutic level range
  tolerance to 270, 272
  toxicity 547–548
  treatment of absences 771
Troxidone, *see* Trimethadione
Tryptophan 70
Tungstic acid 309

Valproic acid (Valproate) 153, 160, 167, 175, 208, 224, 231, 250, 251, 254, 328
  adverse effects 796–797
  antiepileptic activity 508–512

biovailability 520
  in adults 689
chemistry 507–508
combination with
  Methylphenobarbital 785
  phenobarbital 785
  phenytoin 786
  primidone 785
distribution 520
  in adults 690
drug interactions 525
effects on
  aspartate 516
  brain 630
  cyclic nucleotides 517
  GABA metabolism 513–515
  glycine metabolism 516
  monoamine metabolism 517
electrophysiological effects 630–632
elimination 522
excretion 691
half-life and clearance 691
influence on
  GABA synthesis 168
  glycine 169
  phenobarbital levels 836
inhibition of phenytoin metabolism 836
interaction with
  activated charcoal 831
  antipyrine 842
  carbamazepine 833
  diazepam 833
  GABA 630
  intralipid 834
  phenobarbital 833, 839
  phenytoin 833, 839
  primidone 839
kinetic variability 738
metabolism 523–525, 691
monitoring 727
  in tears 747
  of metabolites 750
neurophysiological effects 516
pharmacodynamic properties 519
pharmacokinetics 520–525
  in adults 689–693
  in children 693
  in infants 693
  in neonates 693
plasma protein binding 690, 741
salivary/plasma ratio 746
seizure specifity 768
side effects 738, 770, 771
steady state serum levels 692
suitability 773
therapeutic level range 737–738
tolerance to 272
toxicity 526–527
treatment of
  absences 770
  myoclonic seizures 771
use 780
Veratridine 249
Visually evoked responses 57

West's syndrome 4, 12, 13, 15, 16, 768
  EEG 45
Withdrawal,
  primidone 796

Handbook of Experimental Pharmacology

Continuation of "Handbuch der experimentellen Pharmakologie"

Springer-Verlag
Berlin
Heidelberg
New York
Tokyo

Volume 34
Secretin, Cholecystokinin Pancreozymin and Gastrin

Volume 35: Part 1
Androgene I

Part 2
Androgens II and Antiandrogens/Androgene II und Antiandrogene

Volume 36
Uranium - Plutonium - Transplutonic Elements

Volume 37
Angiotensin

Volume 38: Part 1
Antineoplastic and Immunosuppressive Agents I

Part 2
Antineoplastic and Immunosuppressive Agents II

Volume 39
Antihypertensive Agents

Volume 40
Organic Nitrates

Volume 41
Hypolipidemic Agents

Volume 42
Neuromuscular Junction

Volume 43
Anabolic-Androgenic Steroids

Volume 44
Heme and Hemoproteins

Volume 45: Part 1
Drug Addiction I

Part 2
Drug Addiction II

Volume 46
Fibrinolytics and Antifibronolytics

Volume 47
Kinetics of Drug Action

Volume 48
Arthropod Venoms

Volume 49
Ergot Alkaloids and Related Compounds

Volume 50: Part 1
Inflammation

Part 2
Anti-Inflammatory Drugs

Volume 51
Uric Acid

Volume 52
Snake Venoms

Volume 53
Pharmacology of Ganglionic Transmission

Volume 54: Part 1
Adrenergic Activators and Inhibitors I

Part 2
Adrenergic Activators and Inhibitors II

Handbook of Experimental Pharmacology

Continuation of "Handbuch der experimentellen Pharmakologie"

Springer-Verlag
Berlin
Heidelberg
New York
Tokyo

Volume 55
Psychotropic Agents

Part 1
Antipsychotics and Antidepressants

Part 2
Anxiolytics, Gerontopsychopharmacological Agents and Psychomotor Stimulants

Part 3
Alcohol and Psychotomimetics, Psychotropic Effects of Central Acting Drugs

Volume 56, Part 1 + 2
Cardiac Glycosides

Volume 57
Tissue Growth Factors

Volume 58
Cyclic Nucleotides

Part 1: **Biochemistry**

Part 2: **Physiology and Pharmacology**

Volume 59
Mediators and Drugs in Gastrointestinal Motility

Part 1: **Morphological Basis and Neurophysiological Control**

Part 2: **Endogenous and Exogenous Agents**

Volume 60
Pyretics and Antipyretics

Volume 61
Chemotherapy of Viral Infections

Volume 62
Aminoglycoside Antibiotics

Volume 63
Allergic Reactions to Drugs

Volume 64
Inhibition of Folate Metabolism in Chemotherapy

Volume 65
Teratogenesis and Reproductive Toxicology

Volume 66
Part 1: **Glucagon I**

Part 2: **Glucagon II**

Volume 67
Part 1
Antibiotics Containing the Beta-Lactam Structure I

Part 2
Antibiotics Containing the Beta-Lactam Structure II

Volume 68, Part 1+ 2
Antimalarial Drugs

Volume 69
Pharmacology of the Eye

Volume 70
Part 1
Pharmacology of Intestinal Permeation I

Part 2
Pharmacology of Intestinal Permeation II

Volume 71
Interferons and Their Applications

Volume 72
Antitumor Drug Resistance

Volume 73
Radiocontrast Agents

GPSR Compliance

The European Union's (EU) General Product Safety Regulation (GPSR) is a set of rules that requires consumer products to be safe and our obligations to ensure this.

If you have any concerns about our products, you can contact us on ProductSafety@springernature.com

In case Publisher is established outside the EU, the EU authorized representative is:

Springer Nature Customer Service Center GmbH
Europaplatz 3
69115 Heidelberg, Germany

Batch number: 10838053

Printed by Printforce, the Netherlands